Saunders

Drug Handbook
for
HEALTH PROFESSIONS

NAME/INDICATIONS	DOSAGE/ROUTES	SIDE EFFECTS
permagnesemia (aids in reversing CNS depression)	***Children:*** 0.5–0.7 mEq/kg 3–4 times/day. ***Neonates:*** 2.4 mEq/kg/day in divided doses. ***Cardiopulmonary resuscitation:*** ***IV: Adults, elderly:*** *Calcium gluconate:* 2.3–3.7 mEq. May repeat as needed. *Calcium chloride:* 2.7 mEq. May repeat as needed. ***Children:*** *Calcium chloride:* 0.27 mEq/kg. May repeat in 10 min if needed. ***Hyperkalemia:*** ***IV: Adults, elderly:*** 2.25–14 mEq. Monitor EKG. May repeat after 1–2 min if needed. ***Magnesium intoxication:*** ***IV: Adults, elderly:*** 7 mEq. May repeat based on pt response.	
dextrose Hypoglycemia	***Adults, children >8 yrs:*** 50% 25 g IVP slowly over 2–3 min. ***Children 1–8 yrs:*** 25% 2 ml/kg slow IVP. ***Children<1 yr:*** 12.5% 2 ml/kg slow IVP.	Local venous irritation, tissue necrosis, diuresis. May cause severe neuro signs and symptoms in alcoholics. Intracranial hemorrhage and venous sclerosis in neonates if not diluted
diazepam (Valium) Relief of acute alcohol withdrawal. Adjunct for relief of acute musculoskeletal conditions, treatment of seizures (IV route used for termination of status epilepticus)	***Alcohol withdrawal:*** ***IM/IV: Adults, elderly:*** Initially, 10 mg, followed by 5–10 mg q3–4h. ***Musculoskeletal spasm:*** ***IM/IV: Adults:*** 5–10 mg q3–4h. ***Seizures:*** ***IM/IV: Adults:*** 5–10 mg, repeated at 10–15 min intervals to total of 30 mg. ***Elderly, debilitated:*** 2–5 mg; increase gradually as needed. ***Children:*** 0.5–2 mg.	Drowsiness, sedation, amnesia, ataxia, respiratory depression, respiratory arrest, decreased blood pressure
diphenhydramine (Benadryl) Adjunct to epinephrine in treating severe allergic reactions, including anaphylactic shock. May be used alone in mild to moderate allergic reactions	***IM/IV: Adults:*** 10–50 mg. ***Maximum daily dose:*** 400 mg. ***Children >20 lbs:*** 5 mg/kg/24 hrs 4 times/day.	Drowsiness, headache, confusion, wheezing, palpitations, tachycardia, hypotension, nausea, vomiting

(continued)

NAME/INDICATIONS	DOSAGE/ROUTES	SIDE EFFECTS
epinephrine 1:10,000 Cardiac arrest, profoundly symptomatic bradycardia, anaphylactic shock	***Cardiac arrest:*** 1 mg every 3–5 min. ***Anaphylaxis:*** 0.1–0.5 mg by slow IV infusion. ***Children:*** 0.01 mg/kg.	In noncardiac pts, palpitations, angina, arrhythmias, nausea, vomiting, headache, dizziness
epinephrine 1:1000 Anaphylactic shock, severe allergic reactions, acute bronchial asthma, exacerbation of COPD	***SubQ: Adults:*** 0.3–0.5 mg.	In noncardiac pts, palpitations, angina, arrhythmias, nausea, vomiting, headache, dizziness
fentanyl (Sublimaze) Analgesic	***IV: Adults, elderly:*** 50–100 mcg q1–2h, as needed.	Confusion, blurred vision, chills, orthostatic hypotension, constipation, difficulty urinating. Too rapid IV results in severe respiratory depression, skeletal and thoracic muscle rigidity resulting in apnea, laryngospasm, bronchospasm, cold and clammy skin, cyanosis, coma
furosemide (Lasix) Treatment of edema associated w/CHF, chronic renal failure including nephrotic syndrome, hepatic cirrhosis, acute pulmonary edema	***IV:*** 1 mg/kg. ***Maximum:*** 2 mg/kg.	Postural hypotension, hypokalemia, dehydration, muscle cramps, weakness, blurred vision, nausea, vomiting, diarrhea
ipecac Treatment of poisoning or drug overdose by inducing vomiting in the conscious and alert pt	***Children (<1 yr):*** 5–10 ml, then ½–1 glass water. ***Children (>1 yr to 12 yrs):*** 15 ml followed by 1–2 glasses water. ***Adults:*** 15–30 ml followed by 3–4 glasses water. **Note:** Repeat dose (15 ml) once in pts older than 1 yr if vomiting does not occur within 20–30 min. Perform gastric lavage if vomiting does not occur within 30–45 min after second dose.	Arrhythmias, bradycardia, hypotension, depression, diarrhea
labetalol Treatment of severe hypertension, hypertensive emergency	***IV: Adults:*** Initially, 20 mg. Additional doses of 20–80 mg may be given at 10 min intervals, up to total dose of 300 mg.	Drowsiness, dizziness. May precipitate or aggravate CHF (due to decreased myocardial stimulation)

(continued)

Saunders

Drug Handbook for HEALTH PROFESSIONS

SECOND EDITION

ROBERT J. KIZIOR, BS, RPh
Education Coordinator
Department of Pharmacy
Alexian Brothers Medical Center
Elk Grove Village, Illinois

BARBARA B. HODGSON, RN, OCN
Cancer Institute
St. Joseph's Hospital
Tampa, Florida

W.B. SAUNDERS COMPANY
A Harcourt Health Sciences Company
Philadelphia / London / New York / Sydney / Toronto

W.B. SAUNDERS COMPANY
A Harcourt Health Sciences Company

The Curtis Center
Independence Square West
Philadelphia, Pennsylvania 19106

Library of Congress Cataloging-in-Publication Data

Kizior, Robert J.
Saunders drug handbook for health professions / Robert J. Kizior, Barbara B. Hodgson.—2nd ed.
p. cm.
"ISSN 1524-3591."
Includes index.
ISBN 0-7216-9365-2
1. Drugs—Handbooks, manuals, etc. 2. Pharmacology—Handbooks, manuals, etc. 3. Drugs—Administration—Handbooks, manuals, etc. I. Hodgson, Barbara B. II. Title.

RM301.12.K596 2002
615'.1—dc21

2001020325

Vice President and Publishing Director, Nursing: Sally Schrefer

Acquisitions Editor: Robin Carter

Developmental Editor: Gina Hopf

SAUNDERS DRUG HANDBOOK
FOR HEALTH PROFESSIONS, SECOND EDITION ISBN 0-7216-9365-2

Printed in the United States of America.

Last digit is the print number: 9 8 7 6 5 4 3 2 1

To all health care professionals, who in the expectation of little glory or material reward dedicated themselves to the art and science of healing.

Robert Kizior

To my daughter, Lauren, a true friend, for her unconditional love
To my daughter, Kathryn, always supportive, always encouraging
And to my son, Keith, who is a source of great pride to us all.

Barbara Hodgson

NOTICE

Pharmacology is an ever-changing field. Standard safety precautions must be followed, but as new research and clinical experience broaden our knowledge, changes in treatment and drug therapy become necessary or appropriate. Readers are advised to check the product information currently provided by the manufacturer of each drug to be administered to verify the recommended dose, the method and duration of administration, and contraindications. It is the responsibility of the treating physician, relying on experience and knowledge of the patient, to determine dosages and the best treatment for the patient. Neither the Publisher nor the editor assumes any responsibility for any injury and/or damage to persons or property.

THE PUBLISHER

AUTHOR BIOGRAPHIES

ROBERT (BOB) KIZIOR

Bob graduated from the University of Illinois School of Pharmacy and is licensed to practice in the state of Illinois. He has worked as a hospital pharmacist for thirty-two years at Alexian Brothers Medical Center in Elk Grove Village, Illinois—a suburb of Chicago. Bob is the Clinical Education Coordinator for the Department of Pharmacy where he participates in educational programs for pharmacists, nurses, physicians, and patients. He plays a major role in conducting Drug Utilization Reviews and is co-chair of the Medication Safety Subcommittee that is focused on identifying and preventing medication errors within the medical center. His hospital experience is diverse and includes participation in clinical pharmacy initiatives on inpatient units and in the surgical pharmacy satellite. Bob is a former adjunct faculty member at William Rainey Harper Community College in Palatine, Illinois. It was there that Bob first met Barbara and commenced their long-standing professional association.

An avid fan of Big Ten college athletics, Bob also has eclectic tastes in music that range from classical, big band, rock 'n roll and jazz, to country and western. Bob spends much of his free time reviewing the professional literature to stay current regarding new drug information. He and his wife, Marcia, and their two Labrador retrievers—Caty and Zak—enjoy escape weekends at their year-round lake house in central Wisconsin.

BARBARA HODGSON

Born and raised in Michigan, Barbara was married and raising a young family in Chicago when she decided to fulfill a lifelong dream and become a nurse. After graduation, she started her own business as author and publisher of **Medcards, The Total Medication Reference Guide,** the first of its kind. These drug cards were designed to assist nursing students in understanding drug information to give knowledgeable care to their patients.

In 1981, she met co-author Robert (Bob) Kizior, who was teaching a pharmacology class. After class, Barbara approached him and asked if he would be interested in working on **Medcards** with her. He agreed, and together they became so successful that a few years later Barbara was able to fulfill another dream and move to Florida.

In 1998, Bob approached Barbara to co-author the **Saunders Drug Handbook for Health Professions.** She agreed, and since then Barbara and Bob have worked together on this handbook as well as two other drug references.

Barbara specializes in the field of oncology at the Cancer Institute at St. Joseph's Hospital in Tampa, Florida. Barbara's daughter Lauren and her husband, Jim, are emergency nurses. Her daughter Kathryn is a research biologist. Her son, Keith, is a student and plans to become an emergency nurse.

Barbara's favorite interests are spending time with her very busy, tight-knit family and when she has a rare moment, getting her hands full of dirt working in her garden.

REVIEWERS

Brenda Barnes, RN, LP
Seton Southwest Hospital
Austin, Texas

J. Nile Barnes, BS, LP
Austin Community College
Austin, Texas

Barbara Braband, RN, MA
Mercy College of Health Sciences
Des Moines, Iowa

Christopher L. Carver, BA, LP
Austin Community College
Austin, Texas

Thomas S. Catalina, MPAS, PA-C
Department of Emergency Medicine
Womack Army Medical Center
Ft. Bragg, North Carolina
and
Assistant Professor of Clinical Medicine
Physician Assistant Program
Methodist College
Fayetteville, North Carolina

Heather Davis, MS, NREMT-P
UCLA Center for Prehospital Care
Los Angeles, California

Veda J. Hunt-Scott, CMA
Assistant Professor
Northwestern Business College
School of Health Sciences
Chicago, Illinois

Martha Kelly, PA-C
Department of Physician Assistant Studies
Augsburg College
Minneapolis, Minnesota

Karen A. Kittle, CMA, ASPT, CHUC
Oakland Community College
Waterford, Michigan

David H. Nielsen, PhD, PT
Physical Therapy Graduate Program
University of Iowa
Iowa City, Iowa

Tricia Ann Nixon, PT
University of Bangor
Bangor, Maine

Patricia J. Nunn, RDH, MS
University of Oklahoma
College of Dentistry
Oklahoma City, Oklahoma

Jennifer R. Skeeters, PT
South Arkansas Community College
El Dorado, Arkansas

Shannon Stephens, NREMT-P, CCEMT-P
University of Alabama at Birmingham
Department of Emergency Medicine
Birmingham, Alabama

Dominic A. Steward, NREMT-P
Paramedic
Keystone Quality Transport
Media, Pennsylvania

Larry J. Tillman, PhD
UC Foundation Professor
School of Rehabilitation Professions
Physical Therapy Program
University of Tennessee at Chattanooga
Chattanooga, Tennessee

Rob Theriault, EMCA, RCT (Adv.), CCP(F)
Professor
Department of Paramedic Studies
The Michener Institute
Toronto, Ontario
Canada

Patricia A. Walck, RN, MS, CMA
Assistant Professor and Coordinator of Medical Assisting/Ambulatory Care Technology
Harrisburg Area Community College
Harrisburg, Pennsylvania

PREFACE

Health care professionals face many challenges in today's environment, not the least of which is familiarity with the large number of medications available. New medications are being introduced, and new applications, dosage forms, and different routes of administration for existing medications are increasing at a rapid rate. This voluminous amount of drug information must be quickly integrated into the patient care environment.

Saunders Drug Handbook for Health Professions is designed as an easy–to–use source of the current drug information needed by the busy health care provider. What separates this book from others is that it guides the user through patient care to better practice, and to better care.

This handbook contains:

1. **A handy chart of the 28 most common emergency drugs administered.** The chart is printed on the front and back inside covers and endsheets.
2. **An alphabetical listing of drug entries by generic name.** Color letter tabs help you page through this section quickly. To make scanning pages easier each new entry begins under a color double bar.
3. **The Classification section.** Actions, uses, precautions, interactions, side effects, toxic effects/adverse reactions, and patient considerations are given for some of the most common classes. Unique to this handbook, each class provides an at-a-glance table that compares all the generic drugs within the classification according to dosages, routes of administration, and other characteristics.
4. **A comprehensive reference section.** The reference section is updated and expanded and contains *new* appendixes. The herbal therapies appendix is considerably expanded. The new appendixes include drugs for treatment of arthritis, drugs of abuse, antidotes, guidelines for prehospital emergency treatment of acute coronary syndromes (chest pain), common emergency drugs, and FDA pregnancy categories.
5. **The New Drug Supplement.** The drugs in the supplement are those that have been recently released by the FDA in the years 2000 and 2001. Each New Drug Supplement entry includes the action, use, dosage, and side effects of the generic drug.
6. **The index.** Undoubtedly the most comprehensive tool to help you navigate the handbook, the index is organized by showing generic

drug names in **bold,** trade names capitalized in regular type, and classifications in *italics.*

A detailed guide to the **SAUNDERS DRUG HANDBOOK FOR HEALTH PROFESSIONS:**

The main objective of **Saunders Drug Handbook for Health Professions** is to provide essential drug information in a user-friendly format. The bulk of the handbook contains an alphabetical listing of drug entries by generic name. The following are included within the drug entries:

Generic and Brand Names. The drug entries begin with the generic drug name followed by its pronunciation and U.S. and Canadian brand names.

Fixed-Combination Drugs. Where appropriate, fixed–combinations, or drugs made up of two or more generic medications, are listed with the generic drug.

Pregnancy Category. This vital information is presented at the beginning of each drug entry to help treat pregnant adults. See the *new* appendix at the back of the book for explanations of each category.

Classification. Each entry has this important information up front. Health care providers can review basic information in the classification section in the middle of the book.

Availability. Each drug entry gives the form and availability of the generic drug and indicates whether the drug is obtainable by prescription (Rx) or over the counter (OTC).

Pharmacokinetics. Pharmacokinetics includes the absorption, distribution, metabolism, excretion, and half-life of the medication.

Action/*Therapeutic Effect.* This section describes how the drug is predicted to behave, with the expected therapeutic effect given in *italics.*

Uses/*Unlabeled Uses.* The listing of uses for each drug includes both the FDA uses and unlabeled uses, which appear in *italics.*

Storage/Handling. Instructions on storage and handling are given for each drug monograph. Considerations include, "Does the medication need special storage requirements such as refrigeration?" and "How long is the medication stable once it is reconstituted?"

Administration. Instructions for administration are given for each route of administration, such as Oral, Rectal, Intramuscular (IM), and Intravenous (IV). For all routes of administration, each step is highlighted, and **reconstitution instructions** and **IV flow rates** are provided where necessary.

Indications/Dosage/Routes. Each full entry provides specific dosing guidelines for adults, the elderly, children, and patients with renal and/or hepatic impairment. Dosages are clearly indicated for each approved indication and route.

Contraindications. Each entry lists conditions in which use of the generic drug is contraindicated and should not be used.

Cautions. The cautions warn the health care provider of specific situations in which a drug should be closely monitored because it may exacerbate a patient's pre-existing condition, such as administering gentamicin, which can build up to toxic levels in the blood quickly in elderly patients with renal insufficiency; or giving nonsteroidals (e.g., ibuprofen), which can make patients with a history of peptic ulcer disease more susceptible to future GI problems such as bleeding.

Interactions. This heading enumerates drug and food interactions with the generic drug. As the number of medications a patient receives increases, awareness of drug interactions becomes more important. New information regarding certain foods and their effects on medication make this category a valuable addition to this section. Altered lab values are also included to show what effects the drug may have on lab results.

Side Effects. Side effects are defined as responses that are usually predictable with the drug, are **not** life-threatening, and may or may not require discontinuation of the drug. Unique to this handbook, side effects are grouped by frequency and occurrence percentage so the health care provider can focus on patient care without wading through myriad signs and symptoms of side effects.

Adverse Reactions/Toxic Effects. Adverse reactions and toxic effects are very serious and often life-threatening, undesirable responses that require prompt intervention.

Patient Considerations. Patient considerations are organized as care is organized. That is, "What needs to be done before the first dose is administered?" "What interventions and evaluations are needed during drug therapy?" and "What explicit teaching is needed for the patient and family?" Patient Considerations are presented entirely in color so they are easy to find.

Saunders Drug Handbook for Health Professions is an easy-to-use source of the current drug information for a wide spectrum of health care providers. It is our hope that this handbook will help you provide quality care to your patients.

Robert J. Kizior, BS, RPh
Barbara B. Hodgson, RN, OCN

ACKNOWLEDGMENTS

I offer a special heartfelt thank you to my co-author, Barbara Hodgson, RN, OCN, for her continuing superb work. Without Barbara's effort in this endeavor, this book would not have reached the completeness and excellence it has achieved.

Robert Kizior

ILLUSTRATION CREDITS

Kee JL, Hayes ER (eds.): *Pharmacology: A Nursing Process Approach,* 3rd ed. Philadelphia: WB Saunders Company, 2000.
Lehne RA: *Pharmacology for Nursing Care*, 4th ed. Philadelphia: WB Saunders Company, 2001.

CONTENTS

abacavir

(Ziagen)

See Supplement and Classification section under: Human Immunodeficiency Virus (HIV) Infection

abciximab

ab-**six**-ih-mab

(ReoPro, c7E3 Fab)

CANADIAN AVAILABILITY

ReoPro

PREGNANCY CATEGORY C

CLASSIFICATION

Antiplatelet; antithrombotic

AVAILABILITY (Rx)

Injection: 2 mg/ml (single-use vial)

PHARMACOKINETICS

Absorption: Clears rapidly from plasma. **Half-life:** Following IV bolus administration, half-life decreases <10 min, second phase of half-life within 30 min. Platelet function recovers after 48 hrs. At end of infusion, bleeding time returns to <12 min within 12 hrs in 75% of pts, within 24 hrs in 90% of pts.

ACTION/*THERAPEUTIC EFFECT*

Produces rapid inhibition of platelet aggregation by preventing the binding of fibrinogen to receptor sites on platelets. *Prevents closure of treated coronary arteries. Prevents acute cardiac ischemic complications.*

USES

Adjunctive therapy to prevent cardiac ischemic complications in pts undergoing percutaneous coronary intervention (PCI) and those w/unstable angina not responding to conventional medical therapy when PCI planned within 24 hrs.

STORAGE/HANDLING

Store vials in refrigerator. Do not shake. Discard any unused portion left in vial.

ADMINISTRATION

IV:

- Give in separate IV line; do not add any other medication to infusion.
- Discard any abciximab preparation containing *any* opaque particles.
- Use care when attempting vascular access so only the anterior wall of femoral artery is punctured.
- For bolus injection and continuous infusion, use sterile, nonpyrogenic, low protein-binding 0.2 or 0.22 micron filter.
- While vascular sheath is in position, maintain pt on complete bed rest w/head of bed elevated at 30°.
- Maintain affected limb in straight position.
- Following sheath removal, apply femoral pressure for 30 min, either manually or mechanically; then apply pressure dressing.

INDICATIONS/ROUTES/DOSAGE

Percutaneous coronary intervention (PCI):

IV Bolus: Adults: 0.25 mg/kg, given 10–60 min before the PCI, then give 12-hr IV infusion of 0.125 mcg/kg/min. ***Maximum:*** 10 mcg/min.

PCI (unstable angina):

IV Bolus: Adults: 0.25 mg/kg, follow by 18–24 hr infusion of 10 mcg/min, concluding 1 hr after procedure.

CONTRAINDICATIONS

Active internal bleeding, recent (within 6 wks) GI or GU bleeding, history of CVA <2 yrs or CVA w/residual neurologic defect, oral anticoagulants <7 days unless prothrombin time <1.2 × control, thrombocytopenia (<100,000 cells/mcl), recent surgery or trauma (within 6 wks), intracranial neoplasm, arteriovenous malformation or aneurysm, severe uncontrolled hypertension, history of vasculitis, prior IV dextran use before or during PTCA.

CAUTIONS

Pts who weigh <75 kg, those >65 yrs, those with history of GI disease, those receiving thrombolytics, heparin, aspirin, PTCA <12 hrs of onset of symptoms for acute MI, prolonged PTCA (>70 min), failed PTCA.

INTERACTIONS

DRUG: ***Anticoagulants, heparin*** may increase risk of hemorrhage. ***Platelet aggregation inhibitors*** (e.g., aspirin, dextran, thrombolytic agents) may increase risk of bleeding. **HERBAL:** None known. **FOOD:** None significant. **ALTERED LAB VALUES:** Increases clotting time (ACT), prothrombin time (PT), activated partial thromboplastin time (APTT), platelet count.

SIDE EFFECTS

FREQUENT (10–20%): Hypotension, nausea. **OCCASIONAL (2–9%):** Vomiting, bradycardia, pain in extremities. **RARE (<1%):** Abnormal thinking, pain, peripheral edema, UTI, abnormal vision, dizziness.

ADVERSE REACTIONS/TOXIC EFFECTS

Anticipate a hypersensitivity reaction when medication is given. If symptoms occur, stop infusion immediately. An increase in both major (intracranial hemorrhage, decrease in hemoglobin >5 g/dl) and minor bleeding (spontaneous hematuria, hemoglobin decrease of <4 g/dl).

PATIENT CONSIDERATIONS

BASELINE ASSESSMENT

Heparin should be discontinued 4 hrs prior to arterial sheath removal. Maintain pt on bed rest for 6–8 hrs following sheath removal or drug discontinuation, whichever is later. Check platelet count, PT, APTT before med infusion (assess for preexisting blood abnormalities), 2–4 hrs after treatment, and at 24 hrs or before discharge, whichever is first. Check insertion site, distal pulse of affected limb while femoral artery sheath is in place, and then routinely for 6 hrs after femoral artery sheath removal. Minimize need for numerous injection sites, blood drawings, intubations, catheters.

INTERVENTION/EVALUATION

Stop abciximab and/or heparin infusion if any serious bleeding occurs that is uncontrolled by pressure. Assess skin for bruises, petechiae, particularly femoral arterial access, also catheter insertion, arterial and venous puncture, cutdown, needle site, gastrointestinal sites. Assess clinical response, vital signs (pulse, temperature, respiratory rate, B/P) q4h or per protocol. Handle pt carefully and as infrequently as possible to prevent bleeding. Do not obtain B/P in lower extremities (possible deep vein thrombi). Check stool for occult blood. Assess for decrease in B/P, increase in pulse rate, complaint of abdominal/back pain, severe headache, evidence of hemorrhage, ACT, PT, APTT, platelet count. Question for increase in discharge during menses. Assess urine output for hematuria. Monitor for any occurring hematoma. Use care in removing any dressings.

acarbose

ah-**car**-bose
(Precose)

CANADIAN AVAILABILITY
Prandase

PREGNANCY CATEGORY B

CLASSIFICATION

Antidiabetic: Oral

AVAILABILITY (Rx)

Tablets: 25 mg, 50 mg, 100 mg

PHARMACODYNAMICS

	ONSET	PEAK	DURATION
Oral	—	1 hr	12–24 hrs

PHARMACOKINETICS

Absorption: Not necessary for therapeutic effect. **Metabolism:** Intestinal digestive enzymes/microorganisms. **Elimination:** Through renal and fecal route. **Half-life:** 2.7–9 hrs (increased in impaired renal function).

ACTION/*THERAPEUTIC EFFECT*

Delays glucose absorption and digestion of carbohydrates, *resulting in smaller rise in blood glucose concentration after meals, lowering postprandial hyperglycemia.* Does not enhance insulin secretion.

USES

Use as monotherapy or in combination with a sulfonylurea, insulin, or metformin to lower blood glucose in pts w/type 2 diabetes mellitus when diet plus either acarbose or a sulfonylurea does not give adequate glucose control.

ADMINISTRATION

ORAL:
- Give with the first bite of each main meal.

INDICATIONS/ROUTES/DOSAGE

Diabetes mellitus:
Oral: Adults, elderly: Initially, 25 mg (½ a 50 mg tablet) 3 times/day at the start (w/first bite) of each main meal. ***Range:*** 50–100 mg 3 times/day. ***Maximum:*** <60 kg: 50 mg 3 times/day; >60 kg: 100 mg 3 times/day.

CONTRAINDICATIONS

Significant renal dysfunction (serum creatinine >2mg/dl), hypersensitivity to drug, diabetic ketoacidosis or cirrhosis, inflammatory bowel disease, colonic ulceration, partial intestinal obstruction or predisposition to intestinal obstruction, chronic intestinal diseases associated w/marked disorders of digestion or absorption, conditions that may deteriorate as result of increased gas formation in the intestine.

CAUTIONS

Elderly, malnourished, or debilitated, those w/renal or hepatic dysfunction, cardiac disease. Increased risk for hypoglycemia when given in combination w/insulin.

INTERACTIONS

DRUG: ***Digestive enzymes, intestinal absorbents*** (e.g., charcoal) reduce acarbose effect. Do not use concurrently. ***Sulfonylureas*** may produce hypoglycemia. *Diuretics, corticosteroids, phenytoin, sympathomimetics, phenothiazines, nicotinic acid, thyroid hormones, estrogens, oral contraceptives, calcium channel blockers, isoniazid* may produce hyperglycemia. **HERBAL:** None known. **FOOD:** None significant. **ALTERED LAB VALUES:** May increase serum transaminase levels and slightly reduce hematocrit.

SIDE EFFECTS

FREQUENT: Transient GI disturbances: abdominal pain (21%), diarrhea (33%), flatulence (77%). Symptoms tend to diminish in frequency and intensity over time.

ADVERSE REACTIONS/TOXIC EFFECTS

None significant.

PATIENT CONSIDERATIONS

BASELINE ASSESSMENT

Question for hypersensitivity to acarbose. Check blood glucose level. Discuss lifestyle to determine extent of learning, emotional needs. Assure follow-up instruction if pt/family do not thoroughly understand diabetes management or glucose-testing technique.

INTERVENTION/EVALUATION

Monitor blood glucose, liver function, glycosylated hemoglobin, and food intake. Assess for hypoglycemia (cool wet skin, tremors, dizziness, anxiety, headache, tachycardia, numbness in mouth, hunger, diplopia) or hyperglycemia (polyuria, polyphagia, polydipsia, nausea, vomiting, dim vision, fatigue, deep rapid breathing). Be alert to conditions that alter glucose requirements: fever, increased activity or stress, surgical procedure.

PATIENT/FAMILY TEACHING

Carry oral glucose (dextrose) instead of cane sugar (sucrose) for immediate response to hypoglycemic episode. Prescribed diet is principal part of treatment; do not skip or delay meals. Diabetes mellitus requires lifelong control. Check blood glucose/urine as ordered. Serum transaminase levels should be checked q3 mos during first year of treatment and periodically thereafter. Wear medical alert identification. Check w/physician when glucose demands are altered (e.g., fever, infection, trauma, stress, heavy physical activity). Avoid alcoholic beverages. Do not take other medication w/o consulting physician. Weight control, exercise, hygiene (including foot care), and nonsmoking are an essential part of therapy. Protect skin, limit sun exposure. Avoid exposure to infections. Select clothing, positions that do not restrict blood flow. Notify physician promptly of skin eruptions, itching, bleeding, yellow skin, dark urine. Inform dentist, physician, or surgeon of this medication before any treatment.

---

acebutolol

ah-see-**beaut**-oh-lol
(Sectral)

CANADIAN AVAILABILITY
Monitan, Sectral

PREGNANCY CATEGORY B

CLASSIFICATION

Beta$_1$-adrenergic blocker

AVAILABILITY (Rx)

Capsules: 200 mg, 400 mg

PHARMACODYNAMICS

	ONSET	PEAK	DURATION
Oral (hypotensive)	1–1.5 hrs	2–8 hrs	24 hrs
Oral (antiarrhythmic)	1 hr	4–6 hrs	10 hrs

PHARMACOKINETICS

Absorption: Well absorbed from GI tract. **Metabolism:** Undergoes extensive first-pass liver metabolism to active metabolite. **Excretion:** Eliminated via bile, secreted into GI tract via intestine, excreted in urine. Removed by hemodialysis. **Half-life:** 3–4 hrs; metabolite: 8–13 hrs.

ACTION/*THERAPEUTIC EFFECT*

Predominantly blocks beta$_1$-adrenergic receptors in cardiac tissue, *slowing sinus heart rate, decreasing cardiac output, decreasing B/P.* Large doses may block beta$_2$ receptors, *increasing airway resistance.* Exhibits antiarrhythmic activity, slows AV conduction, reduces rate of spontaneous firing of sinus pacemaker.

USES/*UNLABELED*

Management of mild to moderate hypertension. Used alone or in combination w/diuretics, especially thiazide type. Management of cardiac arrhythmias (primarily PVCs). *Treatment of chronic angina, pectoris, hypertrophic cardiomyopathy, myocardial infarction, pheochromocytoma, tremors, anxiety, thyrotoxicosis, syndrome of mitral valve prolapse.*

ADMINISTRATION

ORAL:

- May be given w/o regard to meals.

INDICATIONS/ROUTES/DOSAGE

Mild to moderate hypertension:
Oral: Adults: Initially, 400 mg/day in 1–2 divided doses. *Maintenance:* 200–800 mg/day.

Severe hypertension:
Oral: Adults: Up to 1,200 mg/day in 2 divided doses.

Ventricular arrhythmias:
Oral: Adults: Initially, 200 mg q12h. Increase gradually up to 600–1,200 mg/day in 2 divided doses.

Usual elderly dosage:
Oral: Initially, 200–400 mg/day. *Maximum:* 800 mg/day.

Dosage in renal impairment:

CREATININE CLEARANCE	% OF NORMAL DOSE
<50 ml/min	50
<25 ml/min	25

CONTRAINDICATIONS

Overt cardiac failure, cardiogenic shock, heart block greater than first degree, severe bradycardia.

CAUTIONS

Impaired renal or hepatic function, peripheral vascular disease, hyperthyroidism, diabetes, inadequate cardiac function, bronchospastic disease.

INTERACTIONS

DRUG: ***Diuretics, other hypotensives*** may increase hypotensive effect; ***sympathomimetics, xanthines*** may mutually inhibit effects; may mask symptoms of hypoglycemia, prolong hypoglycemic effect of ***insulin, oral hypoglycemics; NSAIDs*** may decrease antihypertensive effect; ***Cimetidine*** may increase concentration. **HERBAL:** None known. **FOOD:** None significant.

ALTERED LAB VALUES: May increase ANA titer, SGOT (AST), SGPT (ALT), alkaline phosphatase, LDH, bilirubin, BUN, creatinine, K, uric acid, lipoproteins, triglycerides.

SIDE EFFECTS

Generally well tolerated, w/mild and transient effects. FREQUENT: Hypotension manifested as dizziness, nausea, diaphoresis, headache, cold extremities, fatigue, constipation/diarrhea. OCCASIONAL: Insomnia, flatulence, urinary frequency, impotence or decreased libido. RARE: Rash, arthralgia, myalgia, confusion (especially elderly), change in taste.

ADVERSE REACTIONS/TOXIC EFFECTS

Overdosage may produce profound bradycardia, hypotension. Abrupt withdrawal may result in sweating, palpitations, headache, tremulousness. May precipitate CHF, MI in pts w/cardiac disease, thyroid storm in those w/thyrotoxicosis, peripheral ischemia in those w/existing peripheral vascular disease. Hypoglycemia may occur in previously controlled diabetics. Thrombocytopenia (unusual bruising, bleeding) occurs rarely.

PATIENT CONSIDERATIONS

BASELINE ASSESSMENT

Assess baseline renal/liver function tests. Assess B/P, apical pulse immediately before drug is administered. (If pulse is 60/min or below, or systolic B/P is below 90 mm Hg, withhold medication, contact physician.)

INTERVENTION/EVALUATION

Monitor B/P for hypotension, respiration for shortness of breath. Assess pulse for strength/weakness, irregular rate, bradycardia. Monitor EKG for cardiac arrhythmias, particularly shortening of QT interval, prolongation of PR interval. Assess frequency and consistency of stools. Assist w/ambulation if dizziness occurs. Assess for evidence of CHF: dyspnea (particularly on exertion or lying down), night cough, peripheral edema, distended neck veins, decreased urine output, weight gain. Monitor I&O, daily weight. Assess for nausea, diaphoresis, headache, fatigue.

PATIENT/FAMILY TEACHING

Do not abruptly discontinue medication. Compliance w/therapy regimen is essential to control hypertension, arrhythmias. To avoid hypotensive effect, rise slowly from lying to sitting position; wait momentarily before standing. Avoid tasks that require alertness, motor skills until response to drug is established. Report shortness of breath, excessive fatigue, weight gain, prolonged dizziness, or headache. Do not use nasal decongestants, OTC cold preparations (stimulants) w/o physician approval. Take B/P, pulse before taking medication. (Instruct on proper technique, when to contact physician.) Avoid smoking; follow physician's instructions for weight loss, exercise. Restrict salt, alcohol intake.

---

acetaminophen

ah-see-tah-**min**-oh-fen
(Datril, Tempra, Tylenol)

FIXED-COMBINATION(S)
W/butabarbital, a sedative-hypnotic and caffeine, a stimulant (Fioricet); w/codeine, a narcotic

analgesic **(Tylenol w/codeine)**; w/hydrocodone, a narcotic analgesic **(Vicodin, Zydone)**; w/oxycodone, a narcotic analgesic **(Percocet, Tylox)**; w/propoxyphene, an analgesic **(Darvocet)**.

CANADIAN AVAILABILITY
Abenol, Apo-Acetaminophen, Atasol, Tempra, Tylenol

PREGNANCY CATEGORY B

CLASSIFICATION

Non-narcotic analgesic, antipyretic

AVAILABILITY (OTC)

Capsules: 500 mg. **Elixir:** 120 mg/5 ml, 160 mg/5 ml, 325 mg/5 ml. **Liquid:** 160 mg/5 ml. **Solution:** 100 mg/ml, 120 mg/2.5 ml. **Suppository:** 120 mg, 325 mg, 650 mg. **Tablets (chewable):** 80 mg. **Tablets:** 160 mg, 325 mg, 500 mg, 650 mg.

PHARMACODYNAMICS

	ONSET	PEAK	DURATION
Oral	15–30 min	1–1.5 hrs	4–6 hrs

PHARMACOKINETICS

Absorption: Rapid, completely absorbed from GI tract; rectal absorption variable. **Distribution:** Widely distributed to most body tissues. **Metabolism:** Liver. **Excretion:** Urine. **Half-life:** 1–4 hrs (increased in hepatic disease, elderly, neonates; decreased in children).

ACTION/*THERAPEUTIC EFFECT*

Exact mechanism unknown, but appears to inhibit prostaglandin synthesis in CNS and, to a lesser extent, block pain impulse through peripheral action, *resulting in analgesia.* Acts centrally on hypothalamic heat-regulating center, producing peripheral vasodilation (skin erythema, sweating, heat loss), *resulting in antipyresis.*

USES

Relief of mild to moderate pain, fever.

ADMINISTRATION

ORAL:
- Give w/o regard to meals.
- Tablets may be crushed.

RECTAL:
- Moisten suppository w/cold water before inserting well up into rectum.

INDICATIONS/ROUTES/DOSAGE

Note: Children may repeat doses 4–5 times/day; maximum of 5 doses/24 hrs.

Oral: Adults, elderly: 325–650 mg q4–6h or 1 g 3–4 times/day. ***Maximum:*** 4 g/day. ***Children (11 yrs):*** 480 mg/dose; ***(9–10 yrs):*** 400 mg/dose; ***(6–8 yrs):*** 320 mg/dose; ***(4–5 yrs):*** 240 mg/dose; ***(2–3 yrs):*** 160 mg/dose; ***(1–2 yrs):*** 120 mg/dose; ***(4–11 mos):*** 80 mg/dose; ***(0–3 mos):*** 40 mg/dose.

Rectal: Adults: 650 mg q4–6h. ***Maximum:*** 6 doses/24 hrs. ***Children (6–12 yrs):*** 325 mg q4–6h. ***Maximum:*** 2.6 g/24 hrs. ***Children (3–6 yrs):*** 120 mg q4–6h. ***Maximum:*** 720 mg/24 hrs. ***Children (1–3 yrs):*** 80 g q4h. ***Children (3–11 mos):*** 80 g q6h. ***Children (<3 mos):*** Consult physician.

CONTRAINDICATIONS

Hypersensitivity to acetaminophen.

CAUTIONS

Impaired hepatic function, anemia.

INTERACTIONS

DRUG: *Alcohol* (chronic use), ***liver enzymes inducers*** (e.g., cimetidine), ***hepatotoxic medications*** (e.g., phenytoin) may increase risk of hepatotoxicity w/prolonged high dose or single toxic dose. Regular use may increase risk of bleeding w/*warfarin*. **HERBAL:** None known. **FOOD:** None significant. **ALTERED LAB VALUES:** May increase SGOT (AST), SGPT (ALT), bilirubin, prothrombin levels (may indicate hepatotoxicity).

SIDE EFFECTS

Well tolerated. **RARE:** Hypersensitivity reaction.

ADVERSE REACTIONS/TOXIC EFFECTS

Early signs of acetaminophen toxicity: anorexia, nausea, diaphoresis, generalized weakness within first 12–24 hrs. Later signs of toxicity: vomiting, right upper quadrant tenderness, elevated liver function tests within 48 to 72 hrs after ingestion. *Antidote:* Acetylcysteine.

PATIENT CONSIDERATIONS

Baseline Assessment

Question for sensitivity to acetaminophen. Assess onset, type, location, and duration of pain. Effect of medication is reduced if full pain recurs before next dose.

Fixed-combination
Obtain vital signs before giving medication. If respirations are 12/min or lower (20/min or lower in children), withhold medication, contact physician.

Intervention/Evaluation

Assess for clinical improvement and relief of pain, fever.

Patient/Family Teaching

Do not exceed dosage. Consult physician for use in children <3 yrs, oral use >5 days (children), >10 days (adults), or fever >3 day duration. Severe/recurrent pain or high/continuous fever may indicate serious illness.

Fixed-combination
Avoid tasks that require alertness, motor skills until response to drug is established. Tolerance/dependence may occur w/prolonged use.

acetazolamide

ah-seat-ah-**zole**-ah-myd
(Dazamide, Diamox, AK-Zol)

acetazolamide sodium

(Diamox) [injection]

CANADIAN AVAILABILITY
Apo-Acetazolamide, Diamox

PREGNANCY CATEGORY C

CLASSIFICATION

Carbonic anhydrase inhibitor

AVAILABILITY (Rx)

Capsules (sustained release): 500 mg. **Tablets:** 125 mg, 250 mg. **Powder for Injection:** 500 mg.

PHARMACODYNAMICS

	ONSET	PEAK	DURATION
Oral (tablets)			
	60–90 min	2–4 hrs	8–12 hrs
(capsules)			
	2 hrs	8–18 hrs	18–24 hrs
IV	2 min	15 min	4–5 hrs

PHARMACOKINETICS

Absorption: Well absorbed from GI tract. **Excretion:** Primarily excreted unchanged in urine. **Half-life:** 10–15 hrs.

ACTION/*THERAPEUTIC EFFECT*

Reduces formation of hydrogen and bicarbonate ions from carbon dioxide and water by inhibiting, in proximal renal tubule, the enzyme carbonic anhydrase, thereby promoting renal excretion of sodium, potassium, bicarbonate, water. Ocular: Reduces rate of aqueous humor formation, *lowers intraocular pressure.* Diamox only: Exact mechanism unknown, but may increase CO_2 tension, *producing anticonvulsant activity by retarding neuronal conduction.*

USES / *UNLABELED*

Treatment of open-angle, secondary or angle closure glaucoma, adjunct in managing absence seizures (e.g., petit mal), tonic-clonic, simple, partial and myoclonic seizures. *Lowers intraocular pressure in treatment of malignant glaucoma, treatment of toxicity of weakly acidic medications, prevents uric acid/cystine renal calculi by alkalinizing the urine.*

STORAGE/HANDLING

Store tablets, capsules, parenteral form at room temperature. Syrup suspension mixed w/acetazolamide is stable for 1 week at room temperature. After reconstitution, IV solution is stable for 24 hrs.

ADMINISTRATION

ORAL:

- When oral liquid is needed, tablet may be crushed and mixed w/5 ml cherry, chocolate, raspberry, or other highly flavored carbohydrate syrup. Each tablet may be softened in 2 tsp hot water, then added to 2 tsp honey or syrup (mix just prior to administration). Drug will not dissolve in fruit juice.
- Scored tablets may be crushed; do not crush or break extended-release capsules.
- May give w/food if GI upset occurs.

IV:

- **Note:** IM injection painful due to alkaline pH. IV preferred.
- Reconstitute 500 mg vial w/5 ml sterile water for injection to provide solution containing 100 mg/ml.

INDICATIONS/ROUTES/DOSAGE

Glaucoma:
Oral: Adults: 250 mg 1–4 times/day. ***Extended-Release:*** 500 mg 1–2 times/day usually given in morning and evening.

Secondary glaucoma, preop treatment of acute congestive glaucoma:
Oral/IV: Adults: 250 mg q4h, 250 mg q12h; or 500 mg, then 125–250 mg q4h. ***Oral: Children:*** 10–15 mg/kg/day in divided doses. ***IV: Children:*** 5–10 mg/kg q6h.

Epilepsy:
Oral: Adults, children: 375–1,000 mg/day in 1–4 divided doses.

Acute mountain sickness:
Oral: Adults: 500–1,000 mg/day in divided doses. If possible, begin 24–48 hrs before ascent, continue at least 48 hrs at high altitude.

Usual elderly dosage:
Oral: Initially, 250 mg 2 times/day; use lowest effective dose.

CONTRAINDICATIONS

Hypersensitivity to sulfonamides, severe renal disease, adrenal insufficiency, hypochloremic acidosis.

CAUTIONS

History of hypercalcemia, diabetes mellitus, gout, digitalized patients, obstructive pulmonary disease.

INTERACTIONS

DRUG: May increase ***digoxin*** toxicity (due to hypokalemia). May increase effects/toxicity of ***amphetamines;*** may decrease effects of ***methenamine***. **HERBAL:** None known. **FOOD:** None significant. **ALTERED LAB VALUES:** May increase ammonia, bilirubin, glucose, chloride, uric acid, calcium; may decrease bicarbonate, potassium.

SIDE EFFECTS

FREQUENT: Unusually tired/weak, diarrhea, increased urination/frequency, decreased appetite/weight, altered taste (metallic), nausea, vomiting, numbness in extremities, lips, mouth. **OCCASIONAL:** Depression, drowsiness. **RARE:** Headache, photosensitivity, confusion, tinnitus, severe muscle weakness, loss of taste.

ADVERSE REACTION/TOXIC EFFECTS

Long-term therapy may result in acidotic state. Nephrotoxicity/hepatotoxicity occurs occasionally, manifested as dark urine/stools, pain in lower back, jaundice, dysuria, crystalluria, renal colic/calculi. Bone marrow depression may be manifested as aplastic anemia, thrombocytopenia, thrombocytopenic purpura, leukopenia, agranulocytosis, hemolytic anemia.

PATIENT CONSIDERATIONS

BASELINE ASSESSMENT

Glaucoma

Assess peripheral vision, acuity. Assess affected pupil for dilation, response to light.

Epilepsy

Take history of seizure disorders (length, intensity, duration of seizures, presence of auras, LOC).

INTERVENTION/EVALUATION

Monitor I&O, BUN, electrolytes (particularly serum potassium). Monitor pattern of daily bowel activity and stool consistency. Observe for signs of infection (fever, sore throat, unusual bleeding/bruising, fatigue) due to bone marrow depression. Monitor for acidosis (headache, lethargy progressing to drowsiness, CNS depression, Kussmaul's respiration).

PATIENT/FAMILY TEACHING

Report presence of tingling or tremor in hands or feet, unusual bleeding/bruising, unexplained fever, sore throat, flank pain. Avoid tasks that require alertness, motor skills until response to drug is established.

---

acetohexamide

(Dymelor)

See Classification section under: Antidiabetic

---

acetylcysteine (*N*-acetylcysteine)

ah-sea-tyl-**sis**-teen

(Mucomyst, Mucosil)

CANADIAN AVAILABILITY

Mucomyst, Parvolex

PREGNANCY CATEGORY B

CLASSIFICATION

Antidote, mucolytic

AVAILABILITY (Rx)

Solution: 10%, 20%

PHARMACODYNAMICS

	ONSET	PEAK	DURATION
Inhalant			
	1 min	5 min	—

PHARMACOKINETICS

Absorption: After oral inhalation/intratracheal instillation, most of drug involved in sulfhydryl-disulfide reaction. Remainder absorbed from pulmonary epithelium. After oral administration, readily absorbed from GI tract. **Metabolism:** Liver.

ACTION/*THERAPEUTIC EFFECT*

Splits linkage of mucoproteins, *reducing viscosity of pulmonary secretions, facilitates removal by coughing, postural drainage, mechanical means. Maintains/restores hepatic concentration of glutathione* (necessary for inactivation of hepatotoxic acetaminophen toxicity).

USES

Adjunctive treatment for abnormally viscid mucous secretions present in acute and chronic bronchopulmonary disease and pulmonary complication of cystic fibrosis, tracheostomy care; treatment of acetaminophen overdose.

STORAGE/HANDLING

A light purple color may occur in opened bottle (does not impair safety or effectiveness of medication). After exposure to air, refrigerate solution and use within 96 hrs.

ADMINISTRATION

Note: A slight, disagreeable odor from solution may be noticed during initial administration but disappears quickly

NEBULIZATION:

- 20% solution may be diluted w/0.9% NaCl or sterile water for injection; 10% solution may be used undiluted.
- Avoid contact w/iron, copper, rubber (reacts w/acetylcysteine).
- Use parts made of glass, plastic, aluminum, chromed metal, sterling silver, or stainless steel.

ORAL:

- Give as 5% solution; dilute 1:3 w/cola, soft drink, or juice.
- Prepare fresh; use within 1 hr.
- May give via duodenal tube.

INDICATIONS/ROUTES/DOSAGE

Note: Use 20% solution for oral inhalation or intratracheal instillation.

Bronchopulmonary, tracheostomy:
Nebulization: Adults, elderly: **(20% solution):** 3–5 ml 3–4 times daily. ***Range:*** 1–10 ml q2–6h. ***Adults, elderly:*** **(10% solution):** 6–10 ml 3–4 times daily. ***Range:*** 2–20 ml q2–6hr.
Intratracheal instillation: Adults: 1–2 ml of 10–20% solution instilled into tracheostomy q1–4h.

Acetaminophen overdose:
Oral (5%): Adults, elderly: Loading dose of 140 mg/kg, followed in 4 hrs by maintenance dose of 70 mg/kg q4h for 17 additional doses (unless acetaminophen assay reveals nontoxic level).

CONTRAINDICATIONS

None significant.

CAUTIONS

Bronchial asthma, elderly, debilitated w/severe respiratory insufficiency.

INTERACTIONS

DRUG: None significant. **HERBAL:** None known. **FOOD:** None significant. **ALTERED LAB VALUES:** None significant.

SIDE EFFECTS

FREQUENT: ***Inhalation:*** Stickiness on face, transient unpleasant odor. **OCCASIONAL:** ***Inhalation:*** Increased bronchial secretions, irritated throat, nausea, vomiting, rhinorrhea. RARE: *Inhalation:* Skin rash. *Oral:* Facial edema, bronchospasm, wheezing.

ADVERSE REACTION/TOXIC EFFECTS

Large dosage may produce severe nausea, vomiting.

PATIENT CONSIDERATIONS

BASELINE ASSESSMENT

Mucolytic

Assess pretreatment respirations for rate, depth, rhythm. Place tissue within easy reach of pt.

Antidote

Assess acetominophen plasma level. Determine baselines for AST, ALT, bilirubin, PT, creatinine, BUN, blood sugar, and electrolytes. Assure that the stomach is empty by lavaging or inducing emesis. If activated charcoal has been administered, lavage before administering acetylcysteine.

INTERVENTION/EVALUATION

Mucolytic

Have suction equipment available in case pt cannot clear airway. If bronchospasm occurs, treatment should be discontinued and physician notified; bronchodilator may be added to therapy. Monitor rate, depth, rhythm, type of respiration (abdominal, thoracic). Assess for evidence of stomatitis (erythema of mucous membranes, dry mouth, burning of oral mucosa).Check sputum for color, consistency, amount. Assess lung sounds for rhonchi, wheezing, rales.

Antidote

Continue to monitor lab test results (see Baseline Assessment) daily. Monitor I&O. Assess pt for vomiting (potential is increased due to vomiting from acetaminophen). Treat hypoglycemia as necessary. Avoid diuretics. Vitamin K_1 may be administered if prothombin time ratio exceeds 1.5, fresh frozen plasma if ratio exceeds 3. Monitor vital signs.

PATIENT/FAMILY TEACHING

Mucolytic

A slight, disagreeable odor from solution may be noticed during initial administration but disappears quickly. Explain importance of adequate hydration. Teach proper coughing and deep breathing.

Antidote

Explain purpose of therapy. Report any bleeding at once.

acitretin

ah-sah-**tree**-tin
(Soriatane)

CANADIAN AVAILABILITY
Soriatane

PREGNANCY CATEGORY X

CLASSIFICATION

Antipsoriatic

AVAILABILITY (Rx)

Capsules: 10 mg, 25 mg

PHARMACODYNAMICS:

	ONSET	PEAK	DURATION
Oral	—	2–5 hrs	—

Multiple-dose administration produces steady-state concentration in about 3 wks. A twofold increase in plasma concentration is noted in the elderly, half-life unchanged.

PHARMACOKINETICS

Absorption: Optimal absorption if given with food. Protein binding: 99.9%, primarily albumin. **Metabolism:** Undergoes extensive metabolism. **Excretion:** Excreted in the feces and urine. **Half-life:** 49 hrs.

ACTION/*THERAPEUTIC EFFECT*

May modulate factors influencing epidural proliferation, regulate RNA/DNA synthesis, control glycoprotein formation, or govern immune response, *regulating keratinocyte growth and differentiation.*

USES/*UNLABELED*

Treatment of severe psoriasis, including erythrodermic and generalized pustule types. Reduces severity of scaling, erythema, and epidural induration. *Treatment of Darier's disease, palmoplantar pustulosis, lichen planus; children with lamellar ichthyosis, nonbullous and bullous ichthyosiform erythroderma, Sjogren-Larsson syndrome.*

ADMINISTRATION

ORAL:

- Give as single dose at the main meal.
- Administer whole; do not crush.

INDICATIONS/ROUTES/DOSAGES

Psoriasis:

Oral: Adults, elderly: 25–50 mg day as a single dose with the main meal. ***Maintenance:*** 25–50 mg/day after the initial response is noted. Continue until lesions have resolved.

CONTRAINDICATIONS

Pregnancy, hypersensitivity to acitretin, or parabens (a preservative in the gelatin capsule).

CAUTIONS

Impaired liver or kidney function.

INTERACTIONS

DRUG: ***Methotrexate*** increases risk of hepatotoxicity. ***Tetracycline*** may increase potential for pseudotumor cerebri. **HERBAL:** None known. **FOOD:** None significant. **ALTERED LAB VALUES:** Elevation of SGOT (AST), SGPT (ALT), GGT or LDH, cholesterol occurs in 33% of patients. Increase in triglycerides occurs in 66% of pts. Lowers HDL in 40% of pts.

SIDE EFFECTS

FREQUENT (>75%): Lip inflammation, (50–75%): alopecia, skin peeling, (25–50%): dry skin, pruritus, nail disorder, rhinitis (10–25%): shaking, dry eyes, rash, hyperesthesia, paresthesia, sticky skin, dry mouth, epistaxis, dryness/thickening of conjunctiva. **OCCASIONAL: (1–10%):** Eye irritation, brow and lash loss, sweating, chills, sensation of cold, flushing, edema, blurred vision, diarrhea, nausea, thirst.

ADVERSE REACTIONS/TOXIC EFFECTS

Benign intracranial hypertension (pseudotumor cerebri) occurs rarely. Observe for headache, nausea, vomiting, visual disturbances. Major fetal abnormalities if given during pregnancy; use is contraindicated.

PATIENT CONSIDERATIONS

BASELINE ASSESSMENT

Perform blood lipid, SGOT (AST), SGPT (ALT), and LPH tests levels prior to administration and at intervals of 1–2 wks until response to the drug is established (usually within 4–8 wks). Question for possibility of preg-

nancy prior to initiation of therapy (Pregnancy Category X).

PATIENT/FAMILY TEACHING

Use effective contraception for no less than 1 mo prior to and during drug administration. Contraception should be continued for at least 3 yrs after treatment is stopped. Do not ingest ethanol during therapy and for 2 mos after treatment is stopped. Some birth control methods have failed including tubal ligation and progestin "minipill" preparations. Do not take vitamin A in excess of minimum daily requirement (prevents possible toxic effects). A worsening of psoriasis occurs occasionally during initial treatment. Therapeutic response may not appear for 2–3 mos. A decreased tolerance to contact lenses may occur during treatment. Do not donate blood during and for 3 yrs after treatment has stopped. Avoid sunlamps, excessive exposure to sunlight (UV light is enhanced during therapy).

---

acyclovir

aye-**sigh**-klo-veer

(Zovirax)

CANADIAN AVAILABILITY

Avirax, Zovirax

PREGNANCY CATEGORY C

CLASSIFICATION

Antiviral

AVAILABILITY (Rx)

Tablets: 400 mg, 800 mg. **Capsules:** 200 mg. **Oral Suspension:** 200 mg/5 ml. **Powder for Injection:** 500 mg, 1,000 mg. **Ointment.**

PHARMACOKINETICS

Absorption: Poorly absorbed from GI tract; minimal absorption following topical application. Widely distributed. **Metabolism:** Partially metabolized by cellular enzymes. **Excretion:** Primarily in urine. Removed by hemodialysis. **Half-life:** 2.5 hrs (increased in impaired renal function).

ACTION / *THERAPEUTIC EFFECT*

Converted to acyclovir triphosphate, becoming part of DNA chain, *interfering w/DNA synthesis and viral replication.* Virustatic.

USES

Parenteral: Initial treatment for severe herpes genitalis; herpes zoster ophthalmicus; initial/recurrent mucocutaneous herpes simplex; herpes simplex encephalitis; neonatal herpes simplex; herpes zoster caused by varicella zoster virus (VZV) in immunocompromised pts and disseminated herpes zoster in nonimmunocompromised pts. *Oral:* Initial treatment, management of recurrent and prophylaxis of frequently recurrent herpes genitalis; treatment of herpes zoster (shingles); herpes zoster ophthalmicus; varicella infections (chicken pox) in nonimmunocompromised pts. ***Topical:*** Initial episodes of genital herpes, immunocompromised pts w/limited nonthreatening herpes simplex infections.

STORAGE / HANDLING

Store capsules at room temperature. Solutions of 50 mg/ml stable for 12 hrs at room temperature; may form precipitate when refrigerated. Potency not affected by precipitate and redissolution. IV infusion (piggyback) stable for 24 hrs at room temperature. Yellow discoloration does not affect potency.

ADMINISTRATION

ORAL:

- Give w/o regard to food.
- Do not crush or break capsules.

IV:

- **Note:** Do not administer by IM, Subq, or rapid IV infusion or rapid IV injection.
- Infuse for at least 1 hr.
- Maintain adequate hydration, especially during urine concentration that occurs 2 hrs following IV administration.
- Alternating IV sites, use large veins to reduce risk of phlebitis.

INDICATIONS/ROUTES/DOSAGE

Initial genital herpes infections, intermittent treatment of recurrent episodes:
Oral: Adults, elderly: 200 mg q4h while awake (5 times/day).

Prophylaxis of recurrent episodes:
Oral: Adults, elderly: 400 mg 2 times/day up to 12 mos.

Chicken pox:
Oral: Adults, elderly, children (2–12 yrs): 20 mg/kg (maximum 800 mg) 4 times/day for 5 days.

Mucosal or cutaneous herpes simplex, severe genital herpes:
IV: Adults, elderly: 5 mg/kg q8h. *Children <12 yrs:* 250 mg/m^2 q8h. Continue for 7 days for herpes simplex; 5 days for genital herpes.

Herpes simplex encephalitis:
IV: Adults, elderly: 10 mg/kg q8h for 10 days. *Children, 6 mos-12 yrs:* 500 mg/m^2 q8h for 10 days.

Neonatal herpes simplex:
IV: Neonates: 10 mg/kg q8h for 10 days.

Varicella zoster infections:
IV: Adults, elderly: 10 mg/kg q8h. *Children:* 500 mg/m^2 q8h. Continue for 7 days.

Herpes zoster (acute):
Oral: Adults, elderly: 800 mg q4h (5 times/day) for 7–10 days.

Usual topical dosage:
Topical: Adults, elderly: 3–6 times/day for 7 days.

Dosage in renal impairment:
Dose/frequency is modified based on severity of infection, degree of renal impairment.

Oral: Creatinine clearance of 10 ml/1.73m^2 or less: 200 mg q12h.

IV:

CREATINE CLEARANCE	DOSAGE (ADULTS)	DOSAGE (CHILDREN)
>50 ml/min	5 mg/kg q8h	250 mg/m^2 q8h
25–50 ml/min	5 mg/kg q12h	250 mg/m^2 q12h
10–25 ml/min	5 mg/kg q24h	250 mg/m^2 q24h
0–10 ml/min	2.5 mg/kg q24h	125 mg/m^2 q24h

CONTRAINDICATIONS

Hypersensitivity to acyclovir or components of preparation. Acyclovir reconstituted w/bacteriostatic water containing benzyl alcohol should not be used in neonates.

CAUTIONS

Renal or hepatic impairment, dehydration, fluid/electrolyte imbalance, concurrent use of nephrotoxic agents, neurologic abnormalities.

INTERACTIONS

DRUG: *Probenecid* may increase half-life. *Nephrotoxic medications* (e.g., aminoglycosides) may increase nephrotoxicity. **HERBAL:** None known. **FOOD:** None significant. **ALTERED LAB VALUES:** May increase BUN, serum creatinine concentrations.

SIDE EFFECTS

FREQUENT: *Parenteral:* Phlebitis/inflammation at IV site, anorexia, nausea, vomiting, lightheadedness. *Topical:* Burning, stinging. OCCASIONAL: *Parenteral:* Hypotension, diaphoresis. *Oral:* Nausea, diarrhea, vomiting, abdominal pain, headache, lightheadedness. *Topical:* Itching. RARE: *Parenteral:* Confusion, hallucinations, seizures, tremors. *Topical:* Skin rash.

ADVERSE REACTION/TOXIC EFFECTS

Rapid parenteral administration, excessively high doses, or fluid/electrolyte imbalance may produce renal failure (abdominal pain, decreased urination, decreased appetite, increased thirst, nausea, vomiting). Toxicity not reported w/oral or topical use.

PATIENT CONSIDERATIONS

BASELINE ASSESSMENT

Question history of allergies, particularly to acyclovir. Avoid nephrotoxic drugs if possible. Tissue cultures for HSV should be done before giving first dose (therapy may proceed before results are known).

INTERVENTION/EVALUATION

Monitor I&O, renal function tests if ordered, electrolyte levels. Check food tolerance, vomiting. Assess IV site for phlebitis (heat, pain, red streaking over vein). Evaluate cutaneous lesions. Be alert to neurologic effects: headache, lethargy, confusion, agitation, hallucinations, seizures. Assure adequate ventilation. Manage chicken pox and disseminated herpes zoster with strict isolation. Provide analgesics and comfort measures; especially exhausting to elderly. Encourage fluids. Keep pt's fingernails short, hands clean.

PATIENT/FAMILY TEACHING

Drink adequate fluids. Notify physician if side effects develop. Do not touch lesions with fingers to avoid spreading infection to new site.

Genital herpes
Continue therapy for full length of treatment. Space doses evenly. Use finger cot or rubber glove to apply topical ointment. Avoid sexual intercourse during duration of lesions to prevent infecting partner. Acyclovir does not cure herpes. Notify physician if lesions do not improve or recur. Avoid driving or operating machinery if dizziness is present. Pap smears should be done at least annually due to increased risk of cancer of cervix in women w/genital herpes.

Chicken pox
Unknown whether treatment of childhood chicken pox will have effect on long-term immunity.

adenosine

ah-**den**-oh-seen
(Adenocard)

CANADIAN AVAILABILITY
Adenocard

PREGNANCY CATEGORY C

CLASSIFICATION

Antiarrhythmic

AVAILABILITY (Rx)

Injection: 3 mg/ml

PHARMACOKINETICS

Immediate onset of action. **Metab-**

olism: Rapidly metabolized by enzymes and taken up by erythrocytes and vascular endothelial cells to inosine and adenosine monophosphate.

ACTION/*THERAPEUTIC EFFECT*

Slows impulse formation in SA node, slows conduction time through AV node, *depressing left ventricular function and restoring normal sinus rhythm.*

USES

Treatment of paroxysmal supraventricular tachycardia, including those associated w/accessory bypass tracts (Wolff-Parkinson-White syndrome). Adjunct in myocardial perfusion imaging or stress echocardiography as diagnostic aid.

STORAGE/HANDLING

Store at room temperature. Solution appears clear. Crystallization occurs if refrigerated; if crystallization occurs, dissolve crystals by warming to room temperature. Discard unused portion.

ADMINISTRATION

IV:

- Administer directly into vein, or if using IV line, as proximal as possible. Follow by rapid saline flush.
- Administer rapidly (over 1–2 sec).

INDICATIONS/ROUTES/DOSAGE

Usual adult dosage:
IV: Adults, elderly: Initially, 6 mg (over 1–2 sec). If first dose does not convert within 1–2 min, give 12 mg; may repeat 12 mg dose in 1–2 min if no response has occurred.

Diagnostic testing:
IV Infusion: Adults: 140 mcg/kg/min for 6 min.

CONTRAINDICATIONS

Second- or third-degree AV block or sick-sinus syndrome (w/functioning pacemaker), atrial flutter or fibrillation, ventricular tachycardia.

CAUTIONS

Heart block, arrhythmias at time of conversion, asthma, hepatic/renal failure.

INTERACTIONS

DRUG: ***Methylxanthines*** (e.g., caffeine, theophylline) may decrease effect. ***Dipyridamole*** may increase effect. ***Carbamazepine*** may increase degree of heart block caused by adenosine. **HERBAL:** None known. **FOOD:** None significant. **ALTERED LAB VALUES:** None significant.

SIDE EFFECTS

FREQUENT: Facial flushing, headache, new arrhythmias (e.g., PVCs, sinus bradycardia); pain in chest/arm/jaw/throat; shortness of breath. **OCCASIONAL:** Cough, dizziness, nausea, numbness/tingling in arms.

ADVERSE REACTION/ THERAPEUTIC EFFECTS/ TOXIC EFFECTS

May produce short-lasting heart block.

PATIENT CONSIDERATIONS

BASELINE ASSESSMENT

Identify arrhythmia per cardiac monitor and apical pulse.

INTERVENTION/EVALUATION

Assess cardiac performance per continuous EKG. Monitor B/P, apical pulse (rate, rhythm, and strength), and respirations. Monitor I&O; assess for fluid retention. Check electrolytes.

albumin, human

al-**byew**-min
(Albuminar, Albutein, Buminate, Plasbumin)

CANADIAN AVAILABILITY
Plasbumin

PREGNANCY CATEGORY C

CLASSIFICATION

Blood derivative

AVAILABILITY (Rx)

Injection: 5%, 25%

ACTION/*THERAPEUTIC EFFECT*

Regulates circulating blood volume, tissue fluid balance and maintains pressure, *restoring intravascular volume, plasma volume, and maintaining cardiac output.* Binds and functions as carrier of intermediate metabolites (hormones, enzymes, drugs) in transport and exchange of tissue products.

USES

Symptomatic/supportive treatment of shock due to burns, trauma, surgery, infections. Prevents hemoconcentration and combats water, protein, electrolyte losses in severely burned or hemorrhaging pt, hypoproteinemia, ARDS (adult respiratory distress syndrome), cardiopulmonary bypass surgery (preop blood dilution), acute nephrosis, renal dialysis (treat shock or hypotension), hyperbilirubinemia, and erythroblastosis fetalis.

STORAGE/HANDLING

Store at room temperature. Clear, brownish, odorless, moderate viscous fluid. Do not use if solution has been frozen, solution appears turbid, or contains sediment, or if not used within 4 hrs of opening vial.

ADMINISTRATION

IV:

- Give by IV infusion.
- 5% administered undiluted; 25% may be administered undiluted or diluted w/0.9% NaCl or 5% dextrose.
- May give w/o regard to pt blood group or Rh factor.

INDICATIONS/ROUTES/DOSAGE

Note: Dosage based on pt's condition; duration of administration based on pt's response.

Usual dosage:
IV: Adults, elderly: 25 g by infusion. May be repeated in 15–30 min. ***Maximum:*** 125 g/24 hrs or 250 g/48 hrs.

Shock (greatly reduced blood volume):
IV: Adults, elderly: Administer 5% or 25% fluid as rapidly as possible to improve condition and restore normal blood volume. May be repeated in 15–30 min. ***Infants, neonates:*** 10–20 ml/kg of 5% solution.

Shock (slightly reduced blood volume):
IV: Adults, elderly: **5%:** Give 2–4 ml/min. ***Children:*** Give 0.5–2 ml/min.

IV: Adults, elderly: **25%:** Give 1 ml/min.

Burns (5% or 25%):
IV: Adults, elderly, children: Maintain plasma albumin concentration of 2.5 ± 0.5 g/100 ml (or plasma protein level of 5.2 g/100 ml).

Hypoproteinemia:
IV: Adults, elderly: 50–75 g/day. ***Children:*** 25 g/day. Give at rate not to exceed 5–10 ml/min (5%)

or 2–3 ml/min (25%). This minimizes circulatory overload, pulmonary edema.

Acute nephrosis:
IV: Adults, elderly: **25%:** 100–200 ml (25–50 g) daily for 7–10 days.

Renal dialysis:
IV: Adults, elderly: **25%:** 100 ml (25 g).

Hyperbilirubinemia, erythroblastosis fetalis:
IV: Infants: 1 g/kg 1–2 hrs before transfusion.

CONTRAINDICATIONS

Severe anemia, cardiac failure, history of allergic reaction to albumin, no albumin deficiency.

CAUTIONS

Low cardiac reserve, pulmonary disease, hepatic or renal failure.

INTERACTIONS

DRUG: None significant. **HERBAL:** None known. **FOOD:** None significant. **ALTERED LAB VALUES:** May increase serum alkaline phosphatase concentrations.

SIDE EFFECTS

OCCASIONAL: Hypotension. **RARE:** High dose, repeated therapy may result in altered vital signs; chills, fever, increased salivation, nausea, vomiting, urticaria, tachycardia.

ADVERSE REACTION/TOXIC EFFECTS

Fluid overload (headache, weakness, blurred vision, behavioral changes, incoordination, isolated muscle twitching) and CHF (rapid breathing, rales, wheezing, coughing, increased B/P, distended neck veins) may occur.

PATIENT CONSIDERATIONS

BASELINE ASSESSMENT

Obtain B/P, pulse, respirations immediately before administration. There should be adequate hydration before albumin is administered.

INTERVENTION/EVALUATION

Monitor B/P for hypo/hypertension. Assess frequently for evidence of fluid overload, pulmonary edema (see Adverse Reaction/Toxic Effects). Check skin for flushing, urticaria. Monitor hemoglobin, hematocrit. Monitor I&O ratio (watch for decreased output). Assess for therapeutic response (increased B/P; decreased edema).

---

albuterol

ale-**beut**-er-all
(Proventil, Proventil HFA, Ventolin [inhalation])

albuterol sulfate

(Proventil, Ventolin [syrup, tablets, nebulization], Volmax)

FIXED-COMBINATION(S)
W/ipratropium, a bronchodilator **(Combivent)**

CANADIAN AVAILABILITY
Airomir, Novosalmol, Ventolin

PREGNANCY CATEGORY C

CLASSIFICATION

Bronchodilator

AVAILABILITY (Rx)

Tablets: 2 mg, 4 mg. **Tablets (extended-release):** 4 mg. **Syrup:** 2 mg/5 ml. **Aerosol:** Metered dose inhaler. **Solution for Inhalation:** 0.83 mg/ml, 5 mg/ml. **Capsules for Inhalation:** 200 mcg, 400 mcg.

PHARMACODYNAMICS

	ONSET	PEAK	DURATION
Inhalation	5–15 min	0.5–2 hrs	3–6 hrs
Oral	<30 min	2–3 hrs	4–8 hrs

PHARMACOKINETICS

Absorption: Rapid, well absorbed from GI tract; gradual absorption from bronchi following inhalation. **Metabolism:** Liver. **Excretion:** Primarily excreted in urine. **Half-life:** 3.8 hrs oral; 3.7–5 hrs inhalation.

ACTION/*THERAPEUTIC EFFECT*

Stimulates beta$_2$-adrenergic receptors in the lungs *resulting in relaxation of bronchial smooth muscle. Relieves bronchospasm, reduces airway resistance.*

USES

Relief of bronchospasm due to reversible obstructive airway disease, exercise-induced bronchospasm.

ADMINISTRATION

ORAL:

- Do not crush or break extended-release tablets.

INHALATION:

- Shake container well, exhale completely, then holding mouthpiece 1 inch away from lips, inhale and hold breath as long as possible before exhaling.
- Wait 1–10 min before inhaling second dose (allows for deeper bronchial penetration).
- Rinse mouth w/water immediately after inhalation (prevents mouth/throat dryness).

NEBULIZATION:

- Dilute 0.5 ml of 0.5% solution to final volume of 3 ml w/0.9% NaCl to provide 2.5 mg.
- Administer over 5–15 min.
- Nebulizer should be used w/compressed air or oxygen at rate of 6–10 L/min.

INDICATIONS/ROUTES/DOSAGE

Bronchospasm:

Inhalation (Aerosol): Adults, elderly, children >12 yrs: 2 inhalations q4–6h. One inhalation q4h may be sufficient in some pts. Wait 1–10 min before administering second inhalation.

Inhalation (Capsules): Adults, elderly, children >4 yrs: 200–400 mcg q4–6h.

Inhalation (Solution): Adults, elderly: 2.5 mg 3–4 times/day. By nebulization.

Tablets: Adults, children >12 yrs: 2 or 4 mg 3–4 times/day. Gradually increased to maximum dose of 8 mg 4 times/day (32 mg/day). ***Elderly:*** 2 mg 3–4 times/day. Gradually increased to maximum dose of 8 mg 3–4 times/day. ***Children 6–12 yrs:*** Initially, 2 mg 3–4 times/day. Gradually increase to maximum dose of 24 mg/day in divided doses.

Syrup: Adults, children >14 yrs: 2–4 mg 3–4 times/day. ***Maximum:*** 32 mg/day. ***Children 6–14 yrs:*** 2 mg 3–4 times/day. Dosage may be gradually increased to 24 mg/day in divided doses. ***Children 2–6 yrs:*** Initially, 0.1 mg/kg 3 times/day (do not exceed 2 mg 3 times/day). Gradually increased to 0.2 mg/kg 3 times/day (do not exceed 4 mg 3 times/day).

Extended-Release: Adults, children >12 yrs: 4 or 8 mg q12h.

May be gradually increased to 16 mg daily.

Exercise-induced bronchospasm: *Inhalation: Adults, elderly, children >12 yrs:* 2 inhalations 15 min before exercise.

CONTRAINDICATIONS

History of hypersensitivity to sympathomimetics.

CAUTIONS

Hypertension, cardiovascular disease, hyperthyroidism, diabetes mellitus.

INTERACTIONS

DRUG: *Beta-adrenergic blocking agents (beta blockers)* antagonize effects. May increase risk of arrhythmias w/*digoxin*. *MAO inhibitors, tricyclic antidepressants* may potentiate cardiovascular effects. **HERBAL:** None known. **FOOD:** None significant. **ALTERED LAB VALUES:** May decrease serum potassium levels.

SIDE EFFECTS

FREQUENT (>1%): Trembling, dizziness, shakiness, weakness, hyperactivity, headache, insomnia, nausea, vomiting, GI distress, cough, wheezing, dyspnea, dry throat, altered taste, nasal congestion. **OCCASIONAL (<1%):** Drowsiness, restlessness, diarrhea, dry mouth, sweating, flushing, decreased appetite. ***Inhalation:*** Dry, irritated mouth or throat, coughing, bronchial irritation. **RARE:** Transient increased wheezing, difficulty breathing, chest discomfort.

ADVERSE REACTIONS/TOXIC EFFECTS

Excessive sympathomimetic stimulation may produce palpitations, extrasystoles, tachycardia, chest pain, slight increase in B/P followed by substantial decrease, chills, sweating, blanching of skin. Too frequent or excessive use may lead to loss of bronchodilating effectiveness and/or severe, paradoxical bronchoconstriction.

PATIENT CONSIDERATIONS

BASELINE ASSESSMENT

Offer emotional support (high incidence of anxiety due to difficulty in breathing and sympathomimetic response to drug).

INTERVENTION/EVALUATION

Monitor rate, depth, rhythm, type of respiration; quality and rate of pulse. Assess lung sounds for wheezing (bronchoconstriction) and rales.

PATIENT/FAMILY TEACHING

Instruct on proper use of inhaler. Increase fluid intake (decreases lung secretion viscosity). Do not take more than two inhalations at any one time (excessive use may produce paradoxical bronchoconstriction or a decreased bronchodilating effect). Rinsing mouth with water immediately after inhalation may prevent mouth/throat dryness. Avoid excessive use of caffeine derivatives (chocolate, coffee, tea, cola, cocoa). Do not take OTC medications w/o physician approval: may increase sympathetic stimulation. Avoid smoking, smoke-filled areas.

alclometasone

(Aclovate)

See Classification section under: Corticosteroid: topical

aldesleukin

(Proleukin, Interleukin-2, IL-2)
See Classification section under: Cancer chemotherapy

alendronate sodium

ah-**len**-drew-nate
(Fosamax)

CANADIAN AVAILABILITY
Fosamax

PREGNANCY CATEGORY C

CLASSIFICATION

Bone resorption inhibitor, calcium regulator

AVAILABILITY (Rx)

Tablets: 5 mg, 10 mg, 35 mg, 40 mg, 70 mg

PHARMACOKINETICS

Absorption: Poorly absorbed following oral administration. After oral administration, rapidly taken into bone, w/uptake greatest at sites of active bone turnover. **Excretion:** Primarily in urine. **Terminal half-life:** >10 yrs (reflects release from skeleton as bone is resorbed).

ACTION/*THERAPEUTIC EFFECT*

Inhibits normal and abnormal bone resorption, without retarding mineralization, *leading to significant increased bone mineral density, reversing the progression of osteoporosis.*

USES/*UNLABELED*

Treatment of osteoporosis, glucocorticoid-induced osteoporosis, Paget's disease; prevention of osteoporosis, vertebral compression fractures in postmenopausal women. *Treatment of breast cancer.*

ADMINISTRATION

ORAL:

- Give first thing in morning, at least 30 full min before first food, beverage, or medication of the day.
- Give w/6–8 oz plain water only (mineral water, coffee, tea, juice will decrease absorption).
- Instruct patient *not* to lie down for at least 30 min after administering medication and until eating first food of the day (plain water and not lying down allows medication to reach stomach quickly, minimizes esophageal irritation).

INDICATIONS/ROUTES/DOSAGE

Note: Take with full glass plain water only, 30 min before first food, beverage, or medication.

Treatment of osteoporosis, prevention of fractures:
Oral: Adults, elderly: 10 mg once daily, in the morning or 70 mg once weekly.

Paget's disease:
Oral: Adults, elderly: 40 mg once daily, in the morning.

Prevention of osteoporosis:
Oral: Adults, elderly: 5 mg once daily, in the morning or 35 mg once weekly.

CONTRAINDICATIONS

Hypersensitivity to biphosphonates, renal impairment when serum creatinine clearance 5mg/dl, hypocalcemic. Concurrent use with hormone replacement therapy not recommended.

CAUTIONS

Gastrointestinal diseases (duodenitis, dysphagia, esophagitis, gastritis, ulcers (drug may exacerbate these conditions), hypocalcemia, vitamin D deficiency.

INTERACTIONS

DRUG: Concurrent dietary supplements, food, beverages may interfere with alendronate absorption. IV ***ranitidine*** may double drug bioavailability. ***Aspirin*** may increase GI disturbances. **HERBAL:** None known. **FOOD:** Coffee, orange juice decrease bioavailability. **ALTERED LAB VALUES:** Reduces serum calcium, phosphate concentrations. Significant decrease in serum alkaline phosphatase noted in those w/Paget's disease.

SIDE EFFECTS

FREQUENT (>5%): Abdominal pain, back pain, pain (>20%). **OCCASIONAL (1–5%):** Flatulence, acid regurgitation, esophageal ulcer, headache, musculoskeletal pain, chest pain, constipation, diarrhea, dyspepsia, nausea, flulike symptoms. **RARE (<1%):** Abdominal distension, gastritis, vomiting, altered taste, peripheral edema.

ADVERSE REACTIONS/TOXIC EFFECTS

Hypocalcemia, hypophosphatemia, significant GI disturbances result from overdosage.

PATIENT CONSIDERATIONS

Baseline Assessment

Hypocalcemia, vitamin D deficiency must be corrected before therapy.

Intervention/Evaluation

Check electrolytes (especially calcium and alkaline phosphatase serum levels).

Patient/Family Teaching

Instruct pt that expected benefits occur only when medication is taken w/full glass (6–8 oz) of plain water, first thing in the morning and at least 30 min before first food, beverage, or medication of the day is taken. Any other beverage (mineral water, orange juice, coffee) significantly reduces absorption of medication. Do not lie down for at least 30 min after taking medication (potentiates delivery to stomach, reduces risk of esophageal irritation). If chest pain occurs, discontinue therapy, contact physician. Consider weight-bearing exercise, modify behavioral factors (e.g., cigarette smoking, alcohol consumption).

---

alfentanil

(Alfenta)

See Classification section under: Opioid analgesics

---

alitretinoin

(Panretin)

See Supplement

---

allopurinol

al-low-**pure**-ih-nawl

(Aloprim, Lopurin, Zyloprim)

CANADIAN AVAILABILITY

Apo-Allopurinol, Purinol, Zyloprim

PREGNANCY CATEGORY C

CLASSIFICATION

Antigout

AVAILABILITY (Rx)

Tablets: 100 mg, 300 mg. **Powder for Injection:** 500 mg.

PHARMACOKINETICS

Absorption: Well absorbed from

GI tract. Widely distributed. **Metabolism:** In liver to active metabolite. **Excretion:** Primarily in urine. Removed by hemodialysis. **Half-life:** 1–3 hrs; metabolite: 12–30 hrs.

ACTION / *THERAPEUTIC EFFECT*

Decreases uric acid production by inhibition of xanthine oxidase, an enzyme, *reducing uric acid concentrations in both serum and urine.*

USES / *UNLABELED*

Treatment of chronic gouty arthritis, uric acid nephropathy. Prevents or treats hyperuricemia secondary to blood dyscrasias, cancer chemotherapy. Prevents recurrence of uric acid or calcium stone formation. **Aloprim:** Management of elevated uric acid in cancer pt unable to tolerate oral therapy. *Used in mouthwash following fluorouracil therapy to prevent stomatitis.*

ADMINISTRATION

ORAL:

- May give w/or immediately after meals or milk.
- Instruct pt to drink at least 10–12 eight oz glasses of water/day.
- Doses >300 mg/day to be administered in divided doses.

INDICATIONS / ROUTES / DOSAGE

Gout, hyperuricemia:
Oral: Adults: 200–600 mg/day. *Range:* 100–800 mg/day. *Maximum:* 800 mg/day. *Children (6–10 yrs):* 300 mg/day. *Children (< 6 yrs):* 150 mg/day.

Prevention uric acid nephropathy during neoplastic disease therapy:
Oral: Adults: 600–800 mg/day for 2–3 days (w/high fluid intake).

Reduction acute gouty attacks:
Oral: Adults: Initially, 100 mg/day. May increase by 100 mg/day at weekly intervals (up to maximum of 800 mg/day) until serum uric acid ≤6 mg/dl attained.

Recurrent calcium oxalate stones:
Oral: Adults: 200–300 mg/day.

Usual elderly dosage:
Oral: Initially, 100 mg/day, gradually increased to optimal uric acid level.

Usual parenteral dosage:
IV Infusion: Adults: 200–400 mg/m². *Maximum:* 600 mg/day. *Children:* Initially, 200 mg/m²/day.

Dosage in renal impairment:
Based on creatinine clearance using serum uric acid as index.

CREATININE CLEARANCE	DOSAGE
10–20 ml/min	200 mg/day
3–10 ml/min	100 mg/day maximum
<3 ml/min	100 mg at increased intervals

CONTRAINDICATIONS

Asymptomatic hyperuricemia.

CAUTIONS

Impaired renal, hepatic function.

INTERACTIONS

DRUG: *Thiazide diuretics* may decrease effect. May increase effect *of oral anticoagulants.* May increase effect, toxicity of ***azathioprine, mercaptopurine. Ampicillin, amoxicillin*** may increase incidence of skin rash. **HERBAL:** None known. **FOOD:** None significant. **ALTERED LAB VALUES:** May increase alkaline phosphatase, SGOT (AST), SGPT (ALT), BUN, creatinine.

SIDE EFFECTS

OCCASIONAL: Drowsiness, unusual hair loss, diarrhea, headache, nausea, vomiting, stomach pain. *Injection:* rash, nausea, vomiting, renal insufficiency.

ADVERSE REACTIONS/TOXIC EFFECTS

Pruritic maculopapular rash should be considered a toxic reaction. May be accompanied by malaise, fever, chills, joint pain, nausea, vomiting. Severe hypersensitivity may follow appearance of rash. Bone marrow depression, hepatotoxicity, peripheral neuritis, or acute renal failure occurs rarely.

PATIENT CONSIDERATIONS

BASELINE ASSESSMENT

Question pt for hypersensitivity to allopurinol. Instruct pt to drink 10–12 glasses (8 oz) of fluid daily while on medication.

INTERVENTION/EVALUATION

Discontinue medication immediately if rash or other evidence of allergic reaction appears. Encourage high fluid intake (3,000 ml/day). Monitor I&O (output should be at least 2,000 ml/day). Assess CBC, serum uric acid levels. Assess urine for cloudiness, unusual color, odor. Assess for therapeutic response (reduced joint tenderness, swelling, redness, limitation of motion).

PATIENT/FAMILY TEACHING

May take 1 or more wks for full therapeutic effect. Encourage low purine food intake, drinking 10–12 glasses (8 oz) of fluid daily while on medication. Avoid tasks that require alertness, motor skills until response to drug is established. Contact physician/nurse if rash, irritation of eyes, swelling of lips/mouth occurs.

alpha$_1$-proteinase inhibitor (human, alpha$_1$-PI)

(Prolastin)

CANADIAN AVAILABILITY

Prolastin

PREGNANCY CATEGORY C

CLASSIFICATION

Proteinase inhibitor

AVAILABILITY (Rx)

Powder for Injection: 500 mg, 1,000 mg

ACTION/*THERAPEUTIC EFFECT*

Protects alveolar epithelial lining of lower respiratory tract by alleviating imbalance between elastase (enzyme capable of degrading elastin tissue in lower respiratory tract) and alpha$_1$-proteinase inhibitor (inhibits neutrophil elastase), *allowing for subsequent protection from degradation of elastin tissue.*

USES

Chronic replacement therapy in patients w/clinically demonstrable panacinar emphysema. Do not use in patients w/PiMZ or PiMS phenotypes (small risk of panacinar emphysema).

STORAGE/HANDLING

Store parenteral form in refrigerator. After reconstitution, do not refrigerate. Use within 3 hrs. Discard unused portion.

ADMINISTRATION

IV:

- Reconstitute each vial w/20 or 40 ml sterile water (total functional activity stated in mg is noted on label of each vial); 20 ml = about 500 mg; 40 ml = about 1,000 mg activity.

- May use 0.9% NaCl as diluent.
- Infuse at rate of at least 0.08 ml/kg.

INDICATIONS/ROUTES/DOSAGE

Replacement therapy:
IV Infusion: Adults, elderly: 60 mg/kg once weekly at rate of at least 0.08 ml/kg.

CONTRAINDICATIONS

Pts w/known antibody against IgA (may experience severe reactions including anaphylaxis).

CAUTIONS

Those at risk for circulatory overload. Safety in children not established.

INTERACTIONS

DRUG: None significant. **HERBAL:** None known. **FOOD:** None significant. **ALTERED LAB VALUES:** None significant.

SIDE EFFECTS

RARE (<1%): Delayed fever (occurring 12 hrs after administration, resolves spontaneously), lightheadedness, dizziness.

ADVERSE REACTIONS/TOXIC EFFECTS

Mild leukocytosis occurs rarely.

PATIENT CONSIDERATIONS

BASELINE ASSESSMENT

All patients should be immunized against hepatitis B before initial dose is given.

INTERVENTION/EVALUATION

Maintain blood levels of alpha$_1$-PI at 80 mg/dl. Monitor respiratory status throughout therapy.

PATIENT/FAMILY TEACHING

Explain purpose of medication, importance of hepatitis B vaccine, periodic pulmonary function tests. Avoid smoking. Notify physician of changes in respiratory condition.

---

alprazolam

ale-**praz**-oh-lam
(Xanax)

CANADIAN AVAILABILITY
Apo-Alpraz, Novo-Alprazol, Xanax

PREGNANCY CATEGORY D

CLASSIFICATION

Antianxiety: Benzodiazepine

AVAILABILITY (Rx)

Tablets: 0.25 mg, 0.5 mg, 1 mg, 2 mg. **Oral Solution:** 0.5 mg/5 ml, 1 mg/ml.

PHARMACOKINETICS

Absorption: Well absorbed from GI tract. **Metabolism:** In liver. **Excretion:** Primarily excreted in urine. Minimal removed by hemodialysis. **Half-life:** 11–16 hrs.

ACTION/*THERAPEUTIC EFFECT*

Enhances action of inhibitory neurotransmitters in the brain, *producing anxiolytic effect due to CNS depressant action.*

USES/*UNLABELED*

Management of anxiety disorders associated w/depression, panic disorder. *Improves mood, relieves cramps, insomnia w/premenstrual syndrome.*

ADMINISTRATION

ORAL:

- May be given w/o regard to meals.
- Tablets may be crushed.

INDICATIONS/ROUTES/DOSAGE

Anxiety disorders:
Oral: Adults >18 yrs: Initially, 0.25–0.5 mg 3 times daily. Titrate to maximum of 4 mg daily in divided doses. *Elderly/debilitated/liver disease/low serum albumin:* Initially, 0.25 mg 2–3 times daily. Gradually increase to optimum therapeutic response.

Panic disorder:
Oral: Adults: Initially, 0.5 mg 3 times/day. May increase at 3–4 day intervals at no more than 1 mg/day. *Range:* 1–10 mg/day.

Usual elderly dosage:
Oral: Initially, 0.125–0.25 mg 2 times/day; may increase in 0.125 mg increments until desired effect attained.

Premenstrual syndrome:
Oral: Adults: 0.25 mg 3 times/day.

CONTRAINDICATIONS

Acute narrow-angle glaucoma, acute alcohol intoxication w/depressed vital signs, severe chronic obstructive pulmonary disease, myasthenia gravis, ketoconazole, itraconazole.

CAUTIONS

Impaired renal/hepatic function.

INTERACTIONS

DRUG: Potentiated effects when used w/other *CNS depressants* (including alcohol). **HERBAL:** Kava kava, valerian may increase CNS depressant effects. **FOOD:** None significant. **ALTERED LAB VALUES:** May produce abnormal renal function tests, elevate SGOT (AST), SGPT (ALT), LDH, alkaline phosphatase, serum bilirubin.

SIDE EFFECTS

FREQUENT: Muscular incoordination (ataxia), lightheadedness, transient mild drowsiness, slurred speech (particularly in elderly, debilitated). **OCCASIONAL:** Confusion, depression, blurred vision, constipation/diarrhea, dry mouth, headache, nausea. **RARE:** Behavioral problems (e.g., anger), impaired memory, paradoxical reaction (insomnia, nervousness, irritability).

ADVERSE REACTIONS/TOXIC EFFECTS

Abrupt or too rapid withdrawal may result in pronounced restlessness, irritability, insomnia, hand tremors, abdominal/muscle cramps, sweating, vomiting, seizures. Overdosage results in somnolence, confusion, diminished reflexes, coma. Blood dyscrasias noted rarely.

PATIENT CONSIDERATIONS

Baseline Assessment

Offer emotional support to anxious pt. Assess motor responses (agitation, trembling, tension) and autonomic responses (cold, clammy hands, sweating).

Intervention/Evaluation

For those on long-term therapy, liver/renal function tests, blood counts should be performed periodically. Assess for paradoxical reaction, particularly during early therapy. Assist w/ambulation if drowsiness, lightheadedness occur. Evaluate for thera-

peutic response: calm facial expression, decreased restlessness and/or insomnia.

PATIENT/FAMILY TEACHING

Drowsiness usually disappears during continued therapy. If dizziness occurs, change positions slowly from recumbent to sitting position before standing. Avoid tasks that require alertness, motor skills until response to drug is established. Smoking reduces drug effectiveness. Sour hard candy, gum, or sips of tepid water may relieve dry mouth. Do not abruptly withdraw medication after long-term therapy. Avoid alcohol. Do not take other medications w/o consulting physician.

alprostadil (prostaglandin E_1; PGE_1)

ale-**pros**-tah-dill
(Caverject, Edex, Muse, Prostin VR Pediatric)

CANADIAN AVAILABILITY
Caverject, Prostin VR

CLASSIFICATION

Prostaglandin

AVAILABILITY (Rx)

Injection: 500 mcg/ml. **Powder for Injection:** 5 mcg, 10 mcg, 20 mcg, 40 mcg. **Urethal Suppository** (Muse): 125 mcg, 250 mcg, 500 mcg, 1,000 mcg.

PHARMACOKINETICS

Metabolism: After IV administration, rapidly metabolized in lungs (oxidation). **Excretion:** Primarily in urine. **Half-life:** 5–10 min.

ACTION/*THERAPEUTIC EFFECT*

Vasodilator having direct effect on vascular smooth muscle, ductus arteriosus. *Relaxes cavernous smooth muscle, dilates penile arteries, increases arterial blood flow to penis. Prevents closure of ductus arteriosus.*

USES/*UNLABELED*

Temporarily maintains patency of ductus arteriosus until surgery is performed in those w/congenital heart defects and dependent on patent ductus for survival (e.g., pulmonary atresia or stenosis). Treatment of erectile dysfunction due to neurogenic, vasculogenic, psychogenic causes, adjunct in diagnosis of erectile dysfunction. *Treatment of atherosclerosis, gangrene, pain due to severe peripheral arterial occlusive disease.*

STORAGE/HANDLING

Store parenteral form in refrigerator. Must dilute before use. Prepare fresh every 24 hrs. Discard unused portions. Refrigerate suppositories unless used within 14 days.

ADMINISTRATION

IV:

- Infuse for shortest time, lowest dose possible.
- If significant decrease in arterial pressure is noted via umbilical artery catheter, auscultation, or Doppler transducer, decrease infusion rate immediately.
- Discontinue infusion immediately if apnea or bradycardia occurs (overdosage).
- Dilute 500 mcg amp w/5% dextrose or 0.9% NaCl to volume

appropriate for available pump delivery system.

INDICATIONS/ROUTES/DOSAGE

Note: Give by continuous IV infusion or through umbilical artery catheter placed at ductal opening.

Maintain patency ductus arteriosus:
IV Infusion: Neonate: Initially, 0.05–0.1 mcg/kg/min. After therapeutic response achieved, use lowest dose to maintain response. *Maximum:* 0.4 mcg/kg/min.

Impotence:
Suppository, Intracavernosal: Individualized.

CONTRAINDICATIONS

Respiratory distress syndrome (hyaline membrane disease). Conditions predisposing to priaprism, anatomic deformation of penis, penile implants.

CAUTIONS

Severe liver disease, coagulation defects.

INTERACTIONS

DRUG: ***Anticoagulants, heparin, thrombolytics may increase risk of bleeding. Sympathomimetics*** may decrease effect. ***Vasodilators*** may increase risk of hypotension. **HERBAL:** None known. **HERBAL: None known. FOOD:** None significant. **ALTERED LAB VALUES:** May increase bilirubin. May decrease calcium, glucose, potassium.

SIDE EFFECTS

FREQUENT: *Intracavernosal (1–4%):* Penile pain (37%), prolonged erection, hypertension, local pain, penile fibrosis, injection site hematoma/ecchymosis, headache, respiratory infection, flulike symptoms. *Intraurethral (>3%):* Penile pain (36%), urethral pain/burning, testicular pain, urethral bleeding, headache, dizziness, respiratory infection, flulike symptoms. *Systemic (>1%):* Fever, seizures, flushing, bradycardia, hypotension, tachycardia, apnea, diarrhea, sepsis. OCCASIONAL: *Intracavernosal (<1%):* Hypotension, pelvic pain, back pain, dizziness, cough, nasal congestion. *Intraurethral (<3%):* Fainting, sinusitis, back/pelvic pain. *Systemic (<1%):* Jitteriness, lethargy, stiffness, arrhythmias, respiratory depression, anemia, bleeding, thrombocytopenia, hematuria.

ADVERSE REACTIONS/TOXIC EFFECTS

Systemic: Overdosage manifested as apnea, flushing of face/arms, bradycardia. Cardiac arrest, sepsis occur rarely.

PATIENT CONSIDERATIONS

INTERVENTION/EVALUATION

Monitor arterial pressure by umbilical artery catheter, auscultation, or Doppler transducer. Monitor symptoms of hypotension. If significant decrease in arterial pressure occurs, decrease infusion rate immediately. Maintain continuous cardiac monitoring. Assess heart sounds, femoral pulse (circulation to lower extremities), and respiratory status frequently. Monitor B/P, arterial blood gases, temperature. If apnea or bradycardia occurs, discontinue infusion and notify physician.

PATIENT/FAMILY TEACHING

Explain purpose of this palliative therapy to parents. Erection to occur within 2–5 min. Do not

use if female pregnant (unless using condom barrier). Inform physician if erection >4 hrs or becomes painful or bleeding at injection site persists.

alteplase, recombinant

all-teh-place
(**Activase**)

CANADIAN AVAILABILITY
Activase rt-PA

PREGNANCY CATEGORY C

CLASSIFICATION

Thrombolytic

AVAILABILITY (Rx)

Powder for Injection: 20 mg, 50 mg, 100 mg

PHARMACOKINETICS

Metabolism: Rapidly metabolized in liver. **Excretion:** Primarily excreted in urine. **Half-life:** 35 min.

ACTION/*THERAPEUTIC EFFECT*

Activates fibrinolytic system by directly cleaving bond in plasminogen-producing plasmin, an enzyme that *degrades fibrin clots, fibrinogen, other plasma proteins.* Appears to be more readily clot selective binding within a clot than circulating fibrinogen.

USES

Management of acute myocardial infarction (AMI) for lysis of thrombi obstructing coronary arteries and management of acute massive pulmonary embolus for lysis of acute pulmonary emboli. Treatment acute ischemic stroke (within 5 hrs of symptoms).

STORAGE/HANDLING

Store vials at room temperature. After reconstitution, solutions are colorless to pale yellow. Solution is stable for 8 hrs after reconstitution. Discard unused portions.

ADMINISTRATION

IV:

- Give by IV infusion via infusion pump.
- Reconstitute immediately prior to use w/sterile water for injection.
- Reconstitute 50 mg vial w/50 ml sterile water for injection without preservative (20 ml for 20 mg vial) to provide a concentration of 1 mg/ml. (May be further diluted w/50 ml 5% dextrose or 0.9% NaCl to provide a concentration of 0.5 mg/ml.)
- Avoid excessive agitation; gently swirl or slowly invert vial to reconstitute.
- If minor bleeding occurs at puncture sites, apply pressure for 30 sec; if unrelieved, apply pressure dressing.
- If uncontrolled hemorrhage occurs, discontinue infusion immediately (slowing rate of infusion may produce worsening hemorrhage).
- Avoid undue pressure when drug is injected into catheter (can rupture catheter or expel clot into circulation).

INDICATIONS/ROUTES/DOSAGE

Acute myocardial infarction:
IV Infusion: Adults: 100 mg over 90 min; 15 mg bolus given over 1–2 min; then, 50 mg over 30 min; then, 35 mg over 60 min.

Acute pulmonary emboli:
IV Infusion: Adults: 100 mg over 2

hrs. Institute or reinstitute heparin near end or immediately after infusion (when PTT or thrombin time returns to twice normal or less).

Acute ischemic stroke:
IV Infusion: Adults: 0.9 mg/kg over 60 min (10% total dose as initial IV bolus over 1 min).

CONTRAINDICATIONS

Active internal bleeding, recent (within 2 mos) cerebrovascular accident, intracranial or intraspinal surgery or trauma, intracranial neoplasm, arteriovenous malformation or aneurysm, bleeding diathesis, severe uncontrolled hypertension.

CAUTIONS

Recent (10 days) major surgery or GI bleeding, OB delivery, organ biopsy, recent trauma (cardiopulmonary resuscitation, left heart thrombus, endocarditis, severe hepatic/renal disease, pregnancy, elderly, cerebrovascular disease, diabetic retinopathy, thrombophlebitis, occluded AV cannula at infected site).

INTERACTIONS

DRUG: ***Anticoagulants, heparin, cefotetan, plicamycin, valproic acid*** may increase risk of hemorrhage. ***Platelet aggregation inhibitors*** (e.g., aspirin), ***NSAIDs, ticlodipine*** may increase risk of bleeding. **HERBAL: None known. FOOD:** None significant. **ALTERED LAB VALUES:** Decreases plasminogen and fibrinogen level during infusion, decreasing clotting time (confirms presence of lysis).

SIDE EFFECTS

FREQUENT: Superficial bleeding at puncture sites, decreased B/P. **OCCASIONAL:** Allergic reaction (rash, wheezing), bruising.

ADVERSE REACTIONS/TOXIC EFFECTS

Severe internal hemorrhage may occur. Lysis of coronary thrombi may produce atrial or ventricular dysrhythmias, stroke.

PATIENT CONSIDERATIONS

Baseline Assessment

Obtain baseline B/P, apical pulse. Record weight. Evaluate 12-lead EKG, CPK, CPK-MB, electrolytes. Assess hematocrit, platelet count, thrombin (TT), activated thromboplastin (APTT), prothrombin time (PT), fibrinogen level, before therapy is instituted. Type and hold blood.

Intervention/Evaluation

Continuous cardiac monitoring for arrhythmias, B/P, pulse and respirations q15 min until stable, then hourly. Check peripheral pulses, heart and lung sounds. Monitor chest pain relief and notify physician of continuation or recurrence (note location, type, and intensity). Assess for bleeding: overt blood, blood in any body substance. Monitor PTT per protocol. Maintain B/P; avoid any trauma that might increase risk of bleeding (injections, shaving, etc.). Assess neurologic status.

Patient/Family Teaching

Report any bleeding.

---

altretamine (hexamethylmelamine)

(Hexalen)

See Classification section under: Cancer chemotherapy

aluminum carbonate
(Basaljel)
aluminum hydroxide
(Alternagel, Alu-Cap, Alu-Tab, Amphojel, Dialume)

FIXED-COMBINATION(S)
W/magnesium, an antacid **(Aludrox, Delcid, Gaviscon, Maalox)**; w/magnesium and simethicone, an antiflatulent **(DiGel, Gelusil, Maalox Plus, Mylanta, Silain-Gel)**; w/magnesium and calcium, an antacid **(Camalox)**.

CANADIAN AVAILABILITY
Amphojel, Basaljel

PREGNANCY CATEGORY N/A

CLASSIFICATION

Antacid

AVAILABILITY (OTC)

Aluminum carbonate: Tablets: 500 mg. **Capsules:** 500 mg. **Suspension:** 400 mg/5 ml.

Aluminum hydroxide: Tablets: 300 mg, 500 mg, 600 mg. **Capsules:** 400 mg, 500 mg. **Suspension:** 320 mg/5 ml, 450 mg/5 ml, 675 mg/5 ml. **Liquid:** 600 mg/5 ml.

PHARMACOKINETICS

Absorption: Small amount absorbed from intestine. Onset of action based on solubility in stomach and reaction w/hydrochloric acid. Duration of action based primarily on gastric emptying time (20 min when given ac, up to 3 hrs when given pc).

ACTION/*THERAPEUTIC EFFECT*

Reduces gastric acid, *thereby neutralizing or increasing gastric pH.* Binds w/phosphate in intestine, then excreted in feces *(reduces phosphates in urine, preventing formation of phosphate urinary stones; reduces serum phosphate levels).* May increase absorption of calcium (due to decreased serum phosphate levels). Astringent, adsorbent properties *(decreases fluidity of stools).*

USES

Symptomatic relief of upset stomach associated w/hyperacidity (heartburn, acid indigestion, sour stomach). Hyperacidity associated w/gastric, duodenal ulcers. Symptomatic treatment of gastroesophageal reflux disease. Prophylactic treatment of GI bleeding secondary to gastritis and stress ulceration. In conjunction w/low phosphate diet, prevents formation of phosphate urinary stones, reduces elevated phosphate levels.

ADMINISTRATION

ORAL:
- Usually administered 1–3 hrs after meals.
- Individualize dose (based on neutralizing capacity of antacids).
- Chewable tablets: Thoroughly chew tablets before swallowing (follow w/glass of water or milk).
- If administering suspension, shake well before use.

INDICATIONS/DOSAGE/ROUTES

Note: Usual dose is 30–60 ml.

Aluminum Carbonate:

Antacid:
Oral: Adults, elderly: 2 capsules or 10 ml q2h up to 12 times/day.

Hyperphosphatemia:
Oral: Adults, elderly: 2 capsules or 12.5 ml 3–4 times/day w/meals.

ALUMINUM HYDROXIDE:

Antacid:
Oral: Adults, elderly: 500–1,800 mg 3–6 times/day between meals and bedtime.

Hyperphosphatemia:
Oral: Children: 50–150 mg/kg/24 hrs in divided doses q4–6h.

CONTRAINDICATIONS

Intestinal obstruction.

CAUTIONS

Impaired renal function, gastric outlet obstruction, elderly, dehydration, fluid restriction, Alzheimer's disease, symptoms of appendicitis, GI/rectal bleeding, constipation, fecal impaction, chronic diarrhea.

INTERACTIONS

DRUG: May decrease excretion of ***quinidine, anticholinergics.*** May decrease effects of ***methenamine***. May increase ***salicylate*** excretion. May decrease absorption of ***quinolones, iron preparations, isoniazid, ketoconazole, tetracyclines***. **HERBAL:** None known. **FOOD:** None significant. **ALTERED LAB VALUES:** May increase gastrin, systemic/urinary pH. May decrease serum phosphate.

SIDE EFFECTS

FREQUENT: Chalky taste, mild constipation, stomach cramps. **OCCASIONAL:** Nausea, vomiting, speckling/whitish discoloration of stools.

ADVERSE REACTIONS/TOXIC EFFECTS

Prolonged constipation may result in intestinal obstruction. Excessive or chronic use may produce hypophosphatemia (anorexia, malaise, muscle weakness, bone pain) resulting in osteomalacia, osteoporosis. Prolonged use may produce urinary calculi.

PATIENT CONSIDERATIONS

BASELINE ASSESSMENT

Do not give other oral medication within 1–2 hrs of antacid administration.

INTERVENTION/EVALUATION

Assess pattern of daily bowel activity and stool consistency. Monitor serum phosphate, calcium, uric acid levels. Assess for relief of gastric distress.

PATIENT/FAMILY TEACHING

Chewable tablets: Chew tablets thoroughly before swallowing (may be followed by water or milk). Tablets may discolor stool. Maintain adequate fluid intake.

---

amantadine hydrochloride

ah-**man**-tih-deen
(Symadine, Symmetrel)

CANADIAN AVAILABILITY
Symmetrel

PREGNANCY CATEGORY C

CLASSIFICATION

Antiviral, antiparkinson.

AVAILABILITY (Rx)

Tablets: 100 mg. **Syrup:** 50 mg/5 ml.

PHARMACOKINETICS

Absorption: Rapid, completely absorbed from GI tract. Widely distributed. **Excretion:** Primarily excreted in urine. Minimal removed by hemodialysis. **Half-**

life: 11–15 hrs (increased in elderly, decreased renal function).

ACTION / *THERAPEUTIC EFFECT*

Antiviral action against influenza A virus believed *to prevent uncoating of virus, penetration of host cells, release of nucleic acid into host cells.* Antiparkinsonism *due to increased release of dopamine.* Virustatic.

USES / *UNLABELED*

Prevention, treatment of respiratory tract infections due to influenza virus, Parkinson's disease, drug-induced extrapyramidal reactions. *Treatment of fatigue associated w/multiple sclerosis.*

ADMINISTRATION

ORAL:

- Administer nighttime dose several hours before bedtime (prevents insomnia).

INDICATIONS / ROUTES / DOSAGE

Prophylaxis, symptomatic treatment respiratory illness due to influenza A virus:

Note: Give as single or in 2 divided doses.

Oral: Adults (10–64 yrs): 200 mg daily. ***Adults (>64 yrs):*** 100 mg daily. ***Children (9–12 yrs):*** 100 mg 2 times/day. ***Children (1–9 yrs):*** 4.4–8.8 mg/kg/day (up to 150 mg/day).

Parkinson's disease, extrapyramidal symptoms:
Oral: Adults: 100 mg 2 times/day. May increase up to 400 mg/day in divided doses.

Usual elderly dosage:
Oral: Based on renal function. Ccr 40–50 ml/min: 100 mg/day; Ccr 20 ml/min: 100 mg 3 times/wk.

Dosage in renal impairment:
Dose and/or frequency is modified based on creatinine clearance (Ccr).

CREATININE CLEARANCE	DOSAGE
30–50 ml/min	200 mg first day; 100 mg/day thereafter
15–29 ml/min	200 mg first day; 100 mg on alternate days
<15 ml/min	200 mg every 7 days

CONTRAINDICATIONS

None significant.

CAUTIONS

History of seizures, orthostatic hypotension, CHF, peripheral edema, liver disease, recurrent eczematoid dermatitis, cerebrovascular disease, renal dysfunction, those receiving CNS stimulants.

INTERACTIONS

DRUG: ***Tricyclic antidepressants, antihistamines, phenothiazine, anticholinergics*** may increase anticholinergic effects. ***Hydrochlorothiazide, triamterene*** may increase concentration, toxicity. **HERBAL:** None known. **FOOD:** None significant. **ALTERED LAB VALUES:** None significant.

SIDE EFFECTS

FREQUENT (5–10%): Nausea, dizziness, poor concentration, insomnia, nervousness. **OCCASIONAL (1–5%):** Orthostatic hypotension, anorexia, headache, livedo reticularis (reddish blue, netlike blotching of skin), blurred vision, urinary retention, dry mouth/nose. **RARE (<1%):** Vomiting, depression, irritation/swelling of eyes, skin rash.

ADVERSE REACTIONS/TOXIC EFFECTS

CHF, leukopenia, neutropenia occur rarely. Hyperexcitability, convulsions, ventricular arrhythmias may occur.

PATIENT CONSIDERATIONS

Baseline Assessment

Question history of allergies, especially to amantadine. When treating infections caused by influenza A virus, obtain specimens for viral diagnostic tests before giving first dose (therapy may begin before results are known).

Intervention/Evaluation

Monitor I&O, renal function tests if ordered; check for peripheral edema. Evaluate food tolerance, vomiting. Assess skin for rash, blotching. Be alert to neurologic effects: headache, lethargy, confusion, agitation, blurred vision, seizures. Assess B/P at least twice daily. Determine bowel pattern, modify diet, or administer laxative as needed. Assess for dizziness.

Parkinsonism

Assess for clinical reversal of symptoms (improvement of tremor of head/hands at rest, masklike facial expression, shuffling gait, muscular rigidity).

Patient/Family Teaching

Continue therapy for full length of treatment. Doses should be evenly spaced. Do not take any medications w/o consulting physician. Avoid alcoholic beverages. Do not drive, use machinery, or engage in other activities that require mental acuity if experiencing dizziness, confusion, blurred vision. Get up slowly from a sitting or lying position. Advise physician if no improvement in 2–3 days when taking for viral infection. Inform physician of new symptoms, especially blotching, rash, dizziness, blurred vision, nausea/vomiting. Take nighttime dose several hours before bedtime to prevent insomnia.

---

amcinonide

(Cyclocort)

See Classification section under: Corticosteroid: topical

---

amifostine

am-ih-**fos**-teen

(Ethyol)

CANADIAN AVAILABILITY

Ethyol

PREGNANCY CATEGORY C

CLASSIFICATION

Antineoplastic adjunct, cytoprotective agent

AVAILABILITY (Rx)

Powder for Injection: 500 mg, 500 mg mannitol (10 ml single-use vial)

PHARMACOKINETICS

Rapidly cleared from plasma. Converted in tissue to active free thiol metabolite. Tissue uptake highest in bone marrow, skin, GI mucosa, salivary glands. Following administration, distribution half-life <1 min. Less than 10% remains in plasma 6 min after drug administration.

ACTION/*THERAPEUTIC EFFECT*

Converted by alkaline phosphatase in tissues, allowing its

ability to protect normal tissue relative to tumor tissue, *reducing the toxic effect of chemotherapeutic agent, cisplatin.*

USES/*UNLABELED*

Reduces cumulative renal toxicity associated w/repeated administration of cisplatin in those w/advanced ovarian cancer. Treatment of postoperative radiation-induced dry mouth in pts w/head or neck cancer. *Protects lung fibroblasts from damaging effects of chemotherapeutic agent paclitaxel.*

STORAGE/HANDLING

Reconstituted solution stable for 5 hrs at room temperature, 24 hrs under refrigeration. Do not use if discolored or contains particulate matter.

ADMINISTRATION

IV:

- Reconstitute with 9.5 ml 0.9% NaCl.
- Further dilute w/0.9% NaCl for a concentration of 5–40 mg/ml.
- Administer over 15 min (30 min prior to chemotherapy).
- If hypotension requires interruption of therapy, place pt in Trendelenburg position, give an infusion of normal saline using a separate IV line.
- An antiemetic (dexamethasone 20 mg IV) and serotonin $5HT_3$ (receptor antagonist) should be given prior to and concurrently w/amifostine.

INDICATIONS/ROUTES/DOSAGE

Cytoprotective (chemotherapy):
IV Infusion: Adults: 910 mg/m^2 once daily as 15 min infusion, beginning 30 min prior to chemotherapy (15 min infusion is better tolerated than extended infusions). If full dose cannot be administered, dose for subsequent cycles should be 740 mg/m^2.

Treatment of dry mouth:
IV Infusion: Adults: 200 mg/m^2 daily as 3-min IV infusion starting 15–30 min before radiation therapy.

CONTRAINDICATIONS

Sensitivity to aminothiol compounds or mannitol.

EXTREME CAUTION

Uncorrected dehydration or hypotensive pts, those receiving antihypertensive therapy that cannot be interrupted prior to 24 hrs before amifostine treatment, preexisting cardiovascular or cerebrovascular conditions, i.e., ischemic heart disease, arrhythmias, CHF, history of stroke or TIA, pts receiving chemotherapy for malignancies that are potentially curable (e.g., certain malignancies of germ cell origin).

CAUTIONS

Safety not established in elderly >70 yrs.

INTERACTIONS

DRUG: Pts receiving ***antihypertensive*** medication or drugs that may potentiate hypotension. **HERBAL:** None known. **FOOD:** None significant. **ALTERED LAB VALUES:** May reduce calcium serum levels, especially those w/nephrotic syndrome.

SIDE EFFECTS

FREQUENT (62%): Transient reduction in B/P (62% of pts), w/onset 14 min into infusion, lasts about 6 min. B/P generally returns to normal in 5–15 min, severe nausea, vomiting. **OCCASIONAL (10–20%):** Flushing/feeling of warmth or chills/feeling of coldness, dizziness, hiccups, sneezing, somnolence. **RARE (<1%):**

Clinically relevant hypocalcemia, mild skin rash.

ADVERSE REACTIONS/TOXIC EFFECTS

A pronounced drop in B/P may require temporary cessation of amifostine.

PATIENT CONSIDERATIONS

BASELINE ASSESSMENT

Be sure pt is adequately hydrated prior to infusion. Pt should maintain supine position during the infusion. Monitor B/P q5 min during infusion. Interrupt infusion if systolic B/P decreases significantly from baseline (for baseline of <100, B/P drop by 20 mm Hg; for baseline of 100–119, a drop by 25 mm Hg; for baseline of 120–139, a drop by 30 mm Hg; for baseline of 140–179, a drop by 40 mm Hg; for baseline of >180, a drop by 50 mm Hg). If B/P returns to normal within 5 min and pt appears asymptomatic, begin infusion again so full dose can be administered.

INTERVENTION/EVALUATION

Carefully monitor pt for fluid balance, adequate hydration. Monitor serum calcium levels in those at risk of hypocalcemia (nephrotic syndrome). Monitor B/P every 5 min during infusion.

amikacin sulfate

am-ih-**kay**-sin
(Amikin)

CANADIAN AVAILABILITY
Amikin

PREGNANCY CATEGORY C

CLASSIFICATION

Antibiotic: Aminoglycoside

AVAILABILITY (Rx)

Injection: 50 mg/ml, 250 mg/ml

PHARMACOKINETICS

Absorption: Rapid, complete absorption after IM administration. Widely distributed (does not cross blood-brain barrier, low concentrations in CSF). **Excretion:** Excreted unchanged in urine. Removed by hemodialysis. **Half-life:** 2–4 hrs (increased in decreased renal function, neonates; decreased in cystic fibrosis, burn or febrile pts).

ACTION/*THERAPEUTIC EFFECT*

Irreversibly binds to protein on bacterial ribosome, *interfering in protein synthesis of susceptible microorganisms.*

USES

Treatment of skin/skin structure, bone, joint, respiratory tract, intra-abdominal and complicated urinary tract infections; postop, burns, septicemia, meningitis.

STORAGE/HANDLING

Store vials at room temperature. Solutions appear clear but may become pale yellow (does not affect potency). Intermittent IV infusion (piggyback) stable for 24 hrs at room temperature. Discard if precipitate forms or dark discoloration occurs.

ADMINISTRATION

Note: Coordinate peak and trough lab draws w/administration times.

IM:

- To minimize discomfort, give

deep IM slowly. Less painful if injected into gluteus maximus rather than lateral aspect of thigh.

IV:

- Infuse over 30–60 min for adults, older children, and over 60–120 min for infants, young children.
- Alternating IV sites, use large veins to reduce risk of phlebitis.

INDICATIONS/ROUTES/DOSAGE

Note: Space doses evenly around the clock. Dosage based on ideal body weight. Peak, trough serum level is determined periodically to maintain desired serum concentrations (minimizes risk of toxicity). *Recommended peak level:* 15–30 mcg/ml; *trough level:* 5–10 mcg/ml.

Uncomplicated urinary tract infections:
IM/IV: Adults, elderly: 250 mg q12h.

Moderate to severe infections:
IM/IV: Adults, elderly, children: 15 mg/kg/day in divided doses q8–12h. Do not exceed 15 mg/kg or 1.5 g/day. ***Neonates:*** Loading dose: 10 mg/kg, then 7.5 mg/kg q12h.

Dosage in renal impairment:
Dose and/or frequency is modified based on degree of renal impairment, serum concentration of drug. After loading dose of 5–7.5 mg/kg, maintenance dose/frequency based on serum creatinine or creatinine clearance.

CONTRAINDICATIONS

Sulfite sensitivity (may result in anaphylaxis, especially in asthmatics).

CAUTIONS

Possible cross-sensitivity to other aminoglycosides. Elderly, neonates (potential for renal insufficiency or immaturity); neuromuscular disorders (potential for respiratory depression), prior hearing loss, vertigo, renal impairment.

INTERACTIONS

DRUG: Other ***aminoglycosides, nephrotoxic***- and ***ototoxic***-producing medications may increase toxicity. May increase effects of ***neuromuscular blocking agents.*** **HERBAL:** None known. **FOOD:** None significant. **ALTERED LAB VALUES:** May increase BUN, SGPT (ALT), SGOT (AST), bilirubin, creatinine, LDH concentrations; may decrease serum calcium, magnesium, potassium, sodium concentrations.

SIDE EFFECTS

FREQUENT: Pain, induration at IM injection site; phlebitis, thrombophlebitis w/IV administration. **OCCASIONAL:** Hypersensitivity reactions (rash, fever, urticaria, pruritus). **RARE:** Neuromuscular blockade (difficulty breathing, drowsiness, weakness).

ADVERSE REACTIONS/TOXIC EFFECTS

Frequently occurring nephrotoxicity (evidenced by increased BUN and serum creatinine, decreased creatinine clearance) may be reversible if drug stopped at first sign of symptoms; irreversible ototoxicity (tinnitus, dizziness, ringing/roaring in ears, reduced hearing) and neurotoxicity (headache, dizziness, lethargy, tremors, visual disturbances) occur occasionally. Risk is greater w/higher dosages, prolonged therapy. Superinfections, particularly w/fungi, may result from bacterial imbalance.

PATIENT CONSIDERATIONS

BASELINE ASSESSMENT

Dehydration must be treated before aminoglycoside therapy.

Establish pt's baseline hearing acuity before beginning therapy. Question for history of allergies, especially to aminoglycosides and sulfite. Obtain specimen for culture, sensitivity before giving the first dose (therapy may begin before results are known).

INTERVENTION/EVALUATION

Monitor I&O (maintain hydration), urinalysis (casts, RBC, WBC, decrease in specific gravity). Monitor results of peak/trough blood tests. Be alert to ototoxic and neurotoxic symptoms (see Adverse Reactions/Toxic Effects). Check IM injection site for pain, induration. Evaluate IV site for phlebitis (heat, pain, red streaking over vein). Assess for skin rash. Assess for superinfection, particularly genital/anal pruritus, changes of oral mucosa, diarrhea. When treating those w/neuromuscular disorders, assess respiratory response carefully.

PATIENT/FAMILY TEACHING

Continue antibiotic for full length of treatment. Space doses evenly. Discomfort may occur w/IM injection. Notify physician in event of any hearing, visual, balance, urinary problems even after therapy is completed. Do not take other medication w/o consulting physician. Lab tests are essential part of therapy.

amiloride hydrochloride

ah-**mill**-or-ride
(Midamor)

FIXED-COMBINATION(S)
W/hydrochlorothiazide, a thiazide diuretic **(Moduretic)**

CANADIAN AVAILABILITY
Midamor

PREGNANCY CATEGORY B

CLASSIFICATION

Diuretic: Potassium-sparing

AVAILABILITY (Rx)

Tablets: 5 mg

PHARMACODYNAMICS

	ONSET	PEAK	DURATION
Oral	2 hrs	6–10 hrs	24 hrs

PHARMACOKINETICS

Absorption: Incompletely absorbed from GI tract. **Excretion:** Primarily excreted in urine; partially eliminated in feces. **Half-life:** 6–9 hrs.

ACTION/*THERAPEUTIC EFFECT*

Directly interferes w/sodium reabsorption in distal tubule, *increasing sodium and water excretion and decreasing potassium excretion.* Initial decrease in B/P occurs by decreasing plasma and extracellular fluid volume.

USES/*UNLABELED*

Adjunctive therapy in treatment of diuretic-induced hypokalemia in those w/CHF or hypertension. Used when maintenance of serum potassium levels is necessary (digitalized patients, cardiac arrhythmias). *Reduce lithium-induced polyuria; slow pulmonary function reduction in cystic fibrosis; treatment of edema associated w/CHF, hepatic cirrhosis, nephrotic syndrome; hypertension.*

ADMINISTRATION

ORAL:

- Give w/food to avoid GI distress.

INDICATIONS/ROUTES/DOSAGE

Adjunctive therapy in CHF/hypertension:
Oral: Adults: Initially, 5 mg daily. May be increased to 10 mg daily, as single dose or in divided doses. If hypokalemia persists, dose may be increased to 15 mg, then to 20 mg, w/electrolyte monitoring.

Usual elderly dosage:
Oral: Initially, 5 mg/day or every other day.

CONTRAINDICATIONS

Serum potassium >5.5 mEq/L, pts on other potassium-sparing diuretics, anuria, acute or chronic renal insufficiency, diabetic nephropathy.

CAUTIONS

Those w/BUN >30 mg/dl or serum creatinine >1.5 mg/dl, elderly, debilitated, hepatic insufficiency, those w/cardiopulmonary disease, diabetes mellitus.

INTERACTIONS

DRUG: May decrease effect of ***anticoagulants, heparin. NSAIDs*** may decrease antihypertensive effect. ***ACE inhibitors (e.g., captopril), potassium-containing diuretics, potassium supplements*** may increase potassium. May decrease ***lithium*** clearance, increase toxicity. **HERBAL:** None known. **FOOD:** None significant. **ALTERED LAB VALUES:** May increase BUN, calcium excretion, creatinine, glucose, magnesium, potassium, uric acid. May decrease sodium.

SIDE EFFECTS

Usual elderly dosage:
FREQUENT (>3%): Headache, nausea, diarrhea, vomiting, decreased appetite. **OCCASIONAL (1–3%):** Dizziness, abdominal pain, constipation, cough, dyspnea, weakness, muscle cramps, impotence. **RARE (<1%):** Tremors, vertigo, confusion, nervousness, insomnia, decreased libido, thirst, dry mouth, heartburn, dyspepsia, shortness of breath, pain, increased urination, hypotension, skin rash.

ADVERSE REACTIONS/TOXIC EFFECTS

Severe hyperkalemia may produce irritability, anxiety, heaviness of legs, paresthesia of hands/face/lips, hypotension, bradycardia, tented T waves, widening of QRS, ST depression.

PATIENT CONSIDERATIONS

Baseline Assessment

Assess baseline electrolytes, particularly for low potassium. Assess renal/hepatic functions. Assess edema (note location, extent), skin turgor, mucous membranes for hydration status. Assess muscle strength, mental status. Note skin temperature, moisture. Obtain baseline weight. Initiate strict I&O. Note pulse rate/regularity.

Intervention/Evaluation

Monitor B/P, vital signs, electrolytes (particularly potassium), I&O, weight. Note extent of diuresis. Watch for changes from initial assessment; hyperkalemia may result in muscle strength changes, tremor, muscle cramps, change in mental status (orientation, alertness, confusion), cardiac arrhythmias. Monitor potassium level, particularly during initial therapy.

Weigh daily. Assess lung sounds for rales, wheezing.

PATIENT/FAMILY TEACHING

Expect increase in volume and frequency of urination. Therapeutic effect takes several days to begin and can last for several days when drug is discontinued. High potassium diet/potassium supplements can be dangerous, especially if pt has renal/hepatic problems. Avoid foods high in potassium such as whole grains (cereals), legumes, meat, bananas, apricots, orange juice, potatoes (white, sweet), raisins. Contact physician if confusion, irregular heartbeat, nervousness, numbness of hands/feet/lips, difficulty breathing, unusual tiredness, weakness in legs occurs (hyperkalemia).

aminocaproic acid

ah-meen-oh-kah-**pro**-ick
(Amicar)

CANADIAN AVAILABILITY
Amicar

PREGNANCY CATEGORY C

CLASSIFICATION

Antifibrinolytic, antihemorrhagic

AVAILABILITY (Rx)

Tablets: 500 mg. **Syrup:** 250 mg/5 ml. **Injection:** 250 mg/ml.

PHARMACOKINETICS

Absorption: Rapidly absorbed. **Excretion:** Primarily excreted in urine.

ACTION/*THERAPEUTIC EFFECT*

Inhibits activation of plasminogen, preventing an enzyme (plasmin), *preventing fibrin clots from forming.*

USES/*UNLABELED*

Treatment of excessive bleeding from hyperfibrinolysis or urinary fibrinolysis. Use only in acute life-threatening situations. *Prevents reoccurrence of subarachnoid hemorrhage. Prevents hemorrhage in hemophiliacs following dental surgery.*

ADMINISTRATION

ORAL:

- Scored tablets may be crushed.
- May take w/o regard to food.
- Syrup used by pts unable to take tablets.

IV:

- Give only by IV infusion.
- Dilute w/5% dextrose, 0.9% NaCl, or other compatible solution.
- Monitor for hypotension during infusion. Rapid infusion may produce bradycardia, arrhythmias.

INDICATIONS/ROUTES/DOSAGE

Note: Reduce dosage in presence of cardiac, renal, or hepatic impairment.

Acute bleeding:
Oral/IV Infusion: Adults, elderly: Initially, 4–5 g over 1 hr, then 1–1.25 g/hr. Continue for 8 hrs or until bleeding is controlled. ***Maximum:*** Up to 30 g/24 hrs.

Chronic bleeding:
Oral: Adults, elderly: 5–30 g/day, in divided doses at 3–6 hr intervals.

CONTRAINDICATIONS

Evidence of active intravascular clotting process, disseminated intravascular coagulation w/o concurrent heparin therapy, hematuria of upper urinary tract origin (unless benefits outweigh risk). *Parenteral:* Newborns.

EXTREME CAUTION

Impaired cardiac, hepatic, or renal disease, those w/hyperfibrinolysis.

INTERACTIONS

DRUG: None significant. **HERBAL:** None known. **FOOD:** None significant. **ALTERED LAB VALUES:** May elevate serum potassium level.

SIDE EFFECTS

OCCASIONAL: Nausea, diarrhea, cramps, decreased urination, decreased B/P, dizziness, headache, muscle fatigue/weakness (myopathy), bloodshot eyes.

ADVERSE REACTIONS/TOXIC EFFECTS

Too rapid IV administration produces tinnitus, skin rash, arrhythmias, unusual tiredness, weakness. Rarely, grand mal seizure occurs, generally preceded by weakness, dizziness, headache.

PATIENT CONSIDERATIONS

INTERVENTION/EVALUATION

Monitor serum creatine kinase in those undergoing long-term therapy. If increase is noted in serum creatine kinase test, drug should be discontinued. Question any change in skeletal strength as noted by pt (consider possibility of cardiac damage as a result). Skeletal myopathy characterized by increase in creatine kinase, aldolase, and SGOT (AST) serum levels. Monitor these lab results frequently. Monitor heart rhythm. Assess for decrease in B/P, increase in pulse rate, abdominal or back pain, severe headache (may be evidence of hemorrhage). Assess peripheral pulses, skin for bruises, petechiae. Question for increase in amount of discharge during menses. Check for excessive bleeding from minor cuts, scratches. Assess gums for erythema, gingival bleeding. Assess urine output for hematuria.

PATIENT/FAMILY TEACHING

Use electric razor, soft toothbrush to prevent bleeding. Report any sign of red/dark urine, black/red stool, coffee-ground vomitus, red-speckled mucus from cough. Do not use any OTC medication w/o physician approval (may interfere w/platelet aggregation).

aminophylline (theophylline ethylenediamine)

am-in-**ah**-phil-lin
(Aminophylline, Phyllocontin)

theophylline

Immediate-release: **Aerolate, Slo-Phyllin, Theolair**. Extended-release: **Slo-Bid, Theo-Dur, Theo-24, Uni-Dur, Uniphyl**

CANADIAN AVAILABILITY
Aminophylline: **Phyllocontin;** theophylline: **Theo-Dur, Theolair, Uniphyl**

PREGNANCY CATEGORY C

CLASSIFICATION

Bronchodilator

AVAILABILITY (Rx)

Capsules (immediate-release): 100 mg, 200 mg. **Capsules (extended-release):** 50 mg, 60 mg, 75 mg, 100 mg, 125 mg, 200 mg, 250 mg, 300 mg. **Tablets**

(immediate-release): 100 mg, 125 mg, 200 mg, 250 mg, 300 mg. **Tablets (extended-release):** 100 mg, 200 mg, 250 mg, 300 mg, 400 mg, 450 mg, 500 mg. **Elixir:** 80 mg/15 ml. **Solution:** 80 mg/15 ml, 150 mg/15 ml. **Syrup:** 80 mg/15 ml, 150 mg/15 ml. **Injection:** 25 mg/ml.

PHARMACOKINETICS

Absorption: Well absorbed from GI tract (absorption may vary w/dosage form used). **Metabolism:** Liver. **Excretion:** Primarily in urine. **Half-life:** Dependent on age, liver, cardiac function, lung disease, smoking.

ACTION/ *THERAPEUTIC EFFECT*

Directly relaxes smooth muscle of bronchial airway, pulmonary blood vessels, *relieving bronchospasm, increasing vital capacity. Produces cardiac, skeletal muscle stimulation.*

USES/ *UNLABELED*

Symptomatic relief, prevention of bronchial asthma, reversible bronchospasm due to chronic bronchitis, emphysema, or COPD. *Treatment of apnea in neonates.*

STORAGE/HANDLING

Store solution at room temperature. Discard if solution contains a precipitate.

ADMINISTRATION

ORAL:

- Give w/food to avoid GI distress.
- Do not crush or break extended-release forms.

IV:

- Give loading dose diluted in 100–200 ml of 5% dextrose or 0.9% NaCl. Maintenance dose in larger volume parenteral infusion.
- Do not exceed flow rate of 1 ml/min (25 mg/min) for either piggyback or infusion.
- Administer loading dose over 20–30 min.
- Use infusion pump or micordrip to regulate IV administration.

INDICATIONS/ROUTES/DOSAGE

Note: Dosage calculated on basis of lean body weight. Dosage based on peak serum theophylline concentrations, clinical condition, presence of toxicity.

Chronic bronchospasm:
Oral: Adults, elderly, children: Initially, 16 mg/kg or 400 mg/day (whichever is less) in 2–4 divided doses (6–12 hr intervals). May increase by 25% every 2–3 days up to maximum of 24 mg/kg/day ***(1–9 yrs)***; 20 mg/kg/day ***(9–12 yrs)***; 18 mg/kg/day ***(12–16 yrs)***; 13 mg/kg/day (>16 yrs). Doses above maximum based on serum theophylline concentrations, clinical condition, presence of toxicity.

Acute bronchospasm in pts not currently on theophylline:
IV Loading Dose: Adults, children (>1 yr): Initially, 6 mg/kg (aminophylline), then begin maintenance aminophylline dosage based on patient group.

PT GROUP	MAINTENANCE AMINOPHYLLINE DOSAGE
Neonates	0.2 mg/kg/hr
Children (1–12 mos)	0.2–0.9 mg/kg/hr
Children (1–9 yrs)	1–1.2 mg/kg/hr
Children (9–16 yrs), young adult smokers	0.8–1 mg/kg/hr
Older pts, pts w/cor pulmonale	0.3–0.6 mg/kg/hr
Pts w/CHF, liver disease	0.1–0.5 mg/kg/hr

Oral/Loading Dose: Adults, children >1 yr: Initially, 5 mg/kg (theophylline), then begin maintenance theophylline dosage based on patient group.

PT GROUP	MAINTENANCE THEOPHYLLINE DOSAGE
Children (1–9 yrs)	4 mg/kg q6h
Children (9–16 yrs), young adult smokers	3 mg/kg q6h
Healthy, non-smoking adults	3 mg/kg q8h
Older pts, pts w/cor pulmonale	2 mg/kg q8h
Pts w/CHF, liver disease	1–2 mg/kg q12h

Acute bronchospasm in patients currently on theophylline:

IV/Oral: Adults, children >1 yr: Obtain serum theophylline level. If not possible and pt in respiratory distress and not experiencing toxicity, may give 2.5 mg/kg dose. *Maintenance:* Dosage based on peak serum theophylline concentrations, clinical condition, presence of toxicity.

CONTRAINDICATIONS

History of hypersensitivity to xanthine, caffeine.

CAUTIONS

Impaired cardiac, renal, or hepatic function, hypertension, hyperthyroidism, diabetes mellitus, peptic ulcer, glaucoma, severe hypoxemia, underlying seizure disorder.

INTERACTIONS

DRUG: *Glucocorticoids* may produce hypernatremia. ***Phenytoin, primidone, rifampin*** may increase metabolism. ***Beta blockers*** may decrease effects. ***Cimetidine, ciprofloxacin, erythromycin, norfloxacin*** may increase concentration, toxicity. Smoking may decrease concentration. **HERBAL:** St. John's wort may decrease effect. Ma Huang (Ephedra) may increase toxicity effect. **FOOD:** None significant. **ALTERED LAB VALUES:** None significant.

SIDE EFFECTS

FREQUENT: Momentary change in sense of smell during IV administration; shakiness, restlessness, tachycardia, trembling. **OCCASIONAL:** Heartburn, vomiting, headache, mild diuresis, insomnia, nausea.

ADVERSE REACTIONS/TOXIC EFFECTS

Too rapid rate of IV administration may produce marked fall in B/P w/accompanying faintness and lightheadedness, palpitations, tachycardia, hyperventilation, nausea, vomiting, angina-like pain, seizures, ventricular fibrillation, cardiac standstill.

PATIENT CONSIDERATIONS

BASELINE ASSESSMENT

Offer emotional support (high incidence of anxiety due to difficulty in breathing and sympathomimetic response to drug). Peak serum concentration should be taken 1 hr after IV, 1–2 hrs following immediate-release dose, 3–8 hrs following extended-release. Take trough level just before next dose.

INTERVENTION/EVALUATION

Monitor rate, depth, rhythm, type of respiration; quality and rate of pulse. Assess lung sounds for rhonchi, wheezing, rales. Monitor arterial blood gases. Observe lips, fingernails for blue or dusky color in light-skinned pts; gray in dark-skinned pts. Observe for clavicular retractions, hand tremor. Evaluate for clinical improvement (quieter, slower respirations, relaxed facial expression,

cessation of clavicular retractions). Monitor theophylline blood serum levels (therapeutic level range: 10–20 mcg/ml).

PATIENT/FAMILY TEACHING

Increase fluid intake (decreases lung secretion viscosity). Avoid excessive use of caffeine derivatives (chocolate, coffee, tea, cola, cocoa). Smoking, charcoal-broiled food, high-protein, low-carbohydrate diet may decrease theophylline level. Notify physician if nausea, vomiting, insomnia, nervousness, headache, rash, GI pain, seizures, irregular heartbeat occurs.

amiodarone hydrochloride

ah-me-oh-dah-**roan**
(Cordarone, Pacerone)

CANADIAN AVAILABILITY
Cordarone

PREGNANCY CATEGORY C

CLASSIFICATION

Antiarrhythmic

AVAILABILITY (Rx)

Tablets: 200 mg. **Injection:** 50 mg/ml.

PHARMACOKINETICS

Absorption: Slowly, variably absorbed from GI tract. **Metabolism:** Extensively metabolized in liver to active metabolite. **Excretion:** Excreted via bile; not removed by hemodialysis. **Half-life:** 26–107 days; metabolite: 61 days.

ACTION/*THERAPEUTIC EFFECT*

Prolongs myocardial cell action potential duration and refractory period by direct action on all cardiac tissue, *decreasing AV conduction, sinus node function.*

USES/*UNLABELED*

Treatment of documented, life-threatening, recurrent ventricular fibrillation, and recurrent, hemodynamically unstable ventricular tachycardia in those who have not responded adequately to other antiarrhythmic agents. *Treatment/prophylaxis of supraventricular arrhythmias refractory to conventional treatment.*

ADMINISTRATION

ORAL:
- Give w/meals to reduce GI distress.
- Tablets may be crushed.

IV:
- Administer through central venous catheter (CVC) if possible, using in-line filter.
- Use w/5% dextrose using polyolefin, glass container.
- Infusions >1 hr, concentration not to exceed 2 mg/ml (unless CVC used).
- Does not need protection from light during administration.

INDICATIONS/ROUTES/DOSAGE

Life-threatening ventricular arrhythmias:
Oral: Adults, elderly: Initially, 800–1,600 mg/day in 1–2 divided doses for 1–3 wks. After arrhythmias controlled or side effects occur, reduce to 600–800 mg/day for about 4 wks. ***Maintenance:*** 200–600 mg/day.

IV Infusion: Adults: Initially, 1,050 mg over 24 hrs: 150 mg over 10 min, follow by 360 mg over 6 hrs, follow by 540 mg over 18 hrs. May continue at 0.5 mg/min up to 2–3 wks regardless of age, renal or left ventricular function.

CONTRAINDICATIONS

Severe sinus-node dysfunction, second- and third-degree AV block, bradycardia-induced syncope (except in presence of pacemaker), severe hepatic disease.

CAUTIONS

Thyroid disease

INTERACTIONS

DRUG: May increase cardiac effects w/other ***antiarrhythmics.*** May increase effect of ***beta-blockers, oral anticoagulants***. May increase concentration, toxicity of ***digoxin, phenytoin***. **HERBAL:** None known. **FOOD:** None significant. **ALTERED LAB VALUES:** May increase SGOT (AST), SGPT (ALT), alkaline phosphatase, ANA titer. May cause changes in EKG, thyroid function tests.

SIDE EFFECTS

Corneal microdeposits are noted in almost all pts treated >6 mos (can lead to blurry vision). **FREQUENT (>3%):** ***Parenteral:*** Hypotension, nausea, fever, bradycardia. ***Oral:*** Constipation, headache, decreased appetite, nausea, vomiting, numbness of fingers/toes, photosensitivity, muscular incoordination. **OCCASIONAL (1–3%):** ***Oral:*** Bitter/metallic taste, decreased sexual ability/interest, dizziness, facial flushing, blue-gray coloring of skin of face, arms, neck, blurred vision, slow heartbeat, asymptomatic corneal deposits. **RARE (<1%):** ***Oral:*** Skin rash, vision loss, blindness.

ADVERSE REACTIONS/TOXIC EFFECTS

Serious, potentially fatal pulmonary toxicity (alveolitis, pulmonary fibrosis, pneumonitis, adult respiratory distress syndrome) may begin w/progressive dyspnea and cough w/rales, decreased breath sounds, pleurisy. CHF, hepatotoxicity may be noted. May worsen existing arrhythmias or produce new arrhythmias.

PATIENT CONSIDERATIONS

BASELINE ASSESSMENT

Obtain baseline pulmonary function tests, chest x-ray, liver enzyme tests, SGOT (AST), SGPT (ALT), alkaline phosphatase. Assess B/P, apical pulse immediately before drug is administered (if pulse is 60/min or below, or systolic B/P is below 90 mm Hg, withhold medication, contact physician).

INTERVENTION/EVALUATION

Monitor for symptoms of pulmonary toxicity (progressively worsening dyspnea, cough). Dosage should be discontinued or reduced if toxicity occurs. Assess pulse for strength/weakness, irregular rate, bradycardia. Monitor EKG for cardiac changes, particularly widening of QRS, prolongation of PR and QT intervals. Notify physician of any significant interval changes. Assess for nausea, fatigue, paresthesia, tremor. Monitor for signs of hypothyroidism (periorbital edema, lethargy, pudgy hands/feet, cool/pale skin, vertigo, night cramps) and hyperthyroidism (hot/dry skin, bulging eyes [exophthalmos], frequent urination, eyelid edema, weight loss, breathlessness). Monitor SGOT (AST), SGPT (ALT), alkaline phosphatase for evidence of liver toxicity. Assess skin, cornea for bluish discoloration in those who have been on drug therapy longer than 2 mos. Monitor liver function tests, thyroid test results. If elevated liver enzymes, dose reduction or discontinuation is evident. Monitor for therapeutic serum level (1.5–2.5 mcg/ml).

PATIENT/FAMILY TEACHING

Protect against photosensitivity reaction on skin exposed to sunlight. Bluish skin discoloration gradually disappears when drug is discontinued. Report shortness of breath, cough. Outpatients should monitor pulse before taking medication. Do not abruptly discontinue medication. Compliance w/therapy regimen is essential to control arrhythmias. Do not use nasal decongestants, OTC preparations (stimulants) w/o physician approval. Restrict salt, alcohol intake. Recommend ophthalmic exams every 6 mos. Report any vision changes.

amitriptyline hydrochloride

a-me-**trip**-tih-leen
(Elavil, Endep)

FIXED-COMBINATION(S)
W/chlordiazepoxide, an antianxiety **(Limbitrol)**; w/perphenazine, an antipsychotic **(Etrafon, Triavil)**

CANADIAN AVAILABILITY
Apo-Amitriptyline, Elavil

PREGNANCY CATEGORY D

CLASSIFICATION

Antidepressant: Tricyclic

AVAILABILITY (Rx)

Tablets: 10 mg, 25 mg, 50 mg, 75 mg, 100 mg, 150 mg. **Injection:** 10 mg/ml.

PHARMACOKINETICS

Absorption: Rapid, well absorbed from GI tract. **Metabolism:** In liver, undergoes first pass metabolism. **Excretion:** Primarily excreted in urine. Minimal removal by hemodialysis. **Half-life:** 10–26 hrs.

ACTION/*THERAPEUTIC EFFECT*

Blocks reuptake of neurotransmitters (norepinephrine, serotonin) at presynaptic membranes, increasing synaptic concentration at postsynaptic receptor sites, *resulting in antidepressant effect.* Has strong anticholinergic activity.

USES/*UNLABELED*

Treatment of various forms of depression, exhibited as persistent, prominent dysphoria (occurring nearly every day for at least 2 wks) manifested by 4 of 8 symptoms: appetite change, sleep pattern change, increased fatigue, impaired concentration, feelings of guilt or worthlessness, loss of interest in usual activities, psychomotor agitation or retardation, suicidal tendencies. *Relieves neuropathic pain (e.g., diabetic neuropathy, postherpetic neuralgia, treatment of bulimia nervosa). Treatment of migraine.*

STORAGE/HANDLING

Store parenteral form at room temperature. Protect from light (precipitate may form). Store tablets at room temperature.

ADMINISTRATION

ORAL:

- Give w/food or milk if GI distress occurs.

IM:

- Give by IM only if oral administration is not feasible.
- Crystals may form in injection. Redissolve by immersing ampule in hot water for 1 min.
- Give deep IM slowly.

INDICATIONS/ROUTES/DOSAGE

Note: May give entire daily oral dose at one time (preferably bedtime).

Depression (In-patient):
Oral: Adults: Initially, 75–100 mg/day in 1–4 divided doses. Gradually increase by 25–50 mg increments to maximum of 300 mg/day, then reduce slowly to minimum therapeutic level. ***Elderly, adolescents:*** Initially, 10 mg 3 times/day, plus 20 mg at bedtime. ***Maintenance:*** 40–100 mg/day. ***IM: Adults:*** 20–30 mg 4 times/day.

Depression (outpatient):
Oral: Adults: Initially, 50–100 mg/day. May be gradually increased to 150 mg/day. ***Elderly, adolescents:*** 10 mg 3 times/day, plus 20 mg at bedtime. Dosage should be gradually reduced to minimum therapeutic level (therapeutic effect noted in 2–4 wks).

Usual elderly dosage:
Oral: Initially, 10–25 mg at bedtime; increase at weekly intervals of 10–25 mg. ***Range:*** 25–150 mg/day.

CONTRAINDICATIONS

Acute recovery period following MI, within 14 days of MAO inhibitor ingestion.

CAUTIONS

Prostatic hypertrophy, history of urinary retention or obstruction, glaucoma, diabetes mellitus, history of seizures, hyperthyroidism, cardiac/hepatic/renal disease, schizophrenia, increased intraocular pressure, hiatal hernia.

INTERACTIONS

DRUG: ***CNS depressants (including alcohol, barbiturates, phenothiazines, sedative-hypnotics, anticonvulsants)*** may increase sedation, respiratory depression, hypotensive effects. ***Antithyroid agents*** may increase risk of agranulocytosis. ***Phenothiazines*** may increase sedative, anticholinergic effects. ***Cimetidine, valproic acid*** may increase concentration, toxicity. May decrease effects of ***clonidine, guanadrel***. May increase cardiac effects w/***sympathomimetics***. May increase risk of hypertensive crisis, hyperpyretic, convulsions w/***MAO inhibitors***. **HERBAL:** St. John's wort may decrease effect. May decrease effect of Ma Huang (Ephedra). **FOOD:** None significant. **ALTERED LAB VALUES:** May alter EKG readings (flattens T wave), glucose.

SIDE EFFECTS

FREQUENT: Dizziness, drowsiness, dry mouth, orthostatic hypotension, headache, increased appetite/weight, nausea, unusual tiredness, unpleasant taste. **OCCASIONAL:** Blurred vision, confusion, constipation, hallucinations, delayed micturation, eye pain, arrhythmias, fine muscle tremors, Parkinsonian syndrome, nervousness, diarrhea, increased sweating, heartburn, insomnia. **RARE:** Hypersensitivity, alopecia, tinnitus, breast enlargement.

ADVERSE REACTIONS/TOXIC EFFECTS

High dosage may produce confusion, seizures, severe drowsiness, fast/slow/irregular heartbeat, fever, hallucinations, agitation, shortness of breath, vomiting, unusual tiredness/weakness. Abrupt withdrawal from prolonged therapy may produce headache, malaise, nausea, vomiting, vivid dreams. Rarely, blood dyscrasias, cholestatic jaundice noted.

PATIENT CONSIDERATIONS

Baseline Assessment

For those on long-term therapy, liver/renal function tests, blood counts should be performed periodically. Observe/record behavior. Assess psychological status, thought content, sleep patterns, appearance, interest in environment.

Intervention/Evaluation

Supervise suicidal risk pt closely during early therapy (as depression lessens, energy level improves, increasing suicide potential). Assess appearance, behavior, speech pattern, level of interest, mood. Monitor pattern of daily bowel activity and stool consistency. Monitor B/P, pulse for hypotension, arrhythmias. Assess for urinary retention by bladder palpation.

Patient/Family Teaching

Change positions slowly to avoid hypotensive effect. Tolerance to postural hypotension, sedative and anticholinergic effects usually develops during early therapy. Maximum therapeutic effect may be noted in 2–4 wks. Sensitivity to sun may occur. Dry mouth may be relieved by sugarless gum or sips of tepid water. Report visual disturbances. Do not abruptly discontinue medication. Avoid tasks that require alertness, motor skills until response to drug is established.

---

amlexanox

am-**lecks**-ah-knocks
(Apthasol)

PREGNANCY CATEGORY B

CLASSIFICATION

Antiallergic/antiinflammatory

AVAILABILITY (Rx)

Paste: 5%

PHARMACODYNAMICS

	ONSET	PEAK	DURATION
Topical	—	2.4 hrs	—

PHARMACOKINETICS

Absorption: Most of the systemic absorption is through the GI tract. **Metabolism:** Steady state levels are reached within 1 week. **Excretion:** Eliminated in the urine. **Half-life:** 3.5 hrs.

ACTION/*THERAPEUTIC EFFECT*

Inhibits formation and/or release of inflammatory mediators (e.g., histamine) from mast cells, neutrophils, and mononuclear cells, *alleviating signs/symptoms of aphthous ulcers.*

USES/*UNLABELED*

Treatment of aphthous ulcers in pts with normal immune system.

ADMINISTRATION

TOPICAL:
- Apply paste to ulcer 4 times/day preferably following oral hygiene after meals and at bedtime.
- Gently dab paste onto each mouth ulcer.
- Wash hands immediately following application.

INDICATIONS/ROUTES/DOSAGES

Aphthous ulcers:
Topical: Adults, elderly: Squeeze 0.25 inch (0.5 cm) dab of paste onto a fingertip and place the paste onto each ulcer in the mouth using gentle pressure.

CONTRAINDICATIONS

History of hypersensitivity to amlexanox.

CAUTIONS

None significant.

INTERACTIONS

DRUG: None significant. **HERBAL:** None known. **FOOD:** None significant. **ALTERED LAB VALUES:** None significant.

SIDE EFFECTS

RARE: (1–2%): Stinging, burning at administration site, rash, nausea, vomiting.

ADVERSE REACTIONS/TOXIC EFFECTS

Overdose, i.e., too much paste or if administered more than recommended may result in diarrhea, GI upset or vomiting.

PATIENT CONSIDERATIONS

PATIENT/FAMILY TEACHING

Apply the paste as soon as ulcer symptoms appear. Continue to use the paste 4 times daily, preferably after oral hygiene after breakfast, lunch, dinner and at bedtime. Continue to use the paste until after the ulcer heals. If significant healing or pain reduction is not noted after 10 days, contact physician or dentist.

amlodipine

am-**low**-dih-peen
(Norvasc)

FIXED-COMBINATION(S)
W/benazepril, an angiotensin-converting enzyme inhibitor **(Lotrel)**

CANADIAN AVAILABILITY
Norvasc

PREGNANCY CATEGORY C

CLASSIFICATION

Calcium channel blocker

AVAILABILITY (Rx)

Tablets: 2.5 mg, 5 mg, 10 mg

PHARMACODYNAMICS

	ONSET	PEAK	DURATION
Oral	—	—	**24 hrs**

PHARMACOKINETICS

Absorption: Slowly absorbed from GI tract. **Metabolism:** Undergoes first-pass metabolism in liver. **Excretion:** Excreted primarily in urine. **Half-life:** 30–50 hrs (increased in elderly, pts w/hepatic cirrhosis).

ACTION/*THERAPEUTIC EFFECT*

Inhibits calcium movement across cell membranes of cardiac and vascular smooth muscle, *dilates coronary arteries, peripheral arteries/arterioles. Decreases total peripheral vascular resistance by vasodilation.*

USES

Management of hypertension, chronic stable angina, vasospastic (Prinzmetal's or variant) angina. May be used alone or w/other antihypertensives or antianginals.

ADMINISTRATION

ORAL:

- May take w/o regard to food.

INDICATIONS/ROUTES/DOSAGE

Note: Dosage should be titrated >7–14 days.

Hypertension:
Oral: Adults: Initially, 5 mg/day as single dose. ***Maximum:*** 10 mg/day.

Oral: Small frame, fragile, elderly: Initially, 2.5 mg/day as single dose.

Angina (chronic stable or vasospastic):
Oral: Adults: 5–10 mg. Elderly, hepatic insufficiency: 5 mg.

CONTRAINDICATIONS

Hypersensitivity to amlodipine, severe hypotension.

CAUTIONS

Impaired hepatic function, aortic stenosis, congestive heart failure.

INTERACTIONS

DRUG: None significant. **HERBAL:** None known. **FOOD:** Grapefruit juice may increase concentration. **ALTERED LAB VALUES:** None significant.

SIDE EFFECTS

FREQUENT (>5%): Peripheral edema, headache, flushing. **OCCASIONAL (1–5%):** Dizziness, palpitations, nausea, unusual tiredness/weakness. **RARE (<1%):** Chest pain, slow heartbeat, orthostatic hypotension.

ADVERSE REACTIONS/TOXIC EFFECTS

Overdosage may produce excessive peripheral vasodilation, marked hypotension w/reflex tachycardia.

PATIENT CONSIDERATIONS

BASELINE ASSESSMENT

Assess baseline renal/liver function tests, B/P, and apical pulse.

INTERVENTION/EVALUATION

Assess B/P (if systolic B/P is below 90 mm Hg, withhold medication, contact physician). Assist w/ambulation if lightheadedness, dizziness occurs. Assess for peripheral edema behind medial malleolus (sacral area in bedridden pts). Assess skin for flushing. Monitor liver enzyme tests. Question for headache, asthenia.

PATIENT/FAMILY TEACHING

Do not abruptly discontinue medication. Compliance w/therapy regimen is essential to control hypertension. To avoid hypotensive effect, rise slowly from lying to sitting position, wait momentarily before standing. Avoid tasks that require alertness, motor skills until response to drug is established. Contact physician/nurse if irregular heartbeat, shortness of breath, pronounced dizziness, or nausea occurs. Avoid concomitant ingestion of grapefruit juice.

amoxapine

ah-**mocks**-ah-peen
(Asendin)

CANADIAN AVAILABILITY
Asendin

PREGNANCY CATEGORY C

CLASSIFICATION

Antidepressant: Tricyclic

AVAILABILITY (Rx)

Tablets: 25 mg, 50 mg, 100 mg, 150 mg

PHARMACOKINETICS

Absorption: Rapid, well absorbed from GI tract. **Metabolism:** Metabolized in liver, undergoes first-pass metabolism. **Excretion:** Primarily excreted in urine. Minimal removal by hemodialysis. **Half-life:** 8–30 hrs.

ACTION/*THERAPEUTIC EFFECT*

Blocks reuptake of neurotransmitters (norepinephrine, serotonin) at presynaptic membranes, increasing synaptic concentration at postsynaptic receptor sites, *resulting in antidepressant and antianxiety effect.* Has substantive neuroleptic activity.

USES

Treatment of endogenous depression and anxiety.

ADMINISTRATION

ORAL:

- Give w/food or milk if GI distress occurs.

INDICATIONS/ROUTES/DOSAGE

Note: May give entire daily dose at one time (preferably bedtime).

Depression:

Oral: Adults: Initially, 50 mg 2–3 times/day. May gradually increase to 200–300 mg/day by end of first wk of therapy. If therapeutic response does not occur by end of 2 wks, may increase dose to maximum 400 mg/day for outpatients. Hospitalized pts w/no history of seizures may receive up to 600 mg/day in divided doses.

Usual elderly dosage:

Oral: Initially, 25 mg 2–3 times/day, then increase at 25 mg increments q3days for hospitalized pts; q7days for outpts. ***Range:*** 50–150 mg/day. ***Maximum:*** 300 mg/day.

CONTRAINDICATIONS

Acute recovery period following MI, within 14 days of MAO inhibitor ingestion.

CAUTIONS

Prostatic hypertrophy, history of urinary retention or obstruction, glaucoma, diabetes mellitus, history of seizures, hyperthyroidism, cardiac/hepatic/renal disease, schizophrenia, increased intraocular pressure, hiatal hernia.

INTERACTIONS

DRUG: ***CNS depressants (including alcohol, barbiturates, phenothiazines, sedative-hypnotics, anticonvulsants)*** may increase sedation, respiratory depression, hypotensive effects. ***Antithyroid*** agents may increase risk of agranulocytosis. ***Phenothiazines*** may increase sedative, anticholinergic effects. ***Cimetidine*** may increase concentration, toxicity. May decrease effects of ***clonidine, guanadrel.*** May increase cardiac effects w/***sympathomimetics***. May increase risk of hypertensive crisis, hyperpyretic, convulsions w/***MAO inhibitors***. HERBAL:

None known. **FOOD:** None significant. **ALTERED LAB VALUES:** May alter EKG readings, glucose.

SIDE EFFECTS

FREQUENT: Dizziness, drowsiness, dry mouth, orthostatic hypotension, headache, increased appetite/weight, nausea, unusual tiredness, unpleasant taste. **OCCASIONAL:** Blurred vision, confusion, constipation, hallucinations, delayed micturation, eye pain, arrhythmias, fine muscle tremors, Parkinsonian syndrome, nervousness, diarrhea, increased sweating, heartburn, insomnia. **RARE:** Hypersensitivity, alopecia, tinnitus, neuroleptic malignant syndrome (convulsions, irregular pulse, fever, altered B/P, diaphoresis, severe muscle stiffness).

ADVERSE REACTIONS/TOXIC EFFECTS

High dosage may produce cardiovascular effects (severe postural hypotension, dizziness, tachycardia, palpitations, arrhythmias, altered temperature regulation). Abrupt withdrawal from prolonged therapy may produce headache, malaise, nausea, vomiting, vivid dreams. Rarely, blood dyscrasias, cholestatic jaundice noted.

NURSING IMPLICATIONS

BASELINE ASSESSMENT

For those on long-term therapy, liver/renal function tests, blood counts should be performed periodically. Observe/record behavior. Assess psychological status, thought content, sleep patterns, appearance, interest in environment.

INTERVENTION/EVALUATION

Supervise suicidal risk pt closely during early therapy (as depression lessens, energy level improves, increasing suicide potential). Assess appearance, behavior, speech pattern, level of interest, mood. Monitor pattern of daily bowel activity and stool consistency. Monitor B/P, pulse for hypotension, arrhythmias. Assess for urinary retention by bladder palpation.

PATIENT/FAMILY TEACHING

Change positions slowly to avoid hypotensive effect. Tolerance to postural hypotension, sedative and anticholinergic effects usually develops during early therapy. Maximum therapeutic effect may be noted in 2–4 wks. Sensitivity to sun may occur. Dry mouth may be relieved by sugarless gum or sips of tepid water. Report visual disturbances. Do not abruptly discontinue medication. Avoid tasks that require alertness, motor skills until response to drug is established.

---

amoxicillin

ah-**mocks**-ih-sill-in
(Amoxil, Polymox,Trimox, Wymox)

CANADIAN AVAILABILITY
Amoxil, Apo-Amoxi, Novamoxin

PREGNANCY CATEGORY B

CLASSIFICATION

Antibiotic: Penicillin

AVAILABILITY (Rx)

Tablets (chewable): 125 mg, 200 mg, 250 mg, 400 mg. **Tablets:** 500 mg, 875 mg. **Capsules:** 250 mg,

500 mg. **Powder for Oral Suspension:** 50 mg/ml, 125 mg/5 ml, 200 mg/5 ml, 250 mg/5 ml, 400 mg/5 ml.

PHARMACOKINETICS

Absorption: Well absorbed from GI tract. **Metabolism:** Partially metabolized in liver. **Excretion:** Primarily excreted in urine. Removed by hemodialysis. **Half-life:** 1–1.3 hrs (increased in reduced renal function).

ACTION/*THERAPEUTIC EFFECT*

Bactericidal in susceptible microorganisms by *inhibition of cell wall synthesis.*

USES/*UNLABELED*

Treatment of skin/skin structure, respiratory, GI, and genitourinary infections, otitis media, gonorrhea. Treatment of *H. pylori* associated w/peptic ulcer; *Lyme disease; typhoid fever.*

STORAGE/HANDLING

Store capsules, tablets at room temperature. Oral solution, after reconstitution, is stable for 14 days at either room temperature or refrigeration.

ADMINISTRATION

ORAL:

- Give orally w/o regard to meals.
- Instruct pt to chew or crush chewable tablets thoroughly before swallowing.

INDICATIONS/ROUTES/DOSAGE

Ear, nose, throat, genitourinary, skin/skin structure infections:
Oral: Adults, children >20 kg: 250–500 mg q8h (or 500–875 mg tablets 2 times/day). ***Children <20 kg:*** 20–40 mg/kg/day in divided doses q8–12h.

Lower respiratory tract infections:
Oral: Adults, children >20 kg: 500 mg q8h (or 875 mg tablets 2 times/day). ***Children <20 kg:*** 40 mg/kg/day in divided doses q8–12h.

Acute, uncomplicated gonorrhea, epididymo-orchitis:
Oral: Adults: 3 g one time w/1 g probenecid. Follow w/tetracycline or erythromycin therapy.

Acute otitis media:
Oral: Children: 80–90 mg/kg/day in divided doses.

H. pylori:
Oral: Adults (in combination): 1 g 2 times/day for 10 days.

CONTRAINDICATIONS

Infectious mononucleosis, hypersensitivity to any penicillin.

CAUTIONS

History of allergies (especially cephalosporins), antibiotic-associated colitis.

INTERACTIONS

DRUG: ***Allopurinol*** may increase incidence of rash. ***Probenecid*** may increase concentration, toxicity risk. May decrease effects of ***oral contraceptives***. **HERBAL:** None known. **FOOD:** None significant. **ALTERED LAB VALUES:** May increase SGOT (AST), SGPT (ALT), LDH, bilirubin, creatinine, BUN. May cause positive Coombs' test.

SIDE EFFECTS

FREQUENT: GI disturbances (mild diarrhea, nausea or vomiting), headache, oral/vaginal candidiasis. **OCCASIONAL:** Generalized rash, urticaria.

ADVERSE REACTIONS/TOXIC EFFECTS

Superinfections, potentially fatal

antibiotic-associated colitis (abdominal cramps, watery severe diarrhea, fever) may result from altered bacterial balance. Severe hypersensitivity reactions including anaphylaxis, acute interstitial nephritis occur rarely.

PATIENT CONSIDERATIONS

BASELINE ASSESSMENT

Question for history of allergies, especially penicillins, cephalosporins. Obtain specimen for culture and sensitivity before giving first dose (therapy may begin before results of test are known).

INTERVENTION/EVALUATION

Hold medication and promptly report rash or diarrhea (w/fever, abdominal pain, mucus and blood in stool may indicate antibiotic-associated colitis). Assess food tolerance. Monitor I&O, urinalysis, renal function tests. Be alert for superinfection: increased fever, sore throat onset, vomiting, diarrhea, black/hairy tongue, ulceration or changes of oral mucosa, anal/genital pruritus.

PATIENT/FAMILY TEACHING

Continue antibiotic for full length of treatment. Space doses evenly. Take w/meals if GI upset occurs. Thoroughly chew the chewable tablets before swallowing. Notify physician in event of rash, diarrhea, or other new symptom.

amoxicillin/clavulanate potassium

a-**mocks**-ih-sill-in/klah-view-**lan**-ate

(Augmentin)

CANADIAN AVAILABILITY
Clavulin

PREGNANCY CATEGORY B

CLASSIFICATION

Antibiotic: Penicillin

AVAILABILITY (Rx)

Tablets (chewable): 125 mg, 200 mg, 250 mg, 400 mg. **Tablets:** 250 mg, 500 mg, 875 mg. **Powder for Oral Suspension:** 125 mg/5 ml, 200 mg/5 ml, 250 mg/5 ml, 400 mg/5 ml.

PHARMACOKINETICS

Absorption: Well absorbed from GI tract. **Metabolism:** Partially metabolized in liver. **Excretion:** Primarily excreted in urine. Removed by hemodialysis. **Half-life:** 1–1.3 hrs (increased in decreased renal function).

ACTION/*THERAPEUTIC EFFECT*

Amoxocillin is bactericidal in susceptible microorganisms *by inhibition of cell wall synthesis.* Clavulanate inhibits bacterial beta-lactamase, *protecting amoxicillin from enzymatic degradation.*

USES/*UNLABELED*

Treatment of skin/skin structure, lower respiratory tract and urinary infections, otitis media, sinusitis. *Treatment of bronchitis, chancroid.*

STORAGE/HANDLING

Store tablets at room temperature. Oral suspension, after reconstitution, is stable for 10 days if refrigerated.

ADMINISTRATION

ORAL:

- Give w/o regard to meals.
- Instruct pt to chew or crush chewable tablets thoroughly before swallowing.

INDICATIONS/ROUTES/DOSAGE

Note: Dosage expressed in terms of amoxicillin. Alternative dosing in adults: 500–875 mg 2 times/day; in children: 200–400 mg 2 times/day.

Mild to moderate infections:
Oral: Adults, elderly, children >40 kg: 250 mg q8h. ***Children <40 kg:*** 20 mg/kg/day in divided doses q8h.

Respiratory tract infections, severe infections:
Oral: Adults, elderly, children >40 kg: 500 mg q8h. ***Children <40 kg:*** 40 mg/kg/day in divided doses q8h.

Otitis media, sinusitis, lower respiratory tract infections:
Oral: Children <40 kg: 40 mg/kg/day in divided doses q8h.

CONTRAINDICATIONS

Infectious mononucleosis, hypersensitivity to any penicillin.

CAUTIONS

History of allergies, especially cephalosporins, antibiotic-associated colitis.

INTERACTIONS

DRUG: ***Allopurinol*** may increase incidence of rash. ***Probenecid*** may increase concentration, toxicity risk. May decrease effects of ***oral contraceptive***. HERBAL: None known. FOOD: None significant. ALTERED LAB VALUES: May increase SGOT (AST), SGPT (ALT). May cause positive Coombs' test.

SIDE EFFECTS

FREQUENT: GI disturbances (mild diarrhea, nausea or vomiting), headache, oral/vaginal candidiasis. OCCASIONAL: Generalized rash, urticaria.

ADVERSE REACTIONS/TOXIC EFFECTS

Superinfections, potentially fatal antibiotic-associated colitis (abdominal cramps, watery severe diarrhea, fever) may result from altered bacterial balance. Severe hypersensitivity reactions including anaphylaxis, acute interstitial nephritis occur rarely.

PATIENT CONSIDERATIONS

Baseline Assessment

Question for history of allergies, especially penicillins, cephalosporins. Obtain specimen for culture and sensitivity before giving first dose (therapy may begin before results of test are known).

Intervention/Evaluation

Hold medication and promptly report rash (hypersensitivity) or diarrhea (w/fever, abdominal pain, blood and mucus in stool may indicate antibiotic-associated colitis). Assess food tolerance. Monitor I&O, urinalysis, renal function tests. Be alert for superinfection: increased fever, sore throat onset, vomiting, diarrhea, black/hairy tongue, ulceration or changes of oral mucosa, anal/genital pruritus.

Patient/Family Teaching

Space doses evenly. Take antibiotic for full length of treatment. Take w/meals if GI upset occurs.

Thoroughly chew the chewable tablets before swallowing. Notify physician in event of rash, diarrhea, or other new symptom.

amphotericin B

am-foe-**tear**-ih-sin
(Abelcet, AmBisome, Amphotec, Fungizone)

CANADIAN AVAILABILITY
Fungizone

PREGNANCY CATEGORY B

CLASSIFICATION

Antifungal

AVAILABILITY (Rx)

Injection: 50 mg, 100 mg (Amphotec). **Suspension for Injection:** 5 mg/ml (lipid complex: Abelcet). **Cream, Lotion, Ointment, Oral Suspension:** 100 mg/ml.

PHARMACOKINETICS

Widely distributed. **Metabolism:** Metabolic fate unknown. Cleared by nonrenal pathways. Minimal removal by hemodialysis. **Half-life:** 24 hrs (increased in neonates, children).

ACTION/*THERAPEUTIC EFFECT*

Generally fungistatic but may be fungicidal w/high dosage or very susceptible microorganisms. Binds to sterols in fungal cell membrane, *increasing membrane permeability, allowing loss of potassium, other cellular components.*

USES

Parenteral: Treatment of severe systemic infections/meningitis due to susceptible fungi. Disseminated candidiasis, candidal prophylaxis during immunosuppressive therapy, aspergillosis, histoplasmosis, blastomycosis, coccidioidomycosis, cryptomycosis, sporotrichosis. *Topical:* Treatment of cutaneous/mucocutaneous infections caused by *Candida albicans* (paronychia, oral thrush, perleche, diaper rash, intertriginous candidiasis).

STORAGE/HANDLING

Refrigerate vials (store Amphotec at room temperature). Dilute with D_5W for IV infusion. Solution for IV infusion is stable for 48 hrs (Abelcet: 48 hrs when refrigerated, then 6 hrs at room temperature; AmBisome: 6 hrs). Not necessary to protect IV infusion from light. Discard if precipitate forms.

ADMINISTRATION

IV:

- Give by slow IV infusion. Conventional amphoterecin over 1–6 hrs; Abelcet over 2 hrs (shake contents if infusion >2 hrs); Amphotec over 2–4 hrs; AmBisome over 1 hr.
- Monitor B/P, temperature, pulse, respirations; assess for adverse reactions q15min ×2, then q30min for 4 hrs of initial infusion.
- Potential for thrombophlebitis may be less w/use of pediatric scalp vein needles or (w/physician order) adding dilute heparin solution.
- Observe strict aseptic technique, since no bacteriostatic agent or preservative is present in diluent.

INDICATIONS/ROUTES/DOSAGE

Usual parenteral dosage:
IV Infusion: Adults, elderly:

Dosage based on pt tolerance, severity of infection. Initially, 1 mg test dose is given over 20–30 min. If test dose is tolerated, 5 mg dose may be given the same day. Subsequently, increases of 5 mg/dose are made q12–24h until desired daily dose is reached. Alternatively, if test dose is tolerated, a dose of 0.25 mg/kg is given same day; increased to 0.5 mg/kg the second day. Dose increased until desired daily dose reached. **Total** ***Daily Dose:*** 1 mg/kg/day up to 1.5 mg/kg every other day. Do not exceed maximum total daily dose of 1.5 mg/kg.

Usual AmBisome dosage:
IV Infusion: Adults, children: 1–5 mg/kg over 1 hr.

Usual Amphotec dosage:
IV Infusion: Adults, children: 3–4 mg/kg over 2–4 hrs.

Usual Abelcet dosage:
IV Infusion: Adults,children: 5 mg/kg at rate of 2.5 mg/kg/hr.

Cutaneous infections:
Topical: Adults, elderly, children: Apply liberally and rub in 2–4 times/day.

CONTRAINDICATIONS

Hypersensitivity to amphotericin B, sulfite.

CAUTIONS

Renal impairment, in combination w/antineoplastic therapy. Give only for progressive, potentially fatal fungal infection.

INTERACTIONS

DRUG: **Steroids** may cause severe hypokalemia. **Bone marrow depressants** may increase anemia. May increase **digoxin** toxicity (due to hypokalemia). **Nephrotoxic medications** may increase nephrotoxicity. **HERBAL:** None known. **FOOD:** None significant. **ALTERED LAB VALUES:** May decrease magnesium, potassium; may increase CPK.

SIDE EFFECTS

FREQUENT: *Parenteral:* Anemia, hypokalemia, infusion-related reaction (fever, chills, nausea, vomiting, headache, hypotension), decreased renal function, thrombophlebitis, indigestion, decreased appetite, diarrhea. *Abelcet:* Chills, fever, multiple organ failure, sepsis. OCCASIONAL: *Parenteral:* Blurred vision, arrhythmias, hypersensitivity reaction (rash, shortness of breath, wheezing, tight chest), numbness in hands/feet, seizures, thrombocytopenia. *Topical:* Local irritation, dry skin. RARE: *Topical:* Skin rash.

ADVERSE REACTIONS/TOXIC EFFECTS

Each alternative formulation is less nephrotoxic than conventional amphotericin (Fungizone). Cardiovascular toxicity (hypotension, ventricular fibrillation), anaphylactic reaction occur rarely. Vision and hearing alterations, seizures, hepatic failure, coagulation defects may be noted.

PATIENT CONSIDERATIONS

Baseline Assessment

Question for history of allergies, especially to amphotericin B, sulfite. Avoid, if possible, other nephrotoxic medications. Confirm that a positive culture or histologic test was performed. Check for/obtain orders to reduce adverse reactions during IV therapy (antipyretics, antihistamines, antiemetics, or small doses of cor-

ticosteroids given before or during amphotericin administration may control reactions).

INTERVENTION/EVALUATION

Monitor B/P, temperature, pulse, respirations; assess for adverse reactions q15min, then q30min for 4 hrs of initial infusion (fever, shaking, chills, anorexia, nausea, vomiting, abdominal pain). Slow infusion and administer medication for symptomatic relief. Evaluate IV site for phlebitis (heat, pain, red streaking over vein). Determine pattern of bowel activity and stool consistency. Assess food intake, tolerance. Monitor I&O, renal function tests for nephrotoxicity. Check potassium and magnesium levels, hematologic and hepatic function test results. Assess for bleeding, bruising, soft tissue swelling.

Topical
Assess for itching, irritation, burning.

PATIENT/FAMILY TEACHING

Prolonged therapy (wks or mos) is usually necessary. Discomfort may occur at IV site. Notify physician of bleeding, bruising, soft tissue swelling, other new symptom. Fever reaction may decrease w/continued therapy. Muscle weakness may be noted during therapy (due to hypokalemia).

Topical
Application may cause staining of skin or nails; soap and water or dry cleaning will remove fabric stains. Do not use other preparations or occlusive coverings w/o consulting physician. Keep areas clean, dry; wear light clothing. Separate personal items w/direct contact to area.

ampicillin sodium

amp-ih-**sill**-in
(Omnipen, Polycillin, Principen)

FIXED-COMBINATION(S)
W/probenecid, a uric acid inhibitor **(Principen w/probenecid, Polycillin PRB, Proambicin)**

CANADIAN AVAILABILITY
Apo-Ampi, Novo-Ampicillin, Nu-Ampi

PREGNANCY CATEGORY B

CLASSIFICATION

Antibiotic: Penicillin

AVAILABILITY (Rx)

Capsules: 250 mg, 500 mg. **Powder for Oral Suspension:** 125 mg/5 ml, 250 mg/5 ml, 500 mg/5 ml. **Powder for Injection:** 125 mg, 250 mg, 500 mg, 1 g, 2 g.

PHARMACOKINETICS

Absorption: Moderately absorbed from GI tract. Widely distributed. **Metabolism:** Partially metabolized in liver. **Excretion:** Primarily excreted in urine. Removed by hemodialysis. **Half-life:** 1–1.5 hrs (increase in impaired renal function).

ACTION/*THERAPEUTIC EFFECT*

Bactericidal in susceptible microorganisms by *inhibition of cell wall synthesis.*

USES

Treatment of respiratory, GI and GU tract, skin/skin structure, bone and joint infections, otitis media, gonorrhea, endocarditis, meningitis, septicemia, mild to moderate typhoid fever, perioperative prophylaxis.

STORAGE/HANDLING

Store capsules at room temperature. Oral suspension, after reconstituted, is stable for 7 days at room temperature, 14 days if refrigerated. The IV solution, diluted w/0.9% NaCl, is stable for 3 days if refrigerated. If diluted w/5% dextrose, use immediately (drug inactivation). Discard if precipitate forms.

ADMINISTRATION

ORAL:

- Give orally 1 hr before or 2 hrs after meals for maximum absorption.

IM:

- Reconstitute each vial w/sterile water for injection or bacteriostatic water for injection (consult individual vial for specific volume of diluent).
- Give deeply in large muscle mass.

IV:

- For IV injection, dilute each vial w/5 ml sterile water for injection (10 ml for 1 and 2 g vials) and give over 3–5 min (10–15 min for 1–2 g dose).
- For intermittent IV infusion (piggyback), further dilute w/50–100 ml 0.9% NaCl or 5% dextrose, infuse over 20–30 min.
- Due to potential for hypersensitivity/anaphylaxis, start initial dose at few drops per minute, increase slowly to ordered rate; stay w/pt first 10–15 min, then check q10min.
- Change to oral route as soon as possible.

INDICATIONS/ROUTES/DOSAGE

Respiratory tract, skin/skin structure infections:
Oral: Adults, elderly, children >20 kg: 250 mg q6h. *Children <20 kg:* 50 mg/kg/day in divided doses q6h.

IM/IV: Adults, elderly, children >40 kg: 250–500 mg q6h. *Children <40 kg:* 25–50 mg/kg/day in divided doses q6–8h.

Bacterial meningitis, septicemia:
IM/IV: Adults, elderly: 2 g q4h or 3 g q6h. *Children:* 100–200 mg/kg/day in divided doses q4h.

Gonococcal infections:
Oral: Adults: 3.5 g one time w/1 g probenecid plus tetracycline, erythromycin, or ampicillin.

Perioperative prophylaxis:
IM/IV: Adults, elderly: 2 g 30 min prior to procedure. May repeat in 8 hrs. *Children:* 50 mg/kg using same dosage regimen.

Usual dosage (neonates):
Note: Higher doses may be needed for neonatal meningitis.

IM/IV: Neonates 7–28 days: 75 mg/kg/day in divided doses q8h up to 200 mg/kg/day in divided doses q6h. *Neonates 0–7 days:* 50 mg/kg/day in divided doses q12h up to 150 mg/kg/day in divided doses q8h.

CONTRAINDICATIONS

Infectious mononucleosis, hypersensitivity to any penicillin.

CAUTIONS

History of allergies, particularly cephalosporins, antibiotic-associated colitis.

INTERACTIONS

DRUG: ***Allopurinol*** may increase incidence of rash. ***Probenecid*** may increase concentration, toxicity risk. May decrease effects of ***oral contraceptive***. HERBAL: None known. **FOOD:** None significant. **ALTERED LAB VALUES:** May increase SGOT (AST), SGPT (ALT). May cause positive Coombs' test.

SIDE EFFECTS

FREQUENT: Pain at IM injection site, GI disturbances (mild diarrhea, nausea or vomiting), oral/vaginal candidiasis. **OCCASIONAL:** Generalized rash, urticaria, phlebitis, thrombophlebitis w/IV administration, headache. **RARE:** Dizziness, seizures especially w/IV therapy.

ADVERSE REACTIONS/TOXIC EFFECTS

Superinfections, potentially fatal antibiotic-associated colitis (abdominal cramps, watery severe diarrhea, fever) may result from altered bacterial balance. Severe hypersensitivity reactions including anaphylaxis, acute interstitial nephritis occur rarely.

PATIENT CONSIDERATIONS

Baseline Assessment

Question for history of allergies, especially penicillins, cephalosporins. Obtain specimen for culture and sensitivity before giving first dose (therapy may begin before results are known).

Intervention/Evaluation

Hold medication and promptly report rash (although common w/ampicillin, may indicate hypersensitivity) or diarrhea (w/fever, abdominal pain, mucus and blood in stool may indicate antibiotic-associated colitis). Assess food tolerance. Evaluate IV site for phlebitis (heat, pain, red streaking over vein). Check IM injection site for pain, induration. Monitor I&O, urinalysis, renal function tests. Assess for signs of superinfection: increased fever, sore throat onset, vomiting, diarrhea, anal/genital pruritus, changes in oral mucosa, black/hairy tongue.

Patient/Family Teaching

Space doses evenly. Take antibiotic for full length of treatment. More effective if taken 1 hr before or 2 hrs after food/beverages. Discomfort may occur w/IM injection. Notify physician of rash, diarrhea, or other new symptom.

---

ampicillin/sulbactam sodium

amp-ih-**sill**-in/sull-**bak**-tam
(Unasyn)

PREGNANCY CATEGORY B

CLASSIFICATION

Antibiotic: Penicillin

AVAILABILITY (Rx)

Powder for Injection: 1.5 g, 3 g.

PHARMACOKINETICS

Widely distributed. **Metabolism:** Partially metabolized in liver. **Excretion:** Primarily excreted in urine. Removed by hemodialysis. **Half-life:** 1 hr (increase in decreased renal function).

ACTION/*THERAPEUTIC EFFECT*

Ampicillin is bactericidal in susceptible microorganisms *by inhibition of cell wall synthesis.*

Sulbactam: inhibits bacterial beta-lactamase, protecting ampicillin from enzymatic degradation.

USES

Treatment of intra-abdominal, skin/skin structure, gynecologic infections.

STORAGE/HANDLING

When reconstituted w/0.9% NaCl, IV solution is stable for 8 hrs at room temperature, 48 hrs if refrigerated. Stability may be different w/other diluents. Discard if precipitate forms.

ADMINISTRATION

IM:

- Reconstitute each 1.5 g vial w/3.2 ml sterile water for injection to provide concentration of 250 mg ampicillin/125 mg sulbactam/ml.
- Give deeply into large muscle mass within 1 hr after preparation.

IV:

- For IV injection, dilute w/10–20 ml sterile water for injection. Give slowly over minimum of 10–15 min.
- For intermittent IV infusion (piggyback) further dilute w/50–100 ml 5% dextrose, or NaCl, infuse over 15–30 min.
- Alternating IV sites, use large veins to reduce risk of phlebitis.
- Due to potential for hypersensitivity/anaphylaxis, start initial dose at few drops per minute, increase slowly to ordered rate; stay w/pt first 10–15 min, then check q10min.
- Change to oral antibiotic as soon as possible.

INDICATIONS/ROUTES/DOSAGE

Skin/skin structure, intra-abdominal, gynecologic infections:
IM/IV: Adults, elderly: 1.5 g (1 g ampicillin/500 mg sulbactam) to 3 g (2 g ampicillin/1 g sulbactam) q6h.

Skin/skin structure infections:
IV: Children 1–12 yrs: 300 mg/kg/day in divided doses q6 hrs.

Dosage in renal impairment:
Modification of dose and/or frequency based on creatinine clearance and/or severity of infection.

CREATININE CLEARANCE	DOSAGE
≥30 ml/min	1.5–3 g q6–8h
15–29 ml/min	1.5–3 g q12h
5–14 ml/min	1.5–3 g q24h
<5 ml/min	Not recommended

CONTRAINDICATIONS

Infectious mononucleosis, hypersensitivity to any penicillin.

CAUTIONS

History of allergies, particularly to cephalosporins, antibiotic associated colitis.

INTERACTIONS

DRUG: ***Allopurinol*** may increase incidence of rash. ***Probenecid*** may increase concentration, toxicity risk. May decrease effects ***of oral contraceptive***. **HERBAL:** None known. **FOOD:** None significant. **ALTERED LAB VALUES:** May increase SGOT (AST), SGPT (ALT). May cause positive Coombs' test.

SIDE EFFECTS

FREQUENT: Diarrhea and rash (most common), urticaria, pain at IM injection site; thrombophlebitis w/IV administration; oral/vaginal candidiasis. **OCCASIONAL:** Nausea, vomiting, headache, malaise, urinary retention.

ADVERSE REACTIONS/TOXIC EFFECTS

Severe hypersensitivity reactions, including anaphylaxis, acute interstitial nephritis, blood dyscrasias may be noted. Superinfections, potentially fatal antibiotic-associated colitis (abdominal cramps, watery severe diarrhea, fever) may result from altered bacterial balance. Overdose may produce seizures.

PATIENT CONSIDERATIONS

Baseline Assessment

Question for history of allergies, especially penicillins, cephalosporins. Obtain specimen for culture and sensitivity before giving first dose (therapy may begin before results are known).

Intervention/Evaluation

Hold medication and promptly report rash (although common w/ampicillin, may indicate hypersensitivity) or diarrhea (w/fever, mucus and blood in stool, abdominal pain may indicate antibiotic-associated diarrhea). Assess food tolerance. Evaluate IV site for phlebitis (heat, pain, red streaking over vein). Check IM injection site for pain, induration. Monitor I&O, urinalysis, renal function tests. Assess for initial signs of superinfection: increased fever, sore throat onset, vomiting, diarrhea, anal/genital pruritus, ulceration or changes of oral mucosa.

Patient/Family Teaching

Space doses evenly. Take antibiotic for full length of treatment. Discomfort may occur w/IM injection. Notify physician of rash, diarrhea, or other new symptom.

amprenavir

(Agenerase)

See Supplement and Classification section under: HIV infection

anagrelide

an-**ah**-greh-lyd

(Agrylin)

CANADIAN AVAILABILITY

Agrylin

PREGNANCY CATEGORY C

CLASSIFICATION

Antiplatelet

AVAILABILITY (Rx)

Capsules: 0.5 mg, 1 mg

PHARMACODYNAMICS

	ONSET	PEAK	DURATION
Oral	7–14 days	—	4 days

PHARMACOKINETICS

Absorption: Extensively metabolized. **Excretion:** Eliminated mostly in the urine and, to a lesser extent, in the feces. **Half-life:** 3 days.

ACTION/*THERAPEUTIC EFFECT*

Reduces the megakaryocyte cycle of platelet production during maturation, *decreasing platelet production.* At high doses, *inhibits platelet aggregation.*

USES/*UNLABELED*

Treatment of essential thrombocythemia, thrombocythemia due to myeloproliferative disorders to reduce elevated platelet count, reducing risk of thrombosis. Platelet count decreases during the first 2 wks of therapy.

INDICATIONS/ROUTES/DOSAGES

Thrombocythemia:

Oral: Adults, elderly: 0.5 mg 4 times/day or 1 mg twice/day. *Maintenance:* Maintain same dosage for 1 week to reduce platelet count to <600,000/mcL before decreasing the dosage needed to the maintain the normal platelet count range. May increase the dosage by ≤0.5 mg/day in any 1 wk. *Maximum:* Do not exceed 10 mg/day or 2.5 mg in a single dose.

CONTRAINDICATIONS

History of hypersensitivity to anagrelide.

CAUTIONS

Known or suspected heart disease, impaired renal function, impaired hepatic function.

INTERACTIONS

DRUG: Sucrulfate may interfere with drug absorption. **HERBAL:** None known. **FOOD:** Drug availability is mildly reduced if taken after food and absorption delayed by 2 hrs. **ALTERED LAB VALUES:** None significant.

SIDE EFFECTS

FREQUENT: Headache (44.5%), palpitations (27%), diarrhea, (24%), asthenia (22%). **OCCASIONAL (10–20%):** Edema, abdominal/general pain, nausea, dizziness, dyspnea, flatulence. **RARE (5–7%):** Rash, vomiting, paresthesia, peripheral edema, dyspepsia, back pain, anorexia, malaise.

ADVERSE REACTIONS/TOXIC EFFECTS

Overdosage produces thrombocytopenia. CHF, cardiomyopathy, MI, atrial fibrillation, pericarditis, complete heart block, CVA, pulmonary infiltrates, pulmonary hypertension, pancreatitis, gastric/duodenal ulcer, and seizure may occur in pts with ET or other thrombocythemias of other etiologies.

PATIENT CONSIDERATIONS

BASELINE ASSESSMENT

A cardiovascular exam should be undertaken before treatment and during therapy because therapeutic doses may produce cardiovascular effects. Perform platelet counts prior to drug therapy, every 2 days during the first week of treatment, and weekly thereafter until therapeutic maintenance dose is reached. Abrupt discontinuation of drug therapy produces an elevation of platelet count within 4 days.

INTERVENTION/EVALUATION

Monitor platelet count for evidence of thrombocytopenia. Assess BUN, creatinine, bilirubin, SGOT, SGPT, WBC, Hgb blood tests, signs/symptoms of renal toxicity and hepatic insufficiency during therapy.

PATIENT/FAMILY TEACHING

Notify physician if pregnant or plan to become pregnant.

anastrozole

ah-**nas**-trow-zole
(Arimidex)

CANADIAN AVAILABILITY
Arimidex

PREGNANCY CATEGORY D

CLASSIFICATION

Antineoplastic; hormone

AVAILABILITY (Rx)

Tablets: 1 mg

PHARMACOKINETICS

Absorption: Well absorbed into systemic circulation. Food does not affect extent of absorption. **Metabolism:** Extensively metabolized. **Excretion:** Eliminated by hepatic metabolism and, to a lesser extent, renal excretion. **Half-life:** 50 hrs in postmenopausal women. Plasma concentrations reach steady-state levels at about 7 days.

ACTION / *THERAPEUTIC EFFECT*

Decreases circulating estrogen by inhibiting aromatase, an enzyme that catalyzes the final step in estrogen production. Since growth of many breast cancers are stimulated by estrogens, *drug significantly lowers serum estradiol (estrogen) concentration.*

USES

Treatment of advanced breast cancer in postmenopausal women who have developed progressive disease while receiving tamoxifen therapy. First-line therapy in advanced/ metastatic breast cancer.

INDICATIONS / ROUTES / DOSAGE

Breast cancer:
Oral: Adults, elderly: 1 mg once daily.

CONTRAINDICATIONS

None significant.

CAUTIONS

None significant.

INTERACTIONS

DRUG: None significant. **HERBAL:** None known. **FOOD:** None significant. **ALTERED LAB VALUES:** May elevate serum GGT level in those w/liver metastases. May increase SGOT (AST), SGPT (ALT), alkaline phosphate, total cholesterol, LDL cholesterol.

SIDE EFFECTS

FREQUENT (8–16%): Asthenia, nausea, headache, pain, hot flashes, dyspnea, vomiting, cough, diarrhea. OCCASIONAL (2–8%): Constipation, abdominal pain, decreased appetite, dizziness, rash, dry mouth, depression, peripheral edema.

ADVERSE REACTIONS / TOXIC EFFECTS

Thrombophlebitis, anemia, leukopenia occur rarely.

PATIENT CONSIDERATIONS

PATIENT/FAMILY TEACHING

Notify physician if nausea, asthenia, hot flashes become unmanageable.

---

anistreplase

an-**is**-treh-place
(Eminase)

CANADIAN AVAILABILITY
Eminase

PREGNANCY CATEGORY C

CLASSIFICATION

Thrombolytic

AVAILABILITY (Rx)

Powder for Injection: 30 units

PHARMACODYNAMICS

	ONSET	PEAK	DURATION
IV	—	—	4–6 hrs

PHARMACOKINETICS

Clearance of fibrinolytic activity due to tissue uptake, inactivation by inhibitors, and degradation by circulating antiplasmin. **Half-life:** 70–120 min.

ACTION/*THERAPEUTIC EFFECT*

Activates fibrinolytic system by cleaving bond in plasminogen-producing plasmin, an enzyme *that degrades fibrin clots, fibrinogen, other plasma proteins.* Acts indirectly by competing w/plasminogen. Converted to plasmin complex, which converts residual plasminogen to plasmin.

USES

Management of acute myocardial infarction (AMI) in adults, lysis of thrombi obstructing coronary arteries, reduces infarct size, improves ventricular function following AMI, reduces mortality associated w/AMI.

STORAGE/HANDLING

Refrigerate powder. Reconstituted solutions are colorless to pale yellow. Once reconstituted, discard solution if not used within 30 min.

ADMINISTRATION

IV:

- Reconstitute 30 units vial w/5 ml sterile water for injection (direct fluid against side of vial).
- Gently roll vial, mixing fluid and powder. Do not shake (minimizes foaming).
- Give only by IV injection over 2–5 min into IV line or vein.
- Do not dilute further w/any infusion fluid or add to other medications.
- If minor bleeding occurs at puncture site, apply pressure for 30 min, then apply pressure dressing.
- If uncontrolled hemorrhage occurs, discontinue infusion immediately (slowing rate of infusion may produce worsening hemorrhage).
- Avoid undue pressure when drug is injected into catheter (can rupture catheter or expel clot into circulation).

INDICATIONS/ROUTES/DOSAGE

Management of acute myocardial infarction:

IV: Adults, elderly: 30 units over 2–5 min as soon as possible after onset of symptoms.

CONTRAINDICATIONS

Active internal bleeding, recent (within 2 mos) cerebrovascular accident, intracranial or intraspinal surgery or trauma, intracranial neoplasm, arteriovenous malformation or aneurysm, bleeding diathesis, severe uncontrolled hypertension.

CAUTIONS

Recent (10 days) major surgery or GI bleeding, OB delivery, organ biopsy, recent trauma (cardiopulmonary resuscitation), left heart thrombus, endocarditis, severe hepatic or renal disease, pregnancy, elderly, cerebrovascular disease, diabetic retinopathy, thrombophlebitis, occluded AV cannula at infected site.

INTERACTIONS

DRUG: ***Anticoagulants, heparin, NSAIDs, aspirin, other platelet aggregation inhibitors*** may increase risk of bleeding. ***Antifibrinolytics (e.g., aminocaproic acid)*** may decrease effect. ***Valproic acid*** may increase risk of hemorrhage. **HERBAL:** None known. **FOOD:** None significant. **ALTERED LAB VALUES:** May increase activated partial thromboplastin time (APTT), prothrombin time (PT), thrombin time (TT). May decrease activity of alpha-2 antiplasmin, factor V, VIII, fibrinogen, plasminogen. May decrease hemoglobin, hematocrit.

SIDE EFFECTS

FREQUENT: Superficial or surface bleeding at puncture sites (venous cutdowns; arterial punctures; site of recent surgical intervention; IM, retroperitoneal, or intracerebral site). **OCCASIONAL:** Hypotension, allergic reaction (urticaria, flushing, rash), hematoma, internal bleeding (GI/GU tract, vagina). **RARE:** Severe allergic reactions or anaphylaxis.

ADVERSE REACTIONS/TOXIC EFFECTS

Severe internal hemorrhage (stroke, hemorrhagic, thromboembolic) may occur. Lysis of coronary thrombi may produce atrial or ventricular arrhythmias.

PATIENT CONSIDERATIONS

Baseline Assessment

Avoid arterial invasive technique before and during treatment. If arterial puncture is necessary, use upper extremity vessels. Assess hematocrit, platelet count, thrombin (TT), activated thromboplastin (APTT), prothrombin time (PT), fibrinogen level before therapy is instituted.

Intervention/Evaluation

Handle pt carefully and infrequently as possible to prevent bleeding. Never give via IM injection route. Monitor clinical response, vital signs q4h. Do not obtain B/P in lower extremities (possible deep vein thrombi). Monitor TT, PT, APTT, fibrinogen level q4h after initiation of therapy, stool culture for occult blood. Assess for decrease in B/P, increase in pulse rate, complaint of abdominal or back pain, severe headache (may be evidence of hemorrhage). Question for increase in amount of discharge during menses. Assess area of thromboembolus for color, temperature. Assess peripheral pulses; skin for bruises, petechiae. Check for excessive bleeding from minor cuts, scratches. Assess urine output for hematuria.

antihemophilic factor (factor VIII, AHF)

(AlphaNine SD, Humate P, Koate, Monoclate, ReFacto)

CANADIAN AVAILABILITY
Koate-DVI, Koate-HP, Kogenate

PREGNANCY CATEGORY C

CLASSIFICATION

Hemostatic

AVAILABILITY (Rx)

Injection: 200 IU, 250 IU, 500 IU, 1000 IU, 1250 IU, 1500 IU

PHARMACOKINETICS

Rapidly cleared from plasma. **Half-life:** 4–14 hrs.

ACTION/*THERAPEUTIC EFFECT*

Assists in conversion of prothrombin to thrombin (essential for blood coagulation), *increasing clotting time.* Replaces missing clotting factor, *correcting or preventing bleeding episodes.*

USES/*UNLABELED*

Treatment, prevention of bleeding in patients w/hemophilia A factor XIII deficiency, von Willebrand disease, hypofibrinogenemia. *Treatment of disseminated intravascular coagulation (DIC).*

STORAGE/HANDLING

Refrigerate, avoid freezing. After reconstitution, solution is clear, colorless, or yellow. Stable for 24 hrs at room temperature, but use within 1–3 hrs. Do not refrigerate reconstituted solution.

ADMINISTRATION

IV:

- **Note:** May be given by slow IV injection or infusion.
- Filter before administration. Use only plastic syringes for IV injection.
- Warm concentrate and diluent to room temperature.
- To dissolve, gently agitate or rotate. Do not shake vigorously. Complete dissolution may take 5–10 min.
- Check pulse rate before and during administration. If pulse rate increases, reduce or stop administration.
- After administration, apply prolonged pressure on venipuncture site. Monitor IV site for oozing q5–15 min for 1–2 hrs after administration.

INDICATIONS/ROUTES/DOSAGE

Note: Dosage is highly individualized, based on pt weight, severity of bleeding, coagulation studies.

Prophylaxis of spontaneous hemorrhage:
IV: Adults, elderly, children: 10 AHF/IU/kg as a single infusion.

Moderate hemorrhage, minor surgery:
IV: Adults, elderly, children: Initially, 15–25 AHF/IU/kg. *Maintenance:* 10–15 IU/kg q8–12h.

Severe hemorrhage (near vital organ):
IV: Adults, elderly, children: Initially, 40–50 AHF/IU/kg. *Maintenance:* 20–25 IU/kg q8–12h.

Major surgery:
IV: Adults, elderly, children: 40–50 AHF/IU/kg 1 hr prior to surgery, 20–25 IU/kg 5 hrs later, then 10–15 IU/kg/day for 10–14 days.

von Willebrand disease:
IV: Adults: 40–80 IU/kg q8–12h.

CONTRAINDICATIONS

None significant.

CAUTIONS

Hepatic disease, those w/blood type A, B, AB.

INTERACTIONS

DRUG: None significant. **HERBAL:** None known. **FOOD:** None significant. **ALTERED LAB VALUES:** None significant.

SIDE EFFECTS

OCCASIONAL: Allergic reaction (fever, chills, urticaria [hives], wheezing, slight hypotension, nausea, feeling of chest tightness), stinging at injection site, dizziness, dry mouth, headache, unpleasant taste.

ADVERSE REACTIONS/TOXIC EFFECTS

There is a risk of transmitting viral hepatitis and a slight risk of transmitting AIDS. Possibility of intravascular hemolysis is present if large or frequent doses used in those w/blood group A, B, or AB.

PATIENT CONSIDERATIONS

Baseline Assessment

When monitoring B/P, avoid overinflation of cuff. Remove adhesive tape from any pressure dressing very carefully and slowly.

Intervention/Evaluation

After IV administration, apply prolonged pressure on venipuncture site. Monitor IV site for oozing q5–15min for 1–2 hrs after administration. Assess for allergic reaction (see Side Effects). Report

any evidence of hematuria or change in vital signs immediately. Monitor hematocrit, direct antiglobulin (Coombs') test, CBC, urinalysis, PTT, thromboplastin/prothrombin, AHF test results. Assess for decrease in B/P, increase in pulse rate, complaint of abdominal or back pain, severe headache (may be evidence of hemorrhage). Question for increase in amount of discharge during menses. Assess peripheral pulses; skin for bruises, petechiae. Check for excessive bleeding from minor cuts, scratches. Assess gums for erythema, gingival bleeding. Assess urine for hematuria. Evaluate for therapeutic relief of pain, reduction of swelling, and restricted joint movement.

Patient/Family Teaching

Use electric razor, soft toothbrush to prevent bleeding. Report any sign of red or dark urine, black or red stool, coffee-ground vomitus, red-speckled mucus from cough. Do not use any OTC medication w/o physician approval (may interfere w/platelet aggregation).

---

apraclonidine

(Iopidine)

See Classification section under: Antiglaucoma agents

---

aprotinin

ah-**pro**-tih-nin

(Trasylol)

CANADIAN AVAILABILITY

Trasylol

PREGNANCY CATEGORY B

CLASSIFICATION

Antifibrinolytic; antihemorrhagic, natural proteinase inhibitor

AVAILABILITY (Rx)

Injection: 100 ml, 200 ml vial. Supplied as a solution containing 10,000 KIU/ml (equal to 1.4 mg/ml).

PHARMACOKINETICS

Rapidly distributed into extracellular space, primarily kidney. Actively reabsorbed and accumulated by proximal tubules in kidney. **Excretion:** Excreted in urine as inactive metabolite > 48 hrs. **Initial half-life:** approx. 150 min. Five hrs after dosing, terminal elimination phase w/half-life about 10 hrs.

ACTION/*THERAPEUTIC EFFECT*

Pts undergoing cardiac surgery w/use of a heart-lung machine normally develop adverse changes in blood components. These changes produce hemostatic defect, generally resulting in diffuse bleeding. Aprotinin inhibits coagulation, *directly preventing fibrinolysis, preserving platelet function, thereby decreasing bleeding.*

USES/*UNLABELED*

For prophylactic, perioperative use to reduce blood loss and need for transfusions in pts undergoing cardiopulmonary bypass in repeat coronary artery bypass graft (CABG) surgery and in primary CABG surgery in pts w/high risk of bleeding (e.g., impaired hemostasis) or where access to blood is unavailable or unacceptable. *For reduction in bleeding and transfusion requirements in liver transplant, total hip replacement, colorectal surgery, peripheral vascular surgery, heart and heart-lung transplant.*

STORAGE/HANDLING

Store vials at room temperature. Discard if precipitate is present or contents appear cloudy. Discard any unused portion in vial.

ADMINISTRATION

IV:

- Place pt in supine position.
- Test dose is required before therapy begins. Give 1 ml test dose IV at least 10 min before loading dose.
- Administer all aprotinin doses through central line (do not administer any other drug using the same IV line).
- Give loading dose over 20–30 min after anesthesia induction but before sternotomy (rapid administration can produce fall in B/P). When loading dose is complete, follow by continuous IV infusion until surgery is completed and pt leaves operating room.
- In those who have previously received aprotinin, after a successful test dose, IV diphenhydramine recommended shortly before loading dose of aprotinin.

INDICATIONS/ROUTES/DOSAGE

Note: Regimen A more effective than Regimen B in pts given aspirin operatively.

Regimen A (high dose):
IV: Adults, elderly: Initially, 2 million KIU loading dose, 2 million KIU into pump prime volume, then continuous IV infusion of 500,000 KIU/hr of operation.

Regimen B (low dose):
IV: Adults, elderly: Initially, 1 million KIU loading dose, 1 million KIU into pump prime volume, then continuous IV infusion of 250,000 KIU/hr of operation.

CONTRAINDICATIONS

Allergy to aprotinin.

EXTREME CAUTION

History of allergies, previous aprotinin therapy, those undergoing deep hypothermic circulatory arrest, >65 yrs, surgery of aortic arch.

INTERACTIONS

DRUG: May block hypotensive effect of ***ACE inhibitors (e.g., captopril),*** inhibits effects of ***fibrinolytic agents (alteplase, anistreplase, streptokinase, urokinase),*** increases effect of ***heparin*** (prolonging activated clotting time). **HERBAL:** None known. **FOOD:** None significant. **ALTERED LAB VALUES:** Prolongs whole blood clotting time of heparinized blood, significantly prolongs activated clotting time (ACT) and partial thromboplastin time (PTT), increases serum creatine kinase (CK) levels, serum creatinine, serum transaminase.

SIDE EFFECTS

Side effects reported are frequently seen in open-heart surgery and not necessarily attributed to aprotinin.

ADVERSE REACTIONS/TOXIC EFFECTS

Even after uneventful test dose, loading dose may produce anaphylaxis. Stop infusion immediately and initiate emergency treatment for anaphylaxis. Reactions may range from skin eruptions, itching, dyspnea, nausea, tachycardia, hypotension, bronchospasm to full anaphylactic shock, circulatory failure. Treatment: parenteral epinephrine, O_2, parenteral antihistamines,

IV corticosteroids, airway management (including intubation).

PATIENT CONSIDERATIONS

Baseline Assessment

Question pt regarding previous use of aprotinin (increased risk of anaphylactic reaction to drug).

Intervention/Evaluation

Monitor lab results frequently. Assess for decrease in B/P, increase in pulse rate, abdominal or back pain, severe headache (may be evidence of hemorrhage). Assess peripheral pulses; skin for bruises, petechiae. Question for increase in amount of discharge during menses. Check for excessive bleeding from minor cuts, scratches. Assess gums for erythema, gingival bleeding. Assess urine output for hematuria.

---

ardeparin

ar-deh-**pear**-in
(Normiflo)

PREGNANCY CATEGORY C

CLASSIFICATION

Anticoagulant

AVAILABILITY (Rx)

Injection: 5,000 U/0.5 ml, 10,000 U/0.5 ml

PHARMACODYNAMICS

Absorption: Well absorbed following SubQ administration. **Excretion:** Eliminated primarily in urine. **Half-life:** 2.1–3.3 hrs.

ACTION/*THERAPEUTIC EFFECT*

Binds and accelerates the activity of antithrombin, inhibition of platelets, and bleeding, *producing anticoagulation* by inhibition of factor Xa and thrombin. Does not significantly influence bleeding time, prothrombin time (PT), activated partial thromboplastin time (APTT).

USES/*UNLABELED*

Prevention of postop deep vein thrombosis (DVT) following knee replacement surgery, *preventing possible pulmonary embolism. Treatment of unstable angina, myocardial infarction.*

ADMINISTRATION

Note: Do not mix w/other injections or infusions. Do not give IM.

SubQ:

- Instruct pt to sit or lie down before administering by deep SubQ injection.
- Inject between left and right anterolateral and left and right posterolateral abdominal wall (avoid navel area), the anterior aspect of the thighs or outer upper arms.
- Introduce entire length of needle (½ inch) into skin fold held between thumb and forefinger, holding skin fold during injection.
- Insert the entire length of the needle into the fold at a 45–90° angle.
- Draw back the plunger before injecting (to ensure the needle is not in the intravascular space).
- Do not rub injection site after administration (prevents bruising).
- Vary the administration site with each injection.

INDICATIONS/DOSAGE/ROUTES

Note: Give initial dose as soon as possible after surgery but not more than 24 hrs after surgery.

Prevention of deep vein thrombosis: *SubQ: Adults, elderly:* 50 anti-Xa U/kg q12 hrs. Treatment to begin the evening of the day of surgery or the following morning and continue for <14 days or until the patient is fully ambulatory.

CONTRAINDICATIONS

Active major bleeding, hemorrhagic stroke, severe hypertension, concurrent heparin therapy, thrombocytopenia associated w/positive in vitro test for antiplatelet antibody, hypersensitivity to heparin or pork products.

CAUTIONS

Conditions w/increased risk of hemorrhage, history of heparin-induced thrombocytopenia, impaired renal/liver function, elderly, bacterial endocarditis, history of recent GI ulceration and hemorrhage.

INTERACTIONS

DRUG: *Anticoagulants, platelet inhibitors* may increase bleeding (use w/care). **HERBAL:** Feverfew, garlic, ginko may increase effect. **FOOD:** None significant. **ALTERED LAB VALUES:** Reversible increases in SGOT (AST), SGPT (ALT), alkaline phosphatase, lactic dehydrogenase (LDH).

SIDE EFFECTS

OCCASIONAL (3–8%): Nausea, injection site hematoma, fever. RARE (2%): Pruritus/rash, constipation, confusion, vomiting.

ADVERSE REACTIONS/TOXIC EFFECTS

Accidental overdosage may lead to bleeding complications ranging from minor ecchymosis to major hemorrhage, or anemia. ***Antidote:*** Protamine sulfate (1% solution) should be given by slow IV injection at a dose of 1 mg for every 100 anti-Xa IU of ardeparin injected. A second dose of 0.5 mg protamine sulfate per 100 anti-Xa IU of ardeparin injected may be given if APTT tested 2–4 hrs after the first infusion remains prolonged.

PATIENT CONSIDERATIONS

BASELINE ASSESSMENT

Assess complete blood count, including platelet count. Determine initial B/P.

INTERVENTION/EVALUATION

Periodically monitor CBC, platelet count, stool for occult blood (no need for daily monitoring in pts w/normal presurgical coagulation parameters). Assess for any sign of bleeding: bleeding at surgical site, hematuria, and blood in stool. Bleeding from gums, petechiae, bruising, bleeding from injection sites. Monitor B/P for hypotension.

PATIENT/FAMILY TEACHING

Usual length of therapy is 7–10 days. Report any sign of bleeding (as above). Do not take any OTC medication (especially aspirin) w/o consulting physician.

---

argatroban
(Acova)
See Supplement

---

artificial tears

(Isopto Tears, Liquifilm Forte, Hypotears, Neo-Tears, Just Tears, Tears Naturale, Lacril, Murocel, Lyteers, Isopto Plain, Ultra Tears, Moisture Drops)

CANADIAN AVAILABILITY
Tears Naturale

PREGNANCY CATEGORY C

CLASSIFICATION

Tearlike lubricant

AVAILABILITY (OTC)

Ophthalmic Solution: Many strengths

ACTION/*THERAPEUTIC EFFECT*

Stabilizes/thickens precorneal tear film, lengthening tear film breakup time. *Protects and lubricates the eyes.*

USES/*UNLABELED*

Relief of dryness and irritation due to deficient tear production; ocular lubricant for artificial eyes; some products may be used w/hard contact lenses. *Treatment of recurrent corneal erosions, decreased corneal sensitivity.*

STORAGE/HANDLING

Store at room temperature.

INDICATIONS/ROUTES/DOSAGE

Ophthalmic Lubricant:
Adults, elderly: 1–2 drops 3–4 times/day as needed.

CONTRAINDICATIONS

Hypersensitivity to any component of preparation.

INTERACTIONS

DRUG: None significant. **HERBAL:** None known. **FOOD:** None significant. **ALTERED LAB VALUES:** None significant.

SIDE EFFECTS

OCCASIONAL: Eye irritation, blurred vision, stickiness of eyelashes.

PATIENT CONSIDERATIONS

BASELINE ASSESSMENT

Determine extent of dryness, irritation.

INTERVENTION/EVALUATION

Assess therapeutic response, increased irritation or discomfort.

PATIENT/FAMILY TEACHING

Wash hands thoroughly. Do not touch the tip of the dropper or container to any surface. Cover immediately after administration. Instruct patient on proper instillation. No one else should use the product. Notify physician if condition worsens or redness, irritation is not relieved within 3 days.

---

ascorbic acid (vitamin C)

(Cecon)

CANADIAN AVAILABILITY
Apo-C, Redoxon

PREGNANCY CATEGORY C

CLASSIFICATION

Vitamin

AVAILABILITY (OTC)

Tablets: 100 mg, 250 mg, 500 mg, 1,000 mg. **Tablets (chewable):** 100 mg, 250 mg, 500 mg. **Tablets (time-release):** 500 mg, 1,000 mg, 1,500 mg. **Capsules (time-release):** 500 mg. **Solution:** 100 mg/ml. **Syrup:** 250 mg/ml. **Injection:** 250 mg/ml, 500 mg/ml.

PHARMACOKINETICS

Absorption: Readily absorbed from GI tract. **Metabolism:** In liver. **Excretion:** In urine. Removed by hemodialysis.

ACTION/*THERAPEUTIC EFFECT*

Nutritional supplement necessary

for collagen formation, tissue repair, oxidation-reduction reactions. *Involved in metabolism, carbohydrate utilization, synthesis of lipids, proteins, carnitine. Preserves blood vessel integrity.*

USES/*UNLABELED*

Prophylaxis, treatment of vitamin C deficiency. Increased requirement may be needed in GI disease, malignancy, peptic ulcer, tuberculosis, smokers, oral contraceptive users, hyperthyroidism, prolonged stress, burns, infection, chronic fever, parenteral hyperalimentation, hemodialysis. *Prevention of common cold, urinary acidifier, control idiopathic methemoglobinemia.*

ADMINISTRATION

ORAL:

- Give orally unless infeasible or malabsorption occurs. Incompatible w/potassium penicillin G.

IV:

- Administer IV slowly to avoid dizziness.

INDICATIONS/ROUTES/DOSAGE

Dietary supplement:
Oral: Adults, elderly: 45–60 mg/day. ***Children >4 yrs:*** 30–40 mg/day.

Deficiency:
Oral/IV: Adults, elderly: 75–150 mg/day.

Scurvy:
Oral: Adults, elderly: 300 mg–1 g/day.

Burns:
Oral: Adults, elderly: Up to 2 g/day.

Enhance wound healing:
Oral: Adults, elderly: 300–500 mg/day for 7–10 days.

CONTRAINDICATIONS

None significant.

CAUTIONS

Those on sodium restriction, daily salicylate treatment, warfarin therapy, pts w/diabetes mellitus, hx of renal stones.

INTERACTIONS

DRUG: May increase iron toxicity w/***deferoxamine***. **HERBAL:** None known. **FOOD:** None significant. **ALTERED LAB VALUES:** May decrease bilirubin, urinary pH. May increase uric acid, urine oxalate.

SIDE EFFECTS

RARE: Abdominal cramps, nausea, vomiting, diarrhea, increased urination with doses exceeding 1 g. ***Parenteral:*** Flushing, headache, dizziness, sleepiness or insomnia, soreness at injection site.

ADVERSE REACTIONS/TOXIC EFFECTS

May produce urine acidification leading to crystalluria. Large doses given IV may lead to deep vein thrombosis. Prolonged use of large doses may result in scurvy when dosage is reduced to normal.

PATIENT CONSIDERATIONS

INTERVENTION/EVALUATION

Monitor lab values for improvement of megaloblastic anemia, increased serum ascorbic acid (0.4–1.5 mg/dl), urine acidity. Assess for clinical improvement (improved sense of well-being and sleep patterns). Observe for reversal of deficiency symptoms (gingivitis, bleeding gums, poor wound healing, digestive difficulties, joint pain).

PATIENT/FAMILY TEACHING

Discomfort may occur w/parenteral administration. Report diarrhea (dosage adjustment may be needed). Abrupt vitamin C withdrawal may produce rebound deficiency. Reduce dosage gradually. Foods rich in vitamin C include rose hips, guava, black currant jelly, brussel sprouts, green peppers, spinach, watercress, strawberries, citrus fruits.

asparaginase

(Elspar)

See Classification section under: Cancer chemotherapy

aspirin (acetylsalicylic acid, ASA)

ass-purr-in

(Ascriptin, Bayer, Bufferin, Ecotrin, Halfprin)

FIXED-COMBINATION(S)

W/butabarbital, a barbiturate, and codeine, a narcotic **(Fiorinal)**; w/dipyridamole, an antiplatelet agent **(Aggrenox)**; w/oxycodone, a narcotic **(Percodan)**; w/pentazocine, an analgesic **(Talwin Compound)**; w/caffeine, a stimulant **(Anacin, Midol)**.

CANADIAN AVAILABILITY

Entrophen, Novasen

PREGNANCY CATEGORY C

(D if full dose used in third trimester)

CLASSIFICATION

Nonsteroidal anti-inflammatory: Salicylate

AVAILABILITY (OTC)

Tablets: 325 mg, 500 mg. **Tablets (chewable):** 81 mg. **Tablets (enteric coated):** 81 mg, 165 mg, 325 mg, 500 mg, 650 mg, 975 mg. **Tablets (controlled-release):** 650 mg, 800 mg. **Suppository:** 120 mg, 200 mg, 300 mg, 600 mg.

PHARMACOKINETICS

Absorption: Rapidly, completely absorbed from GI tract; enteric coated absorption delayed; rectal absorption delayed, incomplete. Widely distributed. **Metabolism:** Rapidly hydrolyzed to salicylate. **Half-life:** 15–20 min (aspirin); salicylate: 2–3 hrs at low dose; >20 hrs at high dose.

ACTION/*THERAPEUTIC EFFECT*

Produces analgesic, anti-inflammatory effect by inhibiting prostaglandin synthesis, *reducing inflammatory response and intensity of pain stimulus reaching sensory nerve endings.* Antipyresis produced by drug's effect on hypothalamus, producing vasodilation, *thereby decreasing elevated body temperature.* Inhibits platelet aggregation.

USES/*UNLABELED*

Treatment of mild to moderate pain, fever, inflammatory conditions. Treatment of transient ischemic attack, ischemic stroke, angina, acute myocardial infarction (MI), recurrent MI, specific revascularization procedures, and rheumatologic diseases. *Prophylaxis against thromboembolism, treatment of Kawasaki disease.*

STORAGE/HANDLING

Refrigerate suppositories.

ADMINISTRATION

ORAL:

- Do not crush or break enteric coated or sustained-release form.
- May give w/water, milk, or meals if GI distress occurs.

RECTAL:

- If suppository is too soft, chill for 30 min in refrigerator or run cold water over foil wrapper.
- Moisten suppository w/cold water before inserting well up into rectum.

INDICATIONS/ROUTES/DOSAGE

Pain, fever:
Oral/Rectal: Adults, elderly: 325–650 mg q4h as needed, up to 4 g/day.

Rheumatoid arthritis, osteoarthritis, other inflammatory conditions:
Oral: Adults, elderly: 3.2–6 g/day in divided doses.

Juvenile arthritis:
Oral: Children: 60–110 mg/kg/day in divided doses (q6–8h). May increase dose at 5–7 day intervals.

Acute rheumatic fever:
Oral: Adults, elderly: 5–8 g/day. *Children:* 100 mg/kg/day, then decrease to 75 mg/kg/day for 4–6 wks.

Thrombosis (decrease TIAs):
Oral: Adults, elderly: 1.3 g/day in 2–4 divided doses.

Thrombosis (decrease MI):
Oral: Adults, elderly: 300–325 mg/day.

Usual pediatric dosage:
Oral/Rectal: 10–15 mg/kg/dose q4h up to 60–80 mg/kg/day.

CONTRAINDICATIONS

Chicken pox or flu in children/teenagers, GI bleeding or ulceration, bleeding disorders, history of hypersensitivity to aspirin or NSAIDs, allergy to tartrazine dye, impaired hepatic function.

CAUTIONS

Vitamin K deficiency, chronic renal insufficiency, those w/"aspirin triad" (rhinitis, nasal polyps, asthma).

INTERACTIONS

DRUG: ***Alcohol, NSAIDs*** may increase risk of GI effects (e.g., ulceration). ***Urinary alkalinizers, antacids*** increase excretion. ***Anticoagulants, heparin, thrombolytics*** increase risk of bleeding. Large dose may increase effect of ***insulin, oral hypoglycemics. Valproic acid, platelet aggregation inhibitors*** may increase risk of bleeding. May increase toxicity of ***methotrexate, zidovudine. Ototoxic medications, vancomycin*** may increase ototoxicity. May decrease effect of ***probenecid, sulfinpyrazone***. HERBAL: Feverfew, garlic, ginkgo may increase antiplatelet effect. FOOD: None significant. ALTERED LAB VALUES: May alter SGOT (AST), SGPT (ALT), alkaline phosphatase, uric acid; prolong prothrombin time, bleeding time. May decrease cholesterol, potassium, T_3, T_4.

SIDE EFFECTS

OCCASIONAL: GI distress (cramping, heartburn., abdominal distension, mild nausea), allergic reaction (pruritus, urticaria, bronchospasm).

ADVERSE REACTIONS/TOXIC EFFECTS

High doses may produce GI bleeding and/or gastric mucosal lesions, Low-grade toxicity characterized by ringing in ears, generalized pruritus (may be severe), headache, dizziness, flushing, tachycardia, hyperventilation, sweating, thirst. Febrile, dehydrated children can reach toxic levels quickly. Marked intoxication manifested by hyperthermia, restlessness, abnormal breathing pattern, convulsions, respiratory failure, coma.

PATIENT CONSIDERATIONS

Baseline Assessment

Do not give to children/teenagers who have flu or chicken pox (increases risk of Reye's syndrome). Do not use if vinegarlike odor is noted (indicates chemical breakdown). Assess type, location, duration of pain, inflammation. Inspect appearance of affected joints for immobility, deformities, skin condition. Therapeutic serum level for antiarthritic effect: 20–30 mg/dl (toxicity occurs if levels are over 30 mg/dl).

Intervention/Evaluation

In long-term therapy, monitor plasma salicylic acid concentration. Monitor urinary pH (sudden acidification, pH from 6.5 to 5.5), may result in toxicity. Assess skin for evidence of bruising. If given as antipyretic, assess temperature directly before and 1 hr after giving medication. Evaluate for therapeutic response: relief of pain, stiffness, swelling, increase in joint mobility, reduced joint tenderness, improved grip strength.

Patient/Family Teaching

Do not crush or chew sustained-release or enteric coated form. Therapeutic anti-inflammatory effect noted in 1–3 wks. Take w/food or after meals. Take w/full glass of water (reduces risk of lodging in esophagus). Report ringing in ears or persistent GI pain.

atenolol

ay-**ten**-oh-lol
(Tenormin)

FIXED-COMBINATION(S)
W/chlorthalidone, a diuretic **(Tenoretic)**

CANADIAN AVAILABILITY
Apo-Atenol, Tenormin

PREGNANCY CATEGORY D

CLASSIFICATION

Beta$_1$-adrenergic blocker

AVAILABILITY (Rx)

Tablets: 25 mg, 50 mg, 100 mg. **Injection:** 5 mg/10 ml.

PHARMACODYNAMICS

	ONSET	PEAK	DURATION
PO (heart rate)	1 hr	2–4 hrs	24 hrs
PO (hypotensive)	—	—	24 hrs

PHARMACOKINETICS

Absorption: Incompletely absorbed from GI tract. Minimal liver metabolism. **Excretion:** Primarily excreted unchanged in urine. Removed by hemodialysis. **Half-life:** 6–7 hrs (increase in decreased renal function).

ACTION/*THERAPEUTIC EFFECT*

Blocks beta$_1$-adrenergic receptors in cardiac tissue, *slowing sinus heart rate, decreasing cardiac output, decreasing B/P.* Large doses may block beta$_2$-adrenergic receptors, increasing airway resistance. *Decreases myocardial oxygen demand.*

USES / *UNLABELED*

Management of mild to moderate hypertension. Used alone or in combination w/diuretics, especially thiazide type. Management of chronic stable angina pectoris. Reduces cardiovascular mortality in those w/definite or suspected acute MI. *Hypertrophic cardiomyopathy, pheochromocytoma, prophylaxis of migraine, tremors, thyrotoxicosis, syndrome of mitral valve prolapse. Improves survival in diabetics with heart disease.*

STORAGE/HANDLING

After reconstitution, parenteral form is stable for 48 hrs at room temperature.

ADMINISTRATION

ORAL:

- May be given w/o regard to meals.
- Tablets may be crushed.

IV:

- Dilutions w/5% dextrose or 0.9% NaCl may be used.

INDICATIONSROUTES/DOSAGE

Hypertension:
Oral: Adults: Initially, 25–50 mg once/day. May increase up to 100 mg once/day.

Angina pectoris:
Oral: Adults: Initially, 50 mg once daily. May increase up to 200 mg once daily.

Usual elderly dosage:
Oral: Initially, 25 mg/day for angina/hypertension.

Acute myocardial infarction:
IV: Give 5 mg over 5 min, may repeat in 10 min. In those who tolerate full 10 mg IV dose, begin 50 mg tablets 10 min after last IV dose followed by another 50 mg oral dose 12 hrs later. Thereafter, give 100 mg once/day or 50 mg twice/day for 6–9 days. (Alternatively, for those who do not tolerate full IV dose, give 50 mg orally 2 times/day or 100 mg once/day for at least 7 days.)

Dosage in renal impairment:

CREATININE CLEARANCE	DOSAGE
15–35 ml/min	50 mg daily
<15 ml/min	50 mg q other day

CONTRAINDICATIONS

Overt cardiac failure, cardiogenic shock, heart block greater than first degree, severe bradycardia.

CAUTIONS

Impaired renal or hepatic function, peripheral vascular disease, hyperthyroidism, diabetes, inadequate cardiac function, bronchospastic disease.

INTERACTIONS

DRUG: ***Diuretics, other hypotensives*** may increase hypotensive effect; ***sympathomimetics, xanthines*** may mutually inhibit effects; may mask symptoms of hypoglycemia, prolong hypoglycemic effect of ***insulin, oral hypoglycemics; NSAIDs*** may decrease antihypertensive effect; ***Cimetidine*** may increase concentration. **HERBAL:** None known. **FOOD:** None significant. **ALTERED LAB VALUES:** May increase ANA titer, BUN, creatinine, potassium, uric acid, lipoproteins, triglycerides.

SIDE EFFECTS

Generally well tolerated, w/mild and transient side effects. **FREQUENT:** Hypotension manifested as dizziness, nausea, diaphoresis, headache, cold extremities, fatigue, constipation/diarrhea.

OCCASIONAL: Insomnia, flatulence, urinary frequency, impotence or decreased libido. **RARE:** Rash, arthralgia, myalgia, confusion (especially in elderly), change in taste.

ADVERSE REACTIONS/TOXIC EFFECTS

Overdosage may produce profound bradycardia, hypotension. Abrupt withdrawal may result in sweating, palpitations, headache, tremulousness. May precipitate CHF, MI in those w/cardiac disease, thyroid storm in those w/thyrotoxicosis, peripheral ischemia in those w/existing peripheral vascular disease. Hypoglycemia may occur in previously controlled diabetics. Thrombocytopenia (unusual bruising, bleeding) occurs rarely.

PATIENT CONSIDERATIONS

Baseline Assessment

Assess B/P, apical pulse immediately before drug is administered (if pulse is 60/min or below, or systolic B/P is below 90 mm Hg, withhold medication, contact physician).

Antianginal

Record onset, type (sharp, dull, squeezing), radiation, location, intensity and duration of anginal pain, and precipitating factors (exertion, emotional stress). Assess baseline renal/liver function tests.

Intervention/Evaluation

Monitor B/P for hypotension, pulse for bradycardia, respiration for shortness of breath. Assess pattern of daily bowel activity and stool consistency. Assess for evidence of CHF: dyspnea (particularly on exertion or lying down), night cough, peripheral edema, distended neck veins. Monitor I&O (increase in weight, decrease in urine output may indicate CHF). Assess extremities for coldness. Assist w/ambulation if dizziness occurs. Assess skin for rash, bruising.

Patient/Family Teaching

Do not abruptly discontinue medication. Compliance w/therapy essential to control hypertension, angina. To reduce hypotensive effect, rise slowly from lying to sitting position and permit legs to dangle from bed momentarily before standing. Avoid tasks that require alertness, motor skills until drug reaction is established. Report dizziness, depression, confusion, rash, unusual bruising or bleeding. Do not use nasal decongestants, OTC cold preparations (stimulants) w/o physician approval. Outpatients should monitor B/P, pulse before taking medication (teach correct technique). Restrict salt, alcohol intake. Therapeutic antihypertensive effect noted in 1–2 wks. May change warning signs of hypoglycemia.

---

atorvastatin

ah-tore-**vas**-tah-tin
(Lipitor)

CANADIAN AVAILABILITY
Lipitor

PREGNANCY CATEGORY X

CLASSIFICATION

Antihyperlipoproteinemic

AVAILABILITY (Rx)

Tablets: 10 mg, 20 mg, 40 mg, 80 mg

PHARMACOKINETICS

Absorption: Poorly absorbed from GI tract. **Metabolism:** Metabolized in liver (undergoes first-pass effect). **Excretion:** Minimally eliminated in urine. **Half-life:** 14 hrs.

ACTION/*THERAPEUTIC EFFECT*

Inhibits HMG-CoA reductase, the enzyme that catalyzes the early step in cholesterol synthesis. *Decreases LDL cholesterol, VLDL cholesterol, and plasma triglycerides, increases HDL cholesterol.*

USES

Adjunct to diet therapy to decrease elevated total and LDL cholesterol concentrations in those with primary hypercholesterolemia (types IIa and IIb) and in those w/combined hypercholesterolemia and hypertriglyceridemia.

ADMINISTRATION

ORAL:

- May give w/o regard to food at any time of day.

INDICATIONS/ROUTES/DOSAGES

Hyperlipoproteinemia:
Oral: Adults, elderly: Initially, 10 mg/day given as a single daily dose. ***Dose range:*** Increase at 2–4 wk intervals up to maximum of 80 mg/day.

CONTRAINDICATIONS

Hypersensitivity to atorvastin, active liver disease, unexplained elevated liver function tests, pregnancy, lactation.

CAUTIONS

Anticoagulant therapy, history of liver disease, substantial alcohol consumption, major surgery, severe acute infection, trauma, hypotension, severe metabolic, endocrine, or electrolyte disorders, uncontrolled seizures.

INTERACTIONS

DRUG: ***Antacids, colestipol, propranolol*** decreases atorvastin activity. ***Warfarin, digoxin, oral contraceptives, itraconazole*** levels may increase concentration, producing severe muscle pain, inflammation, weakness. Increased risk of rhabdomyolysis, acute renal failure w/***cyclosporine, erythromycin, gemfibrozil, nicotinic acid***. **HERBAL:** None known. **FOOD:** None significant. **ALTERED LAB VALUES:** May increase creatinine kinase, serum transaminase concentrations.

SIDE EFFECTS

Generally well tolerated. Side effects usually mild and transient. **FREQUENT (16%):** Headache. **OCCASIONAL (2–5%):** Myalgia, rash/pruritus, allergy. **RARE:** Flatulence, dyspepsia.

ADVERSE REACTIONS/TOXIC EFFECTS

Potential for cataracts, photosensitivity.

PATIENT CONSIDERATIONS

BASELINE ASSESSMENT

Question for possibility of pregnancy before initiating therapy (Pregnancy Category X). Question history of hypersensitivity to atorvastin. Assess baseline lab results: cholesterol, triglycerides, liver function tests.

INTERVENTIONS/EVALUATION

Evaluate food tolerance. Determine pattern of bowel activity. Check for headache, dizziness, blurred vision. Assess for rash, pruritus. Monitor cholesterol

and triglyceride lab results for therapeutic response. Be alert for malaise, muscle cramping or weakness. Monitor temperature at least twice a day.

PATIENT/FAMILY TEACHING

Follow special diet (important part of treatment). Periodic lab tests are essential part of therapy. Do not take other medications w/o physician's knowledge. Do not stop medication without consulting physician. Report promptly any muscle pain or weakness, especially if accompanied by fever or malaise. Avoid prolonged exposure to sunlight, use sunscreen, wear protective clothing.

atovaquone

ah-**tow**-vah-quon
(Mepron)

CANADIAN AVAILABILITY
Mepron

PREGNANCY CATEGORY C

CLASSIFICATION

Antiprotozoal

AVAILABILITY (Rx)

Suspension: 750 mg/5 ml

PHARMACOKINETICS

Absorption: Poorly absorbed from GI tract (increased when given w/food, especially high-fat foods). **Excretion:** Primarily eliminated unchanged in feces. **Half-life:** 50–77 hrs.

ACTION/*THERAPEUTIC EFFECT*

Inhibits mitochondrial electron-transport system at the cytochrome bc_1 complex (Complex III). *Interrupts nucleic acid and ATP synthesis.*

USES

Treatment or prevention of mild to moderate *Pneumocystis carinii pneumonia* (PCP) in those intolerant to trimethoprim-sulfamethoxazole (TMP-SMZ).

ADMINISTRATION

ORAL:

- Give w/food (especially high-fat foods).

INDICATIONS/ROUTES/DOSAGE

Pneumocystis carinii pneumonia (PCP):
Oral: Adults: 750 mg w/food 2 times/day for 21 days.

Prevention of PCP:
Oral: Adults: 1,500 mg once daily w/food.

CONTRAINDICATIONS

Development or history of potentially life-threatening allergic reaction to drug.

CAUTIONS

Elderly, pts w/severe PCP, chronic diarrhea, malabsorption syndromes.

INTERACTIONS

DRUG: *Rifampin* may decrease concentration, atovaquone may increase rifampin concentration. **HERBAL:** None known. **FOOD:** None significant. **ALTERED LAB VALUES:** May elevate SGOT (AST), SGPT (ALT), alkaline phosphatase, amylase. May decrease sodium.

SIDE EFFECTS

FREQUENT (>10%): Skin rash,

nausea, diarrhea, headache, vomiting, fever, insomnia, cough. **OCCASIONAL (<10%):** Abdominal discomfort, thrush, asthenia (loss of strength, energy), anemia, neutropenia.

ADVERSE REACTIONS/TOXIC EFFECTS

None significant.

PATIENT CONSIDERATIONS

INTERVENTION/EVALUATION

Assess for GI discomfort, nausea, vomiting. Check consistency and frequency of stools. Assess skin for rash. Monitor I&O, renal function tests, hemoglobin, neutrophil counts. Atovaquone has not been fully evaluated in pts >65 yrs of age; monitor elderly closely because of decreased hepatic, renal, and cardiac function.

PATIENT/FAMILY TEACHING

Continue therapy for full length of treatment. Doses should be evenly spaced. Do not take any other medication unless approved by physician. Notify physician in event of rash, diarrhea, or other new symptom.

---

atracurium

(Tracrium)

See Classification section under: Neuromuscular blockers

---

atropine sulfate

ah-trow-peen

(Atropine Sulfate, Isopto Atropine, Ocu-Tropine)

FIXED-COMBINATION(S)

W/phenobarbital, a sedative-hypnotic **(Antrocol)**; w/diphenoxylate, a constipating meperidine derivative **(Lomotil)**; w/prednisolone, a steroid **(Mydropred Ophthalmic)**.

CANADIAN AVAILABILITY

Atropine Minims, Atropisol, Isopto-Atropine

PREGNANCY CATEGORY C

CLASSIFICATION

Anticholinergic

AVAILABILITY (Rx)

Injection: 0.05 mg/ml, 0.3 mg/ml, 0.4 mg/ml, 0.5 mg/ml, 0.8 mg/ml, 1 mg/ml. **Ophthalmic Ointment:** 1%. **Ophthalmic Solution:** 0.5%, 1%, 2%.

PHARMACODYNAMICS

Mydriatic effect: Peak 30–40 min; recovery 7–12 days. *Cycloplegic effect:* Peak 60–180 min; recovery 6–12 days.

After oral/IM administration, inhibits salivation within 30–60 min (peak 1–2 hrs), duration 4 hrs; increases heart rate within 2–4 min (IV), 5–40 min (IM), or 30–120 min (oral), peak in 0.5–1 hr (IM), 1–2 hrs (oral).

PHARMACOKINETICS

Absorption: Rapidly absorbed after IM, oral administration. **Metabolism:** In liver. **Excretion:** Primarily excreted in urine. **Half-life:** 2–3 hrs.

ACTION/*THERAPEUTIC EFFECT*

Inhibits action of acetylcholine on structures innervated by postganglionic sites (smooth/cardiac muscle, SA/AV nodes, exocrine glands). Larger doses may *decrease motility, secretory activity of GI system, tone of ureter, urinary bladder.* Blocks responses of sphincter muscle and accommodation muscle ciliary body *producing mydriasis, cycloplegia.*

USES

Adjunct in treatment of peptic ulcer disease. Treatment of functional disturbances of GI motility, hypermotility disorders of lower urinary tract, GI hypermotility, diarrhea. Preop medication to prevent or reduce salivation, excessive secretions of respiratory tract. May also prevent cholinergic effects during surgery: cardiac arrhythmias, hypotension, reflex bradycardia. Blocks adverse muscarinic effects of anticholinesterase agents (i.e., neostigmine). Management of sinus bradycardia in those w/acute MI who have hypotension and increased ventricular irritability. For cycloplegic refraction and to dilate pupil in inflammatory conditions of iris and uveal tract.

ADMINISTRATION

ORAL:

- Administer 30 min before meals and at bedtime.

IM:

- May be given SubQ or IM.

IV:

- Generally given rapidly (prevents paradoxical slowing of heart rate).

OPHTHALMIC:

- Place finger on lower eyelid and pull out until pocket is formed between eye and lower lid. Hold dropper above pocket and place prescribed number of drops (¼–½ inch ointment) in pocket. Close eye gently. *Drops:* Apply digital pressure to lacrimal sac for 1–2 min (minimizes drainage into nose and throat, reducing risk of systemic effects). *Ointment:* Close eye for 1–2 min, rolling eyeball (increases contact area of drug to eye). W/either method, remove excess solution or ointment around eye w/tissue.
- Ophthalmic solutions not to be used for injection.

INDICATIONS/ROUTES/DOSAGE

Usual oral dosage:
Oral: Adults, elderly: 0.4–0.6 mg q4–6h. ***Range:*** 0.1–1.2 mg. ***Children:*** 0.01 mg/kg, not to exceed 0.4 mg q4–6h.

Usual parenteral dose:
IM/IV: Adults, elderly: 0.4–0.6 mg q4–6h. ***Range:*** 0.3–1.2 mg. ***Children:*** 0.01 mg/kg, not to exceed 0.4 mg q4–6h.

Bradycardia in advanced cardiac life support:
IV: Adults, elderly: 0.4–1 mg. Repeat at 1–2 hr intervals until desired rate achieved. ***Maximum:*** 2 mg total dose. ***Children:*** 0.01–0.03 mg/kg (minimum dose: 0.1 mg).

Preoperative:
IM/IV: Adults, elderly, children >20 kg: 0.4 mg (***range:*** 0.2–0.6 mg) 30–60 min prior to time of induction of anesthesia or other preanesthetic medications. ***Children (3 kg):*** 0.1 mg; ***(7–9 kg):*** 0.2 mg; ***(12–16 kg):*** 0.3 mg.

Usual ophthalmic dose (mydriasis, cycloplegia):
Ointment: Adults, elderly: 0.3–0.5 cm 1–3 times/day. ***Children:*** 0.3 cm 3 times/day. Administer for 1–3 days prior to procedure.
Solution: Adults, elderly: 1 drop 1% solution. ***Children:*** 1–2 drops

0.5% solution 2 times/day. Administer for 1–3 days prior to and 1 hr before procedure.

Treatment of acute inflammatory ophthalmic conditions:
Solution: Adults, elderly: 1–2 drops of 0.5–1% solution up to 3–4 times/day. ***Children:*** 1–2 drops of 0.5% solution up to 3–4 times/day.

CONTRAINDICATIONS

Narrow-angle glaucoma, severe ulcerative colitis, toxic megacolon, obstructive disease of GI tract, paralytic ileus, intestinal atony, bladder neck obstruction due to prostatic hypertrophy, myasthenia gravis in those not treated w/neostigmine, tachycardia secondary to cardiac insufficiency or thyrotoxicosis, cardiospasm, unstable cardiovascular status in acute hemorrhage.

EXTREME CAUTION

Autonomic neuropathy, known or suspected GI infections, diarrhea, mild to moderate ulcerative colitis.

CAUTIONS

Hyperthyroidism, hepatic or renal disease, hypertension, tachyarrhythmias, CHF, coronary artery disease, gastric ulcer, esophageal reflux or hiatal hernia associated w/reflux esophagitis, infants, elderly, systemic administration in those w/COPD.

INTERACTIONS

DRUG: ***Antacids, antidiarrheals*** may decrease absorption. ***Anticholinergics*** may increase effects. May decrease absorption of ***ketoconazole.*** May increase severity of GI lesions with ***KCl (wax matrix).*** **HERBAL:** None known. **FOOD:** None significant. **ALTERED LAB VALUES:** None significant.

SIDE EFFECTS

Note: Discontinue medication immediately if dizziness, increased pulse, or blurring of vision occurs. **FREQUENT:** Dry mouth/nose/throat (may be severe), decreased sweating, constipation, irritation at IM injection site. **OCCASIONAL:** Swallowing difficulty, blurred vision, bloated feeling, impotence, urinary hesitancy. ***Ophthalmic:*** Blurred vision, eye irritation, eyelid swelling, intolerance to light, headache. **RARE:** Allergic reaction (rash, urticaria), mental confusion/excitement (particularly children), fatigue.

ADVERSE REACTIONS/TOXIC EFFECTS

Overdosage may produce tachycardia, palpitations, hot/dry/flushed skin, absence of bowel sounds, increased respiratory rate, nausea, vomiting, confusion, drowsiness, slurred speech, CNS stimulation, psychosis (agitation, restlessness, rambling speech, visual hallucinations, paranoid behavior, delusions), followed by depression.

PATIENT CONSIDERATIONS

Baseline Assessment

Before giving medication, instruct pt to void (reduces risk of urinary retention).

Intervention/Evaluation

Monitor changes in B/P, pulse, temperature. Assess skin turgor, mucous membranes to evaluate hydration status (encourage adequate fluid intake unless NPO for surgery), bowel sounds for peristalsis. Be alert for fever (increased risk of hyperthermia). Monitor I&O, palpate bladder for urinary retention. Assess stool frequency and consistency.

Patient/Family Teaching

Take oral form 30 min before meals (food decreases absorption of medication). Avoid becoming overheated during exercise in hot weather (may result in heat stroke). Avoid hot baths, saunas. Avoid tasks that require alertness, motor skills until response to drug is established. Sugarless gum, sips of tepid water relieve dry mouth. Do not take antacids or medicine for diarrhea within 1 hr of taking this medication (decreased effectiveness). For preop use, explain that warm, dry, flushing feeling may occur. Remind pt to remain in bed and not eat or drink anything.

---

auranofin

aur-**an**-oh-fin
(Ridaura)

CANADIAN AVAILABILITY
Ridaura

PREGNANCY CATEGORY C

CLASSIFICATION

Antirheumatic: Gold compound

AVAILABILITY (Rx)

Capsule: 3 mg

PHARMACOKINETICS

Absorption: Moderately absorbed from GI tract. **Metabolism:** Rapidly metabolized. **Excretion:** Primarily excreted in urine. **Half-life:** 21–31 days.

ACTION/*THERAPEUTIC EFFECT*

Alters cellular mechanisms, enzyme systems, immune responses, collagen biosynthesis, *suppressing synovitis of the active stage of rheumatoid arthritis.*

USES/*UNLABELED*

Management of rheumatoid arthritis in those w/insufficient therapeutic response to NSAIDs. *Treatment of pemphigus, psoriatic arthritis.*

ADMINISTRATION

ORAL:

- Give w/o regard to food.

INDICATIONS/ROUTES/DOSAGE

Rheumatoid arthritis:
Oral: Adults, elderly: 6 mg/day in 1 or 2 divided doses. May increase to 9 mg/day (in 3 divided doses) if no response in 6 mos. If response still inadequate, discontinue.

CONTRAINDICATIONS

History of gold-induced pathologies (necrotizing enterocolitis, exfoliative dermatitis, pulmonary fibrosis, blood dyscrasias), bone marrow aplasia, severe blood dyscrasias.

CAUTIONS

Renal/hepatic disease, inflammatory bowel disease.

INTERACTIONS

DRUG: ***Bone marrow depressants, hepatotoxic, nephrotoxic medications*** may increase toxicity. ***Penicillamine*** *may increase risk of hematologic or renal adverse effects.* **HERBAL:** None known. **FOOD:** None significant. **ALTERED LAB VALUES:** May decrease hemoglobin, hematocrit, platelets, WBCs. May alter liver function tests. May increase urine protein.

SIDE EFFECTS

FREQUENT (>10%): Diarrhea/loose stools, rash, pruritus, abdominal pain, nausea. **OCCASIONAL (1–10%):** Vomiting, anorexia, flatulence, dyspepsia, constipation, change in sense of taste, glossitis (irritation/soreness of tongue).

ADVERSE REACTIONS/TOXIC EFFECTS

Signs of gold toxicity: decreased hemoglobin, leukopenia (WBC below 4,000/mm^3), reduced granulocyte counts (below 150,000/mm^3), proteinuria, hematuria, stomatitis (ulcers, sores, white spots in mouth, throat), blood dyscrasias (anemia, leukopenia, thrombocytopenia, eosinophilia), glomerulonephritis, nephrotic syndrome, cholestatic jaundice.

PATIENT CONSIDERATIONS

Baseline Assessment

Rule out pregnancy before beginning treatment. CBC, urinalysis, platelet and differential, renal and liver function tests should be performed before therapy begins.

Intervention/Evaluation

Monitor daily bowel activity and stool consistency. Assess urine tests for proteinuria or hematuria. Monitor WBC, hemoglobin, differential, platelet count, renal and hepatic function studies. Question for pruritus (may be first sign of impending rash). Assess skin daily for rash, purpura or ecchymoses. Assess oral mucous membranes, borders of tongue, palate, pharynx for ulceration, complaint of metallic taste sensation (sign of stomatitis). Evaluate for therapeutic response: relief of pain, stiffness, swelling, increase in joint mobility, reduced joint tenderness, improved grip strength.

Patient/Family Teaching

Therapeutic response may be expected in 3–6 mos. Avoid exposure to sunlight (gray to blue pigment may appear). Contact physician if pruritus, rash, sore mouth, indigestion, or metallic taste occurs. Maintain diligent oral hygiene.

aurothioglucose

ah-row-thigh-oh-**glue**-cose
(Solganal)

CANADIAN AVAILABILITY
Solganal

PREGNANCY CATEGORY C

CLASSIFICATION

Antirheumatic: Gold compound

AVAILABILITY (Rx)

Injection: 50 mg/ml suspension

PHARMACOKINETICS

Absorption: Slow, erratic absorption after IM administration. **Metabolism:** Metabolic fate unknown. **Excretion:** Primarily excreted in urine. **Half-life:** 3–27 days (increased w/increased number of doses).

ACTION/*THERAPEUTIC EFFECT*

Alters cellular mechanisms, enzyme systems, immune responses, collagen biosynthesis, *suppressing synovitis of the active stage of rheumatoid arthritis.*

USES

Management of rheumatoid arthritis in those w/insufficient therapeutic response to NSAIDs.

ADMINISTRATION

IM:

- Give in upper outer quadrant of gluteus.

INDICATIONS/ROUTES/DOSAGE

Rheumatoid arthritis:
Note: Give as weekly injections.

IM: Adults, elderly: Initially, 10 mg, then 25 mg for 2 doses, then 50 mg weekly thereafter until total dose of 0.8–1 g given. If pt improved and no signs of toxicity, give 50 mg at 3–4 wk intervals for many mos.

CONTRAINDICATIONS

History of gold-induced pathologies (necrotizing enterocolitis, exfoliative dermatitis, pulmonary fibrosis, blood dyscrasias), bone marrow aplasia, severe blood dyscrasias.

CAUTIONS

Renal/hepatic disease, inflammatory bowel disease.

INTERACTIONS

DRUG: ***Bone marrow depressants, hepatotoxic, nephrotoxic medications may*** increase toxicity. ***Penicillamine*** may increase risk of hematologic or renal adverse effects. **HERBAL:** None known. **FOOD:** None significant. **ALTERED LAB VALUES:** May decrease hemoglobin, hematocrit, platelets, WBCs. May alter liver function tests. May increase urine protein.

SIDE EFFECTS

OCCASIONAL: Rash, pruritus, gingivitis, reddened skin, glossitis (soreness of tongue), metallic taste, stomatitis (ulcers, sores, white spots in mouth/throat). **RARE:** Proteinuria (cloudy urine), joint pain (especially 1–2 days after injection), allergic reaction, abdominal cramping, diarrhea, conjunctivitis, anorexia.

ADVERSE REACTIONS/TOXIC EFFECTS

Signs of gold toxicity: decreased hemoglobin, leukopenia (WBC below 4,000/mm^3), reduced granulocyte counts (below 150,000/mm^3), proteinuria, hematuria, stomatitis, blood dyscrasias (anemia, leukopenia, thrombocytopenia, eosinophilia), glomerulonephritis, nephrotic syndrome, cholestatic jaundice.

PATIENT CONSIDERATIONS

Baseline Assessment

Rule out pregnancy before beginning treatment. CBC, urinalysis, platelet and differential, renal and liver function tests should be performed before therapy begins.

Intervention/Evaluation

Monitor skin for color, rash. Check mouth for sores, white spots, reddened gums. Assess urine tests for proteinuria or hematuria. Monitor WBC, hemoglobin, differential, platelet count, renal, and hepatic function studies. Question for pruritus (may be first sign of impending rash). Assess skin daily for rash, purpura, or ecchymoses. Assess oral mucous membranes, borders of tongue, palate, pharynx for ulceration, complaint of metallic taste sensation (signs of

stomatitis). Evaluate for therapeutic response: relief of pain, stiffness, swelling, increase in joint mobility, reduced joint tenderness, improved grip strength.

PATIENT/FAMILY TEACHING

Therapeutic response may take 6 mos or longer. Avoid exposure to sunlight (gray to blue pigment may appear). Contact physician/nurse if pruritus, rash, sore mouth, indigestion, or metallic taste occures. Maintain diligent oral hygiene. Increased joint pain may continue 1–2 days after injection.

---

azathioprine

asia-**thigh**-oh-preen
(Imuran Oral)

azathioprine sodium

(Imuran Parenteral)

CANADIAN AVAILABILITY
Imuran

PREGNANCY CATEGORY D

CLASSIFICATION

Immunosuppressant

AVAILABILITY (Rx)

Tablet: 50 mg. **Injection:** 100 mg vial.

PHARMACOKINETICS

Absorption: Well absorbed from GI tract. **Metabolism:** Converted to active metabolite. Further metabolized in liver and erythrocytes. **Excretion:** Eliminated via biliary system. Minimal removal by hemodialysis. **Half-life:** 5 hrs.

ACTION/*THERAPEUTIC EFFECT*

Antagonizes metabolism, inhibits RNA, DNA and protein synthesis, *suppressing cell-mediated hypersensitivities, alters antibody production, immune response in transplant recipients. Reduces arthritis severity.*

USES/*UNLABELED*

Adjunct in prevention of rejection in kidney transplantation; treatment of rheumatoid arthritis in those unresponsive to conventional therapy. *Treatment of inflammatory bowel disease, chronic active hepatitis, biliary cirrhosis, systemic lupus erythematosus, glomerulonephritis, nephrotic syndrome, inflammatory myopathy, myasthenia gravis, polymyositis, pemphigus, pemphigoid.*

STORAGE/HANDLING

Store oral, parenteral form at room temperature. After reconstitution, IV solution stable for 24 hrs.

ADMINISTRATION

ORAL:

- Give during or after meal to reduce potential for GI disturbances.

IV:

- Reconstitute 100 mg vial w/10 ml sterile water for injection to provide concentration of 10 mg/ml.
- Further dilute w/5% dextrose or 0.9% NaCl; infuse over 30–60 min.

INDICATIONS/ROUTES/DOSAGE

Note: May give in divided doses if GI disturbance occurs.

Kidney transplantation:
Oral/IV: Adults, elderly, children: Initially, 3–5 mg/kg/day as single

dose on day of transplant. *Maintenance:* 1–3 mg/kg/day.

Rheumatoid arthritis:
Oral/IV: Adults: Initially, 1 mg/kg/day as single or in 2 divided doses. May increase by 0.5 mg/kg/day after 6–8 wks at 4 wk intervals up to maximum dose of 2.5 mg/kg/day. *Maintenance:* Lowest effective dose. May decrease dose by 0.5 mg/kg or 25 mg/day q4wks (other therapy maintained). *Elderly:* Initially, 1 mg/kg/day (50–100 mg); may increase by 25 mg/day until response or toxicity.

CONTRAINDICATIONS

Pregnant rheumatoid arthritis pts.

CAUTIONS

Immunosuppressed pts, those previously treated for rheumatoid arthritis w/alkylating agents (cyclophosphamide, chlorambucil, melphalan), chicken pox (current or recent), herpes zoster, gout, decreased liver/renal function, infection.

INTERACTIONS

DRUG: *Allourinol* may increase activity, toxicity. *Bone marrow depressants* may increase bone marrow depression. *Other immunosuppressants* may increase risk of infection or development of neoplasms. *Live virus vaccines* may potentiate virus replication, increase vaccine side effects, decrease pt's antibody response to vaccine. **HERBAL:** Echinacea may decrease effect. **FOOD:** None significant. **ALTERED LAB VALUES:** May decrease hemoglobin, albumin, uric acid. May increase SGPT (ALT), SGOT (AST), alkaline phosphatase, amylase, bilirubin.

SIDE EFFECTS

FREQUENT: Nausea, vomiting, anorexia, particularly during early treatment and w/large doses, infection, megaloblastic anemia (unusually tired/weak). **OCCASIONAL:** Rash. **RARE:** Severe nausea, vomiting w/diarrhea, stomach pain, hypersensitivity reaction.

ADVERSE REACTIONS/TOXIC EFFECTS

There is an increased risk of neoplasia (new, abnormal growth tumors). Significant leukopenia, thrombocytopenia may occur, particularly in those undergoing kidney rejection. Hepatotoxicity occurs rarely.

PATIENT CONSIDERATIONS

Baseline Assessment

Arthritis
Assess onset, type, location and duration of pain, fever, or inflammation. Inspect appearance of affected joints for immobility, deformities, and skin condition.

Intervention/Evaluation

CBC, platelet count, liver function studies should be performed weekly during first mo of therapy, twice monthly during second and third mos of treatment, then monthly thereafter. If rapid fall in WBC occurs, dosage should be reduced or discontinued. Assess particularly for delayed bone marrow suppression. Report any major change in assessment of pt. Routinely watch for any change from normal.

Arthritis
Evaluate for therapeutic response: relief of pain, stiffness, swelling, increase in joint mobility, reduced

joint tenderness, improved grip strength.

PATIENT/FAMILY TEACHING

Contact physician if unusual bleeding or bruising, sore throat, mouth sores, abdominal pain, or fever occurs. Therapeutic response in rheumatoid arthritis may take up to 12 wks. Women of childbearing age must avoid pregnancy (assure pt has adequate information and resources to comply).

azelaic acid

aye-zeh-**lay**-ick acid
(Azelex)

PREGNANCY CATEGORY B

CLASSIFICATION

Antiacne, hypopigmentation agent

AVAILABILITY (Rx)

Cream: 20%

PHARMOKOKINETICS

Dietary component (whole grain cereals, animal products). **Absorption:** Following application, azelaic acid penetrates into stratum corneum and other viable skin layers; 4% absorbed systemically. **Excretion:** Unchanged in urine.

ACTION/*THERAPEUTIC EFFECT*

Possesses antimicrobial action by inhibiting cellular protein synthesis in aerobic and anaerobic microorganisms, *improving acne vulgaris, normalizing keritin process.* Interrupts hyperactivity of normal melanocytes and their resulting growth in melasma, *reducing macular hyperpigmentation of facial or nuchal (back of neck) hair.*

USES/*UNLABELED*

Treatment of mild to moderate acne vulgaris. *Treatment of melasma (hyperfunctioning melanocytes).*

ADMINISTRATION

TOPICAL:

- Apply thin coating to clean, dry skin, gently but thoroughly rubbing into affected area.
- Wash hands thoroughly following application.
- For external use only.
- Avoid occlusive dressings and wrappings.

INDICATIONS/ROUTES/DOSAGE

Antiacne, hypopigmentation:
Topical: Adults, adolescents: Apply topically to affected area 2 times/day (morning and evening).

CONTRAINDICATIONS

None significant.

CAUTIONS

None significant.

INTERACTIONS

DRUG: None significant. **HERBAL:** None known. **FOOD:** None significant. **ALTERED LAB VALUES:** None significant.

SIDE EFFECTS

OCCASIONAL (1–5%): Pruritus, stinging, burning, tingling. **RARE (<1%):** Erythema, dryness, rash, peeling, irritation, contact dermatitis, small depigmented spots, hypertrichosis, exacerbation of recurrent cold sores.

ADVERSE REACTIONS/TOXIC EFFECTS

None significant.

PATIENT CONSIDERATIONS

Intervention/Evaluation

Assess skin for erythema, dryness. Question pt regarding possible inflammatory reaction (burning, stinging, tingling of skin).

Patient/Family Teaching

Inform pt mild burning, stinging, tingling of skin, and itching may occur at beginning of each treatment, may last 5–20 min but lessens w/continued use. Contact physician if acne worsens, does not improve in first 4 wks or if medication produces excessive redness, dryness, or peeling of skin. Therapeutic improvement noted in about 4 wks. Avoid occlusive dressing. Keep away from mouth, eyes, other mucous membranes. Report abnormal changes in skin color, skin irritation if persists.

---

azelastine

aye-zeh-**las**-teen
(Astelin)

CANADIAN AVAILABILITY
Astelin

PREGNANCY CATEGORY C

CLASSIFICATION

Antihistamine

AVAILABILITY (Rx)

Nasal Spray: 125 mcg/actuation

PHARMACODYNAMICS

	ONSET	PEAK	DURATION
Nasal spray			
	—	2–3 hrs	12 hrs

PHARMACOKINETICS

Absorption: Well absorbed through nasal mucosa. **Excretion:** Excreted by feces. **Half-life:** 22 hrs.

ACTION/*THERAPEUTIC EFFECT*

Prevents activation of basophils, mast cells, eosinophils, macrophages, and monocytes. Blocks synthesis, release, or target receptors of several mediators of immediate inflammatory response (e.g., histamine), *relieving allergic rhinitis.*

USES/*UNLABELED*

Treatment of symptoms of seasonal allergic rhinitis (i.e., rhinorrhea, sneezing, nasal pruritus).

ADMINISTRATION

NASAL SPRAY:

- Clear nasal passages as much as possible before use.
- Tilt head slightly forward.
- Insert spray tip into 1 nostril, pointing toward nasal passage, away from nasal septum
- Spray into 1 nostril while holding the other nostril closed and concurrently inhale through nose to permit medication as high into nasal passages as possible.

INDICATIONS/ROUTES/DOSAGES

Seasonal allergic rhinitis:
Nasal: Adults, elderly, children >12 yrs: 1–2 sprays into each nostril 2 times/day.

CONTRAINDICATIONS

History of hypersensitivity to antihistamines, especially azelastine.

CAUTIONS

Nursing mothers, children <12 yrs of age.

INTERACTIONS

DRUG: *Cimetidine* may increase azelastine level, ***alcohol*** may increase CNS depressant effects. **HERBAL:** None known. **FOOD:** None significant. **ALTERED LAB VALUES:** May suppress wheal and flare reaction to antigen skin testing, unless drug is discontinued 4 days before testing. May increase SGPT.

SIDE EFFECTS

FREQUENT (10–20%): Headache, bitter taste, somnolence. **OCCASIONAL (2–5%):** Nasal burning, paroxysmal sneezing, dry mouth, nausea, fatigue, dizziness, increased weight.

ADVERSE REACTIONS/TOXIC EFFECTS

Epistaxis occurs rarely.

PATIENT CONSIDERATIONS

Baseline Assessment

Question for hypersensitivity to antihistamines, especially azelastine.

Intervention/Evaluation

Assess therapeutic response.

Patient/Family Teaching

Avoid tasks requiring alertness until response to drug is established. Avoid alcohol. Sugarless gum, sips of tepid water may relieve dry mouth. Coffee/tea may decrease drowsiness. Avoid spraying in eyes.

azithromycin

aye-**zith**-row-my-sin
(Zithromax)

CANADIAN AVAILABILITY
Zithromax

PREGNANCY CATEGORY B

CLASSIFICATION

Antibiotic: Macrolide

AVAILABILITY (Rx)

Tablet: 250 mg. **Injection:** 500 mg. **Oral Suspension:** 100 mg/5 ml, 200 mg/5 ml.

PHARMACOKINETICS

Absorption: Rapidly absorbed from GI tract. Widely distributed. **Excretion:** Eliminated primarily unchanged via biliary excretion. **Half-life:** 68 hrs.

ACTION/*THERAPEUTIC EFFECT*

Binds to ribosomal receptor sites of susceptible organisms, *inhibiting protein synthesis.*

USES/*UNLABELED*

Treatment of mild to moderate infections of upper respiratory tract (pharyngitis, tonsillitis), lower respiratory tract (acute bacterial exacerbations, COPD, pneumonia), uncomplicated skin/skin structure infections, and sexually transmitted diseases (nongonococcal urethritis, cervicitis due to *Chlamydia trachomatis*), gonorrhea, chancroid. Prevents disseminated mycobacterium avium complex (MAC). Treatment of mycoplasma pneumonia. Injection: community-acquired pneumonia, PID. *Acne.*

ADMINISTRATION

ORAL:

- May take tablets w/o regard to food.
- May store suspension at room temperature.

IV:

- Infuse over 60 min.

INDICATIONS/ROUTES/DOSAGE

Lower/upper respiratory tract, skin/skin structure infections:
Oral: Adults, elderly: Initially, 500 mg on first day, then 250 mg on days 2–5 (total dose 1.5 g).

Prevention of MAC:
Oral: Adults: 1,200 mg once/week.

Nongonococcal urethritis, cervicitis due to C. trachomatis:
Oral: Adult: 1 g as a single dose.

Usual parenteral dosage:
IV: Adults: 500 mg/day followed by oral therapy.

Usual pediatric dosage:
Oral: 10 mg/kg on day 1; then 5 mg/kg on days 2–5.

CONTRAINDICATIONS

Hypersensitivity to azithromycin, erythromycins, any macrolide antibiotic.

CAUTIONS

Hepatic/renal dysfunction.

INTERACTIONS

DRUG: May increase serum concentrations of ***carbamazepine, cyclosporine, theophylline, warfarin. Aluminum/magnesium-containing antacids*** may decrease concentration (give 1 hr before or 2 hrs after antacid). **HERBAL:** None known. **FOOD:** None significant. **ALTERED LAB VALUES:** May increase serum CPK, SGOT (AST), SGPT (ALT).

SIDE EFFECTS

OCCASIONAL: Nausea, vomiting, diarrhea, abdominal pain. **RARE:** Headache, dizziness, allergic reaction, acute interstitial nephritis.

ADVERSE REACTIONS/TOXIC EFFECTS

Superinfections, especially antibiotic-associated colitis (abdominal cramps, watery severe diarrhea, fever) may result from altered bacterial balance.

PATIENT CONSIDERATIONS

Baseline Assessment

Question pt for history of allergies to azithromycin, erythromycins, hepatitis. Obtain specimens for culture, sensitivity before giving first dose (therapy may begin before results are known).

Intervention/Evaluation

Check for GI discomfort, nausea, vomiting. Determine pattern of bowel activity and stool consistency. Assess skin for rash. Monitor hepatic function tests, assess for hepatotoxicity: malaise, fever, abdominal pain, GI disturbances. Evaluate for superinfection: genital/anal pruritus, sore mouth or tongue, moderate to severe diarrhea.

Patient/Family Teaching

Continue therapy for full length of treatment. Notify physician in event of GI upset, rash, diarrhea, or other new symptom.

aztreonam

az-**tree**-oh-nam
(Azactam)

PREGNANCY CATEGORY B

CLASSIFICATION

Antibiotic: Monobactam

AVAILABILITY (Rx)

Injection: 500 mg, 1 g, 2 g

PHARMACOKINETICS

Absorption: Completely absorbed following IM administration. **Metabolism:** Partially metabolized by hydrolysis. **Excretion:** Primarily excreted unchanged in urine. Removed by hemodialysis. **Half-life:** 1.4–2.2 hrs (increase in decreased renal, liver function).

ACTION/*THERAPEUTIC EFFECT*

Bactericidal effects due to inhibition of cell wall synthesis, *producing cell lysis, death.*

USES/*UNLABELED*

Lower respiratory tract, skin/skin structure, intra-abdominal, gynecologic, complicated/uncomplicated urinary tract infections; septicemia. *Treatment of bone/joint infections.*

STORAGE/HANDLING

Solution appears colorless to light yellow. Following reconstitution for IM injection or IV use, solution stable for 48 hrs at room temperature, or 7 days if refrigerated. Discard if precipitate forms. Discard unused portions.

ADMINISTRATION

Note: Give by deep IM injection, IV injection, intermittent IV infusion (piggyback).

IM:

- Shake immediately, vigorously after adding diluent.
- Inject deeply into large muscle mass.

IV:

- For IV injection, dilute each g w/6–10 ml sterile water, give over 3–5 min.
- For intermittent IV infusion, further dilute w/50–100 ml 5% dextrose or 0.9% NaCl, infuse over 20–60 min.
- Alternating IV sites, use large veins to reduce risk of phlebitis.

INDICATIONS/ROUTES/DOSAGE

Urinary tract infections:
IM/IV: Adults, elderly: 500 mg to 1 g q8–12h.

Moderate to severe systemic infections:
IM/IV: Adults, elderly: 1–2 g q8–12h.

Severe or life-threatening infections:
IV: Adults, elderly: 2 g q6–8h.

Usual pediatric dosage:
IV: 30 mg/kg q6–8h. *Maximum:* 120 mg/kg/day.

Dosage in renal impairment:
Dose and/or frequency is modified based on creatinine clearance, severity of infection:

CREATININE CLEARANCE	DOSAGE
10–30ml/min	1–2 g initially; then 1/2 usual dose at usual intervals
<10 ml/min	1–2 g initially; then 1/4 usual dose at usual intervals

CONTRAINDICATIONS

Hypersensitivity to aztreonam.

CAUTIONS

History of allergy, especially antibiotics, hepatic or renal impairment.

INTERACTIONS

DRUG: None significant. **HERBAL:** None known. **FOOD:** None significant. **ALTERED LAB VALUES:** Positive Coombs' test. May increase

SGOT (AST), SGPT (ALT), LDH, alkaline phosphatase, creatinine.

SIDE EFFECTS

OCCASIONAL (1–3%): Discomfort/swelling at IM injection site, nausea, vomiting, diarrhea, rash. RARE (<1%): Phlebitis/thrombophlebitis at IV injection site, abdominal cramps, headache, hypotension.

ADVERSE REACTIONS/TOXIC EFFECTS

Superinfection, antibiotic-associated colitis (abdominal cramps, watery severe diarrhea, fever) may result from altered bacterial balance. Severe hypersensitivity reactions including anaphylaxis occur rarely.

PATIENT CONSIDERATIONS

BASELINE ASSESSMENT

Question pt for history of allergies, especially to aztreonam, other antibiotics. Obtain culture and sensitivity tests prior to giving first dose (therapy may begin before results are known).

INTERVENTION/EVALUATION

Evaluate for phlebitis (heat, pain, red streaking over vein), pain at IM injection site. Assess for GI discomfort, nausea, vomiting. Monitor stool frequency and consistency. Assess skin for rash. Monitor vital signs. Assess mental status; be alert to tremors, possible seizures. Monitor I&O, renal function tests if indicated. Be alert to superinfection: increased temperature, changes in oral mucosa, sore throat, anal/genital pruritus.

PATIENT/FAMILY TEACHING

Continue therapy for full length of treatment. Doses should be evenly spaced. Notify physician in event of tremors, seizures, rash, diarrhea, other new symptom.

bacampicillin

(Spectrobid)
See Classification section under: Antibiotic: penicillins

bacitracin

bah-cih-**tray**-sin
(Baciguent, Bacitracin, Baci-IM)

FIXED-COMBINATION(S)
W/polymixin B, an antibiotic **(Polysporin)**; w/polymixin B and neomycin, antibiotics **(Mycitracin, Neosporin)**.

CANADIAN AVAILABILITY
Baciguent

PREGNANCY CATEGORY C

CLASSIFICATION

Anti-infective

AVAILABILITY (Rx)

Powder for Injection: 50,000 units. **Ophthalmic Ointment. (OTC) Topical Ointment.**

ACTION/*THERAPEUTIC EFFECT*

Interferes w/plasma membrane permeability in susceptible microorganisms, *inhibiting cell wall synthesis.* Bacteriostatic.

USES

Ophthalmic: Superficial ocular infections (conjunctivitis, keratitis, corneal ulcers, blepharitis). *Topical:* Minor skin abrasions, superficial infections. ***Irrigation:*** Treatment, prophylaxis of surgical procedures.

ADMINISTRATION

OPHTHALMIC:

- Place finger on lower eyelid and pull out until a pocket is formed between eye and lower lid. Place $1/4$–$1/2$ inch ointment in pocket.
- Close eye gently for 1–2 min, rolling eyeball (increases contact area of drug to eye). Remove excess ointment around eye w/tissue.

INDICATIONS/ROUTES/DOSAGE

Usual ophthalmic dosage:
Adults: 1/2 inch ribbon in conjunctival sac q3–4h.

Usual topical dosage:
Adults, children: Apply 1–5 times/day to affected area.

Irrigation:
Adults, elderly: 50,000–150,000 units, as needed.

CONTRAINDICATIONS

Hypersensitivity to bacitracin.

CAUTIONS

None significant.

INTERACTIONS

DRUG: None significant. **HERBAL:** None known. **FOOD:** None significant. **ALTERED LAB VALUES:** None significant.

SIDE EFFECTS

Note: It is important to know side effects of components when bacitracin is used in fixed-combination. **RARE:** *Topical:* Hypersensitivity reaction (itching, burning, inflammation), allergic contact dermatitis. *Ophthalmic:* Burning, itching, redness, swelling, pain.

ADVERSE REACTIONS/TOXIC EFFECTS

Severe hypersensitivity reaction (hypotension, apnea) occurs rarely.

PATIENT CONSIDERATIONS

Baseline Assessment

Question pt for history of allergies, particularly to bacitracin, neomycin.

Intervention/Evaluation

Topical
Evaluate for hypersensitivity: itching, burning, inflammation. W/preparations containing corticosteroids, consider masking effect on clinical signs.

Ophthalmic
Assess eye for therapeutic response or increased redness, swelling, burning, itching.

Patient/Family Teaching

Continue therapy for full length of treatment. Doses should be evenly spaced. Report burning, itching, rash, or increased irritation. Ophthalmic application may cause temporary blurred vision; check w/physician before using eye makeup.

baclofen

back-low-fin
(Lioresal)

CANADIAN AVAILABILITY
Apo-Baclofen, Liotec, Lioresal

PREGNANCY CATEGORY C

CLASSIFICATION

Skeletal muscle relaxant

AVAILABILITY (Rx)

Tablets: 10 mg, 20 mg

PHARMACOKINETICS

Absorption: Well absorbed from GI tract. **Metabolism:** Partially metabolized in liver. **Excretion:** Primarily excreted in urine. **Half-life:** 2.5–4 hrs.

ACTION/*THERAPEUTIC EFFECT*

Acts at spinal cord level *(decreases frequency/amplitude of muscle spasms in patients w/spinal cord lesions)*.

USES/*UNLABELED*

Relief of signs and symptoms of spasticity due to spinal cord injuries or diseases and multiple sclerosis, especially flexor spasms, concomitant pain, clonus, and muscular rigidity. *Treatment of trigeminal neuralgia.*

ADMINISTRATION

ORAL:

- Give w/o regard to meals.
- Tablets may be crushed.

INDICATIONS/ROUTES/DOSAGE

Musculoskeletal spasm:
Oral: Adults: Initially, 5 mg 3 times/day. May increase by 15 mg/day at 3 day intervals. ***Range:*** 40–80 mg/day. Total dose not to exceed 80 mg/day.

Usual elderly dosage:
Oral: Initially, 5 mg 2–3 times/day. May gradually increase dose.

CONTRAINDICATIONS

Skeletal muscle spasm due to rheumatic disorders, stroke, cerebral palsy, Parkinson's disease.

CAUTIONS

Impaired renal function, diabetes mellitus, epilepsy, preexisting psychiatric disorder.

INTERACTIONS

DRUG: Potentiated effects when used w/other ***CNS depressants***

(including alcohol). HERBAL: None known. **FOOD:** None significant. **ALTERED LAB VALUES:** May increase SGOT (AST), alkaline phosphatase, blood sugar.

SIDE EFFECTS

FREQUENT (>10%): Drowsiness, weakness, dizziness, lightheadedness, nausea, vomiting. **OCCASIONAL (1–10%):** Hypotension, headache, insomnia, constipation, urinary frequency, confusion, fatigue. **RARE (<1%):** Slurred speech, blurred vision, seizures.

ADVERSE REACTIONS/TOXIC EFFECTS

Abrupt withdrawal may produce hallucinations, seizures. Overdosage results in blurred vision, convulsions, myosis, mydriasis, severe muscle weakness, strabismus, respiratory depression, vomiting.

PATIENT CONSIDERATIONS

BASELINE ASSESSMENT

Record onset, type, location, and duration of muscular spasm. Check for immobility, stiffness, swelling.

INTERVENTION/EVALUATION

Assess for paradoxical reaction. Assist with ambulation at all times. For those on long-term therapy, liver/renal function tests, blood counts should be performed periodically. Evaluate for therapeutic response: decreased intensity of skeletal muscle pain. Be alert to signs of infection.

Intrathecal
After bolus in screening phase, observe pt closely for decreased muscle spasm (frequency or severity). After implant, monitor carefully for side effects w/resuscitative equipment immediately available. Check pump function and catheter patency.

PATIENT/FAMILY TEACHING

Drowsiness usually diminishes w/continued therapy. Avoid tasks that require alertness, motor skills until response to drug is established. Do not abruptly withdraw medication after long-term therapy. Avoid alcohol and CNS depressants. Notify physician of frequency or painful urination, constipation, headache, nausea, confusion, or insomnia.

---

balsalazide

(Colazal)
See Supplement

---

basiliximab

bay-zul-**ix**-ah-mab
(Simulect)

PREGNANCY CATEGORY B

CLASSIFICATION

Immunosuppressive

AVAILABILITY (Rx)

Powder for injection: 20 mg

PHARMACODYNAMICS

	ONSET	PEAK	DURATION
IV	—	—	36 days

PHARMACOKINETICS

Absorption: Absorbed into the circulation to lymphocytes. **Metabolism:** Peak serum levels must be maintained for therapeutic response to occur. **Half-life:** 7.2 days (children: 11.5 days).

ACTION/*THERAPEUTIC EFFECT*

Binds and blocks interleukin-2 receptor chains found on surface of activated T-lymphocytes, *inhibiting lymphocytic activity and thereby preventing cellular immune response involved in allograft rejection.*

STORAGE/HANDLING

Reconstituted solution is stable for 24 hrs if refrigerated or 4 hrs at room temperature.

USES

Adjunct with cyclosporine, corticosteroids in the prophylaxis of acute organ rejection in patients receiving renal transplant.

INDICATIONS/ROUTES/DOSAGES

Prophylaxis of organ rejection:
IV: Adults, elderly: Two doses of 20 mg each in reconstituted volume of 50 ml and given as IV infusion over 20–30 min. Give first 20 mg dose within 2 hrs before transplant surgery, the second 20 mg dose 4 days after transplant. ***Children:*** 12 mg/m^2 as above. ***Maximum:*** 20 mg dose.

CONTRAINDICATIONS

Hypersensitivity to basiliximab.

CAUTIONS

Those on immunosuppressive therapy, elderly.

INTERACTIONS

DRUG: None significant. **HERBAL:** None known. **FOOD:** None significant. **ALTERED LAB VALUES:** May increase or decrease potassium, increase glucose, uric acid, and cholesterol or decrease phosphates, calcium.

SIDE EFFECTS

FREQUENT (≥10%): GI disturbances, constipation, diarrhea, dyspepsia, CNS (headache, tremor, dizziness, insomnia), respiratory infection, dysuria, acne, leg/back pain, peripheral edema, hypertension. **OCCASIONAL (3–10%):** Angina, neuropathy, abdominal distension, tachycardia, rash, hypotension, urinary disturbances (hematuria, frequent micturation, genital edema), joint pain, increased hair growth, muscle pain.

ADVERSE REACTIONS/TOXIC EFFECTS

None significant.

PATIENT CONSIDERATIONS

BASELINE ASSESSMENT

Obtain baseline BUN, creatinine, potassium, uric acid, glucose, calcium, phosphatase blood serum levels and vital signs, particularly B/P, pulse rate.

INTERVENTION/EVALUATION

Diligently monitor all blood serum levels. Assess B/P for hypertension/hypotension; pulse for evidence of tachycardia. Question for GI disturbances, CNS effects, urinary changes.

PATIENT/FAMILY TEACHING

Headache, tremor may occur as a response to medication.

BCG, intravesical

(TheraCys, Tice BCG)

See Classification section under: Cancer chemotherapy

---

becaplermin

beh-**cap**-lure-min

(Regranex)

PREGNANCY CATEGORY C

CLASSIFICATION

Growth factor

AVAILABILITY (Rx)

Gel: 100 mcg

PHARMACOKINETICS

Absorption: Completely absorbed through skin to tissue involved with wound repair.

ACTION/*THERAPEUTIC EFFECT*

Platelet-derived growth factor that promotes recruitment and proliferation of cells involved in wound repair, *enhancing formation of granulation tissue, wound healing.*

USES

Treatment of lower extremity diabetic neuropathic ulcers that extend into subcutaneous tissue or beyond.

INDICATIONS/ROUTES/DOSAGES

Ulcers:

Topical: Adults, elderly: Apply once daily. Spread gel over entire ulcer and cover with saline-moistened dressing. After 12 hrs, remove dressing and rinse ulcer with saline or water and cover again with saline-moistened gauze dressing (without gel) for remainder of day. Continue to apply once daily until complete healing has taken place. If ulcer does not decrease in size by 30% after 10 wks or has not healed completely by 20 wks, reassess continued treatment.

CONTRAINDICATIONS

Neoplasms at site of application, hypersensitivity to product component (parabens).

CAUTIONS

None significant.

INTERACTIONS

DRUG: None significant. **HERBAL:** None known. **FOOD:** None significant. **ALTERED LAB VALUES:** None significant.

SIDE EFFECTS

RARE (2%): Erythrematous rash.

ADVERSE REACTIONS/TOXIC EFFECTS

None significant.

PATIENT CONSIDERATIONS

BASELINE ASSESSMENT

Measure the length by the width of the ulcer. Each square inch of ulcer surface requires approximately 2/3-inch length of gel to be applied.

INTERVENTIONS/EVALUATION

Assess ulcer site. If ulcer does not decrease in size by 30% after 10 wks or has not healed completely by 20 wks, reassess continued treatment.

PATIENT/FAMILY TEACHING

Wash hands thoroughly before applying medication. Do not allow tip of tube to touch ulcer. Spread gel evenly over ulcerated area to yield a thin layer about 1/16 inch thick.

beclomethasone dipropionate

beck-low-**meth**-ah-sewn

(Beclovent, Beconase, Vanceril, Vancenase)

CANADIAN AVAILABILITY

Beclodisk, Beclovent, Beconase,

Becloforte Inhaler, Vancenase, Vanceril

PREGNANCY CATEGORY C

CLASSIFICATION

Corticosteroid

AVAILABILITY (Rx)

Aerosol for oral, intranasal

PHARMACOKINETICS

Absorption: Rapidly absorbed from pulmonary, nasal, and GI tissue. **Metabolism:** Metabolized in liver, undergoes extensive first-pass effect. **Excretion:** Primarily eliminated in feces. **Half-life:** 15 hrs.

ACTION/*THERAPEUTIC EFFECT*

Inhalation: Decreases number, activity of inflammatory cells into bronchial wall, *inhibits bronchoconstriction, produces smooth muscle relaxation, decreases mucus secretion.* **Intranasal:** Inhibits early-phase allergic reaction, migration of inflammatory cells into nasal tissue, *decreasing response to seasonal and perennial rhinitis.*

USES/*UNLABELED*

Inhalation: Control of bronchial asthma in those requiring chronic steroid therapy. **Intranasal:** Relief of seasonal/perennial rhinitis; prevention of nasal polyps from recurring after surgical removal; treatment of nonallergic rhinitis. ***Nasal: Prophylaxis of seasonal rhinitis.***

ADMINISTRATION

INHALATION:

- Shake container well before use.
- Exhale slowly and as completely as possible through the mouth.
- Place mouthpiece fully into mouth, holding inhaler upright, and close lips fully around mouthpiece.
- Inhale deeply and slowly through mouth while depressing canister.
- Hold breath as long as possible before exhaling.
- Rinse mouth w/water (prevents mouth and throat dryness).

INTRANASAL:

- Blow nose to clear nasal passages as much as possible.
- Tilt head slightly forward for spray, backward for drops.
- Insert tip into 1 nostril, pointing toward inflamed nasal passages, away from nasal septum.
- Apply medication while holding other nostril closed and inspire through nose to permit medication as high into nasal passages as possible.

INDICATIONS/ROUTES/DOSAGE

Usual inhalation dosage:
Inhalation: Adults, elderly: 2 inhalations 3–4 times/day. ***Maximum:*** 20 inhalations/day. ***Children 6–12 yrs:*** 1–2 inhalations 3–4 times/day. ***Maximum:*** 10 inhalations/day. Vanceril DS: 2 inhalations 2 times/day. ***Maximum:*** 5 inhalations/day.

Usual intranasal dosage:
Intranasal: Adults, elderly, children >12 yrs: 1 inhalation each nostril 2–4 times/day. ***Children 6–12 yrs:*** 1 inhalation 3 times/day. Vancenase AQ Forte: 1 inhalation each nostril once daily.

CONTRAINDICATIONS

Hypersensitivity to any corticosteroid or components, primary treatment of status asthmaticus, systemic fungal infections, persistently positive sputum cultures for *Candi-*

da albicans. Untreated localized infections involving nasal mucosa.

CAUTIONS

Glaucoma, ocular herpes simplex, latent/active tuberculosis, recent nasal trauma or surgery.

INTERACTIONS

DRUG:None significant. HERBAL: None known. FOOD: None significant. ALTERED LAB VALUES: None significant.

SIDE EFFECTS

FREQUENT: *Inhalation (4–14%):* Pharyngitis, cough, nasal congestion, sinusitis, viral infections, dysmenorrhea. ***Intranasal:*** Burning, dryness inside nose. OCCASIONAL: *Inhalation (2–3%):* Flulike symptoms, fatigue, pruritus, eczema, sneezing, dyspepsia. ***Intranasal:*** Nasal crusting, nosebleed, sore throat, ulceration nasal mucosa.

ADVERSE REACTIONS/TOXIC EFFECTS

Acute hypersensitivity reaction (urticaria, angioedema, severe bronchospasm) occurs rarely. Transfer from systemic to local steroid therapy may unmask previously suppressed bronchial asthma condition.

PATIENT CONSIDERATIONS

BASELINE ASSESSMENT

Question for hypersensitivity to any corticosteroids, components.

INTERVENTION/EVALUATION

In those receiving bronchodilators by inhalation concomitantly with inhalation of steroid therapy, advise pt to use bronchodilator several min before corticosteroid aerosol (enhances penetration of steroid into bronchial tree).

PATIENT/FAMILY TEACHING

Do not change dose schedule or stop taking drug; must taper off gradually under medical supervision.

Inhalation
Maintain careful mouth hygiene. Rinse mouth w/water immediately after inhalation (prevents mouth/throat dryness, fungal infection of mouth). Contact physician/nurse if sore throat or mouth occurs.

Intranasal
Contact physician if no improvement in symptoms, sneezing or nasal irritation occur. Clear nasal passages prior to use. Improvement seen in several days.

benazepril

ben-**ayz**-ah-prill
(Lotensin)

FIXED-COMBINATION(S)
W/hydrochlorothiazide, a diuretic **(Lotensin-HCT)**; w/amlodipine, a calcium channel blocker **(Lotrel)**.

CANADIAN AVAILABILITY
Lotensin

PREGNANCY CATEGORY D

CLASSIFICATION

Angiotensin-converting enzyme (ACE) inhibitor; antihypertensive

AVAILABILITY (Rx)

Tablets: 5 mg, 10 mg, 20 mg, 40 mg

PHARMACODYNAMICS

	ONSET	PEAK	DURATION
Oral	1 hr	2–4 hrs	24 hrs

PHARMACOKINETICS

Absorption: Partially absorbed from GI tract. **Metabolism:** Metabolized in liver to active metabolite. **Excretion:** Primarily excreted in urine. Minimal removal by hemodialysis. **Half-life:** 35 min; metabolite: 10–11 hrs.

ACTION/*THERAPEUTIC EFFECT*

Decreases rate of conversion of angiotensin I to angiotensin II, a potent vasoconstrictor. Reduces peripheral arterial resistance, *lowers B/P.*

USES/*UNLABELED*

Treatment of hypertension. Used alone or in combination w/other antihypertensives. *Treatment of CHF.*

ADMINISTRATION

ORAL:

- May give w/o regard to food.

INDICATIONS/ROUTES/DOSAGE

Hypertension (used alone):
Oral: Adults: Initially, 10 mg/day. ***Maintenance:*** 20–40 mg/day as single dose. ***Maximum:*** 80 mg/day.

Usual elderly dosage:
Oral: Initially, 10 mg/day. ***Range:*** 20–40 mg/day.

Hypertension (combination therapy):
Note: Discontinue diuretic 2–3 days prior to initiating benazepril therapy.

Oral: Adults: Initially, 5 mg/day titrated to pt's needs.

Dosage in renal impairment (Ccr <30 ml/min):
Initially, 5 mg/day titrated up to maximum of 40 mg/day.

CONTRAINDICATIONS

History of angioedema w/previous treatment w/ACE inhibitors.

CAUTIONS

Renal/liver impairment, those w/sodium depletion or on diuretic therapy, dialysis, hypovolemia, coronary or cerebrovascular insufficiency, diabetes mellitus.

INTERACTIONS

DRUG: ***Alcohol, diuretics, hypotensive agents*** may increase effects. ***NSAIDs*** may decrease effect. ***Potassium-sparing diuretics, potassium supplements*** may cause hyperkalemia. May increase ***lithium*** concentration, toxicity. **HERBAL:** None known. **FOOD:** None significant. **ALTERED LAB VALUES:** May increase potassium, SGOT (AST), SGPT (ALT), alkaline phosphatase, bilirubin, BUN, creatinine. May decrease sodium. May cause positive ANA titer.

SIDE EFFECTS

FREQUENT (3–6%): Cough, headache. **OCCASIONAL (1–2%):** Dizziness, lightheadedness, skin rash, itching, fever, joint pain, diarrhea, loss of taste, fatigue, nausea. **RARE (<1%):** Chest pain, pancreatitis.

ADVERSE REACTIONS/TOXIC EFFECTS

Excessive hypotension ("first-dose syncope") may occur in those w/CHF, severe salt/volume depletion. Angioedema (swelling of face/lips), hyperkalemia occur rarely. Agranulocytosis, neutropenia may be noted in those w/impaired renal function or collagen vascular disease (systemic lupus erythematosus, scleroderma). Nephrotic syndrome may be noted in those w/history of renal disease.

PATIENT CONSIDERATIONS

BASELINE ASSESSMENT

Obtain B/P immediately before

each dose, in addition to regular monitoring (be alert to fluctuations). If excessive reduction in B/P occurs, place pt in supine position w/legs elevated. Perform renal function tests before therapy begins. In those w/renal impairment, autoimmune disease, or taking drugs that affect leukocytes or immune response, perform CBC and differential count before therapy begins and q2wks for 3 mos, then periodically thereafter.

INTERVENTION/EVALUATION

Monitor pattern of daily bowel activity and stool consistency. Assist w/ambulation if dizziness occurs. Monitor B/P, renal function, urinary protein, leukocyte count.

PATIENT/FAMILY TEACHING

To reduce hypotensive effect, rise slowly from lying to sitting position and permit legs to dangle from bed momentarily before standing. Cola, unsalted crackers, dry toast may relieve nausea. Full therapeutic effect may take 2–4 wks. Report any sign of infection (sore throat, fever). Skipping doses or voluntarily discontinuing drug may produce severe rebound hypertension.

benzocaine

(Americaine, Anbesol, Orajel, Cetacaine, Chloroseptic Lozenges, Dermoplast, Hurricane)

See Classification section under: Anesthetics: local

benzonatate

ben-**zow**-nah-tate

(Tessalon Perles)

PREGNANCY CATEGORY C

CLASSIFICATION

Antitussive

AVAILABILITY (Rx)

Capsules: 100 mg

PHARMACODYNAMICS

	ONSET	PEAK	DURATION
Oral	15–20 min	—	3–8 hrs

ACTION/*THERAPEUTIC EFFECT*

Anesthetizes stretch receptors in respiratory passages, lungs, pleura, *thereby reducing cough production.*

USES

Relief of nonproductive cough including acute cough of minor throat/bronchial irritation.

ADMINISTRATION

ORAL:

- Give w/o regard to meals.
- Swallow whole, do not chew/ dissolve in mouth (may produce temporary local anesthesia/choking).

INDICATIONS/ROUTES/DOSAGE

Antitussive:

Oral: Adults, elderly, children >10 yrs: 100 mg 3 times/day, up to 600 mg/day.

CONTRAINDICATIONS

None significant.

CAUTIONS

Productive cough.

INTERACTIONS

DRUG: *CNS depressants* may increase effect. **HERBAL:** None known. **FOOD:** None significant. **ALTERED LAB VALUES:** None significant.

SIDE EFFECTS

OCCASIONAL: Mild drowsiness, mild dizziness, constipation, GI upset, skin eruptions, nasal congestion.

ADVERSE REACTIONS/TOXIC EFFECTS

Paradoxical reaction (restlessness, insomnia, euphoria, nervousness, tremors) has been noted.

PATIENT CONSIDERATIONS

Baseline Assessment

Assess type, severity, frequency of cough, and production.

Intervention/Evaluation

Initiate deep breathing and coughing exercises, particularly in those with impaired pulmonary function. Monitor for paradoxical reaction. Increase fluid intake and environmental humidity to lower viscosity of lung secretions. Assess for clinical improvement and record onset of relief of cough.

Patient/Family Teaching

Avoid tasks that require alertness, motor skills until response to drug is established. Dry mouth, drowsiness, dizziness may be an expected response of drug. Coffee or tea may help reduce drowsiness.

benztropine mesylate

benz-**trow**-peen
(Cogentin)

CANADIAN AVAILABILITY
Apo-Benztropine, Cogentin

PREGNANCY CATEGORY C

CLASSIFICATION

Anticholinergic; antiparkinson

AVAILABILITY (Rx)

Tablets: 0.5 mg, 1 mg, 2 mg. **Injection:** 1 mg/ml.

PHARMACODYAMICS

	ONSET	PEAK	DURATION
Oral	1 hr	—	24 hrs
IM	15 min	—	24 hrs

PHARMACOKINETICS

Absorption: Well absorbed from GI tract.

ACTION/*THERAPEUTIC EFFECT*

Selectively blocks central cholinergic receptors, assists in balancing cholinergic/dopaminergic activity. *Reduces incidence, severity of akinesia, rigidity, and tremor.*

USES

Treatment of Parkinson's disease, drug-induced extrapyramidal reactions, except tardive dyskinesia.

INDICATIONS/ROUTES/DOSAGE

Idiopathic parkinsonism:
Oral/IM: Adults: Initially, 0.5–1 mg/day at bedtime up to 6 mg/day.

Postencephalitic parkinsonism:
Oral/IM: Adults: 2 mg/day as single or divided dose.

Drug-induced extrapyramidal symptoms:
Oral/IM: Adults: 1–4 mg 1–2 times/day.

Acute dystonic reactions:
IM/IV: Adults: 1–2 mg, then 1–2 mg orally 2 times/day to prevent recurrence.

Usual elderly dosage:
Oral: Initially, 0.5 mg 1–2 times/day, may increase by 0.5 mg every 5–6 days. ***Maximum:*** 6 mg/day.

CONTRAINDICATIONS

Angle closure glaucoma, GI obstruction, paralytic ileus, intestinal atony, severe ulcerative colitis, prostatic hypertrophy, myasthenia gravis, megacolon, children <3 yrs.

CAUTIONS

Treated open-angle glaucoma, heart disease, hypertension, pts w/tachycardia, arrhythmias, prostatic hypertrophy, liver/renal impairment, obstructive diseases of the GI or genitourinary tract, urinary retention.

INTERACTIONS

DRUG: *Alcohol, CNS depressants* may increase sedation. ***Amantadine, anticholinergics, MAO inhibitors*** may increase effects. ***Antacids, antidiarrheals*** may decrease absorption, effects. **HERBAL:** None known. **FOOD:** None significant. **ALTERED LAB VALUES:** None significant.

SIDE EFFECTS

Note: Elderly (>60 yrs) tend to develop mental confusion, disorientation, agitation, psychotic-like symptoms. **FREQUENT:** Drowsiness, dry mouth, blurred vision, constipation, decreased sweating/urination, GI upset, photosensitivity. **OCCASIONAL:** Headache, memory loss, muscle cramping, nervousness, peripheral paresthesia, orthostatic hypotension, abdominal cramping. **RARE:** Rash, confusion, eye pain.

ADVERSE REACTIONS/TOXIC EFFECTS

Overdosage may vary from severe anticholinergic effects (unsteadiness, severe drowsiness, severe dryness of mouth/nose/throat, tachycardia, shortness of breath, skin flushing). Also produces severe paradoxical reaction (hallucinations, tremor, seizures, toxic psychosis).

PATIENT CONSIDERATIONS

BASELINE ASSESSMENT

Assess mental status for confusion, disorientation, agitation, psychotic-like symptoms (medication frequently produces such side effects in those >60 yrs). Monitor rate, depth, rhythm, type of respiration; quality and rate of pulse. Assess lung sounds for rhonchi, wheezing, rales.

INTERVENTION/EVALUATION

Be alert to neurologic effects: headache, lethargy, mental confusion, agitation. Assess for clinical reversal of symptoms (improvement of tremor of head/hands at rest, mask-like facial expression, shuffling gait, muscular rigidity). Monitor intra-ocular pressure.

PATIENT/FAMILY TEACHING

Avoid tasks that require alertness, motor skills until response to drug is established. Dry mouth, drowsiness, dizziness may be an expected response of drug. Avoid alcoholic beverages during therapy. Sugarless gum, sips of tepid water may relieve dry mouth. Coffee or tea may help reduce drowsiness. Drowsiness tends to diminish or disappear w/continued therapy.

---

bepridil hydrochloride

beh-prih-dill

(Bepadin, Vascor)

PREGNANCY CATEGORY C

CLASSIFICATION

Calcium channel blocker; antianginal

AVAILABILITY (Rx)

Tablets: 200 mg, 300 mg, 400 mg

PHARMACOKINETICS

Absorption: Rapid, completely absorbed from GI tract. **Metabolism:** Undergoes first-pass metabolism in liver. Metabolized in liver to active metabolite. **Excretion:** Primarily excreted in urine. Not removed by hemodialysis. **Half-life:** <24 hrs.

ACTION/*THERAPEUTIC EFFECT*

Inhibits calcium ion entry across cell membranes of cardiac and vascular smooth muscle *(dilates coronary arteries, peripheral arteries/arterioles);* decreases heart rate, myocardial contractility, slows SA and AV conduction.

USES

Treatment of chronic stable angina (effort-associated angina) in those who have failed to respond or are intolerant to other antianginal drugs. May be used alone or concurrent w/beta blockers, nitrates.

ADMINISTRATION

ORAL:

- Do not crush or break film-coated tablets.
- May give w/o regard to food. May give w/meals and at bedtime (decreases nausea).

INDICATIONS/ROUTES/DOSAGE

Chronic stable angina:
Oral: Adults, elderly: Initially, 200 mg/day; after 10 days, dosage may be adjusted. ***Maintenance:*** 200–400 mg/day.

CONTRAINDICATIONS

Sick-sinus syndrome/second- or third-degree AV block (except in presence of pacemaker), severe hypotension (<90 mm Hg, systolic), history of serious ventricular arrhythmias, uncompensated cardiac insufficiency, congenital QT interval prolongation, use w/other drugs prolonging QT interval.

CAUTIONS

Impaired renal/hepatic function, CHF, extreme bradycardia, hypokalemia, acute myocardial infarction.

INTERACTIONS

DRUG: ***Beta blockers*** may have additive effect. May increase ***digoxin*** concentration. ***Procainamide, quinidine*** may increase risk of QT interval prolongation. ***Hypokalemia-producing agents*** may increase risk of arrhythmias. **HERBAL:** None known. **FOOD:** None significant. **ALTERED LAB VALUES:** QT interval may be increased.

SIDE EFFECTS

FREQUENT (>10%): Dizziness, lightheadedness, nervousness, headache, asthenia (loss of strength), nausea, diarrhea. **OCCASIONAL (2–10%):** Drowsiness, insomnia, tinnitus, tremors, constipation, abdominal discomfort, dry mouth, palpitations, shortness of breath, dyspnea, wheezing, anorexia.

ADVERSE REACTIONS/TOXIC EFFECTS

Can induce serious arrhythmias. CHF, second- and third-degree AV block occur rarely. Overdosage produces nausea, drowsiness, confusion, slurred speech, profound bradycardia.

PATIENT CONSIDERATIONS

Baseline Assessment

Record onset, type (sharp, dull, squeezing), radiation, location, intensity, and duration of anginal pain, and precipitating factors (exertion, emotional stress). Assess baseline renal/liver function tests. Assess pulse rate, EKG for arrhythmias before drug is administered.

Intervention/Evaluation

Assist w/ambulation if lightheadedness, dizziness, drowsiness occur. Question for asthenia, headache, ringing/roaring in ears. Monitor liver enzyme tests. Monitor daily bowel activity and stool consistency. Assess EKG for arrhythmias, lung sounds for rales, wheezing.

Patient/Family Teaching

Do not abruptly discontinue medication. Compliance w/therapy regimen is essential to control anginal pain. To avoid hypotensive effect, rise slowly from lying to sitting position, wait momentarily before standing. Avoid tasks that require alertness, motor skills until response to drug is established. Contact physician/nurse if irregular heartbeat, shortness of breath, pronounced dizziness, nausea, dyspepsia, ringing/roaring in ears, or constipation occurs.

beractant

burr-**act**-tant
(Survanta)

CANADIAN AVAILABILITY
Survanta

CLASSIFICATION

Lung surfactant

AVAILABILITY (Rx)

Suspension: 25 mg/ml vials

ACTION/*THERAPEUTIC EFFECT*

Lowers surface tension on alveolar surfaces during respiration, stabilizes alveoli vs. collapse that may occur at resting transpulmonary pressures. *Replenishes surfactant, restores surface activity to lungs.*

USES

Prevention/treatment (rescue) of respiratory distress syndrome (RDS—hyaline membrane disease) in premature infants. Oxygenation improves within min of administration.

STORAGE/HANDLING

Refrigerate vials. Warm by standing vial at room temperature for 20 min or warm in hand 8 min. If settling occurs, gently swirl vial (do not shake) to redisperse. After warming, may return to refrigerator within 8 hrs. Each vial should be injected w/a needle only one time; discard unused portions. Color is off-white to light brown.

ADMINISTRATION

INTRATRACHEAL:

- Instill through catheter inserted into infant's endotracheal tube. Do not instill into main stem bronchus.
- Monitor for bradycardia, decreased oxygen saturation during administration. Stop dosing procedure if these effects occur; begin appropriate measures before reinstituting therapy.

INDICATIONS/ROUTES/DOSAGE

Usual dosage:
Intratracheal: Infants: 100 mg of phospholipids/kg birth weight (4 ml/kg). Give within 15 min of birth if infant <1,250 g w/evidence of surfactant deficiency; give within 8 hrs when RDS confirmed by x-ray and requiring mechanical ventilation. May repeat no sooner than 6 hrs after preceding dose.

CONTRAINDICATIONS

None significant.

CAUTIONS

Those at risk for circulatory overload.

INTERACTIONS

DRUG: None significant. HERBAL: None known. FOOD: None significant. ALTERED LAB VALUES: None significant.

SIDE EFFECTS

FREQUENT: Transient bradycardia, oxygen desaturation; increased CO_2 tension. OCCASIONAL: Endotracheal tube reflux. RARE: Apnea, endotracheal tube blockage, hypo/hypertension, pallor, vasoconstriction.

ADVERSE REACTIONS/TOXIC EFFECTS

Nosocomial sepsis may occur (not associated w/increased mortality).

PATIENT CONSIDERATIONS

Baseline Assessment

Drug must be administered in highly supervised setting. Clinicians in care of neonate must be experienced w/intubation, ventilator management. Give emotional support to parents.

Intervention/Evaluation

Monitor infant w/arterial or transcutaneous measurement of systemic O_2 and CO_2. Assess lung sounds for rales and moist breath sounds.

betamethasone

bay-tah-**meth**-a-sone
(Celestone)

betamethasone benzoate

(Uticort)

betamethasone sodium phosphate

(Cel-U-Jec, Selestoject)

betamethasone dipropionate

(Alphatrex, Diprolene, Diprosone)

betamethasone valerate

(Valisone, Beta-Val, Betatrex, Luxiq Foam)

FIXED-COMBINATION(S)

Betamethasone sodium phosphate w/betamethasone acetate **(Celestone Soluspan)**. Betamethasone dipropionate w/clotrimazole, an antifungal **(Lotrisone)**.

CANADIAN AVAILABILITY

Beben, Betaderm, Betnesol, Celestone, Diprolene, Diprosone

PREGNANCY CATEGORY C

CLASSIFICATION

Corticosteroid

AVAILABILITY (Rx)

Tablets: 0.6 mg. **Syrup:** 0.6 mg/5 ml. **Injection, Cream:** 0.025%, 0.05%, 0.01%, 0.1%. **Lotion:** 0.025%, 0.05%, 0.1%. **Gel:** 0.025%. **Ointment:** 0.05%, 0.1%. **Aerosol:** 0.1%.

PHARMACOKINETICS

Absorption: Rapid, complete absorption after oral, IM administration. **Metabolism:** Metabolized in liver, kidneys, tissue. **Excretion:** Primarily excreted in urine. **Half-life:** 3–5 hrs.

ACTION / *THERAPEUTIC EFFECT*

Systemic: Inhibits accumulation of inflammatory cells at inflammation sites, inhibits synthesis of mediators of inflammation, *decreases tissue response to inflammatory process.* Topical: Forms complexes that enter cell nucleus stimulating formation of enzymes, *reducing inflammatory effect.*

USES

Substitution therapy in *deficiency states:* acute/chronic adrenal insufficiency, congenital adrenal hyperplasia, adrenal insufficiency secondary to pituitary insufficiency. *Nonendocrine disorders:* arthritis, rheumatic carditis, allergic, collagen, intestinal tract, liver, ocular, renal, and skin diseases, bronchial asthma, cerebral edema, malignancies. *Topical:* Relief of inflammatory and pruritic dermatoses. *Foam:* Relief of inflammation, itching associated w/dermatosis.

ADMINISTRATION

ORAL:

- Give w/milk or food (decreases GI upset).
- Single doses given prior to 9 AM; multiple doses at evenly spaced intervals.

TOPICAL:

- Gently cleanse area prior to application.
- Use occlusive dressings only as ordered.
- Apply sparingly and rub into area thoroughly.
- When using aerosol, spray area 3 sec from 15 cm distance; avoid inhalation.

IM:

- Celestone Soluspan should not be mixed w/diluent or anesthetics containing preservatives.

INDICATIONS / ROUTES / DOSAGE

Usual dosage:
Oral: Adults, elderly: 0.6–7.2 mg/day.

IM/IV: Adults, elderly: Up to 9 mg/day.

Usual topical dosage:
Adults, elderly: 2–4 times/day.
Foam: Apply twice daily.

CONTRAINDICATIONS

Hypersensitivity to any corticosteroid or sulfite, systemic fungal infection. Avoid live virus vaccine such as smallpox. *Topical:* marked circulation impairment.

CAUTIONS

Ocular herpes simplex, diabetes mellitus, esophagitis, gastritis, peptic ulcer, chicken pox, measles, myasthenia gravis, tuberculosis, AIDS/HIV, heart failure, hypertension. ***Topical:*** Cataracts, diabetes mellitus, glaucoma, tuberculosis, infection at treatment site.

INTERACTIONS

DRUG: ***Amphotericin*** may increase hypokalemia. May decrease effect of ***oral hypoglycemics, insulin, diuretics, potassium supplements.*** May increase ***digoxin*** toxicity (due to hypokalemia). ***Hepatic enzyme*** *inducers* may decrease effect. ***Live virus vaccines*** may potentiate virus replication, increase vaccine side effects, decrease pt's antibody response to vaccine. **HERBAL:** None known. **FOOD:** None significant. **ALTERED LAB VALUES:** May decrease calcium, potassium, thyroxine. May increase cholesterol, lipids, glucose, sodium, amylase.

SIDE EFFECTS

FREQUENT: *Systemic:* Increased appetite, abdominal distension, nervousness, insomnia, false sense of well-being. *Foam:* Burning, stinging, itching. **OCCASIONAL:** *Systemic:* Dizziness, facial flushing, diaphoresis, decreased/blurred vision, mood swings. *Topical:* Allergic contact dermatitis, purpura (blood-containing blisters, thinning of skin w/easy bruising), telangiectasis (raised dark red spots on skin). **RARE:** *Systemic:* General allergic reaction (rash, hives), pain/redness/swelling at injection site, hallucinations, mental depression.

ADVERSE REACTIONS/TOXIC EFFECTS

High dose or long-term therapy: acne, Cushing syndrome (moon face), muscle wasting (especially arms, legs), osteoporosis, bone fractures, cataracts, glaucoma, psychosis, diabetes mellitus, pancreatitis, peptic ulcer, amenorrhea, poor healing, hypercalcemia, hypokalemia. Abrupt withdrawal following long-term therapy: anorexia, nausea, fever, headache, joint pain, rebound inflammation, fatigue, weakness, lethargy, dizziness, orthostatic hypotension.

PATIENT CONSIDERATIONS

Baseline Assessment

Question for hypersensitivity to any of the corticosteroids, sulfite. Obtain baselines for height, weight, B/P, glucose, electrolytes. Check results of initial tests, e.g., TB skin test, x-rays, EKG.

Intervention/Evaluation

Monitor I&O, daily weight; assess for edema. Check lab results for blood coagulability and clinical evidence of thromboembolism. Evaluate food tolerance and bowel activity; report hyperacidity promptly. Check B/P, temperature, pulse, respiration at least 2 times/day. Be alert to infection: sore throat, fever, or vague symptoms. Monitor electrolytes. Watch for hypocalcemia (muscle twitching, cramps, positive Trousseau's or Chvostek's signs) or hypokalemia (weakness and muscle cramps, numbness/tingling especially lower extremities, nausea and vomiting, irritability, EKG changes). Assess emotional status, ability to sleep. Provide assistance w/ambulation.

Patient/Family Teaching

Take w/food or milk. Carry identification of drug and dose, physician's name and phone number. Do not change dose/schedule or stop taking drug; must taper off gradually under medical supervision. Notify physician of fever, sore throat, muscle aches, sudden weight gain/swelling. W/dietician give instructions for prescribed diet (usually sodium restricted w/high vitamin D, protein, and potassium). Maintain careful personal hygiene; avoid exposure to disease or trauma. Severe stress (serious infection, surgery, or trauma) may require increased dosage. Do not take aspirin or any other medication w/o consulting physician. Follow-up visits, lab tests are necessary; children must be assessed for growth retardation. Inform dentist or other physicians of betamethasone therapy now or within past 12 mos. Caution against overuse of joints injected for symptomatic relief.

Topical
Apply after shower or bath for best absorption. Do not cover unless physician orders; do not use tight diapers, plastic pants or coverings. Avoid contact w/eyes. Do not expose treated area to sunlight.

betaxolol

beh-**tax**-oh-lol
(Kerlone, Betopic)

CANADIAN AVAILABILITY
Betoptic

PREGNANCY CATEGORY C

CLASSIFICATION

Beta-adrenergic blocker; antihypertensive; antiglaucoma

AVAILABILITY (Rx)

Tablets: 10 mg, 20 mg. **Ophthalmic Solution:** 0.5%. **Ophthalmic Suspension:** 0.25%.

PHARMACODYNAMICS

	ONSET	PEAK	DURATION
Eye-drops	30 min	2 hrs	12 hrs

PHARMACOKINETICS

Absorption: Completely absorbed from GI tract. **Metabolism:** In liver. **Excretion:** Primarily excreted unchanged in urine. Not removed by hemodialysis. **Half-life:** 14–22 hrs (increase in decreased renal function).

ACTION / *THERAPEUTIC EFFECT*

Systemic: Predominantly blocks beta$_1$-adrenergic receptors in cardiac tissue by binding to receptor sites, *slowing sinus heart rate, decreasing cardiac output, decreasing B/P.* Large doses may block beta$_2$ receptors, *increasing airway resistance.* ***Ophthalmic:*** Reduces aqueous humor production, *decreasing intraocular pressure.*

USES / *UNLABELED*

Management of mild to moderate hypertension. Used alone or in combination w/diuretics, especially thiazide type. Reduces intraocular pressure in management of chronic open-angle glaucoma, ocular hypertension. *W/miotics decreases IOP in acute/chronic angle closure glaucoma, treatment of secondary glaucoma, malignant glaucoma, angle closure glaucoma during/after iridectomy.*

STORAGE/HANDLING

Store oral form, ophthalmic solution at room temperature.

ADMINISTRATION

ORAL:

- May be given w/o regard to meals.

OPHTHALMIC:

- Place finger on lower eyelid and pull out until pocket is formed between eye and lower lid. Hold dropper above pocket and place prescribed number of drops in pocket. Instruct pt to close eyes gently so medication will not be squeezed out of sac.
- Apply gentle finger pressure to

the lacrimal sac at inner canthus for 1 min following installation (lessens risk of systemic absorption).

INDICATIONS/ROUTES/DOSAGE

Hypertension:
Oral: Adults: Initially, 10 mg/day alone or added to diuretic therapy. Dose may be doubled if no response in 7–14 days. If used alone, consider addition of another antihypertensive.

Usual elderly dosage:
Oral: Initially, 5 mg/day.

Glaucoma:
Eyedrops: Adults, elderly: 1 drop 2 times/day.

Dosage in renal impairment (dialysis):
Initially 5 mg/day, increase by 5 mg/day q2wks. *Maximum:* 20 mg/day.

CONTRAINDICATIONS

Sinus bradycardia, overt cardiac failure, cardiogenic shock, heart block greater than first degree.

CAUTIONS

Impaired renal or hepatic function, peripheral vascular disease, hyperthyroidism, diabetes, inadequate cardiac function.

INTERACTIONS

DRUG: *Diuretics, other hypotensives* may increase hypotensive effect; *sympathomimetics, xanthines* may mutually inhibit effect; may mask symptoms of hypoglycemia, prolong hypoglycemic effect of *insulin, oral hypoglycemics; NSAIDs* may decrease antihypertensive effect; *cimetidine* may increase concentration. **HERBAL:** None known. **FOOD:** None significant. **ALTERED LAB VALUES:** May increase ANA titer, BUN, creatinine, potassium, uric acid, lipoproteins, triglycerides.

SIDE EFFECTS

Generally well tolerated, w/mild and transient side effects. **FREQUENT:** *Systemic:* Hypotension manifested as dizziness, nausea, diaphoresis, headache, fatigue, constipation/diarrhea; shortness of breath. *Ophthalmic:* Eye irritation, visual disturbances. **OCCASIONAL:** *Systemic:* Insomnia, flatulence, urinary frequency, impotence or decreased libido. *Ophthalmic:* Increased light sensitivity, watering of eye. **RARE:** *Systemic:* Rash, arrhythmias, arthralgia, myalgia, confusion, change in taste, increased urination. *Ophthalmic:* Dry eye, conjunctivitis, eye pain.

ADVERSE REACTIONS/TOXIC EFFECTS

Oral form may produce profound bradycardia, hypotension, bronchospasm. Abrupt withdrawal may result in sweating, palpitations, headache, tremulousness. May precipitate CHF, MI in those w/cardiac disease, thyroid storm in those w/thyrotoxicosis, peripheral ischemia in those w/existing peripheral vascular disease. Hypoglycemia may occur in previously controlled diabetics. Ophthalmic overdosage may produce bradycardia, hypotension, bronchospasm, acute cardiac failure.

PATIENT CONSIDERATIONS

BASELINE ASSESSMENT

Oral

Assess baseline renal/liver function tests. Assess B/P, apical pulse immediately before drug is administered (if pulse is 60/min or below, or systolic B/P is below 90 mm Hg, withhold medication, contact physician).

INTERVENTION/EVALUATION

Monitor B/P for hypotension, respiration for shortness of breath. Assess pulse for strength/weakness, irregular rate, bradycardia. Monitor EKG for cardiac arrhythmias. Monitor daily bowel activity and stool activity. Assist w/ambulation if dizziness occurs. Assess for evidence of CHF: dyspnea (particularly on exertion or lying down), night cough, peripheral edema, distended neck veins. Monitor I&O (increase in weight, decrease in urine output may indicate CHF). Assess for nausea, diaphoresis, headache, fatigue.

PATIENT/FAMILY TEACHING

Do not abruptly discontinue medication. Compliance w/therapy regimen is essential to control glaucoma, hypertension, angina, arrhythmias. To avoid hypotensive effect, rise slowly from lying to sitting position, wait momentarily before standing. Avoid tasks that require alertness, motor skills until response to drug is established. Report shortness of breath, excessive fatigue, prolonged dizziness, or headache. Do not use nasal decongestants, OTC cold preparations (stimulants) w/o physician approval. Monitor B/P, pulse before taking medication. Restrict salt, alcohol intake.

bethanechol chloride

be-**than**-eh-coal
(Duvoid, Urecholine)

CANADIAN AVAILABILITY
Duvoid, Myotonachol, Urecholine

PREGNANCY CATEGORY C

CLASSIFICATION

Cholinergic

AVAILABILITY (Rx)

Tablets: 5 mg, 10 mg, 25 mg, 50 mg. **Injection:** 5 mg/ml.

PHARMACODYNAMICS

	ONSET	PEAK	DURATION
Oral	>30 min	60–90 min	1 hr
SubQ	5–15 min	15–30 min	2 hrs

PHARMACOKINETICS

Large oral doses (300–400 mg) may give up to 6 hrs duration of action. **Absorption:** Poorly absorbed from GI tract.

ACTION/*THERAPEUTIC EFFECT*

Acts directly at cholinergic receptors of smooth muscle of urinary bladder and GI tract. Increases tone of detrusor muscle, *may initiate micturition, bladder emptying. Stimulates gastric, intestinal motility.*

USES/*UNLABELED*

Treatment of acute postop and postpartum nonobstructive urinary retention, neurogenic atony of bladder w/retention. *Treatment of postop gastric atony, congenital megacolon, gastroesophageal reflux.*

STORAGE/HANDLING

Store parenteral form at room temperature. Discard if particulate matter, discoloration occurs.

ADMINISTRATION

ORAL:

- Give on an empty stomach (minimizes risk of GI upset).

SUBQ:

Note: Violent cholinergic reaction if given IM or IV (circulatory collapse, severe hypotension, bloody diarrhea, shock, cardiac arrest). *Antidote:* 0.6–1.2 mg atropine sulfate.

Aspirate syringe before injecting (avoid intra-arterial administration).

INDICATIONS/ROUTES/DOSAGE

Postop/postpartum urinary retention, atony of bladder:
Oral: Adults, elderly: 10–50 mg 3–4 times/day. Minimum effective dose determined by initially giving 5–10 mg, and repeating same amount at 1 hr intervals until desired response achieved, or maximum of 50 mg reached.

SubQ: Adults, elderly: Initially, 2.5–5 mg. Minimum effective dose determined by giving 2.5 mg (0.5 ml), repeating same amount at 15–30 min intervals up to a maximum of 4 doses. Minimum dose repeated 3–4 times/day.

CONTRAINDICATIONS

Hyperthyroidism, peptic ulcer, latent or active bronchial asthma, mechanical GI and urinary obstruction or recent GI resection, acute inflammatory GI tract conditions, anastomosis, bladder wall instability, pronounced bradycardia, hypotension, hypertension, cardiac disease, coronary artery disease, vasomotor instability, epilepsy, Parkinsonism.

CAUTIONS

None significant.

INTERACTIONS

DRUG: *Cholinesterase inhibitors* may increase effects/toxicity. ***Procainamide, quinidine*** may decrease effect. **HERBAL:** None known. **FOOD:** None significant.

ALTERED LAB VALUES: May increase amylase, lipase, SGOT (AST).

SIDE EFFECTS

Note: Effects more noticeable w/SubQ. **OCCASIONAL:** Belching, change in vision, blurred vision, diarrhea, frequent urinary urgency. **RARE:** (SubQ): Shortness of breath, tight chest, bronchospasm.

ADVERSE REACTIONS/TOXIC EFFECTS

Overdosage produces CNS stimulation (insomnia, nervousness, orthostatic hypotension), cholinergic stimulation (headache, increased salivation/sweating, nausea, vomiting, flushed skin, stomach pain, seizures). Cholinergic overstimulation manifested as circulatory collapse, hypotension, bloody diarrhea, sudden cardiac arrest.

PATIENT CONSIDERATIONS

INTERVENTION/EVALUATION

Assess for cholinergic reaction: GI discomfort/cramping, feeling of facial warmth, excessive salivation and sweating, lacrimation, pallor, urinary urgency, blurred vision. Assess eyes for pupillary contraction. Question for complaints of difficulty chewing, swallowing, progressive muscle weakness (see Adverse Reactions/Toxic Effects).

PATIENT/FAMILY TEACHING

Report nausea, vomiting, diarrhea, sweating, increased salivary secretions, irregular heartbeat, muscle weakness, severe abdominal pain, or difficulty in breathing. Dizziness, fainting, lightheadedness may occur especially when getting up from sitting/lying position.

bexarotene

(Targretin)
See Supplement

bicalutamide

by-**kale**-yew-tah-myd
(Casodex)

CANADIAN AVAILABILITY
Casodex

PREGNANCY CATEGORY X

CLASSIFICATION

Antineoplastic: hormone

PHARMACOKINETICS

Absorption: Well absorbed from GI tract. **Metabolism:** Metabolized in liver to inactive metabolite. **Excretion:** Excreted in urine and feces. **Half-life:** 5.8 days.

ACTION/*THERAPEUTIC EFFECT*

Competitively inhibits androgen action by binding to androgen receptors in target tissue. *Decreases growth of prostatic carcinoma.*

USES

Treatment of advanced metastatic prostatic carcinoma (in combination w/LHRH agonistic analogues—i.e., leuprolide). Treatment w/both drugs must be started at same time.

ADMINISTRATION

ORAL:

- May be given with or without food.
- Take at same time each day.

INDICATONS/ROUTES/DOSAGE

Prostatic carcinoma:
Oral: Adults, elderly: 50 mg once daily (morning or evening).

CONTRAINDICATIONS

None significant.

CAUTIONS

Mild-moderate liver impairment.

INTERACTIONS

DRUG: May displace ***warfarin*** from protein-binding sites, increase warfarin effect. **HERBAL:** None known. **FOOD:** None significant. **ALTERED LAB VALUES:** May increase SGOT (AST), SGPT (ALT), alkaline phosphatase, serum creatinine, bilirubin, BUN. May increase WBC, hemoglobin.

SIDE EFFECTS

FREQUENT: Hot flashes (49%), breast pain (38%), muscle pain (27%), constipation (17%), diarrhea (10%), asthenia (15%), nausea (11%). **OCCASIONAL (1–10%):** Nocturia, abdominal pain, peripheral edema. **RARE (<1%):** Vomiting, weight loss, dizziness, insomnia, rash, impotence, iron deficiency anemia, gynecomastia.

ADVERSE REACTIONS/TOXIC EFFECTS

Sepsis, CHF, hypertension may be noted.

PATIENT CONSIDERATIONS

BASELINE ASSESSMENT

Question for possibility of pregnancy (Pregnancy Category X).

INTERVENTION/EVALUATION

Monitor B/P periodically and hepatic function tests in long-term therapy. Check for diarrhea, nausea, and vomiting.

PATIENT/FAMILY TEACHING

Do not stop taking medication (both drugs must be continued). Take medications at same time each day. Explain possible expectancy of frequent side effects. Contact physician if vomiting continues at home.

bisacodyl

bise-ah-**co**-dahl
(Dacody, Dulcolax)

CANADIAN AVAILABILITY
Apo-Bisacodyl, Dulcolax

PREGNANCY CATEGORY C

CLASSIFICATION

Laxative: Stimulant

AVAILABILITY (OTC)

Tablets (enteric coated): 5 mg. **Suppository:** 10 mg.

PHARMACODYNAMICS

	ONSET	PEAK	DURATION
Oral	6–12 hrs	—	—
Rectal	15–60 min	—	—

PHARMACOKINETICS

Absorption: Minimal absorption following oral, rectal administration. **Excretion:** Absorbed drug excreted in urine; remainder eliminated in feces.

ACTION/*THERAPEUTIC EFFECT*

Increases peristalsis by direct effect on colonic smooth musculature (stimulates intramural nerve plexi). *Promotes fluid and ion accumulation in colon to increase laxative effect.*

USES

Facilitates defecation in those w/diminished colonic motor response; for evacuation of colon for rectal, bowel examination, elective colon surgery.

ADMINISTRATION

ORAL:

- Give on empty stomach (faster action).
- Offer 6–8 glasses of water/day (aids stool softening).
- Administer tablets whole; do not chew or crush.
- Avoid giving within 1 hr of antacids, milk, other oral medication.

RECTAL:

- If suppository is too soft, chill for 30 min in refrigerator or run cold water over foil wrapper.
- Moisten suppository w/cold water before inserting well up into rectum.

INDICATIONS/ROUTES/DOSAGE

Laxative:
Oral: Adults: 10–15 mg as needed. *Children >6 yrs:* 5–10 mg (0.3 mg/kg) at bedtime or after breakfast.

Rectal: Adults, children >2 yrs: 10 mg to induce bowel movement. *Children <2 yrs:* 5 mg.

Usual elderly dosage:
Oral: Initially 5 mg/day.

Rectal: 5–10 mg/day.

CONTRAINDICATIONS

Abdominal pain, nausea, vomiting, appendicitis, intestinal obstruction, undiagnosed rectal bleeding.

CAUTIONS

None significant.

INTERACTIONS

DRUG: *Antacids, cimetidine, ranitidine, famotidine;* milk may cause rapid dissolution of bisacodyl (produces abdominal cramping, vomiting). May decrease transit time of concurrently administered oral medication, decreasing absorption. **HERBAL:** None known. **FOOD:** None significant. **ALTERED LAB VALUES:** None significant.

SIDE EFFECTS

FREQUENT: Some degree of abdominal discomfort, nausea, mild cramps, griping, faintness. OCCASIONAL: Rectal administration may produce burning of rectal mucosa, mild proctitis.

ADVERSE REACTIONS/TOXIC EFFECTS

Long-term use may result in laxative dependence, chronic constipation, loss of normal bowel function. Chronic use or overdosage may result in electrolyte disturbances (hypokalemia, hypocalcemia, metabolic acidosis, or alkalosis), persistent diarrhea, malabsorption, weight loss. Electrolyte disturbance may produce vomiting, muscle weakness.

PATIENT CONSIDERATIONS

Intervention/Evaluation

Encourage adequate fluid intake. Assess bowel sounds for peristalsis. Monitor daily bowel activity and stool consistency (watery, loose, soft, semisolid, solid) and record time of evacuation. Assess for abdominal disturbances. Monitor serum electrolytes in those exposed to prolonged, frequent, or excessive use of medication.

Patient/Family Teaching

Cola, unsalted crackers, dry toast may relieve nausea. Institute measures to promote defecation: Increase fluid intake, exercise, high-fiber diet. Do not take antacids, milk, or other medication within 1 hr of taking medication (decreased effectiveness). Report unrelieved constipation, rectal bleeding, muscle pain or cramps, dizziness, weakness.

bismuth subsalicylate

bis-muth sub-sal-**ih**-sah-late
(Pepto-Bismol)

FIXED-COMBINATION(S)
W/ranitidine, an H-2 antagonist **(Tritec)**; kit w/metronidazole and tetracycline, anti-infectives **(Helidac)**

CANADIAN AVAILABILITY
Bismed, PeptoBismol

PREGNANCY CATEGORY C
(Pregnancy Category D during third trimester)

CLASSIFICATION

Antidiarrheal, antinauseant

AVAILABILITY (OTC)

Tablets: 262 mg. **Suspension:** 262 mg/5 ml, 525 mg/5 ml.

PHARMACOKINETICS

Absorption: Hydrolyzed in stomach; nondissociated bismuth subsalicylate reacts to form insoluble bismuth salt; salicylate component rapidly, extensively absorbed from small intestine; bismuth poorly absorbed. **Excretion:** Salicylate primarily excreted in urine; bismuth eliminated in feces.

ACTION/*THERAPEUTIC EFFECT*

Inhibits synthesis of prostaglandins responsible for intestinal inflammation and hypermotility. Binds toxins produced by *Escherichia coli*. Absorbs fluid and electrolytes across intestinal wall, *preventing diarrhea.*

USES/*UNLABELED*

Control of diarrhea. Treatment of indigestion, nausea; relieves gas pain/abdominal cramps, *Helicobac-*

ter pylori-associated duodenal ulcer, gastritis. *Prevents traveler's diarrhea.*

ADMINISTRATION

ORAL:

- Shake suspension before administering.
- Tablets may be chewed or dissolved in mouth.

INDICATIONS/ROUTES/DOSAGE

Diarrhea, gastric distress:
Oral: Adults, elderly: 2 tablets (30 ml) q30–60 min up to 8 doses/24 hrs. ***Children 9–12 yrs:*** 1 tablet or 15 ml q30–60 min up to 8 doses/24 hrs. ***Children 6–9 yrs:*** ⅔ tablet or 10 ml q30–60 min up to 8 doses/24 hrs. ***Children 3–6 yrs:*** ⅓ tablet or 5 ml q30–60 min up to 8 doses/24 hrs.

***H. pylori*-associated duodenal ulcer, gastritis:**
Oral: Adults, elderly: 525 mg 3 times/day 1 hr before meals (w/500 mg amoxicillin and 500 mg metronidazole 3 times/day after meals) for 7–14 days.

CONTRAINDICATIONS

Bleeding ulcers, hemorrhagic states, gout, hemophilia, renal function impairment.

CAUTIONS

Elderly, diabetic pts.

INTERACTIONS

DRUG: ***Anticoagulants, heparin, thrombolytics*** may increase risk of bleeding. Large dose may increase ***oral hypoglycemic, insulin*** effects. Other ***salicylates*** may increase toxicity. May decrease absorption of ***tetracyclines***. **HERBAL:** None known. **FOOD:** None significant. **ALTERED LAB VALUES:** May alter SGPT (ALT), SGOT (AST), alkaline phosphatase, uric acid. May decrease potassium. May prolong prothrombin time.

SIDE EFFECTS

FREQUENT: Darkening of tongue, grayish black stools. **RARE:** Constipation.

ADVERSE REACTIONS/TOXIC EFFECTS

Debilitated pts and infants may develop impaction.

PATIENT CONSIDERATIONS

INTERVENTION/EVALUATION

Encourage adequate fluid intake. Assess bowel sounds for peristaltic activity. Monitor stool frequency and consistency (watery, loose, soft, semisolid, solid).

PATIENT/FAMILY TEACHING

Stool may appear gray/black. If high fever accompanies diarrhea or if diarrhea continues longer than 2 days, contact physician. Dry crackers, cola may help relieve nausea. Chew tablets thoroughly before swallowing

---

bisoprolol fumarate

bye-**sew**-prow-lol
(Zebeta)

FIXED-COMBINATION(S)
W/hydrochlorothiazide, a diuretic **(Ziac)**

PREGNANCY CATEGORY C

CLASSIFICATION

Beta-adrenergic blocker; antihypertensive

AVAILABILITY (Rx)

Tablets: 5 mg, 10 mg

PHARMACOKINETICS

Absorption: Well absorbed from GI tract. **Metabolism:** Metabolized in liver. **Excretion:** Primarily excreted in urine. **Half-life:** 9–12 hrs (increased in decreased renal function).

ACTION/*THERAPEUTIC EFFECT*

Predominantly blocks $beta_1$- adrenergic receptors in cardiac tissue by binding to receptor sites, *slowing sinus heart rate, decreasing cardiac output, decreasing B/P.* Large doses may block $beta_2$ receptors, *increasing airway resistance.*

USES

Management of hypertension, alone or in combination w/diuretics, other medications.

ADMINISTRATION

ORAL:

- May give w/o regard to food.
- Scored tablet may be crushed.

INDICATIONS/ROUTES/DOSAGE

Hypertension:

Oral: Adults, elderly: Initially, 2.5–5 mg/day as single dose either alone or in combination w/diuretic. May increase gradually up to 20 mg/day.

Oral: Renal impairment (<40 ml/min), hepatic impairment (cirrhosis, hepatitis): Initially, 2.5 mg.

CONTRAINDICATIONS

Overt cardiac failure, cardiogenic shock, heart block greater than first degree.

CAUTIONS

Impaired renal or hepatic function, peripheral vascular disease, hyperthyroidism, diabetes, inadequate cardiac function, bronchospastic disease.

INTERACTIONS

DRUG: *Diuretics, other hypotensives* may increase hypotensive effect; ***sympathomimetics, xanthines*** may mutually inhibit effects; may mask symptoms of hypoglycemia, prolong hypoglycemic effect of ***insulin, oral hypoglycemics; NSAIDs*** may decrease antihypertensive effect; ***cimetidine*** may increase concentration. **HERBAL:** None known. **FOOD:** None significant. **ALTERED LAB VALUES:** May increase ANA titer, BUN, creatinine, potassium, uric acid, lipoproteins, triglycerides.

SIDE EFFECTS

Generally well tolerated, w/mild and transient side effects. **FREQUENT:** Hypotension manifested as dizziness, nausea, diaphoresis, headache, cold extremities, fatigue, constipation/diarrhea. **OCCASIONAL:** Insomnia, flatulence, urinary frequency, impotence or decreased libido. **RARE:** Rash, arthralgia, myalgia, confusion (especially elderly), change in taste.

ADVERSE REACTIONS/TOXIC EFFECTS

Overdosage may produce profound bradycardia, hypotension. Abrupt withdrawal may result in sweating, palpitations, headache, tremulousness. May precipitate CHF, MI in those w/cardiac disease, thyroid storm in those w/thyrotoxicosis, peripheral ischemia in those w/existing peripheral vascular disease. Hypoglycemia may occur in previously controlled diabetics. Thrombocytopenia (unusual bruising, bleeding) occurs rarely.

PATIENT CONSIDERATIONS

BASELINE ASSESSMENT

Assess baseline renal/liver func-

tion tests. Assess B/P, apical pulse immediately before drug is administered (if pulse is 60/min or below, or systolic B/P is below 90 mm Hg, withhold medications, contact physician).

INTERVENTION/EVALUATION

Assess pulse for strength/weakness, irregular rate, bradycardia. Monitor EKG for cardiac changes. Assist w/ambulation if dizziness occurs. Assess for peripheral edema of hands, feet (usually, first area of lower extremity swelling is behind medial malleolus in ambulatory, sacral area in bedridden). Monitor stool frequency and consistency. Assess skin for development of rash. Monitor any unusual changes in pt.

PATIENT/FAMILY TEACHING

Do not abruptly discontinue medication. Compliance w/therapy regimen is essential to control hypertension. If dizziness occurs, sit or lie down immediately. Avoid tasks that require alertness, motor skills until response to drug is established. Teach pts how to take pulse properly before each dose and to report excessively slow pulse rate (<60 beats/min), peripheral numbness, di.zziness. Do not use nasal decongestants, OTC cold preparations (stimulants) w/o physician approval. Restrict salt, alcohol intake.

bitolterol mesylate

by-**toll**-ter-all
(Tornalate)

PREGNANCY CATEGORY C

CLASSIFICATION

Bronchodilator

AVAILABILITY (Rx)

Aerosol

PHARMACODYNAMICS

	ONSET	PEAK	DURATION
Inhalation			
	3–4 min	0.5–2 hrs	5–8 hrs 2.5–5 hrs (cortico-steroid - dependent)

PHARMACOKINETICS

Metabolism: Hydrolyzed in tissue/blood to active compound. **Excretion:** Excreted in urine, eliminated in feces. **Half-life:** 3 hrs.

ACTION/*THERAPEUTIC EFFECT*

Stimulates beta$_2$-adrenergic receptors in lungs, *relaxing bronchial smooth muscle. Relieves bronchospasm, reduces airway resistance.*

USES

Prophylaxis, symptomatic treatment of bronchial asthma, acute bronchitis, reversible obstructive airway disease.

ADMINISTRATION

INHALATION:

- Shake container well, exhale completely, then holding mouthpiece 1 inch away from lips, inhale and hold breath as long as possible before exhaling.
- Wait 1–10 min before inhaling second dose (allows for deeper bronchial penetration).
- Rinse mouth w/water immediately after inhalation (prevents mouth/throat dryness).

INDICATIONS/ROUTES/DOSAGE

Symptomatic relief:
Inhalation: Adults, elderly, children >12 yrs: 2 inhalations, sepa-

rated by 1–3 min interval. Third inhalation may be needed.

Prophylaxis:
Inhalation: Adults, elderly, children >12 yrs: 2 inhalations q8h. Do not exceed 3 inhalations q6h, or 2 inhalations q4h.

CONTRAINDICATIONS

History of hypersensitivity to sympathomimetics.

CAUTIONS

Hypertension, cardiovascular disorders, hyperthyroidism, seizure disorders, diabetes mellitus.

INTERACTIONS

DRUG: May decrease effects of ***beta blockers***. May increase risk of arrhythmias w/***digoxin***. **HERBAL:** None known. **FOOD:** None significant. **ALTERED LAB VALUES:** May decrease potassium.

SIDE EFFECTS

FREQUENT (>9%): Trembling. **OCCASIONAL (1–9%):** Coughing, bronchial irritation, dizziness, dry or irritated mouth/throat, flushed face, headache, increased B/P, nausea, nervousness, vomiting, pounding heartbeat, altered taste. **RARE (<1%):** Chest discomfort, irregular/fast heartbeat, paradoxical bronchospasm, insomnia.

ADVERSE REACTIONS/TOXIC EFFECTS

Although tolerance to the bronchodilating effect has not been observed, prolonged or too frequent use may lead to tolerance. Severe paradoxical bronchoconstriction may occur w/excessive use.

PATIENT CONSIDERATIONS

Baseline Assessment

Offer emotional support (high incidence of anxiety due to difficulty in breathing and sympathomimetic response to drug).

Intervention/Evaluation

Monitor rate, depth, rhythm, type of respiration; quality and rate of pulse. Assess lung sounds for wheezing. Monitor arterial blood gases. Observe lips, fingernails for blue or dusky color in light-skinned patients; gray in dark-skinned patients. Observe for clavicular retractions, hand tremor. Evaluate for clinical improvement (quieter, slower respirations, relaxed facial expression, cessation of clavicular retractions).

Patient/Family Teaching

Increase fluid intake (decreases lung secretion viscosity). Instruct pt on proper administration technique. Do not exceed recommended dosage (excessive use may produce paradoxical bronchoconstriction or a decreased bronchodilating effect). Rinsing mouth with water immediately after inhalation may prevent mouth/throat dryness. Avoid excessive use of caffeine derivatives (chocolate, coffee, tea, cola, cocoa). Do not take OTC medications w/o consulting physician. Avoid smoking, smoke-filled environment. Notify physician of dizziness, palpitations/chest pain, or lack of therapeutic response.

---

bivalrudin

(Angiomax)
See Supplement

---

bleomycin sulfate

(Blenoxane)
See Classification section under: Cancer chemotherapy

bretylium tosylate

bre-**till**-ee-um
(Bretylol)

CANADIAN AVAILABILITY
Bretylate

PREGNANCY CATEGORY C

CLASSIFICATION

Antiarrhythmic

AVAILABILITY (Rx)

Injection: 50 mg/ml, 100 mg/ml

PHARMACODYNAMICS

	ONSET	PEAK	DURATION
IM	20–60 min	6–9 hrs	6–24 hrs
IV	5–10 min	6–9 hrs	6–24 hrs

PHARMACOKINETICS

Absorption: Well absorbed after IM administration. **Excretion:** Primarily excreted in urine. Removed by hemodialysis. **Half-life:** 4–17 hrs (increased in decreased renal function).

ACTION/*THERAPEUTIC EFFECT*

Directly affects myocardial cell membrane. Initially, releases norepinephrine, then inhibits its release, *contributing to suppression of ventricular tachycardia.*

USES

Prophylaxis and treatment of ventricular fibrillation in those w/life-threatening ventricular tachyarrhythmias who have not responded to conventional antiarrhythmic therapy.

STORAGE/HANDLING

Solution should appear clear after reconstitution. Discard if precipitate forms. Slight discoloration does not indicate loss of potency.

ADMINISTRATION

IM:

- Do not dilute.
- Do not give more than 5 ml into one site (over 3 ml may cause pain at injection site).
- Rotate injection sites (same-site injection may cause muscular atrophy and necrosis).

IV:

- For injection, give undiluted over 1 min.
- For intermittent IV infusion (piggyback), dilute w/at least 50 ml 5% dextrose or 0.9% NaCl to provide concentration of 10 mg/ml.
- Infuse over at least 8 min (too rapid IV produces nausea, vomiting).

INDICATIONS/ROUTES/DOSAGE

Ventricular arrhythmias, immediate, life threatening:
IV: Adults, elderly: 5 mg/kg undiluted by rapid IV injection. May increase to 10 mg/kg, repeat as needed. ***Maintenance:*** 5–10 mg/kg diluted over >8 min, q6h or IV infusion at 1–2 mg/min. ***Children:*** 5 mg/kg, then 10 mg/kg at 15–30 min interval. ***Maximum:*** 30 mg/kg total dose. ***Maintenance:*** 5–10 mg/kg q6h.

Ventricular arrhythmias, other:
IM: Adults, elderly: 5–10 mg/kg undiluted, may repeat at 1–2 hr intervals. ***Maintenance:*** 5–10 mg/kg q6–8h.

IV: Adults, elderly: 5–10 mg/kg diluted over >8 min, may repeat at 1–2 hr intervals. ***Maintenance:*** 5–10 mg/kg q6h or IV infusion at 1–2 mg/min. ***Children:*** 5–10 mg/kg/dose diluted q6h.

CONTRAINDICATIONS

None significant.

EXTREME CAUTION

Digitalis-induced arrhythmias, fixed cardiac output (severe pulmonary hypertension, aortic stenosis).

CAUTIONS

Impaired renal function, sinus bradycardia. Risk of orthostatic hypotension in the elderly.

INTERACTIONS

DRUG: May increase ***digoxin*** toxicity (due to initial norepinephrine release). ***Procainamide, quinidine*** may decrease inotropic effect, increase hypotension. **HERBAL:** None known. **FOOD:** None significant. **ALTERED LAB VALUES:** None significant.

SIDE EFFECTS

FREQUENT: Transitory hypertension followed by postural and supine hypotension in 50% of pts observed as dizziness, lightheadedness, faintness, vertigo. **OCCASIONAL (1–3%):** Diarrhea, loose stools, nausea, vomiting. **RARE (<1%):** Angina, bradycardia.

ADVERSE REACTIONS/TOXIC EFFECTS

Respiratory depression from possible neuromuscular blockade.

PATIENT CONSIDERATIONS

Baseline Assessment

Have pt in area w/equipment and personnel for constant cardiac and B/P monitoring.

Intervention/Evaluation

Assess for conversion of ventricular arrhythmias and absence of new arrhythmias. Constantly monitor B/P, pulse. Notify physician of systolic B/P <75 mm Hg (dopamine or norepinephrine may be needed, or blood, plasma, or volume correction). Keep pt supine (risk of hypotension) during life-threatening therapy and during infusion until tolerance develops. When permitted, assist w/slow position change and ambulation. Put infusions on continuous infusion pumps. Monitor I&O. Provide emotional support to pt and family.

Patient/Family Teaching

Tolerance to hypotensive effect usually occurs within several days after initial therapy. One hr after dose administration, may rise slowly from lying to sitting position and permit legs to dangle from bed for at least 5 min before standing.

brinzolamide

brin-**zoll**-ah-mide
(Azopt)

PREGNANCY CATEGORY C

CLASSIFICATION

Glaucoma agent

AVAILABILITY (Rx)

Suspension: 1%

PHARMACOKINETICS

Absorption: Absorbed systemically, accumulating in RBCs. **Excretion:** Excreted unchanged primarily in urine. **Half-life:** 3.5–4 mos.

ACTION/*THERAPEUTIC EFFECT*

Inhibits carbonic anhydrase, an enzyme, decreasing aqueous humor secretion, *reducing intraocular pressure (IOP).*

USES

Treatment of elevated intraocular pressure (IOP) in pts with ocular hypertension or open-angle glaucoma.

ADMINISTRATION

OPHTHALMIC:

- Place finger on lower eyelid and pull out until pocket is formed between eye and lower lid. Hold dropper above pocket and place drop into pocket. Close eye gently. Apply digital pressure to lacrimal sac for 1–2 min (minimize drainage into nose and throat, reducing risk of systemic effects). Remove excess solution around eye with tissue.
- If more than one ophthalmic drug is used, give medications at least 10 min apart.
- Do not apply medication while pt is wearing soft contact lenses (absorbs drug preservative). Lenses may be reinserted 15 min after drug is administered.

INDICATIONS/ROUTES/DOSAGES

Elevated intraocular pressure (IOP):
Ophthalmic: Adults, elderly: Apply 1 drop into affected eye 3 times/day.

CONTRAINDICATIONS

History of hypersensitivity to carbonic anhydrase inhibitors.

CAUTIONS

Impaired renal/hepatic function.

INTERACTIONS

DRUG: Increases potential for ***salicylate*** toxicity; ***oral carbonic hydrase inhibitors*** may increase systemic effects. **HERBAL:** None known. **FOOD:** None significant. **ALTERED LAB VALUES:** None significant.

SIDE EFFECTS

FREQUENT (5–10%): Blurred vision, bitter, sour or unusual taste. **OCCASIONAL (1–5%):** Blepharitis, dermatitis, dry eye, foreign body sensation, headache, hyperemia, eye discharge/discomfort, itching eyes, rhinitis. **RARE (<1%):** Allergic reaction, dry mouth, tearing, lid margin crusting, eye fatigue.

ADVERSE REACTIONS/TOXIC EFFECTS

Electrolyte imbalance, acidotic state, CNS effects may occur.

PATIENT CONSIDERATIONS

Baseline Assessment

Monitor serum electrolytes (especially potassium), blood pH levels. Assess physical appearance of eye and pt's perception of vision. Question hypersensitivity to brinzolamide.

Interventions/Evaluation

Monitor for lid reaction (redness, swelling, and discharge), conjunctivitis.Evaluate therapeutic response.

Patient/Family Teaching

Do not apply medication while wearing soft contact lenses (absorbs drug preservative). Reinsert lenses 15 min after drug is administered. Vision may be temporarily blurred. Contact physician if any eye symptoms occur (decreased visual acuity, ocular reactions). Teach proper ophthalmic administration. Do not touch container to any surface; do not allow tip on container to contact eye.

bromocriptine

brom-oh-**crip**-teen
(Parlodel)

CANADIAN AVAILABILITY
Apo-Bromocriptine, Parlodel

PREGNANCY CATEGORY B

CLASSIFICATION

Anti-Parkinson, prolactin inhibitor

AVAILABILITY (Rx)

Tablets: 2.5 mg. **Capsules:** 5 mg.

PHARMACODYNAMICS

	ONSET	PEAK	DURATION
Oral (growth hormone decrease)			
	1–2 hrs	—	4–5 hrs
Oral (prolactin decrease)			
	2 hrs	8 hrs	24 hrs

PHARMACOKINETICS

Absorption: Minimal absorption from GI tract. **Metabolism:** Metabolized in liver. **Excretion:** Excreted in feces via biliary secretion. **Half-life:** 15 hrs.

ACTION/*THERAPEUTIC EFFECT*

Directly inhibits prolactin release from anterior pituitary. Stimulates presynaptic and postsynaptic dopamine receptors. *Suppresses secretion, reduction of elevated growth hormone concentration.*

USES/UNLABELED

Treatment of hyperprolactinemia conditions (amenorrhea w/or w/o galactorrhea, prolactin-secreting adenomas, infertility). Treatment of Parkinson's disease, acromegaly. *Treatment of neuroleptic malignant syndrome, cocaine addiction, hyperprolactemia associated w/pituitary adenomas.*

ADMINISTRATION

ORAL:
- Pt should be lying down before administering first dose.
- Give after food intake (decreases incidence of nausea).

INDICATIONS/ROUTES/DOSAGE

Hyperprolactinemia:
Oral: Adults, elderly: Initially, 1.25–2.5 mg/day. May increase by 2.5 mg/day at 3–7 day intervals. **Range:** 2.5–15 mg/day.

Parkinson's disease:
Oral: Adults, elderly: Initially, 1.25 mg 2 times/day. Increase by 2.5 mg/day every 14–28 days. ***Range:*** 10–40 mg/day.

Acromegaly:
Oral: Adults, elderly: Initially, 1.25–2.5 mg/day at bedtime for 3 days. May increase by 1.25–2.5 mg/day every 3–7 days. ***Range:*** 20–30 mg/day. ***Maximum:*** 100 mg/day.

CONTRAINDICATIONS

Pregnancy, peripheral vascular disease, severe ischemic heart disease, uncontrolled hypertension, hypersensitivity to ergot alkaloids.

CAUTIONS

Impaired hepatic/cardiac function, hypertension, psychiatric disorders.

INTERACTIONS

DRUG: Disulfiram reaction may occur w/***alcohol. Estrogens, progestins*** may decrease effects. ***Phenothiazines, haloperidol, MAO inhibitors*** may decrease prolactin effect. ***Hypotensive agents*** may increase hypotension. ***Levodopa*** may increase effects. **HERBAL:** None known. **FOOD:** None significant. **ALTERED LAB VALUES:** May elevate BUN, SGOT (AST), SGPT

(ALT), CPK, alkaline phosphatase, uric acid.

SIDE EFFECTS

Note: Incidence of side effects is high, especially at beginning of therapy or w/high dosage. **FREQUENT (>10%):** Nausea, headache, dizziness. **OCCASIONAL (4–10%):** Fatigue, lightheadedness, vomiting, abdominal cramps, diarrhea, constipation, nasal congestion, drowsiness, dry mouth.

ADVERSE REACTIONS/TOXIC EFFECTS

Visual or auditory hallucinations noted in parkinsonism syndrome. Long-term, high-dose therapy may produce continuing runny nose, fainting, GI hemorrhage, peptic ulcer, severe abdominal/stomach pain.

PATIENT CONSIDERATIONS

Baseline Assessment

Determine baseline, stability of vital signs. Evaluation of pituitary (rule out tumor) should be done prior to treatment for hyperprolactinemia w/amenorrhea/galactorrhea and infertility. Obtain pregnancy test.

Intervention/Evaluation

Assist w/ambulation if dizziness is noted after administration. Monitor B/P for evidence of hypotension, particularly during early therapy. Assess for therapeutic response (decrease in engorgement, decreases in parkinsonism symptoms). Monitor for constipation.

Patient/Family Teaching

Take w/food. To reduce lightheadedness, rise slowly from lying to sitting position and permit legs to dangle momentarily before standing. Avoid sudden posture changes. Avoid tasks that require alertness, motor skills until response to drug is established. Must use contraceptive measures (other than oral) during treatment. Report any watery nasal discharge to physician. Do not suddenly discontinue the drug. Avoid alcohol. Dry mouth reduced by using sugarless gums/candy. Report to physician if dry mouth continues >2 wks.

---

brompheniramine
(Bromphen, Dimetane)
See Classification section under: Antihistamines

---

budesonide

byew-**des**-oh-nyd
(Pulmicort, Rhinocort)

CANADIAN AVAILABILITY
Entocort, Pulmicort, Rhinocort Aqua

PREGNANCY CATEGORY C

CLASSIFICATION

Corticosteroid: nasal

AVAILABILITY (Rx)

Aerosol for Intranasal: 32 mcg/activation. **Dry Powder for Oral Inhalation:** 200 mcg. **Suspension for Nebulization.**

PHARMACOKINETICS

Absorption: Minimally absorbed from nasal tissue. **Metabolism:** Primarily metabolized in liver. **Half-life:** 2 hrs.

ACTION/*THERAPEUTIC EFFECT*

Decreases/prevents tissue response to inflammatory process, *inhibits accumulation of inflammatory cells.*

USES/*UNLABELED*

Management of symptoms of seasonal or perennial allergic rhinitis in adults and children and nonallergic perennial rhinitis in adults. Maintenance treatment of asthma. *Treatment of vasomotor rhinitis.*

ADMINISTRATION

INTRANASAL:

- Clear nasal passages before use (topical nasal decongestants may be needed 5–15 min before use).
- Tilt head slightly forward.
- Insert spray tip up in 1 nostril, pointing toward inflamed nasal turbinates, away from nasal septum.
- Pump medication into 1 nostril while holding other nostril closed and concurrently inspire through nose.
- Discard used nasal solution after 6 mos.

INHALATION:

- Hold inhaler upright, twist cover off.
- Twist brown grip fully to right, then twist back (you will hear a click).
- Exhale (away from inhaler).
- Do not shake container after loading.
- Place mouthpiece between lips; inhale deeply (inhaler must be held in upright position).
- When finished, rinse with water (do not swallow); prevents hoarseness or dryness.

INDICATIONS/ROUTES/DOSAGE

Usual intranasal dosage:
Adults, children >6 yrs: 32 mcg/spray. Initially, 2 sprays each nostril 2 times/day (morning and evening), or 4 sprays in each nostril in morning. ***Maximum:*** 4 sprays each nostril/day.

Usual inhalation dosage:
Adults: 200–800 mcg 2 times/day. **Note:** May give 200–400 mcg once daily in pts w/mild–moderate asthma well controlled on inhaled corticosteroids.

Children >6 yrs: 200 mcg 2 times/day. ***Maximum:*** 400 mcg 2 times/day.

CONTRAINDICATIONS

Hypersensitivity to any corticosteroid or components, primary treatment of status asthmaticus, systemic fungal infections, persistently positive sputum cultures for *Candida albicans*. Untreated localized infections involving nasal mucosa.

CAUTIONS

Glaucoma, ocular herpes simplex, latent/active tuberculosis, recent nasal trauma or surgery.

INTERACTIONS

DRUG: None significant. **HERBAL:** None known. **FOOD:** None significant. **ALTERED LAB VALUES:** None significant.

SIDE EFFECTS

FREQUENT (>3%): *Inhalation:* Flu-like syndrome, pain, fever, oral candidiasis, respiratory infection, pharyngitis, sinusitis. ***Nasal:*** Mild nasopharyngeal irritation, burning, stinging, dryness, headache, cough. **OCCASIONAL (1–3%):** *Inhalation:* Back pain, vomiting, altered taste/voice, abdominal pain, nausea, dyspepsia. ***Nasal:*** Dry mouth, dyspepsia, rebound congestion, rhinorrhea, loss of sense of taste.

ADVERSE REACTIONS/TOXIC EFFECTS

Acute hypersensitivity reaction (urticaria, angioedema, severe bronchospasm) occurs rarely.

PATIENT CONSIDERATIONS

BASELINE ASSESSMENT

Question for hypersensitivity to any corticosteroids, components.

PATIENT/FAMILY TEACHING

Intranasal
Contact physician if no improvement in symptoms, sneezing or nasal irritation occurs. Clear nasal passages prior to use. Improvement seen 24 hrs; but full effect may take 3–7 days. Do not change dose schedule or stop taking drug; must taper off gradually under medical supervision.

Inhalation
Maintain careful mouth hygiene. Rinse mouth w/water immediately after inhalation (prevents mouth/throat dryness, fungal infection of mouth). Contact physician/nurse if sore throat or mouth occurs.

bumetanide

byew-**met**-ah-nide
(Bumex)

CANADIAN AVAILABILITY
Burinex

PREGNANCY CATEGORY C

CLASSIFICATION

Diuretic: Loop

AVAILABILITY (Rx)

Tablets: 0.5 mg, 1 mg, 2 mg. **Injection:** 0.25 mg/ml.

PHARMACODYNAMICS

	ONSET	PEAK	DURATION
Oral	30–60 min	60–120 min	4–6 hrs
IM	40 min	60–120 min	4–6 hrs
IV	Rapid	15–30 min	2–3 hrs

PHARMACOKINETICS

Absorption: Completely absorbed from GI tract (decreased in CHF, nephrotic syndrome). **Metabolism:** Partially metabolized in liver. **Excretion:** Primarily excreted in urine. **Half-life:** 1–1.5 hrs.

ACTION/*THERAPEUTIC EFFECT*

Enhances excretion of sodium, chloride, and, to lesser degree, potassium, by direct action at ascending limb of loop of Henle and in the proximal tubule, *producing diuresis.*

USES/*UNLABELED*

Treatment of edema associated w/CHF, chronic renal failure including nephrotic syndrome, hepatic cirrhosis w/ascites; treatment of acute pulmonary edema. *Treatment of hypertension, hypercalcemia.*

STORAGE/HANDLING

Store oral, parenteral form at room temperature.

ADMINISTRATION

ORAL:

- Give w/food to avoid GI upset, preferably w/breakfast (may prevent nocturia).

IV:

- May give undiluted but is compatible w/5% dextrose in water, 0.9% sodium chloride or lactated Ringer's.
- Administer direct IV >1–2 min.

- May give through Y tube or 3-way stopcock.

INDICATIONS/ROUTES/DOSAGE

Edema:
Oral: Adults >18 yrs: 0.5–2 mg given as single dose in AM. May repeat at 4–5 hr intervals. ***Elderly:*** 0.5 mg/day, increase as needed.

IM/IV: Adults, elderly: 0.5–1 mg given as single dose. May be repeated at 2–3 hr intervals.

CONTRAINDICATIONS

Anuria, hepatic coma, severe electrolyte depletion.

EXTREME CAUTION

Hypersensitivity to sulfonamides.

CAUTIONS

Impaired renal or hepatic function, diabetes mellitus, elderly/debilitated.

INTERACTIONS

DRUG: ***Amphotericin, ototoxic, nephrotoxic agents*** may increase toxicity. May decrease effect of ***anticoagulants, heparin. Hypokalemia-causing agents*** may increase risk of hypokalemia. May increase risk of ***lithium*** toxicity. **HERBAL:** None known. **FOOD:** None significant. **ALTERED LAB VALUES:** May increase glucose, BUN, uric acid, urinary phosphate. May decrease calcium, chloride, magnesium, potassium, sodium.

SIDE EFFECTS

EXPECTED: Increase in urine frequency/volume. **FREQUENT:** Orthostatic hypotension, dizziness. **OCCASIONAL:** Blurred vision, diarrhea, headache, anorexia, premature ejaculation, impotence, GI upset. **RARE:** Rash, urticaria, pruritus, weakness, muscle cramps, nipple tenderness.

ADVERSE REACTIONS/TOXIC EFFECTS

Vigorous diuresis may lead to profound water/electrolyte depletion, resulting in hypokalemia, hyponatremia, dehydration, coma, circulatory collapse. Acute hypotensive episodes may occur. Ototoxicity manifested as deafness, vertigo, tinnitus (ringing/roaring in ears) may occur, especially in pts w/severe renal impairment or who are on other ototoxic drugs. Blood dyscrasias have been reported.

PATIENT CONSIDERATIONS

Baseline Assessment

Check vital signs, especially B/P for hypotension prior to administration. Assess baseline electrolytes; particularly check for low potassium. Assess edema, skin turgor, mucous membranes for hydration status. Assess muscle strength, mental status. Note skin temperature, moisture. Obtain baseline weight. Initiate I&O.

Intervention/Evaluation

Continue to monitor B/P, vital signs, electrolytes, I&O, weight. Note extent of diuresis. Watch for changes from initial assessment (hypokalemia may result in muscle strength changes, tremor, muscle cramps, change in mental status, cardiac arrhythmias; hyponatremia may result in confusion, thirst, cold/clammy skin).

Patient/Family Teaching

Expect increased frequency and volume of urination. Report irregular heartbeat, signs of electrolyte imbalances (see Adverse Reactions/Toxic Effects), hearing abnormalities (such as sense of fullness in ears, ringing/roaring in ears). Eat foods high in potas-

sium such as whole grains (cereals), legumes, meat, bananas, apricots, orange juice, potatoes (white, sweet), raisins. Avoid sun/sunlamps. Get up slowly from sitting/lying position. Report continued nausea, diarrhea, vomiting.

bupivacaine

(Marcaine, Sensorcaine)

See Classification section under: Anesthetics: local

buprenorphine hydrochloride

byew-**pren**-or-phen

(Buprenex)

PREGNANCY CATEGORY C

CLASSIFICATION

Opioid analgesic **(Schedule V)**

AVAILABILITY (Rx)

Injection: 0.3 mg/ml

PHARMACODYNAMICS

	ONSET	PEAK	DURATION
IM	15 min	1 hr	<6 hrs
IV	Rapid	Rapid	<6 hrs

PHARMACOKINETICS

Absorption: Rapidly absorbed from IM injection. **Metabolism:** Metabolized in liver, undergoes extensive first-pass metabolism. **Excretion:** Primarily eliminated in feces via bile. **Half-life:** 2–3 hrs.

ACTION/*THERAPEUTIC EFFECT*

Binds w/opioid receptors within CNS, *altering pain perception, emotional response to pain.* May displace opioid agonists and competitively inhibit their action (may precipitate withdrawal symptoms).

USES

Relief of moderate to severe pain.

INDICATIONS/ROUTES/DOSAGE

Note: May be given IM or slow IV injection. Do not mix w/diazepam or lorazepam in same syringe.

Analgesia:
IM/IV: Adults, children >13 yrs: 0.3 mg q6h as needed; may repeat 30–60 min after initial dose. May increase to 0.6 mg and/or reduce dosing interval to q4h if necessary. *Children 2–12 yrs:* 2–6 mcg/kg q4–6h.

Usual elderly dosage:
IM/IV: 0.15 mg q6h as needed.

CONTRAINDICATIONS

None significant.

CAUTIONS

Impaired hepatic/renal function, elderly, debilitated, head injury, respiratory disease, hypertension, hypothyroidism, Addison's disease, acute alcoholism, urethral structure.

INTERACTIONS

DRUG: *CNS depressants, MAO inhibitors* may increase CNS or respiratory depression, hypotension. May decrease effects of other *opioid analgesics.* HERBAL: None known. **FOOD:** None significant. **ALTERED LAB VALUES:** May increase amylase, lipase.

SIDE EFFECTS

FREQUENT: Sedation (66%), dizziness (5–10%). **OCCASIONAL:** Headache (1–5%), hypotension (1–5%), nausea/vomiting (1–5%), hypoventilation (1–5%), miosis

(1–5%), sweating (1–5%). RARE: Dry mouth, pallor, visual abnormalities, injection site reaction.

ADVERSE REACTIONS/TOXIC EFFECTS

Overdosage results in cold, clammy skin, weakness, confusion, severe respiratory depression, cyanosis, pinpoint pupils, extreme somnolence progressing to convulsions, stupor, coma.

PATIENT CONSIDERATIONS

Baseline Assessment

Obtain vital signs before giving medication. If respirations are 12/min or lower (20/min or lower in children), withhold medication, contact physician. Assess onset, type, location, duration of pain. Effect of medication is reduced if full pain recurs before next dose.

Intervention/Evaluation

Monitor for change in respirations, B/P, change in rate/quality of pulse. Monitor stool frequency, consistency. Initiate deep breathing, coughing exercises, particularly in those w/impaired pulmonary function. Change pt's position q2–4h. Assess for clinical improvement and record onset of relief of pain.

Patient/Family Teaching

Change positions slowly to avoid dizziness. Avoid tasks that require alertness, motor skills until response to drug is established. Avoid alcohol and benzodiazapines. Do not exceed prescribed dosage.

---

bupropion

byew-**pro**-peon
(Wellbutrin, Zyban)

CANADIAN AVAILABILITY
Wellbutrin SR

PREGNANCY CATEGORY B

CLASSIFICATION

Antidepressant, smoking cessation aid

AVAILABILITY (Rx)

Tablets: 75 mg, 100 mg. **Tablets (sustained-release):** 50 mg, 100 mg, 150 mg.

PHARMACOKINETICS

Absorption: Rapidly absorbed from GI tract. Crosses blood-brain barrier. **Metabolism:** Extensive first-pass metabolism in liver to active metabolite. **Excretion:** Primarily excreted in urine. **Half-life:** 14 hrs.

ACTION/*THERAPEUTIC EFFECT*

Blocks reuptake of neurotransmitters (serotonin, norepinephrine) at CNS presynaptic membranes, increasing availability at postsynaptic receptor sites. Resulting enhancement of synaptic activity *produces antidepressant effect.*

USES

Treatment of depression, particularly endogenous depression, exhibited as persistent and prominent dysphoria (occurring nearly every day for at least 2 wks) manifested by 4 of 8 symptoms: change in appetite, change in sleep pattern, increased fatigue, impaired concentration, feelings of guilt/worthlessness, loss of interest in usual activities, psychomotor agitation/retardation, or suicidal tendencies. Smoking cessation.

ADMINISTRATION

ORAL:

- Avoid bedtime dosage (decreases risk of insomnia).
- Do not crush sustained-release preparations.

INDICATIONS/ROUTES/DOSAGE

Note: Reduce dosage in renal/hepatic impairment, elderly.

Depression:
Oral: Adults: Initially, 75 mg 3 times/day or 100 mg 2 times/day. May increase to 100 mg 3 times/day no sooner than 3 days after initial dosage. Do not exceed dose increase of 100 mg/day in 3 day period. ***Maximum daily dose:*** 150 mg 3 times/day. Do not exceed any single dose of 150 mg.

Usual elderly dosage:
Oral: Initially, 50–100 mg/day. May increase by 50–100 mg/day every 3–4 days.

Smoking cessation:
Oral: Adults: Initially, 150 mg daily for 3 days; then 150 mg 2 times/day.

CONTRAINDICATIONS

Pts w/seizure disorder, current or prior diagnosis of bulimia or anorexia nervosa, concurrent use of MAO inhibitor.

EXTREME CAUTION

History of seizure, cranial trauma; those currently taking antipsychotics, antidepressants.

CAUTIONS

Impaired renal, hepatic function.

INTERACTIONS

DRUG: ***Alcohol, tricyclic antidepressants, lithium, trazodone*** may increase risk of seizures. May increase risk of acute toxicity w/***MAO inhibitors***. **HERBAL:** None known. **FOOD:** None significant. **ALTERED LAB VALUES:** May decrease WBCs.

SIDE EFFECTS

FREQUENT (>10%): Constipation, weight loss, nausea, vomiting, weight gain, anorexia, dry mouth, headache, increased sweating, termor, sedation, insomnia, altered hearing, dizziness, agitation. **OCCASIONAL (5–10%):** Diarrhea, akinesia, blurred vision, tachycardia, confusion, hostility, fatigue.

ADVERSE REACTIONS/TOXIC EFFECTS

Increased risk of seizures w/increase in dosage greater than 150 mg/dose, in pts w/history of bulimia or seizure disorders, w/discontinuing agents that may lower seizure threshold.

PATIENT CONSIDERATIONS

Baseline Assessment

For those on long-term therapy, liver/renal function tests should be performed periodically.

Intervention/Evaluation

Supervise suicidal risk patient closely during early therapy (as depression lessens, energy level improves, increasing suicide potential). Assess appearance, behavior, speech pattern, level of interest, mood. Monitor pattern of daily bowel activity, stool consistency. Monitor B/P, pulse for hypotension, arrhythmias.

Patient/Family Teaching

Full therapeutic effect may be noted in 4 wks. Avoid alcohol (increases risk of seizure). Avoid tasks that require alertness,

motor skills until response to drug is established. Dry mouth may be relieved by sugarless gum/sips of tepid water.

buspirone hydrochloride

byew-spear-own
(BuSpar)

CANADIAN AVAILABILITY
Buspar, Buspirex, Bustab

PREGNANCY CATEGORY B

CLASSIFICATION

Antianxiety

AVAILABILITY (Rx)

Tablets: 5 mg, 10 mg, 15 mg

PHARMACOKINETICS

Absorption: Rapidly and completely absorbed from GI tract. **Metabolism:** Undergoes extensive first-pass metabolism. Metabolized in liver to active metabolite. **Excretion:** Primarily excreted in urine. **Half-life:** 2–3 hrs.

ACTION/*THERAPEUTIC EFFECT*

Binds to serotonin, dopamine at presynaptic neurotransmitter receptors in the CNS, *producing antianxiety effect.*

USES

Short-term relief (up to 4 wks), management of anxiety disorders.

ADMINISTRATION

ORAL:

- Give w/o regard to meals.
- Tablets may be crushed.
- Avoid concomitant administration of grapefruit juice.

INDICATIONS/ROUTES/DOSAGE

Anxiety:

Oral: Adults: 5 mg 2–3 times daily. May increase in 5 mg increments/day at intervals of 2–4 days. *Maintenance:* 15–30 mg/day in 2–3 divided doses. Do not exceed 60 mg/day.

Usual elderly dosage:

Oral: Initially, 5 mg 2 times/day. May increase by 5 mg every 2–3 days. *Maximum:* 60 mg/day.

CONTRAINDICATIONS

Severe renal/hepatic impairment, MAO inhibitor therapy.

CAUTIONS

Renal/hepatic impairment.

INTERACTIONS

DRUG: *Alcohol, CNS depressants* may increase sedation. *MAO inhibitors* may increase B/P. **HERBAL:** Kava kava may increase CNS depression. **FOOD:** Grapefruit juice may increase concentration. **ALTERED LAB VALUES:** May increase SGOT (AST), SGPT (ALT).

SIDE EFFECTS

FREQUENT (6–12%): Dizziness, drowsiness, nausea, headache. OCCASIONAL (2–5%): Nervousness, fatigue, insomnia, dry mouth, lightheadedness, mood swings, blurred vision, poor concentration, diarrhea, numbness in hands/feet. RARE (<2%): Muscle pain/stiffness, nightmares, chest pain, involuntary movements.

ADVERSE REACTIONS/TOXIC EFFECTS

No evidence of tolerance or psychologic and/or physical dependence, no withdrawal syndrome. Overdosage may produce severe nausea, vomiting, dizziness, drowsiness, abdominal distension, excessive pupil contraction.

PATIENT CONSIDERATIONS

BASELINE ASSESSMENT

Offer emotional support to anxious pt. Assess motor responses (agitation, trembling, tension) and autonomic responses (cold, clammy hands; sweating).

INTERVENTION/EVALUATION

For pts on long-term therapy, liver/renal function tests, blood counts should be performed periodically. Assist w/ambulation if drowsiness, lightheadedness occur. Evaluate for therapeutic response: calm, facial expression, decreased restlessness and/or insomnia.

PATIENT/FAMILY TEACHING

Improvement may be noted in 7–10 days, but optimum therapeutic effect generally takes 3–4 wks. Drowsiness usually disappears during continued therapy. If dizziness occurs, change position slowly from recumbent to sitting position before standing. Avoid tasks that require alertness, motor skills until response to drug is established. Avoid alcohol. Do not take other CNS depressants (unless ordered by physician). Do not discontinue drug abruptly. Report any chronic abnormal movement (e.g., motor restlessness).

busulfan

(Myleran)

See Classification section under: Cancer chemotherapy

butorphanol tartrate

byew-**tore**-phen-awl

(Stadol, Stadol NS)

CANADIAN AVAILABILITY

Stadol

PREGNANCY CATEGORY B

(D if used for prolonged time, high dose at term)

CLASSIFICATION

Opioid analgesic **(Schedule IV)**

AVAILABILITY (Rx)

Injection: 1 mg/ml, 2 mg/ml. **Nasal Spray:** 10 mg/ml.

PHARMACODYNAMICS

	ONSET	PEAK	DURATION
IM	10–30 min	30–60 min	3–4 hrs
IV	<1 min	4–5 min	2–4 hrs
Nasal	15 min	1–2 hrs	4–5 hrs

PHARMACOKINETICS

Absorption: Rapidly absorbed from IM injection. **Metabolism:** Extensively metabolized in liver. **Excretion:** Primarily excreted in urine. **Half-life:** 2.5–4 hrs.

ACTION/*THERAPEUTIC EFFECT*

Binds w/opioid receptors within CNS, *altering pain perception, emotional response to pain.* May displace opioid agonists and competitively inhibit their action (may precipitate withdrawal symptoms).

USES

Management of pain (including postop pain). ***Nasal only:*** Migraine headache pain. ***Parenteral only:*** Preop, preanesthetic medication, supplement balanced anesthesia, relief of pain during labor.

ADMINISTRATION

INTRANASAL:

- Clear nasal passages before use (topical nasal decongestants may be needed 5–15 min before use).
- Tilt head slightly forward.
- Insert spray tip up in 1 nostril, pointing toward inflamed nasal turbinates, away from nasal septum.
- Pump medication into 1 nostril while holding other nostril closed and concurrently inspire through nose.

INDICATIONS/ROUTES/DOSAGE

Note: May be given by IM or IV injection.

Analgesia:
IM: Adults: 1–4 mg q3–4h as needed.

IV: Adults: 0.5–2 mg q3–4h as needed.

Nasal: Adults: 1 mg (1 spray in one nostril). May repeat in 60–90 min. May repeat 2 dose sequence q3–4h as needed. Alternatively, 2 mg (1 spray each nostril if pt remains recumbent), may repeat in 3–4h.

Usual elderly dosage:
IM/IV: 1 mg q4–6h as needed.

CONTRAINDICATIONS

Sensitivity to butorphanol.

CAUTIONS

Impaired hepatic/renal function, elderly, debilitated, head injury, respiratory disease, hypertension, prior to biliary tract surgery (produces spasm of sphincter of Oddi), MI w/nausea, vomiting. Not recommended for children <18 yrs.

INTERACTIONS

DRUG: ***Alcohol, CNS depressants*** may increase CNS or respiratory depression, hypotension. ***MAO inhibitors*** may produce severe, fatal reaction (reduce dose to 1/4 usual dose). Effects may be decreased w/***buprenorphine***. **HERBAL:** None known. **FOOD:** None significant. **ALTERED LAB VALUES:** None significant.

SIDE EFFECTS

FREQUENT: *Parenteral:* Drowsiness (43%), dizziness (19%). ***Nasal:*** Nasal congestion (13%), insomnia (11%). **OCCASIONAL (3–9%):** *Parenteral:* Confusion, sweating/clammy skin, lethargy, headache, nausea, vomiting, dry mouth. ***Nasal:*** Vasodilation, constipation, unpleasant taste, dyspnea, epistaxis, nasal irritation, upper respiratory infection, tinnitus. **RARE:** *Parenteral:* Hypotension, pruritus, blurred vision, sensation of heat, CNS stimulation, insomnia. ***Nasal:*** Hypertension, tremor, ear pain, paresthesia, depression, sinusitis.

ADVERSE REACTIONS/TOXIC EFFECTS

Abrupt withdrawal after prolonged use may produce symptoms of narcotic withdrawal (abdominal cramping, rhinorrhea, lacrimation, anxiety, increased temperature, piloerection [goose bumps]). Overdosage results in severe respiratory depression, skeletal muscle flaccidity, cyanosis, extreme somnolence progressing to convulsions, stupor, coma. Tolerance to analgesic effect, physical dependence may occur w/chronic use.

PATIENT CONSIDERATIONS

BASELINE ASSESSMENT

Obtain vital signs before giving medication. If respirations are 12/min or lower (20/min or lower in children), withhold medication, contact physician. Assess onset, type, location, duration of pain. Effect of medication is reduced if full pain recurs before next dose. Protect from falls. During labor, assess fetal heart tones, uterine contractions.

INTERVENTION/EVALUATION

Increase fluid intake and environmental humidity to improve viscosity of lung secretions. Monitor for change in respirations, B/P, change in rate/quality of pulse. Monitor pattern of daily bowel activity, stool consistency. Initiate deep breathing and coughing exercises, particularly in those w/impaired pulmonary function. Change pt's position q2–4h. Assess for clinical improvement and record onset of relief of pain.

PATIENT/FAMILY TEACHING

Change positions slowly to avoid dizziness. Avoid tasks that require alertness, motor skills until response to drug is established. Instruct pt on proper use of nasal spray. Avoid use of alcohol or CNS depressants.

cabergoline

(Dostinex)
See Supplement

caffeine

(Cafcit)
See Supplement

calcipotriene

kal-sih-poe-**tree**-in
(Dovonex)

CANADIAN AVAILABILITY
Dovonex

PREGNANCY CATEGORY C

CLASSIFICATION

Antipsoriatic

AVAILABILITY (Rx)

Cream: 0.005%. **Ointment:** 0.005%. **Scalp Solution:** 0.005%.

PHARMACOKINETICS

Absorption: Absorbed systemically. **Metabolism:** Rapid metabolism. **Excretion:** Excreted in bile.

ACTION/*THERAPEUTIC EFFECT*

A synthetic vitamin D_3 analogue. Regulates skin cell (keratinocyte) production and development, *preventing abnormal growth and production of psoriasis (abnormal keratinocyte growth).*

USES

Treatment of mild to moderate plaque psoriasis. ***Solution:*** Treatment of chronic, moderately severe scalp psoriasis.

INDICATIONS/ROUTES/DOSAGE

Psoriasis:
Topical: Adults, elderly, children >12 yrs: Apply thin layer to affected skin twice daily (morning and evening); rub in gently and completely. ***Solution:*** Apply to lesions after combing hair.

CONTRAINDICATIONS

Hypersensitivity to components of preparation, hypercalcemia or evidence of vitamin D toxicity, use on face.

CAUTIONS

History of nephrolithiasis.

INTERACTIONS

DRUG: None significant. **HERBAL:** None known. **FOOD:** None significant. **ALTERED LAB VALUES:** Excessive use may increase serum calcium level.

SIDE EFFECTS

FREQUENT (10–15%): Burning, itching, skin irritation. **OCCASIONAL (1–10%):** Erythema, dry skin, peeling, rash, worsening of psoriasis dermatitis. **RARE (<1%):** Skin atrophy, hyperpigmentation, folliculitis.

ADVERSE REACTIONS/TOXIC EFFECTS

Potential for hypercalcemia (abdominal pain, depression, easy fatigability, high B/P, anorexia, nausea, thirst) may occur.

PATIENT CONSIDERATIONS

BASELINE ASSESSMENT

Establish baseline electrolytes, particularly serum and urine calcium.

INTERVENTION/EVALUATION

Monitor serum calcium. Assess skin for irritation, erythema, wor-

sening of psoriasis (children, those >65 are at greater risk of reactions than adults). If irritation of lesions or surrounding uninvolved skin develops or if serum calcium level increases outside normal range, medication should be discontinued.

PATIENT/FAMILY TEACHING

Avoid contact w/face or eyes. Wash hands after application. Report any signs of local reactions. Improvement noted usually beginning after 2 wks of therapy, marked improvement after 8 wks of therapy. Follow-up lab tests, office visits are necessary.

calcitonin-salmon

kal-sih-**toe**-nin
(Calcimar, Miacalcin, Osteocalcin, Salmonine)

CANADIAN AVAILABILITY
Calcimar, Caltine

PREGNANCY CATEGORY B

CLASSIFICATION

Calcium regulator, bone resorption inhibitor, osteoporosis therapy

AVAILABILITY (Rx)

Injection: 200 IU/ml. **Nasal Spray:** 200 IU/activation.

PHARMACOKINETICS

Metabolism: Rapidly metabolized (primarily in kidney). **Excretion:** Primarily excreted in urine. **Half-life:** 70–90 min.

ACTION/*THERAPEUTIC EFFECT*

Reduces bone turnover by blocking bone resorption in Paget's disease; directly inhibits bone resorption, decreasing the number/function of osteoclasts in osteoporosis. *Reduces bone turnover, lowers serum calcium concentration.*

USES/*UNLABELED*

Management of moderate to severe Paget's disease of bone, early treatment of hypercalcemic emergencies. Management of postmenopausal osteoporosis to prevent progressive loss of bone mass (w/calcium, vitamin D). *Treatment of secondary osteoporosis due to hormone disturbance, drug therapy.*

STORAGE/HANDLING

Refrigerate. Nasal preparation can be stored at room temperature once pump is activated.

ADMINISTRATION

SUBQ/IM:

- May be administered SubQ or IM. No more than 2 ml dose should be given IM.
- Skin test should be performed before therapy.
- Bedtime administration may reduce nausea, flushing.

INTRANASAL:

- Instruct pt to blow nose to clear nasal passages.
- Tilt head slightly forward. Insert spray tip into 1 nostril, pointing toward nasal passages, away from nasal septum.
- Spray into nostril while holding other nostril closed.

INDICATIONS/ROUTES/DOSAGES

Skin testing:
Prepare a 10 units/ml dilution; withdraw 0.05 ml from 200 IU/ml vial solution in tuberculin syringe; fill up to 1 ml w/0.9% NaCl. Take 0.1 ml and inject intracutaneously on

inner aspect of forearm. Observe after 15 min (positive response: appearance of more than mild erythema or wheal).

Paget's disease:
IM/SubQ: Adults, elderly: Initially, 100 IU/day (improvement in biochemical abnormalities, bone pain seen in first few months; in neurologic lesion, often longer than 1 yr). ***Maintenance:*** 50 IU/day or every other day.

Postmenopausal osteoporosis:
IM/SubQ: Adults, elderly: 100 IU/day (w/adequate calcium and vitamin D intake).

Intranasal: 200 IU as single daily spray, alternating nostrils daily.

Hypercalcemia:
IM/SubQ: Adults, elderly: Initially, 4 IU/kg q12h; may increase to 8 IU/kg q12h if no response in 2 days; may further increase to 8 IU/kg q6h if no response in 2 days.

CONTRAINDICATIONS

Hypersensitivity to calcitonin. Data does not support use in children.

CAUTIONS

History of allergy, renal dysfunction.

INTERACTIONS

DRUG: None significant. **HERBAL:** None known. **FOOD:** None significant. **ALTERED LAB VALUES:** None significant.

SIDE EFFECTS

FREQUENT: *IM/SubQ:* Nausea may occur in 30 min after injection, usually diminishes w/continued therapy. Anorexia, vomiting, diarrhea, flushing of face, ears, hands, feet. ***Nasal:*** Rhinitis, rhinorrhea, facial flushing, nasal dryness, headache, arthralgia, epistaxis, back pain. **OCCASIONAL:** *IM/SubQ:* Tenderness/tingling of palms/soles, local inflammation at injection site, diuresis, unusual taste. ***Nasal:*** Fatigue, rash, hypertension, diarrhea, abdominal pain, angina, cystitis, conjunctivitis. **RARE:** *IM/SubQ:* Headache, chest pressure, nasal congestion, hypersensitivity (including rash, urticaria).

ADVERSE REACTIONS/TOXIC EFFECTS

Potential for hypocalcemic tetany or anaphylaxis w/protein allergy.

PATIENT CONSIDERATIONS

Baseline Assessment

Question for allergies, hypersensitivity to fish, calcitonin. Establish baseline electrolytes.

Intervention/Evaluation

Assess for allergic response: rash, urticaria, swelling, shortness of breath, tachycardia, hypotension. Assure rotation of injection sites; check for inflammation. Monitor electrolytes. Periodic nasal exam. Assess vertebral bone mass (document stabilization /improvement).

Patient/Family Teaching

Instruct pt/family on aseptic technique, proper injection of medication, including rotation of sites. Do not take any other medications w/o consulting physician. Nausea and flushing are transient; nausea and diuresis usually decrease w/continued therapy. Notify physician immediately if rash, urticaria, shortness of breath, significant nasal irritation occur. Follow-up lab tests, office visits are necessary.

calcium acetate
(Phos-Ex, PhosLo)

calcium carbonate
(Dicarbasil, OsCal, Titralac, Tums)

calcium chloride

calcium citrate
(Citracal)

calcium glubionate
(NeoCalglucon)

calcium gluconate

CANADIAN AVAILABILITY

Apo-Cal, Calcijex, Calsan, Caltrate

PREGNANCY CATEGORY C

CLASSIFICATION

Antacid, antihypocalcemic, nutritional supplement

AVAILABILITY (OTC)

Calcium acetate: **Tablets:** 250 mg, 667 mg, 1,000 mg. **Capsules:** 500 mg.

Calcium carbonate: **Tablets:** 500 mg, 650 mg, 1,250 mg, 1,500 mg. **Chewable Tablets:** 350 mg, 500 mg, 750 mg, 1,250 mg. **Capsules:** 1,250 mg.

Calcium chloride (Rx): **Injection:** 10%

Calcium citrate: **Tablets:** 950 mg.

Calcium glubionate: **Syrup.**

Calcium gluconate: **Tablets:** 500 mg, 650 mg, 975 mg, 1,000 mg. **Injection: (Rx):** 10%.

PHARMACOKINETICS

Absorption: Moderately absorbed from small intestine (dependent on presence of vitamin D metabolites, pH). **Excretion:** Primarily eliminated in feces.

ACTION / *THERAPEUTIC EFFECT*

Calcium is essential for function, integrity of nervous, muscular, skeletal systems. Important role in normal cardiac, renal function, respiration, blood coagulation, and cell membrane and capillary permeability. Assists in regulating release/storage of neurotransmitter/hormones. Neutralizes or reduces gastric acid (increases pH). ***Calcium acetate:*** Combines w/dietary phosphate, forming insoluble calcium phosphate. *Replaces calcium in deficiency states, controls hyperphosphatemia in end-stage renal disease.*

USES / *UNLABELED*

Parenteral: Acute hypocalcemia (e.g., neonatal hypocalcemic tetany, alkalosis), electrolyte depletion, cardiac arrest (strengthens myocardial contractions), hyperkalemia (reverses EKG, cardiac depression), hypermagnesemia (aids in reversing CNS depression). ***Oral:*** Chronic hypocalcemia, calcium deficiency, antacid. ***Calcium acetate:*** Controls hyperphosphatemia in end-stage renal disease. ***Calcium carbonate:*** *Treatment of hyperphosphatemia.*

ADMINISTRATION

ORAL:

- Take tablets w/full glass of water 0.5–1 hr after meals. Give syrup before meals (increases absorption), diluted in juice or water.
- Chew chewable tablets well before swallowing.

IV:

- Give by slow IV injection (0.5–1 ml/min for calcium chloride; 1.5–3 ml/min for calcium gluconate).
- Maximum rate for intermittent

infusion is 200 mg/min of calcium gluconate (e.g., 10 ml/min when 1 g diluted w/50 ml diluent).

INDICATIONS/ROUTES/DOSAGES

Calcium Acetate:

Hypophosphatemia:
Oral: Adults, elderly: 2 tablets 3 times/day w/meals.

Calcium Carbonate:

Antihypocalcemic, nutritional supplement:
Oral: Adults, elderly: 0.5–1.25 g (500 mg calcium) 1–3 times/day.

Antacid:
Oral: Adults, elderly: 0.5–1.25 g as needed.

Calcium Citrate:

Antihypocalcemic:
Oral: Adults, elderly: 1–2 tablets 2–4 times/day.

Nutritional supplement:
Oral: Adults, elderly: 4–8 tablets/day in 3–4 divided doses.

Calcium Glubionate:

Antihypocalcemic:
Oral: Adults, elderly: 15 ml 3–4 times/day. *Children 1–4 yrs:* 10 ml 3 times/day. *Children <1 yr:* 5 ml 5 times/day.

Calcium Chloride:

Calcium Gluconate:

Emergency increase of calcium:
IV: Adults, elderly: 7–14 mEq. *Children:* 1–7 mEq. *Infants:* <1 mEq. May repeat dose q1–3 days.

Hypocalcemic tetany:
IV: Adults, elderly: 4.5–16 mEq. May repeat until therapeutic response. *Children:* 0.5–0.7 mEq/kg 3–4 times/day. *Neonates:* 2.4 mEq/kg/day in divided doses.

Cardiopulmonary resuscitation:
IV: Adults, elderly: Calcium gluconate: 2.3–3.7 mEq. May repeat as needed. *Calcium chloride:* 2.7 mEq. May repeat as needed. *Children: Calcium chloride:* 0.27 mEq/kg. May repeat in 10 min if needed.

Hyperkalemia:
IV: Adults, elderly: 2.25–14 mEq. Monitor EKG. May repeat after 1–2 min if needed.

Magnesium intoxication:
IV: Adults, elderly: 7 mEq. May repeat based on pt response.

CONTRAINDICATIONS

Ventricular fibrillation, hypercalcemia, hypercalciuria, calcium renal calculi, sarcoidosis, digoxin toxicity. *Calcium acetate:* Hypoparathyroidism, decreased renal function.

CAUTIONS

Dehydration, history of renal calculi, chronic renal impairment, decreased cardiac function, ventricular fibrillation during cardiac resuscitation.

INTERACTIONS

DRUG: May antagonize ***etidronate, gallium*** effects. May decrease absorption of ***ketoconazole, phenytoin, tetracyclines.*** May decrease effects of ***methenamine, parenteral magnesium.*** May increase risk of arrhythmias w/***digoxin***. **HERBAL:** None known. **FOOD:** None significant. **ALTERED LAB VALUES:** May increase calcium gastrin, pH. May decrease phosphate, potassium.

SIDE EFFECTS

FREQUENT: *Parenteral:* Hypotension, flushing, feeling of warmth, nausea, vomiting; pain, rash, redness, burning at injection site; sweating, decreased B/P. *Oral:* Chalky taste. **OCCASIONAL:** *Oral:* Mild constipation, fecal impaction, swelling of hands/feet, metabolic alkalosis (muscle pain, restlessness, slow breathing, poor taste). ***Calcium carbonate:*** Milk-alkali syndrome (headache, decreased appetite, nausea, vomiting, unusual tiredness). **RARE:** ***Oral:*** Difficult or painful urination.

ADVERSE REACTIONS/TOXIC EFFECTS

Hypercalcemia: Early signs: Constipation, headache, dry mouth, increased thirst, irritability, decreased appetite, metallic taste, fatigue, weakness, depression. Later signs: Confusion, drowsiness, increased B/P, increased light sensitivity, irregular heartbeat, nausea, vomiting, increased urination.

PATIENT CONSIDERATIONS

BASELINE ASSESSMENT

Assess B/P, EKG readings, renal function, magnesium, phosphate, potassium concentrations.

INTERVENTION/EVALUATION

Monitor B/P, EKG, renal function, magnesium, phosphate, potassium, serum and urine calcium concentrations. Monitor for signs of hypercalcemia.

PATIENT/FAMILY TEACHING

Stress importance of diet. Take tablets w/full glass of water, ½–1 hr after meals. Give liquid before meals. Do not take within 1–2 hrs of other oral medications, fiber-containing foods. Avoid excessive alcohol, tobacco, caffeine.

calfactant

cal-**fact**-tant
(Infasurf)

CLASSIFICATION

Lung surfactant

AVAILABILITY (Rx)

Intratracheal Suspension: 35 mg/ml vials

PHARMACOKINETICS

Absorption: Absorbs rapidly to lung alveolar lining and lung tissue.

ACTION/*THERAPEUTIC EFFECT*

Modifies alveolar surface tension, stabilizing the alveoli, *restoring surface activity to infant lungs. Improves lung compliance, respiratory gas exchange.*

USES

Prevention of respiratory distress syndrome (RDS) in premature infants <29 wks of gestational age and for the treatment of premature infants ≤72 hours of age who develop RSD and require endotracheal intubation.

ADMINISTRATION

INTRATRACHEAL:

- Instill through catheter inserted into infant's endotracheal tube.
- Draw dose into syringe from vial using a 20 gauge or larger needle.
- Do *not* shake; gently swirl for redispersion (visible flecks in the suspension and foaming at the surface are normal).
- Administer through a side-port adapter using a 5 French feeding catheter inserted into endotracheal tube while ventilation is continued over 20–30 breaths for each aliquot. Each of 4 aliquots should be administered with the patient in 1 of 4 different positions (prone, supine, right and left lateral).
- Administer repeat doses as

early as 6 hrs after previous dose for up to 4 doses.

INDICATIONS/ROUTES/DOSAGES

Respiratory distress syndrome: ***Endotracheal: Infant:*** Instill 3 ml/kg of birth weight as soon as possible after birth, administered as 2 doses of 1.5 ml/kg. Repeat doses of 3 ml/kg of birth weight, up to total of 3 doses 12 hrs apart.

CONTRAINDICATIONS

None significant.

CAUTIONS

Those at risk for circulatory overload.

INTERACTIONS

DRUG: None significant. **HERBAL:** None known. **FOOD:** None significant. **ALTERED LAB VALUES:** None significant.

SIDE EFFECTS

FREQUENT: Cyanosis **(65%),** airway obstruction **(39%),** bradycardia **(34%),** reflux of surfactant into endotracheal tube **(21%),** requirement of manual ventilation **(16%). OCCASIONAL (3%):** Reintubation.

ADVERSE REACTIONS/TOXIC EFFECTS

Stop calfactant administration if cyanosis, airway obstruction, bradycardia or reflux of surfactant into endotracheal tube occurs. After appropriate measures have been undertaken to reverse the condition, dosing may proceed.

PATIENT CONSIDERATIONS

BASELINE ASSESSMENT

Drug must be administered in a highly supervised setting. Clinicians in care of neonate must be experienced w/intubation, ventilator management. Abrupt discontinuation of drug therapy produces an elevation of platelet count within days. Give emotional support to parents.

INTERVENTION/EVALUATION

Monitor infant with arterial or transcutaneous measurement of systemic O_2 and CO_2. Assess lung sounds for rales and moist breath sounds.

candesartan cilexetil

can-deh-**sar**-tan sill-**ex**-eh-til
(Atacand)

FIXED-COMBINATION(S)
W/hydrochlorothiazide, a diuretic **(Atacand HTZ)**

PREGNANCY CATEGORY C
(Third trimester)

PREGNANCY CATEGORY D
(Second and third trimester)

CLASSIFICATION

Angiotensin II receptor antagonist

AVAILABILITY (Rx)

Tablets: 4 mg, 8 mg, 16 mg, 32 mg.

PHARMACODYNAMICS

	ONSET	PEAK	DURATION
Oral	—	3–4 hrs	24 hrs

PHARMACOKINETICS

Absorption: Rapidly and completely absorbed following oral administration. **Metabolism:** Undergoes minor hepatic metabolism to inactive metabolite. **Excretion:** Excreted unchanged in urine and feces via biliary system. **Half-life:** 9 hrs.

ACTION/*THERAPEUTIC EFFECT*

Potent vasodilator. An angiotensin II receptor (type AT_1) antagonist; blocks vasoconstrictor and aldosterone-secreting effects of angiotensin II, inhibiting the binding of angiotensin II to the AT_1 receptors, *producing vasodilation, decreased peripheral resistance, decrease in B/P.*

USES/*UNLABELED*

Treatment of hypertension alone or in combination with other antihypertensives. *Treatment of heart failure.*

ADMINISTRATION

ORAL:

- Give w/o regard to meals.

INDICATIONS/ROUTES/DOSAGES

Note: If antihypertensive effect using once-daily dosing is inadequate, twice-daily regimen at same total daily dose or an increase in dose may provide therapeutic response. May be given concurrently w/other antihypertensives. If B/P is not controlled by candesartan alone, a diuretic may be added.

Hypertension:

Oral: Adults, elderly, mildly impaired renal or hepatic function: Initially, 16 mg once daily in pts who are not volume depleted. Can be given once or twice daily with total daily doses ranging from 8 to 32 mg. Give lower dose in pts treated with diuretics, severe impaired renal function.

CONTRAINDICATIONS

None significant.

CAUTIONS

Renal/hepatic function impairment, renal arterial stenosis.

INTERACTIONS

DRUG: None significant. **HERBAL:** None known. **FOOD:** None significant. **ALTERED LAB VALUES:** May increase BUN, serum creatinine, SGOT (AST), SGPT (ALT), alkaline phosphatase, bilirubin. May decrease Hgb, Hct.

SIDE EFFECTS

OCCASIONAL: (3–6%): Upper respiratory infection, dizziness, back and leg pain. **RARE: (1–2%):** Pharyngitis, rhinitis, headache, fatigue, diarrhea, nausea, dry cough, peripheral edema.

ADVERSE REACTIONS/TOXIC EFFECTS

Overdosage may manifest as hypotension and tachycardia; bradycardia occurs less often. Institute supportive measures.

PATIENT CONSIDERATIONS

BASELINE ASSESSMENT

Obtain B/P and apical pulse immediately before each dose, in addition to regular monitoring (be alert to fluctuations). If excessive reduction in B/P occurs, place pt in supine position, feet slightly elevated. Question possibility of pregnancy (see Pregnancy Category). Assess medication history (especially diuretic). Question for history of hepatic/renal impairment, renal artery stenosis. Obtain BUN, serum creatinine, SGOT (AST), SGPT (ALT), alkaline phosphatase, bilirubin, Hgb, Hct, and vital signs, particularly B/P, pulse rate.

INTERVENTION/EVALUATION

Maintain hydration (offer fluids frequently). Assess for evidence of upper respiratory infection. Assist with ambulation if dizziness occurs. Monitor all blood serum levels. Assess B/P for hypertension/hypotension.

PATIENT/FAMILY TEACHING

Inform female pt regarding consequences of second- and third-trimester exposure to candesartan. Report pregnancy to physician as soon as possible. Avoid tasks that require alertness, motor skills (possible dizziness effect). Report any sign of infection (sore throat, fever). Do not stop taking medication. Need for lifelong control. Caution against exercising during hot weather (risk of dehydration, hypotension).

---

capecitabine

cap-eh-**sit**-a-bean
(Xeloda)

PREGNANCY CATEGORY D

CLASSIFICATION

Antineoplastic: metabolite

AVAILABILITY (Rx)

Tablets: 150 mg, 500 mg.

PHARMACODYNAMICS

	ONSET	PEAK	DURATION
Oral	—	1.5–2 hrs	—

PHARMACOKINETICS

Absorption: Readily absorbed from GI tract. **Metabolism:** Extensively metabolized in liver. Primarily bound to human albumin. **Excretion:** Eliminated in urine. **Half-life:** 45 min.

ACTION/*THERAPEUTIC EFFECT*

Enzymatically converted to 5-FU. Inhibits enzymes necessary for synthesis of essential cellular components, *interfering with DNA synthesis, RNA processing and protein synthesis.*

USES

Treatment of metastatic breast cancer resistant to other therapy.

ADMINISTRATION

ORAL:

- Give within 30 min after a meal.
- Swallow tablets w/water only.

INDICATIONS/ROUTES/DOSAGES

Metastatic breast cancer:
Oral: Adults, elderly: Initially, 2,500 mg/m^2/day in two equally divided doses 12 hrs apart for 2 wks. Follow with a 2 wk rest period given as 3 wk cycles.

CONTRAINDICATIONS

Hypersensitivity to 5-fluorouracil.

CAUTIONS

Renal function impairment, hepatic dysfunction caused by liver metastases, elderly (higher incidence of adverse events), coronary artery disease.

INTERACTIONS

DRUG: ***Antacids*** increase blood concentration of capecitabine. Concentration of 5-fluorouracil is increased and toxicity of capecitabine may be increased by ***leucovorin***. **HERBAL:** None known. **FOOD:** Food reduces rate, extent of drug absorption in serum blood concentration. **ALTERED LAB VALUES:** May increase bilirubin, alkaline phosphatase, SGOT (AST), SGPT (ALT). May decrease Hgb, WBCs, thrombocytes.

SIDE EFFECTS

FREQUENT: (≥5%): Diarrhea, nausea, vomiting, stomatitis, hand and foot syndrome (palmar-plantar erythema, paresthesia, tingling, swelling, blistering, desquamation), fatigue, anorexia, dermatitis, GI irritation. **OCCASIONAL: (≤5%):**

Constipation, dyspepsia, nail disorder, headache, dizziness, insomnia, dehydration, eye irritation, pyrexia, edema, myalgia, limb pain.

ADVERSE REACTIONS/TOXIC EFFECTS

Blood dyscrasias (neutropenia, thrombocytopenia, anemia, lymphopenia) due to bone marrow depression occur occasionally.

PATIENT CONSIDERATIONS

BASELINE ASSESSMENT

Obtain baseline bilirubin, alkaline phosphatase, SGOT (AST), SGPT (ALT), Hgb, WBCs, thrombocytes. Question for history of hepatic/renal impairment, metastasis.

INTERVENTION/EVALUATION

A grade 2 diarrhea (4–6 stools/day or nocturnal stools, grade 3 diarrhea (7–9 stools/day or incontinence and malabsorption), grade 4 diarrhea (10 stools/day or grossly bloody diarrhea) requires immediately stopping medication until event is resolved or decreased in intensity before treatment can resume. A grade 2 or greater nausea (food intake is significantly increased but able to eat intermittently) requires immediately stopping medication until event is resolved or decreased in intensity before treatment can resume. A grade 2 or greater vomiting (2–5 episodes in 24 hrs) requires immediately stopping medication until event is resolved or decreased in number before treatment can resume. A grade 2 or greater hand and foot syndrome (painful erythema and swelling of hands or feet) requires immediately stopping medication until event is resolved or decreased before treatment can resume. A grade 2 or greater stomatitis (painful erythema, edema or ulcers of mouth or tongue, but able to eat) requires immediately stopping medication until event is resolved or decreased before treatment can resume.

PATIENT/FAMILY TEACHING

Report a fever 100.5° F or any sign of infection (sore throat, chills). Encourage pt to recognize symptoms of grade 2 toxicities associated with treatment (see *Intervention/Evaluation*) and report events promptly to physician.

---

capsaicin

cap-**say**-sin
(Zostrix)

CANADIAN AVAILABILITY
Zostrix

PREGNANCY CATEGORY C

CLASSIFICATION

Topical analgesic

AVAILABILITY (OTC)

Cream: 0.025%, 0.075%

ACTION/*THERAPEUTIC EFFECT*

Depletes and prevents reaccumulation of the chemomediator of pain impulses (substance P) from peripheral sensory neurons to CNS, *relieving pain.*

USES/*UNLABELED*

Treatment of neuralgia (e.g., pain following shingles, painful diabetic neuropathy), osteoarthritis, rheumatoid arthritis. *Treatment of neurogenic pain.*

INDICATIONS/ROUTES/DOSAGE

Usual topical dosage:
Topical: Adults, elderly, children >2 yrs: Apply directly to affected area 3–4 times/day. Continue for 14–28 days for optimal clinical response.

CONTRAINDICATIONS

Hypersensitivity to any component of the preparation.

CAUTIONS

For external use only.

INTERACTIONS

DRUG: None significant. **HERBAL:** None known. **FOOD:** None significant. **ALTERED LAB VALUES:** None significant.

SIDE EFFECTS

FREQUENT: Burning, stinging, erythema at site of application.

PATIENT CONSIDERATIONS

PATIENT/FAMILY TEACHING

For external use only. Avoid contact w/eyes, broken/irritated skin. Transient burning may occur on application, usually disappears after 72 hrs. Wash hands immediately after application. If there is no improvement or condition deteriorates after 28 days, discontinue use and consult physician.

---

captopril

cap-toe-prill
(Capoten)

FIXED-COMBINATION(S)
W/hydrochlorothiazide, a diuretic **(Capozide)**

CANADIAN AVAILABILITY
Capoten, Novo-Captoril

PREGNANCY CATEGORY D

CLASSIFICATION

Angiotensin-converting enzyme (ACE) inhibitor

AVAILABILITY (Rx)

Tablets: 12.5 mg, 25 mg, 50 mg, 100 mg

PHARMACODYNAMICS

	ONSET	PEAK	DURATION
Oral	0.25 hrs	0.5–1.5 hrs	dose related

PHARMACOKINETICS

Absorption: Rapid, well absorbed from GI tract (decreased in presence of food). **Metabolism:** Metabolized in liver. **Excretion:** Primarily excreted in urine. Removed by hemodialysis. **Half-life:** <3 hrs (increased in decreased renal function).

ACTION/*THERAPEUTIC EFFECT*

Suppresses renin-angiotensin-aldosterone system (prevents conversion of angiotensin I to angiotensin II, a potent vasoconstrictor; may also inhibit angiotensin II at local vascular and renal sites). Decreases plasma angiotensin II, increases plasma renin activity, decreases aldosterone secretion. *Reduces peripheral arterial resistance, pulmonary capillary wedge pressure, improves cardiac output, exercise tolerance.*

USES/*UNLABELED*

Treatment of hypertension alone or in combination w/other antihypertensives. Adjunctive therapy for CHF (in combination w/cardiac glycosides, diuretics). Reduces development of severe heart failure following MI in pts w/impaired left ventricular (LV) function. Treats nephropathy/prevents kidney failure in type I diabetes. *Treatment of hypertension/renal crises in scleroderma.*

ADMINISTRATION

ORAL:

- Best taken 1 hr before meals for maximum absorption (food significantly decreases drug absorption).
- Tablets may be crushed.

INDICATIONS/ROUTES/DOSAGE

Hypertension:
Oral: Adults, elderly: Initially, 12.5–25 mg 2–3 times/day. After 1–2 wks, may increase to 50 mg 2–3 times/day. Diuretic may be added if no response in additional 1–2 wks. If taken in combination w/diuretic, may increase to 100–150 mg 2–3 times/day after 1–2 wks. ***Maintenance:*** 25–150 mg 2–3 times/day. ***Maximum:*** 450 mg/day.

CHF:
Oral: Adults, elderly: Initially, 6.25–25 mg 3 times/day. Increase to 50 mg 3 times/day. After at least 2 wks, may increase to 50–100 mg 3 times/day. ***Maximum:*** 450 mg/day.

Post MI, impaired liver function:
Oral: Adults, elderly: 6.25 mg once, then 12.5 mg 3 times/day. Increase to 25 mg 3 times/day over several days up to 50 mg 3 times/day over several wks.

Nephropathy/prevention of kidney failure:
Oral: Adults, elderly: 25 mg 3 times/day.

CONTRAINDICATIONS

History of angioedema w/previous treatment w/ACE inhibitors.

CAUTIONS

Renal impairment, those w/sodium depletion or on diuretic therapy, dialysis, hypovolemia, coronary/cerebrovascular insufficiency.

INTERACTIONS

DRUG: ***Alcohol, diuretics, hypotensive agents*** may increase effect. ***NSAIDs*** may decrease effect. ***Potassium-sparing diuretics, potassium supplements*** may cause hyperkalemia. May increase ***lithium*** concentration, toxicity. **HERBAL:** None known. **FOOD:** None significant. **ALTERED LAB VALUES:** May increase potassium, SGOT (AST), SGPT (ALT), alkaline phosphatase, bilirubin, BUN, creatinine. May decrease sodium. May cause positive ANA titer.

SIDE EFFECTS

FREQUENT: Rash and/or pruritus. **OCCASIONAL:** Headache, cough, insomnia, dizziness, fatigue, paresthesia, malaise, nausea, diarrhea/constipation, dry mouth. **RARE:** Angioedema, tachycardia.

ADVERSE REACTIONS/TOXIC EFFECTS

Excessive hypotension ("first-dose syncope") may occur in those w/CHF, severely salt/volume depleted. Angioedema (swelling of face/lips), hyperkalemia occur rarely. Agranulocytosis, neutropenia may be noted in those w/impaired renal function or collagen vascular disease (systemic lupus erythematosus, scleroderma). Nephrotic syndrome may be noted in those w/history of renal disease.

PATIENT CONSIDERATIONS

BASELINE ASSESSMENT

Obtain B/P immediately before each dose, in addition to regular monitoring (be alert to fluctuations). If excessive reduction in B/P occurs, place pt in supine position w/legs elevated. Renal

function tests should be performed before therapy begins. In pts w/prior renal disease or receiving dosages higher than 150 mg/day, urine test for protein by dipstick method should be made w/first urine of day before therapy begins and periodically thereafter. In those w/renal impairment, autoimmune disease, or taking drugs that affect leukocytes or immune response, CBC and differential count should be performed before therapy begins and q2wks for 3 mos, then periodically thereafter.

INTERVENTION/EVALUATION

Assess skin for rash, hives. Assist w/ambulation if dizziness occurs. Check for urinary frequency. Assess lung sounds for rales, wheezing in those w/CHF. Monitor urinalysis for proteinuria. Assess for anorexia secondary to decreased taste perception. Monitor serum potassium levels in those on concurrent diuretic therapy.

PATIENT/FAMILY TEACHING

To reduce hypotensive effect, rise slowly from lying to sitting position and permit legs to dangle from bed momentarily before standing. Report peripheral edema or any sign of infection (sore throat, fever). Several wks may be needed for full therapeutic effect of B/P reduction. Skipping doses or voluntarily discontinuing drug may produce severe, rebound hypertension. Avoid alcohol.

carbachol

(Isopto-Carbachol)

See Classification section under: Antiglaucoma

carbamazepine

car-bah-**may**-zeh-peen

(Carbatrol, Epitol, Tegretol)

CANADIAN AVAILABILITY

Apo-Carbamazepine, Tegretol

PREGNANCY CATEGORY C

CLASSIFICATION

Anticonvulsant

AVAILABILITY (Rx)

Tablets (chewable): 100 mg. **Tablets:** 200 mg. **Tablets (extended-release):** 100 mg, 200 mg, 300 mg, 400 mg. **Capsules (extended-release):** 200 mg, 300 mg. **Oral Suspension:** 100 mg/5 ml.

PHARMACOKINETICS

Absorption: Slowly, completely absorbed from GI tract. **Metabolism:** Metabolized in liver to active metabolite. **Excretion:** Primarily excreted in urine. **Half-life:** 25–65 hrs (decreased w/chronic use).

ACTION/*THERAPEUTIC EFFECT*

Decreases sodium, calcium ion influx into neuronal membranes, reducing post-tetanic potentiation at synapse; *prevents repetitive discharge.*

USES/*UNLABELED*

Management of generalized tonic-clonic seizures (grand mal), complex partial seizures (temporal lobe, psychomotor), mixed seizures; treatment of trigeminal neuralgia (tic douloureux). *Treatment of neurogenic pain, bipolar disorder, diabetes insipidus, alcohol withdrawal, psychotic disorders.*

STORAGE/HANDLING

Store oral suspension, tablets at room temperature.

ADMINISTRATION

ORAL:

- Give w/meals to reduce risk of GI distress.
- Shake oral suspension well; do not administer simultaneously w/other liquid medicine.
- Do not crush extended-release tablets.

INDICATIONS/ROUTES/DOSAGE

Note: When replacement by another anticonvulsant is necessary, decrease carbamazepine gradually as therapy begins w/low replacement dose. When transferring from tablets to suspension, divide total tablet daily dose into smaller, more frequent doses of suspension. Administer extended-release tablets in 2 divided doses.

Seizure control:
Oral: Adults, elderly, children >12 yrs: Initially, 200 mg 2 times/day. Increase dosage up to 200 mg/day at weekly intervals until response is attained. ***Maintenance:*** 800–1,200 mg/day. Do not exceed 1,000 mg/day in children 12–15 yrs, 1,200 mg/day in pts >15 yrs. ***Children 6–12 yrs:*** Initially, 100 mg 2 times/day. Increase by 100 mg/day until response is attained. ***Maintenance:*** 400–800 mg/day. Give dosage 200 mg or greater/day in 3–4 equally divided doses. ***Syrup: Children 6–12 yrs:*** Initially, 50 mg 4 times/day. Increase dosage slowly (reduces sedation risk). ***Children <6 yrs:*** 10–20 mg/kg/day in 2–4 divided doses.

Trigeminal neuralgia:
Oral: Adults, elderly: 100 mg 2 times/day on day 1. Increase by 100 mg q12h until pain is relieved. ***Maintenance:*** 200–1,200 mg/day. Do not exceed 1,200 mg/day.

CONTRAINDICATIONS

History of bone marrow depression, history of hypersensitivity to tricyclic antidepressants, concomitant use of MAOIs.

CAUTIONS

Impaired cardiac, hepatic, renal function.

INTERACTIONS

DRUG: May decrease effect of ***steroids, anticoagulants.*** May increase metabolism of ***anticonvulsants, barbiturates, benzodiazepines, valproic acid. Tricyclic antidepressants, haloperidol, antipsychotics*** may increase CNS depressant effects. ***Cimetidine*** may increase concentration, toxicity. May decrease effects of ***estrogens, quinidine, clarithromycin, diltiazem, erythromycin, propoxyphene. Verapamil*** may increase toxicity. May increase metabolism of ***isoniazid*** (hepatotoxicity). ***Isoniazid*** may increase concentration, toxicity. ***MAO inhibitors*** may cause hypertensive crises, convulsions. **HERBAL:** None known. **FOOD:** Grapefruit juice increases concentration. **ALTERED LAB VALUES:** May increase BUN, glucose, protein, SGOT (AST), SGPT (ALT), alkaline phosphatase, bilirubin, cholesterol, HDL, triglycerides. May decrease calcium, T_3, T_4, T_4 index.

SIDE EFFECTS

OCCASIONAL: Drowsiness, dizziness, nausea, vomiting, visual abnormalities (spots before eyes, difficulty focusing, blurred vision), dry mouth/pharynx, tongue irritation, headache, water retention, increased sweating, constipation/diarrhea.

ADVERSE REACTIONS/TOXIC EFFECTS

Toxic reactions appear as blood

dyscrasias (aplastic anemia, agranulocytosis, thrombocytopenia, leukopenia, leukocytosis, eosinophilia), cardiovascular disturbances (CHF, hypo/hypertension, thrombophlebitis, arrhythmias), dermatologic effects (rash, urticaria, pruritus, photosensitivity). Abrupt withdrawal may precipitate status epilepticus.

PATIENT CONSIDERATIONS

BASELINE ASSESSMENT

Seizures

Review history of seizure disorder (intensity, frequency, duration, LOC). Provide safety precautions, quiet, dark environment. CBC, platelet count, serum iron determinations, urinalysis, BUN should be performed before therapy begins and periodically during therapy.

INTERVENTION/EVALUATION

Seizures

Observe frequently for recurrence of seizure activity. Assess for clinical improvement (decrease in intensity/frequency of seizures). Monitor for therapeutic serum level (3–14 mcg/ml). Assess for clinical evidence of early toxic signs (fever, sore throat, mouth ulcerations, easy bruising, unusual bleeding, joint pain).

Neuralgia

Avoid triggering tic douloureux (draft, talking, washing face, jarring bed, hot/warm/cold food or liquids).

PATIENT/FAMILY TEACHING

Do not abruptly withdraw medication following long-term use (may precipitate seizures). Strict maintenance of drug therapy is essential for seizure control. Drowsiness usually disappears during continued therapy. Avoid tasks that require alertness, motor skills until response to drug is established. Report visual abnormalities. Blood tests should be repeated frequently during first 3 mos of therapy and at monthly intervals thereafter for 2–3 yrs. Do not take liquid simultaneously w/other liquid medicine. Report unusual bleeding/bruising, fever, sore throat, rash, ulcers in mouth. Avoid giving w/grapefruit juice.

---

carbenicillin

(Geocillin)

See Classification section under: Antibiotic: penicillins

---

carbidopa/levodopa

car-bih-dope-ah/**lev**-oh-dope-ah

(Sinemet)

CANADIAN AVAILABILITY

Sinemet

PREGNANCY CATEGORY C

CLASSIFICATION

Antiparkinson

AVAILABILITY (Rx)

Tablets (expressed as carbidopa/levodopa): 10 mg/100 mg, 25 mg/100 mg, 25 mg/250 mg. **Tablets (extended-release):** 25 mg/100 mg; 50 mg/200 mg.

PHARMACOKINETICS

Carbidopa: **Absorption:** Rapidly, completely absorbed from GI tract. Widely distributed. **Excretion:** Excreted primarily in urine.

Half-life: 1–2 hrs. ***Levodopa:*** Converted to dopamine. **Excretion:** Excreted primarily in urine. **Half-life:** 1–3 hrs.

ACTION/ *THERAPEUTIC EFFECT*

Converted to dopamine in basal ganglia. Increases dopamine concentration in brain, inhibiting hyperactive cholinergic activity, *reducing tremor.* Carbidopa prevents peripheral breakdown of levodopa, allowing more levodopa to be available for transport into brain.

USES

Treatment of idiopathic Parkinson's disease (paralysis agitans), postencephalitic parkinsonism, symptomatic parkinsonism following injury to nervous system by carbon monoxide poisoning, manganese intoxication.

ADMINISTRATION

ORAL:

- Scored tablets may be crushed.
- May be given w/o regard to meals.
- Do not crush sustained-release tablet; may cut in half.

INDICATIONS/ROUTES/DOSAGE

PARKINSONISM:

Not receiving levodopa:
Oral: Adults: 25/100 mg tablet 3 times/day or 10/100 mg tablet 3–4 times/day. May increase by 1 tablet every 1–2 days up to 8 tablets/day.

Usual elderly dosage:
Oral: Initially: 25/100 mg tablet 2 times/day, gradually increased as necessary.

Sustained-release:
Adults: 1 tablet 2 times/day no closer than 6 hrs between doses. ***Range:*** 2–8 tablets at 4–8 hr intervals. May increase dose at intervals not less than 3 days.

Receiving only levodopa:
Note: Discontinue levodopa at least 8 hrs prior to carbidopa/levodopa. Initiate w/dose providing at least 25% of previous levodopa dosage.

Oral: Adults (<1,500 mg levodopa/day): 1 tablet (25/100 mg) 3–4 times/day.

Oral: Adults (>1,500 mg levodopa/day): 1 tablet (25/250 mg) 3–4 times/day.

Sustained-release:
Oral: Adults: 1 tablet 2 times/day.

Receiving carbidopa/levodopa:
Sustained-release:
Oral: Adults: Provide about 10% more levodopa; may increase up to 30% more at 4–8 hr dosing intervals.

CONTRAINDICATIONS

Narrow-angle glaucoma, those on MAO inhibitor therapy.

CAUTIONS

History of MI, bronchial asthma (tartrazine sensitivity), emphysema; severe cardiac, pulmonary, renal, hepatic, endocrine disease; active peptic ulcer; treated open-angle glaucoma.

INTERACTIONS

DRUG: ***Anticonvulsants, benzodiazepines, haloperidol, phenothiazines*** may decrease effect. ***MAO inhibitors*** may increase risk of hypertensive crises. ***Selegiline*** may increase dyskinesias, nausea, orthostatic hypotension, confusion, hallucinations. **HERBAL:** None known. **FOOD:** None significant. **ALTERED LAB VALUES:** May increase alkaline phosphatase,

SGOT (AST), SGPT (ALT), LDH, bilirubin, BUN.

SIDE EFFECTS

FREQUENT: Uncontrolled body movements (including face, tongue, arms, upper body), depression, anxiety, confusion, nervousness. **OCCASIONAL:** Difficulty urinating, irregular heartbeats, nausea, vomiting, dizziness, lightheadedness, decreased appetite, blurred vision, constipation, dry mouth, flushed skin, headache, insomnia, muscle twitching, diarrhea, unusual tiredness, darkening of urine. **RARE:** Hypertension, ulcer, hemolytic anemia (tired/weakness).

ADVERSE REACTIONS/TOXIC EFFECTS

High incidence of involuntary choreiform, dystonic, dyskinetic movements may be noted in pts on long-term therapy. Akinesia (temporary muscular weakness, lasts 1 min to 1 hr, also known as "on-off" phenomenon) may occur. Mental changes (paranoid ideation, psychotic episodes, depression) may be noted. Numerous mild to severe CNS, psychiatric disturbances may include reduced attention span, anxiety, nightmares, daytime somnolence, euphoria, fatigue, paranoia, hallucinations.

PATIENT CONSIDERATIONS

BASELINE ASSESSMENT

Assess symptoms of parkinsonism. Instruct pt to void before giving medication (reduces risk of urinary retention).

INTERVENTION/EVALUATION

Be alert to neurologic effects: headache, lethargy, mental confusion, agitation. Monitor for evidence of dyskinesia (difficulty w/movement). Assess for clinical reversal of symptoms (improvement of tremor of head/hands at rest, mask-like facial expression, shuffling gait, muscular rigidity).

PATIENT/FAMILY TEACHING

Avoid tasks that require alertness, motor skills until response to drug is established. Dry mouth, drowsiness, dizziness may be an expected response to drug. Avoid alcoholic beverages during therapy. Sugarless gum, sips of tepid water may relieve dry mouth. Coffee/tea may help reduce drowsiness. Take w/food to minimize GI upset. Effects may be delayed from several weeks to months. May cause darkening urine/sweat (not harmful). Report any uncontrolled movement of face, eyelids, mouth, tongue, arms, hands, legs, mental changes, palpitations, irregular heartbeats, severe or continuing nausea/vomiting, difficulty in urinating.

---

carboplatin

(Paraplatin)

See classification section under: Cancer chemotherapy

---

carboprost

kar-boe-prost

(Hemabate)

CLASSIFICATION

Prostaglandin

AVAILABILITY (Rx)

Injection: 250 mcg/ml

PHARMACOKINETICS

Metabolism: Metabolized in liver and by enzymes in maternal lung tissues. Mean abortion time: 16 hrs. **Excretion:** Primarily excreted in urine.

ACTION/*THERAPEUTIC EFFECT*

Direct action on myometrium. Stimulates contraction in gravid uterus, *produces cervical dilation and softening.*

USES/*UNLABELED*

To induce abortion between the 13th and 20th wk of pregnancy (as calculated from the first day of the last menstrual period), to treat postpartum hemorrhage related to uterine atony not responsive to conventional therapy. *Treatment of incomplete abortion, benign hydatiform mole, induction of labor, ripen cervix prior to abortion.*

STORAGE/HANDLING

Refrigerate.

ADMINISTRATION

IM:

- Administer only in hospital setting w/emergency equipment available.
- Give deep IM and rotate sites if subsequent doses necessary.
- Avoid skin contact w/carboprost; if spilled on skin, wash thoroughly w/soap and water.

INDICATIONS/ROUTES/DOSAGE

Abortion:
IM: Adults: Initially, 100–250 mcg, may repeat at 1.5–3.5 hr intervals. May increase up to 500 mcg if uterine contractility inadequate. ***Maximum:*** 12 mg total dose or continuous administration >2 days.

Postpartum hemorrhage:
IM: Adults: Initially, 250 mcg, may repeat at 15–90 min intervals. ***Maximum:*** 2 mg total dose.

CONTRAINDICATIONS

Hypersensitivity to carboprost or other prostaglandins; acute pelvic inflammatory disease; active cardiac, pulmonary, renal, or hepatic disease.

CAUTIONS

History of asthma, hypo/hypertension, anemia, jaundice, diabetes, epilepsy, compromised (scarred) uterus, cardiovascular, adrenal, or hepatic disease.

INTERACTIONS

DRUG: ***Oxytocin, oxytocics*** may cause uterine hypertonus, leading to uterine rupture or cervical lacerations. **HERBAL:** None known. **FOOD:** None significant. **ALTERED LAB VALUES:** None significant.

SIDE EFFECTS

FREQUENT: Nausea, vomiting, diarrhea. **OCCASIONAL:** Fever, chills, facial flushing, headache, hyper/hypotension. **RARE:** Wheezing, troubled breathing, tightness in chest (especially asthmatic pts). Stomach cramps/pain, increased uterine bleeding, foul-smelling lochia may indicate postabortion complications.

ADVERSE REACTIONS/TOXIC EFFECTS

Excessive dosage may cause uterine hypertonicity w/spasm and tetanic contraction, leading to cervical laceration/perforation, uterine rupture/hemorrhage.

PATIENT CONSIDERATIONS

BASELINE ASSESSMENT

Question for hypersensitivity to carboprost or other prostagland-

ins. Establish baseline B/P, temperature, pulse, respiration. Obtain orders for antiemetics and antidiarrheals, meperidine or other pain medication for abdominal cramps. Assess any uterine activity/vaginal bleeding.

INTERVENTION/EVALUATION

Check strength, duration, frequency of contractions and monitor vital signs q15min until stable, then hourly until abortion complete. Check resting uterine tone. Administer medications for relief of GI effects if indicated, abdominal cramps. Provide emotional support as necessary.

PATIENT/FAMILY TEACHING

Report fever, chills, foul-smelling/increased vaginal discharge, uterine cramps/pain promptly.

---

carisoprodol

(Soma, Rela)

See Classification section under: Skeletal muscle relaxants

---

carmustine

(BiCNU, Gliadel Wafer)

See Classification section under: Cancer chemotherapy

---

carteolol hydrochloride

cart-**hee**-oh-lol

(Cartrol, Ocupress)

PREGNANCY CATEGORY C

(D if used in second or third trimester)

CLASSIFICATION

Beta-adrenergic blocker

AVAILABILITY (Rx)

Tablets: 2.5 mg, 5 mg. **Ophthalmic Solution:** 1%.

PHARMACOKINETICS

Absorption: Well absorbed from GI tract. **Metabolism:** Minimally metabolized in liver. **Excretion:** Primarily excreted unchanged in urine. **Half-life:** 6 hrs (increased in decreased renal function).

ACTION/*THERAPEUTIC EFFECT*

Blocks effects of adrenergic transmitter by competitive binding to receptor site. Predominantly blocks $beta_1$-adrenergic receptors in cardiac tissue, *slowing sinus heart rate, decreasing cardiac output, decreasing B/P.* Large doses may block $beta_2$-adrenergic receptors, *increasing airway resistance.* ***Ophthalmic:*** Reduces aqueous humor production, *decreasing intraocular pressure.*

USES/*UNLABELED*

Oral: Management of mild to moderate hypertension. Used alone or in combination w/diuretics, especially thiazide type. **Ophthalmic:** Reduces intraocular pressure in management of chronic open-angle glaucoma, ocular hypertension. *W/miotics decreases IOP in acute/chronic angle closure glaucoma, treatment of secondary glaucoma, malignant glaucoma, angle closure glaucoma during/after iridectomy.*

ADMINISTRATION

ORAL:

- May give w/o regard to food.

OPHTHALMIC:

- Place finger on lower eyelid and pull out until pocket is formed between eye and lower lid. Hold dropper above pocket and place prescribed number of drops in pocket.

- Close eye gently. Apply digital pressure to lacrimal sac for 1–2 min (minimized drainage into nose and throat, reducing risk of systemic effects).
- Remove excess solution w/tissue.

INDICATIONS/ROUTES/DOSAGE

Hypertension:
Oral: Adults, elderly: Initially, 2.5 mg/day as single dose either alone or in combination w/diuretic. May increase gradually to 5–10 mg/day as single dose. ***Maintenance:*** 2.5–5 mg/day.

Dosage in renal impairment:

CREATININE CLEARANCE	DOSAGE INTERVAL
>60 ml/min	24 hrs
20–60 ml/min	48 hrs
<20 ml/min	72 hrs

Usual ophthalmic dosage:
Adults, elderly: 1 drop 2 times/day.

CONTRAINDICATIONS

Bronchial asthma, COPD, bronchospasm, overt cardiac failure, cardiogenic shock, heart block greater than first degree, persistently severe bradycardia.

CAUTIONS

Impaired renal/hepatic function, peripheral vascular disease, hyperthyroidism, diabetes, inadequate cardiac function.

INTERACTIONS

DRUG: ***Diuretics, other hypotensives*** may increase hypotensive effect; ***sympathomimetics, xanthines*** may mutually inhibit effects; may mask symptoms of hypoglycemia, prolong hypoglycemic effect of ***insulin, oral hypoglycemics; NSAIDs*** may decrease antihypertensive effect; ***cimetidine*** may increase concentration. **HERBAL:** None known. **FOOD:** None significant. **ALTERED LAB VALUES:** May increase ANA titer, SGOT (AST), SGPT (ALT), alkaline phosphatase, LDH, bilirubin, BUN, creatinine, potassium, uric acid, lipoproteins, triglycerides.

SIDE EFFECTS

Generally well tolerated, w/mild and transient effects. **FREQUENT:** ***Oral:*** Hypotension manifested as dizziness, nausea, diaphoresis, headache, cold extremities, fatigue, constipation/diarrhea. ***Ophthalmic:*** Redness of eye or inside of eyelids, decreased night vision. **OCCASIONAL:** ***Oral:*** Insomnia, flatulence, urinary frequency, impotence or decreased libido. ***Ophthalmic:*** Blepharoconjunctivitis, edema, droopy eyelid, staining of cornea, blurred vision, brow ache, increased light sensitivity, burning, stinging. **RARE:** Rash, arthralgia, myalgia, confusion (especially elderly), change in taste.

ADVERSE REACTIONS/TOXIC EFFECTS

Abrupt withdrawal (particularly in those w/coronary artery disease) may produce angina or precipitate MI. May precipitate thyroid crisis in those w/thyrotoxicosis.

PATIENT CONSIDERATIONS

Baseline Assessment

Assess baseline renal/liver function tests. Assess B/P, apical pulse immediately before drug is administered (if pulse is 60/min or below, or systolic B/P is below 90 mm Hg, withhold medication, contact physician).

Intervention/Evaluation

Assess pulse for strength/weakness, irregular rate, bradycardia. Monitor EKG for cardiac changes. Assist w/ambulation if dizziness occurs. Assess for peripheral

edema of hands, feet (usually, first area of low extremity swelling is behind medial malleolus in ambulatory, sacral area in bedridden). Monitor pattern of daily bowel activity and stool consistency. Assess skin for development of rash. Monitor any unusual changes in pt.

Ophthalmic
Monitor for potential systemic reaction.

PATIENT/FAMILY TEACHING

Do not abruptly discontinue medication (compliance w/therapy regimen is essential to control hypertension). If dizziness occurs, sit or lie down immediately. Full therapeutic response may not occur for up to 2 wks. Avoid tasks that require alertness, motor skills until response to drug is established. Report excessively slow pulse rate (<60 beats/min), peripheral numbness, dizziness. Do not use nasal decongestants, OTC cold preparations (stimulants) w/o physician approval. Outpatients should monitor B/P, pulse before taking medication. Restrict salt, alcohol intake.

Ophthalmic
Instruct pt on proper administration of drops. Do not use after expiration date. Transient stinging or discomfort is common; notify physician of severe or continued discomfort.

carvedilol

car-**veh**-dih-lol
(Coreg)

CANADIAN AVAILABILITY
Coreg

PREGNANCY CATEGORY C

CLASSIFICATION

Beta-adrenergic blocker; antihypertensive

AVAILABILITY (Rx)

Tablets: 3.125 mg, 6.25 mg, 12.5 mg, 25 mg

PHARMACODYNAMICS

	ONSET	PEAK	DURATION
Oral	30 min	1–2 hrs	24 hrs

PHARMACOKINETICS

Absorption: Rapidly and extensively absorbed from GI tract. **Metabolism:** Metabolized in liver. **Excretion:** Excreted primarily via bile into feces. **Half-life:** 7–10 hrs. Food delays rate of absorption.

ACTION/*THERAPEUTIC EFFECT*

Possesses nonselective beta-blocking and alpha-adrenergic blocking activity. *Reduces cardiac output, exercise-induced tachycardia, and reflex orthostatic tachycardia;* causes vasodilation; *reduces peripheral vascular resistance.*

USES/*UNLABELED*

Management of essential hypertension. Used alone or in combination w/diuretics, especially thiazide type. Treatment of CHF. *Treatment of angina pectoris, idiopathic cardiomyopathy.*

ADMINISTRATION

ORAL:

- Give w/food (slows rate of absorption, reduces risk of orthostatic effects).
- Take standing systolic B/P 1 hr after dosing as guide for tolerance.

INDICATIONS/DOSAGE/ROUTES

Hypertension:
Oral: Adults, elderly: Initially, 6.25

mg twice daily. May double at 7–14 day intervals to highest tolerated dose. **Maximum:** 50 mg/day.

CHF:
Oral: Adults, elderly: Initially, 3.125 mg twice daily. May double at 2 wk intervals to highest tolerated dose. **Maximum:** <85 kg: 25 mg twice daily; >85 kg: 50 mg twice daily.

CONTRAINDICATIONS

Class IV decompensated cardiac failure, bronchial asthma or related bronchospastic conditions, second- or third-degree AV block, cardiogenic shock, severe bradycardia.

CAUTIONS

CHF controlled w/digitalis, diuretics, or angiotensin-converting enzyme inhibitor, peripheral vascular disease, anesthesia, diabetes mellitus, hypoglycemia, thyrotoxicosis, impaired hepatic function.

INTERACTIONS

DRUG: ***Diuretics, other hypotensives*** may increase hypotensive effect; may mask symptoms of hypoglycemia, prolong hypoglycemic effect of ***insulin, oral hypoglycemics. Catapres*** may potentiate B/P effects, ***calcium blockers*** increase risk of conduction disturbances, increases ***digoxin*** concentrations. ***Cimetidine*** may increase concentration, ***rifampin*** decreases concentration. HERBAL: None known. FOOD: None significant. ALTERED LAB VALUES: None significant.

SIDE EFFECTS

Generally well tolerated, w/mild and transient side effects. FREQUENT (>10%): Fatigue, upper respiratory tract infection, chest pain. OCCASIONAL: Pain, edema, bradycardia, hypotension, headache, nausea, vomiting, abdominal pain, increased weight, back pain, arthralgia, sinusitis, bronchitis.

ADVERSE REACTIONS/TOXIC EFFECTS

Overdosage may produce profound bradycardia, hypotension, bronchospasm, cardiac insufficiency, cardiogenic shock, cardiac arrest. Abrupt withdrawal may result in sweating, palpitations, headache, tremulousness. May precipitate CHF, MI in those w/cardiac disease, thyroid storm in those w/thyrotoxicosis, peripheral ischemia in those w/existing peripheral vascular disease. Hypoglycemia may occur in previously controlled diabetics.

PATIENT CONSIDERATIONS

Baseline Assessment

Assess B/P, apical pulse immediately before drug is administered (if pulse is 60/min or below, or systolic B/P is below 90 mm Hg, withhold medication, contact physician).

Intervention/Evaluation

Monitor B/P for hypotension, respiration for shortness of breath. Assess pulse for strength/weakness, irregular rate, bradycardia. Monitor EKG for cardiac arrhythmias. Assist w/ambulation if dizziness occurs. Assess for evidence of CHF: dyspnea (particularly on exertion or lying down), night cough, peripheral edema, distended neck veins. Monitor I&O (increase in weight, decrease in urine output may indicate CHF).

Patient/Family Teaching

Full antihypertensive effect noted 1–2 wks. Contact lens wearers

may experience decreased lacrimation. Take w/food. Do not abruptly discontinue medication. Compliance w/therapy regimen is essential to control hypertension. Avoid tasks that require alertness, motor skills until response to drug is established. Report excessive fatigue, prolonged dizziness. Do not use nasal decongestants, OTC cold preparations (stimulants) w/o physician approval. Monitor B/P, pulse before taking medication. Restrict salt, alcohol intake.

cascara sagrada

cass-**care**-ah sah-**graud**-ah
(Cascara Sagrada)

FIXED-COMBINATION(S)
W/milk of magnesia, a saline laxative (Same)

CANADIAN AVAILABILITY
Cascara Sagrada

PREGNANCY CATEGORY C

CLASSIFICATION

Laxative: Stimulant

AVAILABILITY (OTC)

Tablets: 325 mg. **Liquid:** (18% alcohol).

PHARMACODYNAMICS

	ONSET	PEAK	DURATION
Oral	6–12 hrs	—	—

PHARMACOKINETICS

Absorption: Minimal absorption after oral administration. Hydrolyzed by enzymes of colonic flora to active form. **Metabolism:** Absorbed drug metabolized in liver. **Excretion:** Eliminated in feces via biliary system.

ACTION / *THERAPEUTIC EFFECT*

Increases peristalsis by direct effect on colonic smooth musculature (stimulates intramural nerve plexi). *Promotes fluid and ion accumulation in colon to increase laxative effect.*

USES

Facilitates defecation in those w/diminished colonic motor response, for evacuation of colon for rectal, bowel examination, elective colon surgery.

ADMINISTRATION

ORAL:

- Give on empty stomach (faster results).
- Offer 6–8 glasses water/day (aids softening stools).
- Avoid giving within 1 hr of other oral medication (decreases drug absorption).

INDICATIONS/ROUTES/DOSAGE

Laxative:
Oral: Adults, elderly: 1 tablet (or 5 ml) at bedtime.

CONTRAINDICATIONS

Abdominal pain, nausea, vomiting, appendicitis, intestinal obstruction.

CAUTIONS

None significant.

INTERACTIONS

DRUG: May decrease transit time of concurrently administered oral medication, decreasing absorption. **HERBAL:** None known. **FOOD:** None significant. **ALTERED LAB VALUES:** May increase blood glucose. May decrease potassium, calcium.

SIDE EFFECTS

FREQUENT: Pink-red, red-violet, red-brown, or yellow-brown discoloration of urine. OCCASIONAL: Some degree of abdominal discomfort, nausea, mild cramps, griping; faintness.

ADVERSE REACTIONS/TOXIC EFFECTS

Long-term use may result in laxative dependence, chronic constipation, loss of normal bowel function. Chronic use or overdosage may result in electrolyte disturbances (hypokalemia, hypocalcemia, metabolic acidosis or alkalosis), persistent diarrhea, malabsorption, weight loss. Electrolyte disturbance may produce vomiting, muscle weakness.

PATIENT CONSIDERATIONS

INTERVENTION/EVALUATION

Encourage adequate fluid intake. Assess bowel sounds for peristalsis. Monitor daily bowel activity and stool consistency (watery, loose, soft, semisolid, solid) and record time of evacuation. Assess for abdominal disturbances. Monitor serum electrolytes in those exposed to prolonged, frequent, or excessive use of medication.

PATIENT/FAMILY TEACHING

Urine may turn pink-red, red-violet, red-brown, or yellow-brown (only temporary and not harmful). Institute measures to promote defecation: Increase fluid intake, exercise, high-fiber diet. Laxative effect generally occurs in 6–12 hrs, but may take 24 hrs. Do not take other oral medication within 1 hr of taking this medicine (decreased effectiveness due to increased peristalsis). Do not use in presence of nausea, vomiting, abdominal pain longer than 1 wk.

castor oil

(Neoloid)

CANADIAN AVAILABILITY
Castor Oil

PREGNANCY CATEGORY X

CLASSIFICATION

Laxative: Stimulant

AVAILABILITY (OTC)

Liquid. Emulsion.

PHARMACODYNAMICS

	ONSET	PEAK	DURATION
Oral	2–3 hrs	—	—

PHARMACOKINETICS

Absorption: Minimal absorption. **Metabolism:** Converted to ricinoleic acid (active component) in GI tract.

ACTION/*THERAPEUTIC EFFECT*

Increases peristalsis by direct effect on small-bowel musculature (stimulates intramural nerve plexi). *Promotes fluid and ion accumulation in colon to increase laxative effect.*

USES

Facilitates defecation in those w/diminished colonic motor response, for evacuation of colon for rectal, bowel examination, elective colon surgery.

ADMINISTRATION

ORAL:

- Do not give late in day (acts in 2–6 hrs).

- Chill, mix w/juice (improves taste).
- Give on empty stomach (faster action).
- Offer 6–8 glasses of water/day (aids stool softening).
- Avoid giving within 1 hr of other oral medication (decreases drug absorption).

INDICATIONS/ROUTES/DOSAGE

Laxative:
Oral: Adults, elderly: (liquid): 15–60 ml; ***(emulsion):*** 30–60 ml. ***Children 6–12 yrs: (liquid):*** 5–15 ml; ***(emulsion):*** 7.5–30 ml. ***Infants: (emulsion):*** 2.5–5 ml.

CONTRAINDICATIONS

Menstruating/pregnant women, abdominal pain, nausea, vomiting, appendicitis, intestinal obstruction.

CAUTIONS

None significant.

INTERACTIONS

DRUG: May decrease transit time of concurrently administered oral medication, decreasing absorption. **HERBAL:** None known. **FOOD:** None significant. **ALTERED LAB VALUES:** May increase blood glucose. May decrease potassium, calcium.

SIDE EFFECTS

FREQUENT: Some degree of abdominal discomfort, nausea, mild cramps, griping, faintness. **OCCASIONAL:** Excessive colon irritation producing violent purgation. **RARE:** Pelvic congestion.

ADVERSE REACTIONS/TOXIC EFFECTS

Long-term use may result in laxative dependence, chronic constipation, loss of normal bowel function. Chronic use or overdosage may result in electrolyte disturbances (hypokalemia, hypocalcemia, metabolic acidosis or alkalosis), persistent diarrhea, malabsorption, weight loss. Electrolyte disturbance may produce vomiting, muscle weakness.

PATIENT CONSIDERATIONS

BASELINE ASSESSMENT

Question for possibility of pregnancy before initiating therapy (Pregnancy Category X).

INTERVENTION/EVALUATION

Encourage adequate fluid intake. Assess bowel sounds for peristalsis. Monitor daily bowel activity and stool consistency (watery, loose, soft, semisolid, solid) and record time of evacuation. Assess for abdominal disturbances. Monitor serum electrolytes in those exposed to prolonged, frequent, or excessive use of medication.

PATIENT/FAMILY TEACHING

Cola, unsalted crackers, dry toast may relieve nausea. Institute measures to promote defecation: Increase fluid intake, exercise, high-fiber diet. Do not take other oral medication within 1 hr of taking this medicine (decreased effectiveness due to increased peristalsis). Laxative effect generally occurs in 6–12 hrs, but may take 24 hrs. Do not use in presence of nausea, vomiting, abdominal pain longer than 1 wk.

cefaclor

sef-ah-klor
(Ceclor, Ceclor CD)

CANADIAN AVAILABILITY
Apo-Cefaclor, Ceclor

PREGNANCY CATEGORY B

CLASSIFICATION

Antibiotic: Second-generation cephalosporin

AVAILABILITY (Rx)

Capsules: 250 mg, 500 mg. **Tablets (extended-release):** 375 mg, 500 mg. **Oral Suspension:** 125 mg/5 ml, 187 mg/5 ml, 250 mg/5 ml, 375 mg/5 ml.

PHARMACOKINETICS

Absorption: Well absorbed from GI tract. Widely distributed. **Excretion:** Primarily excreted unchanged in urine. Moderately removed by hemodialysis. **Half-life:** 0.6–0.9 hrs (increased in decreased renal function).

ACTION/*THERAPEUTIC EFFECT*

Bactericidal. Binds to bacterial membranes, *inhibiting bacterial cell wall synthesis.*

USES

Treatment of respiratory, skin/skin structure infections, otitis media, UTI. *Extended-Release:* Bacterial infections of acute, chronic bronchitis, skin/skin structure, pharyngitis, tonsillitis.

STORAGE/HANDLING

Oral suspension: after reconstitution, stable for 14 days if refrigerated.

ADMINISTRATION

ORAL:

- Shake oral suspension well before using.
- Give w/o regard to meals; if GI upset occurs, give w/food or milk.
- Do not cut, crush, or chew extended-release tablets.

INDICATIONS/ROUTES/DOSAGE

Mild to moderate infections:
Oral: Adults, elderly: 250 mg q8h. *Children >1 mo:* 20 mg/kg/day in divided doses q8h.

Severe infections:
Oral: Adults, elderly: 500 mg q8h. ***Maximum:*** 4 g/day. ***Children >1 mo:*** 40 mg/kg/day in divided doses q8h. ***Maximum:*** 1 g/day.

Usual dosage for extended-release tablets:
Oral: Adults, children >16 yrs: 375–500 mg q12hrs.

Otitis media:
Oral: Children >1 mo: 40 mg/kg/day in divided doses q8h. ***Maximum:*** 1 g/day.

Dosage in renal impairment:
Reduced dosage may be necessary in those w/creatinine clearance <40 ml/min.

CONTRAINDICATIONS

History of hypersensitivity to cephalosporins, anaphylactic reaction to penicillins.

CAUTIONS

Renal impairment, history of allergies or GI disease (especially ulcerative colitis, antibiotic-associated colitis), concurrent use of nephrotoxic medications.

INTERACTIONS

DRUG: *Probenecid* may increase serum concentrations of cefaclor. **HERBAL:** None known. **FOOD:** None significant. **ALTERED LAB VALUES:** Positive direct/indirect Coombs' test. May increase BUN, serum creatinine, SGPT (ALT), SGOT (AST), alkaline phosphatase, bilirubin, LDH concentrations.

SIDE EFFECTS

FREQUENT: Oral candidiasis (sore mouth/tongue), mild diarrhea, mild abdominal cramping, vaginal candidiasis (itching, discharge). OCCASIONAL: Nausea, serum sickness reaction [joint pain, fever] (usually occurs following second course of therapy, resolves after drug discontinuation). RARE: Allergic reaction (rash, pruritus, urticaria).

ADVERSE REACTIONS/TOXIC EFFECTS

Antibiotic-associated colitis (severe abdominal pain and tenderness, fever, watery and severe diarrhea), other superinfections may result from altered bacterial balance. Nephrotoxicity may occur, especially w/preexisting renal disease. Severe hypersensitivity reaction (severe pruritus, angioedema, bronchospasm, anaphylaxis), particularly those w/history of allergies, especially penicillin.

PATIENT CONSIDERATIONS

Baseline Assessment

Question for history of allergies, particularly cephalosporins, penicillins. Obtain culture and sensitivity test before giving first dose (therapy may begin before results are known).

Intervention/Evaluation

Check mouth for white patches on mucous membranes, tongue. Monitor bowel activity and stool consistency carefully; mild GI effects may be tolerable, but increasing severity may indicate onset of antibiotic-associated colitis. Assess skin for rash. Monitor I&O, urinalysis, renal function reports for nephrotoxicity. Be alert for superinfection: severe genital/anal pruritus, abdominal pain, severe mouth soreness, moderate to severe diarrhea.

Patient/Family Teaching

Continue therapy for full length of treatment. Doses should be evenly spaced. May cause GI upset (may take w/food or milk).

---

cefadroxil

sef-ah-**drocks**-ill
(Duricef, Ultracef)

CANADIAN AVAILABILITY
Duricef

PREGNANCY CATEGORY B

CLASSIFICATION

Antibiotic: First-generation cephalosporin

AVAILABILITY (Rx)

Capsules: 500 mg. **Tablets:** 1,000 mg. **Oral Suspension:** 125 mg/5 ml, 250 mg/5 ml, 500 mg/5 ml.

PHARMACOKINETICS

Absorption: Well absorbed from GI tract. Widely distributed. **Excretion:** Primarily excreted unchanged in urine. Removed by hemodialysis. **Half-life:** 1.2–1.5 hrs (increased in decreased renal function).

ACTION/*THERAPEUTIC EFFECT*

Bactericidal. Binds to bacterial membranes, *inhibiting bacterial cell wall synthesis.*

USES

Treatment of respiratory and GU tract, skin and soft tissue infections; follow-up to parenteral therapy.

STORAGE/HANDLING

Oral suspension: after reconstitution, stable for 14 days if refrigerated.

ADMINISTRATION

ORAL:

- Shake oral suspension well before using.
- Give w/o regard to meals; if GI upset occurs, give w/food or milk.

INDICATIONS/ROUTES/DOSAGE

Note: Space doses evenly around the clock.

Urinary tract infections:
Oral: Adults, elderly: 1–2 g/day in 1–2 divided doses.

Skin/skin structure infections, group A beta-hemolytic streptococcal pharyngitis, tonsillitis:
Oral: Adults, elderly: 500 mg–1 g/day as single or 2 divided doses.

Usual dosage for children:
Oral: Children: 30 mg/kg/day as single or 2 divided doses.

Dosage in renal impairment:
Dose and/or frequency is based on degree of renal impairment and/or severity of infection. After initial 1 g dose:

CREATININE CLEARANCE	DOSAGE INTERVAL
25–50 ml/min	500 mg q12h
10–25 ml/min	500 mg q24h
0–10 ml/min	500 mg q36h

CONTRAINDICATIONS

History of hypersensitivity to cephalosporins, anaphylactic reaction to penicillins.

CAUTIONS

Renal impairment, history of allergies or GI disease (especially ulcerative colitis, antibiotic-associated colitis), concurrent use of nephrotoxic medications.

INTERACTIONS

DRUG: *Probenecid* increases serum concentrations of cefadroxil. **HERBAL:** None known. **FOOD:** None significant. **ALTERED LAB VALUES:** Positive direct/indirect Coombs' test. May increase BUN, serum creatinine, SGPT (ALT), SGOT (AST), alkaline phosphatase, bilirubin, LDH concentrations.

SIDE EFFECTS

FREQUENT: Oral candidiasis (sore mouth/tongue), mild diarrhea, nausea, vaginal candidiasis (itching, discharge). **OCCASIONAL:** Serum sickness reaction (skin rash, joint pain, fever), vomiting. **RARE:** Hemolytic anemia (unusually tired), erythema multiforme (blistering, peeling, loosening of skin), decreased renal function.

ADVERSE REACTIONS/TOXIC EFFECTS

Antibiotic-associated colitis (severe abdominal pain and tenderness, fever, watery and severe diarrhea), other superinfections may result from altered bacterial balance. Nephrotoxicity may occur, especially w/preexisting renal disease. Severe hypersensitivity reaction (severe pruritus, angioedema, bronchospasm, anaphylaxis), particularly those w/history of allergies, especially penicillin.

PATIENT CONSIDERATIONS

BASELINE ASSESSMENT

Question history of allergies, particularly cephalosporins, penicillins. Obtain culture and sensitivity test before giving first dose (therapy may begin before results are known).

INTERVENTION/EVALUATION

Check mouth for white patches on mucous membranes, tongue. Monitor bowel activity and stool consistency carefully; mild GI

effects may be tolerable, but increasing severity may indicate onset of antibiotic-associated colitis. Assess skin for rash. Monitor I&O, urinalysis, renal function reports for nephrotoxicity. Be alert for superinfection: genital/anal pruritus, moniliasis, abdominal pain, sore mouth or tongue, moderate to severe diarrhea.

Patient/Family Teaching

Continue therapy for full length of treatment. Doses should be evenly spaced. May cause GI upset (may take w/food or milk).

cefamandole

(Mandol)

See Classification section under: Antibiotic: cephalosporins

cefazolin sodium

cef-ah-**zoe**-lin

(Ancef, Kefzol, Zolicef)

CANADIAN AVAILABILITY

Ancef, Kefzol

PREGNANCY CATEGORY B

CLASSIFICATION

Antibiotic: First-generation cephalosporin

AVAILABILITY (Rx)

Injection: 500 mg, 1 g. **Ready-to-Hang Infusion:** 1 g/50 ml.

PHARMACOKINETICS

Widely distributed. **Excretion:** Primarily excreted unchanged in urine. Moderately removed by hemodialysis. **Half-life:** 1.4–1.8 hrs (increased in decreased renal function).

ACTION/*THERAPEUTIC EFFECT*

Bactericidal. Binds to bacterial membranes, *inhibiting bacterial cell wall synthesis.*

USES

Treatment of respiratory tract, skin, soft tissue, bone and joint, GU tract, serious intra-abdominal, biliary infections; septicemia. Preferred first-generation cephalosporin for perioperative prophylaxis.

STORAGE/HANDLING

Solutions appear light yellow to yellow. IV infusion (piggyback) stable for 24 hrs at room temperature, 96 hrs if refrigerated. Discard if precipitate forms.

ADMINISTRATION

Note: Give by IM injection, direct IV injection, intermittent IV infusion (piggyback).

IM:

- To minimize discomfort, inject deep IM slowly. Less painful if injected into gluteus maximus rather than lateral aspect of thigh.

IV:

- For direct IV injection, administer over 3–5 min.
- For intermittent IV infusion (piggyback), infuse over 20–40 min.
- Alternating IV sites, use large veins to reduce risk of phlebitis.

INDICATIONS/ROUTES/DOSAGE

Note: Space doses evenly around the clock.

Uncomplicated UTI:
IM/IV: Adults, elderly: 1 g q12h.

Mild to moderate infections:
IM/IV: Adults, elderly: 250–500 mg q8–12h.

Severe infections:
IM/IV: Adults, elderly: 0.5–1 g q6–8h.

Life-threatening infections:
IM/IV: Adults, elderly: 1–1.5 g q6h. *Maximum:* 12 g/day.

Perioperative prophylaxis:
IM/IV: Adults, elderly: 1 g 30–60 min before surgery, 0.5–1 g during surgery, and q6–8h for up to 24 hrs postop.

Usual dosage for children:
IM/IV: Children >1 mo: 25–100 mg/kg/day in 3–4 divided doses.

Dosage in renal impairment:
After initial loading dose of 500 mg, dose and/or frequency modified on basis of creatinine clearance and/or severity of infection.

CREATININE CLEARANCE	CHILDREN'S DOSAGE
40–70 ml/min	60% normal dose q12h
20–40 ml/min	25% normal dose q12h
5–20 ml/mi	10% normal dose q24h
	ADULT DOSAGE
55 ml/min	250–1,000 mg q6–8h
35–54 ml/min	250–1,000 mg q8h
11–34 ml/min	125–500 mg q12h
10 ml/min	125–500 mg q24h

CONTRAINDICATIONS

History of hypersensitivity to cephalosporins, anaphylactic reaction to penicillins.

CAUTIONS

Renal impairment, history of allergies or GI disease (especially ulcerative colitis, antibiotic-associated colitis), concurrent use of nephrotoxic medications.

INTERACTIONS

DRUG: *Probenecid* increases serum concentrations of cefazolin. **HERBAL:** None known. **FOOD:** None significant. **ALTERED LAB VALUES:** Positive direct/indirect Coombs' test. May increase BUN, serum creatinine, SGPT (ALT), SGOT (AST), alkaline phosphatase, bilirubin, LDH concentrations.

SIDE EFFECTS

FREQUENT: Discomfort w/IM administration, oral candidiasis (sore mouth/tongue), mild diarrhea, mild abdominal cramping, vaginal candidiasis (itching, discharge). **OCCASIONAL:** Nausea, serum sickness reaction [joint pain, fever] (usually occurs following second course of therapy, resolves after drug discontinuation). **RARE:** Allergic reaction (rash, pruritus, urticaria), thrombophlebitis (pain, redness, swelling at injection site).

ADVERSE REACTIONS/TOXIC EFFECTS

Antibiotic-associated colitis (severe abdominal pain and tenderness, fever, watery and severe diarrhea), other superinfections may result from altered bacterial balance. Nephrotoxicity may occur, especially w/preexisting renal disease. Severe hypersensitivity reaction (severe pruritus, angioedema, bronchospasm, anaphylaxis), particularly those w/history of allergies, especially penicillin.

PATIENT CONSIDERATIONS

Baseline Assessment

Question for history of allergies, particularly cephalosporins, penicillins. Obtain culture and sensitivity test before giving first dose (therapy may begin before results are known).

Intervention/Evaluation

Evaluate IV site for phlebitis (heat, pain, red streaking over vein). Check IM injection sites for induration, tenderness. Check mouth for white patches on

mucous membranes, tongue. Monitor bowel activity and stool consistency carefully; mild GI effects may be tolerable, but increasing severity may indicate onset of antibiotic-associated colitis. Assess skin for rash. Monitor I&O, urinalysis, renal function reports for nephrotoxicity. Be alert for superinfection: severe genital/anal pruritus, abdominal pain, severe mouth soreness, moderate to severe diarrhea.

PATIENT/FAMILY TEACHING

Discomfort may occur w/IM injection. Doses should be evenly spaced. Continue antibiotic therapy for full length of treatment.

---

cefdinir

cef-din-ur
(Omnicef)

PREGNANCY CATEGORY B

CLASSIFICATION

Antibiotic: Third-generation cephalosporin

AVAILABILITY (Rx)

Capsules: 300 mg. **Oral Suspension:** 125 mg/5 ml

PHARMACOKINETICS

Absorption: Moderately absorbed from GI tract. Widely distributed. **Metabolism:** Not appreciably metabolized. **Excretion:** Primarily excreted unchanged in urine. Minimally removed by hemodialysis. **Half-life:** 1–2 hrs (increased in decreased renal function).

ACTION/ *THERAPEUTIC EFFECT*

Bactericidal. Binds to bacterial membranes, *inhibiting bacterial cell wall synthesis.*

USES

Treatment of community-acquired pneumonia, acute exacerbation of chronic bronchitis, acute maxillary sinusitis, pharyngitis, tonsillitis, uncomplicated skin and skin structure infections, otitis media.

STORAGE/HANDLING

Following reconstitution, oral suspension stable for 10 days at room temperature.

ADMINISTRATION

ORAL:

- Give w/o regard to meals.
- To reconstitute oral suspension, add 39 ml water for the 60 ml bottle; for the 120 ml bottle, add 65 ml water.
- Shake oral suspension well before administering.

INDICATIONS/ROUTES/DOSAGES

Community acquired pneumonia:
Oral: Adults, elderly, children ≥13 yrs: 300 mg q12h for 10 days.

Acute maxillary /acute exacerbations chronic bronchitis:
Oral: Adults, elderly, children ≥13 yrs: 300 mg q12h or 600 mg q24h for 10 days. ***Children 6 mos–12 yrs:*** 7 mg/kg q12h or 14 mg/kg q24h for 10 days.

Pharyngitis/tonsillitis:
Oral: Adults, elderly, children ≥13 yrs: 300 mg q12h for 5–10 days or 600 mg q24h for 10 days. ***Children 6 mos–12 yrs:*** 7 mg/kg q12h for 5–10 days or 14 mg/kg q24h for 10 days.

Uncomplicated skin and skin structure infections:
Oral: Adults, elderly, children ≥13 yrs: 300 mg q12h for 10 days.

Children 6 mos–12 yrs: 7 mg/kg q12h for 10 days.

Acute bacterial otitis media: *Children 6 mos–12 yrs:* 7 mg/kg q12h or 14 mg/kg q24h for 10 days.

Oral Suspension: *Pediatric <20 lbs:* 2.5 ml (½ tsp) q12h or 5 ml (1 tsp) q24h.

Pediatric 20–40 lbs: 5 ml (1 tsp) q12h or 10 ml (2 tsp) q24h.

Pediatric 41–60 lbs: 7.5 ml (1½ tsp) q12h or 15 ml (3 tsp) q24h.

Pediatric 61–80 lbs: 10 ml (2 tsp) q12h or 20 ml (4 tsp) q24h.

Pediatric 81–95 lbs: 12 ml (2½ tsp) q12h or 24 ml (5 tsp) q24h.

Dosage in renal impairment: *Creatinine clearance <30 ml/min:* 300 mg/day as single daily dose. Hemodialysis pts: 300 mg or 7 mg/kg dose every other day.

CONTRAINDICATIONS

Hypersensitivity to cephalosporins.

CAUTIONS

Hypersensitivity to penicillins or other drugs; allergies; history of GI disease (e.g., colitis); renal impairment, impaired hepatic function.

INTERACTIONS

DRUG: *Probenecid* increases serum concentration of cefdinir. *Antacids* decreases cefdinir plasma concentration. HERBAL: None known. FOOD: None significant. ALTERED LAB VALUES: May produce a false-positive reaction for ketones in urine. May increase SGOT (AST), SGOT (ALT), alkaline phosphatase, bilirubin, LDH concentrations.

SIDE EFFECTS

FREQUENT: Diarrhea, abdominal pain, nausea, dyspepsia, flatulence. OCCASIONAL: Hypersensitivity reaction: skin rash, pruritus, urticaria, drug fever; headache, dizziness; genital pruritus; vaginitis.

ADVERSE REACTIONS/TOXIC EFFECTS

Superinfections, especially antibiotic-associated colitis, may result from altered bacterial balance. Blood dyscrasias (transient leukopenia, thrombocytopenia, eosinophilia) occur rarely.

PATIENT CONSIDERATIONS

BASELINE ASSESSMENT

Question for hypersensitivity to cefdinir or other cephalosporins, penicillins. Obtain specimens for culture and sensitivity test (therapy may begin before results are known).

INTERVENTION/EVALUATION

Monitor bowel activity and stool consistency carefully; mild GI effects may be tolerable, but increasing severity may indicate onset of antibiotic-associated colitis. Report hypersensitivity reaction: skin rash, urticaria, pruritus, fever promptly. Be alert for superinfection (e.g., genital-anal pruritus, ulceration or changes in oral mucosa, moderate to severe diarrhea, new or increased fever). Provide symptomatic relief for nausea, flatulence. Monitor hematology reports.

PATIENT/FAMILY TEACHING

Take antacids 2 hrs before or after taking medication. Continue medication for full length of treatment; do not skip doses. Doses should be evenly spaced. Notify physician promptly of onset of diarrhea, rash.

cefepime

sef-eh-**peem**
(Maxipime)

CANADIAN AVAILABILITY
Maxipime

PREGNANCY CATEGORY B

CLASSIFICATION

Antibiotic: Fourth-generation cephalosporin

AVAILABILITY (Rx)

Powder for Injection: 500 mg, 1 g, 2 g

PHARMACOKINETICS

Absorption: Well absorbed after IM administration. Widely distributed. **Excretion:** Primarily excreted unchanged in urine. Removed by hemodialysis. **Half-life:** 2–2.3 hrs (increased in decreased renal function, elderly).

ACTION / *THERAPEUTIC EFFECT*

Bactericidal. Binds to bacterial membrane, *inhibiting bacterial cell wall synthesis.*

USES

Treatment of pneumonia, bronchitis, urinary tract, skin and skin structure, intra-abdominal infections, bacteremia, septicemia, fever and neutropenia in cancer pts, complicated intra-abdominal infections (w/metronidazole).

STORAGE/HANDLING

Solutions stable for 24 hrs at room temperature or 7 days refrigerated.

ADMINISTRATION

Note: May give by IM injection, IV injection, intermittent IV infusion (piggyback).

IM/IV:

- For IM injection, inject into a large muscle mass (e.g., upper gluteus maximus).
- For direct IV injection, administer over 3–5 min.
- For intermittent IV infusion, infuse over 15–30 min.
- Alternating IV sites, use large veins to reduce risk of phlebitis.

INDICATIONS/ROUTES/DOSAGE

Note: Space doses evenly around the clock.

Complicated, uncomplicated UTI:
IM/IV: Adults, elderly: 0.5–1.0 g q12h.

Moderate to severe infections:
IM/IV: Adults, elderly: 1 g q12h.

Severe infections:
IV: Adults, elderly: 2 g q12h.

Life-threatening infections:
IV: Adults, elderly: 2 g q8h.

Usual pediatric dosage:
IM/IV: Children (2 mos–6 yrs): 50 mg/kg q8–12h. Do not exceed the maximum dose for adults.

Dosage in renal impairment:
Dose and/or frequency is based on degree of renal impairment (creatinine clearance) and/or severity of infection.

	CREATININE CLEARANCE 11–30 ML/MIN	<10 ML/MIN
Moderately severe infection	0.5 g q24h	0.25 g q24h
Severe infection	1 g q24h	0.5 g q24h
Life-threatening infection	1 g q12h	1 g q24h

CONTRAINDICATIONS

History of hypersensitivity to cephalosporins, anaphylactic reaction to penicillins.

CAUTIONS

Renal impairment, history of allergies.

INTERACTIONS

DRUG: *Probenecid* may increase concentration of cefepime. **HERBAL:** None known. **FOOD:** None significant. **ALTERED LAB VALUES:** Positive direct/indirect Coombs' test may occur. May increase SGOT (AST), SGPT (ALT), alkaline phosphatase, LDH, bilirubin.

SIDE EFFECTS

FREQUENT: Discomfort w/IM administration, oral candidiasis (sore mouth/tongue), mild diarrhea, mild abdominal cramping, vaginal candidiasis (itching, discharge). **OCCASIONAL:** Nausea, serum sickness reaction [joint pain, fever] (usually occurs following second course of therapy, resolves after drug discontinuation). **RARE:** Allergic reaction (rash, pruritus, urticaria), thrombophlebitis (pain, redness, swelling at injection site).

ADVERSE REACTIONS/TOXIC EFFECTS

Antibiotic-associated colitis (severe abdominal pain and tenderness, fever, watery and severe diarrhea), other superinfections may result from altered bacterial balance. Nephrotoxicity may occur, especially w/preexisting renal disease. Severe hypersensitivity reaction (severe pruritus, angioedema, bronchospasm, anaphylaxis), particularly those w/history of allergies, especially penicillin.

PATIENT CONSIDERATIONS

Baseline Assessment

Question history of allergies, particularly cephalosporins, penicillins. Obtain culture and sensitivity test before giving first dose (therapy may begin before results are known).

Intervention/Evaluation

Monitor IV site for phlebitis (heat, pain, red streaking over vein). Check IM injection sites for induration, tenderness. Check mouth for white patches on mucous membranes, tongue. Monitor bowel activity and stool consistency carefully; mild GI effects may be tolerable, but increasing severity may indicate onset of antibiotic-associated colitis. Assess skin for rash. Monitor I&O, urinalysis, renal function reports for nephrotoxicity. Be alert for superinfection: severe genital/anal pruritus, abdominal pain, severe mouth soreness, moderate to severe diarrhea.

Patient/Family Teaching

Discomfort may occur w/IM injection. Continue therapy for full length of treatment. Doses should be evenly spaced.

---

cefixime

sef-ih-zeem
(Suprax)

CANADIAN AVAILABILITY
Suprax

PREGNANCY CATEGORY B

CLASSIFICATION

Antibiotic: Third-generation cephalosporin

AVAILABILITY (Rx)

Tablets: 200 mg, 400 mg. **Oral Suspension:** 100 mg/5 ml.

PHARMACOKINETICS

Absorption: Moderately absorbed from GI tract. Widely distributed. **Excretion:** Primarily excreted unchanged in urine. Minimally removed by hemodialysis. **Half-life:** 3–4 hrs (increased in decreased renal function).

ACTION/*THERAPEUTIC EFFECT*

Bactericidal. Binds to bacterial membranes, *inhibiting bacterial cell wall synthesis.*

USES

Otitis media, acute bronchitis and acute exacerbations of chronic bronchitis, pharyngitis, tonsillitis, uncomplicated UTI, uncomplicated gonorrhea.

STORAGE/HANDLING

Oral suspension: after reconstitution, stable for 14 days at room temperature. Do not refrigerate.

ADMINISTRATION

ORAL:

- Give w/o regard to meals.
- Shake oral suspension well before administering.

INDICATIONS/ROUTES/DOSAGE

Note: Use oral suspension to treat otitis media (achieves higher peak blood level).

Usual oral dosage:
Oral: Adults, elderly, children >50 kg: 400 mg/day as single or 2 divided doses. ***Children <50 kg:*** 8 mg/kg/day as single or 2 divided doses.

Uncomplicated gonorrhea:
Oral: Adults: 400 mg as single dose.

Dosage in renal impairment:
Creatinine clearance 21–60 ml/min, pt on renal dialysis: 300 mg/day as single or 2 divided doses.

Creatinine clearance <20 ml/min, pt on continuous ambulatory peritoneal dialysis: 200 mg/day as single or 2 divided doses.

CONTRAINDICATIONS

Hypersensitivity to cephalosporins.

CAUTIONS

Hypersensitivity to penicillins or other drugs; allergies; history of GI disease (e.g., colitis); renal impairment.

INTERACTIONS

DRUG: *Probenecid* increases serum concentrations of cefixime. **HERBAL:** None known. **FOOD:** None significant. **ALTERED LAB VALUES:** Positive direct/indirect Coombs' test. May increase BUN, serum creatinine, SGPT (ALT), SGOT (AST), alkaline phosphatase, bilirubin, LDH concentrations.

SIDE EFFECTS

FREQUENT: Oral candidiasis (sore mouth/tongue), mild diarrhea, mild abdominal cramping, vaginal candidiasis (itching, discharge). **OCCASIONAL:** Nausea, serum sickness reaction [joint pain, fever] (usually occurs following second course of therapy, resolves after drug discontinuation). **RARE:** Allergic reaction (rash, pruritus, urticaria).

ADVERSE REACTIONS/TOXIC EFFECTS

Antibiotic-associated colitis (severe abdominal pain and tenderness, fever, watery and severe diarrhea), other superinfections may result from altered bacterial balance. Nephrotoxicity may occur, especially w/preexisting renal disease. Severe hypersensitivity reaction (severe pruritus, angioedema, bronchospasm, anaphylaxis), particularly those w/history of allergies, especially penicillin.

PATIENT CONSIDERATIONS

Baseline Assessment

Question for hypersensitivity to cefixime or other cephalosporins, penicillins, other drugs. Obtain specimens for culture and sensitivity test (therapy may begin before results are known).

Intervention/Evaluation

Check mouth for white patches on mucous membranes, tongue. Monitor bowel activity and stool consistency carefully; mild GI effects may be tolerable, but increasing severity may indicate onset of antibiotic-associated colitis. Assess skin for rash. Monitor I&O, urinalysis, renal function reports for nephrotoxicity. Be alert for superinfection: severe genital/anal pruritus, abdominal pain, severe mouth soreness, moderate to severe diarrhea.

Patient/Family Teaching

Continue medication for full length of treatment; do not skip doses. Doses should be evenly spaced. May cause GI upset (may take we/food or milk).

cefmetazole sodium

cef-**met**-ah-zole
(Zefazone)

PREGNANCY CATEGORY B

CLASSIFICATION

Antibiotic: Second-generation cephalosporin

AVAILABILITY (Rx)

Powder for Injection: 1 g, 2 g

PHARMACOKINETICS

Widely distributed. **Excretion:** Primarily excreted unchanged in urine. Moderately removed by hemodialysis. **Half-life:** 0.8–1.8 hrs (increased in decreased renal function).

ACTION/*THERAPEUTIC EFFECT*

Bactericidal. Binds to bacterial membranes, *inhibiting bacterial cell wall synthesis.*

USES

Treatment of GU, lower respiratory tract, skin and skin structure and intra-abdominal infections. Preop prophylaxis for certain clean, contaminated, or potentially contaminated surgical procedures (cesarean section, abdominal or vaginal hysterectomy, high-risk cholecystectomy, colorectal surgery).

STORAGE/HANDLING

After reconstitution, IV solution stable for 24 hrs at room temperature or 7 days if refrigerated.

ADMINISTRATION

IV:

- Do not use if solution cloudy or insoluble precipitate noted.
- For IV injection, administer over 3–5 min.
- For IV infusion, infuse over 10–60 min.
- Because of potential for hypersensitivity/anaphylaxis, start initial dose at few drops per minute, increase slowly to ordered rate; stay w/pt first 10–15 min, then check every 10 min for first hour.
- Alternating IV sites, use large veins to reduce risk of phlebitis.

INDICATIONS/ROUTES/DOSAGE

Urinary tract infections:
IV: Adults, elderly: 2 g q12h.

Mild to moderate infections:
IV: Adults, elderly: 2 g q8h.

Severe infections:
IV: Adults, elderly: 2 g q6h.

Surgical prophylaxis:
IV: Adults, elderly: 2 g as single dose 30–90 min before surgery or after cord is clamped, or 1–2 g 30–90 min before surgery or after cord is clamped, and repeat 8 and 16 hrs later.

Dosage in renal impairment:
After loading dose of 1–2 g, dosage and/or frequency is modified on basis of creatinine clearance and/or severity of infection.

CREATININE CLEARANCE	DOSAGE
50–90 ml/min	1–2 g q12h
30–49 ml/min	1–2 g q16h
10–29 ml/min	1–2 g q24h
<10 ml/min	1–2 g q48h

CONTRAINDICATIONS

History of hypersensitivity to cefmetazole or cephalosporins.

CAUTIONS

If given to penicillin-sensitive pt, use extreme caution; cross-sensitivity among beta-lactam antibiotics occurs in up to 10% of pts w/history of penicillin allergy. Concurrent use of nephrotoxic medications, history of allergies or GI disease (especially colitis), renal impairment. Safety and effectiveness in children not established.

INTERACTIONS

DRUG: Disulfiram reaction (facial flushing, nausea, sweating, headache, tachycardia) occurs if ***alcohol*** is ingested within 48–72 hrs after dose. ***Probenecid*** increases half-life, duration of action. May increase bleeding risk w/***anticoagulants, heparin, thrombolytics.*** **HERBAL:** None known. **FOOD:** None significant. **ALTERED LAB VALUES:** Positive direct/indirect Coombs' test may occur (interferes w/hematologic tests, cross-matching procedures). May prolong prothrombin times. May increase SGOT (AST), SGPT (ALT), alkaline phosphatase, bilirubin, LDH, BUN, serum creatinine.

SIDE EFFECTS

FREQUENT: Oral candidiasis (sore mouth/tongue), mild diarrhea, mild abdominal cramping, vaginal candidiasis (itching, discharge). **OCCASIONAL:** Nausea, serum sickness reaction [joint pain, fever] (usually occurs following second course **RARE:** Allergic reaction (rash, pruritus, urticaria), thrombophlebitis (pain, redness, swelling at injection site).

ADVERSE REACTIONS/TOXIC EFFECTS

Antibiotic-associated colitis (severe abdominal pain and tenderness, fever, watery and severe diarrhea), other superinfections may result from altered bacterial balance. Nephrotoxicity may occur, especially w/preexisting renal disease. Severe hypersensitivity reaction (severe pruritus, angioedema, bronchospasm, anaphylaxis), particularly those w/history of allergies, especially penicillin.

PATIENT CONSIDERATIONS

Baseline Assessment

Question for history of allergies, especially cefmetazole, cephalosporins, penicillins. Obtain culture and sensitivity test before giving first dose (therapy may begin before results are known).

Intervention/Evaluation

Evaluate IV site for phlebitis

(heat, pain, red streaking over vein). Check mouth for white patches on mucous membranes, tongue. Monitor bowel activity and stool consistency carefully; mild GI effects may be tolerable, but increasing severity may indicate onset of antibiotic-associated colitis. Assess skin for rash. Monitor I&O, urinalysis, renal function reports for nephrotoxicity. Be alert for superinfection: severe genital/anal pruritus, abdominal pain, severe mouth soreness, moderate to severe diarrhea. Monitor PT levels and be alert for signs of bleeding: overt bleeding, bruising or swelling of soft tissue. Check temperature and B/P at least 2 times/day.

PATIENT/FAMILY TEACHING

Doses should be evenly spaced. Continue antibiotic therapy for full length of treatment. Do not take other medications w/o consulting physician. Avoid alcohol and alcohol-containing preparations (salad dressings, sauces, cough syrups—read all labels carefully) during and for 72 hrs after last dose of cefmetazole.

cefonicid sodium

ce-**fon**-oh-sid
(Monocid)

PREGNANCY CATEGORY B

CLASSIFICATION

Antibiotic: Second-generation cephalosporin

AVAILABILITY (Rx)

Powder for Injection: 500 mg, 1 g

PHARMACOKINETICS

Widely distributed. **Excretion:** Primarily excreted unchanged in urine. Moderately removed by hemodialysis. **Half-life:** 4.5 hrs (increased in decreased renal function).

ACTION/*THERAPEUTIC EFFECT*

Bactericidal. Binds to bacterial membranes, *inhibiting bacterial cell wall synthesis.*

USES

Treatment of respiratory, GU tract, skin and bone infections, septicemia, perioperative prophylaxis.

STORAGE/HANDLING

Solutions appear colorless to light amber. Solutions may darken (slight yellow color change does not indicate loss of potency). IV infusion (piggyback) stable for 24 hrs at room temperature, 72 hrs if refrigerated. Discard if precipitate forms.

ADMINISTRATION

Note: Give IM, direct IV injection, intermittent IV infusion (piggyback).

IM:

- Inject deep IM into gluteus maximus or lateral aspect of thigh. For 2 g dose, use 2 separate injection sites.

IV:

- For direct IV injection, administer over 3–5 min.
- For intermittent IV infusion (piggyback), infuse over 20–30 min.
- Alternating IV sites, use large veins to reduce risk of phlebitis.

INDICATIONS/ROUTES/DOSAGE

Uncomplicated UTI:
IM/IV: Adults, elderly: 500 mg q24h.

Mild to moderate infections:
IM/IV: Adults, elderly: 1 g q24h.

Severe or life-threatening infections:
IM/IV: Adults, elderly: 2 g q24h.

Perioperative prophylaxis:
IM/IV: Adults, elderly: 1 g before surgery (in pts undergoing cesarean section, only after umbilical cord is clamped) up to 1 g daily for 2 days postop.

Dosage in renal impairment:
After loading dose of 7.5 mg/kg, dose and/or frequency based on creatinine clearance and/or severity of infection.

CREATININE CLEARANCE	MILD TO MODERATE INFECTIONS	SEVERE INFECTIONS
60–79 ml/min	10 mg/kg q24h	25 mg/kg q24h
40–59 ml/min	8 mg/kg q24h	20 mg/kg q24h
20–39 ml/min	4 mg/kg q24h	15 mg/kg q24h
10–19 ml/min	4 mg/kg q48h	15 mg/kg q48h
5–9 ml/min	4 mg/kg q3–5days	15 mg/kg q3–5days
<5 ml/min	3 mg/kg q3–5days	4 mg/kg q3–5days

CONTRAINDICATIONS

History of hypersensitivity to cephalosporins, anaphylactic reaction to penicillins.

CAUTIONS

Renal impairment, history of allergies or GI disease (especially ulcerative colitis, antibiotic-associated colitis), concurrent use of nephrotoxic medications.

INTERACTIONS

DRUG: *Probenecid* increases serum concentrations of cefonicid. HERBAL: None known. FOOD: None significant. **ALTERED LAB VALUES:** Positive direct/indirect Coombs' test may occur (interferes w/hematologic tests, cross-matching procedures). May increase SGOT (AST), SGPT (ALT), alkaline phosphatase, bilirubin, LDH, BUN, serum creatinine concentrations.

SIDE EFFECTS

FREQUENT: Oral candidiasis (sore mouth/tongue), mild diarrhea, nausea, vaginal candidiasis, discomfort w/IM administration. **OCCASIONAL:** Serum sickness reaction (skin rash, joint pain, fever), vomiting. **RARE:** Hemolytic anemia (unusually tired), erythema multiforme (blistering, peeling, loosening of skin), thrombophlebitis (pain, redness, swelling at injection site).

ADVERSE REACTIONS/TOXIC EFFECTS

Nephrotoxicity has occurred w/high dosages or preexisting renal impairment. Antibiotic-associated colitis, other superinfections may result from altered bacterial balance. Hypersensitivity reactions (ranging from rash, urticaria, fever to anaphylaxis) may occur, particularly those w/history of allergies, especially penicillin.

PATIENT CONSIDERATIONS

Baseline Assessment

Question for history of allergies, particularly cephalosporins, penicillins. Obtain culture and sensitivity test before giving first dose (therapy may begin before results are known).

Intervention/Evaluation

Evaluate IV site for phlebitis (heat, pain, red streaking over vein). Check IM injection sites for induration, tenderness. Moni-

tor bowel activity and stool consistency carefully; mild GI effects may be tolerable, but increasing severity may indicate onset of antibiotic-associated colitis. Assess skin for rash. Monitor I&O, urinalysis, renal function reports for nephrotoxicity. Be alert for superinfection: nausea, diarrhea, vaginal discharge, genital/anal pruritus, ulceration or changes in oral mucosa.

PATIENT/FAMILY TEACHING

Discomfort may occur w/IM injection. Doses should be evenly spaced. Continue antibiotic therapy for full length of treatment.

cefoperazone sodium

sef-o-**pear**-a-zone
(Cefobid)

PREGNANCY CATEGORY B

CLASSIFICATION

Antibiotic: Third-generation cephalosporin

AVAILABILITY (Rx)

Powder for Injection: 1 g, 2 g

PHARMACOKINETICS

Widely distributed. Achieves high biliary concentration. **Excretion:** Primarily excreted unchanged in bile (excreted primarily in urine in pts w/severe liver impairment). Minimally removed by hemodialysis. **Half-life:** 1.6–2.6 hrs (increased in decreased liver and/or biliary function).

ACTION/*THERAPEUTIC EFFECT*

Bactericidal. Binds to bacterial membranes, *inhibiting bacterial cell wall synthesis.*

USES

Treatment of intra-abdominal, biliary, pelvic inflammatory infections; respiratory, GU tract, skin and bone infections; septicemia.

STORAGE/HANDLING

Solutions appear colorless to light yellow. IV infusion (piggyback) stable for 24 hrs at room temperature, 5 days if refrigerated. Discard if precipitate forms.

ADMINISTRATION

Note: Give by IM injection or intermittent IV infusion (piggyback).

IM:

- To minimize discomfort, inject deep IM slowly. Less painful if injected into gluteus maximus rather than lateral aspect of thigh.

IV:

- For intermittent IV infusion (piggyback), infuse over 15–30 min.
- Alternating IV sites, use large veins to reduce risk of phlebitis.

INDICATIONS/ROUTES/DOSAGE

Note: Space doses evenly around the clock.

Mild to moderate infections:
IM/IV: Adults, elderly: 2–4 g/day in divided doses q12h.

Severe or life-threatening infections:
IM/IV: Adults, elderly: Total daily dose and/or frequency may be increased to 6–12 g/day divided into 2, 3, or 4 equal doses of 1.5–4 g per dose.

Dosage in renal and/or hepatic impairment:
Do not exceed 4 g/day in those w/liver disease and/or biliary

obstruction. Modification of dose usually not necessary in those w/renal impairment. Dose should not exceed 1–2 g/day in those w/both hepatic and substantial renal impairment.

CONTRAINDICATIONS

History of hypersensitivity to cephalosporins, anaphylactic reaction to penicillins.

CAUTIONS

History of allergies, GI disease (especially ulcerative colitis, antibiotic-associated colitis), hepatic or renal impairment.

INTERACTIONS

DRUG: Disulfiram reaction (facial flushing, nausea, sweating, headache, tachycardia) may occur when ***alcohol*** is ingested. May increase bleeding risk w/***anticoagulants, heparin, thrombolytics***. **HERBAL:** None known. **FOOD:** None significant. **ALTERED LAB VALUES:** Positive direct/indirect Coombs' test may occur (interferes w/hematologic tests, cross-matching procedures). Prothrombin times may be increased. May increase BUN, serum creatinine, SGOT (AST), SGPT (ALT), alkaline phosphatase concentrations.

SIDE EFFECTS

FREQUENT: Discomfort w/IM administration, oral candidiasis (sore mouth/tongue), mild diarrhea, mild abdominal cramping, vaginal candidiasis (itching, discharge). **OCCASIONAL:** Nausea, unusual bruising/bleeding, serum sickness reaction [joint pain, fever] (usually occurs following second course of therapy, resolves after drug discontinuation). **RARE:** Allergic reaction (rash, pruritus, urticaria), thrombophlebitis (pain, redness, swelling at injection site).

ADVERSE REACTIONS/TOXIC EFFECTS

Antibiotic-associated colitis (severe abdominal pain and tenderness, fever, watery and severe diarrhea), other superinfections may result from altered bacterial balance. Nephrotoxicity may occur, especially w/preexisting renal disease. Severe hypersensitivity reaction (severe pruritus, angioedema, bronchospasm, anaphylaxis), particularly those w/history of allergies, especially penicillin.

PATIENT CONSIDERATIONS

Baseline Assessment

Question for history of allergies, particularly cephalosporins, penicillins. Obtain culture and sensitivity test before giving first dose (therapy may begin before results are known).

Intervention/Evaluation

Evaluate IV site for phlebitis (heat, pain, red streaking over vein). Check IM injection sites for induration, tenderness. Check mouth for white patches on mucous membranes, tongue. Monitor bowel activity and stool consistency carefully; mild GI effects may be tolerable, but increasing severity may indicate onset of antibiotic-associated colitis. Assess skin for rash. Monitor I&O, urinalysis, renal function reports for nephrotoxicity. Be alert for superinfection: severe genital/anal pruritus, abdominal pain, severe mouth soreness, moderate to severe diarrhea.

Patient/Family Teaching

Discomfort may occur w/IM

injection. Doses should be evenly spaced. Continue antibiotic therapy for full length of treatment. Avoid alcohol and alcohol-containing preparations (salad dressings, sauces, cough syrups—read all labels carefully) during and for 72 hrs after last dose of cefoperazone.

cefotaxime sodium

seh-fo-**tax**-eem
(Claforan)

CANADIAN AVAILABILITY
Claforan

PREGNANCY CATEGORY B

CLASSIFICATION

Antibiotic: Third-generation cephalosporin

AVAILABILITY (Rx)

Powder for Injection: 1 g, 2 g

PHARMACOKINETICS

Widely distributed (including CSF). **Metabolism:** Partially metabolized in liver to active metabolite. **Excretion:** Primarily excreted in urine. Moderately removed by hemodialysis. **Half-life:** 1 hr (increased in decreased renal function).

ACTION/*THERAPEUTIC EFFECT*

Bactericidal. Binds to bacterial membranes, *inhibiting bacterial cell wall synthesis.*

USES/*UNLABELED*

Treatment of respiratory, GU tract, skin and bone infections; septicemia, gonorrhea; gynecologic, intra-abdominal, biliary infections; meningitis; perioperative prophylaxis. *Treatment of Lyme disease.*

STORAGE/HANDLING

Solutions appear light yellow to amber. IV infusion (piggyback) may darken in color (does not indicate loss of potency). IV infusion (piggyback) stable for 24 hrs at room temperature, 5 days if refrigerated. Discard if precipitate forms.

ADMINISTRATION

Note: Give by IM injection, direct IV injection, intermittent IV infusion (piggyback).

IM:

- To minimize discomfort, inject deep IM slowly. Less painful if injected into gluteus maximus rather than lateral aspect of thigh. For 2 g IM dose, give at 2 separate sites.

IV:

- For direct IV injection, administer over 3–5 min.
- For intermittent IV infusion (piggyback), infuse over 20–30 min.
- Alternating IV sites, use large veins to reduce risk of phlebitis.

INDICATIONS/ROUTES/DOSAGE

Note: Space doses evenly around the clock.

Uncomplicated infections:
IM/IV: Adults, elderly: 1 g q12h.

Mild to moderate infections:
IM/IV: Adults, elderly: 1–2 g q8h.

Severe infections:
IM/IV: Adults, elderly: 2 g q6–8h.

Life-threatening infections:
IM/IV: Adults, elderly: 2 g q4h.

Uncomplicated gonorrhea:
IM: Adults: 1 g one time.

Perioperative prophylaxis:
IM/IV: Adults, elderly: 1 g 30–90 min before surgery.

Cesarean section:
IV: Adults: 1 g as soon as umbilical cord is clamped, then 1 g 6 and 12 hrs after first dose.

Usual dosage for children:
IM/IV: Children >1 mo: 50–180 mg/kg/day in 4 to 6 divided doses. *Neonates 1–4 wks:* 25–50 mg/kg q8h. *Neonates 0–7 days:* 25–50 mg/kg q12h.

Dosage in renal impairment:
Creatinine clearance <20 ml/min: Give 1/2 dose at usual dosage intervals.

CONTRAINDICATIONS

History of hypersensitivity to cephalosporins, anaphylactic reaction to penicillins.

CAUTIONS

Concurrent use of nephrotoxic medications, history of allergies or GI disease (especially ulcerative colitis, antibiotic-associated colitis), renal impairment w/creatinine clearance <20 ml/min.

INTERACTIONS

DRUG: *Probenecid* increases serum concentration of ***cefotaxime***. **HERBAL:** None known. **FOOD:** None significant. **ALTERED LAB VALUES:** Positive direct/indirect Coombs' test may occur. May increase liver function tests.

SIDE EFFECTS

FREQUENT: Discomfort w/IM administration, oral candidiasis (sore mouth/tongue), mild diarrhea, mild abdominal cramping, vaginal candidiasis (itching, discharge). **OCCASIONAL:** Nausea, serum sickness reaction [joint pain, fever] (usually occurs following second course of therapy, resolves after drug discontinuation). **RARE:** Allergic reaction (rash, pruritus, urticaria), thrombophlebitis (pain, redness, swelling at injection site).

ADVERSE REACTIONS/TOXIC EFFECTS

Antibiotic-associated colitis (severe abdominal pain and tenderness, fever, watery and severe diarrhea), other superinfections may result from altered bacterial balance. Nephrotoxicity may occur, especially w/preexisting renal disease. Severe hypersensitivity reaction (severe pruritus, angioedema, bronchospasm, anaphylaxis), particularly those w/history of allergies, especially penicillin.

PATIENT CONSIDERATIONS

BASELINE ASSESSMENT

Question for history of allergies, particularly cephalosporins, penicillins. Obtain culture and sensitivity test before giving first dose (therapy may begin before results are known).

INTERVENTION/EVALUATION

Evaluate IV site for phlebitis (heat, pain, red streaking over vein). Check IM injection sites for induration, tenderness. Check mouth for white patches on mucous membranes, tongue. Monitor bowel activity and stool consistency carefully; mild GI effects may be tolerable, but increasing severity may indicate onset of antibiotic-associated colitis. Assess skin for rash. Monitor I&O, urinalysis, renal function reports for nephrotoxicity. Be alert for superinfection: severe genital/anal pruritus, abdominal pain, severe mouth soreness, moderate to severe diarrhea.

PATIENT/FAMILY TEACHING

Discomfort may occur w/IM injection. Doses should be evenly spaced. Continue antibiotic therapy for full length of treatment.

cefotetan disodium

seh-fo-**teh**-tan
(Cefotan)

CANADIAN AVAILABILITY
Cefotan

PREGNANCY CATEGORY B

CLASSIFICATION

Antibiotic: Second-generation cephalosporin

AVAILABILITY (Rx)

Powder for Injection: 1 g, 2 g

PHARMACOKINETICS

Widely distributed. **Excretion:** Primarily excreted unchanged in urine. Minimally removed by hemodialysis. **Half-life:** 3–4.6 hrs (increased in decreased renal function).

ACTION/*THERAPEUTIC EFFECT*

Bactericidal. Binds to bacterial membranes, *inhibiting bacterial cell wall synthesis.*

USES

Treatment of respiratory, GU tract, skin, bone, gynecologic, intra-abdominal infections; perioperative prophylaxis.

STORAGE/HANDLING

Solutions appear colorless to light yellow. Color change to deep yellow does not indicate loss of potency. IV infusion (piggyback) stable for 24 hrs at room temperature, 96 hrs if refrigerated. Discard if precipitate forms.

ADMINISTRATION

Note: Give by IM injection, direct IV injection, intermittent IV infusion (piggyback).

IM:

- To minimize discomfort, inject deep IM slowly. Less painful if injected into gluteus maximus rather than lateral aspect of thigh.

IV:

- For direct IV injection, administer over 3–5 min.
- For intermittent IV infusion (piggyback), infuse over 20–30 min.
- Alternating IV sites, use large veins to reduce risk of phlebitis.

INDICATIONS/ROUTES/DOSAGE

Note: Space doses evenly around the clock.

Urinary tract infections:
IM/IV: Adults, elderly: 500 mg q12h, or 1–2 g q12–24h.

Mild to moderate infections:
IM/IV: Adults, elderly: 1–2 g q12h.

Severe infections:
IM/IV: Adults, elderly: 2 g q12h.

Life-threatening infections:
IM/IV: Adults, elderly: 3 g q12h.

Perioperative prophylaxis:
IV: Adults, elderly: 1–2 g 30–60 min before surgery.

Cesarean section:
IV: Adults: 1–2 g as soon as umbilical cord is clamped.

Dosage in renal impairment:
Dose and/or frequency modified on basis of creatinine clearance and/or severity of infection.

CREATININE CLEARANCE	DOSAGE INTERVAL
10–30 ml/min	Usual dose q24h
<10 ml/min	Usual dose q48h

CONTRAINDICATIONS

History of hypersensitivity to cephalosporins, anaphylactic reaction to penicillins.

CAUTIONS

Renal impairment, history of allergies or GI disease (especially ulcerative colitis, antibiotic-associated colitis), concurrent use of nephrotoxic medications.

INTERACTIONS

DRUG: Disulfiram reaction (facial flushing, nausea, sweating, headache, tachycardia) may occur when ***alcohol*** is ingested. May increase bleeding risk w/***anticoagulants, heparin, thrombolytics***. **HERBAL:** None known. **FOOD:** None significant. **ALTERED LAB VALUES:** Positive direct/indirect Coombs' test may occur (interferes w/hematologic tests, cross-matching procedures). Prothrombin times may be increased. May increase BUN, serum creatinine, SGOT (AST), SGPT (ALT), alkaline phosphatase concentrations.

SIDE EFFECTS

FREQUENT: Discomfort w/IM administration, oral candidiasis (sore mouth/tongue), mild diarrhea, mild abdominal cramping, vaginal candidiasis (itching, discharge). **OCCASIONAL:** Nausea, unusual bruising/bleeding, serum sickness reaction [joint pain, fever] (usually occurs following second course of therapy, resolves after drug discontinuation). **RARE:** Allergic reaction (rash, pruritus, urticaria), thrombophlebitis (pain, redness, swelling at injection site).

ADVERSE REACTIONS/TOXIC EFFECTS

Antibiotic-associated colitis (severe abdominal pain and tenderness, fever, watery and severe diarrhea), other superinfections may result from altered bacterial balance. Nephrotoxicity may occur, especially w/preexisting renal disease. Severe hypersensitivity reaction (severe pruritus, angioedema, bronchospasm, anaphylaxis), particularly those w/history of allergies, especially penicillin.

PATIENT CONSIDERATIONS

BASELINE ASSESSMENT

Question for history of allergies, particularly cephalosporins, penicillins. Obtain culture and sensitivity test before giving first dose (therapy may begin before results are known).

INTERVENTION/EVALUATION

Evaluate IV site for phlebitis (heat, pain, red streaking over vein). Check IM injection sites for induration, tenderness. Check mouth for white patches on mucous membranes, tongue. Monitor bowel activity and stool consistency carefully; mild GI effects may be tolerable, but increasing severity may indicate onset of antibiotic-associated colitis. Assess skin for rash. Monitor I&O, urinalysis, renal function reports for nephrotoxicity. Be alert for superinfection: severe genital/anal pruritus, abdominal pain, severe mouth soreness, moderate to severe diarrhea.

PATIENT/FAMILY TEACHING

Discomfort may occur w/IM injection. Doses should be evenly spaced. Continue antibiotic therapy for full length of treatment.

Avoid alcohol and alcohol-containing preparations (salad dressings, sauces, cough syrups—read all labels carefully) during and for 72 hrs after last dose of cefotetan.

cefoxitin sodium

seh-**fox**-ih-tin
(Mefoxin)

CANADIAN AVAILABILITY
Mefoxin

PREGNANCY CATEGORY B

CLASSIFICATION

Antibiotic: Second-generation cephalosporin

AVAILABILITY (Rx)

Powder for Injection: 1 g, 2 g

PHARMACOKINETICS

Widely distributed. **Excretion:** Primarily excreted unchanged in urine. Moderately removed by hemodialysis. **Half-life:** 0.7–1.1 hrs (increased in decreased renal function).

ACTION/*THERAPEUTIC EFFECT*

Bactericidal. Binds to bacterial membranes, *inhibiting bacterial cell wall synthesis.*

USES

Treatment of respiratory, GU tract, skin, bone, intra-abdominal, gynecologic infections; gonorrhea, septicemia, perioperative prophylaxis.

STORAGE/HANDLING

Solutions appear colorless to light amber but may darken (does not indicate loss of potency). IV infusion (piggyback) stable for 24 hrs at room temperature, 48 hrs if refrigerated. Discard if precipitate forms.

ADMINISTRATION

Note: Give IM, direct IV injection, or intermittent IV infusion (piggyback).

IM:

- To minimize discomfort, inject deep IM slowly. Less painful if injected into gluteus maximus rather than lateral aspect of thigh.

IV:

- For direct IV injection, administer over 3–5 min.
- For intermittent IV infusion (piggyback), infuse over 30 min.
- Alternating IV sites, use large veins to reduce potential for phlebitis.

INDICATIONS/ROUTES/DOSAGE

Note: Space doses evenly around the clock.

Mild to moderate infections:
IM/IV: Adults, elderly: 1–2 g q6–8h.

Severe infections:
IM/IV: Adults, elderly: 1 g q4h or 2 g q6–8h up to 2 g q4h.

Uncomplicated gonorrhea:
IM: Adults: 2 g one time w/1 g probenecid.

Perioperative prophylaxis:
IM/IV: Adults, elderly: 2 g 30–60 min before surgery and q6h up to 24 hrs postop. *Children >3 mos:* 30–40 mg/kg 30–60 min before surgery and q6h postop for no more than 24 hrs.

Cesarean section:
IV: Adults: 2 g as soon as umbilical cord is clamped, then 2 g 4 and 8 hrs after first dose, then q6h for no more than 24 hrs.

Usual dosage for children:
IM/IV: Children >3 mos: 80–160 mg/kg/day in 4–6 divided doses. *Maximum:* 12 g/day.

Dosage in renal impairment:
After loading dose of 1–2 g, dosage and/or frequency is modified on basis of creatinine clearance and/or severity of infection.

CREATININE CLEARANCE	DOSAGE
30–50 ml/min	1–2 g q8–12h
10–29 ml/min	1–2 g q12–24h
5–9 ml/min	500 mg-1 g q12–24h
<5 ml/min	500 mg-1 g q24–48h

CONTRAINDICATIONS

History of hypersensitivity to cephalosporins, anaphylactic reaction to penicillins.

CAUTIONS

Renal impairment, history of allergies or GI disease (especially ulcerative colitis, antibiotic-associated colitis), concurrent use of nephrotoxic medications.

INTERACTIONS

DRUG: *Probenecid* increases serum concentrations of cefoxitin. **HERBAL:** None known. **FOOD:** None significant. **ALTERED LAB VALUES:** Positive direct/indirect Coombs' test may occur (interferes w/hematologic tests, cross-matching procedures). May increase BUN, serum creatinine, SGOT (AST), SGPT (ALT), alkaline phosphatase concentrations.

SIDE EFFECTS

FREQUENT: Discomfort w/IM administration, oral candidiasis (sore mouth/tongue), mild diarrhea, mild abdominal cramping, vaginal candidiasis (itching, discharge). **OCCASIONAL:** Nausea, serum sickness reaction [joint pain, fever] (usually occurs following second course of therapy, resolves after drug discontinuation). **RARE:** Allergic reaction (rash, pruritus, urticaria), thrombophlebitis (pain, redness, swelling at injection site).

ADVERSE REACTIONS/TOXIC EFFECTS

Antibiotic-associated colitis (severe abdominal pain and tenderness, fever, watery and severe diarrhea), other superinfections may result from altered bacterial balance. Nephrotoxicity may occur, especially w/preexisting renal disease. Severe hypersensitivity reaction (severe pruritus, angioedema, bronchospasm, anaphylaxis), particularly those w/history of allergies, especially penicillin.

PATIENT CONSIDERATIONS

Baseline Assessment

Question for history of allergies, particularly cephalosporins, penicillins. Obtain culture and sensitivity test before giving first dose (therapy may begin before results are known).

Intervention/Evaluation

Evaluate IV site for phlebitis (heat, pain, red streaking over vein). Check IM injection sites for induration, tenderness. Check mouth for white patches on mucous membranes, tongue. Monitor bowel activity and stool consistency carefully; mild GI effects may be tolerable, but increasing severity may indicate onset of antibiotic-associated colitis. Assess skin for rash. Monitor I&O, urinalysis, renal function reports for nephrotoxicity. Be alert for superinfection: severe genital/anal pruritus, abdominal pain, severe mouth

soreness, moderate to severe diarrhea.

PATIENT/FAMILY TEACHING

Discomfort may occur w/IM injection. Doses should be evenly spaced. Continue antibiotic therapy for full length of treatment.

cefpodoxime proxetil

sef-poe-**docks**-em
(Vantin)

PREGNANCY CATEGORY B

CLASSIFICATION

Antibiotic: Second-generation cephalosporin

AVAILABILITY (Rx)

Tablets: 100 mg, 200 mg. **Oral Suspension:** 50 mg/5 ml, 100 mg/5 ml.

PHARMACOKINETICS

Absorption: Well absorbed from GI tract (food increases absorption). Widely distributed. **Excretion:** Primarily excreted unchanged in urine. Partially removed by hemodialysis. **Half-life:** 2.3 hrs (increased in decreased renal function, elderly).

ACTION/*THERAPEUTIC EFFECT*

Bactericidal. Binds to bacterial membrane, *inhibiting bacterial cell wall synthesis.*

USES

Treatment of lower respiratory tract infections (pneumonia, chronic bronchitis), upper respiratory tract (otitis media, pharyngitis/tonsillitis), acute maxillary sinusitis, sexually transmitted diseases (urethral and cervical gonorrhea, anorectal infection), skin and skin structure, urinary tract infections.

STORAGE/HANDLING

Oral suspension: after reconstitution, stable for 14 days if refrigerated.

ADMINISTRATION

ORAL:

- Administer w/food to enhance absorption.

INDICATIONS/ROUTES/DOSAGE

Pneumonia, chronic bronchitis:
Oral: Adults, elderly, children >13 yrs: 200 mg q12h for 10–14 days.

Gonorrhea, rectal gonococcal infection (women only):
Oral: Adults, children >13 yrs: 200 mg as single dose.

Skin/skin structure infections:
Oral: Adults, elderly, children >13 yrs: 400 mg q12h for 7–14 days.

Pharyngitis/tonsillitis:
Oral: Adults, elderly, children >13 yrs: 100 mg q12h for 5–10 days. *Children 6 mos-12 yrs:* 5 mg/kg q12h for 5–10 days. *Maximum:* 100 mg/dose.

Acute maxillary sinusitus:
Oral: Adults, children >13 yrs: 200 mg twice daily for 10 days. *Children 2 mos–12 yrs:* 5 mg/kg q12h for 10 days.

Urinary tract infection:
Oral: Adults, elderly, children >13 yrs: 100 mg q12h for 7 days.

Acute otitis media:
Oral: Children 6 mos–12 yrs: 5 mg/kg q12h for 5 days. *Maximum:* 400 mg/dose.

Dosage in renal impairment:
Dose and/or frequency is based on

degree of renal impairment (creatinine clearance). Creatinine clearance <30 ml/min: dose q24h; on hemodialysis: 3 times/wk after dialysis.

CONTRAINDICATIONS

History of hypersensitivity to cephalosporins, anaphylactic reaction to penicillins.

CAUTIONS

Renal impairment, history of allergies or GI disease (especially ulcerative colitis, antibiotic-associated colitis), concurrent use of nephrotoxic medications.

INTERACTIONS

DRUG: ***Antacids, H_2 antagonists*** may decrease absorption. ***Probenecid*** may increase concentration. **HERBAL:** None known. **FOOD:** None significant. **ALTERED LAB VALUES:** Positive direct/indirect Coombs' test may occur. May increase SGOT (AST), SGPT (ALT), alkaline phosphatase, LDH, bilirubin, BUN, serum creatinine.

SIDE EFFECTS

FREQUENT: Oral candidiasis (sore mouth/tongue), mild diarrhea, mild abdominal cramping, vaginal candidiasis (itching, discharge). **OCCASIONAL:** Nausea, serum sickness reaction [joint pain, fever] (usually occurs following second course of therapy, resolves after drug discontinuation). **RARE:** Allergic reaction (rash, pruritus, urticaria).

ADVERSE REACTIONS/TOXIC EFFECTS

Antibiotic-associated colitis (severe abdominal pain and tenderness, fever, watery and severe diarrhea), other superinfections may result from altered bacterial balance. Nephrotoxicity may occur, especially w/preexisting renal disease. Severe hypersensitivity reaction (severe pruritus, angioedema, bronchospasm, anaphylaxis), particularly those w/history of allergies, especially penicillin.

PATIENT CONSIDERATIONS

BASELINE ASSESSMENT

Shake oral suspension well before using. Question history of allergies, particularly cephalosporins, penicillins. Obtain culture and sensitivity test before giving first dose (therapy may begin before results are known).

INTERVENTION/EVALUATION

Check mouth for white patches on mucous membranes, tongue. Monitor bowel activity and stool consistency carefully; mild GI effects may be tolerable, but increasing severity may indicate onset of antibiotic-associated colitis. Assess skin for rash. Monitor I&O, urinalysis, renal function reports for nephrotoxicity. Be alert for superinfection: severe genital/anal pruritus, abdominal pain, severe mouth soreness, moderate to severe diarrhea.

PATIENT/FAMILY TEACHING

Doses should be evenly spaced. Continue antibiotic therapy for full length of treatment. Take w/food.

---

cefprozil

sef-**proz**-ill
(Cefzil)

CANADIAN AVAILABILITY
Cefzil

PREGNANCY CATEGORY B

CLASSIFICATION

Antibiotic: Second-generation cephalosporin

AVAILABILITY (Rx)

Tablets: 250 mg, 500 mg. **Oral Suspension:** 125 mg/5 ml, 250 mg/5 ml.

PHARMACOKINETICS

Absorption: Well absorbed from GI tract. Widely distributed. **Excretion:** Primarily excreted unchanged in urine. Moderately removed by hemodialysis. **Half-life:** 1.3 hrs (increased in decreased renal function).

ACTION/*THERAPEUTIC EFFECT*

Bactericidal. Binds to bacterial membranes, *inhibiting bacterial cell wall synthesis.*

USES

Treatment of pharyngitis/tonsillitis, otitis media, secondary bacterial infection of acute bronchitis and acute bacterial exacerbation of chronic bronchitis, uncomplicated skin/skin structure infections, acute sinusitis.

STORAGE/HANDLING

Oral suspension: after reconstitution, stable for 14 days if refrigerated.

ADMINISTRATION

ORAL:

- Shake oral suspension well before using.
- Give w/o regard to meals; if GI upset occurs, give w/food or milk.

INDICATIONS/ROUTES/DOSAGE

Note: Space doses evenly around the clock.

Pharyngitis, tonsillitis:
Oral: Adults, elderly: 500 mg q24h for 10 days. ***Children (2–12 yrs):*** 7.5 mg/kg q12h for 10 days.

Secondary bacterial infection of acute bronchitis; acute bacterial exacerbation of chronic bronchitis:
Oral: Adults, elderly: 500 mg q12h for 10 days.

Skin/skin structure infections:
Oral: Adults, elderly: 250–500 mg q12h for 10 days. ***Children:*** 20 mg/kg q24h.

Acute sinusitis:
Oral: Adults, elderly: 250–500 mg q12h. ***Children (6 mos–12 yrs):*** 7.5–15 mg/kg q12h.

Otitis media:
Oral: Children (6 mos–12 yrs): 15 mg/kg q12h for 10 days.

Dosage in renal impairment:
Dose and/or frequency is based on degree of renal impairment (creatinine clearance). Creatinine clearance <30 ml/min: 50% dosage at usual interval.

CONTRAINDICATIONS

History of hypersensitivity to cephalosporins, anaphylactic reaction to penicillins.

CAUTIONS

Renal impairment, history of allergies or GI disease (especially ulcerative colitis, antibiotic-associated colitis), concurrent use of nephrotoxic medications.

INTERACTIONS

DRUG: ***Probenecid*** increases serum concentrations of cefprozil. **HERBAL:** None known. **FOOD:** None significant. **ALTERED LAB VALUES:** Positive direct/indirect Coombs' test may occur (interferes w/hematologic tests, cross-matching procedures). May increase liver function tests.

SIDE EFFECTS

FREQUENT: Oral candidiasis (sore mouth/tongue), mild diarrhea, mild abdominal cramping, vaginal candidiasis (itching, discharge). OCCASIONAL: Nausea, serum sickness reaction [joint pain, fever] (usually occurs following second course of therapy, resolves after drug discontinuation). RARE: Allergic reaction (rash, pruritus, urticaria).

ADVERSE REACTIONS/TOXIC EFFECTS

Antibiotic-associated colitis (severe abdominal pain and tenderness, fever, watery and severe diarrhea), other superinfections may result from altered bacterial balance. Nephrotoxicity may occur, especially w/preexisting renal disease. Severe hypersensitivity reaction (severe pruritus, angioedema, bronchospasm, anaphylaxis), particularly those w/history of allergies, especially penicillin.

PATIENT CONSIDERATIONS

BASELINE ASSESSMENT

Question history of allergies, particularly cephalosporins, penicillins. Obtain culture and sensitivity test before giving first dose (therapy may begin before results are known).

INTERVENTION/EVALUATION

Check mouth for white patches on mucous membranes, tongue. Monitor bowel activity and stool consistency carefully; mild GI effects may be tolerable, but increasing severity may indicate onset of antibiotic-associated colitis. Assess skin for rash. Monitor I&O, urinalysis, renal function reports for nephrotoxicity. Be alert for superinfection: severe genital/anal pruritus, abdominal pain, severe mouth soreness, moderate to severe diarrhea.

PATIENT/FAMILY TEACHING

Doses should be evenly spaced. Continue antibiotic therapy for full length of treatment. May cause GI upset (may take w/food or milk).

ceftazidime

sef-**taz**-ih-deem
(Ceptaz, Fortaz, Tazicef, Tazidime)

CANADIAN AVAILABILITY
Ceptaz, Fortaz, Tazidime

PREGNANCY CATEGORY B

CLASSIFICATION

Antibiotic: Third-generation cephalosporin

AVAILABILITY (Rx)

Powder for Injection: 500 mg, 1 g, 2 g

PHARMACOKINETICS

Widely distributed (including CSF). **Excretion:** Primarily excreted unchanged in urine. Removed by hemodialysis. **Half-life:** 2 hrs (increased in decreased renal function).

ACTION/*THERAPEUTIC EFFECT*

Bactericidal. Binds to bacterial membranes, *inhibiting bacterial cell wall synthesis.*

USES

Treatment of intra-abdominal, biliary tract infections, respiratory, GU tract, skin, bone infections; meningitis, septicemia.

STORAGE/HANDLING

Solutions appear light yellow to amber, tend to darken (color change does not indicate loss of potency). IV infusion (piggyback) stable for 18 hrs at room temperature, 7 days if refrigerated. Discard if precipitate forms.

ADMINISTRATION

Note: Give by IM injection, direct IV injection, intermittent IV infusion (piggyback).

IM:

- To minimize discomfort, inject deep IM slowly. Less painful if injected into gluteus maximus rather than lateral aspect of thigh.

IV:

- For direct IV injection, administer over 3–5 min.
- For intermittent IV infusion (piggyback), infuse over 15–30 min.
- Alternating IV sites, use large veins to reduce risk of phlebitis.

INDICATIONS/ROUTES/DOSAGE

Note: Space doses evenly around the clock.

Urinary tract infections:
IM/IV: Adults: 250–500 mg q8–12h.

Mild to moderate infections:
IM/IV: Adults: 1 g q8–12h.

Uncomplicated pneumonia, skin or skin structure infection:
IM/IV: Adults: 0.5–1 g q8h.

Bone and joint infection:
IM/IV: Adults: 2 g q12h.

Meningitis, serious gynecologic, intra-abdominal infections:
IM/IV: Adults: 2 g q8h.

Pseudomonal pulmonary infections in pts w/cystic fibrosis:
IV: Adults: 30–50 mg/kg q8h. *Maximum:* 6 g/day.

Usual elderly dosage:
IM/IV: Normal renal function q12h.

Usual dosage for children:
IV: Children >1 mo: 30–50 mg/kg q8h. *Children <1 mo:* 30 mg/kg q12h (increase to 50 mg/kg for meningitis).

Dosage in renal impairment:
After initial 1 g dose, dose and/or frequency is modified on basis of creatinine clearance and/or severity of infection.

CREATININE CLEARANCE	DOSAGE
31–50 ml/min	1 g q12h
16–30 ml/min	1 g q24h
6–15 ml/min	500 mg q24h
<5 ml/min	500 mg q48h

CONTRAINDICATIONS

History of hypersensitivity to cephalosporins, anaphylactic reactions to penicillins.

CAUTIONS

Renal impairment, history of GI disease (especially ulcerative colitis, antibiotic-associated colitis) or allergies, concurrent use of nephrotoxic medications.

INTERACTIONS

DRUG: None significant. **HERBAL:** None known. **FOOD:** None significant. **ALTERED LAB VALUES:** Positive direct/indirect Coombs' test may occur (interferes w/hematologic tests, cross-matching procedures). May increase BUN, serum creatinine, SGOT (AST), SGPT (ALT), alkaline phosphatase, LDH concentrations.

SIDE EFFECTS

FREQUENT: Discomfort w/IM administration, oral candidiasis (sore mouth/tongue), mild diarrhea, mild abdominal cramping, vaginal candidiasis (itching, discharge). **OCCASIONAL:** Nausea, serum sickness reaction [joint pain, fever] (usually occurs following second course of therapy, resolves after drug discontinuation). **RARE:** Allergic reaction (rash, pruritus, urticaria), thrombophlebitis (pain, redness, swelling at injection site).

ADVERSE REACTIONS/TOXIC EFFECTS

Antibiotic-associated colitis (severe abdominal pain and tenderness, fever, watery and severe diarrhea), other superinfections may result from altered bacterial balance. Nephrotoxicity may occur, especially w/preexisting renal disease. Severe hypersensitivity reaction (severe pruritus, angioedema, bronchospasm, anaphylaxis), particularly those w/history of allergies, especially penicillin.

PATIENT CONSIDERATIONS

Baseline Assessment

Question for history of allergies, particularly cephalosporins, penicillins. Obtain culture and sensitivity test before giving first dose (therapy may begin before results are known).

Intervention/Evaluation

Evaluate IV site for phlebitis (heat, pain, red streaking over vein). Check IM injection sites for induration, tenderness. Check mouth for white patches on mucous membranes, tongue. Monitor bowel activity and stool consistency carefully; mild GI effects may be tolerable, but increasing severity may indicate onset of antibiotic-associated colitis. Assess skin for rash. Monitor I&O, urinalysis, renal function reports for nephrotoxicity. Be alert for superinfection: severe genital/anal pruritus, abdominal pain, severe mouth soreness, moderate to severe diarrhea.

Patient/Family Teaching

Discomfort may occur w/IM injection. Doses should be evenly spaced. Continue antibiotic therapy for full length of treatment.

ceftibuten

sef-tih-**byew**-ten
(Cedax)

PREGNANCY CATEGORY B

CLASSIFICATION

Antibiotic: Third-generation cephalosporin

AVAILABILITY (Rx)

Capsules: 400 mg. **Oral Suspension:** 90 mg/5 ml, 180 mg/5 ml.

PHARMACOKINETICS

Absorption: Moderately absorbed from GI tract. Widely distributed to most tissues and fluids. **Excretion:** Primarily excreted unchanged in urine. Minimally removed by hemodialysis. **Half-life:** 2–3 hrs (increased in impaired renal function).

ACTION/THERAPEUTIC EFFECT

Bactericidal. Binds to bacterial cell membranes, *inhibiting bacterial cell wall synthesis.*

USES

Acute bacterial exacerbations of chronic bronchitis, acute bacterial otitis media, pharyngitis, tonsillitis.

STORAGE/HANDLING

After reconstitution, refrigerate oral suspension. Stable for 14 days. Discard unused portion after 14 days.

ADMINISTRATION

ORAL:

Capsule:

- Give capsules w/o regard to meals.

Oral suspension:

- Shake oral suspension well before administering.
- Administer suspension at least 2 hrs before or 1 hr after a meal.

INDICATIONS/ROUTES/DOSAGE

Note: Use oral suspension to treat otitis media (achieves higher peak blood level).

Usual oral dosage:
Oral: Adults, elderly, children >12 yrs: 400 mg/day as single daily dose for 10 days. ***Children <12 yrs:*** 9 mg/kg/day as single dose for 10 days. ***Maximum:*** 400 mg/day.

Dosage in renal impairment:
Based on creatinine clearance.

CREATININE CLEARANCE	DOSAGE
>50 ml/min	400 mg or 9 mg/kg q24h
30–49 ml/min	200 mg or 4.5 mg/kg q24h
<30 ml/min	100 mg or 2.25 mg/kg q24h

CONTRAINDICATIONS

Hypersensitivity to cephalosporins.

CAUTIONS

Hypersensitivity to penicillins or other drugs; allergies; history of GI disease (e.g., colitis); renal impairment.

INTERACTIONS

DRUG: ***Probenecid*** increases cephalosporin serum levels. Increased risk of nephrotoxicity w/concurrent use of ***aminoglycosides***. **HERBAL:** None known. **FOOD:** None significant. **ALTERED LAB VALUES:** Positive direct/indirect Coombs' test. May increase BUN, serum creatinine, SGPT (ALT), SGOT (AST), alkaline phosphatase, bilirubin, LDH concentrations.

SIDE EFFECTS

FREQUENT: Oral candidiasis (sore mouth/tongue), mild diarrhea, nausea, vaginal candidiasis. **OCCASIONAL:** Serum sickness reaction (skin rash, joint pain, fever), vomiting. **RARE:** Hemolytic anemia (unusually tired), erythema multiforme (blistering, peeling, loosening of skin), decreased renal function.

ADVERSE REACTIONS/TOXIC EFFECTS

Antibiotic-associated colitis, other superinfections may result from altered bacterial balance. Hypersensitivity reactions (ranging from rash, urticaria, fever to anaphylaxis) may occur, particularly those w/history of allergies, especially penicillin.

PATIENT CONSIDERATIONS

BASELINE/ASSESSMENT

Question for hypersensitivity to ceftibuten or other cephalosporins, penicillins, other drugs. Obtain specimens for culture and sensitivity test (therapy may begin before results are known).

INTERVENTION/EVALUATION

Monitor bowel activity and stool consistency carefully; mild GI effects may be tolerable, but

increasing severity may indicate onset of antibiotic-associated colitis. Report hypersensitivity reaction: skin rash, urticaria, pruritus, fever promptly. Be alert for superinfection (e.g., genital/anal pruritus, ulceration or changes in oral mucosa, moderate to severe diarrhea, new or increased fever). Provide symptomatic relief for nausea, flatulence. Monitor hematology reports.

PATIENT/FAMILY TEACHING

Continue medication for full length of treatment; do not skip doses. Doses should be evenly spaced. Take w/meals if GI upset occurs. Notify physician promptly of onset of diarrhea, rash, bleeding or bruising, or other symptom.

---

ceftizoxime sodium

cef-tih-**zox**-eem
(Cefizox)

CANADIAN AVAILABILITY
Cefizox

PREGNANCY CATEGORY B

CLASSIFICATION

Antibiotic: Third-generation cephalosporin

AVAILABILITY (Rx)

Powder for Injection: 1 g, 2 g

PHARMACOKINETICS

Widely distributed (including CSF). **Excretion:** Primarily excreted unchanged in urine. Moderately removed by hemodialysis. **Half-life:** 1.7 hrs (increased in decreased renal function).

ACTION/*THERAPEUTIC EFFECT*

Bactericidal. Binds to bacterial membranes, *inhibiting bacterial cell wall synthesis.*

USES

Treatment of intra-abdominal, biliary tract, respiratory, GU tract, skin, bone infections; gonorrhea, meningitis, septicemia, pelvic inflammatory disease (PID).

STORAGE/HANDLING

Solutions appear clear to pale yellow. Color change from yellow to amber does not indicate loss of potency. IV infusion (piggyback) stable for 24 hrs at room temperature, 96 hrs if refrigerated. Discard if precipitate forms.

ADMINISTRATION

Note: Give by IM injection, direct IV injection, intermittent IV infusion (piggyback).

IM:

- Inject deep IM slowly to minimize discomfort.
- When giving 2 g dose, divide dose, give in different large muscle masses.

IV:

- For direct IV injection, administer over 3–5 min.
- For intermittent IV infusion (piggyback), infuse over 15–30 min.
- Alternating IV sites, use large veins to reduce risk of phlebitis.

INDICATIONS/ROUTES/DOSAGE

Uncomplicated UTI:
IM/IV: Adults, elderly: 500 mg q12h.

Mild to moderate to severe infection:
IM/IV: Adults, elderly: 1–2 g q8–12h.

PID:
IV: Adults: 2 g q4–8h.

Life-threatening infections:
IV: Adults, elderly: 3–4 g q8h, up to 2 g q4h.

Uncomplicated gonorrhea:
IM: Adults: 1 g one time.

Usual dosage for children:
IM/IV: Children >6 mos: 50 mg/kg q6–8h.

Dosage in renal impairment:
After loading dose of 0.5–1 g, dose and/or frequency is modified on basis of creatinine clearance and/or severity of infection.

CREATININE CLEARANCE	DOSAGE
50–79 ml/min	500 mg–1.5 g q8h
5–49 ml/min	250 mg–1 g q12h
<5 ml/min	250–500 mg q24h

CONTRAINDICATIONS

History of hypersensitivity to cephalosporins, anaphylactic reaction to penicillins.

CAUTIONS

History of allergies, GI disease (especially ulcerative colitis, antibiotic-associated colitis), hepatic and renal impairment.

INTERACTIONS

DRUG: *Probenecid* increases serum concentration of ceftizoxime. **HERBAL:** None known. **FOOD:** None significant. **ALTERED LAB VALUES:** Positive direct/indirect Coombs' test may occur. May increase BUN, serum creatinine, SGOT (AST), SGPT (ALT), alkaline phosphatase concentrations.

SIDE EFFECTS

FREQUENT: Discomfort w/IM administration, oral candidiasis (sore mouth/tongue), mild diarrhea, mild abdominal cramping, vaginal candidiasis (itching, discharge). **OCCASIONAL:** Nausea, serum sickness reaction [joint pain, fever] (usually occurs following second course of therapy, resolves after drug discontinuation). **RARE:** Allergic reaction (rash, pruritus, urticaria), thrombophlebitis (pain, redness, swelling at injection site).

ADVERSE REACTIONS/TOXIC EFFECTS

Antibiotic-associated colitis (severe abdominal pain and tenderness, fever, watery and severe diarrhea), other superinfections may result from altered bacterial balance. Nephrotoxicity may occur, especially w/preexisting renal disease. Severe hypersensitivity reaction (severe pruritus, angioedema, bronchospasm, anaphylaxis) particularly those w/history of allergies, especially penicillin.

PATIENT CONSIDERATIONS

BASELINE ASSESSMENT

Question for history of allergies, particularly cephalosporins, penicillins. Obtain culture and sensitivity test before giving first dose (therapy may begin before results are known).

INTERVENTION/EVALUATION

Evaluate IV site for phlebitis (heat, pain, red streaking over vein). Check IM injection sites for induration, tenderness. Check mouth for white patches on mucous membranes, tongue. Monitor bowel activity and stool consistency carefully; mild GI effects may be tolerable, but increasing severity may indicate onset of antibiotic-associated colitis. Assess skin for rash. Monitor I&O, urinalysis, renal function

reports for nephrotoxicity. Be alert for superinfection: severe genital/anal pruritus, abdominal pain, severe mouth soreness, moderate to severe diarrhea.

PATIENT/FAMILY TEACHING

Discomfort may occur w/IM injection. Doses should be evenly spaced. Continue antibiotic therapy for full length of treatment.

ceftriaxone sodium

cef-try-**ax**-zone
(Rocephin)

CANADIAN AVAILABILITY
Rocephin

PREGNANCY CATEGORY B

CLASSIFICATION

Antibiotic: Third-generation cephalosporin

AVAILABILITY (Rx)

Powder for Injection: 1 g, 2 g

PHARMACOKINETICS

Widely distributed (including CSF). **Excretion:** Primarily excreted unchanged in urine. Not removed by hemodialysis. **Half-life:** 4.3–4.6 hrs IV; 5.8–8.7 hrs IM (increased in decreased renal function).

ACTION/*THERAPEUTIC EFFECT*

Bactericidal. Binds to bacterial membranes, *inhibiting bacterial cell wall synthesis.*

USES

Treatment of respiratory, GU tract, skin, bone, intra-abdominal, biliary tract infections; septicemia, meningitis, gonorrhea, Lyme disease, acute bacterial otitis media.

STORAGE/HANDLING

Solution appears light yellow to amber. IV infusion (piggyback) stable for 3 days at room temperature, 10 days if refrigerated. Discard if precipitate forms.

ADMINISTRATION

Note: Give by IM injection, intermittent IV infusion (piggyback).

IM:
- To minimize discomfort, inject deep IM slowly. Less painful if injected into gluteus maximus rather than lateral aspect of thigh.

IV:
- Administer over 2–4 min.
- For intermittent IV infusion (piggyback), infuse over 15–30 min for adults, 10–30 min in children, neonates.
- Alternating IV sites, use large veins to reduce potential for phlebitis.

INDICATIONS/ROUTES/DOSAGE

Mild to moderate infections:
IM/IV: Adults, elderly: 1–2 g given as single dose or 2 divided doses.

Serious infections:
IM/IV: Adults, elderly: Up to 4 g/day in 2 divided doses. *Children:* 50–75 mg/kg/day in divided doses q12h. *Maximum:* 2 g/day.

Skin/skin structure infections:
IM/IV: Children: 50–75 mg/kg/day as single or 2 divided doses. *Maximum:* 2 g/day.

Meningitis:
IV: Children: Initially, 75 mg/kg, then 100 mg/kg/day as single or in divided doses q12h. *Maximum:* 4 g/day.

Acute bacterial otitis media:
IM: Children: 50 mg/kg as single dose. *Maximum:* 1 g.

Lyme disease:
IV: Adults, elderly: 2–4 g daily for 10–14 days.

Perioperative prophylaxis:
IM/IV: Adults, elderly: 1 g 0.5–2 hrs before surgery.

Uncomplicated gonorrhea:
IM: Adults: 250 mg one time plus doxycycline.

Dosage in renal impairment:
Dosage modification usually unnecessary, but should be monitored in those w/both renal and hepatic impairment or severe renal impairment.

CONTRAINDICATIONS

History of hypersensitivity to cephalosporins, anaphylactic reactions to penicillins.

CAUTIONS

Renal or hepatic impairment, history of GI disease (especially ulcerative colitis, antibiotic-associated colitis), concurrent administration of nephrotoxic medications.

INTERACTIONS

DRUG: None significant. **HERBAL:** None known. **FOOD:** None significant. **ALTERED LAB VALUES:** Positive direct/indirect Coombs' test may occur (interferes w/hematologic tests, cross-matching procedures). May increase BUN, serum creatinine, SGOT (AST), SGPT (ALT), alkaline phosphatase, bilirubin concentrations.

SIDE EFFECTS

FREQUENT: Discomfort w/IM administration, oral candidiasis (sore mouth/tongue), mild diarrhea, mild abdominal cramping, vaginal candidiasis (itching, discharge). **OCCASIONAL:** Nausea, serum sickness reaction [joint pain, fever] (usually occurs following second course of therapy, resolves after drug discontinuation). **RARE:** Allergic reaction (rash, pruritus, urticaria), thrombophlebitis (pain, redness, swelling at injection site).

ADVERSE REACTIONS/TOXIC EFFECTS

Antibiotic-associated colitis (severe abdominal pain and tenderness, fever, watery and severe diarrhea), other superinfections may result from altered bacterial balance. Nephrotoxicity may occur, especially w/preexisting renal disease. Severe hypersensitivity reaction (severe pruritus, angioedema, bronchospasm, anaphylaxis), particularly those w/history of allergies, especially penicillin.

PATIENT CONSIDERATIONS

BASELINE ASSESSMENT

Question for history of allergies, particularly cephalosporins, penicillins. Obtain culture and sensitivity test before giving first dose (therapy may begin before results are known).

INTERVENTION/EVALUATION

Evaluate IV site for phlebitis (heat, pain, red streaking over vein). Check IM injection sites for induration, tenderness. Check mouth for white patches on mucous membranes, tongue. Monitor bowel activity and stool consistency carefully; mild GI effects may be tolerable, but increasing severity may indicate onset of antibiotic-associated colitis. Assess skin for rash. Mon-

itor I&O, urinalysis, renal function reports for nephrotoxicity. Be alert for superinfection: severe genital/anal pruritus, abdominal pain, severe mouth soreness, moderate to severe diarrhea.

Patient/Family Teaching

Discomfort may occur w/IM injection. Doses should be evenly spaced. Continue antibiotic therapy for full length of treatment.

---

cefuroxime axetil

sef-yur-**ox**-ime

(Ceftin)

cefuroxime sodium

(Kefurox, Zinacef)

CANADIAN AVAILABILITY

Ceftin, Kefurox, Zinacef

PREGNANCY CATEGORY B

CLASSIFICATION

Antibiotic: Second-generation cephalosporin

AVAILABILITY (Rx)

Tablets: 125 mg, 250 mg, 500 mg. **Oral Suspension:** 125 mg/5 ml, 250 mg/5 ml. **Powder for Injection:** 750 mg, 1.5 g.

PHARMACOKINETICS

Absorption: Rapidly absorbed from GI tract. Oral form rapidly hydrolyzed to cefuroxime. Widely distributed (including CSF). **Excretion:** Primarily excreted unchanged in urine. Moderately removed by hemodialysis. **Half-life:** 1.3 hrs (increased in decreased renal function).

ACTION/*THERAPEUTIC EFFECT*

Bactericidal. Binds to bacterial membranes, *inhibiting bacterial cell wall synthesis.*

USES

Treatment of otitis media, respiratory, GU tract, gynecologic, skin, bone infections; septicemia, bacterial meningitis, gonorrhea and other gonococcal infections; ampicillin-resistant influenza, perioperative prophylaxis, impetigo, acute bacterial maxillary sinusitis, early Lyme disease.

STORAGE/HANDLING

Solutions appear light yellow to amber; may darken, but color change does not indicate loss of potency. IV infusion (piggyback) stable for 24 hrs at room temperature, 7 days if refrigerated. Discard if precipitate forms.

ADMINISTRATION

Note: Give orally, IM, direct IV injection, intermittent IV infusion (piggyback).

ORAL:

- Give w/o regard to meals. If GI upset occurs, give w/food or milk.
- Tablets may be crushed, mixed w/food.
- Suspension must be given w/food.

IM:

- To minimize discomfort, inject deep IM slowly. Less painful if injected into gluteus maximus rather than lateral aspect of thigh.

IV:

- For direct IV injection, dilute 750 mg in 8 ml (1.5 g in 14 ml) sterile water for injection to provide a concentration of 100 mg/ml. Administer over 3–5 min.

- For intermittent IV infusion (piggyback), further dilute w/50–100 ml 5% dextrose or 0.9% NaCl, infuse over 15–60 min.
- Alternating IV sites, use large veins to reduce risk of phlebitis.

INDICATIONS/ROUTES/DOSAGE

Pharyngitis/tonsillitis:
Oral: Adults, elderly: 250 mg 2 times/day. *Children:* 125 mg 2 times/day or 20 mg/kg/day in 2 divided doses.

Acute otitis media:
Oral: Children: 250 mg 2 times/day or 30 mg/kg/day in 2 divided doses.

Acute/chronic bronchitis:
Oral: Adults: 250–500 mg 2 times/day.

Acute bacterial maxillary sinusitis:
Oral: Adults, children >13 yrs: 250 mg 2 times/day for 10 days. *Children: 3 mos–12 yrs:* 30 mg/kg in 2 divided doses.

Impetigo:
Oral: Children: 30 mg/kg/day in 2 divided doses.

Skin/skin structure infections:
Oral: Adults: 250–500 mg 2 times/day.

IM/IV: Adults: 750 mg–1.5 g q8h.

Early Lyme disease:
Oral: Adults: 500 mg 2 times/day.

Urinary tract infections:
Oral: Adults: 125–250 mg 2 times/day.

IM/IV: Adults: 750 mg–1.5 g q8h.

Pneumonia:
IM/IV: Adults: 750 mg–1.5 g q8h.

Uncomplicated gonorrhea:
Oral: Adults: 1 g as single dose.

IM: Adults: 1.5 g as single dose.

Disseminated gonococcal infection:
IM/IV: Adults: 750 mg to 1.5 g q8h.

Bone/joint infections:
IM/IV: Adults, elderly: 1.5 g q8h.

Life-threatening infections:
IV: Adults, elderly: 1.5 g q8h. *Children:* 150 mg/kg/day in 3 divided doses.

Bacterial meningitis:
IV: Adults: Up to 3 g q8h. *Children:* Initially, 200–240 mg/kg/day in 3–4 divided doses; then, 100 mg/kg/day w/clinical improvement.

Perioperative prophylaxis:
IV: Adults, elderly: 1.5 g 30–60 min before surgery and 750 mg q8h postop.

Dosage in renal impairment:
Adult dosage is modified on basis of creatinine clearance and/or severity of infection.

CREATININE CLEARANCE	DOSAGE
10–20 ml/min	750 mg q12h
<10 ml/min	750 mg q24h

CONTRAINDICATIONS

History of hypersensitivity to cephalosporins, anaphylactic reaction to penicillins.

CAUTIONS

Renal impairment, history of allergies or GI disease (especially ulcerative colitis, antibiotic-associated colitis), concurrent use of nephrotoxic medications.

INTERACTIONS

DRUG: *Probenecid* increases serum concentration of cefuroxime. **HERBAL:** None known. **FOOD:** None significant. **ALTERED LAB VALUES:** Positive direct/indirect Coombs' test may occur (interferes w/hematologic tests, cross-matching procedures). May increase SGOT (AST), SGPT (ALT), alkaline phosphatase, bilirubin, LDH concentrations.

SIDE EFFECTS

FREQUENT: Discomfort w/IM administration, oral candidiasis (sore mouth/tongue), mild diarrhea, mild abdominal cramping, vaginal candidiasis (itching, discharge). **OCCASIONAL:** Nausea, serum sickness reaction [joint pain, fever] (usually occurs following second course of therapy, resolves after drug discontinuation). **RARE:** Allergic reaction (rash, pruritus, urticaria), thrombophlebitis (pain, redness, swelling at injection site).

ADVERSE REACTIONS/TOXIC EFFECTS

Antibiotic-associated colitis (severe abdominal pain and tenderness, fever, watery and severe diarrhea), other superinfections may result from altered bacterial balance. Nephrotoxicity may occur, especially w/preexisting renal disease. Severe hypersensitivity reaction (severe pruritus, angioedema, bronchospasm, anaphylaxis), particularly those w/history of allergies, especially penicillin.

PATIENT CONSIDERATIONS

Baseline Assessment

Question for history of allergies, particularly cephalosporins, penicillins. Obtain culture and sensitivity test before giving first dose (therapy may begin before results are known).

Intervention/Evaluation

Evaluate IV site for phlebitis (heat, pain, red streaking over vein). Check IM injection sites for induration, tenderness. Check mouth for white patches on mucous membranes, tongue. Monitor bowel activity and stool consistency carefully; mild GI effects may be tolerable, but increasing severity may indicate onset of antibiotic-associated colitis. Assess skin for rash. Monitor I&O, urinalysis, renal function reports for nephrotoxicity. Be alert for superinfection: severe genital/anal pruritus, abdominal pain, severe mouth soreness, moderate to severe diarrhea.

Patient/Family Teaching

Discomfort may occur w/IM injection. Doses should be evenly spaced. Continue antibiotic therapy for full length of treatment. May cause GI upset (may take w/food or milk).

---

celecoxib

seal-ee-**cox**-ib
(Celebrex)

PREGNANCY CATEGORY C

CLASSIFICATION

Cyclo-oxygenase-2 inhibitor

AVAILABILITY (Rx)

Capsules: 100 mg, 200 mg

PHARMACOKINETICS

Absorption: Widely distributed. **Metabolism:** Metabolized in liver. **Excretion:** Primarily eliminated in feces. **Half-life:** 11.2 hrs.

ACTION/*THERAPEUTIC EFFECT*

Selectively inhibits cyclo-oxygenase-2, which produces prostaglandins that cause pain and inflammation *producing anti-inflammatory and analgesic effects.*

USES/ *UNLABELED*

Treatment of pain, arthritis.

ADMINISTRATION

ORAL:

- May take w/o regard to food.

INDICATIONS/ROUTES/DOSAGES

Arthritis:

Oral: Adults, elderly: 100–400 mg/day.

CONTRAINDICATIONS

Sensitivity to celecoxib.

CAUTIONS

Pts w/past history of peptic ulcer, >60 yrs of age, pts receiving anticoagulant therapy, steroids, alcohol consumption, smoking. Allergy to aspirin, NSAIDs, sulfa.

INTERACTIONS

DRUG: May increase risk of bleeding with ***warfarin.*** **HERBAL:** Feverfew, ginkgo may increase risk of bleeding. **FOOD:** None significant. **ALTERED LAB VALUES:** May increase liver function tests.

SIDE EFFECTS

FREQUENT (>5%): Diarrhea, dyspepsia, headache, upper respiratory tract infection. **OCCASIONAL (1–5%):** Abdominal pain, flatus, nausea, back pain. peripheral edema, dizziness, pharyngitis, rhinitis, rash.

ADVERSE REACTIONS/TOXIC EFFECTS

None significant.

PATIENT CONSIDERATIONS

BASELINE ASSESSMENT

Assess onset, type, location and duration of pain/inflammation. Inspect appearance of affected joints for immobility, deformities, skin condition.

INTERVENTIONS/EVALUATION

Evaluate for therapeutic response: pain relief, stiffness, swelling, increased joint mobility, decreased tenderness, improved grip strength.

PATIENT/FAMILY TEACHING

If GI upset occurs, take w/food. Avoid aspirin, alcohol (increases risk of GI bleeding). Report any fluid retention, or signs of GI bleeding.

---

cephalexin

cef-ah-**lex**-in

(Keflet, Keflex)

cephalexin hydrochloride

(Keftab)

CANADIAN AVAILABILITY

Apo-Cephalex, Keflex, Novolexin

PREGNANCY CATEGORY B

CLASSIFICATION

Antibiotic: First-generation cephalosporin

AVAILABILITY (Rx)

Capsules: 250 mg, 500 mg. **Tablets:** 250 mg, 500 mg, 1 g. **Oral Suspension:** 125 mg/5 ml, 250 mg/5 ml.

PHARMACOKINETICS

Absorption: Rapidly absorbed from GI tract. Widely distributed. **Excretion:** Primarily excreted unchanged in urine. Moderately removed by hemodialysis. **Half-life:** 0.9–1.2 hrs (increased in decreased renal function).

ACTION/*THERAPEUTIC EFFECT*

Bactericidal. Binds to bacterial membranes, *inhibiting bacterial cell wall synthesis.*

USES

Treatment of respiratory tract, GU tract, skin, soft tissue, bone infections; otitis media, rheumatic fever prophylaxis; follow-up to parenteral therapy.

STORAGE/HANDLING

Oral suspension: after reconstitution, stable for 14 days if refrigerated.

ADMINISTRATION

ORAL:

- Shake oral suspension well before using.
- Give w/o regard to meals. If GI upset occurs, give w/food or milk.

INDICATIONS/ROUTES/DOSAGE

Note: Space doses evenly around the clock.

Usual dosage for adults:
Oral: Adults, elderly: 250–500 mg q6h up to 4 g/day.

Streptococcal pharyngitis, skin/skin structure infections, uncomplicated cystitis:
Oral: Adults elderly: 500 mg q12h.

Usual dosage for children:
Oral: Children: 25–100 mg/kg/day in 2–4 divided doses.

Otitis media:
Oral: Children: 75–100 mg/kg/day in 4 divided doses.

Dosage in renal impairment:
After usual initial dose, dose and/or frequency is modified on basis of creatinine clearance and/or severity of infection.

CREATININE CLEARANCE	DOSAGE
11–40 ml/min	500 mg q8–12h
5–10 ml/min	250 mg q12h
<5 ml/min	250 mg q12–24h

CONTRAINDICATIONS

History of hypersensitivity to cephalosporins, anaphylactic reaction to penicillins.

CAUTIONS

Renal impairment, history of allergies or GI disease (especially ulcerative colitis, antibiotic-associated colitis), concurrent use of nephrotoxic medications.

INTERACTIONS

DRUG: ***Probenecid*** increases serum concentration of cephalexin. **HERBAL:** None known. **FOOD:** None significant. **ALTERED LAB VALUES:** Positive direct/indirect Coombs' test may occur (interferes w/hematologic test, cross-matching procedures). May increase SGOT (AST), SGPT (ALT), alkaline phosphatase concentrations.

SIDE EFFECTS

FREQUENT: Oral candidiasis (sore mouth/tongue), mild diarrhea, nausea, vaginal candidiasis. **OCCASIONAL:** Serum sickness reaction (skin rash, joint pain, fever), vomiting. **RARE:** Hemolytic anemia (unusually tired), erythema multiforme (blistering, peeling, loosening of skin), decreased renal function.

ADVERSE REACTIONS/TOXIC EFFECTS

Antibiotic-associated colitis, other superinfections may result from altered bacterial balance. Nephrotoxicity may occur, especially w/preexisting renal disease. Hypersensitivity reactions (ranging from rash, urticaria, fever to anaphylaxis) occur in those w/history of allergies, especially penicillin.

PATIENT CONSIDERATIONS

BASELINE ASSESSMENT

Question history of allergies, particularly cephalosporins, penicillins. Obtain culture and sensitivity test before giving first dose (therapy may begin before results are known).

INTERVENTION/EVALUATION

Check mouth for white patches on mucous membranes, tongue. Monitor bowel activity and stool consistency carefully; mild GI effects may be tolerable, but increasing severity may indicate onset of antibiotic-associated colitis. Assess skin for rash. Monitor I&O, urinalysis, renal function reports for nephrotoxicity. Be alert for superinfection: genital/anal pruritus, moniliasis, abdominal pain, sore mouth or tongue, moderate to severe diarrhea.

PATIENT/FAMILY TEACHING

Continue therapy for full length of treatment. Doses should be evenly spaced. May cause GI upset (may take w/food).

---

cephalothin

(Keflin)

See Classification section under: Antibiotic: cephalosporins

---

cerivastatin

sara-vah-**stah**-tin

(Baycol)

CANADIAN AVAILABILITY

Baycol

PREGNANCY CATEGORY X

CLASSIFICATION

Antihyperlipidemic

AVAILABILITY (Rx)

Tablets: 0.2 mg, 0.3 mg, 0.4 mg, 0.8 mg

PHARMACOKINETICS

Absorption: Poorly absorbed from GI tract. **Metabolism:** Metabolized in liver. **Excretion:** Primarily excreted in feces via biliary system and to a lesser extent in the urine. **Half-life:** 2–3 hrs. Half-life increased in moderate to severe renal impairment.

ACTION/*THERAPEUTIC EFFECT*

Inhibits HMG-CoA reductase, the enzyme that catalyzes the early step in cholesterol synthesis. *Decreases LDL cholesterol, VLDL cholesterol, and plasma triglycerides; increases HDL cholesterol.*

USES

Adjunct to diet therapy to decrease elevated total and LDL cholesterol concentrations in those with primary hypercholesterolemia (types IIa and IIb) and in those w/combined hypercholesterolemia and hypertriglyceridemia.

ADMINISTRATION

ORAL:

- May give without regard to food.

INDICATIONS/ROUTES/DOSAGES

Hyperlipidemia:

Oral: Adults, elderly: 0.3 mg once daily in the evening. ***Moderate to severe renal function impairment:*** 0.2 mg once daily in the evening. When used in combination therapy, give ≥2 hrs after a bile acid sequestrant is given.

CONTRAINDICATIONS

Hypersensitivity to cerivastatin, active liver disease, unexplained elevated liver function tests, pregnancy, lactation.

CAUTIONS

Anticoagulant therapy, history of liver disease, substantial alcohol consumption, major surgery, severe acute infection, trauma, hypotension, severe metabolic, endocrine, or electrolyte disorders, uncontrolled seizures.

INTERACTIONS

DRUG: Increased risk of rhabdomyolysis, severe myopathy with *cyclosporine, erythromycin, gemfibrozil, nicotinic acid*. May increase *digoxin, warfarin* levels. *Propranolol* may decrease hyperlipidemic effect. **HERBAL:** None known. **FOOD:** None significant. **ALTERED LAB VALUES:** May increase creatinine kinase, serum transaminase concentrations.

SIDE EFFECTS

Generally well tolerated. Side effects usually mild and transient. **FREQUENT (11–13%):** Rhinitis, headache. **OCCASIONAL (4–7%):** Arthralgia, dyspepsia, back pain, diarrhea, abdominal cramping, flatulence, asthenia. **RARE (2–3%):** Myalgia, cough, nausea/vomiting, dizziness, insomnia, leg pain, constipation.

ADVERSE REACTIONS/TOXIC EFFECTS

Potential for cataracts, photosensitivity.

PATIENT CONSIDERATIONS

Baseline Assessment

Question for possibility of pregnancy before initiating therapy (Pregnancy Category X). Before initiating therapy, assess baseline lab results: cholesterol, triglycerides, liver function tests.

Interventions/Evaluation

Determine pattern of bowel activity. Check for headache, dizziness, nasal symptoms. Monitor cholesterol and triglyceride lab results for therapeutic response. Be alert for headache, rhinitis. Pay attention to elevated serum transaminase levels (drug should be discontinued if level rises above 3 times normal level).

Patient/Family Teaching

Follow special diet (important part of treatment). Periodic lab tests are essential part of therapy. Do not take other medications without physician's knowledge. Do not stop medication without consulting physician. Report promptly any muscle pain or weakness, especially if accompanied by fever or malaise. Avoid prolonged exposure to sunlight, use sunscreen, wear protective clothing.

cetirizine

sih-**tier**-eh-zeen
(Zyrtec)

CANADIAN AVAILABILITY
Reactine, Zyrtec

PREGNANCY CATEGORY B

CLASSIFICATION

Antihistamine

AVAILABILITY (Rx)

Tablets: 5 mg, 10 mg. **Syrup:** 5 mg/5 ml.

PHARMACODYNAMICS

	ONSET	PEAK	DURATION
Oral	<1 hr	4–8 hrs	<24 hrs

PHARMACOKINETICS

Absorption: Rapidly, almost completely absorbed from GI tract. Food has no effect on absorption. **Metabolism:** Undergoes low first-pass metabolism; not extensively metabolized. **Excretion:** Primarily excreted in urine (>80% as unchanged drug). **Half-life:** 6.5–10 hrs.

ACTION / *THERAPEUTIC EFFECT*

Competes w/histamine at histaminic receptor sites on effector cells, *preventing allergic response (urticaria, pruritus). Also produces mild bronchodilation, blocks histamine-induced bronchoconstriction in asthmatic patients.* Minimal anticholinergic effects.

USES / *UNLABELED*

Relief of symptoms (sneezing, rhinorrhea, postnasal discharge, nasal pruritus, ocular pruritus, tearing) of seasonal and perennial allergic rhinitis (hay fever). Treatment of chronic urticaria (hives). *Treatment of bronchial asthma.*

ADMINISTRATION

ORAL:

- May give w/o regard to meals.

INDICATIONS/ROUTES/DOSAGE

Allergic rhinitis, hives:
Oral: Adults, elderly: 5–10 mg /day. May increase up to 20 mg/day. ***Children 6–11 yrs:*** 5–10 mg once daily. ***Children 2–5 yrs:*** Initially, 2.5 mg once daily. ***Maximum:*** 5 mg once daily or 2.5 mg q12h.

Renal impairment (creatinine clearance 11–31 ml/min), hemodialysis (creatinine clearance <7 ml/min), hepatic impairment:
Oral: Adults, elderly: 5 mg once daily.

CONTRAINDICATIONS

None significant.

CAUTIONS

Impaired hepatic impairment, symptomatic prostatic hypertrophy, urinary retention, angle closure glaucoma.

INTERACTIONS

DRUG: *Alcohol, CNS depressants* may increase CNS depression. **HERBAL:** None known. **FOOD:** None significant. **ALTERED LAB VALUES:** May suppress wheal and flare reactions to antigen skin testing, unless antihistamines are discontinued 4 days before testing.

SIDE EFFECTS

Minimal anticholinergic effects. **OCCASIONAL (2–10%):** Pharyngitis, dry mouth, nose, throat, nausea, vomiting, abdominal pain, headache, dizziness, fatigue, thickening mucus, drowsiness, increased sensitivity of skin to sun.

ADVERSE REACTIONS/TOXIC EFFECTS

Children may experience dominant paradoxical reaction (restlessness, insomnia, euphoria, nervousness, tremors). Dizziness, sedation, confusion more likely to occur in elderly pts.

PATIENT CONSIDERATIONS

BASELINE ASSESSMENT

Assess lung sound, rhinitis, urticaria, or other symptoms, liver function tests.

INTERVENTION/EVALUATION

For upper respiratory allergies, increase fluids to maintain thin secretions and offset thirst, loss of fluids from increased sweating. Monitor symptoms for therapeutic response.

PATIENT/FAMILY TEACHING

Generally does not cause drowsiness; however, if blurred vision or eye pain occurs, do not drive or perform activities requiring visual acuity. Avoid alcohol during antihistamine therapy. May take w/food (may cause GI upset). Avoid prolonged exposure to sunlight.

cetrorelix

(Cetrotide)

See Supplement

cevimeline

(Evoxac)

See Supplement

charcoal, activated

(Actidose, Charcocaps)

CANADIAN AVAILABILITY

Aqueous Charcodote

PREGNANCY CATEGORY C

CLASSIFICATION

Antidote

AVAILABILITY (OTC)

Tablets: 260 mg, 325 mg, 650 mg. **Capsules:** 250 mg, 260 mg. **Suspension:** 12.5 g, 15 g, 25 g, 30 g, 50 g.

PHARMACOKINETICS

Absorption/metabolism: Not absorbed or metabolized. **Excretion:** Eliminated via intestinal tract.

ACTION

Adsorbs (detoxifies) ingested toxic substances, irritants, intestinal gas.

USES

Emergency antidote in treatment of poisoning. Reduces volume of intestinal gas, diarrhea.

ADMINISTRATION

ORAL:

- Give 2 hrs before or 1 hr after other oral medication.
- Shake suspension well before using.

INDICATIONS/ROUTES/DOSAGE

Antidote:

Oral: Adults, elderly: Can give 30–100 g as slurry (30 g in at least 8 oz H_2O) or 12.5–50 g in aqueous or sorbitol suspension. Usually given as single dose.

Antidiarrheal:

Oral: Adults, elderly: 520 mg, repeat q30min–1h up to 4.16 g/day.

Antiflatulent:

Oral: Adults, elderly: 1.04–3.9 g 3 times/day after meals.

CONTRAINDICATIONS

None significant.

CAUTIONS

None significant.

INTERACTIONS

DRUG: May decrease absorption, effects of orally administered medications. **HERBAL:** None known. **FOOD:** None significant. **ALTERED LAB VALUES:** None significant.

SIDE EFFECTS

OCCASIONAL: Diarrhea, GI discomfort, intestinal gas.

ADVERSE REACTIONS/TOXIC EFFECTS

None significant.

PATIENT CONSIDERATIONS

INTERVENTION/EVALUATION

Monitor bowel pattern, stool consistency. Assess bowel sounds for peristalsis. When using activated charcoal as an antidote, monitor vital signs, LOC, and other clinical signs related to specific drug ingested.

chloral hydrate

klor-al **high**-drate
(Noctec, Aquachloral Supprettes)

CANADIAN AVAILABILITY
PMS-Chloral Hydrate

PREGNANCY CATEGORY C

CLASSIFICATION

Sedative, hypnotic

AVAILABILITY (Rx)

Capsules: 250 mg, 500 mg. **Syrup:** 250 mg/5 ml, 500 mg/5 ml. **Suppository:** 324 mg, 500 mg, 648 mg.

PHARMACODYNAMICS

	ONSET	PEAK	DURATION
Oral	30–60 min	—	4–8 hrs
Rectal	30–60 min	—	4–8 hrs

PHARMACOKINETICS

Absorption: Readily absorbed from GI tract. **Metabolism:** Metabolized in liver, erythrocytes to active metabolite. **Excretion:** Excreted in urine. **Half-life:** 7–10 hrs.

ACTION/*THERAPEUTIC EFFECT*

Produces CNS depression (mechanism unknown). *Induces quiet, deep sleep, w/only slight decrease in respiration, B/P.*

USES

Treatment of insomnia (replaced by other medications), adjunct to anesthesia preoperatively to produce sedation/relieve anxiety.

ADMINISTRATION

ORAL:
- May be given w/o regard to meals.
- Capsules may be emptied and mixed w/food.
- Mix syrup form with ½ glass (4 oz) water, fruit juice, ginger ale.

RECTAL:
- If suppository is too soft, chill for 30 min in refrigerator or run cold water over foil wrapper.
- Moisten suppository w/cold water before inserting well up into rectum.

INDICATIONS/ROUTES/DOSAGE

Premedication for dental/ medical procedures:
*Oral/Rectal: **Adults:*** 0.5–1 g. ***Children:*** 75 mg/kg up to 1 g total.

Premedication for EEG:
*Oral/Rectal: **Adults:*** 0.5–1.5 g. ***Children:*** 25 mg/kg.

CONTRAINDICATIONS

Marked hepatic, renal impairment, severe cardiac disease, presence of gastritis. ***Oral form:*** Esophagitis, gastritis, gastric/duodenal ulcer.

CAUTIONS

History of drug abuse, mental depression.

INTERACTIONS

DRUG: *Alcohol, CNS depressants* may increase effects. May increase effect of ***warfarin***. IV ***furosemide*** given within 24 hrs following chloral hydrate may alter B/P, cause diaphoresis. **HERBAL:** None known. **FOOD:** None significant. **ALTERED LAB VALUES:** None significant.

SIDE EFFECTS

FREQUENT: Nausea, vomiting, stomach pain. **OCCASIONAL:** Skin rash, hives, diarrhea, dizziness, drowsiness, unsteadiness. **RARE:** Confusion, paradoxical excitement, paradoxical CNS hyperactivity/nervousness in children, excitement/restlessness in elderly (particularly noted when given in presence of pain).

ADVERSE REACTIONS/TOXIC EFFECTS

Overdosage may produce somnolence, confusion, slurred speech, severe incoordination, respiratory depression, coma. Tolerance and psychological dependence may occur by second week of therapy. Abrupt withdrawal of drug after long-term use may produce weakness, facial flushing, sweating, vomiting, tremor.

PATIENT CONSIDERATIONS

BASELINE ASSESSMENT

Assess B/P, pulse, respirations immediately before administration. Raise bed rails. Provide environment conducive to sleep (back rub, quiet environment, low lighting).

INTERVENTION/EVALUATION

Assess sleep pattern of pt. Assess elderly/children for paradoxical reaction. Evaluate for therapeutic response to insomnia: a decrease in number of nocturnal awakenings, increase in length of sleep.

PATIENT/FAMILY TEACHING

Do not abruptly withdraw medication after long-term use. Avoid tasks that require alertness, motor skills until response to drug is established. Tolerance/dependence may occur w/prolonged use of high doses.

---

chlorambucil

(Leukeran)

See Classification section under: Cancer chemotherapy

---

chloramphenicol

klor-am-**fen**-ih-call

(Chloromycetin, Chloroptic)

chloramphenicol palmitate

(Chloromycetin oral suspension)

chloramphenicol sodium succinate

(Chloromycetin)

FIXED-COMBINATION(S)

W/polymyxin B, an antibiotic, and hydrocortisone, acetate **(Ophthocort)**

CANADIAN AVAILABILITY

Chloromycetin

PREGNANCY CATEGORY C

CLASSIFICATION

Antibiotic

AVAILABILITY (Rx)

Capsule: 250 mg. **Oral Suspension:** 150 mg/5 ml. **Powder for Injection:** 100 mg/ml. **Oph-**

thalmic Solution: 5 mg/ml. **Ophthalmic Ointment:** 10 mg/g. **Otic Solution:** 0.5%.

PHARMACOKINETICS

Absorption: Rapidly, completely absorbed after oral, IM administration. Widely distributed (including CSF). **Metabolism:** Metabolized in liver. **Excretion:** Primarily excreted in urine. Minimally removed by hemodialysis. **Half-life:** 1.5–3.5 hrs (increased in decreased renal, liver function, children, neonates).

ACTION / *THERAPEUTIC EFFECT*

Bacteriostatic (may be bactericidal in high concentrations). Binds to ribosomal receptor sites, *inhibiting protein synthesis.*

USES

Intra-abdominal, soft tissue, or orificial infections, typhoid fever, osteomyelitis, septic arthritis, cellulitis, septicemia, meningitis; adjunctive therapy for cerebral abscesses or other CNS infections, rickettsial infections when tetracyclines are contraindicated. Treatment of superficial ocular infections, superficial infections of external auditory canal.

STORAGE/HANDLING

Store capsules, oral suspension at room temperature. Solution for injection is stable for 30 days at room temperature. Discard if cloudy or precipitate forms.

ADMINISTRATION

ORAL:

- Change therapy from IV to oral as soon as possible.
- Administer oral doses on empty stomach 1 hr before or 2 hrs after meals (may give w/food if GI upset occurs).

IV:

- **Note:** Give by IV injection or intermittent IV infusion (piggyback).
- For IV injection, administer dose over at least 1 min.
- Dosage adjusted to maintain plasma concentration at 5–20 mcg/ml.
- For intermittent IV infusion (piggyback), infuse >30 min.
- Pts should be hospitalized during chloramphenicol therapy for close observation, adequate blood studies.

OPHTHALMIC:

- Place finger on lower eyelid and pull out until a pocket is formed between eye and lower lid.
- Hold dropper above pocket and place correct number of drops ($\frac{1}{4}$–$\frac{1}{2}$ inch ointment) into pocket. Close eye gently.
- *Solution:* Apply digital pressure to lacrimal sac for 1–2 min (minimizes drainage into nose and throat, reducing risk of systemic effects).
- *Ointment:* Close eye for 1–2 min, rolling eyeball (increases contact area of drug to eye).
- Remove excess solution or ointment around eye w/tissue.

INDICATIONS/ROUTES/DOSAGE

Mild to moderate infections:
Oral/IV: Adults, elderly, children: 50 mg/kg/day in divided doses q6h.

Severe infections, infections due to moderately resistant organisms:
Oral/IV: Adults, elderly, children: 50–100 mg/kg/day in divided doses q6h.

Dosage in renal or hepatic impairment:
Dosage is reduced on basis of

degree of renal impairment, plasma concentration of drug. Initially, 1 g, then 500 mg q6h.

Usual dosage for neonates:
Oral/IV: Newborn infants: 25 mg/kg/day in 4 doses q6h. ***Infants >2 wks:*** 50 mg/kg/day in 4 doses q6h. ***Neonates <2 kg:*** 25mg/kg once daily. ***Neonates <7 days, >2 kg:*** 25 mg/kg once daily. ***Neonates >7 days, >2 kg:*** 50 mg/kg/day in divided doses q12h.

Usual ophthalmic dosage:
Ointment: Adults, elderly, children: Apply thin strip to conjunctiva q3–4h.

Drops: Adults, elderly, children: 1–2 drops 4–6 times/day.

Usual otic dosage:
Otic: Adults, elderly, children: 2–3 drops into ear 3 times/day.

CONTRAINDICATIONS

Hypersensitivity to chloramphenicol or other components in fixed combination. Not for use in infections when less toxic drugs can be used. Prolonged treatment or frequent application should be avoided w/topical application.

CAUTIONS

Hepatic or renal impairment, infants/children <2 yrs, bone marrow depression, previous cytotoxic drug therapy, radiation therapy.

INTERACTIONS

DRUG: ***Anticonvulsants, bone marrow depressants*** may increase bone marrow depression. May increase effect of ***oral hypoglycemics.*** May antagonize effects of ***clindamycin, erythromycin.*** May increase concentration of ***phenobarbital, phenytoin, warfarin.*** **HERBAL:** None known. **FOOD:** None significant. **ALTERED LAB VALUES:** None significant.

SIDE EFFECTS

OCCASIONAL: ***Systemic:*** Nausea, vomiting, diarrhea. ***Ophthalmic:*** Blurred vision, burning, stinging, hypersensitivity reaction. ***Otic:*** Hypersensitivity reaction. **RARE:** "Gray baby" syndrome [neonates]: (abdominal distension, blue gray skin color, cardiovascular collapse, unresponsiveness), rash, shortness of breath, confusion, headache, optic neuritis (eye pain, blurred vision), peripheral neuritis (numbness/weakness in hands/feet).

ADVERSE REACTIONS/TOXIC EFFECTS

Superinfection due to bacterial or fungal overgrowth. Narrow margin between effective therapy and toxic levels producing blood dyscrasias: bone marrow depression w/resulting aplastic anemia, hypoplastic anemia, pancytopenia (may occur wks or months later).

PATIENT CONSIDERATIONS

Baseline Assessment

Question pt for history of allergies, particularly to chloramphenicol. Avoid, if possible, other drugs that cause bone marrow depression. Obtain specimens for culture and sensitivity test before giving first dose (therapy may begin before results are known). Establish baseline blood studies before therapy.

Intervention/Evaluation

Monitor hematology reports carefully. Coordinate w/lab for drawing of chloramphenicol plasma levels. Assess for appetite, vomiting. Evaluate mental status. Check for visual disturbances. Assess skin for rash. Determine pattern of bowel activity and stool consistency.

Monitor I&O, renal function tests if indicated. Watch for superinfection: diarrhea, anal/genital pruritus, change in oral mucosa, increased fever.

Patient/Family Teaching

Continue therapy for full length of treatment; ophthalmic treatment should continue at least 48 hrs after eye returns to normal appearance. Doses should be evenly spaced. Take oral doses on empty stomach, 1 hr before or 2 hrs after meals (may take w/food if GI upset occurs, but not w/iron or vitamins). Notify physician in event of unusual bleeding or bruising, blurred vision, tired/weak feeling, or other new symptom; w/ophthalmic use report any increased irritation, burning, itching.

chlordiazepoxide

klor-dye-az-eh-**pox**-eyd

(Libritabs)

chlordiazepoxide hydrochloride

(Librium, Lipoxide)

FIXED-COMBINATION(S)

W/clidinium bromide, an anticholinergic **(Librax)**; w/estrogen **(Menrium)**; w/amitriptyline hydrochloride, an antidepressant **(Limbitrol)**.

CANADIAN AVAILABILITY

Apo-Chlordiazepoxide, Novopoxide

PREGNANCY CATEGORY D

CLASSIFICATION

Antianxiety: Benzodiazepine

AVAILABILITY (Rx)

Capsules: 5 mg, 10 mg, 25 mg. **Tablets:** 5 mg, 10 mg, 25 mg. **Injection:** 100 mg ampul.

PHARMACODYNAMICS

	ONSET	PEAK	DURATION
IV	1–5 min	—	15 min–1 hr

PHARMACOKINETICS

Absorption: Well absorbed from GI tract; slow, erratic after IM administration. **Metabolism:** Metabolized in liver to active metabolite. **Excretion:** Excreted in urine. **Half-life:** 5–30 hrs.

ACTION/THERAPEUTIC EFFECT

Enhances action of gamma aminobutyric acid (GABA) neurotransmission at CNS, *producing anxiolytic effect.*

USES/*UNLABELED*

Management of anxiety disorders, acute alcohol withdrawal symptoms; short-term relief of symptoms of anxiety, preop anxiety, tension. *Treatment of panic disorder, tension headache, tremors.*

STORAGE/HANDLING

Store unreconstituted parenteral form at room temperature. Refrigerate diluent; do not use if hazy or opalescent. Prepare immediately before administration; discard unused portions. Do not mix w/infusion fluids.

ADMINISTRATION

ORAL:

- Give w/o regard to meals.
- Tablets may be crushed (do not crush combination form).

- Capsules may be emptied and mixed w/food.

IM:

- Do not use IV preparation for IM injection (produces pain at injection site).
- Add 2 ml of diluent provided to 100 mg ampule to yield 50 mg/ml. Add diluent carefully to minimize air bubbles. Agitate gently to dissolve.
- Inject deep IM slowly into upper outer quadrant of gluteus maximus.

IV:

- Do not use IM diluent solution for IV injection (air bubbles form during reconstitution of diluent).
- Dilute each 100 mg ampule w/5 ml of 0.9% NaCl or sterile water for injection administration to yield 20 mg/ml. Agitate gently until dissolved.
- Use Y tube or 3-way stopcock to control infusion rate.
- Administer 100 mg or fraction thereof over at least 1 min.
- A too rapid IV may produce hypotension, respiratory depression.

INDICATIONS/ROUTES/DOSAGE

Note: Use smallest effective dose in elderly or debilitated, those w/liver disease, low serum albumin.

Parenteral form: Do not exceed 300 mg/24 hrs.

Mild to moderate anxiety:
Oral: Adults: 5–10 mg 3–4 times/day. ***Elderly/debilitated:*** 5 mg 2–4 times/day. Do not exceed 10 mg/day initially. ***Children >6 yrs:*** 5 mg 2–4 times/day. Do not exceed 10 mg/day initially.

Severe anxiety:
Oral: Adults: 20–25 mg 3–4 times/day.

IM/IV: Adults: Initially, 50–100 mg, then 25–50 mg 3–4 times/day. ***Elderly:*** 25–50 mg 3–4 times/day.

Preoperative:
IM/IV: Adults: 50–100 mg 1 hr before surgery. ***Elderly/debilitated, children 12–18 yrs:*** 25–50 mg 1 hr before surgery.

Alcohol withdrawal:
Oral: Adults: 50–100 mg followed by repeated doses until agitation is controlled. Do not exceed 300 mg/day.

IM/IV: Adults: Initially, 50–100 mg. May repeat in 2–4 hrs, if necessary.

CONTRAINDICATIONS

Acute narrow-angle glaucoma, acute alcohol intoxication.

CAUTIONS

Impaired kidney/liver function.

INTERACTIONS

DRUG: ***Alcohol, CNS depressants*** may increase CNS depressant effect. **HERBAL:** Kava kava, valerian may increase CNS depression. **FOOD:** None significant. **ALTERED LAB VALUES:** None significant.

SIDE EFFECTS

FREQUENT: Pain w/IM injection; drowsiness, ataxia, dizziness, confusion w/oral dose, particularly in elderly, debilitated. **OCCASIONAL:** Rash, peripheral edema, GI disturbances. **RARE:** Paradoxical CNS hyperactivity/nervousness in children, excitement/restlessness in elderly (generally noted during first 2 wks of therapy, particularly noted in presence of uncontrolled pain).

ADVERSE REACTIONS/TOXIC EFFECTS

IV route may produce pain, swelling, thrombophlebitis, carpal tunnel syndrome. Abrupt or too rapid withdrawal may result in pronounced restlessness, irritability, insomnia, hand tremors, abdominal/muscle cramps, sweating, vomiting, seizures. Overdosage results in somnolence, confusion, diminished reflexes, coma.

PATIENT CONSIDERATIONS

BASELINE ASSESSMENT

Assess B/P, pulse, respirations immediately before administration. Pt must remain recumbent for up to 3 hrs (individualized) after parenteral administration to reduce hypotensive effect. Assess autonomic response (cold, clammy hands, sweating) and motor response (agitation, trembling, tension). Offer emotional support to anxious pt.

INTERVENTION/EVALUATION

Assess motor responses (agitation, trembling, tension) and autonomic responses (cold, clammy hands, sweating). Assess children, elderly for paradoxical reaction, particularly during early therapy. Assist w/ambulation if drowsiness, ataxia occur. For those on long-term therapy, liver/renal function tests, blood counts should be performed periodically.

PATIENT/FAMILY TEACHING

Discomfort may occur w/IM injection. Drowsiness usually disappears during continued therapy. If dizziness occurs, change positions slowly from recumbent to sitting before standing. Avoid tasks that require alertness, motor skills until response to drug is established. Smoking reduces drug effectiveness. Do not abruptly withdraw medication after long-term therapy.

---

chloroprocaine

(Nesacaine)

See Classification section under: Anesthetics: local

---

chloroquine hydrochloride

klor-oh-kwin

(Aralen hydrochloride)

chloroquine phosphate

(Aralen phosphate)

CANADIAN AVAILABILITY

Aralen

PREGNANCY CATEGORY C

CLASSIFICATION

Antimalarial, amebecide

AVAILABILITY (Rx)

Tablets: 500 mg. **Injection:** 50 mg/ml.

PHARMACOKINETICS

Absorption: Readily absorbed from GI tract. Widely distributed. **Metabolism:** Partially metabolized in liver to active metabolite. **Excretion:** Excreted slowly in urine. Removed by hemodialysis. **Half-life:** 1–2 mos.

ACTION/*THERAPEUTIC EFFECT*

Concentrates in parasite acid vesicles, *increases pH (inhibits parasite growth)*. May interfere w/parasite protein synthesis.

USES/*UNLABELED*

Treatment of *Plasmodium falciparum* malaria (terminates acute attacks, cures nonresistant strains), suppression of acute attacks, prolongation of interval between treatment/relapse in *P. vivax, P. ovale, P. malariae* malaria. Adjunctive therapy for extraintestinal amebiasis (including liver abscess). In combination w/primaquine cure for *P. vivax* and *P. ovale* malaria. *Treatment of sarcoid-associated hypercalcemia, juvenile arthritis, rheumatoid arthritis, systemic lupus erythematosus, solar urticaria, chronic cutaneous vasculitis.*

ADMINISTRATION

ORAL:

- Administer w/meals to reduce adverse GI effects.
- Tablets have bitter taste; may be crushed and mixed w/food or encased in gelatin capsule.

INDICATIONS/ROUTES/DOSAGE

Note: Chloroquine PO_4 500 mg = 300 mg base; chloroquine HCl 50 mg = 40 mg base.

Chloroquine Phosphate:

Treatment of malaria (acute attack): Dose (mg base)

DOSE TIME	ADULTS	CHILDREN
Initial Day 1	600 mg	10 mg/kg
Second 6 hrs later	300 mg	5 mg/kg
Third Day 2	300 mg	5 mg/kg
Fourth Day 3	300 mg	5 mg/kg

Suppression of malaria:
Oral: Adults: 300 mg (base)/wk on same day each week beginning 2 wks before exposure; continue for 6–8 wks after leaving endemic area. ***Children:*** 5 mg base/kg/wk. If therapy is not begun prior to exposure, then: ***Oral: Adults:*** 600 mg base initially given in 2 divided doses 6 hrs apart. ***Children:*** 10 mg base/kg.

Amebiasis:
Oral: Adults: 1 g (600 mg base) daily for 2 days; then, 500 mg (300 mg base)/day for at least 2–3 wks.

Chloroquine HCl:

Treatment of malaria:
IM: Adults: Initially, 160–200 mg base (4–5 ml), repeat in 6 hrs. ***Maximum:*** 800 mg base in first 24 hrs. Begin oral therapy as soon as possible and continue for 3 days until approximately 1.5 g base given. ***Children:*** Initially, 5 mg base/kg, repeat in 6 hrs. Do not exceed 10 mg base/kg/24 hrs.

Amebiasis:
IM: Adults: 160–200 mg base (4–5 ml) daily for 10–12 days. Change to oral therapy as soon as possible.

CONTRAINDICATIONS

Hypersensitivity to 4-aminoquinolones, retinal or visual field changes, psoriasis, porphyria.

CAUTIONS

Alcoholism, hepatic disease, G-6-PD deficiency, severe blood disorders, liver disease, or neurologic disorders. Children are especially susceptible to chloroquine fatalities.

INTERACTIONS

DRUG: May increase concentration of ***penicillamine***, increase risk of hematologic/renal or severe skin reaction. **HERBAL:** None known. **FOOD:** None significant. **ALTERED LAB VALUES:** Acute decrease in Hct, Hgb, RBC count may occur.

SIDE EFFECTS

FREQUENT: Difficulty reading, diarrhea, decreased appetite, nausea, vomiting, stomach pain, headache, pruritus. **OCCASIONAL:** Bleaching of hair, increased hair loss, blurred vision, skin rash, blue-black skin discoloration. **RARE:** Hypotension, change in personality, increased muscle weakness, seizures.

ADVERSE REACTIONS/TOXIC EFFECTS

Ocular toxicity (tinnitus), ototoxicity (reduced hearing). ***Prolonged therapy:*** peripheral neuritis and neuromyopathy, hypotension, EKG changes, agranulocytosis, aplastic anemia, thrombocytopenia, convulsions, psychosis. ***Overdosage:*** headache, vomiting, visual disturbance, drowsiness, convulsions, hypokalemia followed by cardiovascular collapse, death.

PATIENT CONSIDERATIONS

Baseline Assessment

Question for hypersensitivity to chloroquine or hydroxychloroquine sulfate. Evaluate CBC, hepatic function results.

Intervention/Evaluation

Check for and promptly report any visual disturbances. Evaluate for GI distress: Give dose w/food, discuss w/physician dividing dose into separate days during week. Monitor hepatic function tests and check for fatigue, jaundice, or other signs of hepatic effects. Assess skin and buccal mucosa, inquire about pruritus. Check vital signs and be alert to signs/symptoms of overdosage (especially w/parental administration, children). Monitor CBC results for adverse hematologic effects. Notify physician of tinnitus, reduced hearing. W/prolonged therapy, test for muscle weakness. Parenteral therapy should be converted to oral therapy as soon as possible.

Patient/Family Teaching

IM administration may cause local pain. Continue drug for full length of treatment. Notify physician of *any* new symptom, visual difficulties or decreased hearing, tinnitus immediately. Do not take any other medication w/o consulting physician. Periodic lab and visual tests are important part of therapy. Keep out of reach of children (small amount can cause serious effects, death).

---

chlorothiazide

(Diuril)

See Classification section under: Diuretics

---

chlorotrianisene

(TACE)

See Classification section under: Cancer chemotherapy

---

chlorpheniramine

(Teldrin, Chlor-Trimeton)

See Classification section under: Antihistamines

---

chlorpromazine

klor-**pro**-mah-zeen

(Thorazine)

chlorpromazine hydrochloride

(Thorazine)

CANADIAN AVAILABILITY

Chlorpromanyl, Largactil

PREGNANCY CATEGORY C

CLASSIFICATION

Antipsychotic

AVAILABILITY (Rx)

Tablets: 10 mg, 25 mg, 50 mg, 100 mg, 200 mg. **Capsules (sustained-release):** 30 mg, 75 mg, 150 mg, 200 mg, 300 mg. **Syrup:** 10 mg/5 ml. **Oral Concentrate:** 30 mg/ml, 100 mg/ml. **Injection:** 25 mg/ml. **Suppository:** 25 mg, 100 mg.

PHARMACODYNAMICS

	ONSET	PEAK	DURATION
Oral	30–60 min	—	4–6 hrs
Extended-release	30–60 min	—	10–12 hrs
IM	Rapid	—	—
IV	Rapid	—	—
Rectal	>60 min	—	3–4 hrs

PHARMACOKINETICS

Absorption: Variably absorbed after oral administration; well absorbed after IM administration. **Metabolism:** Metabolized in liver to some active metabolites. **Excretion:** Excreted in urine, eliminated in feces. **Half-life:** 30 hrs.

ACTION/*THERAPEUTIC EFFECT*

Blocks dopamine neurotransmission at postsynaptic dopamine receptor sites. Possesses strong anticholinergic, sedative, antiemetic effects, moderate extrapyramidal effects, slight antihistamine action. *Reduces psychosis, relieves nausea and vomiting, controls intractable hiccups, porphyria.*

USES/*UNLABELED*

Management of psychotic disorders, manic phase of manic-depressive illness, severe nausea or vomiting, preop sedation, severe behavioral disturbances in children. Relief of intractable hiccups, acute intermittent porphyria. *Treatment of choreiform movement of Huntington's disease.*

STORAGE/HANDLING

Store at room temperature (including suppositories), protect from light (darkens on exposure). Yellow discoloration of solution does not affect potency, but discard if markedly discolored or if precipitate forms.

ADMINISTRATION

ORAL:

- Dilute oral concentrate solution w/tomato, fruit juice, milk, orange syrup, carbonated beverages, coffee, tea, water. May also mix w/semisolid food.

IM:

- **Note:** After parenteral administration, pt must remain recumbent for 30–60 min in head-low position w/legs raised to minimize hypotensive effect.
- Inject slow, deep IM. If irritation occurs, further injections may be diluted w/0.9% NaCl or 2% procaine hydrochloride.
- Massage IM injection site to reduce discomfort.

IV:

- **Note:** Give by direct IV injection or IV infusion.
- Direct IV used only during surgery to control nausea and vomiting.
- For direct IV, dilute w/0.9% NaCl to concentration not exceeding 1 mg/ml.
- Administer direct IV at rate not exceeding 1 mg/min for adults and 0.5 mg/min for children.
- IV infusion used only for intractable hiccups.

- For IV infusion, add chlorpromazine hydrochloride to 500–1,000 ml of 0.9% NaCl.

RECTAL:
- If suppository is too soft, chill for 30 min in refrigerator or run cold water over foil wrapper.
- Moisten suppository w/cold water before inserting well up into rectum.

INDICATIONS/ROUTES/DOSAGE

Outpatient: mild psychotic disorders, acute anxiety:
Oral: Adults: 30–75 mg/day in 2–4 divided doses.

IM: Adults: 25 mg initially. May repeat in 1 hr.

Outpatient: moderate to severe psychotic disorders:
Oral: Adults: 25 mg 3 times/day. Increase twice weekly by 20–25 mg until therapeutic response is achieved. Maintain dosage for 2 wks, then gradually reduce to maintenance level.

Hospitalized: acute psychotic disorders:
Oral: Children: 0.55 mg/kg q4–6h.

IM: Adults: 25 mg. May give an additional 25–50 mg in 1 hr if needed. Gradually increase over several days to maximum 400 mg q4–6h.

Rectal: Adults: 50–100 mg 3–4 times/day. ***Children:*** 1.1 mg/kg q6–8h (severe cases).

Nausea, vomiting:
Oral: Adults: 10–25 mg q4–6h.

Rectal: Adults: 50–100 mg q6–8h. ***Children:*** 1.1 mg/kg q6–8h.

IM: Adults: 25 mg. Give additional 25–50 mg q3–4h if hypotension does not occur. ***Children:*** 0.55 mg/kg q6–8h.

Porphyria:
Oral: Adults: 25–50 mg 3–4 times/day.

IM: Adults: 25 mg 3–4 times/day.

Intractable hiccups:
Oral: Adults: 25–50 mg 3 times/day. If symptoms continue, administer by IM or slow IV infusion.

Preop:
Oral: Adults: 25–50 mg 2–3 hrs before surgery. ***Children:*** 0.55 mg/kg.

IM: Adults: 12.5–25 mg 1–2 hrs before surgery. ***Children:*** 0.55 mg/kg.

Usual elderly dosage (nonpsychotic):
Oral: Initially, 10–25 mg 1–2 times/day. May increase by 10–25 mg/day every 4–7 days. ***Maximum:*** 800 mg/day.

CONTRAINDICATIONS

Severe CNS depression, comatose states, severe cardiovascular disease, bone marrow depression, subcortical brain damage.

CAUTIONS

Impaired respiratory/hepatic/renal/cardiac function, alcohol withdrawal, history of seizures, urinary retention, glaucoma, prostatic hypertrophy, hypocalcemia (increases susceptibility to dystonias).

INTERACTIONS

DRUG: ***Alcohol, CNS depressants*** may increase CNS, respiratory depression, hypotensive effects. ***Tricyclic antidepressants, MAO inhibitors*** may increase sedative, anticholinergic effects. ***Antithyroid agents*** may increase risk of agranulocytosis. Increased risk of extrapyramidal symptoms (EPS) w/***EPS-producing medications.***

Hypotensives may increase hypotension. May decrease ***levodopa*** effects. ***Lithium*** may decrease absorption, produce adverse neurologic effects. **HERBAL:** None known. **FOOD:** None significant. **ALTERED LAB VALUES:** May produce false-positive pregnancy test, phenylketonuria (PKU). EKG changes may occur, including Q and T wave disturbances.

SIDE EFFECTS

FREQUENT: Drowsiness, blurred vision, hypotension, defective color vision, difficulty in night vision, dizziness, decreased sweating, constipation, dry mouth, nasal congestion. **OCCASIONAL:** Difficulty urinating, increased skin sensitivity to sun, skin rash, decreased sexual ability, swelling or pain in breasts, increased weight, nausea, vomiting, stomach pain, tremors.

ADVERSE REACTIONS/TOXIC EFFECTS

Extrapyramidal symptoms appear dose related (particularly high dosage), and divided into 3 categories: akathisia (inability to sit still, tapping of feet, urge to move around); parkinsonian symptoms (mask-like face, tremors, shuffling gait, hypersalivation); and acute dystonias: torticollis (neck muscle spasm), opisthotonos (rigidity of back muscles), and oculogyric crisis (rolling back of eyes). Dystonic reaction may also produce profuse sweating, pallor. Tardive dyskinesia (protrusion of tongue, puffing of cheeks, chewing/puckering of the mouth) occurs rarely (may be irreversible). Abrupt withdrawal after long-term therapy may precipitate nausea, vomiting, gastritis, dizziness, tremors. Blood dyscrasias, particularly agranulocytosis, mild leukopenia may occur. May lower seizure threshold.

PATIENT CONSIDERATIONS

BASELINE ASSESSMENT

Avoid skin contact w/solution (contact dermatitis).

Antiemetic

Assess for dehydration (poor skin turgor, dry mucous membranes, longitudinal furrows in tongue).

Antipsychotic

Assess behavior, appearance, emotional status, response to environment, speech pattern, thought content.

INTERVENTION/EVALUATION

Monitor B/P for hypotension. Assess for extrapyramidal symptoms. Monitor WBC, differential count for blood dyscrasias. Monitor for fine tongue movement (may be early sign of tardive dyskinesia). Supervise suicidal risk pt closely during early therapy (as depression lessens, energy level improves, increasing suicide potential). Assess for therapeutic response (interest in surroundings, improvement in self-care, increased ability to concentrate, relaxed facial expression).

PATIENT/FAMILY TEACHING

Full therapeutic response may take up to 6 wks. Urine may darken. Do not abruptly withdraw from long-term drug therapy. Report visual disturbances. Sugarless gum or sips of tepid water may relieve dry mouth. Drowsiness generally subsides during continued therapy. Avoid tasks that require alertness, motor skills until response to drug is established. Avoid alcohol.

C

chlorpropamide
(Diabinese)
See Classification section under: Antidiabetic agents

chlorthalidone
klor-**thal**-ih-doan
(Hygroton, Thalitone)

FIXED-COMBINATION(S)
W/clonidine, an antihypertensive **(Combipres);** w/atenolol, an antihypertensive **(Tenoretic);** w/reserpine, an antihypertensive **(Demi-Regroton, Regroton).**

CANADIAN AVAILABILITY
Apo-Chlorthalidone, Hygroton

PREGNANCY CATEGORY B

CLASSIFICATION
Diuretic: Thiazide

AVAILABILITY (Rx)
Tablets: 15 mg, 25 mg, 50 mg, 100 mg

PHARMACODYNAMICS

	ONSET	PEAK	DURATION
Oral (diuretic)			
	2 hrs	2–6 hrs	Up to 36 hrs

PHARMACOKINETICS
Absorption: Rapidly absorbed from GI tract. **Excretion:** Excreted unchanged in urine. **Half-life:** 35–50 hrs. Onset antihypertensive effect: 3–4 days; optimal therapeutic effect: 3–4 wks.

ACTION/*THERAPEUTIC EFFECT*
Diuretic: Blocks reabsorption of sodium, potassium, chloride at distal convoluted tubule, *promoting renal excretion.* **Antihypertensive:** Reduces plasma, extracellular fluid volume, peripheral vascular resistance, *lowering B/P.*

USES
Adjunctive therapy in edema associated w/CHF, hepatic cirrhosis, corticoid or estrogen therapy, renal impairment. In treatment of hypertension, may be used alone or w/other antihypertensive agents.

ADMINISTRATION
ORAL:
- Give w/food or milk if GI upset occurs, preferably w/breakfast (may prevent nocturia). Scored tablets may be crushed.

INDICATIONS/ROUTES/DOSAGE
Note: Fixed-combination medication should not be used for initial therapy but for maintenance therapy.

Edema:
Oral: Adults: 50–100 mg 1 time/day in morning or 100 mg every other day. May require 150–200 mg every day or every other day. Reduce dose to lowest maintenance level when dry weight is achieved (nonedematous state).

Hypertension:
Oral: Adults: Initially, 25 mg/day. May increase to 50 mg/day. ***Maintenance:*** 25–50 mg/day.

Usual elderly dosage:
Oral: Initially, 12.5–25 mg/day or every other day.

CONTRAINDICATIONS
History of hypersensitivity to sulfonamides or thiazide diuretics, renal decompensation, anuria.

CAUTIONS

Severe renal disease, impaired hepatic function, diabetes mellitus, elderly/debilitated, gout, pts w/hypercholesterolemia.

INTERACTIONS

DRUG: *Cholestyramine, colestipol* may decrease absorption, effects. May increase ***digoxin*** toxicity (due to hypokalemia). May increase ***lithium*** toxicity. **HERBAL:** None known. **FOOD:** None significant. **ALTERED LAB VALUES:** May increase bilirubin, serum calcium, LDL, cholesterol, triglycerides, creatinine, glucose, uric acid. May decrease urinary calcium, magnesium, potassium, sodium.

SIDE EFFECTS

EXPECTED: Increase in urine frequency/volume. **FREQUENT:** Potassium depletion (rarely produces symptoms). **OCCASIONAL:** Anorexia, impotence, diarrhea, orthostatic hypotension, GI upset, photosensitivity. **RARE:** Rash.

ADVERSE REACTIONS/TOXIC EFFECTS

Vigorous diuresis may lead to profound water loss and electrolyte depletion, resulting in hypokalemia, hyponatremia, dehydration. Acute hypotensive episodes may occur. Hyperglycemia may be noted during prolonged therapy. Overdosage can lead to lethargy, coma w/o changes in electrolytes or hydration.

PATIENT CONSIDERATIONS

BASELINE ASSESSMENT

Check vital signs, especially B/P for hypotension before administration. Assess baseline electrolytes, particularly check for low potassium. Assess edema, skin turgor, mucous membranes for hydration status. Evaluate muscle strength, mental status. Note skin temperature, moisture. Obtain baseline weight. Initiate I&O.

INTERVENTION/EVALUATION

Continue to monitor B/P, vital signs, electrolytes, I&O, weight. Note extent of diuresis. Watch for electrolyte disturbances (hypokalemia may result in weakness, tremor, muscle cramps, nausea, vomiting, change in mental status, tachycardia; hyponatremia may result in confusion, thirst, cold/clammy skin). Periodically check blood sugar for hyperglycemia in prolonged therapy.

PATIENT/FAMILY TEACHING

Expect increased frequency and volume of urination. To reduce hypotensive effect, rise slowly from lying to sitting position and permit legs to dangle momentarily before standing. Eat foods high in potassium such as whole grains (cereals), legumes, meat, bananas, apricots, orange juice, potatoes (white, sweet), raisins. May take w/food or milk. Avoid prolonged exposure to sunlight. Report muscle pain, weakness, cramps, nausea, vomiting, excessive thirst, tiredness, drowsiness, diarrhea, dizziness.

---

chlorzoxazone

(Paraflex, Parafon Forte DSC)

See Classification section under: Skeletal muscle relaxants

cholestyramine resin

coal-es-**tie**-rah-mean
(Prevalite, Questran Lite)

CANADIAN AVAILABILITY
Novo-Cholamine, Questran

PREGNANCY CATEGORY B

CLASSIFICATION

Antihyperlipoproteinemic

AVAILABILITY (Rx)

Powder: 4 g

PHARMACOKINETICS

Absorption: Not absorbed from GI tract. Decreases in LDL apparent in 5–7 days, serum cholesterol in 1 mo. Serum cholesterol returns to baseline levels about 1 mo after discontinuing drug.

ACTION/*THERAPEUTIC EFFECT*

Binds w/bile acids in intestine forming insoluble complex. Binding results in partial removal of bile acid from enterohepatic circulation, *removing low density lipoproteins (LDL) and cholesterol from plasma.*

USES/*UNLABELED*

Adjunct to dietary therapy to decrease elevated serum cholesterol levels in those w/primary hypercholesterolemia. Relief of pruritus associated w/partial biliary obstruction. *Treatment of diarrhea (due to bile acids); hyperoxaluria.*

ADMINISTRATION

ORAL:

- Give other drugs at least 1 hr before or 4–6 hrs after cholestyramine (capable of binding drugs in GI tract).
- Do not give in dry form (highly irritating). Mix w/3–6 oz water, milk, fruit juice, soup. Place powder on surface for 1–2 min (prevents lumping), then mix thoroughly. Excessive foaming w/carbonated beverages; use extra large glass and stir slowly.
- Administer before meals.

INDICATIONS/ROUTES/DOSAGE

Primary hypercholesterolemia:
Oral: Adults, elderly: Initially: 4 g 1–2 times/day before meals. ***Maintenance:*** 4 g 1–6 times/day before meals and at bedtime.

CONTRAINDICATIONS

Hypersensitivity to cholestyramine or tartrazine (frequently seen in aspirin hypersensitivity), complete biliary obstruction.

CAUTIONS

GI dysfunction (especially constipation), hemorrhoids, bleeding disorders, osteoporosis.

INTERACTIONS

DRUG: May increase effects of ***anticoagulants*** by decreasing vitamin K. May decrease ***warfarin*** absorption. May bind, decrease absorption of ***digoxin, thiazides, penicillins, propranolol, tetracyclines, folic acid, thyroid hormones, troglitazone,*** other medications. Binds, decreases effect of ***oral vancomycin.*** **HERBAL:** None known. **FOOD:** None significant. **ALTERED LAB VALUES:** May increase SGOT (AST), SGPT (ALT), alkaline phosphatase, magnesium. May decrease calcium, potassium, sodium. May prolong prothrombin time.

SIDE EFFECTS

FREQUENT: Constipation (may lead to fecal impaction), nausea, vomiting, stomach pain, indigestion. **OCCASIONAL:** Diarrhea, belching, bloating, headache, dizziness. **RARE:** Gallstones, pancreatitis, peptic ulcer, malabsorption syndrome.

ADVERSE REACTIONS/TOXIC EFFECT

GI tract obstruction, hyperchloremic acidosis, osteoporosis secondary to calcium excretion. High dosage may interfere w/fat absorption, resulting in steatorrhea.

PATIENT CONSIDERATIONS

Baseline Assessment

Question for history of hypersensitivity to cholestyramine, tartrazine, aspirin. Obtain specimens for baseline levels: serum cholesterol, serum triglyceride, electrolytes.

Intervention/Evaluation

Determine pattern of bowel activity. Evaluate food tolerance, abdominal discomfort, and flatulence. Monitor lab results for electrolytes, serum cholesterol, and periodically serum triglyceride (may increase w/prolonged therapy). Assess skin and mucous membranes for rash/irritation. Encourage several glasses of water between meals.

Patient/Family Teaching

Complete full course; do not omit or change doses. Take other drugs at least 1 hr before or 4–6 hrs after cholestyramine. Check w/physician before taking any other medication. Never take in dry form; mix w/3–6 oz water, milk, fruit juice, soup (place powder on surface for 1–2 min to prevent lumping, then mix well). Use extra large glass and stir slowly when mixing w/carbonated beverages due to foaming. Take before meals and drink several glasses of water between meals. Reduce fats, sugars, and cholesterol per diet determined by physician. Eat high-fiber foods (whole grain cereals, fruits, vegetables) to reduce potential for constipation. Notify physician immediately of bleeding, constipation, or development of new symptom.

---

chorionic gonadotropin, HCG

kore-ee-**on**-ik goe-nad-oh-**troe**-pin
(Novarel, Pregnyl, APL, Profasai HP)

CANADIAN AVAILABILITY
APL, Profasi HP

PREGNANCY CATEGORY C

CLASSIFICATION

Gonadotropin

AVAILABILITY (Rx)

Powder for Injection: 5,000 unit, 10,000 unit, 20,000 unit vials

ACTION/*THERAPEUTIC EFFECT*

Stimulates production of gonadal steroid hormones by stimulating interstitial cells (Leydig cells) of the testes to produce androgen, and the corpus luteum of the ovary to produce progesterone. Androgen stimulation in the male *causes production of secondary sex characteristics and may stimulate descent of testes when no anatomic impediment exists.* In women of childbearing age w/normally functioning ovaries, *causes maturation of corpus luteum and triggers ovulation.*

USES / *UNLABELED*

Treatment of prepubertal cryptorchidism w/o obstruction, selected cases of hypogonadotropic hypogonadism. To induce ovulation and pregnancy in women w/secondary anovulation (after pretreatment w/menotropin). *Diagnosis of male hypogonadism, treatment of corpus luteum dysfunction.*

ADMINISTRATION

IM:
- For IM use only.
- Follow manufacturer's directions for reconstitution.
- Use completely or refrigerate after reconstitution.

INDICATIONS / ROUTES / DOSAGE

Prepubertal cryptorchidism, hypogonadotropic hypogonadism:
IM: Adults: Dosage is individualized based on indication, age and weight of pt, and physician preference.

Induction of ovulation and pregnancy:
IM: Adults: (After pretreatment w/menotropins), 5,000–10,000 IU 1 day after last dose of menotropins.

CONTRAINDICATIONS

Prior allergic reaction to chorionic gonadotropin, precocious puberty, carcinoma of the prostate or other androgen-dependent neoplasia. Not for adjunctive therapy in obesity.

CAUTIONS

Prepubertal males, conditions aggravated by fluid retention (cardiac or renal disease, epilepsy, migraine, asthma).

INTERACTIONS

DRUG: None significant. **HERBAL:** None known. **FOOD:** None significant. **ALTERED LAB VALUES:** None significant.

SIDE EFFECTS

FREQUENT: Pain at injection site. ***Induction ovulation:*** Ovarian cysts, uncomplicated ovarian enlargement. **OCCASIONAL:** Enlarged breasts, headache, irritability, fatigue, depression. ***Induction ovulation:*** Severe ovarian hyperstimulation, peripheral edema. ***Cryptorchidism:*** Precocious puberty (acne, deepening voice, penile growth, pubic/axillary hair).

ADVERSE REACTIONS / TOXIC EFFECTS

When used w/menotropins: increased risk of arterial thromboembolism, ovarian hyperstimulation w/high incidence (20%) of multiple births (premature deliveries and neonatal prematurity), ruptured ovarian cysts.

PATIENT CONSIDERATIONS

BASELINE ASSESSMENT

Question for prior allergic reaction to drug. Obtain baseline weight, B/P.

INTERVENTION / EVALUATION

Assess for edema: weigh every 2–3 days, report >5 lbs gain/wk; monitor B/P periodically during treatment; check for decreased urinary output, swelling of ankles, fingers.

PATIENT / FAMILY TEACHING

Report promptly abdominal pain, vaginal bleeding, signs of precocious puberty in males (deepening of voice; axillary, facial, and pubic hair; acne, penile growth)

or signs of edema. In anovulation treatment, proper method of taking/recording daily basal temperature; advise intercourse daily beginning the day preceding HCG treatment. Possibility of multiple births.

ciclopirox

(Loprox)

See Classification section under: Antifungals: Topical

cidofovir

sid-dough-**foe**-vir

(Vistide)

PREGNANCY CATEGORY C

CLASSIFICATION

Antiviral

AVAILABILITY (Rx)

Injection: 75 mg/ml (5 ml amp)

PHARMACOKINETICS

Excretion: Excreted primarily unchanged in urine. **Half-life:** 1.4–3.8 hrs.

ACTION/*THERAPEUTIC EFFECT*

Suppresses cytomegalovirus (CMV) replication *by inhibition of viral DNA synthesis.* Incorporation of cidofovir in growing viral DNA chain *results in reduction in rate of viral DNA synthesis.*

USES

Treatment of cytomegalovirus (CMV) retinitis in those w/acquired immunodeficiency syndrome (AIDS).

STORAGE/HANDLING

Store at controlled room temperature (68°–77° F). Admixtures may be refrigerated for no more than 24 hrs. Allow refrigerated admixtures to warm to room temperature before use.

ADMINISTRATION

Note: Do not exceed the recommended dosage, frequency or infusion rate.

IV:

- Dilute in 100 ml 0.9% saline solution prior to administration.
- Infuse over 1 hr.
- IV hydration with normal saline and probenecid therapy *must* be used w/each cidofovir infusion (minimizes risk of nephrotoxicity).
- Ingestion of food before each dose of probenecid may reduce nausea and vomiting. An antiemetic may also reduce potential for nausea.

INDICATIONS/ROUTES/DOSAGE

Probenecid:

Oral: Adults: Give 2 g 3 hrs prior to cidofovir dose, and 1 g given at 2 and again at 8 hrs after completion of the 1 hr cidofovir infusion (total of 4 g).

Hydration:

IV: Adults: 1 L 0.9% NaCl given over 1–2 hrs immediately before cidofovir infusion. If tolerated, a 2nd liter may be given at start or immediately after cidofovir infusion and infused over 1–3 hrs.

Usual dosage:

IV Infusion: Adults (Induction): 5 mg/kg at constant rate over 1 hr once weekly for 2 consecutive wks. ***Maintenance:*** 5 mg/kg at constant rate over 1 hr once every 2 wks.

Renal function impairment:
Dose based on creatinine clearance.

CREATININE CLEARANCE	INDUCTION DOSE	MAINTENANCE DOSE
(ml/min)		
41–55	2 mg/kg	2 mg/kg
30–40	1.5 mg/kg	1.5 mg/kg
20–29	1 mg/kg	1 mg/kg
≤19	0.5 mg/kg	0.5 mg/kg

CONTRAINDICATIONS

Hypersensitivity to cidofovir; history of clinically severe hypersensitivity to probenecid or other sulfa-containing medication; direct intraocular injection renal function impairment (serum creatinine >1.5 mg/dl or creatinine clearance ≤55 ml/min or urine protein >100 mg/dl.

CAUTIONS

Preexisting diabetes.

INTERACTIONS

DRUG: Avoid concurrent administration of cidofovir and medication w/nephrotoxic risk ***(amphotericin B, aminoglycosides, foscarnet, IV pentamidine)***. **HERBAL:** None known. **FOOD:** None significant. **ALTERED LAB VALUES:** May decrease neutrophil count, serum phosphate, uric acid, and bicarbonate; elevate serum creatinine.

SIDE EFFECTS

FREQUENT: Nausea, vomiting (65%), fever (57%), asthenia (46%), rash (30%), diarrhea (27%), headache (27%), alopecia (25%), chills (24%), anorexia (22%), dyspnea (22%), abdominal pain (17%).

ADVERSE REACTIONS/TOXIC EFFECTS

Proteinuria (80%), nephrotoxicity (53%), neutropenia (31%), serum creatinine elevations (29%), infection (24%), anemia (20%), ocular hypotony (12%) (decrease in intraocular pressure), pneumonia (9%). Probenecid may produce hypersensitivity reaction (rash, fever, chills, anaphylaxis), acute renal failure.

PATIENT CONSIDERATIONS

BASELINE ASSESSMENT

Establish baseline electrolytes. For those taking zidovudine, temporarily discontinue zidovudine administration or decrease zidovudine dose by 50% on days of infusion (probenecid reduces metabolic clearance of zidovudine). Emphasize need for close monitoring of renal function (urinalysis, serum creatinine) during therapy.

INTERVENTION/EVALUATION

Monitor serum creatinine, urine protein, and WBC counts w/differential prior to each dose. In those w/proteinuria, give IV hydration and repeat test. Periodically monitor intraocular pressure (IOP), visual acuity, and ocular symptoms. Monitor for proteinuria (may be early indicator of dose-dependent nephrotoxicity).

PATIENT/FAMILY TEACHING

Obtain regular follow-up ophthalmologic exams. Advise that cidofovir is not cure for CMV retinitis, and condition may progress in spite of treatment. Those of child-bearing age should use effective contraception during and for 1 mo following treatment. Men should practice barrier contraceptive methods during and for 3 mos following treatment. Do not take any medications w/o physician approval. Emphasize renal monitoring (urinalysis, serum creatinine). Must complete full course of probenecid w/each cidofovir dose.

cilostazol

sill-oh-**stay**-zole
(Pletal)

PREGNANCY CATEGORY C

CLASSIFICATION

Antiplatelet

AVAILABILITY (Rx)

Tablets: 100 mg

PHARMACOKINETICS

Absorption: Moderately absorbed from GI tract. Primarily bound to albumin.

ACTION/*THERAPEUTIC EFFECT*

Inhibits platelet aggregation, direct arterial vasodilator, *improving walking distance in pts w/intermittent claudication.*

USES

Treatment of symptomatic intermittent claudication.

ADMINISTRATION

ORAL:

- Take at least 1/2 hr before or 2 hrs after meals.
- Do no take with grapefruit juice.

INDICATIONS/ROUTES/DOSAGES

Intermittent claudication:
Oral: Adults, elderly: 100 mg 2 times/day.

CONTRAINDICATIONS

Congestive heart failure of any severity.

CAUTIONS

Sensitivity to cilostazol.

INTERACTIONS

DRUG: None significant. **HERBAL:** None known. **FOOD:** Do not take with grapefruit juice. **ALTERED LAB VALUES:** No information presently available.

SIDE EFFECTS

OCCASIONAL: Headache, diarrhea, abnormal stools, dizziness, palpitations.

ADVERSE REACTIONS/TOXIC EFFECTS

None significant.

PATIENT CONSIDERATIONS

Take on empty stomach (1/2 hr before or 2 hrs after meals). Do not take with grapefruit juice.

cimetidine

sih-**met**-ih-deen
(Tagamet, Tagamet HB)

CANADIAN AVAILABILITY
Apo-Cimetidine, Novocimetine, Peptol, Tagamet

PREGNANCY CATEGORY B

CLASSIFICATION

H_2 receptor antagonist

AVAILABILITY (Rx)

Tablets: 100 mg (OTC), 200 mg, 300 mg, 400 mg, 800 mg. **Oral Liquid:** 300 mg/5 ml. **Injection:** 300 mg/2 ml. **Suspension:** 200 mg/5 ml.

PHARMACOKINETICS

Absorption: Well absorbed from GI tract. Widely distributed.

Metabolism: Metabolized in liver. **Excretion:** Primarily excreted in urine. **Half-life:** 2 hrs (increased in decreased renal function).

ACTION / *THERAPEUTIC EFFECT*

Inhibits histamine action at H_2 receptor sites of parietal cells, *inhibiting gastric acid secretion.*

USES / *UNLABELED*

Short-term treatment of active duodenal ulcer. Prevention of duodenal ulcer recurrence, upper GI bleeding in critically ill pts. Treatment of active benign gastric ulcer, pathologic GI hypersecretory conditions, gastroesophageal reflux disease (GERD). *Treatment of upper GI bleeding, prophylaxis of aspiration pneumonia, acute urticaria, chronic warts.*

STORAGE/HANDLING

Store tablets, liquid, parenteral form at room temperature. Reconstituted IV is stable for 48 hrs at room temperature.

ADMINISTRATION

ORAL:

- Give w/o regard to meals. Best given with meals and at bedtime.
- Do not administer within 1 hr of antacids.

IM:

- Administer undiluted.
- Inject deep into large muscle mass.

IV:

- For direct IV injection, administer over not less than 2 min (prevents arrhythmias, hypotension).
- For intermittent IV (piggyback) administration, infuse over 15–20 min.
- For IV infusion, dilute w/100 to 1,000 ml 0.9% NaCl or 5% dextrose. Infuse over 24 hrs.

INDICATIONS/ROUTES/DOSAGE

Active duodenal ulcer:
Oral: Adults, elderly: 300 mg 4 times/day, or 400 mg 2 times/day (morning and at bedtime), or 800 mg at bedtime.

Prophylaxis of recurrent duodenal ulcer:
Oral: Adults, elderly: 400 mg at bedtime.

Benign active gastric ulcer:
Oral: Adults, elderly: 300 mg 4 times/day or 800 mg at bedtime.

Pathologic gastric hypersecretory conditions:
Oral: Adults, elderly: 300 mg 4 times/day up to 2,400 mg/day.

Gastroesophageal reflux disease:
Oral: Adults, elderly: 1,600 mg/day in divided doses (800 mg 2 times/day or 400 mg 4 times/day) for 12 wks.

Usual parenteral dosage:
IM/IV: Adults, elderly: 300 mg q6–8h. *Maximum:* 2,400 mg/day.

IV Infusion: Adults, elderly: 900 mg/day.

Prevent upper GI bleeding:
IV Infusion: Adults, elderly: 1,200 mg/day (50 mg/hr).

Dosage in renal impairment:
Oral/IM/IV: Adults, elderly: 300 mg q8–12h.

CONTRAINDICATIONS

None significant.

CAUTIONS

Impaired renal/hepatic function, elderly.

INTERACTIONS

DRUG: *Antacids* may decrease absorption (do not give within ½–1 hr). May decrease absorption of

ketoconazole(give at least 2 hrs after). May decrease metabolism, increase concentration of ***oral anticoagulants, tricyclic antidepressants, oral hypoglycemics, metoprolol, metronidazole, phenytoin, propranolol, theophylline, calcium channel blockers, cyclosporine, lidocaine.*** **HERBAL:** None known. **FOOD:** None significant. **ALTERED LAB VALUES:** Interferes w/skin tests using allergen extracts. May increase creatinine, prolactin, transaminase. May decrease parathyroid hormone concentration.

SIDE EFFECTS

OCCASIONAL (2–4%): Diarrhea, dizziness, headache, drowsiness, nausea, vomiting, skin rash, confusion, psychosis, disorientation, hallucinations (effects reverse in 3–4 days after discontinuation). **RARE (<2%):** Agranulocytosis (fever, sore throat), fever, neutropenia, fast pounding heartbeat, thrombocytopenia (unusual bleeding/bruising), gynecomastia, arthralgia, myalgia.

ADVERSE REACTIONS/TOXIC EFFECTS

Rapid IV may produce cardiac arrhythmias, hypotension.

PATIENT CONSIDERATIONS

Baseline Assessment

Do not administer antacids concurrently (separate by 1 hr).

Intervention/Evaluation

Monitor B/P for hypotension during IV infusion. Assess for GI bleeding: hematemesis, blood in stool. Check mental status in elderly, severely ill, those w/impaired renal function.

Patient/Family Teaching

IM may produce transient discomfort at injection site. Do not take antacids within 1 hr of cimetidine administration. Avoid tasks that require alertness, motor skills until drug response is established. Avoid smoking. Report any blood in vomitus or stool, or dark, tarry stool. Avoid food, beverages, alcohol, other medications that may cause GI irritation. Report if condition does not improve or worsens.

---

ciprofloxacin hydrochloride

sip-row-**flocks**-ah-sin
(Ciloxan, Cipro)

FIXED-COMBINATION(S): W/hydrocortisone, a glucocorticoid **(Cipro HC Otic)**

CANADIAN AVAILABILITY
Ciloxan, Cipro

PREGNANCY CATEGORY C

CLASSIFICATION

Anti-infective: Quinolone

AVAILABILITY (Rx)

Tablets: 100 mg, 250 mg, 500 mg, 750 mg. **Oral Suspension. Injection:** 200 mg, 400 mg. **Ophthalmic Solution:** 0.03%.

PHARMACOKINETICS

Absorption: Well absorbed from GI tract (delayed by food). Widely distributed (including CSF). **Metabolism:** Metabolized in liver to active metabolite. **Excretion:** Primarily excreted in urine. Minimal removal by hemodialysis. **Half-life:** 4–6 hrs (increased in decreased renal function, elderly).

ACTION / *THERAPEUTIC EFFECT*

Inhibits DNA enzyme in susceptible microorganisms, *interfering w/bacterial DNA replication.* Bactericidal.

USES / *UNLABELED*

Treatment of infections of urinary tract, chronic bacterial prostatitis skin/skin structure, GI tract, bone/joint, lower respiratory tract, infectious diarrhea, uncomplicated gonorrhea, empiric treatment of febrile neutropenia, acute sinusitis. ***Ophthalmic:*** Treatment of corneal ulcers, conjunctivitis.

ADMINISTRATION

ORAL:

- May be given w/o regard to meals (preferred dosing time: 2 hrs after meals).
- Do not administer antacids (aluminum, magnesium) within 2 hrs of ciprofloxacin.
- Encourage cranberry juice, citrus fruits (to acidify urine).
- Suspension may be stored for 14 days at room temperature.

IV:

- Use large vein to reduce venous irritation.
- Infuse over 60 min.

OPHTHALMIC:

- Tilt pt's head back; place solution in conjunctival sac.
- Have pt close eyes; press gently on lacrimal sac for 1 min.
- Do not use ophthalmic solutions for injection.
- Unless infection very superficial, systemic administration generally accompanies ophthalmic.

INDICATIONS / ROUTES / DOSAGE

Mild to moderate urinary tract infections:
Oral: Adults, elderly: 250 mg q12h.

IV: Adults, elderly: 200 mg q12h.

Complicated urinary tract, mild to moderate respiratory tract infections, skin/skin structure, bones and joint, infectious diarrhea:
Oral: Adults, elderly: 500 mg q12h.

IV: Adults, elderly: 400 mg q12h.

Severe, complicated infections:
Oral: Adults, elderly: 750 mg q12h.

IV: Adults, elderly: 400 mg q12h.

Prostatitis:
Oral: Adults, elderly: 500 mg q12h for 28 days.

Uncomplicated bladder infection:
Oral: Adults: 100 mg 2 times/day for 3 days.

Acute sinusitis:
Oral: Adults: 500 mg q12h.

Uncomplicated gonorrhea:
Oral: Adults: 250 mg as single dose.

Dosage in renal impairment:
The dose and/or frequency is modified in pts based on severity of infection and degree of renal impairment.

CREATININE CLEARANCE	DOSAGE
>50 ml/min (Oral); >30 ml/min (IV)	No change
30–50 ml/min	250–500 mg q12h
5–29 ml/min	250–500 mg Oral q18h; 200–400 mg IV q18–24h
Hemodialysis, peritoneal dialysis	250–500 mg q24h (after dialysis)

Corneal ulcers:
Adults, elderly: 2 drops q15min for 6 hrs, then 2 drops q30min remainder first day; 2 drops q1h second day; then 2 drops q4h days 3–14.

Conjunctivitis:
Adults, elderly: 1–2 drops q2h for 2 days, then q4h for next 5 days.

CONTRAINDICATIONS

Hypersensitivity to ciprofloxacin, quinolones, any component of the preparation. ***Ophthalmic:*** Vaccinia, varicella, epithelial herpes simplex, keratitis, mycobacterial infection, fungal disease of ocular structure. Not for use after uncomplicated removal of foreign body.

CAUTIONS

Renal impairment, CNS disorders, seizures, those taking theophylline or caffeine. Suspension not for use in an NG tube.

INTERACTIONS

DRUG: ***Antacids, iron preparations, sucralfate*** may decrease absorption. Decreases clearance, may increase concentration, toxicity of ***theophylline***. May increase effects of ***oral anticoagulants***. **HERBAL:** None known. **FOOD:** None significant. **ALTERED LAB VALUES:** May increase SGOT (AST), SGPT (ALT), alkaline phosphatase, LDH, bilirubin, BUN, creatinine.

SIDE EFFECTS

FREQUENT (2–5%): Dizziness, lightheadedness, headache, insomnia, drowsiness, nausea, vomiting, diarrhea, stomach pain or discomfort, nervousness. ***Ophthalmic:*** Burning, crusting in corner of eye. **OCCASIONAL (1–2%):** Photosensitivity. ***Ophthalmic:*** Bad taste, sense of something in eye, redness of eyelids, eyelid itching. **RARE (<1%):** Confusion, tremors, hallucinations, hypersensitivity reaction, interstitial nephritis, pain at injection site. May cause inflamed/ruptured tendons.

ADVERSE REACTIONS/TOXIC EFFECTS

Superinfection (especially enterococcal, fungal), nephropathy, cardiopulmonary arrest, cerebral thrombosis may occur. Arthropathy may occur. ***Ophthalmic:*** Sensitization may contraindicate later systemic use of ciprofloxacin.

PATIENT CONSIDERATIONS

BASELINE ASSESSMENT

Question for history of hypersensitivity to ciprofloxacin, quinolones, any component of preparation. Obtain specimen for diagnostic tests before giving first dose (therapy may begin before results are known).

INTERVENTION/EVALUATION

Evaluate food tolerance. Determine pattern of bowel activity; be alert to blood in feces. Check for dizziness, headache, visual difficulties, tremors. Monitor B/P at least twice daily. Assess for chest, joint pain.

Ophthalmic

Check for therapeutic response, side effects (see Adverse Reactions/Toxic Effects).

PATIENT/FAMILY TEACHING

Do not skip dose; take full course of therapy. Take w/8 oz water; drink several glasses of water between meals. Eat/drink high sources of ascorbic acid to prevent crystalluria (cranberry juice, citrus fruits). Do not take antacids (reduces/destroys effectiveness). Shake suspension well before using; do not chew microcapsules in suspension. Avoid tasks that require alertness, motor skills until response to drug is established. Avoid sunlight/ultraviolet exposure; wear sunscreen, protective clothing if photosensitivity develops. Sugarless gum or hard candy may relieve bad taste. Report inflammation or tendon pain. Notify nurse/physician if new symptoms occur. Shake suspension

well before use; do not chew microcapsules in suspension.

Ophthalmic
Explain possibility of crystal precipitate forming, and usual resolution. Report any increased burning, itching, or other discomfort promptly.

cisapride

sis-ah-pride
(Propulsid)

CANADIAN AVAILABILITY
Prepulsid

PREGNANCY CATEGORY C

CLASSIFICATION

GI stimulant

AVAILABILITY (Rx)

Tablets: 10 mg, 20 mg. **Suspension:** 1 mg/ml.

PHARMACODYNAMICS

	ONSET	PEAK	DURATION
Oral	30–60 min	—	—

PHARMACOKINETICS

Absorption: Rapid, completely absorbed from GI tract. Widely distributed. **Metabolism:** Metabolized in liver. **Excretion:** Excreted in urine, eliminated in feces. **Half-life:** 6–12 hrs.

ACTION/*THERAPEUTIC EFFECT*

Enhances release of acetylcholine at the muscular coat of the intestine, *increasing GI motility, peristalsis, accelerates gastric emptying.*

USES/*UNLABELED*

Treatment of nocturnal heartburn due to gastroesophageal reflux disease (GERD). *Treatment of gastroparesis.*

ADMINISTRATION

ORAL:
- Tablets may be crushed.

INDICATIONS/ROUTES/DOSAGE

Symptomatic gastroesophageal reflux:
Oral: Adults, elderly: 10 mg 4 times/day 15 min before meals and at bedtime. May increase up to 20 mg 4 times/day.

CONTRAINDICATIONS

GI hemorrhage, mechanical obstruction, perforation, history of QT prolongation, bradycardia.

CAUTIONS

None significant.

INTERACTIONS

DRUG: ***Clarithromycin, erythromycin, fluconazole, indinavir, itraconazole, ketoconazole, miconazole, nefazodone, ritonavir*** may decrease metabolism, increase concentration of cisapride (may cause serious arrhythmias). **HERBAL:** None known. **FOOD:** Avoid grapefruit juice. **ALTERED LAB VALUES:** None significant.

SIDE EFFECTS

FREQUENT (>10%): Diarrhea, abdominal discomfort, headache. OCCASIONAL (5–10%): Nausea, constipation, drowsiness. **RARE (<5%):** Rhinitis, flatulence, sinusitis.

ADVERSE REACTIONS/TOXIC EFFECTS

Acute overdosage results in tremors, convulsions, dyspnea, catatonia, hypotonia.

PATIENT CONSIDERATIONS

BASELINE ASSESSMENT

Consider effect of accelerated gastric emptying on rate of absorption of other drugs being administered.

INTERVENTION/EVALUATION

Monitor stool frequency and consistency.

PATIENT/FAMILY TEACHING

Elevate head of bed to reduce potential for aspiration w/nocturnal gastroesophageal reflux. Sedative effects of alcohol may be accelerated. Do not take grapefruit juice.

---

cisatracurium

(Nimbex)

See Classification section under: Neuromuscular blockers

---

cisplatin

(Platinol-AQ)

See Classification section under: Cancer chemotherapy

---

citalopram hydrobromide

sigh-**tail**-oh-pram high-dro-**broh**-mide

(Celexa)

PREGNANCY CATEGORY C

CLASSIFICATION

Antidepressant

AVAILABILITY (Rx)

Tablets: 20 mg, 40 mg

PHARMACOKINETICS

Absorption: Well absorbed following oral administration. **Metabolism:** Primarily metabolized in liver. **Excretion:** Primarily excreted in urine. **Half-life:** 35 hrs.

ACTION / *THERAPEUTIC EFFECT*

Blocks uptake of the neurotransmitter serotonin at CNS neuronal presynaptic membranes, increasing availability at postsynaptic receptor sites. *Resulting enhancement of postsynaptic activity produces antidepressant effect.*

USES

Treatment of major depressive disorder.

ADMINISTRATION

ORAL:

- May give w/o regard to food.

INDICATIONS/ROUTES/DOSAGES

Depression:

Oral: Adults: Initially, 20 mg once daily in the morning or evening. Dosage may be increased in increments of 20 mg at intervals of no less than 1 wk. ***Maximum:*** Do not exceed 40 mg/day. ***Elderly, impaired hepatic function:*** 20 mg/day. May titrate to 40 mg/day only for nonresponding pts.

CONTRAINDICATIONS

Sensitivity to citalopram, concurrent use of MAO inhibitors.

CAUTIONS

Liver, renal impairment, history of seizures, mania or hypomania.

INTERACTIONS

DRUG: ***MAO inhibitors*** may cause serotonergic syndrome (excitement, diaphoresis, rigidity, hyperthermia, autonomic hyperactivity, coma). ***Antifungals, macrolide antibiotics, cimetidine*** may increase plasma levels; ***carbamazepine*** may decrease plasma levels. Increases ***metoprolol*** plasma levels. **HERBAL:** St. John's wort may increase adverse effects. Ma Huang (Ephedra) may decrease effect. **FOOD:** None significant. **ALTERED LAB VALUES:** None significant.

SIDE EFFECTS

FREQUENT: Sexual dysfunction (e.g., decreased libido, impotence), drowsiness, dry mouth, nausea, insomnia. **OCCASIONAL:** Blurred vision, loss of memory, apathy, confusion, trouble breathing, fever, increased urination, skin rash/itching, abdominal pain, decreased appetite, anxiety, muscle pain, diarrhea, dizziness, increased sweating, trembling or shakiness, vomiting.

ADVERSE REACTIONS/TOXIC EFFECTS

Signs of overdose: dizziness, drowsiness, nausea, increased heart rate, sweating, tremors, vomiting.

PATIENT CONSIDERATIONS

Baseline Assessment

For those on long-term therapy, liver/renal function tests, blood counts should b e performed periodically. Observe/record behavior. Assess psychological status, thought content, sleep patterns, appearance, interest in environment.

Interventions/Evaluation

Supervise suicidal risk pt closely during early therapy (as energy level improves, suicide potential increases). Assess appearance, behavior, speech pattern, level of interest, mood.

Patient/Family Teaching

Do not stop taking medication or increase dosage. Avoid use of alcohol. Caution driving, jobs requiring alertness until effect of medication known.

citrates potassium citrate

(Urocit K)

potassium citrate and citric acid

(Polycitra K)

sodium citrate and citric acid

(Bicitra)

tricitrates

(Polycitra syrup)

CANADIAN AVAILABILITY
Polycitra-K

PREGNANCY CATEGORY C

CLASSIFICATION

Antiurolithic, alkalizer

AVAILABILITY (Rx)

Tablets: 5 mEq, 10 mEq. **Syrup. Oral Solution.**

PHARMACOKINETICS

Metabolism: Oxidized to form potassium or sodium bicarbonate. **Excretion:** Primarily excreted in urine.

ACTION/*THERAPEUTIC EFFECT*

Increases urinary pH, increasing solubility of cystine in urine and ionization of uric acid to urate ion. Increasing urinary pH and urinary citrate decreases calcium ion activity and decreases saturation of calcium oxalate. Increases plasma bicarbonate, buffers excess hydrogen ion concentration, *increasing blood pH and reversing acidosis.*

USES

Treats/prevents uric acid/cystine lithiasis, prevents urate crystallization (increased urinary pH). Treats/prevents calcium phosphate, calcium oxalate or uric acid kidney stones (increase urinary citrate). Treats chronic metabolic acidosis. Neutralizes/buffers excess quantities of gastric hydrochloric acid.

ADMINISTRATION

ORAL:

- Take after meals.
- ***Tablets:*** Swallow whole; do not crush, chew; take w/full glass of water or juice.
- ***Liquid:*** Dilute w/6 oz water or juice; chilling may increase palatability.

INDICATIONS/ROUTES/DOSAGE

Potassium Citrate:

Antiurolithic, urinary alkalizer:
Oral: Adults, elderly: 10 mEq 3 times/day up to 15 mEq 4 times/day or 20 mEq 3 times/day.

Potassium Citrate and Citric Acid:

Antiurolithic, urinary/systemic alkalizer:
Oral: Adults, elderly: 20–30 mEq 4 times/day. ***Children:*** 10–30 mEq 4 times/day.

Sodium Citrate and Citric Acid:

Antiurolithic, urinary/systemic alkalizer:
Oral: Adults, elderly: 10–30 mEq 4 times/day. ***Maximum:*** 150 mEq/day. ***Children:*** 5–15 mEq 4 times/day.

Tricitrates:

Antiurolithic, urinary alkalizer:
Oral: Adults, elderly: 15–30 mEq 4 times/day. ***Children:*** 5–10 mEq 4 times/day.

CONTRAINDICATIONS

Aluminum toxicity, severe myocardial damage, heart failure, severe renal impairment, active urinary tract infection, hyperkalemia, peptic ulcer.

CAUTIONS

Severe renal tubular acidosis.

INTERACTIONS

DRUG: May increase ***quinidine*** excretion. ***Antacids*** may increase risk of systemic alkalosis. ***NSAIDs, angiotensin-converting enzyme inhibitors, potassium-sparing diuretics, potassium-containing medication*** may increase risk of hyperkalemia. May decrease effect of ***methenamine.*** **HERBAL:** None known. **FOOD:** None significant. **ALTERED LAB VALUES:** None significant.

SIDE EFFECTS

OCCASIONAL: Diarrhea, loose bowel movements, mild abdominal pain, nausea, vomiting. **RARE:** Metabolic alkalosis, bowel obstruction/perforation, hyperkalemia, hypernatremia.

ADVERSE REACTIONS/TOXIC EFFECTS

None significant.

PATIENT CONSIDERATIONS

Baseline Assessment

Assess urinary pH determination, EKG in pts w/cardiac dis-

ease, serum acid-base balance, CBC, hemoglobin, hematocrit, serum creatinine.

INTERVENTION/EVALUATION

Monitor urinary pH, EKG in pts w/cardiac disease, serum acid-base balance, CBC, hemoglobin, hematocrit, serum creatinine.

PATIENT/FAMILY TEACHING

Take after meals. Mix in water or juice and follow w/additional liquid if desired. Notify physician if diarrhea, nausea/vomiting, abdominal pain, or seizures occur. Check w/physician if black, tarry stools or other signs of GI bleeding are observed.

cladribine

(Leustatin)

See Classification section under: Cancer chemotherapy

clarithromycin

clair-**rith**-row-my-sin

(Biaxin)

CANADIAN AVAILABILITY

Biaxin

PREGNANCY CATEGORY C

CLASSIFICATION

Antibiotic: macrolide

AVAILABILITY (Rx)

Tablets: 250 mg, 500 mg. **Oral Suspension:** 125 mg/5 ml, 250 mg/5 ml.

PHARMACOKINETICS

Absorption: Well absorbed from GI tract. Widely distributed. **Metabolism:** Metabolized in liver to active metabolite. **Excretion:** Primarily excreted in urine. **Half-life:** 3–7 hrs; metabolite: 5–7 hrs (increased in decreased renal function).

ACTION/*THERAPEUTIC EFFECT*

Bacteriostatic. Binds to ribosomal receptor sites, *inhibiting protein synthesis. May be bactericidal w/high dosage or very susceptible microorganisms.*

USES/*UNLABELED*

Treatment of mild to moderate infections of upper respiratory tract (pharyngitis, tonsillitis, sinusitis), lower respiratory tract (acute exacerbation of chronic bronchitis, pneumonia), and uncomplicated skin/skin structure infections, disseminated mycobacterium complex in AIDS, *H. pylori*-associated peptic ulcer disease. Prevents disseminated Mycobacterium avium (MAC). *Treatment of Legionnaire's disease.*

ADMINISTRATION

ORAL:

- May give w/o regard to food.
- Do not crush/break tablets.

INDICATIONS/ROUTES/DOSAGE

Note: Space doses evenly around the clock.

Lower respiratory tract infections:
Oral: Adults, elderly: 250–500 mg q12h for 7–14 days.

Upper respiratory tract infections:
Oral: Adults, elderly: 250–500 mg q12h for 10–14 days.

Uncomplicated skin/skin structure infections:
Oral: Adults, elderly: 250 mg q12h for 7–14 days.

H. pylori:
Oral: Adults (in combination): 500 mg 2 times/day for 10–14 days.

Prevent MAC:
Oral: Adults: 500 mg 2 times/day. *Children:* 7.5 mg/kg 2 times/day up to 500 mg 2 times/day.

Usual pediatric dosage:
Oral: Children: (6 mos–12 yrs): 7.5–15 mg/kg q12h.

Disseminated mycobacterium complex:
Oral: Adults: 500 mg q12h.

CONTRAINDICATIONS

Hypersensitivity to clarithromycin, erythromycins, any macrolide antibiotic.

CAUTIONS

Hepatic and renal dysfunction, elderly w/severe renal impairment.

INTERACTIONS

DRUG: May increase concentration, toxicity of ***astemizole, carbamazepine, cisapride, digoxin, terfenadine, theophylline.*** May cause serious arrhythmias w/***cisapride.*** May decrease concentration of ***zidovudine.*** May increase ***warfarin*** effects. ***Rifampin*** may decrease clarithromycin concentrations. HERBAL: None known. FOOD: None significant. ALTERED LAB VALUES: May rarely increase SGOT (AST), SGPT (ALT), BUN.

SIDE EFFECTS

FREQUENT (3–6%) : Diarrhea, nausea, altered taste, vomiting, abdominal pain, rash. OCCASIONAL (1–2%): Headache, dyspepsia. RARE (<1%): Hypersensitivity reaction.

ADVERSE REACTIONS/TOXIC EFFECTS

Superinfections, especially antibiotic-associated colitis may occur. Hepatotoxicity, thrombocytopenia occur rarely.

PATIENT CONSIDERATIONS

BASELINE ASSESSMENT

Question pt for history of hepatitis or allergies to clarithromycin, erythromycins. Obtain specimens for culture and sensitivity before giving first dose (therapy may begin before results are known).

INTERVENTION/EVALUATION

Check for GI discomfort, nausea. Determine pattern of bowel activity and stool consistency. Monitor hepatic function tests, assess for hepatotoxicity: malaise, fever, abdominal pain, GI disturbances. Evaluate for superinfection: genital/anal pruritus, sore mouth or tongue, moderate to severe diarrhea.

PATIENT/FAMILY TEACHING

Continue therapy for full length of treatment. Doses should be evenly spaced. Take medication w/8 oz water w/o regard to food. Notify physician in event of GI upset, rash, diarrhea, or other new symptom.

---

clemastine fumarate

klem-**ass**-teen
(Tavist, Tavist-1)

FIXED-COMBINATION(S)
W/phenylpropanolamine, a nasal decongestant **(Tavist-D)**

CANADIAN AVAILABILITY
Tavist

PREGNANCY CATEGORY B

CLASSIFICATION

Antihistamine

AVAILABILITY (Rx)

Tablets: 1.34 mg, 2.68 mg. **Syrup:** 0.67 mg/5 ml.

PHARMACODYNAMICS

	ONSET	PEAK	DURATION
Oral	15–60 min	5–7 hrs	10–12 hrs

PHARMACOKINETICS

Absorption: Well absorbed from GI tract. **Metabolism:** Metabolized in liver. **Excretion:** Excreted primarily in urine.

ACTION/*THERAPEUTIC EFFECT*

Competes w/histamine at histaminic receptor sites, *relieving allergic conditions (urticaria, pruritus).* Anticholinergic effects cause drying of nasal mucosa.

USES

Relief of allergic conditions (nasal allergies, allergic dermatitis), cold symptoms, hypersensitivity reaction.

ADMINISTRATION

ORAL:

- Give w/o regard to meals.
- Scored tablets may be crushed (do not crush extended-release or film-coated forms).

INDICATIONS/ROUTES/DOSAGE

Allergic rhinitis:
Oral: Adults, children >12 yrs: 1.34 mg 2 times/day. May increase dose to maximum 8.04 mg/day, if needed. ***Children 6–11 yrs:*** 0.67 mg 2 times/day. May increase dose to maximum 4.02 mg/day, if needed.

Allergic urticaria, angioedema:
Oral: Adults, children >12 yrs: 2.68 1–3 times/day. Do not exceed 8.04 mg/day. ***Children 6–11 yrs:*** 1.34 mg 2 times/day. Do not exceed 4.02 mg/day.

Usual elderly dosage:
Oral: 1.34 mg 1–2 times/day.

CONTRAINDICATIONS

Acute asthmatic attack, those receiving MAO inhibitors.

CAUTIONS

Narrow-angle glaucoma, peptic ulcer, prostatic hypertrophy, pyloroduodenal or bladder neck obstruction, asthma, COPD, increased intraocular pressure, cardiovascular disease, hyperthyroidism, hypertension, seizure disorders.

INTERACTIONS

DRUG: ***Alcohol, CNS depressants*** may increase CNS depressant effects. ***MAO inhibitors*** may increase anticholinergic, CNS depressant effects. **HERBAL:** None known. **FOOD:** None significant. **ALTERED LAB VALUES:** May suppress wheal, flare reactions to antigen skin testing, unless antihistamines discontinued 4 days prior to testing.

SIDE EFFECTS

Note: Fixed-combination form (Tavist-D) may produce mild CNS stimulation. **FREQUENT:** Thickening of bronchial secretions. ***Elderly:*** Sedation, dizziness, hypotension. **OCCASIONAL:** Drowsiness, confusion, difficulty urinating, dizziness, decreased appetite, paradoxical excitement, increased sensitivity of skin to sunlight, skin rash, ringing in ears, dry mouth, nose, throat.

ADVERSE REACTIONS/TOXIC EFFECTS

Children may experience dominant paradoxical reaction (restlessness, insomnia, euphoria, nervousness, tremors). Overdosage in children may result in hallucinations, convulsions, death. Hypersensitivity reaction (eczema, pruritus, rash, cardiac disturbances, angioedema, photosensitivity) may occur. Overdosage may vary from CNS depression (sedation, apnea, cardiovascular collapse, death) to severe paradoxical reaction (hallucinations, tremor, seizures).

PATIENT CONSIDERATIONS

Baseline Assessment

If pt is undergoing allergic reaction, obtain history of recently ingested foods, drugs, environmental exposure, recent emotional stress. Monitor rate, depth, rhythm, type of respiration; quality and rate of pulse. Assess lung sounds for rhonchi, wheezing, rales.

Intervention/Evaluation

Monitor B/P, especially in elderly (increased risk of hypotension). Monitor children closely for paradoxical reaction.

Patient/Family Teaching

Tolerance to antihistaminic effect generally does not occur; tolerance to sedative effect may occur. Avoid tasks that require alertness, motor skills until response to drug is established. Dry mouth, drowsiness, dizziness may be an expected response of drug. Avoid alcoholic beverages during antihistamine therapy. Sugarless gum, sips of tepid water may relieve dry mouth. Coffee or tea may help reduce drowsiness.

clindamycin hydrochloride

klin-da-**my**-sin
(Cleocin HCL)

clindamycin palmitate hydrochloride

(Cleocin Pediatric)

clindamycin phosphate

(Cleocin phosphate, Cleocin T)

CANADIAN AVAILABILITY
Dalacin

PREGNANCY CATEGORY B

CLASSIFICATION

Antibiotic

AVAILABILITY (Rx)

Capsules: 75 mg, 150 mg, 300 mg. **Oral Solution:** 75 mg/5 ml. **Injection:** 150 mg/ml. **Vaginal Cream:** 2%. **Vaginal Suppository. Lotion. Topical Solution.**

PHARMACOKINETICS

Absorption: Rapidly absorbed from GI tract. Widely distributed. **Metabolism:** Metabolized in liver to some active metabolites. **Excretion:** Primarily excreted in urine. Not removed by hemodialysis. **Half-life:** 2.4–3 hrs (increased in decreased renal function, premature infants).

ACTION/*THERAPEUTIC EFFECT*

Bacteriostatic. Binds to ribosomal receptor sites, *inhibiting protein synthesis*. Topically, decreases fatty acid concentration on skin, preventing acne vulgaris breakout.

USES / *UNLABELED*

Treatment of respiratory tract, skin/soft tissue, chronic bone/joint infections, septicemia, intra-abdominal, female genitourinary infections, bacterial vaginosis, endocarditis. ***Topical:*** Acne vulgaris. *Treatment of malaria, otitis media, PCP, toxoplasmosis.*

STORAGE/HANDLING

Store capsules at room temperature. After reconstitution, oral solution is stable for 2 wks at room temperature. Do not refrigerate oral solution (avoids thickening). IV infusion (piggyback) stable for 16 days at room temperature.

ADMINISTRATION

Note: Space doses evenly around the clock. May be given by IM injection, intermittent IV infusion (piggyback).

ORAL:

- Give w/8 oz water.
- May take w/o regard to food.

IM:

- Do not exceed 600 mg/dose.
- Administer deep IM.

IV:

- Dilute 300–600 mg w/50 ml 5% dextrose or 0.9% NaCl (900–1,200 mg w/100 ml). 50 ml piggyback is infused >10–20 min; 100 ml piggyback is infused >30–40 min.
- No more than 1.2 g should be given in one infusion.
- Do not administer IV push.
- Alternating IV sites, use large veins to reduce risk of phlebitis.
- Avoid prolonged use of indwelling IV catheters.

INDICATIONS/ROUTES/DOSAGE

Mild to moderate infections:
Oral: ***Adults, elderly:*** 150–300 mg q6h. ***Children:*** 8–16 mg/kg/day in 3–4 divided doses.

IM/IV: ***Adults, elderly:*** 600–1,200 mg/day in 2–4 divided doses. ***Children >1 mo:*** 15–25 mg/kg/day in 3–4 divided doses. ***Children <1 mo:*** 15–20 mg/kg/day in 3–4 divided doses.

Serious infections:
Oral: ***Adults, elderly:*** 300–450 mg q6h. ***Children:*** 13–25 mg/kg/day in 3–4 divided doses. ***Children <10 kg: Minimum:*** 37.5 mg 3 times/day.

IM/IV: ***Adults, elderly:*** 1.2–2.7 g/day in 2–4 divided doses. ***Children:*** 25–40 mg/kg/day in 3–4 divided doses.

Life-threatening infections:
IV: ***Adults, elderly:*** Up to 4.8 g/day in divided doses.

Bacterial vaginosis:
Intravaginal: ***Adults:*** One applicatorful at bedtime for 3–7 days, or 1 suppository at bedtime for 3 days.

Acne vulgaris:
Topical: ***Adults:*** Apply thin film 2 times/day to affected area.

CONTRAINDICATIONS

Hypersensitivity to clindamycin or lincomycin, known allergy to tartrazine dye, history of ulcerative colitis, regional enteritis, or antibiotic-associated colitis.

CAUTIONS

Severe renal or hepatic dysfunction, concomitant use of neuromuscular blocking agents, neonates. Topical preparations should not be applied to abraded areas or near eyes.

INTERACTIONS

DRUG: *Adsorbent antidiarrheals* may delay absorption. ***Chloram-***

phenicol, erythromycin may antagonize effects. May increase effect of ***neuromuscular blockers.*** **HERBAL:** None known. **FOOD:** None significant. **ALTERED LAB VALUES:** May increase SGOT (AST), SGPT (ALT), alkaline phosphatase.

SIDE EFFECTS

FREQUENT: Abdominal pain, nausea, vomiting, diarrhea. ***Vaginal:*** Vaginitis, itching. ***Topical:*** Dry scaly skin. **OCCASIONAL:** Phlebitis, thrombophlebitis w/IV administration; pain, induration at IM injection site; allergic reaction, urticaria, pruritus. ***Vaginal:*** Headache, dizziness, nausea, vomiting, abdominal pain. ***Topical:*** Contact dermatitis, abdominal pain, mild diarrhea, stinging/burning. **RARE:** ***Vaginal:*** Hypersensitivity reaction.

ADVERSE REACTIONS/TOXIC EFFECTS

Antibiotic-associated colitis during and several wks after therapy (including topical), superinfection (especially fungal) due to bacterial imbalance may occur. Blood dyscrasias (leukopenia, thrombocytopenia), nephrotoxicity (proteinuria, azotemia, oliguria) occur rarely.

PATIENT CONSIDERATIONS

Baseline Assessment

Question pt for history of allergies, particularly to clindamycin, lincomycin, aspirin. Avoid, if possible, concurrent use of neuromuscular blocking agents. Obtain specimens for culture and sensitivity, Gram's stain for vaginitis, before giving first dose (therapy may begin before results are known).

Intervention/Evaluation

Monitor bowel activity, stool consistency, report diarrhea promptly due to potential for serious colitis. Monitor periodic renal, hepatic, blood cell reports. Assess for ability to swallow, vomiting. Check I&O. Assess skin for rash (dryness, irritation w/topical application). Observe for phlebitis: pain, heat, red streaking over vein. Check for pain, induration at IM site. W/all routes of administration, assess for superinfection: severe diarrhea, anal/genital pruritus, increased fever, change of oral mucosa.

Patient/Family Teaching

Continue therapy for full length of treatment. Doses should be evenly spaced. Take oral doses w/ 8 oz water. Caution should be used when applying topical clindamycin concurrently w/peeling, abrasive acne agents, soaps, or alcohol-containing cosmetics to avoid cumulative effect. Do not apply topical preparations near eyes or abraded areas. Notify physician immediately in event of diarrhea; report onset of new symptoms.

Vaginal

Avoid contact w/eyes. In event of accidental contact w/eyes, rinse w/copious amounts of cool tap water. Do not engage in sexual intercourse during treatment. Instruct pt on correct application (manufacturer's insert).

---

clobetasol

(Temovate)

See Classification section under: Corticosteroids: topical

---

clofibrate

(Atromid-S)

See Classification section under: Antihyperlipidemics

clomipramine hydrochloride

klow-**mih**-prah-meen
(Anafranil)

CANADIAN AVAILABILITY
Anafranil

PREGNANCY CATEGORY C

CLASSIFICATION

Antidepressant: tricyclic

AVAILABILITY (Rx)

Capsules: 25 mg, 50 mg, 75 mg

PHARMACOKINETICS

Absorption: Well absorbed from GI tract. **Metabolism:** Metabolized in liver, undergoes first-pass metabolism. **Excretion:** Primarily excreted in urine. Minimal removal by hemodialysis. **Half-life:** 21–31 hrs.

ACTION/*THERAPEUTIC EFFECT*

Blocks reuptake of neurotransmitters (norepinephrine, serotonin) at CNS presynaptic membranes, increasing availability at postsynaptic receptor sites, *reducing obsessive-compulsive behavior.* Strong anticholinergic activity.

USES/*UNLABELED*

Treatment of obsessive-compulsive disorder manifested as repetitive tasks producing marked distress, time consuming, or significantly interfering w/social or occupational behavior. *Treatment of mental depression, panic disorder, neurogenic pain, cataplexy associated w/narcolepsy, bulimia.*

ADMINISTRATION

ORAL:

- Give w/food or milk if GI distress occurs.

INDICATIONS/ROUTES/DOSAGE

Obsessive-compulsive disorder: *Oral: Adults:* Initially, 25 mg/day. Gradually increase over 2 wks to 100 mg/day in divided doses. May further increase over several wks to 250 mg/day in divided doses. After titration, may give as single bedtime dose (reduces daytime sedation). ***Children >10 yrs:*** Initially, 25 mg/day. Gradually increase over 2 wks to 3 mg/kg or 100 mg/day in divided doses (whichever is less). May then increase over several wks up to 3 mg/kg or 200 mg (whichever is less). ***Maintenance:*** Lowest effective dose.

CONTRAINDICATIONS

Acute recovery period following MI, within 14 days of MAO inhibitor ingestion.

CAUTIONS

Prostatic hypertrophy, history of urinary retention or obstruction, glaucoma, diabetes mellitus, history of seizures, hyperthyroidism, cardiac/hepatic/renal disease, schizophrenia, increased intraocular pressure, hiatal hernia.

INTERACTIONS

DRUG: *Alcohol, CNS depressants* may increase CNS, respiratory depression, hypotensive effects. ***Antithyroid agents*** may increase risk of agranulocytosis. ***Phenothiazines*** may increase sedative, anticholinergic effects. ***Cimetidine*** may increase concentration, toxicity. May decrease effects of ***clonidine, guanadrel***. May increase cardiac effects w/***sympathomimetics***. May increase risk of hypertensive crisis, hyperpyretic, convulsions w/***MAO inhibitors***. **HERBAL:** None known. **FOOD:** None significant. **ALTERED LAB VALUES:** May alter EKG readings, glucose.

SIDE EFFECTS

FREQUENT: Drowsiness, fatigue, dry mouth, blurred vision, constipation, sexual dysfunction (42%), ejaculatory failure (20%), impotence; weight gain (18%), delayed micturition, postural hypotension, excessive sweating, disturbed concentration, increased appetite, urinary retention. **OCCASIONAL:** GI disturbances (nausea, GI distress, metallic taste), asthenia, aggressiveness, muscle weakness. **RARE:** Paradoxical reactions (agitation, restlessness, nightmares, insomnia, extrapyramidal symptoms, particularly fine hand tremor), laryngitis, seizures.

ADVERSE REACTIONS/TOXIC EFFECTS

High dosage may produce confusion, seizures, severe drowsiness, fast/slow/irregular heartbeat, fever, hallucinations, agitation, shortness of breath, vomiting, unusual tiredness/weakness. Abrupt withdrawal from prolonged therapy may produce headache, malaise, nausea, vomiting, vivid dreams. Rarely, blood dyscrasias, cholestatic jaundice noted.

PATIENT CONSIDERATIONS

Baseline Assessment

For those on long-term therapy, liver/renal function tests, blood counts should be performed periodically.

Intervention/Evaluation

Supervise suicidal risk pt closely during early therapy (as depression lessens, energy level improves, increasing suicide potential). Assess appearance, behavior, speech pattern, level of interest, mood. Monitor pattern of daily bowel activity and stool consistency. Monitor B/P, pulse for hypotension, arrhythmias. Assess for urinary retention by bladder palpation.

Patient/Family Teaching

Change positions slowly to avoid hypotensive effect. Tolerance to postural hypotension, sedative, and anticholinergic effects usually develops during early therapy. Maximum therapeutic effect may be noted in 2–4 wks. Photosensitivity to sun may occur. Dry mouth may be relieved by sugarless gum, sips of tepid water. Report visual disturbances. Do not abruptly discontinue medication. Avoid tasks that require alertness, motor skills until response to drug is established. Avoid alcohol.

---

clonazepam

klon-**nah**-zih-pam
(Klonopin)

CANADIAN AVAILABILITY
Rivotril

PREGNANCY CATEGORY C

CLASSIFICATION

Anticonvulsant

AVAILABILITY (Rx)

Tablets: 0.125 mg, 0.25 mg, 0.5 mg, 1 mg, 2 mg

PHARMACOKINETICS

Absorption: Well absorbed from GI tract. **Metabolism:** Metabolized in liver. **Excretion:** Excreted in urine. **Half-life:** 18–50 hrs.

ACTION / *THERAPEUTIC EFFECT*

Elevates seizure threshold in response to electrical/chemical stimulation by enhancing presynaptic inhibition in CNS, *suppressing seizure activity.*

USES / *UNLABELED*

Adjunct in treatment of Lennox-Gastaut syndrome (petit mal variant epilepsy), akinetic, and myoclonic seizures, absence seizures (petit mal). Treatment of panic disorder. *Adjunct treatment of seizures, treatment of simple/complex partial seizures, tonic-clonic seizures.*

ADMINISTRATION

ORAL:

- Give w/o regard to meals.
- Tablets may be crushed.

INDICATIONS / ROUTES / DOSAGE

Anticonvulsant:
Note: When replacement by another anticonvulsant is necessary, decrease clonazepam gradually as therapy begins w/low replacement dose.
Oral: Adults, elderly: 1.5 mg daily. Dosage may be increased in 0.5–1 mg increments at 3 day intervals until seizures are controlled. Do not exceed maintenance dose of 20 mg daily. ***Infants, children <10 yrs, or <66 lbs:*** 0.01–0.03 mg/kg daily in 2–3 divided doses. Dosage may be increased in up to 0.5 mg increments at 3 day intervals until seizures are controlled. Do not exceed maintenance dose of 0.2 mg/kg daily.

Panic disorder:
Oral: Adults: Initially 0.25 mg 2 times/day. Increase up to target dose of 1 mg/day after 3 days.

CONTRAINDICATIONS

Significant liver disease, narrow-angle glaucoma.

CAUTIONS

Impaired kidney/liver function, chronic respiratory disease.

INTERACTIONS

DRUG: ***Alcohol, CNS depressants*** may increase CNS depressant effect. **HERBAL:** Kava kava, valerian may increase CNS depression. **FOOD:** None significant. **ALTERED LAB VALUES:** None significant.

SIDE EFFECTS

FREQUENT: Muscular incoordination (ataxia), lightheadedness, transient mild drowsiness, slurred speech (particularly in elderly, debilitated). **OCCASIONAL:** Confusion, depression, blurred vision, constipation/diarrhea, dry mouth, headache, nausea. **RARE:** Behavioral problems (e.g., anger), impaired memory, paradoxical reaction (insomnia, nervousness, irritability).

ADVERSE REACTIONS / TOXIC EFFECTS

Abrupt withdrawal may result in pronounced restlessness, irritability, insomnia, hand tremors, abdominal/muscle cramps, sweating, vomiting, status epilepticus. Overdosage results in somnolence, confusion, diminished reflexes, coma.

PATIENT CONSIDERATIONS

BASELINE ASSESSMENT

Review history of seizure disorder (frequency, duration, intensity, LOC). Implement safety measures and observe frequently for recurrence of seizure activity.

INTERVENTION/EVALUATION

Assess children, elderly for paradoxical reaction, particularly during early therapy. Assist w/ambulation if drowsiness, ataxia occur. For those on long-term therapy, liver/renal function tests, blood counts should be performed periodically. Evaluate for therapeutic response: a decrease in intensity/frequency of seizures.

PATIENT/FAMILY TEACHING

Drowsiness usually diminishes w/continued therapy. Avoid tasks that require alertness, motor skills until response to drug is established. Smoking reduces drug effectiveness. Do not abruptly withdraw medication after long-term therapy. Strict maintenance of drug therapy is essential for seizure control. Avoid alcohol.

clonidine

klon-ih-deen
(Catapres TTS)

clonidine hydrochloride

(Catapres, Duraclon)

FIXED-COMBINATION(S)
W/chlorthalidone, a diuretic **(Combipres)**

CANADIAN AVAILABILITY
Catapres, Dixarit

PREGNANCY CATEGORY C

CLASSIFICATION

Antihypertensive

AVAILABILITY (Rx)

Tablets: 0.1 mg, 0.2 mg, 0.3 mg. **Transdermal Patch:** 2.5 mg (release at 0.1 mg/24 hrs), 5 mg (release at 0.2 mg/24hrs, 7.5 mg (release at 0.3 mg/24 hrs).

PHARMACODYNMICS

	ONSET	PEAK	DURATION
Oral	0.5–1 hr	2–4 hrs	Up to 8 hrs

PHARMACOKINETICS

Absorption: Well absorbed from GI tract. Transdermal best absorbed from chest, upper arm; least absorbed from thigh. **Metabolism:** Metabolized in liver. **Excretion:** Primarily excreted in urine. Minimal removal by hemodialysis. **Half-life:** 12–16 hrs (increased in decreased renal function).

ACTION/*THERAPEUTIC EFFECT*

Stimulates $alpha_2$-adrenergic receptors in CNS (inhibits sympathetic cardioaccelerator and vasoconstrictor center); decreases sympathetic outflow from CNS. *Reduces peripheral resistance, decreases B/P, heart rate.*

USES/*UNLABELED*

Treatment of hypertension alone or in combination w/other antihypertensive agents. Treatment of severe pain in cancer pts. *Diagnosis of pheochromocytoma, prevents migraine headaches, treatment of dysmenorrhea/menopausal flushing, opioid withdrawal.*

ADMINISTRATION

ORAL:

- May give w/o regard to food.
- Tablets may be crushed.
- Give last oral dose just before retiring.

TRANSDERMAL:

- Apply transdermal system to dry, hairless area of intact skin on upper arm or chest.
- Rotate sites (prevents skin irritation).
- Do not trim patch to adjust dose.

INDICATIONS/ROUTES/DOSAGE

Hypertension:
Oral: Adults: Initially, 0.1 mg 2 times/day. Increase by 0.1–0.2 mg every 2–4 days. ***Maintenance:*** 0.2–1.2 mg/day in 2–4 divided doses up to maximum of 2.4 mg/day. ***Children:*** 5–25 mcg/kg/day in divided doses q6h; increase at 5–7 day intervals.

Transdermal: Adults, elderly: System delivering 0.1 mg/24 hrs up to 0.6 mg/24 hrs every 7 days.

Usual elderly dosage:
Oral: Initially, 0.1 mg at bedtime. May increase gradually.

Severe pain:
Epidural: Adults, elderly: 30 mcg/hr.

CONTRAINDICATIONS

None significant.

CAUTIONS

Severe coronary insufficiency, recent MI, cerebrovascular disease, chronic renal failure, Raynaud's disease, thromboangiitis obliterans.

INTERACTIONS

DRUG: *Tricyclic antidepressants* may decrease effect. Discontinuing concurrent ***beta blockers*** may increase risk of clonidine-withdrawal hypertensive crisis. **HERBAL:** None known. **FOOD:** None significant. **ALTERED LAB VALUES:** None significant.

SIDE EFFECTS

FREQUENT (>10%): Itching, red skin (Transdermal), constipation, dizziness, drowsiness (33%), dry mouth (40%), unusual tiredness. **OCCASIONAL (1–5%):** Depression, swelling of feet, loss of appetite, decreased sexual ability, itching eyes, dizziness, nausea, vomiting, nervousness. ***Transdermal:*** Darkening of skin. **RARE (<1%):** Nightmares, vivid dreams, cold feeling in finger/toes.

ADVERSE REACTIONS/TOXIC EFFECTS

Overdosage produces profound hypotension, irritability, bradycardia, respiratory depression, hypothermia, miosis (pupillary constriction), arrhythmias, apnea. Abrupt withdrawal may result in rebound hypertension associated w/nervousness, agitation, anxiety, insomnia, hand tingling, tremor, flushing, sweating.

PATIENT CONSIDERATIONS

Baseline Assessment

Obtain B/P immediately before each dose is administered, in addition to regular monitoring (be alert to B/P fluctuations).

Intervention/Evaluation

Assist w/ambulation if dizziness occurs. Monitor pattern of daily bowel activity and stool consistency. If clonidine is to be withdrawn, discontinue concurrent beta-blocker therapy several days before discontinuing clonidine (prevents clonidine withdrawal hypertensive crisis). Slowly reduce clonidine dose over 2–4 days.

Patient/Family Teaching

Sugarless gum, sips of tepid water may relieve dry mouth. If nausea occurs, unsalted crackers, noncola beverages, or dry toast may relieve effect. To

reduce hypotensive effect, rise slowly from lying to sitting position and permit legs to dangle momentarily before standing. Skipping doses or voluntarily discontinuing drug may produce severe, rebound hypertension. Side effects tend to diminish during therapy.

clopidogrel

klow-**pih**-duh-grel
(Plavix)

CANADIAN AVAILABILITY
Plavix

PREGNANCY CATEGORY B

CLASSIFICATION

Antiplatelet

AVAILABILITY (Rx)

Tablets: 75 mg

PHARMACODYNAMICS

	ONSET	PEAK	DURATION
Oral	1 hr	2 hrs	—

PHARMACOKINETICS

Absorption: Rapidly absorbed; binds to plasma proteins. **Metabolism:** Extensively metabolized by the liver. **Excretion:** Eliminated equally in the urine and feces. **Half-life:** 8 hrs.

ACTION/*THERAPEUTIC EFFECT*

Inhibits binding of the enzyme adenosine phosphate (ADP) to its platelet receptor and subsequent ADP-mediated activation of a glycoprotein complex, *inhibiting platelet aggregation.*

USES

Reduces risk of myocardial infarction (MI), stroke, vascular death in pts with atherosclerosis documented by recent stroke, MI, or established peripheral arterial disease.

ADMINISTRATION

ORAL:

- May be given w/o regard to food.

INDICATIONS/ROUTES/DOSAGES

Inhibition of platelet aggregation: *Oral: Adults, elderly:* 75 mg once daily.

CONTRAINDICATIONS

History of hypersensitivity to clopidogrel, active pathologic bleeding (peptic ulcer, intracranial hemorrhage).

CAUTIONS

Neutropenic pts, hepatic function impairment, those at risk of increased bleeding from trauma, surgery, or other pathologic conditions.

INTERACTIONS

DRUG: May interfere with metabolism of ***phenytoin, tamoxifen, tolbutamide, warfarin, torsemide, fluvastatin,*** other ***nonsteroidal anti-inflammatory*** agents. ***Aspirin, NSAIDs*** may increase risk of GI bleeding. **HERBAL:** Feverfew, garlic, ginkgo may increase antiplatelet effect, bleeding. **FOOD:** None significant. **ALTERED LAB VALUES:** May increase bilirubin, liver enzymes, cholesterol; may decrease platelet count.

SIDE EFFECTS

FREQUENT (15%): Skin disorders. **OCCASIONAL (6–8%):** Upper respiratory tract infection, chest pain, flu-like symptoms, headache, dizziness, arthralgia. **RARE (3–5%):** Fatigue, edema, hypertension, abdominal pain, dyspepsia, diarrhea, nausea, epistaxis, dyspnea, rhinitis.

ADVERSE REACTIONS/TOXIC EFFECTS

None significant.

PATIENT CONSIDERATIONS

Baseline Assessment

Perform platelet counts prior to drug therapy, every 2 days during the first week of treatment and weekly thereafter until therapeutic maintenance dose is reached. Abrupt discontinuation of drug therapy produces an elevation of platelet count within 5 days.

Intervention/Evaluation

Monitor platelet count for evidence of thrombocytopenia. Assess BUN, creatinine, bilirubin, SGOT, SGPT, WBC, Hgb blood tests, signs/symptoms of hepatic insufficiency during therapy.

Patient/Familyteaching

Inform patient it may take longer to stop bleeding during drug therapy. Report any unusual bleeding. Patients should inform all physicians and dentists they are taking clopidogrel before surgery is scheduled or before taking any new drug.

clorazepate dipotassium

klor-**az**-eh-payt

(Tranxene)

CANADIAN AVAILABILITY

Novoclopate, Tranxene

PREGNANCY CATEGORY D

CLASSIFICATION

Antianxiety, anticonvulsant

AVAILABILITY (Rx)

Capsules: 3.75 mg, 7.5 mg, 15 mg. **Tablets:** 3.75 mg, 7.5 mg, 15 mg. **Tablets (single dose):** 11.25 mg, 22.5 mg.

PHARMACOKINETICS

Absorption: Rapidly, well absorbed from GI tract. Widely distributed. **Metabolism:** Metabolized in stomach and liver (first-pass metabolism) to active metabolites. **Excretion:** Excreted in urine. **Half-life:** metabolite: 48–96 hrs.

ACTION/*THERAPEUTIC EFFECT*

Enhances gamma-aminobutyric acid (GABA) neurotransmission at CNS, *producing anxiolytic effect.* Elevates seizure threshold in response to electrical/chemical stimulation by enhancing presynaptic inhibition in CNS, *suppressing seizure activity.*

USES

Management of anxiety disorders, short-term relief of anxiety symptoms, partial seizures, acute alcohol withdrawal symptoms.

ADMINISTRATION

ORAL:

- Give w/o regard to meals.
- Tablets may be crushed.
- Capsules may be emptied and mixed w/food.

INDICATIONS/ROUTES/DOSAGE

Note: When replacement by another anticonvulsant is necessary, decrease clorazepate gradually as therapy begins w/low-replacement dose.

Anxiety:

Oral: Adults: 30 mg daily in divided doses. ***Elderly, debilitated:*** 7.5–15 mg in divided doses or single bedtime dose. ***Daily dose range:*** 15–60 mg.

Partial seizures:
Oral: Adults, children >12 yrs: Initially, up to 7.5 mg 3 times daily. Do not increase dosage more than 7.5 mg/wk or exceed 90 mg/day.

Alcohol withdrawal:
Oral: Adults: Day 1: 30 mg followed by 30–60 mg in divided doses. ***Day 2:*** 45–90 mg in divided doses. ***Day 3:*** 22.5–45 mg in divided doses. ***Day 4:*** 15–30 mg in divided doses, then gradually reduce to 7.5–15 mg daily.

CONTRAINDICATIONS

Acute narrow-angle glaucoma.

CAUTIONS

Impaired renal/hepatic function, acute alcohol intoxication.

INTERACTIONS

DRUG: ***Alcohol, CNS depressants*** may increase CNS depressant effect. **HERBAL:** Kava kava, valerian may increase CNS depression. **FOOD:** None significant. **ALTERED LAB VALUES:** None significant.

SIDE EFFECTS

FREQUENT: Muscular incoordination (ataxia), lightheadedness, transient mild drowsiness, slurred speech (particularly in elderly, debilitated). **OCCASIONAL:** Confusion, depression, blurred vision, constipation/diarrhea, dry mouth, headache, nausea. **RARE:** Behavioral problems (e.g., anger), impaired memory, paradoxical reaction (insomnia, nervousness, irritability).

ADVERSE REACTIONS/TOXIC EFFECTS

Abrupt or too rapid withdrawal may result in pronounced restlessness, irritability, insomnia, hand tremors, abdominal/muscle cramps, sweating, vomiting, seizures. Overdosage results in somnolence, confusion, diminished reflexes, coma.

PATIENT CONSIDERATIONS

BASELINE ASSESSMENT

Anxiety
Assess autonomic response (cold, clammy hands, sweating) and motor response (agitation, trembling, tension). Offer emotional support to anxious pt.

Seizures
Review history of seizure disorder (intensity, frequency, duration, LOC). Observe frequently for recurrence of seizure activity. Initiate seizure precautions.

INTERVENTION/EVALUATION

For those on long-term therapy, liver/renal function tests, blood counts should be performed periodically. Assess for paradoxical reaction, particularly during early therapy. Assist w/ambulation if drowsiness, dizziness occur. Evaluate for therapeutic response:

Anxiety
A calm facial expression; decreased restlessness.

Seizures
A decrease in intensity or frequency of seizures.

PATIENT/FAMILY TEACHING

Do not abruptly withdraw medication following long-term use (may precipitate seizures). Strict maintenance of drug therapy is essential for seizure control. Drowsiness usually disappears during continued therapy. If dizziness occurs, change positions slowly from recumbent to sitting position before standing.

Avoid tasks that require alertness, motor skills until response to drug is established. Smoking reduces drug effectiveness. Avoid alcohol.

clotrimazole

kloe-**try**-mah-zole
(Mycelex, Mycelex-G, Lotrimin, Gyne-Lotrimin)

FIXED-COMBINATION(S)
W/betamethasone dipropionate, a corticosteroid **(Lotrisone)**

CANADIAN AVAILABILITY
Canesten, Clotrimaderm

PREGNANCY CATEGORY B

CLASSIFICATION

Antifungal

AVAILABILITY (Rx)

Troches: 10 mg. **Vaginal Tablets:** 100 mg, 500 mg. **Vaginal Cream:** 1%. **Topical Cream:** 1%. **Topical Solution:** 1%. **Lotion:** 1%.

PHARMACOKINETICS

Absorption: Poorly, erratically absorbed from GI tract. Bound to oral mucosa. **Metabolism:** Absorbed portion metabolized in liver. **Excretion:** Eliminated in feces. ***Topical:*** Minimal systemic absorption (highest concentration in stratum corneum). ***Intravaginal:*** Small amount systemically absorbed.

ACTION/*THERAPEUTIC EFFECT*

Binds w/phospholipids in fungal cell membrane. The altered cell membrane permeability *inhibits yeast growth.*

USES/*UNLABELED*

Oral lozenges: Treatment/prophylaxis oropharyngeal candidiasis due to *Candida* sp. ***Topical:*** Treatment of tinea pedis, tinea cruris, tinea corporis, tinea versicolor, cutaneous candidiasis (moniliasis) due to *Candida albicans.* ***Intravaginally:*** Treatment of vulvovaginal candidiasis (moniliasis) due to *Candida* sp. ***Topical:*** *Treatment of paronychia, tinea barbae, tinea capitas.*

ADMINISTRATION

ORAL:

- Lozenges must be dissolved in mouth >15–30 min for oropharyngeal therapy.
- Swallow saliva.

TOPICAL:

- Rub well into affected, surrounding areas.
- Do not apply occlusive covering or other preparations.

VAGINAL:

- Use vaginal applicator; insert high in vagina.

INDICATIONS/ROUTES/DOSAGE

Oral-local/oropharyngeal:
Oral: Adults, elderly: 10 mg 5 times/day for 14 days.

Prophylaxis vs. oropharyngeal candidiasis:
Oral: Adults, elderly: 10 mg 3 times/day.

Usual topical dosage:
Topical: Adults, elderly: 2 times/day. Therapeutic effect may take up to 8 wks.

Vulvovaginal candidiasis:
Vaginal: (Tablets) Adults, elderly: 1 tablet (100 mg) at bedtime for 7 days; 2 tablets (200 mg) at bedtime for 3 days; or 500 mg tablet one time.

Vaginal: (Cream) Adults, elderly: 1 applicatorful at bedtime for 7–14 days.

CONTRAINDICATIONS

Hypersensitivity to clotrimazole or any ingredient in preparation, children <3 yrs.

CAUTIONS

Hepatic disorder w/oral therapy.

INTERACTIONS

DRUG: None significant. **HERBAL:** None known. **FOOD:** None significant. **ALTERED LAB VALUES:** May increase SGOT (AST).

SIDE EFFECTS

FREQUENT: *Oral:* Nausea, vomiting, diarrhea, abdominal pain. **OCCASIONAL:** *Topical:* Itching, burning, stinging, erythema, urticaria. *Vaginal:* Mild burning (tablets/cream); irritation, cystitis (cream). **RARE:** *Vaginal tablets:* Itching, rash, lower abdominal cramping, headache.

ADVERSE REACTIONS/TOXIC EFFECTS

None significant.

PATIENT CONSIDERATIONS

BASELINE ASSESSMENT

Question for history of hypersensitivity to clotrimazole. Assess pt's ability to understand and follow directions regarding use of oral lozenges.

INTERVENTION/EVALUATION

W/oral therapy, assess for nausea, vomiting; monitor hepatic function tests especially w/preexisting hepatic disorder. Check skin for erythema, urticaria, blistering; inquire about itching, burning, stinging. W/vaginal therapy, evaluate for vulvovaginal irritation, abdominal cramping, urinary frequency, discomfort.

PATIENT/FAMILY TEACHING

Continue for full length of therapy. Inform physician of increased irritation. Avoid contact w/eyes.

Topical
Keep areas clean, dry; wear light clothing to promote ventilation. Separate personal items, linens.

Vaginal
Continue use during menses. Refrain from sexual intercourse or advise partner to use condom during therapy.

cloxacillin sodium

clocks-ah-sill-in
(Cloxapen, Tegopen)

CANADIAN AVAILABILITY
ApoCloxi, Novocloxin, Tegopen

PREGNANCY CATEGORY B

CLASSIFICATION

Antibiotic: penicillin

AVAILABILITY (Rx)

Capsules: 250 mg, 500 mg. **Oral Solution:** 125 mg/5 ml.

PHARMACOKINETICS

Absorption: Moderately absorbed from GI tract. **Metabolism:** Partially metabolized in liver. **Excretion:** Primarily excreted in urine. Not removed by hemodialysis. **Half-life:** 0.5–1.1 hrs (increased in decreased renal function).

ACTION/*THERAPEUTIC EFFECT*

Bactericidal in susceptible microorganisms by *inhibition of cell wall synthesis.*

USES

Treatment of mild to moderate infections of respiratory tract and skin/skin structure, chronic osteomyelitis, urinary tract infections; follow-up to parenteral therapy for acute, severe infections. Predominantly treatment of infections caused by penicillinase-producing staphylococci.

STORAGE/HANDLING

Store capsules at room temperature; oral solution, after reconstitution, is stable for 3 days at room temperature, 14 days if refrigerated.

ADMINISTRATION

ORAL:

- Space doses evenly around clock.
- Give 1 hr before or 2 hrs after meals.

INDICATIONS/ROUTES/DOSAGE

Mild to moderate upper respiratory, localized skin/skin structure infections:
Oral: Adults, elderly, children >20 kg: 250 mg q6h. *Children <20 kg:* 50 mg/kg/day in divided doses q6h.

Severe infections, lower respiratory tract, disseminated infections:
Oral: Adults, elderly, children >20 kg: 500 mg q6h. *Children <20 kg:* 100 mg/kg/day in divided doses q6h.

CONTRAINDICATIONS

Hypersensitivity to any penicillin.

CAUTIONS

History of allergies, particularly cephalosporins.

INTERACTIONS

DRUG: *Probenecid* may increase concentration, toxicity risk. **HERBAL:** None known. **FOOD:** None significant. **ALTERED LAB VALUES:** May increase SGOT (AST), SGPT (ALT), alkaline phosphatase, LDH. May cause positive Coombs' test.

SIDE EFFECTS

FREQUENT: Mild diarrhea, nausea, vomiting, headache, oral/vaginal candidiasis. **OCCASIONAL:** Mild hypersensitivity reaction (fever, rash, pruritus).

ADVERSE REACTIONS/TOXIC EFFECTS

Superinfections, antibiotic-associated colitis (abdominal cramps, watery severe diarrhea, fever) may result from altered bacterial balance. Hematologic effects, severe hypersensitivity reactions, anaphylaxis occur rarely.

PATIENT CONSIDERATIONS

Baseline Assessment

Question for history of allergies, especially penicillins, cephalosporins. Obtain specimen for culture and sensitivity before giving first dose (therapy may begin before results are known).

Intervention/Evaluation

Hold medication and promptly report rash (hypersensitivity) or diarrhea (w/fever, abdominal pain, mucus or blood in stool may indicate antibiotic-associated colitis). Assess food tolerance. Check hematology reports (especially WBCs), periodic renal or hepatic reports in prolonged therapy. Be alert for superinfection: increased fever, onset sore throat, diarrhea, ulceration or changes of oral mucosa, vaginal discharge, anal/genital pruritus.

Patient/Family Teaching

Space doses evenly. Continue antibiotic for full length of treatment. Notify physician in event of diarrhea, rash, other new symptom.

clozapine

klow-zah-peen
(Clozaril)

CANADIAN AVAILABILITY
Clozaril

PREGNANCY CATEGORY B

CLASSIFICATION

Antipsychotic

AVAILABILITY (Rx)

Tablets: 25 mg, 100 mg

PHARMACOKINETICS

Absorption: Rapid, almost completely absorbed from GI tract. Widely distributed. **Metabolism:** Extensively metabolized by first-pass liver metabolism. **Excretion:** Primarily excreted in urine. **Half-life:** 8–12 hrs.

ACTION/*THERAPEUTIC EFFECT*

Interferes with the binding of dopamine at dopamine receptor sites (binds primarily at non-dopamine receptor sites), *diminishing schizophrenic behavior.* Unlike other antipsychotics, produces few extrapyramidal effects.

USES

Management of severely ill schizophrenic pts who fail to respond to other antipsychotic therapy.

ADMINISTRATION

ORAL:

- May give w/o regard to meals.

INDICATIONS/ROUTES/DOSAGE

Schizophrenic disorders:
Oral: Adults: Initially, 25 mg 1–2 times/day. May increase by 25–50 mg/day over 2 wks until dose of 300–450 mg/day achieved. May further increase dose by 50–100 mg/day no more frequently than 1–2 times/wk. ***Range:*** 200–600 mg/day. ***Maximum:*** 900 mg/day.

Usual elderly dosage:
Oral: Initially, 25 mg/day. May increase by 25 mg/day. ***Maximum:*** 450 mg/day.

CONTRAINDICATIONS

Myeloproliferative disorders, history of clozapine-induced agranulocytosis or severe granulocytopenia, concurrent administration w/other drugs having potential to suppress bone marrow function, severe CNS depression, comatose state.

CAUTIONS

History of seizures, cardiovascular disease, impaired respiratory, hepatic, renal function, alcohol withdrawal, urinary retention, glaucoma, prostatic hypertrophy.

INTERACTIONS

DRUG: ***Alcohol, CNS depressants*** may increase CNS depressant effects. ***Bone marrow depressants*** may increase myelosuppression. ***Lithium*** may increase risk of seizures, confusion, dyskinesias. Phenobarbital decreases concentration. **HERBAL:** None known. **FOOD:** None significant. **ALTERED LAB VALUES:** None significant.

SIDE EFFECTS

FREQUENT: Drowsiness (39%), salivation (31%), tachycardia (25%), dizziness (19%), constipation (14%). **OCCASIONAL:** Hypotension (9%), headache (7%); tremor, syncope, sweating, dry mouth (6%); nausea, visual disturbances (5%); nightmares, restlessness, akinesia, agitation, hypertension, abdominal discomfort/ heartburn, weight gain (4%). **RARE:** Rigidity, confusion, fatigue, insomnia, diarrhea, rash.

ADVERSE REACTIONS/TOXIC EFFECTS

Seizures occur occasionally (3%). Overdosage produces CNS depression (sedation, coma, delirium), respiratory depression, hypersalivation. Blood dyscrasias, particularly agranulocytosis, mild leukopenia may occur.

PATIENT CONSIDERATIONS

BASELINE ASSESSMENT

Obtain baseline WBC and differential count before initiating treatment and WBC count every week for first 6 mos of continuous therapy, then biweekly for those w/acceptable WBC counts. Assess behavior, appearance, emotional status, response to environment, speech pattern, thought content.

INTERVENTION/EVALUATION

Monitor B/P for hyper/hypotension. Assess pulse for tachycardia (common side effect). Monitor WBC, differential count for blood dyscrasias. Question bowel activity for evidence of constipation. Supervise suicidal risk pt closely during early therapy (as depression lessens, energy level improves, increasing suicide potential). Assess for therapeutic response (interest in surroundings, improvement in self-care, increased ability to concentrate, relaxed facial expression).

PATIENT/FAMILY TEACHING

Do not abruptly withdraw from long-term drug therapy. Report visual disturbances. Sugarless gum or sips of tepid water may relieve dry mouth. Drowsiness generally subsides during continued therapy. Avoid tasks that require alertness, motor skills until response to drug is established. Avoid alcohol.

---

cocaine

koe-**kane**
(Cocaine HCl)

CANADIAN AVAILABILTY
Cocaine

PREGNANCY CATEGORY C
(X if nonmedical use)

CLASSIFICATION

Topical anesthetic

AVAILABILITY (Rx)

Topical Solution: 4%, 10%

PHARMACODYNAMICS

	ONSET	PEAK	DURATION
Topical	1 min	2–5 min	0.5–2 hrs

PHARMACOKINETICS

Absorption: Readily absorbed from all mucous membranes. **Metabolism:** Hydrolyzed by plasma and liver cholinesterases to active metabolite. **Excretion:** Primarily excreted in urine. **Half-life:** 1–1.5 hrs.

ACTION/*THERAPEUTIC EFFECT*

Blocks conduction of nerve impulses by decreasing membrane permeability, increases norepinephrine at postsynaptic receptor sites, producing intense vasoconstriction.

USES

Topical anesthesia for mucous membranes of oral laryngeal, nasal areas.

ADMINISTRATION

TOPICAL:

- Avoid inhalation of any sprays. Do not puncture spray container or use near open flame.
- Do not get preparations near eyes.
- When used for anesthesia of throat, NPO until sensation returns (failure to protect from aspiration, difficulty w/swallowing).

INDICATIONS/ROUTES/DOSAGE

Usual topical dosage:
Topical: Adults, elderly: 1–10% solution. ***Maximum single dose:*** 1 mg/kg.

CONTRAINDICATIONS

Hypersensitivity to cocaine or local anesthetics. Systemic or ophthalmic use.

CAUTIONS

History of drug sensitivities or drug abuse (can cause strong psychologic dependence and some tolerance); has been abused for cortical stimulant effect. Severe trauma or sepsis in area to be anesthetized. Limit to office and surgical procedures; prolonged use can cause ischemic damage to nasal mucosa. Safety in children not established.

INTERACTIONS

DRUG: ***Tricyclic antidepressants, digoxin, methyldopa*** may increase arrhythmias. May decrease effects of ***beta blockers. Cholinesterase inhibitors*** may increase effects, risk of toxicity. ***CNS stimulation-producing agents*** may increase effects. ***Sympathomimetics*** increase CNS stimulation, risk of cardiovascular effects. **HERBAL:** None known. **FOOD:** None significant. **ALTERED LAB VALUES:** None significant.

SIDE EFFECTS

FREQUENT: Loss of sense of smell/taste. **OCCASIONAL:** Repeated nasal application: stuffy nose, chronic rhinitis.

ADVERSE REACTIONS/TOXIC EFFECTS

Nasal: None significant. ***Systemic: Overdose, early signs:*** Increased B/P, increased pulse, irregular heartbeat, chills/fever, agitation, nervousness, confusion, inability to remain still, nausea, vomiting, abdominal pain, increased sweating, rapid breathing, large pupils. ***Advanced:*** Arrhythmias, CNS hemorrhage, CHF, convulsions, delirium, hyperreflexia, loss of bladder/bowel control, respiratory weakness. ***Late stage:*** Loss of reflexes, muscle paralysis, dilated pupils, LOC, cyanosis, pulmonary edema, cardiac/respiratory failure.

PATIENT CONSIDERATIONS

BASELINE ASSESSMENT

Question for hypersensitivity to cocaine. Obtain baseline vital signs.

INTERVENTION/EVALUATION

Monitor for anesthetic response. Be alert to CNS stimulation:

assess for euphoria, restlessness, increased B/P, pulse, respirations. Be prepared to provide ventilatory support and emergency medications in event of progression of CNS response—death from overdose will occur within minutes, up to 3 hrs after initial reaction.

PATIENT/FAMILY TEACHING

NPO until sensation returns when used for throat anesthesia. One-time or infrequent use for procedures will not cause dependence. Report feelings of euphoria, restlessness, or rapid heartbeat if these develop during procedure.

codeine phosphate

koe-**deen**

codeine sulfate

FIXED-COMBINATION(S)
W/aspirin, butalbital, a barbiturate, and caffeine **(Fiorinal)**; w/acetaminophen **(Phenaphen, Tylenol w/codeine)**; w/aspirin **(Empirin w/codeine)**

CANADIAN AVAILABILITY
Codeine Contin

PREGNANCY CATEGORY C
(D if used for prolonged periods or at high doses at term)

CLASSIFICATION

Opioid analgesic: **Schedule II;** fixed-combination form: **Schedule III**

AVAILABILITY (Rx)

Tablets: 15 mg, 30 mg, 60 mg. **Soluble Tablets:** 15 mg, 30 mg, 60 mg. **Injection:** 30 mg, 60 mg.

PHARMACODYNAMICS

	ONSET	PEAK	DURATION
Oral	15–30 min	1–1.5 hrs	4–6 hrs
IM	15–30 min	30–60 min	4–6 hrs
SubQ	15–30 min	—	4–6 hrs

PHARMACOKINETICS

Absorption: Moderately absorbed from GI tract; completely after IM administration. Widely distributed. **Metabolism:** Metabolized in liver. **Excretion:** Excreted in urine. **Half-life:** 2.5–4 hrs.

ACTION/*THERAPEUTIC EFFECT*

Binds at opiate receptor sites in CNS. *Reduces intensity of pain stimuli incoming from sensory nerve endings, suppresses cough reflex, decreases intestinal motility.*

USES/*UNLABELED*

Relief of mild to moderate pain and/or nonproductive cough. *Treatment of diarrhea.*

STORAGE/HANDLING

Store oral, parenteral form at room temperature.

ADMINISTRATION

ORAL:
- Give w/o regard to meals.
- Shake oral suspension well.

SUBQ/IM:
- Parenteral form incompatible w/aminophylline, ammonium chloride, amobarbital, chlorothiazide, heparin, methicillin, nitrofurantoin, pentobarbital, phenobarbital, sodium bicarbonate, sodium iodide, thiopental.
- Pt should be recumbent before drug is administered.
- Assess for wheals at injection

site (sign of local tissue irritation, induration).
- Those w/circulatory impairment may experience overdosage due to delayed absorption of repeated administration.

INDICATIONS/ROUTES/DOSAGE

Note: Reduce initial dosage in those w/hypothyroidism, concurrent CNS depressants, Addison's disease, renal insufficiency, elderly/debilitated.

Analgesia:
Oral/SubQ/IM: Adults, elderly: 30 mg q4–6h. ***Range:*** 15–60 mg daily. ***Children:*** 0.5 mg/kg q4–6h.

Antitussive:
Oral: Adults, elderly, children >12 yrs: 10–20 mg q4–6h. ***Children 6–11 yrs:*** 5–10 mg q4–6h. ***Children 2–5 yrs:*** 2.5–5 mg q4–6h.

CONTRAINDICATIONS

None significant.

EXTREME CAUTION

CNS depression, anoxia, respiratory depression, seizures, acute alcoholism, diarrhea associated w/pseudomembranous colitis/poisoning (until toxic substance eliminated from GI tract), acute respiratory depression/dysfunction, acute asthma attack, severe inflammatory bowel disease.

CAUTIONS

Increased intracranial pressure, impaired hepatic function, acute abdominal conditions, hypothyroidism, prostatic hypertrophy, urethral stricture, COPD, cardiac arrhythmias, history of seizures, drug abuse, alcoholism, gallbladder disease, increased intracranial pressure, head injury, decreased renal/liver function, hypothyroidism, prostatic hypertrophy/obstruction.

INTERACTIONS

DRUG: ***Alcohol, CNS depressants*** may increase CNS or respiratory depression, hypotension. ***MAO inhibitors*** may produce severe, fatal reaction (reduce dose to $\frac{1}{4}$ usual dose). **HERBAL:** None known. **FOOD:** None significant. **ALTERED LAB VALUES:** May increase amylase, lipase.

SIDE EFFECTS

Note: Ambulatory pts, those not in severe pain may experience dizziness, nausea, vomiting, hypotension more frequently than those in supine position or w/severe pain. **FREQUENT:** Constipation, drowsiness, nausea, vomiting. **OCCASIONAL:** Paradoxical excitement, confusion, pounding heartbeat, facial flushing, decreased urination, blurred vision, dizziness, dry mouth, headache, hypotension, decreased appetite, redness/burning/pain at injection site. **RARE:** Hallucinations, depression, stomach pain, insomnia.

ADVERSE REACTIONS/TOXIC EFFECTS

Too frequent use may result in paralytic ileus. Overdosage results in cold/clammy skin, confusion, convulsions, decreased B/P, restlessness, pinpoint pupils, bradycardia, respiratory depression, LOC, severe weakness. Tolerance to analgesic effect, physical dependence may occur w/repeated use.

PATIENT CONSIDERATIONS

Baseline Assessment

Obtain vital signs before giving medication. If respirations are 12/min or lower (20/min or lower in children), withhold medication, contact physician.

Analgesic
Assess onset, type, location, and duration of pain. Effect of medication is reduced if full pain recurs before next dose.

Antitussive
Assess type, severity, frequency of cough, and production. Increase fluid intake and environmental humidity to lower viscosity of lung secretions.

INTERVENTION/EVALUATION

Monitor vital signs q15–30min after parenteral administration (monitor for decreased B/P, change in rate or quality of pulse). Increase fluid intake and environmental humidity to improve viscosity of lung secretions. Palpate bladder for urinary retention. Monitor pattern of daily bowel activity and stool consistency. Initiate deep breathing and coughing exercises, particularly in those w/impaired pulmonary function. Assess for clinical improvement; record onset of relief of pain or cough.

PATIENT/FAMILY TEACHING

Discomfort may occur w/injection. Change positions slowly to avoid orthostatic hypotension. Avoid tasks that require alertness, motor skills until response to drug is established. Tolerance/dependence may occur w/prolonged use of high doses. Avoid alcohol. Report shortness of breath or breathing difficulty.

colchicine

coal-cheh-seen
(Colchicine)

CANADIAN AVAILABILITY
Colchicine

PREGNANCY CATEGORY D

CLASSIFICATION

Antigout

AVAILABILITY (Rx)

Tablets: 0.5 mg, 0.6 mg. **Injection:** 1 mg.

PHARMACOKINETICS

Absorption: Rapidly absorbed from GI tract. Highest concentration in liver, spleen, kidney. Reenters intestinal tract (biliary secretion), reabsorbed from intestines. **Metabolism:** Partially metabolized in liver. **Excretion:** Eliminated primarily in feces.

ACTION/*THERAPEUTIC EFFECT*

Decreases leukocyte motility, phagocytosis, lactic acid production, *resulting in decreased urate crystal deposits, inflammatory process.*

USES/*UNLABELED*

Treatment of attacks of acute gouty arthritis, prophylaxis of recurrent gouty arthritis. *Reduce frequency of familial Mediterranean fever, treatment of acute attacks of calcium pyrophosphate, deposition, sarcoid arthritis, amyloidosis, biliary cirrhosis, recurrent pericarditis.*

ADMINISTRATION

ORAL:
- May give w/o regard to meals.

IV:
- **Note:** SubQ or IM administration produces severe local reaction. Use via IV route only.
- Administer over 2–5 min.

- May dilute w/0.9% NaCl or sterile water for injection.
- Do not dilute w/5% dextrose.

INDICATIONS/ROUTES/DOSAGE

Acute gouty arthritis:
Oral: Adults, elderly: 0.5–1.2 mg, then 0.5–0.6 mg q1–2h or 1–1.2 mg q2h until pain relieved or nausea, vomiting, or diarrhea occurs. *Total dose:* 4–8 mg.

IV: Adults, elderly: Initially, 2 mg, then 0.5 mg q6h until satisfactory response. *Maximum:* 4 mg/24 hrs or 4 mg/one course of treatment. *Note:* If pain recurs, may give 1–2 mg/day for several days but no sooner than 7 days after a full course of IV therapy (4 mg).

Chronic gouty arthritis:
Oral: Adults, elderly: 0.5–0.6 mg once weekly up to once daily (dependent on number of attacks per year).

CONTRAINDICATIONS

Severe gastrointestinal, renal, hepatic, or cardiac disorders; blood dyscrasias.

CAUTIONS

Impaired hepatic function, elderly, debilitated.

INTERACTIONS

DRUG: *NSAIDs* may increase risk of neutropenia, thrombocytopenia, bone marrow depression. *Bone marrow depressants* may increase risk of blood dyscrasias. **HERBAL:** None known. **FOOD:** None significant. **ALTERED LAB VALUES:** May decrease platelet count. May increase SGOT (AST), alkaline phosphatase.

SIDE EFFECTS

Note: Those w/impaired renal function may exhibit myopathy and neuropathy manifested as generalized weakness. **FREQUENT:** *Oral:* Nausea, vomiting, abdominal discomfort. **OCCASIONAL:** *Oral:* Anorexia. **RARE:** Hypersensitivity reaction, including angioedema. *Parenteral only:* Nausea, vomiting, diarrhea, abdominal discomfort, pain/redness at injection site, neuritis in injected arm.

ADVERSE REACTIONS/TOXIC EFFECTS

Bone marrow depression (aplastic anemia, agranulocytosis, thrombocytopenia) may occur w/long-term therapy. Overdose: *Initially:* Burning feeling in throat/skin, severe diarrhea, abdominal pain. *Secondly:* Fever, seizures, delirium, renal damage (hematuria, oliguria). *Third stage:* Hair loss, leukocytosis, stomatitis.

PATIENT CONSIDERATIONS

Baseline Assessment

Instruct pt to drink 8–10 glasses (8 oz) of fluid daily while on medication. Medication should be discontinued if any GI symptoms occur. Periodic CBC should be performed routinely in those receiving long-term therapy.

Intervention/Evaluation

Discontinue medication immediately if GI symptoms occur. Encourage high fluid intake (3,000 ml/day). Monitor I&O (output should be at least 2,000 ml/day). Assess CBC, serum uric acid levels. Assess for therapeutic response (reduced joint tenderness, swelling, redness, limitation of motion).

Patient/Family Teaching

Encourage low-purine food intake; drink 8–10 glasses (8 oz) of fluid daily while on medication. Report skin rash, sore throat, fever, unusual bruising/bleeding, weakness, tiredness, numbness. Stop medication as soon as gout pain relieved or first sign of nausea, vomiting, or diarrhea.

colesevelam

(Welchol)
See Supplement

colestipol

(Cholestid)
See Classification section under: Antihyperlipidemics

colfosceril palmitate

kol-**foss**-er-ill
(Exosurf)

CANADIAN AVAILABILITY
Exosurf

CLASSIFICATION

Lung surfactant

AVAILABILITY (Rx)

Powder for Injection: 108 mg

ACTION/*THERAPEUTIC EFFECT*

Lowers surface tension on alveolar surfaces during respiration, stabilizes alveoli vs. collapse that may occur at resting pulmonary pressures. *Replenishes surfactant, restores surface activity to lungs.*

USES

Prophylactic use in infants <1,350 g at risk of developing RDS, infants >1,350 g w/evidence of pulmonary immaturity; treatment in infants w/RDS.

STORAGE/HANDLING

Store vials at room temperature. After reconstitution, stable for 12 hrs.

ADMINISTRATION:

INTRATRACHEAL:

- Reconstitute immediately prior to use w/8 ml preservative-free sterile water for injection. Refer to manufacturer's instructions.
- Do not use if vacuum in vial not present.
- Instill through catheter inserted into infant's endotracheal tube. Do not instill into main stem bronchus.
- Stop administration if reflux into endotracheal tube occurs. If needed, increase peak inspiratory pressure on ventilator by 4–5 cm H_2O until tube clears.
- Stop administration if transcutaneous oxygen saturation decreases. If needed, increase peak inspiratory pressure on ventilator by 4–5 cm H_2O for 1–2 min. May also need to increase FiO_2 for 1–2 min.

INDICATIONS/ROUTES/DOSAGE

Prophylaxis for RDS:
Intratracheal: Neonates: 5 ml/kg given as two 2.5 ml/kg doses as soon as possible after birth. May repeat 12 and 24 hrs later in infants remaining on mechanical ventilator.

RDS rescue:
Intratracheal: Neonates: 5 ml/kg given as two 2.5 ml/kg doses. Repeat in 12 hrs in all infants remaining on ventilator.

CONTRAINDICATIONS

None significant.

CAUTIONS

Those at risk for circulatory overload.

INTERACTIONS

DRUG: None significant. **HERBAL:** None known. **FOOD:** None significant. **ALTERED LAB VALUES:** None significant.

SIDE EFFECTS

OCCASIONAL: Gagging. **RARE:** Apnea, bradycardia, tachycardia.

ADVERSE REACTIONS/TOXIC EFFECTS

Failure to reduce peak ventilator inspiratory pressures after chest expansion, after dosing, may result in lung overdistension and fatal pulmonary air leak. Failure to reduce transcutaneous oxygen saturation if in excess of 95% by decreasing FiO_2 in small but repeated steps until saturation is 90% to 95% may result in hyperoxia. Failure to reduce ventilator if arterial or transcutaneous CO_2 measurements are <30 may result in hypocarbia, reducing blood-brain flow.

PATIENT CONSIDERATIONS

BASELINE ASSESSMENT

Drug must be administered in highly supervised setting. Clinicians in care of neonate must be experienced w/intubation, ventilator management. Give emotional support to parents. Suctioning infant before dosing may decrease chance of mucous plugs obstructing endotracheal tube.

INTERVENTION/EVALUATION

Monitor infant w/arterial or transcutaneous measurement of systemic O_2 and CO_2. Maintain vigilant clinical attention to neonate prior to, during, and after drug administration. Assess lung sounds for rales and moist breath sounds. If chest expansion improves dramatically after dosing, reduce peak ventilator inspiratory pressures immediately (failure to do so may result in lung overdistension and fatal pulmonary air leak). If transcutaneous oxygen saturation >95% and neonate appears pink, reduce FiO_2 in small but repeated steps until saturation is 90% to 95% (failure to do so may result in hyperoxia). If arterial or transcutaneous CO_2 measurements are <30, reduce ventilator immediately (failure to do so may result in hypocarbia, reducing brain-blood flow).

---

conjugated estrogens

ess-troe-jenz
(Cenestin, Premarin)

FIXED-COMBINATION(S)
W/meprobamate, a tranquilizer **(Milprem);** Premarin w/methyltestosterone, an androgen, w/medroxyprogesterone, a progestin **(Premphase, Prempro)**.

CANADIAN AVAILABILITY
C.E.S., Congest, Premarin

PREGNANCY CATEGORY X

CLASSIFICATION

Estrogen

AVAILABILITY (Rx)

Tablets: 0.3 mg, 0.625 mg, 0.9 mg, 1.25 mg, 2.5 mg. **Injection:** 25 mg. **Vaginal Cream.**

PHARMACOKINETICS

Absorption: Well absorbed from GI tract. Widely distributed. **Metabolism:** Metabolized in liver.

Excretion: Primarily excreted in urine.

ACTION/*THERAPEUTIC EFFECT*

Increases synthesis of DNA, RNA, and various proteins in responsive tissues. Reduces release of gonadotropin-releasing hormone, reducing follicle-stimulating hormone (FSH) and leuteinizing hormone (LH). *Promotes vasomotor stability, maintains genitourinary function, normal growth, development of female sex organs. Prevents accelerated bone loss by inhibiting bone resorption, restoring balance of bone resorption and formation. Inhibits LH, decreases serum concentration of testosterone.*

USES/*UNLABELED*

Management of moderate to severe vasomotor symptoms associated w/menopause. Treatment of atrophic vaginitis, kraurosis vulvae, female hypogonadism and castration, primary ovarian failure. Retardation of osteoporosis in postmenopausal women. Palliative treatment of inoperable, progressive cancer of the prostate in men and of the breast in postmenopausal women. *Prevents estrogen deficiency-induced premenopausal osteoporosis.* ***Cream:*** *Prevention of nosebleeds.*

STORAGE/HANDLING

Keep tablets at room temperature. Refrigerate vials for IV use. Reconstituted solution stable for 60 days refrigerated. Do not use if solution darkens or precipitate forms.

ADMINISTRATION

ORAL:

- Administer at the same time each day.
- Give w/milk or food if nausea occurs.

IV:

- Reconstitute w/5 ml sterile water for injection containing benzyl alcohol (diluent provided).
- Slowly add diluent, shaking gently. Avoid vigorous shaking.
- Give slowly to prevent flushing reaction.

INDICATIONS/ROUTES/DOSAGE

Vasomotor symptoms associated w/menopause, atrophic vaginitis, kraurosis vulvae:
Oral: Adults, elderly: 0.3–1.25 mg/day cyclically (21 days on; 7 days off). If pt is menstruating, begin on 5th day of cycle; if pt not menstruating within previous 2 mos, start arbitrarily.

Intravaginal: Adults, elderly: 2–4 g/day cyclically.

Female hypogonadism:
Oral: Adults: 2.5–7.5 mg/day in divided doses for 20 days; rest 10 days. If bleeding occurs prior to 10th drug-free day, a 20 day estrogen-progestin regimen given for 20 days, w/progestin given during last 5 days of estrogen therapy. If menstruation begins prior to completing the estrogen-progestin regimen, discontinue therapy, reinstitute on 5th day of menstruation.

Female castration, primary ovarian failure:
Oral: Adults: Initially, 1.25 mg/day cyclically.

Osteoporosis:
Oral: Adults, elderly: 0.3–0.625 mg/day, cyclically.

Breast cancer:
Oral: Adults, elderly: 10 mg 3 times/day for at least 3 mos.

Prostate cancer:
Oral: Adults, elderly: 1.25–2.5 mg 3 times/day.

Abnormal uterine bleeding:
IM/IV: Adults: 25 mg, may repeat once in 6–12 hrs.

CONTRAINDICATIONS

Known or suspected breast cancer (except select pts w/metastasis), estrogen-dependent neoplasia; undiagnosed abnormal genital bleeding; active thrombophlebitis or thromboembolic disorders; history of thrombophlebitis, thrombosis, or thromboembolic disorders w/previous estrogen use, hypersensitivity to estrogen.

CAUTIONS

Conditions that may be aggravated by fluid retention: cardiac, renal, or hepatic dysfunction, epilepsy, migraine, mental depression, metabolic bone disease w/potential hypercalcemia, history of jaundice during pregnancy, strong family history of breast cancer, fibrocystic disease or breast nodules, children in whom bone growth is not complete.

INTERACTIONS

DRUG: May interfere w/effects of ***bromocriptine***. May increase concentration of ***cyclosporine,*** increase hepatic, nephrotoxicity. ***Hepatotoxic medications*** may increase hepatotoxicity. **HERBAL:** Saw palmetto can interfere w/therapy. **FOOD:** None significant. **ALTERED LAB VALUES:** May affect metapyrone, thyroid function tests. May decrease cholesterol, LDH. May increase calcium, glucose, HDL, triglycerides.

SIDE EFFECTS

FREQUENT: Loss of appetite, nausea, swelling of breasts, edema.

OCCASIONAL: Vomiting (especially w/high doses), intolerance to contact lenses, headache or migraine, increased B/P, changes in vaginal bleeding (spotting, breakthrough, or prolonged bleeding), glucose intolerance, brown spots on exposed skin, libido changes. **RARE:** Chorea, cholestatic jaundice, loss of scalp hair, depression.

ADVERSE REACTIONS/TOXIC EFFECTS

Prolonged administration may increase risk of gallbladder, thromboembolic disease, and breast, cervical, vaginal, endometrial, and liver carcinoma.

PATIENT CONSIDERATIONS

Baseline Assessment

Question hypersensitivity to estrogen, previous jaundice, or thromboembolic disorders associated w/pregnancy or estrogen therapy. Establish baseline B/P, blood glucose.

Intervention/Evaluation

Assess blood pressure periodically. Check for swelling; weigh daily. Monitor blood glucose 4 times/day for pts w/diabetes. Promptly report signs and symptoms of thromboembolic or thrombotic disorders: sudden severe headache, shortness of breath, vision or speech disturbance, weakness or numbness of an extremity, loss of coordination, pain in chest, groin, or leg. Note estrogen therapy on specimens.

Patient/Family Teaching

Need for medical supervision. Avoid smoking due to increased risk of heart attack or blood clots. Explain importance of diet

and exercise when taken to retard osteoporosis. Do not take other medications w/o physician approval. Teach how to perform Homan's test, signs and symptoms of blood clots (report these to physician immediately). Also notify physician of abnormal vaginal bleeding, depression, other symptoms. Teach female pts to perform breast self-exam. Avoid exposure to sun or ultraviolet light. Check weight daily; report weekly gain of >5 lbs. Stop taking medication and contact physician if suspect pregnancy. Give labeling from drug package.

---

corticorelin
(Acthrel)
See Supplement

---

corticotropin injection

kore-tih-koe-**troe**-pin
(ACTH, Acthar)

corticotropin repository

(Cortigel, Cortrophin-Gel, Acthar Gel)

PREGNANCY CATEGORY C

CLASSIFICATION

Adrenocorticotropic hormone

AVAILABILITY (Rx)

Powder for Injection: 25 units, 40 units. **Repository Injection:** 40 units/ml, 80 units/ml.

PHARMACOKINETICS

Absorption: Rapid absorption from IM/SubQ sites (respiratory forms have delayed absorption). Widely distributed.

ACTION / *THERAPEUTIC EFFECT*

Stimulates adrenal cortex to secrete cortisol, corticosterone, aldosterone and androgenic substances. Acts to stimulate synthesis of adrenocortical hormones. *Suppresses immune response, inflammation.*

USES

Diagnostic testing of adrenocortical function. Limited therapeutic value in conditions responsive to corticosteroid therapy. May be used in hypercalcemia of cancer, acute exacerbations of multiple sclerosis, nonsuppurative thyroiditis.

STORAGE/HANDLING

Refrigerate repository dosage forms. After reconstitution, corticotropin injection is stable for 24 hrs if refrigerated.

ADMINISTRATION

Assess for hypersensitivity reaction during first 15 min of IV administration or immediately following IM or SubQ injection.

IM/SubQ:

- Repository corticotropin may be given SubQ or IM for prolonged effects.
- Reconstitute in 0.9% sodium chloride solution or sterile water for injection to produce final volume of 1–2 ml.

IV:

- Give IV only for diagnostic use or in adults w/idiopathic thrombocytopenic purpura.
- For IV infusion, further dilute in

0.9% NaCl, 5% dextrose, or 5% dextrose in 0.9% NaCl solutions.

INDICATIONS/ROUTES/DOSAGE

Note: May give IM, SubQ. IV only for corticotropin injection; IM only for corticotropin zinc hydroxide.

Diagnostic testing:
IV: Adults: 10–25 units in 500 ml D_5W infused over 8 hrs.

IM/SubQ: Adults: 20 units 4 times/day.

Acute exacerbation of multiple sclerosis:
IM: Adults: 80–120 units/day for 2–3 wks.

Infantile spasms:
IM: Infants: 20–40 units/day or 80 units every other day for 3 mos (or 1 mo after cessation of seizures).

Usual repository injection dosage:
IM/SubQ: Adults: 40–80 units q24–72h.

CONTRAINDICATIONS

Hypersensitivity to any corticosteroid or porcine proteins, systemic fungal infection, peptic ulcers (except life-threatening situations), scleroderma, primary adrenocortical insufficiency. Avoid live virus vaccine; long-term therapy in children.

CAUTIONS

Thromboembolic disorders, history of tuberculosis (may reactivate disease), hypothyroidism, cirrhosis, nonspecific ulcerative colitis, CHF, hypertension, psychosis, renal insufficiency, seizures. Prolonged therapy should be discontinued slowly.

INTERACTIONS

DRUG: ***Amphotericin*** may increase hypokalemia. May decrease effect of ***oral hypoglycemics, insulin, diuretics, potassium supplements.*** May increase ***digoxin*** toxicity (due to hypokalemia). ***Hepatic enzyme inducers*** may decrease effect. ***Live virus vaccines*** may potentiate virus replication, increase vaccine side effects, decrease pt's antibody response to vaccine. **HERBAL:** None known. **FOOD:** None significant. **ALTERED LAB VALUES:** May decrease calcium, potassium, thyroxine. May increase cholesterol, lipids, glucose, sodium, amylase.

SIDE EFFECTS

FREQUENT: Insomnia, heartburn, nervousness, abdominal distension, increased sweating, acne, mood swings, increased appetite, facial flushing, delayed wound healing, increased susceptibility to infection, diarrhea/constipation. **OCCASIONAL:** Headache, edema, change in skin color, frequent urination. **RARE:** Tachycardia, allergic reaction (rash, hives), pain, redness, swelling at injection site, psychic changes, hallucinations, depression.

ADVERSE REACTIONS/TOXIC EFFECTS

Long-term therapy: Hypocalcemia, hypokalemia, muscle wasting (especially arms, legs), osteoporosis, spontaneous fractures, amenorrhea, cataracts, glaucoma, peptic ulcer, CHF. ***Abrupt withdrawal following long-term therapy:*** Anorexia, nausea, fever, headache, joint pain, rebound inflammation, fatigue, weakness, lethargy, dizziness, orthostatic hypertension.

PATIENT CONSIDERATIONS

BASELINE ASSESSMENT

Question for hypersensitivity to any of the corticosteroids. Obtain

baseline values for weight, B/P, glucose, cholesterol, electrolytes. Check results of initial tests, (e.g., TB skin test, x-rays, EKG).

INTERVENTION/EVALUATION

Monitor I&O, daily weight; assess for edema. Check B/P, temperature, respirations, pulse at least 2 times/day. Be alert to infection (reduced immune response): sore throat, fever, or vague symptoms. Evaluate bowel activity. Monitor electrolytes. Watch for hypocalcemia (muscle twitching, cramps, positive Trousseau's or Chvostek's signs) or hypokalemia (weakness and muscle cramps, numbness/tingling especially lower extremities, nausea and vomiting, irritability, EKG changes.) Assess emotional status, ability to sleep.

PATIENT/FAMILY TEACHING

Carry identification of drug and dose, physician's name and phone number. Do not change dose/schedule or stop taking drug, *must* taper off under medical supervision. Notify physician of fever, sore throat, muscle aches, sudden weight gain/swelling. W/dietician, give instructions for prescribed diet (usually sodium restricted w/high vitamin D, protein, and potassium). Maintain careful personal hygiene, avoid exposure to disease or trauma. Severe stress (serious infection, surgery, or trauma) may require increased dosage. Do not take aspirin or any other medication w/o consulting physician. Follow-up visits, lab tests are necessary; children must be assessed for growth retardation. Inform dentist or other physicians of cortisone therapy now or within past 12 mos.

C

cortisone acetate

kore-tih-zone
(Cortone Acetate)

CANADIAN AVAILABILITY
Cortone

PREGNANCY CATEGORY D

CLASSIFICATION

Corticosteroid

AVAILABILITY (Rx)

Tablets: 5 mg, 10 mg, 25 mg

PHARMACOKINETICS

Absorption: Rapid, complete absorption from GI tract. Widely distributed. **Metabolism:** Primarily metabolized in liver to hydrocortisone. **Excretion:** Primarily excreted in urine. **Half-life:** 30 min.

ACTION/*THERAPEUTIC EFFECT*

Inhibits accumulation of inflammatory cells at inflammation sites, phagocytosis, lysosomal enzyme release and synthesis and/or release of mediators of inflammation. *Prevents/suppresses cell-mediated immune reactions. Decreases/prevents tissue response to inflammatory process.*

USES

Substitution therapy in deficiency states: acute/chronic adrenal insufficiency, congenital adrenal hyperplasia, adrenal insufficiency secondary to pituitary insufficiency. **Nonendocrine disorders:** arthritis, rheumatic carditis, allergic, collagen, intestinal tract, liver, ocular, renal, and skin diseases, bronchial asthma, cerebral edema, malignancies.

ADMINISTRATION

ORAL:

- Give w/milk or food (decreases GI upset).
- Single doses given prior to 9 AM; multiple doses at evenly spaced intervals.

INDICATIONS/ROUTES/DOSAGE

Note: Individualize dose based on disease, pt, and response.

Usual oral dosage:
Oral: Adults: Initially 25–300 mg/day. ***Maintenance:*** Lowest dosage that maintains adequate clinical response.

Usual elderly dosage:
Oral: Use lowest effective dosage.

CONTRAINDICATIONS

Hypersensitivity to any corticosteroid, systemic fungal infection, peptic ulcers (except life-threatening situations). Avoid live virus vaccine.

CAUTIONS

Thromboembolic disorders, history of tuberculosis (may reactivate disease), hypothyroidism, cirrhosis, nonspecific ulcerative colitis, CHF, hypertension, psychosis, renal insufficiency, seizure disorders. Prolonged therapy should be discontinued slowly.

INTERACTIONS

DRUG: ***Amphotericin*** may increase hypokalemia. May decrease effect of ***oral hypoglycemics, insulin, diuretics, potassium supplements.*** May increase ***digoxin*** toxicity (due to hypokalemia). ***Hepatic enzyme inducers*** may decrease effect. ***Live virus vaccines*** may potentiate virus replication, increase vaccine side effects, decrease pt's antibody response to vaccine. **HERBAL:** Ginseng may decrease effect. **FOOD:** None significant. **ALTERED LAB VALUES:** May decrease calcium, potassium, thyroxine. May increase cholesterol, lipids, glucose, sodium, amylase.

SIDE EFFECTS

FREQUENT: Insomnia, heartburn, nervousness, abdominal distension, increased sweating, acne, mood swings, increased appetite, facial flushing, delayed wound healing, increased susceptibility to infection, diarrhea/constipation. **OCCASIONAL:** Headache, edema, change in skin color, frequent urination. **RARE:** Tachycardia, allergic reaction (rash, hives), psychic changes, hallucinations, depression.

ADVERSE REACTIONS/TOXIC EFFECTS

Long-term therapy: Hypocalcemia, hypokalemia, muscle wasting (especially arms, legs), osteoporosis, spontaneous fractures, amenorrhea, cataracts, glaucoma, peptic ulcer, CHF. ***Abrupt withdrawal following long-term therapy:*** Anorexia, nausea, fever, headache, joint pain, rebound inflammation, fatigue, weakness, lethargy, dizziness, orthostatic hypertension.

PATIENT CONSIDERATIONS

Baseline Assessment

Question for hypersensitivity to any of the corticosteroids. Obtain baseline values for weight, B/P, glucose, cholesterol, electrolytes. Check results of initial tests, (e.g., TB skin test, x-rays, EKG).

Intervention/Evaluation

Monitor I&O, daily weight; assess for edema. Check B/P, temperature, respirations, pulse at least 2 times/day. Be alert to infection (reduced immune response):

sore throat, fever, or vague symptoms. Evaluate bowel activity. Monitor electrolytes. Watch for hypocalcemia (muscle twitching, cramps, positive Trousseau's or Chvostek's signs) or hypokalemia (weakness and muscle cramps, numbness/tingling especially lower extremities, nausea and vomiting, irritability, EKG changes). Assess emotional status, ability to sleep.

Patient/Family Teaching

Carry identification of drug and dose, physician's name and phone number. Do not change dose/schedule or stop taking drug, *must* taper off under medical supervision. Notify physician of fever, sore throat, muscle aches, sudden weight gain/swelling. W/dietician, give instructions for prescribed diet (usually sodium restricted w/high vitamin D, protein, and potassium). Maintain careful personal hygiene, avoid exposure to disease or trauma. Severe stress (serious infection, surgery, or trauma) may require increased dosage. Do not take aspirin or any other medication w/o consulting physician. Follow-up visits, lab tests are necessary; children must be assessed for growth retardation.Inform dentist or other physicians of cortisone therapy now or within past 12 mos.

---

cosyntropin

koe-syn-**troe**-pin
(Cortrosyn)

CANADIAN AVAILABILITY
Cortrosyn

PREGNANCY CATEGORY C

CLASSIFICATION

Adrenocorticotropic hormone

AVAILABILITY (Rx)

Powder for Injection: 0.25 mg

PHARMACOKINETICS

Absorption: Rapid absorption from IM/SubQ sites. Widely distributed.

ACTION

Increases endogenous corticoid synthesis. Stimulates initial reaction in synthesis of adrenal steroids from cholesterol. Other effects due to generated endogenous corticosteroids.

USES

Diagnostic testing of adrenocortical function.

ADMINISTRATION

IM/IV:

- Reconstitute by adding 1 ml of 0.9% NaCl injection to a 0.25 mg vial of cosyntropin to produce solution of 0.25 mg/ml.
- For IV infusion, dilute w/5% dextrose or 0.9% NaCl and infuse at rate of 0.04 mg/hr over 6 hrs.

INDICATIONS/ROUTES/DOSAGE

Screening test for adrenal function:
IM: Adults: 0.25–0.75 mg one time. *Children (<2 yrs):* 0.125 mg one time.

IV infusion: Adults: 0.25 mg in 5% dextrose or 0.9% NaCl, infuse at rate of 0.04 mg/hr.

CONTRAINDICATIONS

Hypersensitivity to cosyntropin or corticotropin.

CAUTIONS

Short duration for diagnostic use

does not produce effects of long-term corticotropin therapy.

INTERACTIONS

DRUG: None significant. **HERBAL:** None known. **FOOD:** None significant. **ALTERED LAB VALUES:** None significant.

SIDE EFFECTS

OCCASIONAL: Nausea, vomiting. **RARE:** Hypersensitivity reaction (fever, pruritus).

ADVERSE REACTIONS/TOXIC EFFECTS

None significant.

PATIENT CONSIDERATIONS

Baseline Assessment

Question for hypersensitivity to cosyntropin or corticotropin. Hold cortisone, hydrocortisone, or spironolactone on the test day. Assure that baseline plasma cortisol concentration has been drawn prior to start of test, or 24 hr urine for 17-KS or 17-OHCS is initiated.

Intervention/Evaluation

Assess for pruritus, rash, or other sign of hypersensitivity reaction. Adhere to time frame for blood draws; monitor collection of urine if indicated.

Patient/Family Teaching

Explain the procedure and purpose of the test.

co-trimoxazole (sulfamethoxazole-trimethoprim)

koe-try-**mox**-oh-zole

(Bactrim, Cotrim, Septra, Sulfamethoprim)

FIXED-COMBINATION(S)

W/sulfamethoxazole, a sulfonamide and trimethoprim, a folate antagonist

CANADIAN AVAILABILITY

Apo-Sulfatrim, Bactrim, Novo-trimel, Septra

PREGNANCY CATEGORY C

CLASSIFICATION

Anti-infective

AVAILABILITY (Rx)

Tablets: 80 mg trimethoprim/400 mg sulfamethoxazole; 160 mg/800 mg. **Oral Suspension:** 40 mg/200 mg/5 ml. **Injection:** 80 mg/400 mg per 5 ml.

PHARMACOKINETICS

Absorption: Rapid, well absorbed from GI tract. Widely distributed. **Metabolism:** Metabolized in liver. **Excretion:** Excreted in urine. **Half-life:** 6–12 hrs (trimethoprim 8–10 hrs). Half-life increased in decreased renal function.

ACTION/*THERAPEUTIC EFFECT*

Blocks bacterial synthesis of essential nucleic acids, *producing bactericidal action in susceptible microorganisms.*

USES/*UNLABELED*

Acute/complicated and recurrent/chronic urinary tract infection, *Pneumocystis carinii* pneumonia, shigellosis, enteritis, otitis media, chronic bronchitis, traveler's diarrhea. Prophylaxis of *Pneumocystis carinii* pneumonia. *Treatment of biliary tract, bone/joint, chancroid, bacterial endocarditis, chlamydial infection, gonorrhea, intra-abdominal, meningitis, sinusitis, septicemia, skin/soft tissue.*

STORAGE/HANDLING

Store tablets, suspension at room temperature. IV infusion (piggyback) stable for 2–6 hrs (use immediately); discard if cloudy or precipitate forms.

ADMINISTRATION

Note: Space doses evenly around the clock.

ORAL:

- Administer on empty stomach w/8 oz water.
- Give several extra glasses of water/day.

IV:

- For IV infusion (piggyback), dilute each 5 ml w/75–125 ml 5% dextrose.
- Do not mix w/other drugs or solutions.
- Infuse over 60–90 min. Must avoid bolus or rapid infusion.
- Do not give IM.
- Assure adequate hydration.

INDICATIONS/ROUTES/DOSAGE

Note: Potency expressed in terms of trimethoprim content.

UTI, enteritis, acute otitis media:
Oral: Adults, elderly: 160 mg q12h for 7–14 days. ***Children >2 mos:*** 7.5–8 mg/kg/day q12h for 5–10 days.

Severe UTI, enteritis:
IV: Adults, elderly, children >2 mos: 8–10 mg/kg/day in 2–4 equally divided doses q6–12h for 5–14 days. ***Maximum:*** 960 mg/day.

Pneumocystis carinii pneumonia:
Oral: Adults, elderly, children >2 mos: 20 mg/kg/day in 4 divided doses q6h.

IV: Adults, elderly, children >2 mos: 15–20 mg/kg/day in 3–4 divided doses q6–8h.

Prevention of Pneumocystis carinii pneumonia:
Oral: Adults: 160 mg/day. ***Children:*** 150 mg/m^2/day on 3 consecutive days/wk.

Traveler's diarrhea:
Oral: Adults, elderly: 160 mg q12h for 5 days.

Acute exacerbation of chronic bronchitis:
Oral: Adults, elderly: 160 mg q12h for 14 days.

Dosage in renal impairment:
The dose and/or frequency is modified based on severity of infection, degree of renal impairment, and serum concentration of drug. For those w/creatinine clearance of 15–30 ml/min, a reduction in dose of 50% is recommended.

CONTRAINDICATIONS

Hypersensitivity to trimethoprim or any sulfonamides, megaloblastic anemia due to folate deficiency, infants <2 mos. Not for treatment of streptococcal pharyngitis.

CAUTIONS

Elderly, impaired renal or hepatic function, history of severe allergy or bronchial asthma (allergic reaction to metabisulfite in injection more likely), AIDS (higher incidence of adverse reactions).

INTERACTIONS

DRUG: May increase, prolong effects, increase toxicity w/***warfarin, hydantoin anticonvulsants, oral hypoglycemics.*** May increase risk of toxicity w/other ***hemolytics. Hepatotoxic medications*** may increase risk of hepatotoxicity. ***Methenamine*** may form precipitate. May increase effect of ***methotrexate.*** **HERBAL:** None known. **FOOD:** None significant. **ALTERED LAB VALUES:** May increase SGOT (AST), SGPT (ALT), alkaline phosphatase, BUN, creatinine, potassium.

SIDE EFFECTS

FREQUENT: Anorexia, nausea, vomiting, rash (generally 7–14 days after therapy begins), urticaria. OCCASIONAL: Diarrhea, abdominal pain, local pain/irritation at IV site. RARE: Headache, vertigo, insomnia, seizures, hallucinations, depression.

ADVERSE REACTIONS/TOXIC EFFECTS

Rash, fever, sore throat, pallor, purpura, cough, shortness of breath may be early signs of serious adverse reactions. Fatalities are rare but have occurred in sulfonamide therapy following Stevens-Johnson syndrome, toxic epidermal necrolysis, fulminant hepatic necrosis, agranulocytosis, aplastic anemia, other blood dyscrasias. Elderly are at increased risk of adverse reactions: bone marrow suppression, decreased platelets, severe dermatologic reactions.

PATIENT CONSIDERATIONS

Baseline Assessment

Check history for hypersensitivity to trimethoprim or any sulfonamide, sulfite sensitivity, severe allergy or bronchial asthma. Obtain specimens for diagnostic tests before giving first dose (therapy may begin before results are known). Determine renal, hepatic, hematologic baselines.

Intervention/Evaluation

Evaluate food tolerance. Determine pattern of bowel activity. Assess skin for rash, pallor, purpura. Check IV site, flow rate. Monitor renal, hepatic, hematology reports. Assess I&O. Check for CNS symptoms: headache, vertigo, insomnia, hallucinations. Monitor vital signs at least twice a day. Watch for cough or shortness of breath. Assess for overt bleeding, bruising, or swelling.

Patient/Family Teaching

Continue medication for full length of therapy. Space doses evenly around the clock. Take oral doses w/8 oz water and drink several extra glasses of water daily. Notify physician of new symptoms immediately, especially rash or other skin changes, bleeding or bruising, fever, sore throat.

cromolyn sodium

krom-oh-lin
(Crolom, Gastrocom, Intal, Nasalcrom, Opticrom)

CANADIAN AVAILABILITY
Apo-Cromolyn, Intal, Nalcrom, Opticrom

PREGNANCY CATEGORY B

CLASSIFICATION

Antiasthmatic, antiallergic, mast cell stabilizer

AVAILABILITY (Rx)

Oral Concentrate, Capsules for Inhalation: 20 mg. **Solution for Nebulization:** 20 mg amp. **Aerosol Spray:** 800 mcg/spray. **Nasal Spray (OTC):** 40 mg/ml. **Capsules (oral):** 100 mg. **Ophthalmic Solution:** 4%.

PHARMACOKINETICS

Absorption: Minimal absorption following oral, inhalation, or nasal administration. **Excretion:** Absorbed portion excreted in urine or via biliary elimination.

ACTION/*THERAPEUTIC EFFECT*

Possesses no direct antihistaminic, anti-inflammatory properties. *Prevents release of mast cells (e.g., histamine) after exposure to allergens that produces allergic reaction.*

USES

Prophylactic management of severe bronchial asthma, exercise-induced bronchospasm, perennial or seasonal allergic rhinitis, symptomatic treatment of systemic mastocytosis. ***Ophthalmic:*** conjunctivitis.

ADMINISTRATION

INHALATION:
- Shake container well; exhale completely; then holding mouthpiece 1 inch away from lips, inhale and hold breath as long as possible before exhaling.
- Wait 1–10 min before inhaling 2nd dose (allows for deeper bronchial penetration).
- Rinse mouth w/water immediately after inhalation (prevents mouth/throat dryness).

NEBULIZATION, INHALATION CAPSULES:
- Inhalation capsules are not to be swallowed; instruct pt on use of Spinhaler.

OPHTHALMIC:
- Place finger on lower eyelid and pull out until pocket is formed between eye and lower lid. Hold dropper above pocket and place prescribed number of drops in pocket. Instruct pt to close eyes gently so medication will not be squeezed out of sac.
- Apply gentle finger pressure to the lacrimal sac at inner canthus for 1 min following installation (lessens risk of systemic absorption).

ORAL CAPSULES:
- Give at least 30 min before meals.
- Pour contents of capsule in hot water, stirring until completely dissolved; add equal amount cold water while stirring.
- Do not mix w/fruit juice, milk, or food.

NASAL:
- Nasal passages should be clear (may require nasal decongestant).
- Inhale through nose.

INDICATIONS/ROUTES/DOSAGE:

Asthma:
Oral Inhalation: Adults, elderly, children >2 yrs (oral solution), children >5 yrs (oral powder): 20 mg 4 times/day.

Prevention of bronchospasm:
Oral Inhalation: Adults, elderly, children >2 yrs (oral solution), children >5 yrs (oral powder): 20 mg not longer than 1 hr before exercise or exposure to precipitating factor.

Allergic rhinitis:
Intranasal: Adults, elderly, children >6 yrs: 1 spray each nostril 3–4 times/day. May increase up to 6 times/day.

Systemic mastocytosis:
Oral: Adults, elderly, children >12 yrs: 200 mg 4 times/day. ***Children 2–12 yrs:*** 100 mg 4 times/day. ***Children <2 yrs:*** 20 mg/kg/day in 4 divided doses.

Usual ophthalmic dose:
Ophthalmic: Adults, elderly: 1–2 drops in both eyes 4–6 times/day.

CONTRAINDICATIONS

None significant.

CAUTIONS

Impaired renal or hepatic function.

INTERACTIONS

DRUG: None significant. HERBAL: None known. FOOD: None significant. ALTERED LAB VALUES: None significant.

SIDE EFFECTS

FREQUENT: *Inhalation:* Cough, dry mouth/throat, stuffy nose, throat irritation, unpleasant taste. *Nasal:* Burning, stinging, irritation of nose, increased sneezing. *Ophthalmic:* Burning, stinging of eye. *Oral:* Headache, diarrhea. OCCASIONAL: *Inhalation:* Bronchospasm, hoarseness, watering eyes. *Nasal:* Cough, headache, unpleasant taste, postnasal drip. *Ophthalmic:* Increased watering/itching of eye. *Oral:* Skin rash, abdominal pain, joint pain, nausea, insomnia. RARE: *Inhalation:* Anaphylactic reaction, angioedema, dizziness, painful urination, muscle/joint pain, skin rash. *Nasal:* Nosebleeds, skin rash. *Ophthalmic:* Chemosis (edema of conjunctiva), eye irritation.

ADVERSE REACTIONS/TOXIC EFFECTS

Nasal, oral: Anaphylaxis occurs rarely.

PATIENT CONSIDERATIONS

Baseline Assessment

Offer emotional support (high incidence of anxiety due to difficulty in breathing and sympathomimetic response to drug).

Intervention/Evaluation

Monitor rate, depth, rhythm, type of respiration; quality and rate of pulse. Assess lung sounds for rhonchi, wheezing, rales. Monitor arterial blood gases. Observe lips, fingernails for blue or dusky color in light-skinned patients; gray in dark-skinned patients. Observe for clavicular retractions, hand tremor. Evaluate for clinical improvement (quieter, slower respirations, relaxed facial expression, cessation of clavicular retractions).

Patient/Family Teaching

Increase fluid intake (decreases lung secretion viscosity). Do not take more than 2 inhalations at any one time (excessive use may produce paradoxical bronchoconstriction or a decreased bronchodilating effect). Rinsing mouth with water immediately after inhalation may prevent mouth/throat dryness. Effect of therapy dependent on administration at regular intervals.

cyanocobalamin (vitamin B_{12})

sye-ah-no-koe-**bal**-a-min
(Rubramin PC, Crysti-12, Cyanoject, Cyomin, Nascobal)

FIXED-COMBINATION(S)

W/liver extract, 10 mcg/ml **(liver injection)**; w/liver excrete crude, 2 mcg/ml; vitamin B_{12} w/intrinsic factor **(Ciopar Forte)**.

CANADIAN AVAILABILITY

Rubramin

PREGNANCY CATEGORY A

(C if used at doses greater than RDA)

CLASSIFICATION

Vitamin, antianemic

AVAILABILITY (Rx)

Tablets: 25 mcg, 50 mcg, 100 mcg, 250 mcg, 500 mcg, 1,000 mcg. **Injection:** 100 mcg/ml, 1,000 mcg/ml. **Nasal Gel:** 500 mcg/spray.

PHARMACOKINETICS

Absorption: Absorbed in lower half of ileum in presence of calcium. Initially bound to intrinsic factor; this complex passes down intestine, binding to receptor sites on ileal mucosa. In presence of calcium, absorbed systemically. **Metabolism:** Metabolized in liver. **Excretion:** Eliminated via biliary excretion. **Half-life:** 6 days.

ACTION/*THERAPEUTIC EFFECT*

Coenzyme for metabolic functions (fat, carbohydrate metabolism, protein synthesis). *Necessary for growth, cell replication, hematopoiesis, and myelin synthesis.*

USES

Prophylaxis, treatment of pernicious anemia, vitamin B_{12} deficiency due to inadequate diet or intestinal malabsorption, hemolytic anemia, hyperthyroidism, malignancy of pancreas, bowel, gastrectomy, GI lesions, neurologic damage, malabsorption syndrome, vegetarians, breast-fed infants, metabolic disorders, prolonged stress, chronic fever, renal disease. Deficiency generally occurs concurrently w/other B-vitamin deficiencies.

ADMINISTRATION

ORAL:

- Give w/meals (increases absorption).

INDICATIONS/ROUTES/DOSAGE

Deficiency:
*SubQ/IM: **Adults, elderly:*** Initially, 100 mcg/day for 6–7 days, then every other day for 7 doses, then every 3–4 days for 2–3 wks. ***Maintenance:*** 100–200 mcg every month. ***Children:*** Initially, 30–50 mcg/day for at least 2 wks. ***Maintenance:*** 100 mcg every month.

Usual nasal dosage:
Adults, elderly: 500 mcg (1 spray) every week (after deficiency corrected).

Supplement:
Oral: Adults, elderly: 1–25 mcg/day. ***Children >1 yr:*** 1 mcg/day. ***Children <1 yr:*** 0.3 mcg/day.

CONTRAINDICATIONS

History of allergy to cobalamin, folate deficient anemia, hereditary optic nerve atrophy.

CAUTIONS

None significant.

INTERACTIONS

DRUG: ***Alcohol, colchicine*** may decrease absorption. ***Ascorbic acid*** may destroy vitamin B_{12}. ***Folic acid*** (large doses) may decrease concentration. **HERBAL:** None known. **FOOD:** None significant. **ALTERED LAB VALUES:** None significant.

SIDE EFFECTS

OCCASIONAL: Diarrhea, itching.

ADVERSE REACTIONS/TOXIC EFFECTS

Rare allergic reaction generally due to impurities in preparation. May produce peripheral vascular thrombosis, pulmonary edema, hypokalemia, CHF.

PATIENT CONSIDERATIONS

INTERVENTION/EVALUATION

Assess for CHF, pulmonary

edema, hypokalemia in cardiac pts receiving SubQ/IM therapy. Monitor potassium levels (3.5–5 mEq/L), serum B_{12} (200–800 pg/ml), rise in reticulocyte count (peaks in 5–8 days). Assess for reversal of deficiency symptoms: hyporeflexia, loss of positional sense, ataxia, fatigue, irritability, insomnia, anorexia, pallor, palpitation on exertion. Therapeutic response to treatment usually dramatic within 48 hrs.

PATIENT/FAMILY TEACHING

Lifetime treatment may be necessary w/pernicious anemia. Report symptoms of infection. Foods rich in vitamin B_{12} include organ meats, clams, oysters, herring, red snapper, muscle meats, fermented cheese, dairy products, egg yolks.

cyclobenzaprine hydrochloride

cy-klow-**benz**-ah-preen
(Flexeril)

CANADIAN AVAILABILITY
Flexeril, Novo-Cycoprine

PREGNANCY CATEGORY B

CLASSIFICATION

Skeletal muscle relaxant

AVAILABILITY (Rx)

Tablets: 10 mg

PHARMACODYNAMICS

	ONSET	PEAK	DURATION
Oral	1 hr	3–4 hrs	12–24 hrs

PHARMACOKINETICS

Absorption: Well (slow) absorbed from GI tract. **Metabolism:** Metabolized in GI tract, liver. **Excretion:** Primarily excreted in urine. **Half-life:** 1–3 days.

ACTION / *THERAPEUTIC EFFECT*

Acts within CNS at brain stem, *relieving local skeletal muscle spasm.*

USES / *UNLABELED*

For short-term (2–3 wks) use as adjunct to rest, physical therapy, other measures for relief of discomfort due to acute, painful musculoskeletal conditions. *Treatment of fibromyalgia.*

INDICATIONS/ROUTES/DOSAGE

Note: Do not use longer than 2–3 wks.

Acute, painful musculoskeletal conditions:
Oral: Adults, elderly: 10 mg 3 times/day. ***Range:*** 20–40 mg/day in 2–4 divided doses. ***Maximum:*** 60 mg/day.

CONTRAINDICATIONS

Concurrent use of MAO inhibitors or within 14 days after their discontinuation, acute recovery phase of MI, those w/arrhythmias, heart blocks or conduction disturbances, CHF, hyperthyroidism.

CAUTIONS

Impaired renal or hepatic function, history of urinary retention, angle closure glaucoma, increased intraocular pressure.

INTERACTIONS

DRUG: *Tricyclic antidepressants, CNS depression–producing medications* may increase CNS depression. *MAO inhibitors* may increase risk of hypertensive crisis, severe seizures. **HERBAL:** None known. **FOOD:** None signifi-

cant. **ALTERED LAB VALUES:** None significant.

SIDE EFFECTS

FREQUENT (>10%): Drowsiness, dizziness, dry mouth. **OCCASIONAL (1–10%):** Fatigue, unusually tired, blurred vision, headache, nervousness, confusion, nausea, constipation, dyspepsia, altered taste.

ADVERSE REACTIONS/TOXIC EFFECTS

Overdosage may result in visual hallucinations, hyperactive reflexes, muscle rigidity, vomiting, hyperpyrexia.

PATIENT CONSIDERATIONS

Baseline Assessment

Record onset, type, location, and duration of muscular spasm. Check for immobility, stiffness, swelling.

Intervention/Evaluation

Assist w/ambulation at all times. Evaluate for therapeutic response: decreased intensity of skeletal muscle pain/tenderness, improved mobility, decrease in stiffness.

Patient/Family Teaching

Drowsiness usually diminishes w/continued therapy. Avoid tasks that require alertness, motor skills until response to drug is established. Avoid alcohol or other depressants while taking medication. Avoid sudden changes in posture. Sugarless gum, sips of water may relieve dry mouth.

cyclophosphamide

(Cytoxan, Neosar)

See Classification section under: Cancer chemotherapy

cyclosporine

sigh-klo-**spore**-in

(Neoral, Sandimmune, SangCya)

CANADIAN AVAILABILITY

Neoral, Sandimmune

PREGNANCY CATEGORY C

CLASSIFICATION

Immunosuppressant

AVAILABILITY (Rx)

Capsules: 25 mg, 100 mg. **Oral Solution:** 100 mg/ml (in 50 ml calibrated liquid measuring device). **IV Solution:** 50 mg/ml (5 ml amps). **Ophthalmic Emulsion:** 0.05%.

PHARMACOKINETICS

Absorption: Variably absorbed from GI tract. Widely distributed. **Metabolism:** Metabolized in liver. **Excretion:** Eliminated primarily by biliary/fecal excretion. **Half-life:** adults 10–27 hrs, children 7–19 hrs.

ACTION/*THERAPEUTIC EFFECT*

Inhibits interleukin-2, a proliferative factor needed for T cell activity. *Inhibits both cellular and humoral immune responses.*

USES/*UNLABELED*

Prevents rejection of kidney, liver, heart in combination w/steroid therapy. Treatment of chronic allograft rejection in those previously treated w/other immunosuppressives. Capsules/solution: Treatment of severe, active rheumatoid arthritis, psoriasis. *Treatment of alopecia areata, aplastic anemia, atopic dermatitis, Behçet's disease, biliary cirrhosis, corneal transplantation.*

STORAGE/HANDLING

Store capsules, oral solution, parenteral form at room temperature. Protect IV solution from light. After diluted, stable for 24 hrs. Avoid refrigeration of oral solution (separation of solution may occur). Discard oral solution after 2 mos once bottle is opened.

ADMINISTRATION

Note: Oral solution available in bottle form w/calibrated liquid measuring device. Oral form should replace IV administration as soon as possible.

ORAL:

- Oral solution may be mixed in glass container w/milk, chocolate milk, or orange juice (preferably at room temperature). Stir well. Drink immediately.
- Add more diluent to glass container and mix w/remaining solution to ensure total amount is given.
- Dry outside of calibrated liquid measuring device before replacing in cover. Do not rinse w/water.
- Avoid concomitant grapefruit/grapefruit juice.

IV:

- Dilute each ml concentrate w/20–100 ml 0.9% NaCl or 5% dextrose.
- Infuse over 2–6 hrs.
- Monitor pt continuously for first 30 min after instituting infusion and frequently thereafter for hypersensitivity reaction (see Side Effects).

INDICATIONS/ROUTES/DOSAGE

Note: May be given w/adrenal corticosteroids, but not w/other immunosuppressive agents (increases susceptibility to infection, development of lymphoma).

Psoriasis, rheumatoid arthritis: *Oral: Adults:* 2.5 mg/kg daily in 2 divided doses.

Prevention of allograft rejection: *Oral: Adults, elderly, children:* Initially, 15 mg/kg as single dose 4–12 hrs prior to transplantation, continue daily dose of 10–14 mg/kg/day for 1–2 wks. Taper dose by 5%/wk over 6–8 wks. *Maintenance:* 5–10 mg/kg/day.

IV: Adults, elderly, children: Give about one-third of oral dose: 5–6 mg/kg as single dose; 4–12 hrs prior to transplantation, continue this daily single dose until pt is able to take oral medication.

CONTRAINDICATIONS

History of hypersensitivity to cyclosporine or polyoxyethylated castor oil.

CAUTIONS

Impaired hepatic, renal, cardiac function, malabsorption syndrome, pregnancy, chicken pox, herpes zoster, infection, hyperkalemia.

INTERACTIONS

DRUG: ***Cimetidine, danazol, diltiazem, erythromycin, ketoconazole*** may increase concentration, risk of hepatotoxicity, nephrotoxicity; ***ACE inhibitors, potassium-sparing diuretics, potassium supplements*** may cause hyperkalemia. ***Immunosuppressants*** may increase risk of infection, lymphoproliferative disorders. ***Lovastatin*** may increase risk of rhabdomyolysis, acute renal failure. ***Live virus vaccines*** may potentiate virus replication, increase vaccine side effects, decrease pt's antibody response to vaccine. **HERBAL:** St. John's wort may reduce concentration, effect. **FOOD:** Grapefruit/grapefruit juice may interfere w/metabolism. **ALTERED LAB VAL-**

UES: May increase BUN, creatinine, SGOT (AST), SGPT (ALT), alkaline phosphatase, amylase, bilirubin, uric acid, potassium. May decrease magnesium.

SIDE EFFECTS

FREQUENT (>5%): Gingival hyperplasia (bleeding tender gums), hypertension, increased hair growth, tremors. **OCCASIONAL (1–5%):** Acne, oily skin, headache, nausea, vomiting, cramping of legs, convulsions, infection (fever, chills). **RARE (<1%):** Anaphylactic reaction, pancreatitis (severe stomach pain, w/nausea, vomiting).

ADVERSE REACTIONS/TOXIC EFFECTS

Mild nephrotoxicity occurs in 25% of renal transplants after transplantation, 38% in cardiac transplants, and 37% of liver transplants, respectively. Hepatotoxicity occurs in 4% of renal, 7% of cardiac, and 4% of liver transplants, respectively. Both toxicities usually responsive to dosage reduction. Severe hyperkalemia, hyperuricemia occur occasionally.

PATIENT CONSIDERATIONS

Baseline Assessment

Note that if nephrotoxicity occurs, mild toxicity is generally noted 2–3 mos after transplantation; more severe toxicity noted early after transplantation; hepatotoxicity may be noted during first month after transplantation.

Intervention/Evaluation

Diligently monitor BUN, creatinine, bilirubin, SGOT (AST), SGPT (ALT), LDH blood serum levels for evidence of hepatotoxicity or nephrotoxicity (mild toxicity noted by slow rise in serum levels; more overt toxicity noted by rapid rise in levels; hematuria also noted). Assess potassium level for evidence of hyperkalemia. Encourage diligent oral hygiene (gum hyperplasia). Monitor B/P for evidence of hypertension.

Patient/Family Teaching

Essential to repeat blood testing on a routine basis while receiving medication. Headache, tremor may occur as a response to medication. Repeat lab tests while receiving medication. Avoid grapefruit/grapefruit juice. May dilute oral solution w/milk, chocolate milk, orange or apple juice to improve flavor. Report fever, sore throat, tiredness, unusual bleeding/bruising. Take at same time of day w/relation to meals. Maintain good dental hygiene. Avoid immunizations unless approved by physician. Avoid grapefruit, grapefruit juice.

cyproheptadine hydrochloride

sigh-pro-**hep**-tah-deen
(Periactin)

CANADIAN AVAILABILITY
Periactin

PREGNANCY CATEGORY B

CLASSIFICATION

Antihistamine

AVAILABILITY (Rx)

Tablets: 4 mg. **Syrup:** 2 mg/5 ml.

PHARMACOKINETICS

Absorption: Well absorbed from GI tract. **Metabolism:** Metabolized in liver. **Excretion:** Primarily eliminated in feces.

ACTION/*THERAPEUTIC EFFECT*

Competes w/histamine at histaminic receptor sites, *relieving allergic conditions (urticaria, pruritus)*. Anticholinergic effects cause drying of nasal mucosa.

USES/*UNLABELED*

Relief of nasal allergies, allergic dermatitis, cold urticaria, hypersensitivity reactions. *Stimulates appetite in underweight pts, those w/anorexia nervosa. Treatment of vascular cluster headaches.*

ADMINISTRATION

ORAL:

- Give w/o regard to meals.
- Scored tablets may be crushed.

INDICATIONS/ROUTES/DOSAGE

Allergic condition:

Oral: Adults, children >15 yrs: 4 mg 3 times/day. May increase dose but do not exceed 0.5 mg/kg/day. ***Children 7–14 yrs:*** 4 mg 2–3 times/day, or 0.25 mg/kg daily in divided doses. ***Children 2–6 yrs:*** 2 mg 2–3 times/day, or 0.25 mg/kg daily in divided doses.

Usual elderly dosage:

Oral: Initially, 4 mg 2 times/day.

CONTRAINDICATIONS

Acute asthmatic attack, pts receiving MAO inhibitors.

CAUTIONS

Narrow-angle glaucoma, peptic ulcer, prostatic hypertrophy, pyloroduodenal or bladder neck obstruction, asthma, COPD, increased intraocular pressure, cardiovascular disease, hyperthyroidism, hypertension, seizure disorders.

INTERACTIONS

DRUG: *Alcohol, CNS depressants* may increase CNS depressant effects. ***MAO inhibitors*** may increase anticholinergic, CNS depressant effects. **HERBAL:** None known. **FOOD:** None significant. **ALTERED LAB VALUES:** May suppress wheal, flare reactions to antigen skin testing, unless antihistamines discontinued 4 days prior to testing.

SIDE EFFECTS

FREQUENT: Drowsiness, dizziness, muscular weakness, dry mouth/nose/throat/lips, urinary retention, thickening of bronchial secretions. Sedation, dizziness, hypotension more likely noted in elderly. **OCCASIONAL:** Epigastric distress, flushing, visual disturbances, hearing disturbances, paresthesia, sweating, chills.

ADVERSE REACTIONS/TOXIC EFFECTS

Children may experience dominant paradoxical reaction (restlessness, insomnia, euphoria, nervousness, tremors). Overdosage in children may result in hallucinations, convulsions, death. Hypersensitivity reaction (eczema, pruritus, rash, cardiac disturbances, angioedema, photosensitivity) may occur. Overdosage may vary from CNS depression (sedation, apnea, cardiovascular collapse, death) to severe paradoxical reaction (hallucinations, tremor, seizures).

PATIENT CONSIDERATOINS

BASELINE ASSESSMENT

If pt is undergoing allergic reaction, obtain history of recently ingested foods, drugs, environmental exposure, recent emotional

stress. Monitor rate, depth, rhythm, type of respiration; quality and rate of pulse. Assess lung sounds for rhonchi, wheezing, rales.

INTERVENTION/EVALUATION

Monitor B/P, especially in elderly (increased risk of hypotension). Monitor children closely for paradoxical reaction.

PATIENT/FAMILY TEACHING

Tolerance to antihistaminic effect generally does not occur; tolerance to sedative effect may occur. Avoid tasks that require alertness, motor skills until response to drug is established. Dry mouth, drowsiness, dizziness may be an expected response of drug. Avoid alcoholic beverages during antihistamine therapy. Sugarless gum, sips of tepid water may relieve dry mouth. Coffee or tea may help reduce drowsiness.

cysteamine

(Cystagon)

See Supplement

cytarabine

(ARA-C, Cytosar-U)

See Classification section under: Cancer chemotherapy

dacarbazine

(DTIC-Dome)

See Classification section under: Cancer chemotherapy

daclizumab

day-slih-zu-mab

(Zenapax)

PREGNANCY CATEGORY C

CLASSIFICATION

Immunosuppressive

AVAILABILITY (Rx)

Powder for Injection: 25 mg/5 ml

PHARMACOKINETICS

Absorption: Absorbed into the circulation to activated lymphocytes. **Metabolism:** Peak serum levels must be maintained for therapeutic response to occur. **Half-life:** 11–38 days (children: 11.5 days).

ACTION/*THERAPEUTIC EFFECT*

Binds to interleukin-2 (IL-2) receptors found on surface of activated lymphocytes, *inhibiting lymphocytic activity thereby preventing cellular immune response involved in allograft rejection.*

USES

Adjunct with cyclosporine, corticosteroids in the prophylaxis of acute organ rejection in pts receiving renal transplant.

ADMINISTRATION

IV:

- Mix calculated volume of daclizumab with 50 ml sterile 0.9% NaCl solution.
- To prevent foaming, invert the bag; do not shake.
- After reconstitution, give within 4 hrs. If it must be held longer may be refrigerated for up to 24 hrs. After 24 hrs refrigeration, solution must be discarded.
- Do not add or infuse any other drug through the same IV line.
- Administer by peripheral or central vein over a 15 min period.

INDICATIONS/ROUTES/DOSAGES

Prophylaxis of organ rejection:
IV: Adults, elderly: The standard course of therapy is 5 doses. Administer 1 mg/kg and give over 15 min. Give first dose 24 hrs before transplant. Give four remaining doses at intervals of 14 days.

CONTRAINDICATIONS

Hypersensitivity to daclizumab.

CAUTIONS

Those on immunosuppressive therapy, elderly, diabetes mellitus, infection, history of or current malignancy.

INTERACTIONS

DRUG: None significant. **HERBAL:** None known. **FOOD:** None significant. **ALTERED LAB VALUES:** May increase blood glucose.

SIDE EFFECTS

Because all patients receive concurrent corticosteroids and cyclosporine, side effects reported include those of adjunctive therapy. **OCCASIONAL (>2%):** Shortness of breath, hypertension, dizziness, nausea, peripheral edema (swelling of feet), coughing, tachycardia, tremors, vomiting, weakness, wound infection, joint pain, constipation, diarrhea, headache, insomnia, muscle pain. **RARE (<2%):** Increased urination.

ADVERSE REACTIONS/TOXIC EFFECTS

None significant.

PATIENT CONSIDERATIONS

Baseline Assessment

Obtain all baseline blood serum levels, radiology reports, cardiac test results, vital signs, respiratory function tests in order to monitor any change from baseline results.

Intervention/Evaluation

Diligently monitor all ongoing test results, weight, electrolytes (especially potassium, calcium, glucose). Be alert to signs and symptoms of impending infection; recognize that glucocorticoids may mask evidence of developing illness. Question for GI disturbances, CNS effects, urinary changes, difference in respiratory function, weight change.

Patient/Family Teaching

Report any new symptom to physician immediately. Self-monitor for sore throat, fever or any sign of infection. Do not take any other medication, including OTC medicine, without consulting physician. Diligently take all medication as scheduled for you.

---

dactinomycin

(Cosmegen)

See Classification section under: Cancer chemotherapy

---

dalteparin sodium

dawl-teh-**pear**-in

(Fragmin)

CANADIAN AVAILABILITY

Fragmin

PREGNANCY CATEGORY B

CLASSIFICATION

Anticoagulant

AVAILABILITY (Rx)

Solution: 2,500 anti-Factor Xa IU per 0.2 ml. **Single-Dose Syringe:** 5,000 IU single-dose syringe. **Multidose Vial:** 95,000 IU.

PHARMACODYNAMICS

	ONSET	PEAK	DURATION
SubQ	—	4 hrs	—

PHARMACOKINETICS

Half-life: Terminal half-life following SubQ administration: 3–5 hrs.

ACTION/*THERAPEUTIC EFFECT*

Antithrombin; in presence of low molecular weight heparin, *produces anticoagulation* by inhibition of factor Xa and thrombin by antithrombin. Only slightly influences platelet aggregation, prothrombin time (PT), activated partial thromboplastin time (APTT).

USES

Treatment of unstable angina and non-Q-wave myocardial infarction to prevent ischemia events. Prevention of deep vein thrombosis (DVT) in pts undergoing hip replacement or abdominal surgery who are at risk of thrombolic complications. Those at risk are >40 yrs, obese, undergoing surgery under general anesthesia lasting >30 min, malignancy or history of DVT or pulmonary embolism.

STORAGE/HANDLING

Store at room temperature.

ADMINISTRATION

Note: Do not mix w/other injections or infusions. Do not give IM.

SubQ:

- Instruct pt to lie down before administering by deep SubQ injection.
- Inject in U-shaped area around the navel, upper outer side of

thigh, or upper outer quadrangle of buttock.

- Introduce entire length of needle (1/2 inch) into skin fold held between thumb and forefinger, holding skin fold during injection at a 45°–90° angle.
- Vary injection site daily.

INDICATIONS/DOSAGE/ROUTES

Prevention of deep vein thrombosis:
SubQ: Adults: 2,500–5,000 IU each day, starting 1–2 hrs before surgery. Repeat once daily for 5–10 days postop.

Prevention of ischemic events:
SubQ: Adults, elderly: 120 IU/kg q12h (w/concurrent aspirin). ***Maximum:*** 10,000.

CONTRAINDICATIONS

Active major bleeding, concurrent heparin therapy, thrombocytopenia associated w/positive in vitro test for antiplatelet antibody, hypersensitivity to dalteparin, heparin, or pork products.

CAUTIONS

Conditions w/increased risk of hemorrhage, bacterial endocarditis, history of heparin-induced thrombocytopenia, impaired renal or hepatic function, uncontrolled arterial hypertension, history of recent GI ulceration and hemorrhage, hypertensive or diabetic retinopathy.

INTERACTIONS

DRUG: *Anticoagulants, platelet inhibitors* may increase bleeding (use w/care). **HERBAL:** Feverfew, garlic, ginkgo may increase risk of bleeding. **FOOD:** None significant. **ALTERED LAB VALUES:** Reversible increases in SGOT (AST), SGPT (ALT), alkaline phosphatase, lactate dehydrogenase (LDH).

SIDE EFFECTS

FREQUENT: Bleeding (0.5–16%), injection site hematoma (0.2–7%), wound hematoma (0.3–3.5%).

ADVERSE REACTIONS/TOXIC EFFECTS

Accidental overdosage may lead to bleeding complications ranging from local ecchymoses to major hemorrhage. Thrombocytopenia occurs rarely.

PATIENT CONSIDERATIONS

BASELINE ASSESSMENT

Assess complete blood count, including platelet count. Determine initial B/P.

INTERVENTION/EVALUATION

Periodically monitor CBC, platelet count, stool for occult blood (no need for daily monitoring in pts w/normal presurgical coagulation parameters). Assess for any sign of bleeding: bleeding at surgical site, hematuria, blood in stool, bleeding from gums, petechiae, bruising, bleeding from injection sites.

PATIENT/FAMILY TEACHING

Usual length of therapy is 5–10 days. Report any sign of bleeding, bruising, dizziness or lightheadedness, rash, itching, fever, swelling, breathing difficulty. Do not take any OTC medication (especially aspirin) w/o consulting physician. Rotate injection site daily. Teach proper injection technique. Excessive bruising at injeciton site may be lessened by ice massage prior to injection.

---

danaparoid

dan-ah-**pear**-oid
(Organan)

CANADIAN AVAILABILITY
Organan

PREGNANCY CATEGORY B

CLASSIFICATION

Antithrombotic (heparinoid)

AVAILABILITY (Rx)

Injection: 750 anti-Xa units/0.6 ml

PHARMACODYNAMICS

	ONSET	PEAK	DURATION
SubQ	—	2–5 hrs	—

PHARMACODYNAMICS

Absorption: Well absorbed following SubQ administration. **Excretion:** Eliminated primarily by kidneys. **Half-life:** 24 hrs. Half-life prolonged in those with severely impaired renal function.

ACTION/*THERAPEUTIC EFFECT*

Inhibits thrombin formation through factor anti-Xa and anti II-A effects, *producing anthrombotic activity, anticoagulation.* Does not significantly influence bleeding time, prothrombin time (PT), activated partial thromboplastin time (APTT), platelet function. Possesses greater antithrombotic activity than anticoagulant activity.

USES/*UNLABELED*

Prophylaxis of postop deep vein thrombosis (DVT) following elective hip replacement surgery. *Treatment of thromboembolism, to produce anticoagulation during hemodialysis, hemofiltration during cardiovascular operation, and in pregnant patients at increased risk of thrombosis.*

ADMINISTRATION

SubQ:

- Instruct pt to sit lie down before administering by deep SubQ injection.
- Inject between left and right anterolateral and left and right posterolateral abdominal wall (avoid navel area).
- Use a fine needle (25 to 26 gauge) to minimize tissue trauma.
- Introduce entire length of needle into skin fold held between thumb and forefinger, holding skin fold during injection.
- Do not pinch or rub injection site after administration (prevents bruising).
- Alternate the administration site with each injection.

INDICATIONS/DOSAGE/ROUTES

Note: Give initial dose as soon as possible after surgery but not more than 24 hrs after surgery.

Prevention of deep vein thrombosis:
SubQ: Adults, elderly: 750 anti-Xa units twice daily beginning 1–4 hours preoperatively, and then not sooner than 2 hrs after surgery. Continue treatment throughout postop care until risk of DVT has diminished (average duration 7–14 days).

CONTRAINDICATIONS

Severe hemorrhagic diathesis (hemophilia, idiopathic thrombocytopenic purpura), active major bleeding state, including hemorrhagic stroke in the acute phase, Type II phase thrombocytopenia associated with positive in vitro test for antiplatelet antibody in presence of danaparoid, hypersensitivity to pork products, danaparoid.

CAUTIONS

Conditions w/increased risk of hemorrhage, acute bacterial endocarditis, congenital or acquired bleeding disorders, active ulcerative and angiodysplastic GI disease, nonhemorrhagic stroke, shortly after brain, spinal, or ophthalmological surgery, postop indwelling epidural catheter use, severe uncontrolled hypertension, renal/hepatic function impairment, those with sulfite sensitivity (more frequently seen in asthmatics).

INTERACTIONS

DRUG: *Anticoagulants, platelet inhibitors* may increase bleeding (use w/care). **HERBAL:** Feverfew, garlic, ginkgo may increase risk of bleeding. **FOOD:** None significant. **ALTERED LAB VALUES:** None significant.

SIDE EFFECTS

FREQUENT: (13%): Injection site pain. **OCCASIONAL (4–9%):** Fever, pain, nausea, urinary tract infection, constipation. **RARE (≤2%):** Rash, pruritus, infection.

ADVERSE REACTIONS/TOXIC EFFECTS

Accidental overdosage may lead to bleeding complications ranging from minor ecchymosis to major hemorrhage. ***Antidote:*** Protamine sulfate only partially neutralizes danaparoid activity and is incapable of reducing severe nonsurgical bleeding during treatment. If serious bleeding occurs, discontinue danaparoid, give blood or blood product transfusions.

PATIENT CONSIDERATIONS

BASELINE ASSESSMENT

Assess complete blood count, including platelet count.

INTERVENTION/EVALUATION

Periodically monitor CBC, platelet count, stool for occult blood. Assess for any sign of bleeding: bleeding at surgical site, hematuria, and blood in stool, bleeding from gums, petechiae, bruising, bleeding from injection sites. In those with renal function impairment, monitor with serum creatinine 2 mg/dl. Monitor for signs/symptoms of neurologic impairment.

PATIENT/FAMILY TEACHING

Usual length of therapy is 7–14 days. Report any sign of bleeding (as above). Do not take any OTC medication (especially aspirin) w/o consulting physician.

---

danazol

dan-ah-zole
(Danocrine)

CANADIAN AVAILABILITY
Cyclomen

PREGNANCY CATEGORY X

CLASSIFICATION

Gonadotropin inhibitor

AVAILABILITY (Rx)

Capsules: 50 mg, 100 mg, 200 mg

PHARMACOKINETICS

Metabolism: Metabolized in liver. **Excretion:** Excreted in urine. **Half-life:** 4.5 hrs.

ACTION/*THERAPEUTIC EFFECT*

As a gonadotropin inhibitor, suppresses the pituitary-ovarian axis *by inhibiting the output of pituitary gonadotropins.* In endometriosis, *causes atrophy of both normal and ectopic endometrial tissue, producing anovulation and amenorrhea.* For fibrocystic breast disease, follicle-stimulating hormone (FSH) and luteinizing hormone (LH) are depressed, *reducing the production of estrogen;* inhibits steroid synthesis and binding of steroids to their receptors in breast tissue. Increases serum levels of esterase inhibitor, *correcting biochemical deficiency as seen in hereditary angioedema.*

USES / *UNLABELED*

Palliative treatment of endometriosis, fibrocystic breast disease; prophylactic treatment of hereditary angioedema. *Treatment of gynecomastia, menorrhagia, precocious puberty.*

INDICATIONS / ROUTES / DOSAGE

Note: Initiate therapy during menstruation or when pt not pregnant.

Endometriosis:
Oral: Adults: 200–800 mg/day in 2 divided doses for 3–9 mos.

Fibrocystic breast disease:
Oral: Adults: 100–400 mg/day in 2 divided doses.

Hereditary angioedema:
Oral: Adults: Initially, 200 mg 2–3 times/day. Decrease dose by 50% or less at 1–3 mo intervals. If attack occurs, increase dose by up to 200 mg/day.

CONTRAINDICATIONS

Hypersensitivity to danazol or ingredients. Undiagnosed abnormal genital bleeding; severe hepatic, renal, or cardiac impairment.

CAUTIONS

Conditions aggravated by fluid retention (cardiac or renal disease, epilepsy, migraine, asthma). Possibility of carcinoma of the breast should be excluded prior to therapy.

INTERACTIONS

DRUG: May increase effect of ***oral anticoagulants.*** May decrease effect of ***insulin, oral hypoglycemics.*** May increase concentration, toxicity of ***cyclosporine.*** **HERBAL:** None known. **FOOD:** None significant. **ALTERED LAB VALUES:** May increase SGOT (AST), SGPT (ALT), glucose, LDL. May decrease HDL. May alter thyroid function tests.

SIDE EFFECTS

FREQUENT: ***Females:*** Amenorrhea, breakthrough bleeding/spotting, decreased breast size, increased weight, irregular menstrual period. **OCCASIONAL:** ***Males/females:*** Edema, rhabdomyolysis (muscle cramps, unusual fatigue), virilism (acne, oily skin), flushed skin, altered moods. **RARE:** ***Males/females:*** Hematuria, gingivitis, carpal tunnel syndrome, cataracts, severe headache, vomiting, rash, photosensitivity. ***Females:*** Enlarged clitoris, hoarseness, deepening voice, hair growth, monilial vaginitis. ***Males:*** Decreased testicle size.

ADVERSE REACTIONS / TOXIC EFFECTS

Jaundice may occur in those receiving 400 mg/day or more. Liver dysfunction, eosinophilia, thrombocytopenia, pancreatitis occur rarely.

PATIENT CONSIDERATIONS

Baseline Assessment

Inquire about menstrual cycle. Therapy should begin during menstruation. Establish baseline weight, B/P.

Intervention/Evaluation

Weigh 2–3 times/week; report >5 lbs/wk gain or swelling of fingers or feet. Monitor B/P peri-

odically.Check for jaundice (yellow eyes or skin, dark urine, clay-colored stools).

Patient/Family Teaching

Patient should use nonhormonal contraceptive during therapy. Do not take drug, check w/physician if suspect pregnancy (risk to fetus).Importance of full length of therapy, regular visits to physician's office (hepatic function tests, etc.). Notify physician promptly of masculinizing effects (may not be reversible), weight gain, muscle cramps, or fatigue. Spotting or bleeding may occur in first months of therapy for endometriosis (does not mean lack of efficacy). In fibrocystic breast disease, irregular menstrual periods and amenorrhea may occur w/ or w/o ovulation.

dantrolene sodium

dan-trow-lean
(Dantrium)

CANADIAN AVAILABILITY
Dantrium

PREGNANCY CATEGORY C

CLASSIFICATION

Skeletal muscle relaxant

AVAILABILITY (Rx)

Capsules: 25 mg, 50 mg, 100 mg. **Powder for Injection:** 20 mg vial.

PHARMACOKINETICS

Absorption: Poorly absorbed from GI tract. **Metabolism:** Metabolized in liver. **Excretion:** Primarily excreted in urine. **Half-life:** IV 4–8 hrs; oral 8.7 hrs.

ACTION/*THERAPEUTIC EFFECT*

Reduces muscle contraction by interfering w/release of calcium ion, *dissociating excitation-contraction coupling.* Reduced calcium ion concentration, *interfering w/catabolic process associated w/malignant hyperthermic crisis.*

USES/*UNLABELED*

Oral: Relief of signs and symptoms of spasticity due to spinal cord injuries, stroke, cerebral palsy, multiple sclerosis, especially flexor spasms, concomitant pain, clonus, and muscular rigidity. ***Parenteral:*** Management of fulminant hypermetabolism of skeletal muscle due to malignant hyperthermia crisis. *Treatment of neuroleptic malignant syndrome, relief of exercise-induced pain in patients w/muscular dystrophy, treatment of flexor spasms.*

STORAGE/HANDLING

Store oral, parenteral form at room temperature. Use within 6 hrs after reconstitution. Solution is clear, colorless. Discard if cloudy, precipitate formed.

ADMINISTRATION

ORAL:
- Give w/o regard to meals.

IV:
- Diligently monitor for extravasation (high pH of IV preparation). May produce severe complications.
- Reconstitute 20 mg vial w/60 ml sterile water for injection to provide concentration of 0.33 mg/ml.
- For IV infusion, administer over 1 hr.

INDICATIONS/ROUTES/DOSAGE

Spasticity:
Note: Best to begin w/low-dose

therapy, then increase gradually at 4–7 day intervals (reduces incidence of side effects).

Oral: Adults, elderly: Initially, 25 mg/day. Increase to 25 mg 2–4 times/day, then by 25 mg increments up to 100 mg 2–4 times/day. *Children >5 yrs:* Initially, 0.5 mg/kg 2 times/day. Increase to 0.5 mg/kg 3–4 times/day, then increase by 0.5 mg/kg/day up to 3 mg/kg 2–4 times/day.

Prevention of malignant hyperthermia crisis:
Oral: Adults, elderly, children: 4–8 mg/kg/day in 3–4 divided doses 1–2 days prior to surgery (last dose 3–4 hrs prior to surgery).

IV Infusion: Adults, elderly, children: 2.5 mg/kg about 1.25 hrs prior to surgery.

Management of hyperthermia crisis:
IV: Adults, elderly, children: Initially (minimum), 1 mg/kg rapid IV; may repeat up to total maximum dose of 10 mg/kg. May follow w/4–8 mg/kg/day orally in 4 divided doses up to 3 days after crisis.

CONTRAINDICATIONS

Oral: Active liver disease (i.e., hepatitis, cirrhosis), when spasticity is needed to maintain upright posture and balance when walking or to achieve or support increased function, severely impaired cardiac function, previous liver disease/dysfunction.

CAUTIONS

Females, those >35 yrs of age, impaired liver or pulmonary function.

INTERACTIONS

DRUG: *CNS depressants* may increase CNS depression (short-term use). *Hepatotoxic medications* may increase risk of hepatotoxicity (chronic use). **HERBAL:** None known. **FOOD:** None significant. **ALTERED LAB VALUES:** May alter liver function tests.

SIDE EFFECTS

Note: Effects are generally transient and appear during early treatment. **FREQUENT:** Drowsiness, dizziness, weakness, general malaise, diarrhea. **OCCASIONAL:** Confusion, headache, insomnia, constipation, urinary frequency. **RARE:** Paradoxical CNS excitement/restlessness, paresthesia, tinnitus, slurred speech, tremor, blurred vision, dry mouth, diarrhea, nocturia, impotence.

ADVERSE REACTIONS/TOXIC EFFECTS

Risk of hepatotoxicity, most notably in females, those >35 yrs of age, those taking other medications concurrently. Overt hepatitis noted most frequently between 3rd and 12th mo of therapy. Overdosage results in vomiting, muscular hypotonia, muscle twitching, respiratory depression, seizures.

PATIENT CONSIDERATIONS

Baseline Assessment

Obtain baseline liver function tests (SGOT [AST], SGPT [ALT], alkaline phosphatase, total bilirubin). Record onset, type, location, and duration of muscular spasm. Check for immobility, stiffness, swelling.

Intervention/Evaluation

Assist w/ambulation at all times. For those on long-term therapy, liver/renal function tests, blood counts should be performed periodically. Evaluate for thera-

peutic response: decreased intensity of skeletal muscle pain.

PATIENT/FAMILY TEACHING

Drowsiness usually diminishes w/continued therapy. Avoid tasks that require alertness, motor skills until response to drug is established. Avoid alcohol or other depressants while taking medication. Report continued weakness, fatigue, nausea or diarrhea, skin rash, itching, bloody black stools.

daunorubicin

(Cerubidine, DaunoXome)

See Classifcation section under: Cancer chemotherapy

deferoxamine

deaf-er-**ox**-ah-meen

(Desferal Mesylate)

CANADIAN AVAILABILITY

Desferal

PREGNANCY CATEGORY C

CLASSIFICATION

Antidote

AVAILABILITY (Rx)

Injection: 500 mg

PHARMACOKINETICS

Absorption: Well absorbed after IM, SubQ administration. Widely distributed. **Metabolism:** Rapidly metabolized in tissues, plasma. **Excretion:** Excreted in urine, eliminated in feces via biliary excretion. Removed by hemodialysis. **Half-life:** 6 hrs.

ACTION/*THERAPEUTIC EFFECT*

Binds w/iron to form complex, *promoting urine excretion of acute iron poisoning.*

USES/*UNLABELED*

Treatment of acute iron toxicity, chronic iron toxicity secondary to multiple transfusions associated w/some chronic anemia (e.g., thalassemia). *Treatment/diagnosis of aluminum toxicity.*

STORAGE/HANDLING

Store parenteral powder at room temperature.

ADMINISTRATION

Note: Reconstitute each 500 mg vial w/2 ml sterile water to provide a concentration of 250 mg/ml.

SUBQ:

- Administer SubQ very slowly; may give undiluted.

IM:

- Inject deeply into upper outer quadrant of buttock.
- May give undiluted.

IV:

- For IV infusion, further dilute w/0.9% NaCl, 5% dextrose, and administer at maximum rate of 15 mg/ kg/hr.
- A too-rapid IV administration may produce skin flushing, urticaria, hypotension, shock.

INDICATIONS/ROUTES/DOSAGE

Acute iron intoxication:

IM: Adults: Initially, 90 mg/kg, then 45 mg/kg up to 1 g q4–12h. ***Maximum:*** 6 g/day.

IV: Adults: 15 mg/kg/hr up to 90 mg/kg q8hrs. ***Maximum:*** 6 g/day. ***Children:*** 15 mg/kg/hr.

Chronic iron overload:
SubQ: Adults: 1–2 g/day (20–40 mg/kg) over 8–24 hrs. *Children:* 10 mg/kg/day.

IM: Adults: 0.5–1 g/day. *IV:* In addition to IM, 2 g infused at rate not to exceed 15 mg/kg/hr.

CONTRAINDICATIONS

Severe renal disease, anuria, primary hemochromatosis.

CAUTIONS

None significant.

INTERACTIONS

DRUG: *Vitamin C* may increase effect. HERBAL: None known. FOOD: None significant. ALTERED LAB VALUES: May cause a falsely high total iron-binding capacity (TIBC).

SIDE EFFECTS

FREQUENT: Pain, induration at injection site, urine color change (to orange-rose). OCCASIONAL: Abdominal discomfort, diarrhea, leg cramps, impaired vision.

ADVERSE REACTIONS/TOXIC EFFECTS

Neurotoxicity, including high-frequency hearing loss, has been noted.

PATIENT CONSIDERATIONS

BASELINE ASSESSMENT

Inform pt injection may produce discomfort at IM or SubQ injection site. Assess serum iron levels, iron binding capacity before and during therapy.

INTERVENTION/EVALUATION

Question pt for evidence of hearing loss (neurotoxicity). Periodic slit-lamp ophthalmic exams should be obtained in those treated for chronic iron overload. If using SubQ technique, monitor for pruritus, erythema, skin irritation, and swelling.

PATIENT/FAMILY TEACHING

Urine will appear reddish. Discomfort may occur at site of injection.

delavirdine mesylate

del-all-**vur**-dean **mess**-eh-late
(Rescriptor)

PREGNANCY CATEGORY X

CLASSIFICATION

Antiviral

AVAILABILITY (Rx)

Tablets: 100 mg

PHARMACODYNAMICS

	ONSET	PEAK	DURATION
Oral	—	1 hr	—

PHARMACOKINETICS

Absorption: Rapidly absorbed following oral administration. **Metabolism:** Extensively bound to plasma proteins, primarily albumin. Metabolized by liver. **Excretion:** Eliminated in urine and feces. **Half-life:** 5.8 hrs.

ACTION/*THERAPEUTIC EFFECT*

Inhibits catalytic reaction of HIV reverse transcriptase (RT), blocking RNA dependent and DNA-dependent polymerase activities, *interrupting HIV replication, slowing progression of HIV infection.*

USES

Treatment of HIV infection in combination with other appropriate antiretoviral agents.

ADMINISTRATION

ORAL:

- May be given without regard to meals.
- Pts with achlorhydria should take tablets with an acidic drink (orange or cranberry juice).
- May be prepared as a slurry prior to administration (increases drug bioavailability).
- Add four tablets to 3 oz water. Allow to stand for a few minutes, then stir until a uniform suspension occurs.

INDICATIONS/ROUTES/DOSAGES

HIV infection:

Oral: Adults, elderly: 400 mg (four 100 mg tablets) 3 times/day.

CONTRAINDICATIONS

History of hypersensitivity to delalvirdine or its component, pregnancy, breastfeeding.

CAUTIONS

Impaired hepatic function.

INTERACTIONS

DRUG: Concurrent use with ***antihistamines (terfenadine, astemizole), antimicrobial agents (clarithromycin, dapsone, rifabutin), benzodiazepines, cisapride, nifedipine, ergot derivatives, indinavir, saquinavir, quinidine, warfarin*** may produce serious or life-threatening events including cardiac arrhythmias. ***Antacids*** reduce delavirdine absorption. **HERBAL:** St. John's wort may decrease effect. **FOOD:** None significant. **ALTERED LAB VALUES:** May increase SGOT (AST), SGPT (ALT).

SIDE EFFECTS

FREQUENT: (5–10%): Rash, headache, nausea, diarrhea, increased liver enzymes. **OCCASIONAL (2%):** Fatigue, vomiting, pruritus.

ADVERSE REACTIONS/TOXIC EFFECTS

Major toxicity is rash. May be accompanied by fever, blistering, oral lesions, conjunctivitis, muscle/joint aches.

PATIENT CONSIDERATIONS

Baseline Assessment

Offer emotional support. Obtain baseline SGOT (AST), SGPT (ALT) prior to initiating therapy and at intervals during therapy.

Intervention/Evaluation

Closely monitor for evidence of rash (toxicity). May be accompanied by fever, blistering, oral lesions, conjunctivitis, muscle/joint aches. Drug may be discontinued. Monitor liver enzyme studies for abnormalities. Assess for headache, nausea, diarrhea.

Patient/Family Teaching

If rash appears, contact physician immediately. Take medication every day as prescribed. If taking antacids, separate medications at least 1 hr apart. Delavirdine is not a cure for HIV infection, nor does it reduce risk of transmission to others.

---

demecarium

(Humorsol)

See Classification section under: Antiglaucoma agents

demeclocycline hydrochloride

deh-meh-clo-**sigh**-clean
(Declomycin)

CANADIAN AVAILABILITY
Declomycin

PREGNANCY CATEGORY D

CLASSIFICATION

Antibiotic: Tetracycline

AVAILABILITY (Rx)

Capsules: 150 mg. **Tablets:** 150 mg, 300 mg.

PHARMACOKINETICS

Absorption: Readily absorbed from GI tract (food decreases absorption). Widely distributed. **Excretion:** Primarily excreted unchanged in urine. **Half-life:** 10–17 hrs (increased in decreased renal function).

ACTION/*THERAPEUTIC EFFECT*

Bacteriostatic due to binding to ribosomes, *inhibiting protein synthesis.* Inhibits ADH-induced water reabsorption, *producing water diuresis.*

USES

Treatment of respiratory and urinary tract infections, uncomplicated gonorrhea, brucellosis, rheumatic fever prophylaxis, trachoma, Rocky Mountain spotted fever, typhus, Q fever, rickettsialpox, psittacosis, ornithosis, granuloma inguinale, lymphogranuloma venereum. Treatment of syndrome of inappropriate ADH secretion (SIADH).

ADMINISTRATION

ORAL:

- Give w/full glass of water 1 hr before or 2 hrs after meals/milk.

INDICATIONS/ROUTES/DOSAGE

Note: Space doses evenly around the clock.

Mild to moderate infections:
Oral: Adults, elderly: 600 mg/day in 2–4 divided doses. *Children >8 yrs:* 6–12 mg/kg/day in 2–4 divided doses.

Uncomplicated gonorrhea:
Oral: Adults: Initially, 600 mg, then 300 mg q12h for 4 days for total of 3 g.

Chronic form of SIADH:
Oral: Adults, elderly: 600 mg-1.2 g/day in 3–4 divided doses, or 3.25–3.75 mg/kg q6h.

CONTRAINDICATIONS

Hypersensitivity to tetracyclines, last half of pregnancy, infants–8 yrs.

CAUTIONS

Renal impairment, sun or ultraviolet exposure (severe photosensitivity reaction).

INTERACTIONS

DRUG: ***Antacids*** containing aluminum/calcium/magnesium, ***laxatives*** containing magnesium, ***oral iron*** preparations, ***dairy products*** impair absorption of tetracyclines (give 1–2 hrs before or after tetracyclines). ***Cholestyramine, colestipol*** may decrease absorption. May decrease effect of ***oral contraceptives.*** **HERBAL:** St. John's wort may increase risk of photosensitivity. **FOOD:** Dairy products may impair absorption. **ALTERED LAB VALUES:** May increase BUN, SGOT (AST), SGPT (ALT), alkaline phosphatase, amylase, bilirubin concentrations.

SIDE EFFECTS

FREQUENT: Anorexia, nausea, vomiting, diarrhea, dysphagia, exaggerated sunburn reaction w/moderate to high dosage. OCCASIONAL: Urticaria, rash. Long-term therapy may result in diabetes insipidus syndrome: polydipsia, polyuria, weakness.

ADVERSE REACTIONS/TOXIC EFFECTS

Superinfection (especially fungal) anaphylaxis, increased intracranial pressure, bulging fontanelles occur rarely in infants.

PATIENT CONSIDERATIONS

Baseline Assessment

Question for history of allergies, especially to tetracyclines. Obtain culture, sensitivity test before giving first dose (therapy may begin before results are known).

Intervention/Evaluation

Determine pattern of bowel activity and stool consistency. Check food intake, tolerance. Monitor I&O, renal function test results. Assess for rash. Be alert to superinfection: diarrhea, ulceration or changes of oral mucosa, tongue, anal/genital pruritus. Monitor B/P and LOC because of potential for increased intracranial pressure.

Patient/Family Teaching

Continue antibiotic for full length of treatment. Space doses evenly. Take oral doses on empty stomach w/full glass of water. Avoid bedtime doses. Notify physician in event of diarrhea, rash, other new symptom. Avoid sun/ultraviolet light exposure. Consult physician before taking any other medication.

desipramine hydrochloride

deh-**sip**-rah-meen
(Norpramin)

CANADIAN AVAILABILITY
Norpramin

PREGNANCY CATEGORY C

CLASSIFICATION

Antidepressant: Tricyclic

AVAILABILITY (Rx)

Tablets: 10 mg, 25 mg, 50 mg, 75 mg, 100 mg, 150 mg. **Capsules:** 25 mg, 50 mg.

PHARMACOKINETICS

Absorption: Rapid, well absorbed from GI tract. **Metabolism:** Metabolized in liver. **Excretion:** Primarily excreted in urine. **Half-life:** 12–27 hrs.

ACTION/*THERAPEUTIC EFFECT*

Increases synaptic concentration of norepinephrine and/or serotonin (inhibits reuptake by presynaptic membrane), *producing antidepressant effect.* Strong anticholinergic activity.

USES/*UNLABELED*

Treatment of various forms of depression, often in conjunction w/ psychotherapy. *Treatment of panic disorder, neurogenic pain, attention deficit hyperactivity disorder, narcolepsy/cataplexy, bulimia nervosa, cocaine withdrawal.*

D

ADMINISTRATION

ORAL:

- Give w/food or milk if GI distress occurs.

INDICATIONS/ROUTES/DOSAGE

Depression:
Oral: Adults: Initially, 75–150 mg daily as single daily dose, or in divided doses. Gradually increase to lowest effective therapeutic level. Do not exceed 300 mg daily.

Usual elderly dosage:
Oral: 25–100 mg/day. *Maximum:* 150 mg/day.

CONTRAINDICATIONS

Acute recovery period following MI, within 14 days of MAO inhibitor ingestion.

CAUTIONS

Prostatic hypertrophy, history of urinary retention or obstruction, glaucoma, diabetes mellitus, history of seizures, hyperthyroidism, cardiac/hepatic/ renal disease, schizophrenia, increased intraocular pressure, hiatal hernia.

INTERACTIONS

DRUG: *Alcohol, CNS depressants* may increase CNS, respiratory depression, hypotensive effects. *Antithyroid agents* may increase risk of agranulocytosis. *Phenothiazines* may increase sedative, anticholinergic effects. *Cimetidine* may increase concentration, toxicity. May decrease effects of *clonidine, guanadrel*. May increase cardiac effects w/*sympathomimetics*. May increase risk of hypertensive crisis, hyperpyrexia, convulsions w/*MAO inhibitors*. *Phenytoin* may decrease desipramine concentration. HERBAL: None known. FOOD: None significant. ALTERED LAB VALUES: May alter EKG readings, glucose serum level.

SIDE EFFECTS

FREQUENT: Dizziness, drowsiness, dry mouth, orthostatic hypotension, headache, increased appetite/ weight, nausea, unusual tiredness, unpleasant taste. OCCASIONAL: Blurred vision, confusion, constipation, hallucinations, delayed micturation, eye pain, arrhythmias, fine muscle tremors, Parkinsonian syndrome, nervousness, diarrhea, increased sweating, heartburn, insomnia. RARE: Hypersensitivity, alopecia, tinnitus, breast enlargement.

ADVERSE REACTIONS/TOXIC EFFECTS

High dosage may produce confusion, seizures, severe drowsiness, fast/slow/irregular heartbeat, fever, hallucinations, agitation, shortness of breath, vomiting, unusual tiredness/weakness. Abrupt withdrawal from prolonged therapy may produce severe headache, malaise, nausea, vomiting, vivid dreams.

PATIENT CONSIDERATIONS

BASELINE ASSESSMENT

For those on long-term therapy, liver/renal function tests, blood counts should be performed periodically.

INTERVENTION/EVALUATION

Supervise suicidal risk pt closely during early therapy (as depression lessens, energy level improves, increasing suicide potential). Assess appearance, behavior, speech pattern, level of interest, mood. Monitor pattern of daily bowel activity and stool consistency. Monitor B/P, pulse for hypotension, arrhythmias. Assess for urinary retention by monitoring I&O and by bladder palpation.

PATIENT/FAMILY TEACHING

Change positions slowly to avoid hypotensive effect. Tolerance to postural hypotension, sedative, and anticholinergic effects usually develops during early therapy. Maximum therapeutic effect may be noted in 2–4 wks. Photosensitivity to sun may occur. Dry mouth may be relieved by sugarless gum or sips of tepid water. Do not abruptly discontinue medication. Report visual disturbances. Avoid tasks that require alertness, motor skills until response to drug is established. Avoid alcohol.

desmopressin

des-moe-**press**-in
(DDAVP, Stimate)

CANADIAN AVAILABILITY
DDAVP, Octostim

PREGNANCY CATEGORY B

CLASSIFICATION

Antidiuretic

AVAILABILITY (Rx)

Tablets: 0.1 mg, 0.2 mg. **Nasal Solution:** 0.1 mg/ml, 1.5 mg/ml. **Nasal Spray. Injection:** 4 mcg/ml.

PHARMACODYNAMICS

	ONSET	PEAK	DURATION
Oral	1 hr	4–7 hrs	—
Intranasal	15 min–1 hr	1–5 hrs	5–21 hrs
IV	15–30 min	1.5–3 hrs	—

PHARMACOKINETICS

Absorption: 10–20% from nasal administration. **Metabolism:** Metabolized renally. **Half-life:** 75 min.

ACTION / *THERAPEUTIC EFFECT*

Increases reabsorption of water by increasing permeability of collecting ducts of the kidneys, *decreasing urinary output. Increases plasma factor VIII (antihemophilic factor),* plasminogen activator.

USES

DDAVP ***Intranasal:*** Primary nocturnal enuresis, central cranial diabetes insipidus. ***Parenteral:*** Central cranial diabetes insipidus, hemophilia A, von Willebrand's disease (type I).

Stimate ***Intranasal:*** Hemophilia A, von Willebrand's disease (type I).

Oral: Central cranial diabetes insipidus.

STORAGE/HANDLING

Refrigerate nasal solution, injection. Nasal solution stable for up to 3 wks at room temperature. Nasal spray stored at room temperature.

ADMINISTRATION

SUBQ:

- Evening dosage should consider satisfactory sleep response.
- Morning and evening doses should be adjusted separately.

IV:

- For preop use, administer 30 min before procedure.
- Monitor B/P and pulse during IV infusion.
- IV dose = 1/10 intranasal dose.
- IV infusion: dilute in 10–50 ml 0.9% NaCl; infuse over 15–30 min.

INTRANASAL:

- A calibrated catheter (rhinyle) is used to draw up a measured quantity of desmopressin; w/one end inserted in the nose, the pt blows on the other end to deposit the solution deep in the nasal cavity.

- For infants, young children, obtunded pts, an air-filled syringe may be attached to the catheter to deposit the solution.

INDICATIONS/ROUTES/DOSAGE

Primary nocturnal enuresis:
Intranasal: Adults, elderly, children 6 yrs or greater: Initially, 20 mcg (0.2 ml) at bedtime (1/2 dose each nostril). Adjust up to 40 mcg.

Central cranial diabetes insipidus:
Oral: Adults, elderly: Initially, 0.05 mg 2 times/day. ***Range:*** 0.1–1.2 mg/day in 2–3 divided doses. ***Children:*** 0.05 mg initially.

Intranasal: Adults, elderly: 0.1–0.4 ml/day as single or 2–3 divided doses. ***Children (3 mos–12 yrs):*** 0.05–0.3 ml/day as single or 2 divided doses.

SubQ/IV: Adults, elderly: 0.5–1 ml/day in 2 divided doses.

Hemophilia A, von Willebrand's disease (type I):
IV Infusion: Adults, elderly, children >10 kg: 0.3 mcg/kg diluted in 50 ml 0.9% NaCl. ***Children <10 kg:*** 0.3 mcg/kg diluted in 10 ml 0.9% NaCl.

Intranasal: Adults, elderly >50 kg: 300 mcg (1 spray each nostril). ***Adults, elderly <50 kg:*** 150 mcg as single spray.

CONTRAINDICATIONS

Hypersensitivity to desmopressin; type IIB or platelet-type von Willebrand's disease; nasal scarring, blockage, or other impairment w/intranasal administration. Intranasal administration with impaired level of consciousness.

CAUTIONS

Coronary artery insufficiency, hypertensive cardiovascular disease, infants, and children <6 yrs.

INTERACTIONS

DRUG: ***Carbamazepine, chlorpropamide, clofibrate*** may increase effect. ***Demeclocycline, lithium, norepinephrine*** may decrease effect. **HERBAL:** None known. **FOOD:** None significant. **ALTERED LAB VALUES:** None significant.

SIDE EFFECTS

OCCASIONAL: *IV:* Pain/redness/swelling at injection site, headache, abdominal cramps, vulval pain, flushed skin; mild elevation of B/P; nausea w/high doses. *Nasal:* Runny/stuffy nose; slight elevation of B/P.

ADVERSE REACTIONS/TOXIC EFFECTS

Water intoxication or hyponatremia (coma, confusion, drowsiness, headache, decreased urination, seizures, rapid weight gain) may occur in overhydration. Elderly, infants, children are especially at risk.

PATIENT CONSIDERATIONS

BASELINE ASSESSMENT

Question for hypersensitivity to desmopressin. Establish baselines for B/P, pulse, weight, electrolytes, urine specific gravity. Check lab values for factor VIII coagulant concentration for hemophilia A and von Willebrand's disease; bleeding times, ristocetin colactor, and Willebrand factor for von Willebrand's disease.

INTERVENTION/EVALUATION

Monitor I&O closely, restrict intake as necessary to prevent water intoxication.Weigh daily if indicated. Check B/P and pulse q15min during IV administration, 2 times/day for other routes. Monitor electrolytes, urine specific gravity, and other lab results (see Baseline Assessment). Evaluate parenteral injection site for erythema, pain. Report side effects to physician for dose reduction. Assess bleeding as appropriate. Check for nasal mucosa changes w/intranasal route. Be alert for early signs of water intoxication: drowsiness, listlessness, headache.

PATIENT/FAMILY TEACHING

Teach pt/family proper technique for intranasal administration. Report headache, nausea, shortness of breath, or other symptoms promptly. Stress importance of I&O.Notify physician if bleeding not controlled.

desonide

(Otic Tridesilon, Tridesilon)

See Classification section under: Corticosteroids: topical

desoximetasone

(Topicort)

See Classification section under: Corticosteroids: topical

dexamethasone

dex-a-**meth**-a-sone

(Decadron, Hexadrol)

dexamethasone acetate

(Dalalone L.A., Decadron L.A., Dexone L.A.)

dexamethasone sodium phosphate

(Decadron, Respihaler)

FIXED-COMBINATION(S)

Dexamethasone phosphate w/neomycin sulfate, an anti-infective **(NeoDecadron)**; dexamethasone sodium phosphate w/lidocaine, a local anesthetic

CANADIAN AVAILABILITY

Decadron, Dexasone, Maxidex

PREGNANCY CATEGORY C

CLASSIFICATION

Corticosteroid

AVAILABILITY (Rx)

Tablets: 0.25 mg, 0.5 mg, 0.75 mg, 1 mg, 1.5 mg, 2 mg, 4 mg, 6 mg. **Elixir:** 0.5 mg/5 ml. **Oral Solution:** 0.5 mg/5 ml, 0.5 mg/0.5 ml. **Injection:** 4 mg/ml, 8 mg/ml (suspension), 10 mg/ml, 16 mg/ml (suspension), 20 mg/ml, 24 mg/ml. ***Inhalant, Intranasal, Ophthalmic:*** Solution, suspension, ointment. *Topical:* Aerosol, cream.

PHARMACOKINETICS

Absorption: Rapid, complete absorption from GI tract, after IM administration. Widely distributed. **Metabolism:** Metabolized in liver. **Excretion:** Primarily excreted in urine. **Half-life:** 3–4.5 hrs.

ACTION / *THERAPEUTIC EFFECT*

Inhibits accumulation of inflammatory cells at inflammation sites, phagocytosis, lysosomal enzyme release and synthesis and/or release of mediators of inflammation. *Prevents/suppresses cell and tissue immune reactions, inflammatory process.*

USES

Substitution therapy in deficiency states: acute/chronic adrenal insufficiency, congenital adrenal hyperplasia, adrenal insufficiency secondary to pituitary insufficiency.

Nonendocrine disorders: arthritis, rheumatic carditis, allergic, collagen, intestinal tract, liver, ocular, renal, and skin diseases, bronchial asthma, cerebral edema, malignancies.

Ophthalmic: Treatment of responsive inflammatory conditions of palpebral and bulbar conjunctiva, cornea, and anterior segment of globe. ***Nasal:*** Maintenance treatment of asthma. Allergic/inflammatory nasal conditions and nasal polyps. ***Topical:*** Relief of inflammatory/pruritic conditions of steroid-responsive dermatoses. ***Respiratory:*** Control of bronchial asthma in pts requiring chronic steroid therapy.

ADMINISTRATION

ORAL:

- Give w/milk or food.

IM:

- Give deep IM, preferably in gluteus maximus.

IV:

- **Note:** Dexamethasone sodium phosphate may be given by direct IV injection or IV infusion.
- For IV infusion, mix w/0.9% NaCl or 5% dextrose.
- For neonate, solution must be preservative free.
- IV solution must be used within 24 hrs.

OPHTHALMIC:

- Place finger on lower eyelid and pull out until a pocket is formed between eye and lower lid. Hold dropper above pocket and place correct number of drops ($^1/_4$–$^1/_2$ inch ointment) into pocket. Close eye gently. ***Solution:*** Apply digital pressure to lacrimal sac for 1–2 min (minimizes drainage into nose and throat, reducing risk of systemic effects). ***Ointment:*** Close eye for 1–2 min, rolling eyeball (increases contact area of drug to eye). Remove excess solution or ointment around eye w/tissue.
- Ointment may be used at night to reduce frequency of solution administration.
- As w/other corticosteroids, taper dosage slowly when discontinuing.

TOPICAL:

- Gently cleanse area prior to application.
- Use occlusive dressings only as ordered.
- Apply sparingly and rub into area thoroughly.

INDICATIONS/ROUTES/DOSAGE

Dexamethasone, oral:
Oral: Adults, elderly: 0.75–9 mg/day.

Dexamethasone acetate:
IM: Adults, elderly: 8–16 mg, may repeat in 1–3 wks. ***Intralesional: Adults, elderly:*** 0.8–1.6 mg.

Intra-Articular and Soft Tissues: Adults, elderly: 4–16 mg; may repeat ql–3 wks.

Dexamethasone sodium phosphate:
IM/IV: Adults, elderly: Initially, 0.5–9 mg/day.

Intra-Articular, Intralesional, or Soft Tissue: 0.4–6 mg.

Usual topical dosage:
Topical: Adults, elderly: 2–4 times/day.

Respiratory inhalant:
Respiratory Inhalation: Adults, elderly: 3 inhalations 3–4 times/day; *Maximum:* 12/day. *Children:* 2 inhalations 3–4 times/day. *Maximum:* 8/day.

Usual intranasal dosage:
Adults, elderly: 2 sprays each nostril 2–3 times/day. *Maximum:* 12/day. *Children:* 1–2 sprays 2 times/day. *Maximum:* 8/day.

CONTRAINDICATIONS

Hypersensitivity to any corticosteroid or components, systemic fungal infection, peptic ulcers (except life-threatening situations). Avoid live virus vaccine such as smallpox. *Topical:* Marked circulation impairment. Do not instill ocular solutions when topical corticosteroids are being used on eyelids or surrounding skin.

CAUTIONS

Thromboembolic disorders, history of tuberculosis (may reactivate disease), hypothyroidism, cirrhosis, nonspecific ulcerative colitis, CHF, hypertension, psychosis, renal insufficiency, seizure disorders. Prolonged therapy should be discontinued slowly. *Topical:* Do not apply to extensive areas.

INTERACTIONS

DRUG: ***Amphotericin*** may increase hypokalemia. May decrease effect of ***oral hypoglycemics, insulin, diuretics, potassium supplements***. May increase ***digoxin*** toxicity (due to hypokalemia). ***Hepatic enzyme inducers*** may decrease effect. ***Live virus vaccines*** may potentiate virus replication, increase vaccine side effects, decrease pt's antibody response to vaccine. **HERBAL:** Ginseng, Ma Huang (Ephedra) may decrease effect. **FOOD:** None significant. **ALTERED LAB VALUES:** May decrease calcium, potassium, thyroxine. Increases cholesterol, glucose, lipids, sodium, amylase serum levels.

SIDE EFFECTS

FREQUENT: *Inhalation:* Cough, dry mouth, hoarseness, throat irritation. *Intranasal:* Burning, dryness inside nose. *Ophthalmic:* Blurred vision. *Systemic:* Insomnia, facial swelling ("moon face"), moderate abdominal distension, indigestion, increased appetite, nervousness, facial flushing, increased sweating. OCCASIONAL: *Inhalation:* Localized fungal infection (thrush). *Intranasal:* Crusting inside nose, nosebleed, sore throat, ulceration of nasal mucosa. *Ophthalmic:* Decreased vision, watering of eyes, eye pain, nausea, vomiting, burning, stinging, redness of eyes. *Systemic:* Dizziness, decreased/blurred vision. *Topical:* Allergic contact dermatitis, purpura (blood-containing blisters), thinning of skin w/easy bruising, telangiectasis (raised dark red spots on skin). RARE: *Inhalation:* Increased bronchospasm, esophageal candidiasis. *Intranasal:* Nasal/pharyngeal candidiasis, eye pain. *Systemic:* General allergic reaction (rash, hives), pain, redness, swelling at injection site, psychic changes, false sense of well-being, hallucinations, depression.

ADVERSE REACTIONS/TOXIC EFFECTS

Long-term therapy: Muscle wasting (especially arms, legs), osteoporosis, spontaneous fractures, amenorrhea, cataracts, glaucoma, peptic ulcer, CHF. *Abrupt withdrawal following long-term therapy:* Severe joint pain, severe headache, anorexia, nausea, fever, rebound inflammation, fatigue, weakness, lethargy, dizziness, orthostatic hypotension. *Ophthalmic:* Glaucoma, ocular hypertension, cataracts.

PATIENT CONSIDERATIONS

BASELINE ASSESSMENT

Question for hypersensitivity to any of the corticosteroids, components. Obtain baselines for height, weight, B/P, glucose, electrolytes. Check results of initial tests (e.g., TB skin test, x-rays, EKG).

INTERVENTION/EVALUATION

Monitor I&O, daily weight. Assess for edema. Check lab results for blood coagulability and clinical evidence of thromboembolism. Evaluate food tolerance and bowel activity: report hyperacidity promptly. Check B/P, temperature, respirations, pulse at least 2 times/day. Be alert to infection: sore throat, fever, or vague symptoms. Monitor electrolytes. Watch for hypercalcemia (muscle twitching. cramps, positive Trousseau's or Chvostek's signs), hypokalemia (weakness and muscle cramps, numbness/tingling especially lower extremities, nausea and vomiting, irritability, EKG changes). Assess emotional status, ability to sleep. Provide assistance w/ambulation.

PATIENT/FAMILY TEACHING

Take w/food or milk. Carry identification of drug and dose, physician's name and phone number. Do not change dose/schedule or stop taking drug. *Must* taper off gradually under medical supervision. Notify physician of fever, sore throat, muscle aches, sudden weight gain/swelling. W/dietician give instructions for prescribed diet (usually sodium-restricted w/high vitamin D, protein, and potassium). Maintain careful personal hygiene, avoid exposure to disease or trauma. Severe stress (serious infection, surgery, or trauma) may require increased dosage. Do not take any other medication w/o consulting physician. Follow-up visits, lab tests are necessary; children must be assessed for growth retardation. Inform dentist or other physicians of dexamethasone therapy now or within past 12 mos. Caution against overuse of joints injected for symptomatic relief.

Topical

Apply after shower or bath for best absorption. Do not cover unless physician orders; do not use tight diapers, plastic pants, or coverings. Avoid contact w/eyes. Do not expose treated area to sunlight.

---

dexmedetomidine

(Precedex)

See Supplement

---

dexrazoxane

dex-**rah**-zox-ann

(Zinecard)

CANADIAN AVAILABILITY

Zinecard

PREGNANCY CATEGORY C

CLASSIFICATION

Antineoplastic adjunct, cardioprotective agent

AVAILABILITY (Rx)

Powder for Injection: 250 mg (10

mg/ml reconstituted in 25 ml single-use vial), 500 mg (10 mg/ml reconstituted in 50 ml single-use vial)

PHARMACOKINETICS

Rapidly distributed following IV administration. **Excretion:** Primarily excreted in urine. **Half-life:** 2.1–2.5 hrs.

ACTION/*THERAPEUTIC EFFECT*

Readily penetrates cell membranes converting intracellularly to a chelating agent, *binding iron and preventing free radical formation by anthracycline, protecting against anthracycline-induced cardiomyopathy.*

USES

Reduction of incidence and severity of cardiomyopathy associated w/doxorubicin therapy in women w/metastatic breast cancer. Not recommended w/initiation of doxorubicin therapy.

STORAGE/HANDLING

Store vials at room temperature. Reconstituted solution stable for 6 hrs at room temperature or refrigeration. Discard unused solution.

ADMINISTRATION

Note: Do not mix w/other drugs. Use caution in handling and preparation of reconstituted solution (glove use recommended).

IV:

- Reconstitute w/0.167 molar (M/6) sodium lactate injection to give concentration of 10 mg dexrazoxane for each ml of sodium lactate.
- Give reconstituted solution by slow IV push or rapid drip IV infusion from a bag.
- After infusion is completed, and before a total elapsed time of 30 min from beginning of dexrazoxane infusion, give IV injection of doxorubicin.

INDICATIONS/ROUTES/DOSAGE

Note: Dexrazoxane should only be used in those who have received a cumulative doxorubicin dose of 300 mg/m^2 and are continuing w/doxorubicin therapy. The reconstituted dexrazoxane solution may be diluted w/0.9% NaCl injection or 5% dextrose injection to a concentration range of 1.3 to 5 mg/ml in IV infusion bags.

Cardioprotective:

IV: Adults: Recommended dosage ratio of dexrazoxane:doxorubicin is 10:1 (e.g., 500 mg/m^2 dexrazoxane: 50 mg/m^2 doxorubicin).

CONTRAINDICATIONS

Chemotherapy regimens that do not contain an anthracycline.

CAUTIONS

Chemotherapeutic agents that are additive to myelosuppression, concurrent FAC therapy (fluorouracil, doxorubicin, cyclophosphamide).

INTERACTIONS

DRUG: Concurrent FAC therapy ***(fluorouracil, doxorubicin, cyclophosphamide)*** may produce severe blood dyscrasias. **HERBAL:** None known. **FOOD:** None significant. **ALTERED LAB VALUES:** Concurrent FAC (fluorouracil, doxorubicin, cyclophosphamide) therapy may produce abnormal hepatic or renal function tests.

SIDE EFFECTS

FREQUENT (>10%): Alopecia, nausea, vomiting, fatigue, malaise, anorexia, stomatitis, fever, infection, diarrhea. **OCCASIONAL (1–10%):** Pain w/injection, neurotoxicity, phlebitis, dysphagia, streaking/erythema. **RARE (<1%):** Urticaria, skin reaction.

ADVERSE REACTIONS/TOXIC EFFECTS

FAC therapy w/dexrazoxane may produce more severe leukopenia, granulocytopenia, and thrombocytopenia than those receiving FAC w/o dexrazoxane. Overdosage can be removed w/peritoneal or hemodialysis.

PATIENT CONSIDERATIONS

Baseline Assessment

Use gloves when preparing solution. If powder or solution comes in contact w/skin, wash immediately w/soap and water. Antiemetics may be effective in preventing, treating nausea.

Intervention/Evaluation

Frequently monitor blood counts for evidence of blood dyscrasias. Monitor for stomatitis (burning/erythema of oral mucosa at inner margin of lips, sore throat, difficulty swallowing). Monitor hematologic status, renal/hepatic function studies, cardiac function. Assess pattern of daily bowel activity, stool consistency. Monitor for hematologic toxicity (fever, signs of local infection, easy bruising, unusual bleeding from any site).

Patient/Family Teaching

Alopecia is reversible, but new hair growth may have different color or texture. New hair growth resumes 2–3 mos after last therapy dose. Maintain fastidious oral hygiene. Do not have immunizations w/o physician approval (drug lowers body's resistance). Avoid those who have recently taken live virus vaccine. Promptly report fever, sore throat, signs of local infection. Contact physician if nausea/vomiting continues at home.

dextran, low molecular weight (dextran 40)

dex-tran
(Gentran, Rheomacrodex)

dextran, high molecular weight (dextran 75)

(Macrodex)

CANADIAN AVAILABILITY
Hyskon, Rheomacrodex

PREGNANCY CATEGORY C

CLASSIFICATION

Plasma volume expander

AVAILABILITY (Rx)

Injection: 10% dextran 40 in NaCl or D_5W, 6% dextran 75 in NaCl or D_5W.

PHARMACOKINETICS

Evenly distributed in vascular circulation. **Metabolism:** Enzymatically degraded to glucose. **Excretion:** Excreted in urine, feces.

ACTION/*THERAPEUTIC EFFECT*

Draws fluid from interstitial to intravascular space (colloidal osmotic effect) *resulting in increased central venous pressure, cardiac output, stroke volume, B/P, urine output, capillary perfusion, pulse pressure, and decreased heart rate, peripheral resistance, blood viscosity.* Reduces aggregation of erythrocytes. Enhances blood flow *(corrects hypovolemia, improves circulation).*

USES

Adjunctive treatment of shock or impending shock (due to burns, surgery, hemorrhage); primary fluid in pump oxygenation during extracorporeal circulation. Prophylaxis against deep vein thrombosis, pulmonary embolism in those having procedures associated w/high risk of thromboembolic complications.

STORAGE/HANDLING

Store at room temperature. Use only clear solutions. Discard partially used containers.

ADMINISTRATION

IV:

- Give by IV infusion only.
- Monitor pt closely during first minutes of infusion for anaphylactoid reaction. Monitor vital signs q5min.
- Monitor urine flow rates during administration (if oliguria or anuria occurs, dextran 40 should be discontinued and osmotic diuretic given—minimizes vascular overloading).
- Monitor central venous pressure (CVP) when given by rapid infusion. If there is a precipitous rise in CVP, immediately discontinue drug (overexpansion of blood volume).
- Monitor B/P diligently during infusion; if marked hypotension occurs, stop infusion immediately (imminent anaphylactoid reaction).
- If evidence of blood volume overexpansion occurs, discontinue IV until blood volume adjusts via urine output.

INDICATIONS/ROUTES/DOSAGE

Usual Low Molecular Weight Dextran Dosages:

Adjunct to shock therapy:
IV: Adults, elderly: Total dose for first 24 hrs not to exceed 20 ml/kg. Infuse first 10 ml/kg rapidly. Therapy beyond 24 hrs not to exceed 10 ml/kg/day or 5 days duration.

Hemodilution in extracorporeal solutions:
IV: Adults, elderly: 10–20 ml/kg added to perfusion circuit. Do not exceed 20 ml/kg.

Prophylactic use in deep vein thrombosis and pulmonary embolism:
IV: Adults, elderly: 500–1,000 ml (10 ml/kg) on day of surgery; continue 500 ml/day for 2–3 additional days. Thereafter, continue therapy at 500 ml q2–3days up to 2 wks (based on risk of complications).

Usual High Molecular Weight Dextran Dosages:

IV: Adults, elderly: 500–1,000 ml given up to 20–40 ml/min. ***Maximum:*** 20 ml/kg in first 24 hrs, then 10 ml/kg/24 hrs thereafter. ***Children:*** 20 ml/kg in first 24 hrs, then 10 ml/kg/24 hrs.

CONTRAINDICATIONS

Marked hemostatic defects, including drug-induced, marked cardiac decompensation, renal disease with severe oliguria or anuria, hypervolemic conditions, severe bleeding disorders, when use of sodium or chloride could be detrimental.

CAUTIONS

Those w/thrombocytopenia, CHF, pulmonary edema, severe renal insufficiency, those on corticosteroids or corticotropin, presence of edema w/sodium retention, impaired renal clearance, chronic liver disease, pathologic abdominal conditions, those undergoing bowel surgery.

INTERACTIONS

DRUG: None significant. **HERBAL:** None known. **FOOD:** None significant. **ALTERED LAB VALUES:** Prolongs bleeding time, increases bleeding tendency, depresses platelet count. Decreases factor VIII, factor V, factor IX.

SIDE EFFECTS

OCCASIONAL: Mild hypersensitivity reaction (urticaria, nasal congestion, wheezing).

ADVERSE REACTIONS/TOXIC EFFECTS

Severe or fatal anaphylaxis (marked hypotension, cardiac/respiratory arrest) may occur, noted early during IV infusion, generally in those not previously exposed to IV dextran.

PATIENT CONSIDERATIONS

Intervention/Evaluation

Monitor urine output closely (increase in output generally occurs in oliguric pts after dextran administration). If no increase is observed after 500 ml dextran is infused, discontinue drug until diuresis occurs. Monitor for fluid overload (peripheral and/or pulmonary edema, impending CHF symptoms). Assess lung sounds for rales. Monitor central venous pressure (detects overexpansion of blood volume). Observe closely for allergic reaction. Assess for bleeding, especially following surgery or those on anticoagulant therapy (overt bleeding especially at surgical site and bruising, petechiae development).

dextroamphetamine sulfate

dex-tro-am-**fet**-ah-meen
(Dexedrine)

CANADIAN AVAILABILITY
Dexedrine

PREGNANCY CATEGORY C

CLASSIFICATION

CNS stimulant

AVAILABILITY (Rx)

Tablets: 5 mg, 10 mg. **Capsules (sustained-release):** 5 mg, 10 mg, 15 mg. **Elixir:** 5 mg/5 ml.

PHARMACODYNAMICS

	ONSET	PEAK	DURATION
Oral	1–2 hrs	—	2–10 hrs

PHARMACOKINETICS

Absorption: Well absorbed from GI tract. Widely distributed. **Excretion:** Primarily excreted in urine. **Half-life:** 10–12 hrs (children 6–8 hrs).

ACTION/*THERAPEUTIC EFFECT*

Enhances release, action of catecholamine (dopamine, norepinephrine) by blocking reuptake, inhibiting MAO. *Increases motor activity, mental alertness, decreases drowsiness, fatigue.*

USES

Treatment of narcolepsy; treatment of attention deficit disorder in hyperactive children; short-term treatment to assist caloric restriction in exogenous obesity.

STORAGE/HANDLING

Store elixir form at room temperature.

ADMINISTRATION

ORAL:

- Give single daily dose, initial daily dose upon awakening.
- When given in 2–3 divided doses/day, give at 4–6 hr intervals.
- Give last dose at least 6 hrs before retiring (prevents insomnia).
- Give sustained-release form (one capsule daily), 10–14 hrs before bedtime.
- If used as anorexic, give dose 30–60 min before meals.
- Do not break capsule or tablet form.

INDICATIONS/ROUTES/DOSAGE

Narcolepsy:

Oral: Adults, children >12 yrs: Initially, 10 mg/day. Increase by 10 mg at weekly intervals until therapeutic response achieved. Usual dose: 5–60 mg/day. *Children 6–12 yrs:* Initially, 5 mg/day. Increase by 5 mg/day at weekly intervals until therapeutic response achieved.

Attention deficit disorder:

Oral: Children >6 yrs: Initially, 5 mg 1–2 times/day. Increase by 5 mg/day at weekly intervals until therapeutic response achieved. *Maximum daily dose:* 40 mg. *Children 3–5 yrs:* Initially, 2.5 mg/day. Increase by 2.5 mg/day at weekly intervals until therapeutic response achieved.

Appetite suppressant:

Oral: Adults: 5–30 mg daily in divided doses of 5–10 mg each dose, given 30–60 min before meals. *Extended-Release:* 1 capsule in morning.

CONTRAINDICATIONS

Hyperthyroidism, advanced arteriosclerosis, agitated states, moderate to severe hypertension, symptomatic cardiovascular disease, history of drug abuse, glaucoma, history of hypersensitivity to sympathomimetic amines, within 14 days of MAO inhibitor ingestion.

CAUTIONS

Elderly, debilitated, tartrazine-sensitive pts.

INTERACTIONS

DRUG: ***Tricyclic antidepressants*** may increase cardiovascular effects. ***Beta blockers*** may increase risk of hypertension, bradycardia, heart block. ***CNS stimulants*** may increase effects. May increase risk of arrhythmias w/***digoxin. Meperidine*** may increase risk of hypotension, respiratory depression, convulsions, vascular collapse. ***MAO inhibitors*** may prolong, intensify effects. May increase effects of ***thyroid hormone. Thyroid hormones*** may increase effects. **HERBAL:** Ma Huang (Ephedra) may increase CNS stimulation. **FOOD:** None significant. **ALTERED LAB VALUES:** May increase plasma corticosteroid concentrations.

SIDE EFFECTS

FREQUENT: Irregular heartbeat, CNS stimulation, false sense of well-being, nervousness, insomnia. Increased motor activity, talkativeness, nervousness, mild euphoria, insomnia. **OCCASIONAL:** Headache, chilliness, dry mouth, GI distress, increased depression in depressed pts, tachycardia, palpitations, chest pain.

ADVERSE REACTIONS/TOXIC EFFECTS

Overdose may produce pallor or

flushing, cardiac irregularities, psychotic syndrome. Abrupt withdrawal following prolonged administration of high dosage may produce lethargy (may last for weeks). Prolonged administration to children w/ADD may produce a temporary suppression of weight and/or height patterns.

PATIENT CONSIDERATIONS

PATIENT/FAMILY TEACHING

Normal dosage levels may produce tolerance to drug's anorexic mood-elevating effects within a few weeks. Avoid tasks that require alertness, motor skills until response to drug is established. Dry mouth may be relieved by sugarless gum, sips of tepid water. Take early in day. May mask extreme fatigue. Report pronounced nervousness, dizziness, decreased appetite, dry mouth.

dezocine

dez-oh-seen
(Dalgan)

PREGNANCY CATEGORY C

CLASSIFICATION

Opioid analgesic **(Schedule V)**

AVAILABILITY (Rx)

Injection: 5 mg/ml, 10 mg/ml, 15 mg/ml

PHARMACODYNAMICS

	ONSET	PEAK	DURATION
IM	<30 min	30–45 min	2–4 hrs
IV	<15 min	30 min	2–4 hrs

PHARMACOKINETICS

Absorption: Rapid, complete absorption after IM administration. **Metabolism:** Metabolized in liver. **Excretion:** Primarily excreted in urine. **Half-life:** IM 2.2 hrs; IV 2.4–2.6 hrs.

ACTION/*THERAPEUTIC EFFECT*

Binds w/opiate receptors in CNS (probably in limbic system), *producing impaired pain perception.*

USES

Relief of moderate to severe pain.

STORAGE/HANDLING

Store parenteral form at room temperature. Discard if solution contains a precipitate.

INDICATIONS/ROUTES/DOSAGE

Analgesia:
IM: Adults, >18 yrs, elderly: 5–20 mg q3–6h as needed. *Maximum:* 120 mg/day.

IV: Adults, >18 yrs, elderly: 2.5–10 mg q2–4h as needed.

CONTRAINDICATIONS

None significant.

CAUTIONS

Impaired hepatic/renal function, elderly, debilitated, head injury, respiratory disease, hypertension, hypothyroidism, acute alcoholism, urethral stricture.

INTERACTIONS

DRUG: ***CNS depressants, MAO inhibitors*** may increase CNS or respiratory depression, hypotensive effects. May decrease effects of other ***opioid analgesics,*** may also precipitate withdrawal symptoms. **HERBAL:** None known. **FOOD:** None significant. **ALTERED LAB VALUES:** May increase SGOT (AST), alkaline phosphatase.

SIDE EFFECTS

FREQUENT (3–9%): Drowsiness,

nausea, vomiting. **OCCASIONAL (1–3%):** Anxiety, confusion, dizziness, slurred speech, flushed skin, abdominal pain, diarrhea, constipation, altered vision. **RARE (<1%):** Coughing, difficulty breathing, chest pain, delirium skin rash, irregular heartbeat, thrombophlebitis.

ADVERSE REACTIONS/TOXIC EFFECTS

Overdosage results in acute respiratory depression, skeletal muscle flaccidity, cyanosis, extreme somnolence progressing to convulsions, stupor, coma. Naloxone given as antidote.

PATIENT CONSIDERATIONS

Baseline Assessment

Raise bed rails. Obtain vital signs before giving medication. If respirations are 12/min or lower (20/min or lower in children), withhold medication, contact physician. Assess onset, type, location, and duration of pain. Effect of medication is reduced if full pain recurs before next dose.

Intervention/Evaluation

Increase fluid intake and environmental humidity to improve viscosity of lung secretions. Monitor for change in respirations, B/P, change in rate or quality of pulse. Monitor daily bowel activity and prevent constipation. Initiate deep breathing and coughing exercises, particularly in those w/impaired pulmonary function. Change pt's position q2–4h and ambulate w/assistance. Assess for clinical improvement and record onset of relief of pain.

Patient/Family Teaching

Change positions slowly to avoid dizziness. Avoid tasks that require alertness, motor skills until response to drug is established. Avoid alcohol.

---

diazepam

dye-**az**-eh-pam

(Diastat, Dizac, Valium, Valrelease)

CANADIAN AVAILABILITY

Apo-Diazepam, Diazemuls, Valium, Vivol

PREGNANCY CATEGORY D

CLASSIFICATION

Antianxiety: Benzodiazepine **(Schedule IV)**

AVAILABILITY (Rx)

Tablets: 2 mg, 5 mg, 10 mg. **Capsules (sustained-release):** 15 mg. **Oral Solution:** 5 mg/5 ml, 5 mg/ml. **Injection:** 5 mg/ml. **Injectable Emulsion:** 5 mg/ml. **Rectal Gel:** 2.5 mg, 10 mg, 15 mg, 20 mg.

PHARMACODYNAMICS

	ONSET	PEAK	DURATION
IV	1–5 min	—	15–60 min

PHARMACOKINETICS

Absorption: Well absorbed from GI tract. Widely distributed. **Metabolism:** Metabolized in liver to active metabolite. **Excretion:** Excreted in urine. **Half-life:** 20–70 hrs (increased in elderly, liver dysfunction).

ACTION/*THERAPEUTIC EFFECT*

Enhances action of neurotransmitter

gamma-aminobutyric acid (GABA) neurotransmission at CNS, *producing anxiolytic effect*. Enhances presynaptic inhibition, *elevating seizure threshold* in response to electrical/chemical stimulation. Inhibits spinal afferent pathways, *producing skeletal muscle relaxation.*

USES/*UNLABELED*

Short-term relief of anxiety symptoms, preanesthetic medication, relief of acute alcohol withdrawal. Adjunct for relief of acute musculoskeletal conditions, treatment of seizures (IV route used for termination of status epilepticus). ***Gel:*** Control of increased seizure activity in refractory epilepsy in those on stable regimens. *Treatment of panic disorders, tension headache, tremors.*

STORAGE/HANDLING

Store tablets, extended-release capsules, oral/parenteral solutions at room temperature.

ADMINISTRATION

ORAL:

- Give w/o regard to meals.
- Dilute oral concentrate w/ water, juice, carbonated beverages; may also be mixed in semisolid food (applesauce, pudding).
- Tablets may be crushed.
- Do not crush or break capsule.

PARENTERAL FORM:

- Do not mix w/other injections (produces precipitate).

IM:

- Injection may be painful. Inject deeply into deltoid muscle.

IV:

- Give by direct IV injection.
- Administer directly into a large vein (reduces risk of thrombosis/phlebitis). If not possible, administer into tubing of a flowing IV solution as close to the vein insertion point as possible. Do not use small veins (e.g., wrist/dorsum of hand).
- Administer IV rate not exceeding 5 mg/min. For children, give over a 3 min period (a too rapid IV may result in hypotension, respiratory depression).
- Monitor respirations q5–15 min for 2 hrs. May produce arrhythmias when used prior to cardioversion.

INDICATIONS/ROUTES/DOSAGE

Note: Use smallest effective dose in those w/liver disease, low serum albumin.

Anxiety:

Oral/IM/IV: Adults: 2–10 mg 2–4 times/day. ***Elderly/debilitated:*** 2.5 mg 2 times/day. ***Children >6 mos:*** 1–2.5 mg 3–4 times/day.

Preanesthesia:

IV: Adults, elderly: 5–15 mg 5–10 min prior to procedure.

Alcohol withdrawal:

Oral: Adults, elderly: 10 mg 3–4 times during first 24 hrs, then reduce to 5–10 mg 3–4 times/day as needed.

IM/IV: Adults, elderly: Initially, 10 mg, followed by 5–10 mg q3–4h.

Musculoskeletal spasm:

Oral: Adults: 2–10 mg 2–4 times/day. ***Elderly:*** 2–5 mg 2–4 times/day.

IM/IV: Adults: 5–10 mg q3–4h.

Seizures:

Oral: Adults: 2–10 mg 2–4 times/day. ***Elderly, debilitated:*** 2.5 mg 2 times/day.

IM/IV: Adults: 5–10 mg, repeated at 10–15 min intervals to total of 30 mg. ***Elderly, debilitated:*** 2–5 mg. Increase gradually as needed.

Gel: Adults, elderly, children: 0.2–0.5 mg/kg depending on age. May repeat in 4–12 hrs.

CONTRAINDICATIONS

Acute narrow-angle glaucoma, acute alcohol intoxication.

CAUTIONS

Impaired kidney/liver function.

INTERACTIONS

DRUG: *Alcohol, CNS depressants* may increase CNS depressant effect. **HERBAL:** Kava kava, valerian may increase CNS depression. **FOOD:** None significant. **ALTERED LAB VALUES:** May produce abnormal renal function tests, elevate SGOT (AST), SGPT (ALT), LDH, alkaline phosphatase, serum bilirubin.

SIDE EFFECTS

FREQUENT: Pain w/IM injection, drowsiness, fatigue, ataxia (muscular incoordination). **OCCASIONAL:** Slurred speech, orthostatic hypotension, headache, hypoactivity, constipation, nausea, blurred vision. **RARE:** Paradoxical CNS hyperactivity/nervousness in children, excitement/restlessness in elderly/debilitated (generally noted during first 2 wks of therapy, particularly noted in presence of uncontrolled pain).

ADVERSE REACTIONS/TOXIC EFFECTS

IV route may produce pain, swelling, thrombophlebitis, carpal tunnel syndrome. Abrupt or too rapid withdrawal may result in pronounced restlessness, irritability, insomnia, hand tremors, abdominal/muscle cramps, sweating, vomiting, seizures. Abrupt withdrawal in pts w/epilepsy may produce increase in frequency and/or severity of seizures. Overdosage results in somnolence, confusion, diminished reflexes, coma.

PATIENT CONSIDERATIONS

BASELINE ASSESSMENT

Assess B/P, pulse, respirations immediately before administration. Pt must remain recumbent for up to 3 hrs (individualized) after parenteral administration to reduce hypotensive effect.

Anxiety
Assess autonomic response (cold, clammy hands, sweating) and motor response (agitation, trembling, tension). Offer emotional support to anxious pt.

Musculoskeletal spasm
Record onset, type, location, duration of pain. Check for immobility, stiffness, swelling.

Seizures
Review history of seizure disorder (length, intensity, frequency, duration, LOC). Observe frequently for recurrence of seizure activity. Initiate seizure precautions.

INTERVENTION/EVALUATION

Monitor IV site for swelling, phlebitis (heat, pain, red streaking of skin over vein, hardness to vein). Assess children, elderly for paradoxical reaction, particularly during early therapy. Assist w/ambulation if drowsiness, ataxia occur. For those on long-term therapy, liver/renal function tests, blood counts should be performed periodically. Evaluate for therapeutic response: a decrease in intensity/frequency of seizures; a calm facial expression, decreased restlessness; decreased intensity of skeletal muscle pain.

Patient/Family Teaching

Discomfort may occur w/IM injection. Drowsiness usually diminishes w/continued therapy. Avoid tasks that require alertness, motor skills until response to drug is established. Smoking reduces drug effectiveness. Do not abruptly withdraw medication after long-term therapy. Strict maintenance of drug therapy is essential for seizure control. Avoid alcohol.

diazoxide

dye-ah-**zocks**-eyd
(Hyperstat, Proglycem)

CANADIAN AVAILABILITY
Hyperstat, Proglycem

PREGNANCY CATEGORY C

CLASSIFICATION

Antihypertensive, antihypoglycemic

AVAILABILITY (Rx)

Capsules: 50 mg. **Oral Suspension:** 50 mg/ml. **Injection:** 15 mg/ml.

PHARMACODYNAMICS

	ONSET	PEAK	DURATION
Oral: hypoglycemia	1 hr	—	Up to 8 hrs
IV: hypotensive	1 min	2–5 min	3–12 hrs

PHARMACOKINETICS

Absorption: Readily absorbed from GI tract. **Metabolism:** Metabolized in liver. **Excretion:** Excreted in urine. Removed by hemodialysis. **Half-life:** 21–36 hrs (increased in decreased renal function).

ACTION/*THERAPEUTIC EFFECT*

Directly relaxes smooth muscle in peripheral arterioles, *reducing peripheral vascular resistance, B/P.* Inhibits insulin release from pancreas, *increasing blood glucose.*

USES

Emergency lowering of B/P in adults w/severe, nonmalignant and malignant hypertension; children w/acute severe hypertension. Management of hypoglycemia caused by hyperinsulinism associated w/islet cell adenoma, carcinoma, or extrapancreatic malignancy.

STORAGE/HANDLING

Store capsules, oral suspension at room temperature. Parenteral forms should appear clear, colorless. Discard darkened solution (may be subpotent), or if precipitate is present.

ADMINISTRATION

ORAL:

- Shake well before using oral suspension.
- May give w/o regard to food.

IV:

- **Note:** IV form frequently produces a feeling of warmth along injection vein. Extravasation produces severe burning, cellulitis, phlebitis.
- Place pt in supine position during and for 1 hr after IV dosing, monitor B/P diligently, follow by standing B/P in ambulatory pts.
- Administer only in peripheral vein.
- Give over 30 sec or less.
- Do not use longer than 10 days.

INDICATIONS/ROUTES/DOSAGE

Severe hypertension:

IV: Adults, elderly, children: 1–3 mg/kg (up to maximum of 150 mg). Repeat q5–15min until adequate decrease in B/P occurs. Thereafter, give at intervals of 4–24 hrs.

Hypoglycemia:
*Oral: **Adults, elderly, children:*** Initially, 3 mg/kg/day in 3 divided doses q8h. ***Maintenance:*** 3–8 mg/kg/day in 2–3 divided doses at 12 or 8 hr intervals. ***Maximum:*** Up to 15 mg/kg/day. ***Infants, neonates:*** Initially, 10 mg/kg/day in 3 divided doses q8h. ***Maintenance:*** 8–15 mg/kg/day in 2–3 divided doses at 12 or 8 hr intervals.

CONTRAINDICATIONS

History of hypersensitivity to thiazide derivatives. *IV:* Hypertension associated w/aortic coarctation, arteriovenous shunt. *Oral:* Management of functional hypoglycemia.

CAUTIONS

Impaired renal function, cardiac reserve; caution when reducing severely elevated B/P.

INTERACTIONS

DRUG: *Beta blockers, vasodilators, hypotension-producing medications* may increase hypotensive effect. *Oral:* May decrease effect of ***phenytoin.*** HERBAL: None known. **FOOD:** None significant. **ALTERED LAB VALUES:** May increase SCOT (AST), alkaline phosphatase, free fatty acids, sodium, uric acid, glucose, BUN. May decrease hemoglobin, hematocrit, creatinine clearance.

SIDE EFFECTS

FREQUENT: Edema (increased weight, swelling of feet). OCCASIONAL: Tachycardia, altered taste, constipation, anorexia, nausea, vomiting, abdominal pain. *Parenteral:* Back pain, tinnitus, facial flushing, headache, pain/warmth along injection site. **RARE:** *IV/Oral:* Sensitivity reaction (rash, fever), confusion, paresthesia, orthostatic hypotension.

ADVERSE REACTIONS/TOXIC EFFECTS

Overdose may cause hyperglycemia/ketoacidosis (increased urination, thirst, fruitlike breath). Angina, myocardial infarction, thrombocytopenia occur rarely.

PATIENT CONSIDERATIONS

BASELINE ASSESSMENT

Establish baseline B/P, blood glucose. When administering IV, achieve desired B/P over as long a period of time as possible.

INTERVENTION/EVALUATION

If excessive reduction in B/P occurs, place pt in supine position w/legs elevated. If parenteral form leaks in SubQ tissue, apply warm compresses to decrease pain sensation. Monitor for development of hyperglycemia, particularly in those w/renal or liver disease, diabetes mellitus, concurrent therapy that may increase blood glucose concentrations. Monitor blood glucose concentrations daily in those receiving IV therapy. Monitor serum uric acid in those w/history of gout, hyperuricemia.

PATIENT/FAMILY TEACHING

Blood glucose or daily urine testing should be attained in those on chronic oral therapy. Report increases in urinary frequency, thirst, or fruity breath odor. Inform physician if pregnant.

D

dibucaine

(Nupercainal)

See Classification section under: Anesthetics: local

diclofenac sodium

dye-**klo**-feh-nak

(Voltaren, Voltaren XR)

diclofenac potassium

(Cataflam)

FIXED-COMBINATION(S)

W/misoprostil, an antisecretory gastric protectant **(Arthrotec)**

CANADIAN AVAILABILITY

Diclotec, Novo-Difenac, Voltaren

PREGNANCY CATEGORY B

(D if used in third trimester or near delivery)

CLASSIFICATION

Nonsteroidal anti-inflammatory

AVAILABILITY (Rx)

Tablets: 50 mg (Cataflam). **Tablets (delayed-release):** 25 mg, 50 mg, 75 mg. **Tablets (extended-release):** 100 mg. **Ophthalmic Solution:** 0.1%.

PHARMACODYNAMICS

	ONSET	PEAK	DURATION
Oral	—	2–3 hrs	—

PHARMACOKINETICS

Absorption: Completely absorbed from GI tract, penetrates cornea after ophthalmic administration (may be systemically absorbed). Widely distributed. **Metabolism:** Metabolized in liver. **Excretion:** Primarily excreted in urine. **Half-life:** 1.2–2 hrs.

ACTION / *THERAPEUTIC EFFECT*

Inhibits prostaglandin synthesis, reducing inflammatory response and intensity of pain stimulus reaching sensory nerve endings, *producing analgesic and anti-inflammatory effect.* Constricts iris sphincter, *preventing miosis during cataract surgery.*

USES / *UNLABELED*

Symptomatic treatment of acute and/or chronic rheumatoid arthritis, osteoarthritis, ankylosing spondylitis; postop inflammation of cataract extraction; analgesic, primary dysmenorrhea. Treatment of photophobia, relief of pain in incisional refractive surgery. *Ophthalmic: Reduces occurrence/severity of cystoid macular edema post cataract surgery. Oral: Treatment of vascular headaches.*

ADMINISTRATION

ORAL:

- Do not crush or break enteric-coated form.
- May give w/food, milk, or antacids if GI distress occurs.

OPHTHALMIC:

- Place finger on lower eyelid and pull out until pocket is formed between eye and lower lid. Hold dropper above pocket and place prescribed number of drops in pocket.
- Close eye gently. Apply digital pressure to lacrimal sac for 1–2 min (minimized drainage into nose and throat, reducing risk of systemic effects).
- Remove excess solution w/tissue.

INDICATIONS / DOSAGE / ROUTES

Osteoarthritis:

Oral: Adults, elderly: 100–150 mg/day in 2–3 divided doses.

Extended release: 100 mg/day as single dose.

Rheumatoid arthritis:
Oral: Adults, elderly: 150–200 mg/day in 2–4 divided doses. *Extended-release:* 100 mg/day.

Ankylosing spondylitis:
Oral: Adults, elderly: 100–125 mg/day in 4–5 divided doses.

Analgesic, primary dysmenorrhea:
Oral: Adults: 150 mg/day in 3 divided doses.

Usual ophthalmic dosage:
Adults, elderly: Apply 1 drop to eye 4 times/day commencing 24 hrs after cataract surgery. Continue for 2 wks after surgery.

Photophobia:
Adults, elderly: 1 drop to affected eye 1 hr preop, within 15 min postop, then 4 times/day for 3 days.

CONTRAINDICATIONS

Nasal polyps associated w/bronchospasm induced by aspirin, history of hypersensitivity to aspirin or NSAIDs, bone marrow depression, blood dyscrasias.

CAUTIONS

History of inflammatory or ulcerative disease of GI tract (e.g., peptic ulcer, Crohn's disease), hemophilia or other bleeding problems, impaired renal/liver function, stomatitis.

INTERACTIONS

DRUG: May increase effects of ***oral anticoagulants, heparin, thrombolytics.*** May decrease effect of ***antihypertensives, diuretics. Salicylates, aspirin*** may increase risk of GI side effects, bleeding. ***Bone marrow depressants*** may increase risk of hematologic reactions. May increase concentration, toxicity of ***lithium.*** May increase ***methotrexate*** toxicity. ***Probenecid*** may increase concentration. ***Ophthalmic:*** May decrease effect of ***acetylcholine, carbachol.*** May decrease antiglaucoma effect of ***epinephrine,*** other ***antiglaucoma medications.*** **HERBAL:** Feverfew, ginkgo may increase risk of bleeding. **FOOD:** None significant. **ALTERED LAB VALUES:** May increase alkaline phosphatase, LDH, serum transaminase, potassium urine protein, BUN, serum creatinine. May decrease uric acid.

SIDE EFFECTS

FREQUENT (3–9%): *Oral:* Headache, abdominal cramps, constipation, diarrhea, nausea, indigestion. *Ophthalmic:* Burning, stinging on instillation, ocular discomfort. **OCCASIONAL (1–3%):** *Oral:* Chest pain, arrhythmias, itching, skin rash, abdominal distension, ringing in ears, dizziness. *Ophthalmic:* Itching, tearing. **RARE (<1%):** *Oral:* Rash, peripheral edema/fluid retention, visual disturbances, vomiting, drowsiness.

ADVERSE REACTIONS/TOXIC EFFECTS

Overdosage may result in acute renal failure. In those treated chronically, peptic ulcer, GI bleeding, gastritis, severe hepatic reaction (jaundice), nephrotoxicity (hematuria, dysuria, proteinuria), severe hypersensitivity reaction (bronchospasm, angiofacial edema) occur rarely.

PATIENT CONSIDERATIONS

BASELINE ASSESSMENT

Anti-inflammatory
Assess onset, type, location, and duration of pain or inflammation. Inspect appearance of affected

joints for immobility, deformities, and skin condition.

INTERVENTION/EVALUATION

Monitor for headache, dyspepsia. Monitor pattern of daily bowel activity and stool consistency. Evaluate for therapeutic response: relief of pain, stiffness, swelling, increase in joint mobility, reduced joint tenderness, improved grip strength.

PATIENT/FAMILY TEACHING

Swallow tablet whole; do not crush or chew. Avoid aspirin, alcohol during therapy (increases risk of GI bleeding). If GI upset occurs, take w/food, milk. GI distress, visual disturbances, rash, edema, headache. Report skin rash, itching, increased weight, changes in vision, black stools, persistent headache. Avoid tasks requiring alertness, motor skills until response to drug is established.

dicloxacillin sodium

dye-**clocks**-ah-sill-in
(Dynapen, Dycill, Pathocil)

PREGNANCY CATEGORY B

CLASSIFICATION

Antibiotic: Penicillin

AVAILABILITY (Rx)

Capsules: 250 mg, 500 mg. **Oral Solution:** 125 mg/5 ml.

PHARMACOKINETICS

Absorption: Moderately absorbed from GI tract (food decreases absorption). **Metabolism:** Metabolized in liver. **Excretion:** Primarily excreted in urine. Not removed by hemodialysis. **Half-life:** 0.5–1.1 hrs (increase in decreased renal function).

ACTION/*THERAPEUTIC EFFECT*

Inhibits cell wall synthesis by binding to bacterial membranes, *producing bactericidal effect.*

USES

Treatment of mild to moderate infections of respiratory tract and skin/skin structure, chronic osteomyelitis, urinary tract infection; follow-up to parenteral therapy for acute, severe infections. Predominantly treatment of infections caused by penicillinase-producing *Staphylococcus.*

STORAGE/HANDLING

Store capsules at room temperature. Oral solution, after reconstitution, is stable for 7 days at room temperature, 14 days if refrigerated.

ADMINISTRATION

ORAL:

- Give 1 hr before or 2 hrs after meals.
- Space doses evenly around the clock.

INDICATIONS/ROUTES/DOSAGE

Mild to moderate upper respiratory, localized skin/skin structure infections:
Oral: Adults, elderly, children >40 kg: 125 mg q6h. ***Children <40 kg:*** 12.5 mg/kg/day in divided doses q6h.

Severe infections, lower respiratory tract, disseminated infections:
Oral: Adults, elderly, children >40 kg: 250 mg q6h. ***Maximum:*** 4 g/day. ***Children <40 kg:*** 25 mg/kg/day in divided doses q6h.

CONTRAINDICATIONS

Hypersensitivity to any penicillin.

CAUTIONS

History of allergies, particularly cephalosporins.

INTERACTIONS

DRUG: *Probenecid* may increase concentration, toxicity risk. **HERBAL:** None known. **FOOD:** None significant. **ALTERED LAB VALUES:** May increase SGOT (AST), SGPT (ALT), alkaline phosphatase, LDH. May cause positive Coombs' test.

SIDE EFFECTS

FREQUENT: Mild hypersensitivity reaction (fever, rash, pruritus), nausea, vomiting, diarrhea, flatulence.

ADVERSE REACTIONS/TOXIC EFFECTS

Superinfections, potentially fatal antibiotic-associated colitis may result from altered bacterial balance. Hematologic effects, severe hypersensitivity reactions, anaphylaxis occur rarely.

PATIENT CONSIDERATIONS

Baseline Assessment

Question for history of allergies, especially penicillins, cephalosporins. Obtain specimen for culture and sensitivity before giving first dose (therapy may begin before results are known).

Intervention/Evaluation

Hold medication and promptly report rash (may indicate hypersensitivity) or diarrhea (w/fever, abdominal pain, mucus and blood in stool may indicate antibiotic-associated colitis). Assess food tolerance. Check hematology reports (especially WBCs), periodic renal or hepatic reports in prolonged therapy. Be alert for superinfection: increased fever, sore throat, diarrhea, ulceration or changes of oral mucosa, vaginal discharge, anal/genital pruritus.

Patient/Family Teaching

Continue antibiotic for full length of treatment. Space doses evenly. Notify physician in event of diarrhea, rash, other new symptom.

dicyclomine hydrochloride

dye-**sigh**-clo-meen
(Antispaz, Bentyl, Dibent, Di-Spaz, Neoquess, OrTyl, Spasmoject)

CANADIAN AVAILABILITY
Bentylol, Formulex, Lomine

PREGNANCY CATEGORY B

CLASSIFICATION

Antispasmodic

AVAILABILITY (Rx)

Capsules: 10 mg, 20 mg. **Tablets:** 20 mg. **Syrup:** 10 mg/5 ml. **Injection:** 10 mg/ml.

PHARMACOKINETICS

Absorption: Readily absorbed from GI tract. Widely distributed. **Metabolism:** Metabolized in liver. **Half-life:** 9–10 hrs.

ACTION/ *THERAPEUTIC EFFECT*

Direct relaxant action on smooth muscle, *reducing tone, motility of GI tract.*

USES

Treatment of functional disturbances of GI motility (i.e., irritable bowel syndrome).

STORAGE/HANDLING

Store capsules, tablets, syrup, parenteral form at room temperature. Injection should appear colorless.

ADMINISTRATION

ORAL:

- Dilute oral solution w/equal volume of water just before administration.
- May give w/o regard to meals (food may slightly decrease absorption).

IM:

- Do not administer IV or SubQ.
- Inject deep into large muscle mass.
- Do not give longer than 2 days.

INDICATIONS/ROUTES/DOSAGE

Functional disturbances of GI motility:

Oral: Adults: 10–20 mg 3–4 times/day up to 40 mg 4 times/day. ***Children 6 mos–2 yrs:*** 5–10 mg 3–4 times/day. ***Children >2 yrs:*** 10 mg 3–4 times/day.

IM: Adults: 20 mg q4–6h.

Usual elderly dosage:

Oral: 10–20 mg 4 times/day. May increase up to 160 mg/day.

CONTRAINDICATIONS

Narrow-angle glaucoma, severe ulcerative colitis, toxic megacolon, obstructive disease of GI tract, paralytic ileus, intestinal atony, bladder neck obstruction due to prostatic hypertrophy, myasthenia gravis in those not treated w/neostigmine, tachycardia secondary to cardiac insufficiency or thyrotoxicosis, cardiospasm, unstable cardiovascular status in acute hemorrhage.

EXTREME CAUTION

Autonomic neuropathy, known or suspected GI infections, diarrhea, mild to moderate ulcerative colitis.

CAUTIONS

Hyperthyroidism, hepatic or renal disease, hypertension, tachyarrhythmias, CHF, coronary artery disease, gastric ulcer, esophageal reflux or hiatal hernia associated w/reflux esophagitis, infants, elderly, those w/COPD.

INTERACTIONS

DRUG: ***Antacids, antidiarrheals*** may decrease absorption. ***Anticholinergics*** may increase effects. May decrease absorption of ***ketoconazole.*** May increase severity of GI lesions with ***KCl*** (wax matrix). **HERBAL:** None known. **FOOD:** None significant. **ALTERED LAB VALUES:** None significant.

SIDE EFFECTS

FREQUENT: Dry mouth (sometimes severe), decreased sweating, constipation. **OCCASIONAL:** Blurred vision, bloated feeling, urinary hesitancy, drowsiness (w/high dosage), headache, intolerance to light, loss of taste, nervousness, flushing, insomnia, impotence, mental confusion/excitement (particularly in elderly, children). IM may produce temporary lightheadedness, local irritation. **RARE:** Dizziness, faintness.

ADVERSE REACTIONS/TOXIC EFFECTS

Overdosage may produce temporary paralysis of ciliary muscle, pupillary dilation, tachycardia, palpitation, hot/dry/flushed skin, absence of bowel sounds, hyperthermia, increased respiratory rate, EKG abnormalities, nausea, vomiting, rash over face/upper trunk, CNS stimulation, psychosis (agitation, restlessness, rambling speech, visual hallucination, paranoid behavior, delusions), followed by depression.

PATIENT CONSIDERATIONS

BASELINE ASSESSMENT

Before giving medication, instruct pt to void (reduces risk of urinary retention).

INTERVENTION/EVALUATION

Monitor daily bowel activity and stool consistency. Assess for urinary retention. Monitor changes in B/P, temperature. Assess skin turgor, mucous membranes to evaluate hydration status (encourage adequate fluid intake), bowel sounds for peristalsis. Be alert for fever (increased risk of hyperthermia).

PATIENT/FAMILY TEACHING

Do not become overheated during exercise in hot weather (may result in heat stroke). Avoid hot baths, saunas. Avoid tasks that require alertness, motor skills until response to drug is established. Sugarless gum, sips of tepid water may relieve dry mouth. Do not take antacids or medicine for diarrhea within 1 hr of taking this medication (decreased effectiveness).

didanosine

dye-**dan**-oh-sin
(Videx)

CANADIAN AVAILABILITY
Videx

PREGNANCY CATEGORY B

CLASSIFICATION

Antiviral

AVAILABILITY (Rx)

Tablets: 25 mg, 50 mg, 100 mg, 150 mg. **Powder for Oral Solution (packets):** 100 mg, 167 mg, 250 mg, 375 mg. **Powder for Oral Solution (bottles):** 2 g, 4 g.

PHARMACOKINETICS

Absorption: Variably absorbed from GI tract. **Metabolism:** Rapidly metabolized intracellularly to active form. **Excretion:** Primarily excreted in urine. **Half-life:** 1.5 hrs; metabolite: 8–24 hrs.

ACTION/*THERAPEUTIC EFFECT*

Intracellularly converted into a triphosphate, interfering w/RNA-directed DNA polymerase (reverse transcriptase). *Virustatic,* inhibiting replication of retroviruses, including human immunodeficiency virus (HIV).

USES

Management (not cure) of advanced HIV disease in pts who cannot tolerate zidovudine or who have had clinically or immunologically significant deterioration during zidovudine therapy. Initial therapy in AIDS.

STORAGE/HANDLING

Store at room temperature. If tablets dispersed in water, stable for 1 hr at room temperature; after reconstitution of buffered powder, oral solution stable for 4 hrs at room temperature. Pediatric powder for oral solution after reconstitution as directed, stable for 30 days refrigerated.

ADMINISTRATION

ORAL:

- Give 1 hr before or 2 hrs after meals (food decreases rate and extent of absorption).
- Chewable tablets: thoroughly crushed and dispersed in at least 30 ml water before swallowing. Mixture should be stirred well (2–3 min) and swallowed immediately.
- Buffered powder for oral solution: Reconstitute prior to administration by pouring contents of packet into about 4 oz water; stir until completely dissolved (up to 2–3 min). Do not mix w/fruit juice or other acidic liquid because didanosine is unstable at acidic pH.
- Unbuffered pediatric powder: add 100–200 ml water to 2 or 4 g, respectively, to provide concentration of 20 mg/ml. Immediately mix w/equal amount of antacid to provide concentration of 10 mg/ml. Shake thoroughly prior to removing each dose.

INDICATIONS/DOSAGE/ROUTES

Note: Each dose consists of 2 tablets (prevents degradation of drug). Children <1 yr need only 1 tablet/dose.

HIV infections (adults):
Oral (Tablets): Adults >60 kg: 200 mg q12h. ***<60 kg:*** 125 mg q12h. ***(Buffered oral solution): Adults >60 kg:*** 250 mg q12h. ***<60 kg:*** 167 mg q12h.

HIV infections (children):
Oral (Tablets): Children BSA 1.1–1.4 m²: 100 mg q12h; ***BSA 0.8–1.0 m²:*** 75 mg q12h; ***BSA 0.5–0.7 m²:*** 50 mg q12h; ***BSA <0.4 m²:*** 25 mg q12h. ***(Pediatric oral solution): Children BSA 1.1–1.4 m²:*** 125 mg q12h; ***BSA 0.8–1.0 m²:*** 94 mg q12h; ***BSA 0.5–0.7 m²:*** 62 mg q12h; ***BSA <0.4 m²:*** 31 mg q12h.

CONTRAINDICATIONS

Hypersensitivity to drug or any component of preparation.

CAUTIONS

Renal or hepatic dysfunction, alcoholism, elevated triglycerides, T cell counts less than 100 cells/mm^3; extreme caution w/history of pancreatitis. Phenylketonuria and sodium-restricted diets due to phenylalanine and sodium content of preparations.

INTERACTIONS

DRUG: May increase risk of pancreatitis, peripheral neuropathy ***w/medications producing pancreatitis, peripheral neuropathy,*** respectively. May decrease absorption of ***dapsone, itraconazole, ketoconazole, tetracyclines, fluoroquinolones.*** **HERBAL:** None known. **FOOD:** Decreases rate/extent of absorption. **ALTERED LAB VALUES:** May increase alkaline phosphatase, SGOT (AST), SGPT (ALT), bilirubin, amylase, lipase, triglycerides, uric acid. May decrease potassium.

SIDE EFFECTS

FREQUENT (>10%): ***Adults:*** Diarrhea, neuropathy, chills/fever. **(>25%):** ***Children:*** Chills, fever, decreased appetite, pain, malaise, nausea, diarrhea, vomiting, abdominal pain, headache, nervousness, cough, rhinitis, dyspnea, asthma, rash, itching. **OCCASIONAL (2–9%):** ***Adults:*** Rash, itching, headache, abdominal pain, nausea, vomiting, pneumonia, myopathy, decreased appetite, dry mouth, dyspnea. (10–25%): *Children:* Failure to thrive, decreased weight, stomatitis, oral thrush, ecchymosis, arthritis, myalgia, insomnia, epistaxis, pharyngitis.

ADVERSE REACTIONS/TOXIC EFFECTS

Pneumonia, opportunistic infection occur occasionally. Peripheral neuropathy, potentially fatal pancreatitis are the major toxicities.

PATIENT CONSIDERATIONS

BASELINE ASSESSMENT

Obtain baseline values for CBC, renal and hepatic function tests, vital signs, weight. Question for hypersensitivity to didanosine or components of preparation.

INTERVENTION/EVALUATION

In event of abdominal pain and nausea, vomiting, or elevated serum amylase, triglycerides, contact physician before administering medication (potential pancreatitis). Be alert to burning feet, "restless leg syndrome" (unable to find comfortable position for legs and feet), lack of coordination and other signs of peripheral neuropathy. Check food intake and assure availability of desired foods. Monitor consistency and frequency of stools. Check skin for rash, eruptions. Assess temperature, respiration, pulse, B/P at least 2 times/day. Assess for opportunistic infections: onset of fever, oral mucosa changes, cough, or other respiratory symptoms. Monitor lab values carefully. Assess children for epistaxis or other bleeding, petechiae. Evaluate for dehydration (especially children): decreased skin turgor, dry skin and mucous membranes, decreased urinary output. Check weight at least twice a week. Assess for visual or hearing difficulty; provide protection from light if photophobia develops. Auscultate lungs and assess for difficult breathing. If dizziness occurs, provide assistance w/ambulation.

PATIENT/FAMILY TEACHING

Explain correct administration of medication. Small, frequent meals of favorite foods to offset anorexia, vomiting. Accurate I&O record. Report development of fever or any new symptom promptly.

dienestrol

dye-en-**ess**-troll
(Ortho Dienestrol)

CANADIAN AVAILABILITY
Ortho Dienestrol

PREGNANCY CATEGORY X

CLASSIFICATION

Estrogen

AVAILABILITY (Rx)

Vaginal Cream: 0.01%

PHARMACOKINETICS

Absorption: Extensively absorbed into systemic circulation. Widely distributed. **Metabolism:** Metabolized in liver. **Excretion:** Primarily excreted in urine.

ACTION/*THERAPEUTIC EFFECT*

Increases synthesis of DNA, RNA, and various proteins in responsive tissues, *alleviating signs and symptoms of vulvovaginal epithelial atro-*

phy (atrophic vaginitis), kraurosis vulvae associated w/menopause.

USES

Treatment of atrophic vaginitis, kraurosis vulvae.

ADMINISTRATION

VAGINAL:
- Apply at bedtime for best absorption.
- Assemble and fill applicator per manufacturer's directions.
- Insert end of applicator into vagina, direct slightly toward sacrum; push plunger down completely.
- Avoid skin contact w/cream due to absorption.

INDICATIONS/ROUTES/DOSAGE

Atrophic vaginitis, kraurosis vulvae:
Intravaginal: Adults, elderly: Initially, 1–2 applicatorsful/day for 7–14 days. Reduce dose by 1/2 for additional 1–2 wks. ***Maintenance:*** 1 applicatorful 1–3 times/wk.

CONTRAINDICATIONS

Known or suspected breast cancer, estrogen-dependent neoplasia; undiagnosed abnormal genital bleeding; active thrombophlebitis or thromboembolic disorders; history of thrombophlebitis, thrombosis, or thromboembolic disorders w/previous estrogen use, hypersensitivity to estrogen or ingredients of cream.

CAUTIONS

Conditions that may be aggravated by fluid retention: cardiac, renal, or hepatic dysfunction, epilepsy, migraine. Mental depression, hypercalcemia, history of jaundice during pregnancy, or strong family history of breast cancer, fibrocystic disease, or breast nodules.

INTERACTIONS

DRUG: May interfere w/effects of ***bromocriptine.*** May increase concentration of ***cyclosporine,*** increase hepatic, nephrotoxicity. ***Hepatotoxic medications*** may increase hepatotoxicity. **HERBAL:** None known. **FOOD:** None significant. **ALTERED LAB VALUES:** May affect metapyrone, thyroid function tests. May decrease cholesterol, LDH. May increase calcium, glucose, HDL, triglycerides.

SIDE EFFECTS

FREQUENT: Breast pain/tenderness, enlarged breasts, edema (swelling of feet, increased weight), decreased appetite, abdominal cramping. **OCCASIONAL:** Diarrhea, dizziness, headache, increased libido, abnormal vaginal bleeding, breast tumors, liver, gallbladder obstruction, local irritation (itching, redness).

ADVERSE REACTIONS/TOXIC EFFECTS

Prolonged administration increases risk of gallbladder, thromboembolic disease, and breast, cervical, vaginal, endometrial, and liver carcinoma.

PATIENT CONSIDERATIONS

Baseline Assessment

Question hypersensitivity to estrogen or ingredients of cream, previous jaundice or thromboembolic disorders associated w/pregnancy or estrogen therapy. Establish baseline B/P, blood glucose.

Intervention/Evaluation

Initially assess B/P, weight daily. Monitor blood glucose 4 times/

day for pts w/diabetes. Check for swelling. Assess for vaginal discharge, local irritation. Promptly report signs and symptoms of thromboembolic or thrombotic disorders: weakness, pain or numbness of an extremity, chest pain, shortness of breath. Note estrogen therapy on specimens.

Patient/Family Teaching

Importance of medical supervision. W/systemic absorption, smoking may increase risk of heart attack or blood clots. Notify physician of abnormal vaginal bleeding pain or numbness of an extremity, other symptoms. Teach breast self-exam. Use protection from sun or ultraviolet light. Check weight weekly; report weekly gain of 5 lbs or more. Remain recumbent at least 30 min after application and do not use tampons. Stop using dienestrol, contact physician at once if suspect pregnancy. Give labeling from drug package.

diethylstilbestrol

dye-eth-ill-still-**bess**-trole
(DES, Stilphostrol)

diethylstilbestrol diphosphate

(Stilphostrol)

CANADIAN AVAILABILITY
Honvol

PREGNANCY CATEGORY X

CLASSIFICATION

Antineoplastic, estrogen

AVAILABILITY (Rx)

Tablets: 1 mg, 5 mg. **Tablets (as diphosphate):** 50 mg. **Injection (as diphosphate):** 250 mg.

PHARMACOKINETICS

Absorption: Well absorbed from GI tract. Widely distributed. **Metabolism:** Metabolized in liver. **Excretion:** Primarily excreted in urine.

ACTION/*THERAPEUTIC EFFECT*

Increases synthesis of DNA, RNA, and various proteins in responsive tissues. Reduces release of gonadotopin-releasing hormone, *reducing follicle-stimulating hormone (FSH) and luteinizing hormone (LH); decreases serum concentration of testosterone.*

USES/*UNLABELED*

Palliative therapy for inoperable cancer of the prostate and advanced metastatic cancer of the breast in men and postmenopausal women. *Prophylaxis of postmenopausal osteoporosis, estrogen deficiency–induced premenopausal osteoporosis.*

STORAGE/HANDLING

:Injection is colorless to light yellow solution. Discard if solution is cloudy or precipitate forms.

ADMINISTRATION

ORAL:

- Enteric tablets should not be crushed.
- Give w/food to reduce nausea.

IV:

- Dilute in 300 ml normal saline or 5% dextrose for injection.
- Administer slowly (12 ml/min) the first 10–15 min, then increase rate to infuse over 1 hr.

INDICATIONS/ROUTES/DOSAGE

Breast carcinoma:
Oral: Adults, elderly: 15 mg/day.

Prostatic carcinoma:
Oral: Adults, elderly: Initially, 1–3 mg/day. ***Maintenance:*** 1 mg/day.

Usual dosage for diethylstilbestrol diphosphate:
Oral: Adults, elderly: Initially, 50 mg 3 times/day; increase to 200 mg 3 times/day.

IV: Adults, elderly: Initially, 500 mg, then 1 g/day for 5 or more days. ***Maintenance:*** 250–500 mg 1–2 times/wk.

CONTRAINDICATIONS

Known or suspected breast cancer (except select cases), estrogen-dependent neoplasia; undiagnosed abnormal genital bleeding; active thrombophlebitis or thromboembolic disorders; history of thrombophlebitis, thrombosis, or thromboembolic disorders w/previous estrogen use, hypersensitivity to estrogen. Stilphostrol (diethylstilbestrol diphosphate) is not for use in women.

CAUTIONS

Conditions that may be aggravated by fluid retention: cardiac, renal, or hepatic dysfunction, epilepsy, migraine. Metabolic bone disease w/potential hypercalcemia, mental depression, history of jaundice during pregnancy, or strong family history of breast cancer, fibrocystic disease, or breast nodules, young pts in whom bone growth is not complete.

INTERACTIONS

DRUG: May interfere w/effects of ***bromocriptine.*** May increase concentration of ***cyclosporine,*** increase hepatic, nephrotoxicity. ***Hepatotoxic medications*** may increase hepatotoxicity. **HERBAL:** None known. **FOOD:** None significant. **ALTERED LAB VALUES:** May affect metapyrone, thyroid function tests. May decrease cholesterol, LDH. May increase calcium, glucose, HDL, triglycerides.

SIDE EFFECTS

FREQUENT: Loss of appetite, nausea, swelling of breasts, edema. **OCCASIONAL:** Vomiting (especially w/high doses), intolerance to contact lenses, headache or migraine, increased B/P, changes in vaginal bleeding (spotting, breakthrough, or prolonged bleeding), glucose inolerance, brown spots on exposed skin, libido changes. **RARE:** Chorea, cholestatic jaundice, loss of scalp hair, depression.

ADVERSE REACTIONS/TOXIC EFFECTS

Prolonged administration may have possibility of increased risk of gallbladder, thromboembolic disease, and cervical, vaginal, endometrial, and liver carcinoma.

PATIENT CONSIDERATIONS

Baseline Assessment

Question for possibility of pregnancy before initiating therapy. Question hypersensitivity to estrogen, previous jaundice, or thromboembolic disorders associated w/pregnancy or estrogen therapy. Establish baseline B/P, blood glucose.

Intervention/Evaluation

Assess B/P at least daily. Monitor blood glucose 4 times/day in diabetic pts. Check for swelling; weigh daily. Promptly report signs and symptoms of thromboembolic or thrombotic disor-

ders: sudden severe headache, shortness of breath, vision or speech disturbance, weakness or numbness of an extremity, loss of coordination, pain in chest, groin, or leg. Estrogen therapy should be noted on specimens.

PATIENT/FAMILY TEACHING

Importance of medical supervision. Avoid smoking due to increased risk of heart attack or blood clots. Do not take other medications w/o physician approval. Teach how to perform Homan's test, signs and symptoms of blood clots (report these to physician immediately). Notify physician of vaginal discharge or bleeding, difficulty or discomfort w/urination, other symptoms. Teach female patients to perform breast self-exam. Cyclic treatment of atrophic vaginitis may take several years. Avoid exposure to sun or ultraviolet light. Check weight daily; report weekly gain of 5 lbs or more. Use nonhormonal contraceptive or inform physician if suspect pregnancy. Libido improves, gynecomastia is reduced when medication stopped.

diflunisal

dye-**flew**-neh-sol
(Dolobid)

CANADIAN AVAILABILITY
Apo-Diflunisal, Dolobid, Novo-Diflunisal

PREGNANCY CATEGORY C
(D if used in third trimester or near delivery)

CLASSIFICATION

Nonsteroidal anti-inflammatory

AVAILABILITY (Rx)

Tablets: 250 mg, 500 mg

PHARMACODYNAMICS

	ONSET	PEAK	DURATION
Oral	1 hr	2–3 hrs	—

PHARMACOKINETICS

Absorption: Completely absorbed from GI tract. Widely distributed. **Metabolism:** Metabolized in liver. **Excretion:** Primarily excreted in urine. **Half-life:** 8–12 hrs.

ACTION / *THERAPEUTIC EFFECT*

Inhibits prostaglandin synthesis, reducing inflammatory response and intensity of pain stimulus reaching sensory nerve endings, *producing analgesic and anti-inflammatory effect.*

USES / *UNLABELED*

Treatment of acute or long-term mild to moderate pain associated w/acute and/or chronic rheumatoid arthritis, osteoarthritis. *Treatment of psoriatic arthritis, vascular headache.*

ADMINISTRATION

ORAL:

- May give w/water, milk, or meals.
- Do not crush or break film-coated tablets.

INDICATIONS/ROUTES/DOSAGE

Mild to moderate pain:
Oral: Adults, elderly: Initially, 0.5–1 g, then 250–500 mg q8–12h.

Rheumatoid arthritis, osteoarthritis:
Oral: Adults, elderly: 0.5–1 g/day in 2 divided doses.

CONTRAINDICATIONS

Nasal polyps associated w/bronchospasm induced by aspirin, history of hypersensitivity to aspirin or NSAIDs, bone marrow depression, blood dyscrasias.

CAUTIONS

History of inflammatory or ulcerative disease of GI tract (e.g., peptic ulcer, Crohn's disease), hemophilia or other bleeding problems, impaired renal/liver function, stomatitis.

INTERACTIONS

DRUG: May increase effects of ***oral anticoagulants, heparin, thrombolytics.*** May decrease effect of ***antihypertensives, diuretics. Salicylates, aspirin*** may increase risk of GI side effects, bleeding. ***Bone marrow depressants*** may increase risk of hematologic reactions. May increase concentration, toxicity of ***lithium.*** May increase ***methotrexate*** toxicity. ***Probenecid*** may increase concentration. HERBAL: Feverfew, ginkgo may increase risk of bleeding. FOOD: None significant. ALTERED LAB VALUES: May increase serum transaminase activity. May decrease uric acid.

SIDE EFFECTS

FREQUENT (3–9%): Skin rash, headache, abdominal pain/discomfort, diarrhea, nausea, indigestion. OCCASIONAL (1–3%): Ringing in ears, dizziness, drowsiness, insomnia, unusual weakness, constipation, bloated, vomiting, dry, sore mouth. RARE (<1%): Confusion, depression, itching, GI bleeding, gastritis.

ADVERSE REACTIONS/TOXIC EFFECTS

Overdosage may produce drowsiness, vomiting, nausea, diarrhea, hyperventilation, tachycardia, sweating, stupor, coma. Peptic ulcer, GI bleeding, gastritis, severe hepatic reaction (cholestasis, jaundice) occur rarely. Nephrotoxicity (dysuria, hematuria, proteinuria, nephrotic syndrome) and severe hypersensitivity reaction (bronchospasm, angiofacial edema) occur rarely.

PATIENT CONSIDERATIONS

Baseline Assessment

Assess onset, type, location, and duration of pain or inflammation. Inspect appearance of affected joints for immobility, deformities, and skin condition.

Intervention/Evaluation

Monitor for nausea, dyspepsia. Assess skin for evidence of rash. Monitor pattern of daily bowel activity and stool consistency. Evaluate for therapeutic response: relief of pain, stiffness, swelling, increase in joint mobility, reduced joint tenderness, improved grip strength.

Patient/Family Teaching

Swallow tablet whole; do not crush or chew. If GI upset occurs, take w/food, milk. Avoid aspirin, alcohol during therapy (increases risk of GI bleeding). Report GI distress, headache, rash.

---

digoxin

di-**jox**-in

(Lanoxin, Lanoxicaps)

CANADIAN AVAILABILITY

Lanoxin

PREGNANCY CATEGORY C

CLASSIFICATION

Antiarrhythmic, cardiotonic

AVAILABILITY (Rx)

Tablets: 0.125 mg, 0.25 mg, 0.5 mg. **Capsules:** 0.05 mg, 0.1 mg, 0.2 mg. **Elixir:** 0.05 mg/ml. **Injection:** 0.25 mg/ml, 0.1 mg/ml.

PHARMACOKINETICS

Absorption: Readily absorbed from GI tract. Widely distributed. **Metabolism:** Partially metabolized in liver. **Excretion:** Primarily excreted in urine. **Half-life:** 36–48 hrs (increased in decreased renal function, elderly).

ACTION/*THERAPEUTIC EFFECT*

Direct action on cardiac muscle, conduction system. Decreases conduction rate through SA, AV node. *Increases force, velocity of myocardial contraction.*

USES

Prophylactic management and treatment of CHF, control of ventricular rate in pts w/atrial fibrillation. Treatment and prevention of recurrent paroxysmal atrial tachycardia.

ADMINISTRATION

Note: IM rarely used (produces severe local irritation, erratic absorption). If no other route possible, give deep into muscle followed by massage. Give no more than 2 ml at any one site.

ORAL:

- May be given w/o regard to meals.
- Tablets may be crushed.

IV:

- May give undiluted or dilute w/at least a 4-fold volume of sterile water for injection, or 5% dextrose (less than this may cause a precipitate). Use immediately.
- Give IV slowly over at least 5 min.

INDICATIONS/ROUTES/DOSAGE

Note: Adjust dose in elderly, pts w/renal dysfunction. Larger doses often required for adequate control of ventricular rate in pts w/atrial fibrillation or flutter. Administer loading dosage in several doses at 4–8 hr intervals.

USUAL DOSAGE FOR ADULTS:

Rapid loading dosage:
IV: Adults, elderly: 0.6–1 mg.

Oral: Adults, elderly: 0.75–1.25 mg.

Maintenance dosage:
Oral/IV: Adults, elderly: 0.125–0.375 mg/day.

USUAL DOSAGE FOR CHILDREN:

Rapid loading dosage:
IV: Children (>10 yrs): 8–12 mcg/kg; ***(5–10 yrs):*** 15–30 mcg/kg; ***(2–5 yrs):*** 25–35 mcg/kg; ***(1–24 mos):*** 30–50 mcg/kg; ***(Full term):*** 20–30 mcg/kg; ***(Premature):*** 15–25 mcg/kg.

Oral: Children (>10 yrs): 10–15 mcg/kg; ***(5–10 yrs):*** 20–35 mcg/kg; ***(2–5 yrs):*** 30–40 mcg/kg; ***(1–24 mos):*** 35–60 mcg/kg; ***(Full term):*** 25–35 mcg/kg; ***(Premature):*** 20–30 mcg/kg.

Maintenance dosage:
Oral/IV: Children: 25–35% loading dose (20–30% for premature).

CONTRAINDICATIONS

Ventricular fibrillation, ventricular tachycardia unrelated to CHF.

CAUTIONS

Impaired renal function, impaired hepatic function, hypokalemia, advanced cardiac disease, acute myocardial infarction, incomplete AV block, cor pulmonale, hypothyroidism, pulmonary disease.

INTERACTIONS

DRUG: *Glucocorticoids, amphotericin, potassium-depleting diuretics* may increase toxicity (due to hypokalemia). ***Amiodarone*** may increase concentration, toxicity; additive effect on SA, AV nodes. ***Antiarrhythmics, parenteral calcium, sympathomimetics*** may increase risk of arrhythmias. ***Antidiarrheals, cholestyramine, colestipol, sucralfate*** may decrease absorption. ***Diltiazem, fluoxetine, verapamil, quinidine*** may increase concentration. ***Parenteral magnesium*** may cause conduction changes, heart block. **HERBAL:** Siberian ginseng may increase concentration; Ma Huang (Ephedra) may cause arrhythmias. **FOOD:** None significant. **ALTERED LAB VALUES:** None significant.

SIDE EFFECTS

None significant; however, there is a very narrow margin of safety between a therapeutic and toxic result. See Adverse Reactions/Toxic Effects.

ADVERSE REACTIONS/TOXIC EFFECTS

The most common early manifestations of toxicity are GI disturbances (anorexia, nausea, vomiting) and neurologic abnormalities (fatigue, headache, depression, weakness, drowsiness, confusion, nightmares). Facial pain, personality change, ocular disturbances (photophobia, light flashes, halos around bright objects, yellow or green color perception) may be noted.

PATIENT CONSIDERATIONS

BASELINE ASSESSMENT

Assess apical radial pulse for 60 sec (30 sec if on maintenance therapy). If pulse is 60/min or below (70/min or below for children), withhold drug and contact physician. Blood samples are best taken 6–8 hrs after dose or just prior to next dose.

INTERVENTION/EVALUATION

Monitor pulse for bradycardia, EKG for arrhythmias for 1–2 hrs after administration (excessive slowing of pulse may be a first clinical sign of toxicity). Assess for GI disturbances, neurologic abnormalities (signs of toxicity) q2–4h during digitalization (daily during maintenance). Monitor serum potassium, magnesium levels. Monitor for therapeutic plasma level (0.5–2.0 ng/ml).

PATIENT/FAMILY TEACHING

Importance of follow-up visits, tests. Teach pt to take pulse correctly and to report pulse below 60/min (or as indicated by physician). Assure pt understands signs of toxicity and need to notify physician if any occur. Wear/carry identification of digoxin therapy and inform dentist or other physician of taking digoxin. Take medication as directed; do not increase or skip doses. Do not take OTC medications w/o consulting physician. Chronic therapy may produce mammary gland enlargement in women but is reversible when drug is withdrawn.

digoxin immune FAB

(Digibind)

CANADIAN AVAILABILITY

Digibind

PREGNANCY CATEGORY C

CLASSIFICATION

Antidote

AVAILABILITY (Rx)

Powder for Injection: 38 mg vial

PHARMACODYNAMICS

	ONSET	PEAK	DURATION
IV	30 min	—	3–4 days

PHARMACOKINETICS

Widely distributed into extracellular space. **Excretion:** Excreted in urine. **Half-life:** 15–20 hrs.

ACTION/*THERAPEUTIC EFFECT*

Acts in extracellular space. Binds molecules of digoxin, *making digoxin unavailable for binding at its site of action on cells in the body.*

USES

Treatment of potentially life-threatening digoxin intoxication.

STORAGE/HANDLING

Refrigerate vials. After reconstitution, stable for 4 hrs if refrigerated. Use immediately after reconstitution.

ADMINISTRATION

IV:

- Reconstitute each 38 mg vial w/4 ml sterile water for injection to provide a concentration of 9.5 mg/ml.
- Further dilute w/50 ml 0.9% NaCl and infuse over 30 min (recommended that solution be infused through a 0.22 micron filter).
- If cardiac arrest imminent, may give IV push.

INDICATIONS/ROUTES/DOSAGE

Dosage varies according to amount of digoxin to be neutralized. Refer to manufacturer's dosing guidelines.

CONTRAINDICATIONS

None significant.

CAUTIONS

Impaired cardiac, renal function.

INTERACTIONS

DRUG: None significant. **HERBAL:** None known. **FOOD:** None significant. **ALTERED LAB VALUES:** May alter potassium concentration. Serum digoxin concentration may increase precipitously and persist for up to 1 wk (until FAB/digoxin complex is eliminated from body).

SIDE EFFECTS

None significant.

ADVERSE REACTIONS/TOXIC EFFECTS

As result of digitalis intoxication, hyperkalemia may present (diarrhea, paresthesia of extremities, heaviness of legs, decreased B/P, cold skin, grayish pallor, hypotension, mental confusion, irritability, flaccid paralysis, tented T waves, widening QRS, ST depression). When effect of digitalis is reversed, hypokalemia may develop rapidly (muscle cramping, nausea, vomiting, hypoactive bowel sounds, abdominal distension, difficulty breathing, postural hypotension). Rarely, low cardiac output, CHF may occur.

PATIENT CONSIDERATIONS

BASELINE ASSESSMENT

Obtain serum digoxin level before administering drug. If drawn <6 hrs before last digoxin dose, serum digoxin level may be unreliable. Those w/impaired

renal function may require >1 wk before serum digoxin assay is reliable. Assess baseline electrolytes, particularly potassium levels. Assess muscle strength, mental status. Note skin temperature, moisture. Obtain baseline weight. Initiate I&O.

INTERVENTION/EVALUATION

Closely monitor temperature, B/P, EKG, and potassium serum level during and after drug is administered. Watch for changes from initial assessment (hypokalemia may result in muscle strength changes, tremor, muscle cramps, change in mental status, cardiac arrhythmias; hyponatremia may result in confusion, thirst, cold/clammy skin).

diltiazem hydrochloride

dill-**tie**-ah-zem
(Cardizem, Cardizem CD, Dilacor XR, Tiazac)

FIXED-COMBINATION(S)
W/enalapril, an ACE inhibitor **(Teczem)**

CANADIAN AVAILABILITY
Apo-Diltiaz, Cardizem, Novo-Diltiazem, Tiazac

PREGNANCY CATEGORY C

CLASSIFICATION

Calcium channel blocker

AVAILABILITY (Rx)

Tablets: 30 mg, 60 mg, 90 mg, 120 mg. **Capsules (sustained-release):** 60 mg, 90 mg, 120 mg, 180 mg, 240 mg, 300 mg, 360 mg. **Injection:** 5 mg/ml vials, 100 mg Monovial.

PHARMACODYNAMICS

	ONSET	PEAK	DURATION
Oral	30–60 min	—	—

PHARMACOKINETICS

Absorption: Well absorbed from GI tract. **Metabolism:** Undergoes first-pass metabolism in liver. Metabolized in liver to active metabolite. **Excretion:** Primarily excreted in urine. Not removed by hemodialysis. **Half-life:** 3–8 hrs.

ACTION/*THERAPEUTIC EFFECT*

Inhibits calcium movement across cell membranes of cardiac and vascular smooth muscle (dilates coronary arteries, peripheral arteries/arterioles); *decreases heart rate, myocardial contractility, slows SA and AV conduction. Decreases total peripheral vascular resistance by vasodilation.*

USES

Oral: Treatment of angina due to coronary artery spasm (Prinzmetal's variant angina), chronic stable angina (effort-associated angina). ***Extended-release:*** Treatment of essential hypertension, angina. ***Parenteral:*** Temporary control of rapid ventricular rate in atrial fibrillation/flutter. Rapid conversion of PSVT to normal sinus rhythm.

ADMINISTRATION

ORAL:

- Give before meals and at bedtime.
- Tablets may be crushed.
- Do not crush sustained-release capsules.

IV:

- Add 125 mg to 100 ml 5% dextrose, 0.9% NaCl, or 5% dextrose/0.45% NaCl to provide a concentration of 1 mg/ml. Add 250 mg to 250 or 500 ml diluent to provide a concentration of 0.83 mg/ml or 0.45 mg/ml, respectively.

- After dilution, stable for 24 hrs.
- Infuse per dilution/rate chart provided by manufacturer.

INDICATIONS/ROUTES/DOSAGE

Angina:
Oral: Adults, elderly: Initially, 30 mg 4 times/day. Increase up to 180–360 mg/day in 3–4 divided doses at 1–2 day intervals.

(CD capsules): Adults, elderly: Initially, 120–180 mg/day; titrate over 7–14 days. *Range:* Up to 480 mg/day.

Essential hypertension:
Oral (Extended-release): Adults, elderly: Initially, 60–120 mg 2 times/day.

(CD capsules): Adults, elderly: Initially, 180–240 mg/day. *Range:* 240–360 mg in 2 divided doses.

(Dilacor XR): Adults, elderly: Initially, 180–240 mg/day. *Range:* 180–480 mg/day.

Usual parenteral dosage:
IV Push: Adults, elderly: Initially, 0.25 mg/kg actual body weight over 2 min. May repeat in 15 min at dose of 0.35 mg/kg actual body weight. Subsequent doses individualized.

IV Infusion: Adults, elderly: After initial bolus injection, 5–10 mg/ hr, may increase at 5 mg/hr up to 15 mg/hr. Maintain over 24 hrs.

Note: Refer to manufacturer's information for dose concentration/infusion rates.

CONTRAINDICATIONS

Sick-sinus syndrome/second- or third-degree AV block (except in presence of pacemaker), severe hypotension (<90 mm Hg, systolic), acute MI, pulmonary congestion.

CAUTIONS

Impaired renal/hepatic function, CHF.

INTERACTIONS

DRUG: ***Beta blockers*** may have additive effect. May increase ***digoxin*** concentration. ***Procainamide, quinidine*** may increase risk of QT interval prolongation. ***Carbamazepine, quinidine, theophylline*** may increase concentration, toxicity. **HERBAL:** None known. **FOOD:** None significant. **ALTERED LAB VALUES:** PR interval may be increased.

SIDE EFFECTS

FREQUENT (5–10%): Dizziness, lightheadedness, headache, peripheral edema, AV block, bradycardia. **OCCASIONAL (1–5%):** Shakiness, somnolence, asthenia, insomnia, nausea, constipation, abdominal discomfort, altered EKG, rash, flushing, increased urination. **RARE (<1%):** Altered sleep, nervousness, psychiatric disturbances (e.g., depression), ringing in ears, tremors, diarrhea, vomiting, dry mouth.

ADVERSE REACTIONS/TOXIC EFFECTS

Abrupt withdrawal may increase frequency/duration of angina. CHF, second- and third-degree AV block occur rarely. Overdosage produces nausea, drowsiness, confusion, slurred speech, profound bradycardia.

PATIENT CONSIDERATIONS

BASELINE ASSESSMENT

Concurrent therapy of sublingual nitroglycerin may be used

for relief of anginal pain. Record onset, type (sharp, dull, squeezing), radiation, location, intensity, and duration of anginal pain, and precipitating factors (exertion, emotional stress). Assess baseline renal/liver function tests. Assess B/P, apical pulse immediately before drug is administered.

INTERVENTION/EVALUATION

Assist w/ambulation if dizziness occurs. Assess for peripheral edema behind medial malleolus (sacral area in bedridden patients). Monitor pulse rate for bradycardia. Question for asthenia, headache.

PATIENT/FAMILY TEACHING

Do not abruptly discontinue medication. Compliance w/therapy regimen is essential to control anginal pain. To avoid hypotensive effect rise slowly from lying to sitting position, wait momentarily before standing. Avoid tasks that require alertness, motor skills until response to drug is established. Contact physician/nurse if irregular heartbeat, shortness of breath, pronounced dizziness, nausea, or constipation occurs.

dimenhydrinate

(Dramamine)

See Classification section under: Antihistamines

dinoprostone

dye-noe-**pros**-tone

(Cervidil, Prepidil Gel, Prostaglandin E_2, Prostin E_2)

CANADIAN AVAILABILITY

Cervidil, Prepidil Gel, Prostin E_2

PREGNANCY CATEGORY C

CLASSIFICATION

Prostaglandin

AVAILABILITY (Rx)

Vaginal Suppository: 20 mg. **Vaginal Gel:** 0.5 mg (Prepidil). **Vaginal Inserts:** 10 mg (Cervidil).

PHARMACOKINETICS

Metabolism: Undergoes rapid enzymatic deactivation primarily in maternal lungs. **Excretion:** Primarily excreted in urine.

ACTION/*THERAPEUTIC EFFECT*

Direct action on myometrium. Direct softening, dilation effect on cervix. *Stimulates myometrial contractions in gravid uterus.*

USES/*UNLABELED*

Suppository: To induce abortion from the 12th wk of pregnancy through the second trimester; to evacuate uterine contents in missed abortion or intrauterine fetal death up to 28 wks gestational age (as calculated from the first day of the last normal menstrual period), benign hydatidiform mole. ***Gel:*** Ripening of unfavorable cervix in pregnant women at or near term w/medical or obstetrical need for labor induction. ***Suppository:*** *Treatment of postpartum/postabortion hemorrhage, induction of labor at or near term.* ***Gel:*** *Induction of labor at or near term.*

STORAGE/HANDLING

Suppository: Keep frozen (<4°F); bring to room temperature just prior to use. ***Gel:*** Refrigerate.

ADMINISTRATION

INTRAVAGINAL (SUPPOSITORY):

- Administer only in hospital setting w/emergency equipment available.
- Warm suppository to room temperature before removing foil wrapper.
- Avoid skin contact because of risk of absorption.
- Insert high in vagina.
- Pt should remain supine for 10 min after administration.

INTRACERVICAL (GEL):

- Use caution in handling, prevent skin contact. Wash hands thoroughly w/soap and water after administration.
- Bring to room temperature just before use (avoid forcing the warming process).
- Assemble dosing apparatus as described in manufacturer insert.
- Have pt in dorsal position w/cervix visualized using a speculum.
- Introduce gel into cervical canal just below level of internal os.
- Have pt remain in supine position at least 15–30 min (minimizes leakage from cervical canal).

INDICATIONS/ROUTES/DOSAGE

Abortifacient:
Intravaginal: Adults: 20 mg (one suppository) high into vagina. May repeat at 3–5 hr intervals until abortion occurs. Do not administer >2 days.

Ripening of unfavorable cervix:
Intracervical: (Prepidil): Adults: Initially, 0.5 mg (2.5 ml); if no cervical/uterine response, may repeat 0.5 mg dose in 6 hrs. ***Maximum:*** 1.5 mg (7.5 ml) for a 24 hr period. *(Cervidil): Adults:* 10 mg over 12 hr period. Remove upon onset of active labor or 12 hrs after insertion.

CONTRAINDICATIONS

Hypersensitivity to dinoprostone or other prostaglandins; acute pelvic inflammatory disease; active cardiac, renal, hepatic, or pulmonary disease; fetal malpresentation or significant cephalopelvic disproportion.

CAUTIONS

Cervicitis, infected endocervical lesions or acute vaginitis, history of asthma, hypo/hypertension, anemia, jaundice, diabetes, epilepsy, uterine fibroids, compromised (scarred) uterus, cardiovascular, renal, or hepatic disease.

INTERACTIONS

DRUG: *Oxytocics* may cause uterine hypertonus, possibly causing uterine rupture or cervical laceration. **HERBAL:** None known. **FOOD:** None significant. **ALTERED LAB VALUES:** None significant.

SIDE EFFECTS

FREQUENT: Abdominal/stomach cramps, diarrhea, fever, nausea, vomiting. **OCCASIONAL:** Headache, chills/shivering, hives, shortness of breath, wheezing, bradycardia, bronchoconstriction, increased uterine pain accompanying abortion, peripheral vasoconstriction. **RARE:** Flushing, ileus, vulvae edema.

ADVERSE REACTIONS/TOXIC EFFECTS

Excessive dosage may cause uterine hypertonicity w/spasm and tetanic contraction, leading to cervical laceration/perforation, uterine rupture or hemorrhage.

PATIENT CONSIDERATIONS

BASELINE ASSESSMENT

Suppository
Question for hypersensitivity to dinoprostone or other prostaglandins. Establish baseline B/P, temperature, respirations, pulse. Obtain orders for antiemetics and antidiarrheals, meperidine or other pain medication for abdominal cramps. Assess any uterine activity or vaginal bleeding.

Gel
Question pt regarding conditions where prolonged uterine contractions are inappropriate. Assess Bishop score. Assess degree of effacement (determines size of shielded endocervical catheter).

INTERVENTION/EVALUATION

Suppository
Check strength, duration, and frequency of contractions and monitor vital signs q15min until stable, then hourly until abortion complete. Check resting uterine tone. Administer medications for relief of GI effects if indicated, abdominal cramps. Provide emotional support as necessary.

Gel
Monitor uterine activity (onset of uterine contractions), fetal status (heart rate), character of cervix (dilation, effacement). Have pt remain recumbent 12 hrs after application w/continuous electronic monitoring of fetal heart rate and uterine activity. Record maternal vital signs at least hourly in presence of uterine activity. Reassess Bishop score.

PATIENT/FAMILY TEACHING

Suppository
Report fever, chills, foul smelling/increased vaginal discharge, uterine cramps, or pain promptly.

diphenhydramine hydrochloride

dye-phen-**high**-dra-meen
(Benadryl)

FIXED-COMBINATION(S)
W/calamine, an astringent, and camphor, a counterirritant **(Caladryl)**

CANADIAN AVAILABILITY
Allerdryl, Benadryl, Nytol

PREGNANCY CATEGORY B

CLASSIFICATION

Antihistamine

AVAILABILITY (OTC)

Capsules: 25 mg, 50 mg. **Tablets:** 25 mg, 50 mg. **Elixir:** 12.5 mg/5 ml. **Injection (Rx):** 10 mg/ml, 50 mg/ml.

PHARMACODYNAMICS

	ONSET	PEAK	DURATION
Oral			
	15–30 min	1–4 hrs	4–6 hrs
IM/IV			
	<15 min	1–4 hrs	4–6 hrs

PHARMACOKINETICS

Absorption: Well absorbed following oral, parenteral administration. Widely distributed. **Metabolism:** Metabolized in liver. **Excretion:** Primarily excreted in urine. **Half-life:** 1–4 hrs.

ACTION/ *THERAPEUTIC EFFECT*

Competes w/histamine at histaminic receptor sites, *resulting in anticholinergic, antipruritic, antitussive, antiemetic effects.* Inhibits central acetylcholine, *producing antidyskinetic, sedative effect.*

USES

Treatment of allergic reactions, parkinsonism, prevention and treatment of nausea, vomiting, vertigo due to motion sickness; antitussive, short-term management of insomnia. Topical form used for relief of pruritus, insect bites, skin irritations.

STORAGE/HANDLING

Store oral, elixir, topical, parenteral forms at room temperature. Powder slowly darkens on exposure to light (does not alter effectiveness).

ADMINISTRATION

ORAL:
- Give w/o regard to meals.
- Scored tablets may be crushed.
- Do not crush capsules or film-coated tablets.

IM:
- Give deep IM into large muscle mass.

IV:
- May be given undiluted.
- Give IV injection over at least 1 min.

INDICATIONS/ROUTES/DOSAGE

Allergic reaction, parkinsonism, treatment of motion sickness:
Oral: Adults: 25–50 mg 3–4 times/day q4–6h. ***Elderly:*** Initially, 25 mg 2–3 times/day. May increase as needed. ***Children >20 lbs:*** 5 mg/kg/24 hrs in divided doses 4 times/day.
IM/IV: Adults: 10–50 mg. ***Maximum daily dose:*** 400 mg. ***Children >20 lbs:*** 5 mg/kg/24 hrs 4 times/day.

Prevention of motion sickness:
Oral: Adults: 25–50 mg 30 min before exposure to motion. Give subsequent doses q4–6h.

Nighttime sleep aid:
Oral: Adults: 50 mg 20 min before bedtime.

Cough:
Oral: Adults: 25 mg q4h. ***Syrup: Children:*** 6.25–12.5 mg q4h.

Pruritus relief:
Topical: Adults: Apply to affected area 3–4 times/day.

CONTRAINDICATIONS

Acute asthmatic attack, those receiving MAO inhibitors.

CAUTIONS

Narrow-angle glaucoma, peptic ulcer, prostatic hypertrophy, pyloroduodenal or bladder neck obstruction, asthma, COPD, increased intraocular pressure, cardiovascular disease, hyperthyroidism, hypertension, seizure disorders.

INTERACTIONS

DRUG: ***Alcohol, CNS depressants*** may increase CNS depressant effects. ***MAO inhibitors*** may increase anticholinergic, CNS depressant effects. ***Anticholinergics*** may increase anticholinergic effects. **HERBAL:** None known. **FOOD:** None significant. **ALTERED LAB VALUES:** May suppress wheal and flare reactions to antigen skin testing unless antihistamines are discontinued 4 days prior to testing.

SIDE EFECTS

FREQUENT: Drowsiness, dizziness, muscular weakness, hypotension, dry mouth/nose/throat/lips, urinary retention, thickening of bronchial secretions. Sedation, dizziness, hypotension more likely noted in elderly. **OCCASIONAL:** Epigastric distress, flushing, visual disturbances, hearing disturbances, paresthesia, sweating, chills.

ADVERSE REACTIONS/TOXIC EFFECTS

Children may experience dominant paradoxical reactions (restlessness, insomnia, euphoria, nervousness, tremors). Overdosage in children may result in hallucinations, convulsions, death. Hypersensitivity reaction (eczema, pruritus, rash, cardiac disturbances, photosensitivity) may occur. Overdosage may vary from CNS depression (sedation, apnea, cardiovascular collapse, death) to severe paradoxical reaction (hallucinations, tremor, seizures).

PATIENT CONSIDERATIONS

Baseline Assessment

If pt is undergoing allergic reaction, obtain history of recently ingested foods, drugs, environmental exposure, recent emotional stress. Monitor rate, depth, rhythm, type of respiration, and quality and rate of pulse. Assess lung sounds for rhonchi, wheezing, rales.

Intervention/Evaluation

Monitor B/P, especially in elderly (increased risk of hypotension). Monitor children closely for paradoxical reaction.

Patient/Family Teaching

Tolerance to antihistaminic effect generally does not occur; tolerance to sedative effect may occur. Avoid tasks that require alertness, motor skills until response to drug is established. Dry mouth, drowsiness, dizziness may be an expected response of drug. Avoid alcoholic beverages during antihistamine therapy. Sugarless gum, sips of tepid water may relieve dry mouth. Coffee or tea may help reduce drowsiness.

diphenoxylate hydrochloride w/atropine sulfate

dye-pen-**ox**-e-late
(Lofene, Logen, Lomanate, Lomotil)

CANADIAN AVAILABILITY
Lomotil

PREGNANCY CATEGORY C

CLASSIFICATION

Antidiarrheal

AVAILABILITY (Rx)

Tablets: 2.5 mg. **Liquid:** 2.5 mg/5 ml.

PHARMACOKINETICS

Absorption: Well absorbed from GI tract. **Metabolism:** Metabolized in liver to active metabolite. **Excretion:** Primarily eliminated in feces. **Half-life:** 2.5 hrs; metabolite: 12–24 hrs.

ACTION/*THERAPEUTIC EFFECT*

Acts locally, centrally *to reduce intestinal motility.*

USES

Adjunctive treatment of acute, chronic diarrhea.

ADMINISTRATION

ORAL:

- Give w/o regard to meals. If GI irritation occurs, give w/food or meals.
- Use liquid for children under 12 yrs (use dropper for administration of liquids).

INDICATIONS/ROUTES/DOSAGE

Antidiarrheal:

Oral: Adults, elderly: Initially, 2.5 mg 4 times/day. ***Maintenance:*** 2.5 mg 2–3 times/day. ***Children:*** Initially, 0.3–0.4 mg/kg/day in 4 divided doses. ***Maintenance:*** As low as 1/4 initial dose (0.075–0.1 mg/kg/day in divided doses).

CONTRAINDICATIONS

Obstructive jaundice, diarrhea associated w/pseudomembranous enterocolitis due to broad-spectrum antibiotics or w/organisms that invade intestinal mucosa (*E. coli, Shigella, Salmonella*), acute ulcerative colitis (may produce toxic megacolon).

CAUTIONS

Advanced hepatorenal disease, abnormal liver function.

INTERACTIONS

DRUG: ***Alcohol, CNS depressants*** may increase effect. ***Anticholinergics*** may increase effect of atropine. ***MAO inhibitors*** may precipitate hypertensive crisis. **HERBAL:** None known. **FOOD:** None significant. **ALTERED LAB VALUES:** May increase amylase.

SIDE EFFECTS

OCCASIONAL: Paralytic ileus or toxic megacolon (constipation, decreased appetite, severe stomach pain w/nausea/vomiting), blurred vision, dry mouth, dizziness, drowsiness, depression, confusion, headache, numbness of hands/feet, rash, itching, swelling of gums. **RARE:** Increased sweating, muscle or stomach cramps, nausea, vomiting, trembling.

ADVERSE REACTIONS/TOXIC EFFECTS

Dehydration may predispose to toxicity. Paralytic ileus, toxic megacolon (constipation, decreased appetite, stomach pain w/nausea/vomiting) occurs rarely. Severe anticholinergic effects (severe drowsiness, hypotonic reflexes, hyperthermia) may result in severe respiratory depression, coma.

PATIENT CONSIDERATIONS

Baseline Assessment

Check baseline hydration status: skin turgor, mucous membranes for dryness, urinary status.

Intervention/Evaluation

Encourage adequate fluid intake. Assess bowel sounds for peristalsis. Monitor daily bowel activity, stool consistency (watery, loose, soft, semisolid, solid) and record time of evacuation. Assess for abdominal disturbances. Discontinue medication if abdominal distension occurs. Check I&O. Monitor for paradoxical reaction.

Patient/Family Teaching

Avoid tasks that require alertness, motor skills until response to drug is established. Do not ingest alcohol or barbiturates. Contact physician if fever, palpitations occur or diarrhea persists. Cola, unsalted crackers, dry toast may relieve nausea. Dry mouth may be relieved by sugarless gum, sips of tepid water.

dipivefrin

(Propine)

See Classification section under: Antiglaucoma agents

dipyridamole

die-pie-**rid**-ah-mole

(Persantine)

FIXED-COMBINATION(S)

W/aspirin, an antiplatelet, Aggrenox

CANADIAN AVAILABILITY

Apo-Dipyridamole, Novodipiradol, Persantine

PREGNANCY CATEGORY C

CLASSIFICATION

Antiplatelet

AVAILABILITY (Rx)

Tablets: 25 mg, 50 mg, 75 mg. **Injection:** 10 mg.

PHARMACOKINETICS

Absorption: Slow, variably absorbed from GI tract. Widely distributed. **Metabolism:** Metabolized in liver. **Excretion:** Primarily eliminated via biliary excretion. **Half-life:** 10–15 hrs.

ACTION/*THERAPEUTIC EFFECT*

Direct action on small vessels of coronary vascular bed, *increasing coronary blood flow, coronary sinus oxygen saturation.*

USES/*UNLABELED*

Adjunct to coumarin anticoagulant in prevention of postop thromboembolic complications of cardiac valve replacement. **IV use:** alternative to exercise in thallium myocardial perfusion imaging for evaluation of coronary artery disease. *Prophylaxis of myocardial reinfarction, treatment of transient ischemic attacks (TIAs).*

ADMINISTRATION

ORAL:

- Best taken on empty stomach w/full glass of water.

IV:

- Dilute to at least 1:2 ratio w/0.9% NaCl or 5% dextrose in water for total volume of 20–50 ml (undiluted may cause irritation).
- Infuse over 4 min.
- Inject thallium within 5 min after dipyridamole infusion.

INDICATIONS/ROUTES/DOSAGE

Prevention of thromboembolic disorders:

Oral: Adults, elderly: 75–100 mg 4 times/day in combination w/other medications.

Diagnostic:

IV: Adults, elderly (based on weight): 0.142 mg/kg/min infused over 4 min; doses >60 mg not needed for any pt.

CONTRAINDICATIONS

None significant.

CAUTIONS

Those w/hypotension.

INTERACTIONS

DRUG: May increase risk of bleeding w/ ***anticoagulants, heparin, thrombolytics, aspirin, salicylates.*** **HERBAL:** Feverfew, garlic, ginkgo may increase effect, risk of bleeding. **FOOD:** None significant. **ALTERED LAB VALUES:** None significant.

SIDE EFFECTS

FREQUENT (5–10%): Dizziness, GI irritation, diarrhea, nausea, cramping, vomiting, headache. OCCASIONAL (1–5%): Skin rash, itching, dyspnea, flushing, weakness.

ADVERSE REACTIONS/TOXIC EFFECTS

Overdosage produces peripheral vasodilation, resulting in hypotension.

PATIENT CONSIDERATIONS

Baseline Assessment

Assess chest pain, B/P, pulse. When used as antiplatelet, check hematologic levels.

Intervention/Evaluation

Assist w/ambulation if dizziness occurs. Monitor heart sounds by auscultation. Assess B/P for hypotension. Assess skin for flushing, rash.

Patient/Family Teaching

If nausea occurs, cola, unsalted crackers, or dry toast may relieve effect. Therapeutic response may not be achieved before 2–3 mos of continuous therapy.

dirithromycin

dih-**rith**-row-my-sin
(Dynabac)

PREGNANCY CATEGORY C

CLASSIFICATION

Antibiotic: Macrolide

AVAILABILITY (Rx)

Tablets, enteric coated: 250 mg

PHARMACOKINETICS

Absorption: Rapidly absorbed from GI tract. Widely distributed into tissues and within cells. **Excretion:** Eliminated primarily unchanged via biliary excretion. **Half-life:** 30–44 hrs.

ACTION / *THERAPEUTIC EFFECT*

Binds to ribosomal receptor sites of susceptible organisms, *inhibiting protein synthesis.*

USES

Treatment of mild to moderate infections of upper respiratory tract (pharyngitis, tonsillitis), acute bronchitis, chronic bronchitis, uncomplicated skin/skin structure infections, community-acquired pneumonia.

ADMINISTRATION

ORAL:

- Administer w/food or within an hour of having eaten (food increases absorption).
- Swallow whole (tablets not to be cut, crushed, or chewed).

INDICATIONS/ROUTES/DOSAGE

Pharyngitis/tonsillitis:
Oral: Adults, elderly, children ≥12 yrs: 500 mg once daily for 10 days.

Acute bronchitis, chronic bronchitis:
Oral: Adults, elderly, children ≥12 yrs: 500 mg once daily for 7 days.

Community-acquired pneumonia:
Oral: Adults, elderly, children ≥12 yrs: 500 mg once daily for 14 days.

Skin, skin structure infections:
Oral: Adults, elderly, children ≥12 yrs: 500 mg once daily for 7 days.

CONTRAINDICATIONS

Hypersensitivity to dirithromycin, erythromycins, any macrolide antibiotic, concurrent terfenadine therapy, electrolyte disturbances (may cause cardiac dysrhythmias), bacteremia.

CAUTIONS

Hepatic/renal dysfunction.

INTERACTIONS

DRUG: *H_2 antagonists* increase dirithromycin absorption. ***Aluminum/magnesium***-containing antacids may decrease concentration (give 1 hr before or 2 hrs after antacid). **HERBAL:** None known. **FOOD:** None significant. **ALTERED LAB VALUES:** May increase platelet count, potassium CPK, eosinophils, neutrophils. Decreases bicarbonate level.

SIDE EFFECTS

FREQUENT: Abdominal pain (10%), headache (9%), nausea, diarrhea (8%). **OCCASIONAL:** Vomiting, dyspepsia (3%), dizziness, nonspecific pain, asthenia (2%). **RARE:** Increased cough, flatulence, rash, dyspnea, pruritus/urticaria, insomnia.

ADVERSE REACTIONS/TOXIC EFFECTS

Superinfections, especially antibiotic-associated colitis (abdominal cramps, watery severe diarrhea, fever) may result from altered bacterial balance.

PATIENT CONSIDERATIONS

Baseline Assessment

Question pt for history of allergies to dirithromycin, erythromycins. Obtain specimens for culture, sensitivity before giving first dose (therapy may begin before results are known).

Intervention/Evaluation

Check for GI discomfort, nausea, headache, diarrhea. Determine pattern of bowel activity and stool consistency. Evaluate for superinfection: genital/anal pruritus, sore mouth or tongue, moderate to severe diarrhea.

Patient/Family Teaching

Continue therapy for full length of treatment. Doses should be evenly spaced. Take medication w/food or within an hour of having eaten.

disopyramide phosphate

dye-so-**peer**-ah-myd
(Norpace)

CANADIAN AVAILABILITY
Rythmodan

PREGNANCY CATEGORY C

CLASSIFICATION

Antiarrhythmic

AVAILABILITY (Rx)

Capsules: 100 mg, 150 mg. **Capsules (extended-release):** 100 mg, 150 mg.

PHARMACODYNAMICS

	ONSET	PEAK	DURATION
Oral			
	0.5–3.5 hrs	—	1.5–8.5 hrs

PHARMACOKINETICS

Absorption: Rapidly, completely absorbed from GI tract. **Metabolism:** Metabolized in liver. **Excretion:** Primarily excreted in urine. Removed by hemodialysis. **Half-life:** 7 hrs (increased in reduced renal function).

D

ACTION/*THERAPEUTIC EFFECT*

Prolongs refractory period by direct effect, decreasing myocardial excitability and conduction velocity. *Depresses myocardial contractility. Has anticholinergic, negative inotropic effects.*

USES/*UNLABELED*

Suppression and prevention of unifocal/multifocal premature ventricular contractions (ectopic), paired ventricular contractions (couplets), episodes of ventricular tachycardia. *Prophylaxis/treatment of supraventricular tachycardia.*

ADMINISTRATION

ORAL:

- May be given w/o regard to meals but best absorbed 1 hr before or 2 hrs after meals.
- Do not crush or break extended-release capsules.

INDICATIONS/ROUTES/DOSAGE

Usual dosage:
Oral: Adults, elderly >50 kg: 150 mg q6h (300 mg ql2h w/extended-release). ***Adults, elderly <50 kg:*** 100 mg q6h (200 mg q12h w/extended-release). ***Children 12–18 yrs:*** 6–15 mg/kg/day in divided doses q6h. ***Children 4–12 yrs:*** 10–15 mg/kg/day in divided doses q6h. ***Children 1–4 yrs:*** 10–20 mg/kg/day in divided doses q6h. ***Children <1 yr:*** 10–30 mg/kg/day in divided doses q6h.

Rapid control of arrhythmias:
Note: Do not use extended-release capsules.

Oral: Adults, elderly >50 kg: Initially, 300 mg, then 150 mg q6h.

Adults, elderly <50 kg: Initially, 200 mg, then 100 mg q6h.

Severe refractory arrhythmias:
Oral: Adults, elderly: Up to 400 mg q6h.

Dosage in renal impairment:
W/ or w/o loading dose of 150 mg:

CREATININE CLEARANCE	DOSAGE
>40 ml/min	100 mg q6h (extended-release 200 mg q12h)
30–40 ml/min	100 mg q8h
15–30 ml/min	100 mg q12h
<15 ml/min	100 mg q24h

Dosage in hepatic impairment:
100 mg q6h (200 mg q12h w/extended-release).

Dosage in cardiomyopathy, decompensated myocardium:
No loading dose; 100 mg q6–8h w/gradual dosage adjustments.

CONTRAINDICATIONS

Preexisting urinary retention, preexisting second- or third-degree AV block, cardiogenic shock, narrow-angle glaucoma, unless pt is undergoing cholinergic therapy.

CAUTIONS

CHF, myasthenia gravis, narrow-angle glaucoma, prostatic hypertrophy, sick-sinus syndrome (bradycardia/tachycardia), Wolff-Parkinson-White syndrome, bundle-branch block, impaired renal/hepatic function.

INTERACTIONS

DRUG: Other ***antiarrhythmics (e.g., propranolol, diltiazem, verapamil)*** may prolong conduction, decrease cardiac output. ***Pimozide*** may increase cardiac arrhythmias. **HERBAL:** None known. **FOOD:** None significant. **ALTERED LAB VALUES:** May decrease glucose. May cause EKG changes.

SIDE EFFECTS

FREQUENT (>9%): Dry mouth (32%), urinary hesitancy, constipation. OCCASIONAL (3–9%): Blurred vision, dry eyes, nose, throat, urinary retention, frequency, urgency, headache, dizziness, fatigue, nausea. RARE (1–3%): Impotence, hypotension, edema, increased weight, shortness of breath, syncope, chest pain, nervousness, diarrhea, vomiting, decreased appetite, rash, itching.

ADVERSE REACTIONS/TOXIC EFFECTS

May produce or aggravate CHF. May produce severe hypotension, compounded w/shortness of breath, chest pain, syncope (especially in those w/primary cardiomyopathy or in inadequately compensated CHF). Hepatic toxicity occurs rarely.

PATIENT CONSIDERATIONS

BASELINE ASSESSMENT

Assess baseline hepatic, renal function studies. Before giving medication, instruct pt to void (reduces risk of urinary retention).

INTERVENTION/EVALUATION

Monitor EKG for cardiac changes, particularly widening of QRS complex, prolongation of PR and QT intervals. Notify physician of any significant interval changes. Assess pattern of daily bowel activity, stool consistency. Monitor I&O (be alert to urinary retention). Assess for evidence of CHF (cough, dyspnea [particularly on exertion], rales at base of lungs, fatigue). Assess for edema directly behind medial malleolus in ambulatory pts, sacral area in bedridden pts (usually first areas showing impending edema). Assist w/ambulation if dizziness occurs. Monitor for therapeutic serum level (2–8 mcg/ml).

PATIENT/FAMILY TEACHING

Report shortness of breath, productive cough. Compliance w/therapy regimen is essential to control cardiac dysrhythmias. Do not use nasal decongestants, OTC cold preparations (stimulants) w/o physician approval. Restrict salt, alcohol intake. Sugarless gum, sips of tepid water may relieve dry mouth. Report visual disturbances, headache, dizziness.

---

disulfiram

dye-**sul**-fi-ram
(Antabuse)

CANADIAN AVAILABILITY
Antabuse

PREGNANCY CATEGORY C

CLASSIFICATION

Alcohol deterrent

AVAILABILITY (Rx)

Tablets: 250 mg, 500 mg

PHARMACOKINETICS

Absorption: Slowly absorbed from GI tract. **Metabolism:** Metabolized in liver. **Excretion:** Primarily excreted in urine. Up to 20% of dose remains in body for at least 1 wk.

ACTION/*THERAPEUTIC EFFECT*

Inhibits enzyme aldehyde dehydrogenase, responsible for breakdown of ethanol metabolite acetaldehyde. Increased acetaldehyde responsible for *disulfiram reaction after alcohol ingestion.*

USES

Adjunct in management of selected chronic alcoholic pts who want to remain in state of enforced sobriety.

ADMINISTRATION

ORAL:

- Scored tablets may be crushed.
- Give w/o regard to meals.

INDICATIONS/ROUTES/DOSAGE

Note: Pts must abstain from alcohol for at least 12 hrs before initial dose is administered.

Oral: Adults, elderly: Initially, administer maximum of 500 mg daily given as a single dose for 1–2 wks. ***Maintenance:*** 250 mg daily (normal range: 125–500 mg). Do not exceed maximum daily dose of 500 mg.

CONTRAINDICATIONS

Severe heart disease, psychosis.

CAUTIONS

Alcoholic disease.

INTERACTIONS

DRUG: ***Alcohol*** within 14 days results in disulfiram/alcohol reaction. ***Oral anticoagulant*** effect may be increased. May increase concentration, toxicity of ***phenytoin. Isoniazid*** may increase CNS effects. ***Metronidazole*** may increase toxicity. **HERBAL:** None known. **FOOD:** None significant. **ALTERED LAB VALUES:** May increase cholesterol concentrations. May decrease VMA concentrations.

SIDE EFFECTS

FREQUENT: Drowsiness. **OCCASIONAL:** Neurotoxicity, including optic neuritis (eye pain, change in vision), peripheral neuritis (numbness of hands/feet), mental changes, headache, impotence, metallic/garlic taste, skin rash, unusual tiredness. **RARE:** Encephalopathy (mental changes), liver toxicity (hepatitis).

ADVERSE REACTIONS/TOXIC EFFECTS

Disulfiram-alcohol reaction to ingestion of alcohol in any form: flushing/throbbing in head and neck, throbbing headache, nausea, copious vomiting, diaphoresis, dyspnea, hyperventilation, tachycardia, hypotension, marked uneasiness, vertigo, blurred vision, confusion. Can produce death.

PATIENT CONSIDERATIONS

Intervention/Evaluation

Do not give w/o pt's knowledge. Fully inform pt of consequences of alcohol ingestion. Therapy cannot be started until a minimum of 12 hrs has elapsed since pt's last ingestion of alcohol.

Patient/Family Teaching

Avoid cough syrups, vinegars, fluid extracts, elixirs because of their alcohol content. Even external application of liniments, shaving or body lotion may precipitate a crisis. Effects of medication may occur several days after discontinuance. Use caution driving, performing tasks requiring alertness.

dobutamine hydrochloride

do-**byew**-ta-meen

(Dobutrex)

CANADIAN AVAILABILITY
Dobutrex

PREGNANCY CATEGORY C

CLASSIFICATION

Sympathomimetic

AVAILABILITY (Rx)

Injection: 250 mg vial. **Infusion:** 500 mg/250 ml solution.

PHARMACODYNAMICS

	ONSET	PEAK	DURATION
IV	1–2 min	10 min	Length of infusion

PHARMACOKINETICS

Metabolism: Metabolized in liver. **Excretion:** Primarily excreted in urine. **Half-life:** 2 min.

ACTION/*THERAPEUTIC EFFECT*

Direct acting inotropic agent acting primarily on $beta_1$-adrenergic receptors, *enhancing myocardial contractility, stroke volume, cardiac output.* Decreases preload, afterload. Excessive doses *increase heart rate. Improves renal blood flow, urine output.*

USES

Prophylaxis/treatment of acute hypotension, shock (associated w/myocardial infarction, trauma, renal failure, cardiac decompensation, open heart surgery), treatment of low cardiac output, CHF.

STORAGE/HANDLING

Store at room temperature. Freezing produces crystallization. Pink discoloration of solution (due to oxidation) does not indicate loss of potency if used within recommended time period. Reconstituted, concentrated solution maintains potency for 6 hrs at room temperature, 48 hrs if refrigerated. Further diluted solutions for infusion must be used within 24 hrs.

ADMINISTRATION

Note: Correct hypovolemia w/volume expanders before dobutamine infusion. Those w/atrial fibrillation should be digitalized prior to infusion. Administer by IV infusion only.

IV:

- Dilute 250 mg ampule w/10 ml sterile water for injection or 5% dextrose for injection. Resulting solution: 25 mg/ml. Add additional 10 ml of diluent if not completely dissolved (resulting solution: 12.5 mg/ml).
- Dilute further to at least 50 ml w/5% dextrose, 0.9% NaCl, or sodium lactate injection before administration.
- Use infusion pump to control flow rate.
- Titrate dosage to individual response.

INDICATIONS/ROUTES/DOSAGE

Note: Dosage determined by pt response.

IV Infusion: Adults, elderly: 2.5–10 mcg/kg/min. Rarely, infusion rate up to 40 mcg/kg/min to increase cardiac output.

CONTRAINDICATIONS

Idiopathic hypertrophic subaortic stenosis, hypovolemic pts, sulfite sensitivity.

CAUTIONS

Atrial fibrillation, hypertension. Safety in children not established.

INTERACTIONS

DRUG: *Tricyclic antidepressants, MAO inhibitors, oxytocics* may increase effect (arrhythmias, hypertension), *beta blockers* may antagonize effects, *digoxin* may increase risk of arrhythmias, additional inotropic effect. **HERBAL:** None known. **FOOD:** None significant. ALTERED LAB VALUES: Decreases potassium serum levels.

SIDE EFFECTS

FREQUENT (>5%): Increased heart rate, blood pressure, hypotension, PVCs. OCCASIONAL (3–5%): Pain at injection site. RARE (1–3%): Nausea, headache, anginal pain, shortness of breath, fever.

ADVERSE REACTIONS/TOXIC EFFECTS

Overdosage may produce marked increase in heart rate (30 beats/min or greater), marked increase in systolic B/P (50 mm Hg or greater), anginal pain, premature ventricular beats.

PATIENT CONSIDERATIONS

Baseline Assessment

Pt must be on continuous cardiac monitoring. Determine weight (for dosage calculation). Obtain initial B/P, heart rate, and respirations.

Intervention/Evaluation

Continuously monitor for cardiac rate, arrhythmias. W/physician, establish parameters for adjusting rate or stopping infusion. Maintain accurate I&O; measure urine output frequently. Assess potassium levels and dobutamine plasma level (therapeutic range = 40–190 ng/ml). Check cardiac output. Monitor B/P continuously (hypertension greater risk in pts w/preexisting hypertension) and pulmonary wedge pressure or central venous pressure frequently. Immediately notify physician of decreased urine output, cardiac arrhythmias, significant increase in B/P or heart rate, and less commonly hypotension.

Patient/Family Teaching

Explain rationale for therapy. Report chest pain, discomfort at IV site.

---

docetaxel

(Taxotere)
See Classification section under: Cancer chemotherapy

---

docosanol

(Abreva)
See Supplement

---

docusate calcium

dock-cue-sate
(Pro-Cal-Sof, Surfak)

docusate potassium

(Dialose, Diocto-K, Kasof)

docusate sodium

(Colace, Doxinate, Modane Soft)

FIXED-COMBINATION(S)
W/casanthranol, a stimulant laxative **(Peri-colace)**; w/phenolphthalein, a laxative **(Correctol, Doxidan)**

CANADIAN AVAILABILITY
Colace, Surfak

PREGNANCY CATEGORY C

CLASSIFICATION

Laxative: Stool softener

AVAILABILITY (OTC)

Calcium: Capsules: 50 mg, 240 mg

Potassium: Capsules: 100 mg, 240 mg

Sodium: Tablets: 100 mg. **Capsules:** 50 mg, 100 mg, 240 mg, 250 mg. **Syrup:** 60 mg/15 ml, 50 mg/15 ml. **Liquid:** 150 mg/15 ml. **Solution:** 50 mg/ml.

PHARMACOKINETICS

Absorption: Minimal absorption from GI tract. Acts in small/large intestine. Results occur 1–2 days after first dose (may take 3–5 days).

ACTION/*THERAPEUTIC EFFECT*

Decreases surface film tension by mixing liquid and bowel contents, *increasing infiltration of liquid to form a softer stool.*

USES

Prophylaxis/treatment of constipation.

ADMINISTRATION

ORAL:

- Drink 6–8 glasses of water/day (aids stool softening).
- Give each dose w/glass of water or fruit juice.

INDICATIONS/ROUTES/DOSAGE

Stool Softener:

Calcium docusate:
Oral: Adults, elderly: 240 mg/day until evacuation. *Children >6 yrs:* 50–150 mg/day.

Potassium docusate:
Oral: Adults, elderly: 100–300 mg/day until evacuation. *Children >6 yrs:* 100 mg at bedtime.

Sodium docusate:
Oral: Adults, elderly: 50–500 mg/day. *Children 6–12 yrs:* 40–120 mg/day. *Children 3–6 yrs:* 20–60 mg/day. *Children <3 yrs:* 10–40 mg/day.

CONTRAINDICATIONS

Abdominal pain, nausea, vomiting, appendicitis.

CAUTIONS

None significant.

INTERACTIONS

DRUG: May increase absorption of ***mineral oil, danthron, phenolphthalein.*** **HERBAL:** None known. **FOOD:** None significant. **ALTERED LAB VALUES:** None significant.

SIDE EFFECTS

OCCASIONAL: Mild GI cramping, throat irritation (liquid preparation). **RARE:** Rash.

ADVERSE REACTIONS/TOXIC EFFECTS

None significant.

PATIENT CONSIDERATIONS

Intervention/Evaluation

Encourage adequate fluid intake. Assess bowel sounds for peristalsis. Monitor daily bowel activity and stool consistency (watery, loose, soft, semisolid, solid) and record time of evacuation.

Patient/Family Teaching

Institute measures to promote defecation: increase fluid intake, exercise, high-fiber diet.

---

dofetilade

(Tikosyn)
See Supplement

---

dolasetron

dole-**ah**-stron
(Anzemet)

CANADIAN AVAILABILITY
Anzemet

PREGNANCY CATEGORY B

CLASSIFICATION

Antiemetic

AVAILABILITY (Rx)

Tablets: 50 mg, 100 mg. **Injection:** 20 mg/ml.

PHARMACOKINETICS

Absorption: Oral form readily absorbed from GI tract. **Metabolism:** Metabolized in liver. **Excretion:** Primarily excreted in urine. **Half-life:** 7.5 hrs.

ACTION / *THERAPEUTIC EFFECT*

Exhibits selective 5-HT_3 receptor antagonism for *preventing nausea/vomiting associated w/cancer chemotherapy.* Action may be central (CTZ) or peripheral (vagus nerve terminal).

USES / *UNLABELED*

Prevention of nausea/vomiting associated with cancer chemotherapy, including high-dose cisplatin; prevention of postop nausea/vomiting. *Injection:* Treatment of postop nausea/vomiting. *Radiotherapy-induced nausea and vomiting.*

ADMINISTRATION

- Can be infused as rapidly as 100 mg/30 secs.
- May dilute in compatible IV solution (0.9% normal saline, D_5W, D_5W and 0.45% normal saline, D_5W and lactated Ringer's, lactated Ringer's, 10% mannitol injection) to 50 ml and infuse over a period of up to 15 min.
- For children, injection may be mixed in apple or apple-grape juice.

INDICATIONS / ROUTES / DOSAGES

Prevention of chemotherapy-induced nausea/vomiting:
IV: Adults, children (1–16 yrs): 1.8 mg/kg as a single dose 30 min before chemotherapy. ***Maximum:*** 100 mg for children.

Oral: Adults: 100 mg within 1 hr of chemotherapy. ***Children (2–16 yrs):*** 1.8 mg/kg within 1 hr before chemotherapy. ***Maximum:*** 100 mg.

Treatment/prevention of postop nausea/vomiting:
IV: Adults: 12.5 mg. ***Children (2–16 yrs):*** 0.35 mg/kg. ***Maximum:*** 12.5 mg. Give approximately 15 min before cessation of anesthesia or as soon as nausea/vomiting presents.

Oral: Adults: 100 mg. ***Children (2–16 yrs):*** 1.2 mg/kg. ***Maximum:*** 100 mg within 2 hrs of surgery.

CONTRAINDICATIONS

None significant.

CAUTIONS

Those who have or may have prolongation of cardiac conduction intervals, hypokalemia, hypomagnesemia, those taking diuretics with potential for inducing electrolyte disturbances, congenital QT syndrome, those taking antiarrhythmics that may lead to QT prolongation and cumulative high-dose anthracycline therapy.

INTERACTIONS

DRUG: None significant. **HERBAL:** None known. **FOOD:** None significant. **ALTERED LAB VALUES:** May alter liver function tests.

SIDE EFFECTS

FREQUENT (5–10%): Headache, diarrhea, fatigue. **OCCASIONAL (1–5%):** Fever, dizziness, tachycardia, dyspepsia.

ADVERSE REACTIONS/TOXIC EFFECTS

Overdose may produce combination of CNS stimulation and depressant effects.

PATIENT CONSIDERATIONS

BASELINE ASSESSMENT

Assess for dehydration if excessive vomiting occurs (poor skin turgor, dry mucous membranes, longitudinal furrows in tongue). Provide emotional support.

INTERVENTIONS/EVALUATION

Monitor for therapeutic relief from nausea/vomiting. Maintain quiet, supportive atmosphere.

PATIENT/FAMILY TEACHING

Relief from nausea/vomiting generally occurs shortly after drug administration.

donepezil hydrochloride

doh-**neh**-peh-zil
(Aricept)

CANADIAN AVAILABILITY
Aricept

PREGNANCY CATEGORY C

CLASSIFICATION

Cholinergic

AVAILABILITY (Rx)

Tablets: 5 mg, 10 mg

PHARMACOKINETICS

Absorption: Well absorbed following oral administration. **Metabolism:** Extensively metabolized in liver; binds to plasma proteins, mainly albumin. **Excretion:** Eliminated in urine and feces. **Half-life:** 50–70 hrs.

ACTION/*THERAPEUTIC EFFECT*

Enhances cholinergic function by increasing the concentration of acetylcholine through inhibition of the hydrolysis of acetylcholine by the enzyme acetycholinesterase, *slowing the progression of Alzheimer's disease.*

USES

Treatment of mild to moderate dementia of Alzheimer's disease.

ADMINISTRATION

ORAL:

- May be given w/o regard to meals or time of administration (morning vs. evening dose), although it is suggested dose be given in the evening, just prior to bedtime.

INDICATIONS/ROUTES/DOSAGE

Alzheimer's disease:
Oral: Adults, elderly: 5–10 mg/day as a single dose. If initial dose is 5 mg, do not increase to 10 mg for 4–6 weeks.

CONTRAINDICATIONS

History of hypersensitivity to donepezil or piperidine derivatives.

CAUTIONS

Asthma, COPD, bladder outflow obstruction, history of ulcer disease, those on concurrent nonsteroidal anti-inflammatory drugs (NSAIDs), "sick-sinus syndrome" or other supraventricular cardiac conduction conditions, seizures.

INTERACTIONS

DRUG: ***Ketoconazole, quinidine*** inhibits donepezil metabolism.

Decreases effect of **anticholinergics**. Synergistic effects with ***succinylcholine, neuromuscular blocking agents, cholinergic agonists*** may occur. **HERBAL:** None known. **FOOD:** None significant. **ALTERED LAB VALUES:** May decrease potassium, increase creatine kinase, blood sugar, lactate dehydrogenase.

SIDE EFFECTS

FREQUENT (8–11%): Nausea, diarrhea, headache, insomnia, pain in various locations, dizziness. **OCCASIONAL (3–6%):** Mild muscle cramps, fatigue, vomiting, anorexia, ecchymosis. **RARE (2–3%):** Depression, abnormal dreams, weight decrease, arthritis, somnolence, syncope, frequent urination.

ADVERSE REACTIONS/TOXIC EFFECTS

Overdosage may result in cholinergic crisis characterized by severe nausea, increased salivation/sweating, bradycardia, hypotension, flushed skin, stomach pain, respiratory depression, seizures, collapse. Increasing muscle weakness may occur, resulting in death if respiratory muscles are involved. ***Antidote:*** 1–2 mg IV atropine sulfate with subsequent doses based on therapeutic response.

PATIENT CONSIDERATIONS

Baseline Assessment

Obtain baseline vital signs. Obtain history of peptic ulcer, urinary obstruction, asthma, COPD.

Intervention/Evaluation

Monitor for cholinergic reaction: GI discomfort/cramping, feeling of facial warmth, excessive salivation and sweating, lacrimation, pallor, urinary urgency, dizziness. Assess eyes for pupillary contraction. Monitor for nausea, diarrhea, headache, insomnia.

Patient/Family Teaching

Report nausea, vomiting, diarrhea, sweating, increased salivary secretions, severe abdominal pain, dizziness.

dopamine hydrochloride

dope-a-meen
(Intropin, Dopastat)

CANADIAN AVAILABILITY
Intropin

PREGNANCY CATEGORY C

CLASSIFICATION

Sympathomimetic

AVAILABILITY (Rx)

Injection: 40 mg/ml, 80 mg/ml, 160 mg/ml. **Injection w/Dextrose:** 80 mg/100 ml, 160 mg/100 ml, 320 mg/100 ml.

PHARMACODYNAMICS

	ONSET	PEAK	DURATION
IV	1–2 min	<5 min	<10 min

PHARMACOKINETICS

Widely distributed. Does not cross blood-brain barrier. **Metabolism:** Metabolized in liver, kidney, plasma. **Excretion:** Primarily excreted in urine. **Half-life:** 2 min.

ACTION/*THERAPEUTIC EFFECT*

Stimulates adrenergic receptors; effects are dose dependent. ***Low doses:*** Stimulates dopaminergic receptors causing renal vasodilation *(increases renal blood flow, urine flow, sodium excretion)*. ***Low to moderate doses:*** Positive inotropic effect by direct action, release of norepinephrine *(increases myocardial contractility, stroke volume, cardiac output)*. ***High doses:*** Stimulates alpha receptors *(increased peripheral resistance, renal vasoconstriction, increases systolic and diastolic B/P)*.

USES

Prophylaxis/treatment of acute hypotension, shock (associated w/myocardial infarction, trauma, renal failure, cardiac decompensation, open heart surgery), treatment of low cardiac output, CHF.

STORAGE/HANDLING

Do not use solutions darker than slightly yellow or discolored to yellow, brown, or pink to purple (indicates decomposition of drug).

ADMINISTRATION

Note: Blood volume depletion must be corrected before administering dopamine (may be used concurrently with fluid replacement).

IV:

- Dilute each 5 ml (200 mg) ampule in 250–500 ml of compatible solution (concentration is dependent on dosage and fluid requirement of pt); 250 ml solution yields 800 mcg/ml; 500 ml solution yields 400 mcg/ml.
- Administer into large vein (antecubital fossa) to prevent extravasation.
- Use infusion pump to control rate of flow.
- Titrate each pt to the desired hemodynamic or renal response.

INDICATIONS/ROUTES/DOSAGE

IV: Adults, elderly: Begin with rate of 1–5 mcg/kg/min in those likely to respond to minimal treatment. May be gradually increased in 1–4 mcg/kg/min increments at 10–30 min intervals until optimum response achieved. Most pts are maintained on dose of 20 mcq/kg/min or less.

Seriously ill:

IV: Adults, elderly: Begin with 5 mcg/kg/min rate; gradually increase in 5–10 mcg/kg/min increments up to rate of 20–50 mcg/kg/min. Those who do not respond may require further increments.

Pts with occlusive vascular disease:

IV: Adults, elderly: Begin with rate of 1 mcg/kg/min.

Pts on MAO inhibitors:

IV: Adults, elderly: Reduce dose to one-tenth the calculated amount.

CONTRAINDICATIONS

Pheochromocytoma, uncorrected tachyarrhythmias, ventricular fibrillation, sulfite sensitivity.

CAUTIONS

Ischemic heart disease, occlusive vascular disease. Safety and efficacy for use in children has not been established.

INTERACTIONS

DRUG: ***Tricyclic antidepressants*** may increase cardiovascular effects. ***Beta blockers*** may decrease effects. May increase risk of arrhythmias w/***digoxin.***

Ergot alkaloids may increase vasoconstriction. *MAO inhibitors* may increase cardiac stimulation, vasopressor effects. **HERBAL:** None known. **FOOD:** None significant. **ALTERED LAB VALUES:** Increases urea nitrogen in blood.

SIDE EFFECTS

FREQUENT: Headache, ectopic beats, tachycardia, anginal pain, palpitations, vasoconstriction, hypotension, nausea, vomiting, dyspnea. **OCCASIONAL:** Piloerection (goose bumps), bradycardia, widening of QRS complex. **RARE:** Increased urination.

ADVERSE REACTIONS/TOXIC EFFECTS

High doses may produce ventricular arrhythmias. Pts with occlusive vascular disease are high-risk candidates for further compromise of circulation to extremities, which may result in gangrene. Extravasation resulting in tissue necrosis with sloughing may occur w/IV administration.

PATIENT CONSIDERATIONS

Baseline Assessment

Check for MAO inhibitor therapy within last 2–3 wks (dosage reduction). Pt must be on continuous cardiac monitoring. Determine weight (for dosage calculation). Obtain initial B/P, heart rate, and respirations.

Intervention/Evaluation

Continuously monitor for cardiac arrhythmias. W/physician, establish parameters for adjusting rate or stopping infusion. Maintain accurate I&O. Measure urine output frequently. Assure proper placement of IV catheter. If extravasation occurs, immediately infiltrate the affected tissue w/10–15 ml 0.9% NaCl solution containing 5–10 mg phentolamine mesylate. Monitor B/P, heart rate, and respirations every 15 min during administration (or more often if indicated). Assess cardiac output, pulmonary wedge pressure or central venous pressure frequently. Assess peripheral circulation (palpate pulses, note color and temperature of extremities). Immediately notify physician of decreased urine output, cardiac arrhythmias, significant changes in B/P or heart rate (or failure to respond to increase/decrease in infusion rate), decreased peripheral circulation (cold, pale, or mottled extremities). Taper dosage before discontinuing because abrupt cessation of therapy may result in marked hypotension. Be alert to excessive vasoconstriction (as evidenced by decreased urine output, increased heart rate or arrhythmias, and a disproportionate increase in diastolic B/P and decrease in pulse pressure); slow or temporarily stop the infusion and notify physician at once.

Patient/Family Teaching

Explain rationale for therapy. Report cold extremities, chest pain, difficulty breathing, or discomfort at IV site.

dornase alfa

door-**naze**-al-fah

(Pulmozyme)

CANADIAN AVAILABILITY

Pulmozyme

PREGNANCY CATEGORY B

CLASSIFICATION

Enzyme

AVAILABILITY (Rx)

Solution for Inhalation: 1 mg/ml

PHARMACODYNAMICS

	ONSET	PEAK	DURATION
Inhalant			
	15 min	3 days	—

PHARMACOKINETICS

Minimal systemic absorption after inhalation.

ACTION / *THERAPEUTIC EFFECT*

Selectively splits, hydrolyzes DNA in sputum, *reducing sputum viscid elasticity.*

USES

Management (w/standard therapy) of cystic fibrosis pts (including pts w/advanced disease) to reduce frequency of respiratory infections, improve pulmonary function.

STORAGE/HANDLING

Refrigerate. Ampules are clear, colorless (discard if cloudy, discolored, or left at room temperature for a total time >24 hrs).

ADMINISTRATION

Note: Administer only w/compressed-air-driven nebulizers and compressors. Do not mix/dilute w/other drugs.

NEBULIZATION:

- Wash hands thoroughly w/soap and water before preparation.
- Pour entire contents of one single-use ampule into nebulizer.
- Hold tab at base of ampule firmly, twist off top, and squeeze contents into nebulizer cup (use full dose of drug).
- Attach nebulizer cup, connect plastic T to nebulizer cup.
- Connect open end to port at bottom of nebulizer cup.
- Instruct pt to breathe normally by inhaling and exhaling through mouth only.

INDICATIONS/ROUTES/DOSAGE

Management of pulmonary function:
Nebulization: Adults, children >5 yrs: 2.5 mg (1 ampule) once daily via recommended nebulizer. (Twice daily dosing may be beneficial for some pts.)

CONTRAINDICATIONS

None significant.

CAUTIONS

None significant.

INTERACTIONS

DRUG: None significant. **HERBAL:** None known. **FOOD:** None significant. **ALTERED LAB VALUES:** None significant.

SIDE EFFECTS

Note: Effects are generally mild and disappear within a few weeks after therapy begins. **FREQUENT:** Chest pain/discomfort (18%), sore throat, change in voice (12%), pharyngitis (36%). **OCCASIONAL (3–10%):** Conjunctivitis, hoarseness, skin rash.

ADVERSE REACTIONS/TOXIC EFFECTS

None significant.

PATIENT CONSIDERATIONS

BASELINE ASSESSMENT

Assess ABGs, lung sounds, dyspnea and fatigue, pulmonary secretions (amount, color, viscosity).

INTERVENTION/EVALUATION

Provide emotional support to pt, family, parents. Encourage activity within limits of physical ability. Assess for relief of dyspnea, fatigue. Monitor ABGs, lung sounds, and observe for decreased viscosity of pulmonary secretions. Encourage fluid intake.

PATIENT/FAMILY TEACHING

Refrigerate. Do not dilute/mix w/other medications. Treatment lasts 10–15 min. Inhale full-treatment dose. May have hoarseness or other upper airway irritation. Not a replacement for other components of therapy (e.g., antibiotics, bronchodilators, and daily physical exercise) or a cure.

dorzolamide

(Trusopt)

See Classification section under: Antiglaucoma agents

doxacurium chloride

(Nuromax)

See Classification section under: Neuromuscular blockers

doxazosin mesylate

docks-ah-**zoe**-sin

(Cardura)

CANADIAN AVAILABILITY

Cardura

PREGNANCY CATEGORY B

CLASSIFICATION

Antihypertensive

AVAILABILITY (Rx)

Tablets: 1 mg, 2 mg, 4 mg, 8 mg

PHARMACODYNAMICS

	ONSET	PEAK	DURATION
Oral	—	2–6 hrs	—

PHARMACOKINETICS

Absorption: Well absorbed from GI tract. **Metabolism:** Metabolized in liver. **Excretion:** Primarily eliminated in feces. **Half-life:** 19–22 hrs.

ACTION/*THERAPEUTIC EFFECT*

Selectively blocks alpha$_1$-adrenergic receptors, decreasing peripheral vascular resistance. Resulting peripheral vasodilation *lowers B/P, relaxes smooth muscle of bladder/prostate.*

USES

Treatment of mild to moderate hypertension. Used alone or in combination w/other antihypertensives. Treatment of benign prostatic hyperplasia.

ADMINISTRATION

ORAL:

- May give w/o regard to food.

INDICATIONS/ROUTES/DOSAGE

Hypertension:

Oral: Adults: Initially, 1 mg/day. May increase to 2, 4, 8, and 16 mg if necessary. ***Elderly:*** Initially, 0.5 mg/day.

Note: Doses >4 mg increase potential postural effects.

Benign prostatic hyperplasia:

Oral: Adults, elderly: 2–16 mg/day.

CONTRAINDICATIONS

None significant.

CAUTIONS

Chronic renal failure, impaired hepatic function.

INTERACTIONS

DRUG: *NSAIDs, estrogen* may decrease effect. *Hypotension-producing medications* may increase effect. **HERBAL:** None known. **FOOD:** None significant. **ALTERED LAB VALUES:** None significant.

SIDE EFFECTS

FREQUENT (10–20%): Dizziness, asthenia, headache, edema. **OCCASIONAL (3–9%):** Nausea, pharyngitis, rhinitis, extremity pain, somnolence. **RARE (1–3%):** Palpitations, arrhythmias, diarrhea, constipation, dyspnea, myalgia, altered vision, vertigo, nervousness.

ADVERSE REACTIONS/TOXIC EFFECTS

First-dose syncope (hypotension w/sudden loss of consciousness) generally occurs 30–90 min after giving initial dose of 2 mg or greater, a too rapid increase in dose, or addition of another hypotensive agent to therapy. May be preceded by tachycardia (120–160 beats/min).

PATIENT CONSIDERATIONS

Baseline Assessment

Give first dose at bedtime. If initial dose is given during daytime, pt must remain recumbent for 3–4 hrs. Assess B/P, pulse immediately before each dose, and q15–30min until stabilized (be alert to B/P fluctuations).

Intervention/Evaluation

Monitor pulse diligently (first-dose syncope may be preceded by tachycardia). Monitor pattern of daily bowel activity and stool consistency. Assist w/ambulation if dizziness, lightheadedness occurs.

Patient/Family Teaching

Dry mouth may be relieved by sugarless gum, sips of tepid water. Cola, unsalted crackers, dry toast may relieve nausea. Nasal congestion may occur. Full therapeutic effect may not occur for 3–4 wks. May cause syncope (fainting). Avoid driving for 12–24 hrs after receiving first dose on increase in dosage. Use caution when rising from sitting or lying position. Report dizziness, palpitations if bothersome. Use caution driving or operating machinery.

doxepin hydrochloride

dox-eh-pin

(Adapin, Sinequan, Zonalon)

CANADIAN AVAILABILITY

Novo-Doxepin, Sinequan, Zonalon

PREGNANCY CATEGORY C

Topical: Pregnancy Category B.

CLASSIFICATION

Antidepressant: Tricyclic

AVAILABILITY (Rx)

Capsules: 10 mg, 25 mg, 50 mg, 75 mg, 100 mg, 150 mg. **Oral Concentrate:** 10 mg/ml. **Cream:** 5%.

PHARMACOKINETICS

Oral: **Absorption:** Rapid, well absorbed from GI tract. **Metabo-**

lism: Metabolized in liver to active metabolite. **Excretion:** Primarily excreted in urine. **Half-life:** 11–23 hrs. ***Topical:*** **Absorption:** Absorbed through skin, distributed to body tissues. **Metabolism:** Metabolized to active metabolite. **Excretion:** Eliminated renally.

ACTION/*THERAPEUTIC EFFECT*

Increases synaptic concentration of norepinephrine and/or serotonin (inhibits reuptake by presynaptic membrane), *producing antidepressant, anxiolytic effect.* Strong anticholinergic activity. Topical may produce antihistamine/sedative effect.

USES/*UNLABELED*

Treatment of various forms of depression, often in conjunction w/psychotherapy. Treatment of anxiety. ***Topical:*** Treatment of pruritus associated w/eczema. *Treatment of panic disorder, neurogenic pain, prophylaxis vascular headache, pruritus in idiopathic cold urticaria.*

ADMINISTRATION

ORAL:

- Give w/food or milk if GI distress occurs.
- Dilute concentrate in 8 oz glass of water, milk, orange, grapefruit, tomato, prune, pineapple juice. Incompatible w/carbonated drinks.

INDICATIONS/ROUTES/DOSAGE

Mild to moderate depression/anxiety:
Oral: Adults: 25 mg 3 times/day (75 mg/day). ***Usual therapeutic range:*** 75–150 mg/day. Alternately, 150 mg/day as single dose at bedtime.

Severe depression/anxiety:
Oral: Adults: 50 mg 3 times/day. Gradually increase to 300 mg/day, if needed.

Emotional symptoms accompanying organic brain disease:
Oral: Adults: 25–50 mg/day.

Usual elderly dosage:
Oral: Initially, 10–25 mg at bedtime. May increase by 10–25 mg/day every 3–7 days. ***Maximum:*** 75 mg/day.

Usual topical dosage:
Topical: Adults, elderly: Apply thin film 4 times/day.

CONTRAINDICATIONS

Acute recovery period following myocardial infarction, within 14 days of MAO inhibitor ingestion.

CAUTIONS

Prostatic hypertrophy, history of urinary retention/obstruction, glaucoma, diabetes mellitus, history of seizures, hyperthyroidism, cardiac/hepatic/renal disease, schizophrenia, increased intraocular pressure, hiatal hernia.

INTERACTIONS

DRUG: ***Alcohol, CNS depressants*** may increase CNS, respiratory depression, hypotensive effects. ***Antithyroid agents*** may increase risk of agranulocytosis. ***Phenothiazines*** may increase sedative, anticholinergic effects. ***Cimetidine*** may increase concentration, toxicity. May decrease effects of ***clonidine, guanadrel.*** May increase cardiac effects w/***sympathomimetics.*** May increase risk of hypertensive crisis, hyperpyretic, convulsions w/***MAO inhibitors.*** **HERBAL:** None known. **FOOD:** None significant. **ALTERED LAB VALUES:** May alter EKG readings, glucose.

SIDE EFFECTS

FREQUENT: *Oral:* Orthostatic hypotension, drowsiness, dry mouth, headache, increased appetite/weight, nausea, unusual tiredness, unpleasant taste. ***Topical:*** Edema at application site, increased itching/eczema, burning, stinging of skin, altered taste, dizziness, drowsiness, dry skin, dry mouth, fatigue, headache, thirst. OCCASIONAL: *Oral:* Blurred vision, confusion, constipation, hallucinations, difficult urination, eye pain, irregular heartbeat, fine muscle tremors, Parkinson syndrome, nervousness, impaired sexual function, diarrhea, increased sweating, heartburn, insomnia. ***Topical:*** Anxiety, skin irritation/cracking, nausea. RARE: Allergic reaction, alopecia, tinnitus, breast enlargement. ***Topical:*** Fever.

ADVERSE REACTIONS/TOXIC EFFECTS

High dosage may produce confusion, seizures, severe drowsiness, fast/slow/irregular heartbeat, fever, hallucinations, agitation, shortness of breath, vomiting, unusual tiredness/weakness. Abrupt withdrawal from prolonged therapy may produce headache, malaise, nausea, vomiting, vivid dreams.

PATIENT CONSIDERATIONS

Baseline Assessment

For those on long-term therapy, liver/renal function tests, blood counts should be performed periodically.

Intervention/Evaluation

Supervise suicidal risk pt closely during early therapy (as depression lessens, energy level improves, increasing suicide potential). Assess appearance, behavior, speech pattern, level of interest, mood. Monitor pattern of daily bowel activity, stool consistency. Monitor B/P, pulse for hypotension, arrhythmias. Assess for urinary retention by bladder palpation. Avoid alcohol.

Patient/Family Teaching

Change positions slowly to avoid hypotensive effect. Tolerance to postural hypotension, sedative and anticholinergic effects usually develops during early therapy. Therapeutic effect may be noted within 2–5 days, maximum effect within 2–3 wks. Photosensitivity to sun may occur. Dry mouth may be relieved by sugarless gum, sips of tepid water. Report visual disturbances. Do not abruptly discontinue medication. Avoid tasks that require alertness, motor skills until response to drug is established.

---

doxorubicin

(Adriamycin, Doxil, Rubex)

See Classification section under: Cancer chemotherapy

---

doxycycline calcium

dock-see-**sigh**-clean

(Vibramycin Calcium syrup)

doxycycline hyclate, monohydrate

(Doryx, Periostat, Vibra-Tabs, Vibramycin)

CANADIAN AVAILABILITY

Apo-Doxy, Doxycin, Vibra-Tabs

PREGNANCY CATEGORY D

CLASSIFICATION

Antibiotic: Tetracycline

AVAILABILITY (Rx)

Capsules: 20 mg, 50 mg, 100 mg. **Tablets:** 50 mg, 100 mg. **Powder for Oral Suspension:** 25 mg/5 ml, 50 mg/5 ml. **Syrup:** 50 mg/5 ml. **Powder for Injection:** 100 mg, 200 mg.

PHARMACOKINETICS

Absorption: Well absorbed from GI tract (may give w/food). Widely distributed. **Metabolism:** Partially inactivated in intestine. **Excretion:** Excreted in urine, eliminated in feces via biliary secretion. Not removed by hemodialysis. **Half-life:** 12–22 hrs.

ACTION/*THERAPEUTIC EFFECT*

Bacteriostatic due to binding to ribosomes, *inhibiting protein synthesis.*

USES/*UNLABELED*

Treatment of periodonitis, respiratory, skin/ soft tissue, urinary tract infections, syphilis, uncomplicated gonorrhea, pelvic inflammatory disease, rheumatic fever prophylaxis, brucellosis, trachoma, Rocky Mountain spotted fever, typhus, Q fever, rickettsia, smallpox, psittacosis, ornithosis, granuloma inguinale, lymphogranuloma venereum, adjunctive treatment of intestinal amebiasis. *Treatment of gonorrhea, malaria, atypical mycobacterial infections, prophylaxis/treatment of traveler's diarrhea, rheumatoid arthritis.*

STORAGE/HANDLING

Store capsules, tablets at room temperature. Oral suspension stable for 2 wks at room temperature. After reconstitution, IV infusion (piggyback) is stable for 12 hrs at room temperature, 72 hrs if refrigerated. Protect from direct sunlight. Discard if precipitate forms.

ADMINISTRATION

Note: Do not administer IM or SubQ. Space doses evenly around clock.

ORAL:
- Give w/full glass of fluid.
- May take w/food or milk.

IV:
- **Note:** Give by intermittent IV infusion (piggyback).
- Reconstitute each 100 mg vial w/10 ml sterile water for injection for concentration of 10 mg/ml.
- Further dilute each 100 mg w/at least 100 ml 5% dextrose, 0.9% NaCl, or other compatible IV fluid. Infuse >1–4 hrs.

INDICATIONS/DOSAGE/ROUTES

Usual dosage:
Oral: Adults, elderly: Initially, 200 mg (100 mg ql2h), then 100 mg/day as single dose or in 2 divided doses (100 mg q12h in severe infections). ***Children >8 yrs, >45 kg:*** Initially, 4.4 mg/kg divided in 2 doses, then 2.2 mg/kg as single dose or in 2 divided doses (4.4 mg/kg in severe infections).

IV: Adults, elderly: Initially, 200 mg as 1–2 infusions; then 100–200 mg/day (200 mg as 1–2 infusions). ***Children:*** Initially, 4.4 mg/kg on first day as 1–2 infusions; then 2.2–4.4 mg/kg as 12 infusions.

Acute gonococcal infections:
Oral: Adults: Initially, 200 mg, then 100 mg at bedtime on first day; then 100 mg 2 times/day for 3 days.

Syphilis:
Oral/IV: Adults: 300 mg/day in divided doses for 10 days.

Traveler's diarrhea:
Oral: Adults, elderly: 100 mg daily during a period of risk (up to 14 days) and for 2 days after returning home.

Periodonitis:
Oral: Adults: 20 mg 2 times/day.

CONTRAINDICATIONS

Hypersensitivity to tetracyclines, sulfite, last half of pregnancy, children <8 yrs.

CAUTIONS

Sun/ultraviolet light exposure (severe photosensitivity reaction).

INTERACTIONS

DRUG: *Antacids* containing aluminum/calcium/magnesium, *laxatives* containing magnesium, *oral iron preparations* impair absorption of tetracyclines (give 1–2 hrs before or after tetracyclines). *Barbiturates, phenytoin, carbamazepine* may decrease doxycycline concentrations. *Cholestyramine, colestipol* may decrease absorption. May decrease effect of *oral contraceptives.* HERBAL: St. John's wort may increase photosensitivity risk. FOOD: None significant. ALTERED LAB VALUES: May increase SGOT (AST), SGPT (ALT), alkaline phosphatase, amylase, bilirubin concentrations; alter CBC.

SIDE EFFECTS

FREQUENT: Anorexia, nausea, vomiting, diarrhea, dysphagia, photosensitivity. OCCASIONAL: Rash, urticaria.

ADVERSE REACTIONS/TOXIC EFFECTS

Superinfection (especially fungal), benign intracranial hypertension (headache, visual changes). Liver toxicity, fatty degeneration of liver, pancreatitis occur rarely.

PATIENT CONSIDERATIONS

BASELINE ASSESSMENT

Question for history of allergies, especially to tetracyclines, sulfite. Obtain culture and sensitivity test before giving first dose (therapy may begin before results are known).

INTERVENTION/EVALUATION

Check IV site for phlebitis (heat, pain, red streaking over vein). Determine pattern of bowel activity, stool consistency. Monitor food intake, tolerance. Assess skin for rash. Monitor B/P and LOC because of potential for increased intracranial pressure. Be alert for superinfection: diarrhea, ulceration or changes of oral mucosa, anal/genital pruritus.

PATIENT/FAMILY TEACHING

Continue antibiotic for full length of treatment. Space doses evenly. Drink full glass of water w/capsules or tablets. Notify physician in event of diarrhea, rash, or other new symptoms. Protect skin from sun/ultraviolet light exposure. Consult physician before taking any other medication. May take w/food or milk.

dronabinol

drow-**nab**-in-all
(Marinol)

CANADIAN AVAILABILITY
Marinol

PREGNANCY CATEGORY B

CLASSIFICATION

Antinausea, antiemetic **(Schedule III)**

AVAILABILITY (Rx)

Capsules: 2.5 mg, 5 mg, 10 mg

PHARMACOKINETICS

Absorption: Poorly absorbed from GI tract. **Metabolism:** Metabolized in liver. **Excretion:** Primarily eliminated via biliary excretion. **Half-life:** 15–18 hrs (metabolite).

ACTION

May inhibit vomiting control mechanisms in medulla oblongata.

USES

Prevention, treatment of nausea, vomiting due to cancer chemotherapy; appetite stimulant in AIDS pts.

INDICATIONS/ROUTES/DOSAGE

Nausea, vomiting:
Oral: Adults: Initially, 5 mg/m^2, 1–3 hrs before chemotherapy, then q2–4h after chemotherapy for total of 4–6 doses/day. May increase by 2.5 mg/m^2 up to 15 mg/m^2/dose.

Appetite stimulant:
Oral: Adults: Initially, 2.5 mg 2 times/day (before lunch, dinner). *Range:* 2.5–20 mg/day.

CONTRAINDICATIONS

Nausea, vomiting other than due to chemotherapy.

CAUTIONS

Hypertension, heart disease; manic, depressive, or schizophrenic pts. Not recommended in children.

INTERACTIONS

DRUG: *CNS depressants* may enhance sedative effects. **HERBAL:** None known. **FOOD:** None significant. **ALTERED LAB VALUES:** None significant.

SIDE EFFECTS

FREQUENT (3–10%): Nausea, vomiting, euphoria (24%), dizziness, somnolence, paranoid reactions. **OCCASIONAL (1–3%):** Asthenia, ataxia, confusion, abnormal thinking, altered vision. **RARE (<1%):** Diarrhea, depression, nightmares, speech difficulties, headache, anxiety, tinnitus, flushing of skin.

ADVERSE REACTIONS/TOXIC EFFECTS

Overdosage may produce increased sensory awareness (e.g., taste, smell, sound), altered time perception, reddened conjunctiva, memory impairment, urinary retention, constipation, slurred speech.

PATIENT CONSIDERATIONS

Baseline Assessment

Assess for dehydration if excessive vomiting occurs (poor skin turgor, dry mucous membranes, decreased urine output).

Intervention/Evaluation

Provide emotional support. Supervise closely for serious mood and behavior responses. Do not continue drug after a psychotic episode until pt and situation have been fully evaluated.

Patient/Family Teaching

Potentially abusable drug—take only as directed. Report visual disturbances. Dry mouth is expected response to medication. Relief from nausea/vomiting generally occurs within 15 min of drug administration. Avoid alcohol, barbiturates. Avoid tasks that require alertness, motor skills until response to drug is established. Remain under supervision of a responsible adult because mood alterations and adverse behavioral effects can occur. For appetite stimulation take before lunch and dinner.

droperidol

droe-**pear**-ih-dall
(Inapsine)

FIXED-COMBINATION(S)
W/fentanyl, a narcotic **(Innovar)**

PREGNANCY CATEGORY C

CLASSIFICATION

Antiemetic

AVAILABILITY (Rx)

Injection: 2.5 mg/ml

PHARMACODYNAMICS

	ONSET	PEAK	DURATION
IM	3–10 min	30 min	2–4 hrs
IV	3–10 min	30 min	2–4 hrs

PHARMACOKINETICS

Absorption: Well absorbed after IM administration. Crosses blood-brain barrier. **Metabolism:** Metabolized in liver. **Excretion:** Primarily excreted in urine.

ACTION/*THERAPEUTIC EFFECT*

Antagonizes dopamine neurotransmission at synapses by blocking postsynaptic dopamine receptor sites; partially blocks adrenergic receptor binding sites, *producing tranquilization, antiemetic effect.*

USES

Tranquilization, control of nausea/vomiting during surgical, diagnostic procedures. Used preoperatively w/opiate analgesics during general anesthesia as anxiolytic, to increase analgesic effect of opiate.

STORAGE/HANDLING

Store parenteral form at room temperature. Precipitate occurs if mixed w/barbiturate.

ADMINISTRATION

Note: Pt must remain recumbent for 30–60 min in head-low position w/legs raised, to minimize hypotensive effect.

IM: Inject slow, deep IM into upper outer quadrant of gluteus maximus.

IV: Dose for high-risk pts should be added to 5% dextrose or lactated Ringer's injection to a concentration of 1 mg/50 ml; give by slow IV infusion.

INDICATIONS/ROUTES/DOSAGE

Preop:
IM/IV: Adults, elderly: 2.5–10 mg 30–60 min before induction of general anesthesia. *Children 2–12 yrs:* 0.088–0.165 mg/kg.

Adjunct for induction of general anesthesia:
IV: Adults, elderly: 0.22–0.275 mg/kg. *Children 2–12 yrs:* 0.088–0.165 mg/kg.

Adjunct for maintenance of general anesthesia:
IV: Adults, elderly: 1.25–2.5 mg.

Diagnostic procedures w/o general anesthesia:
IM: Adults, elderly: 2.5–10 mg 30–60 min before procedure. If needed, may give additional doses of 1.25–2.5 mg (usually by IV injection).

Adjunct to regional anesthesia:
IM/IV: Adults, elderly: 2.5–5 mg.

CONTRAINDICATIONS

Known intolerance to drug.

CAUTIONS

Impaired hepatic/renal/cardiac function.

INTERACTIONS

DRUG: *CNS depressants* may increase CNS depressant effect. *Hypotensives* may increase hypotension. **HERBAL:** None known. **FOOD:** None significant. **ALTERED LAB VALUES:** None significant.

SIDE EFFECTS

FREQUENT: Mild to moderate hypotension. **OCCASIONAL:** Tachycardia, postop drowsiness, dizziness, chills, shivering. **RARE:** Postop nightmares, facial sweating, bronchospasm.

ADVERSE REACTIONS/TOXIC EFFECTS

Extrapyramidal symptoms may appear as akathisia (motor restlessness) and dystonias: torticollis (neck muscle spasm), opisthotonos (rigidity of back muscles), and oculogyric crisis (rolling back of eyes).

PATIENT CONSIDERATIONS

BASELINE ASSESSMENT

Assess vital signs. Have pt void. Prepare for surgery. Raise side rails. Instruct to remain recumbent.

INTERVENTION/EVALUATION

Monitor B/P and pulse diligently for hypotensive reaction during and after procedure. Assess pulse for tachycardia. Monitor for extrapyramidal symptoms. Evaluate for therapeutic response from anxiety: a calm facial expression, decreased restlessness.

edetate calcium disodium (calcium EDTA)

ed-eh-tate
(Calcium Disodium Versenate)

PREGNANCY CATEGORY C

CLASSIFICATION

Antidote

AVAILABILITY (Rx)

Injection: 200 mg/ml

PHARMACODYNAMICS

	ONSET	PEAK	DURATION
IV	1 hr	24–48 hrs	—

PHARMACOKINETICS

Absorption: Well absorbed after parenteral administration. Primarily distributed in extracellular fluid. **Excretion:** Excreted unchanged in urine. **Half-life:** 20–90 min.

ACTION/*THERAPEUTIC EFFECT*

Reduces blood concentration of heavy metals, especially lead, forming stable complexes, *allowing heavy metal excretion in urine.*

USES

Acute and chronic lead poisoning, lead encephalopathy.

STORAGE/HANDLING

Store parenteral form at room temperature.

ADMINISTRATION

IM:

- Add 1 ml 1% procaine to each ml calcium EDTA prior to administration.

IV:

- Dilute each calcium EDTA ampule (1 g) w/5% dextrose or 0.9% NaCl to provide a concentration of 2–4 mg/ml.
- For intermittent IV administration, solution containing ½ daily dose infused over 1–2 hrs; second dose infused at least 6 hrs after first infusion.
- For IV infusion, give over 12–24 hrs. **Note:** Interrupt infusion for 1 hr before blood lead concentration measured (avoids falsely elevated reading).

INDICATIONS/ROUTES/DOSAGE

Note: When administered IV, calcium EDTA may be given in 2 divided doses at 12 hr intervals or 12–24 hr infusions; when administered IM and used alone, may be given in divided doses at 8–12 hr intervals; when given IM w/dimercaprol in divided doses, administer at 4 hr intervals.

Diagnosis of lead poisoning:
IM/IV Infusion: Adults, elderly: 500 mg/m^2. ***Maximum:*** 1 g.

IV Infusion: Children: 500 mg/m^2.

IM: Children: 500 mg/m^2 as single dose or 500 mg/m^2 each at 12 hr intervals.

Lead poisoning (w/o encephalopathy):
Note: Total dose dependent on severity of lead poisoning, pt response/tolerance to medication. Consult specific protocols.

IM/IV: Adults, elderly, children: 1–1.5 g/m^2 daily for 3–5 days. (If blood lead concentration >100 mcg/dl, calcium edetate usually given w/dimercaprol.) Allow at least 2–4 days, up to 2–3 wks between courses of therapy. Adults should not be given more than 2 courses of therapy.

Lead poisoning (w/encephalopathy):
IM: Adults, elderly, children: Initially, dimercaprol 4 mg/kg; then give dimercaprol 4 mg/kg and calcium EDTA 250 mg/m^2; then 4 hrs later and q4h for 5 days.

CONTRAINDICATIONS

Anuria.

CAUTIONS

None significant.

INTERACTIONS

DRUG: May decrease effects of *zinc.* **HERBAL:** None known. **FOOD:** None significant. **ALTERED LAB VALUES:** None significant.

SIDE EFFECTS

FREQUENT: Chills, fever, anorexia, headache, histaminelike reaction (sneezing, stuffy nose, watery eyes), decreased B/P, nausea, vomiting, thrombophlebitis. **OCCASIONAL:** Transient anemia/bone marrow depression, hypercalcemia (constipation, drowsiness, dry mouth, metallic taste). **RARE:** Frequent urination, secondary gout (severe pain in feet, knees, elbows).

ADVERSE REACTIONS/TOXIC EFFECTS

Renal tubular necrosis.

PATIENT CONSIDERATIONS

Baseline Assessment

Assure urine flow before start of therapy. Determine serum and urine, lead levels, BUN. Assess family members for lead poisoning.

Intervention/Evaluation

Monitor EKG during therapy. Assess vital signs, neurologic status. Maintain careful I&O. Avoid rapid IV infusion (may be lethal due to increased ICP). Periodically check serum and urine lead levels, BUN; obtain daily urinalysis. Stop drug immediately and notify physician of anuria or urinalysis report of increased proteinuria, increased erythrocytes, or presence of large renal epithelial cells.

Patient/Family Teaching

Necessity of follow-up visits for tests and possible further therapy. Evaluation of home to prevent future poisoning.

---

efavirenz

eh-fah-vir-enz
(Sustiva)

PREGNANCY CATEGORY C

CLASSIFICATION

Antiviral

AVAILABILITY (Rx)

Capsules: 50 mg, 100 mg, 200 mg

PHARMACOKINETICS

Absorption: Rapidly absorbed following oral administration. **Metabolism:** Highly bound to plasma proteins, primarily albumin. Metabolized to major isoenzymes in liver. **Excretion:** Eliminated in urine and feces. **Half-life:** 40–55 hrs.

ACTION/*THERAPEUTIC EFFECT*

Inhibits activity of HIV reverse transcriptase (RT) of human immunodeficiency virus type 1 (HIV-1), *interrupting HIV replication, slowing progression of HIV infection.*

USES

Treatment of HIV infection in combination with other appropriate antiretoviral agents.

ADMINISTRATION

ORAL:

- May be taken w/o regard to meals but a high-fat meal may increase absorption of medication and should be avoided.

INDICATIONS/ROUTES/DOSAGE

HIV infection:

Oral: Adults, elderly: 600 mg once/day in combination with a protease inhibitor or nucleoside analog reverse transcriptase inhibitors (NRTIs). Bedtime dosing is recommended during first 2–4 wks of therapy (temporary nervous system side effects). ***Children 3 yrs: 88 lbs:*** 600 mg once/day. ***71.5–88 lbs:*** 400 mg once/day. ***55–71.5 lbs:*** 350 mg once/day. ***55 lbs:*** 300 mg once/day. ***33–44 lbs:*** 250 mg once/day. ***22–33 lbs:*** 200 mg once/day.

CONTRAINDICATIONS

History of hypersensitivity to medication, monotherapy, concurrent administration with astemizole, cisapride, midazolam, triazolam, ergot derivatives.

CAUTIONS

History of mental illness or substance abuse, hepatic impairment.

INTERACTIONS

DRUG: ***Astemizole, cisapride, midazolam, triazolam, ergot derivatives*** may create serious or life-threatening events (cardiac arrhythmias, prolonged sedation, respiration depression. ***Alcohol, psychoactive drugs*** may produce additive CNS effects. ***Phenobarbital, rifampin, rifabutin*** lowers efavirenz plasma concentration. Decreases ***clarithromycin*** plasma levels. Decreases ***indinavir, saquinavir*** plasma concentration, increases ***nelfinavir, ritonavir*** plasma concentration, alters ***warfarin*** plasma concentration. **HERBAL:** St. John's wort may decrease concentration, effect. **FOOD:** None significant. **ALTERED LAB VALUES:** May produce false-positive urine cannabinoid test results, increase total cholesterol, triglycerides, increase SGOT (AST), SGPT (ALT) liver enzymes.

SIDE EFFECTS

FREQUENT (52%, mild to severe symptoms): Dizziness, abnormal dreaming, insomnia, confusion, abnormal thinking, impaired concentration, amnesia, agitation, depersonalization, hallucinations, euphoria. **OCCASIONAL (27%):** Maculopapular ash, mild to moderate degree. **(<26%):** Nausea, fatigue, headache, diarrhea, fever, cough.

ADVERSE REACTIONS/TOXIC EFFECTS

None significant.

PATIENT CONSIDERATIONS

Baseline Assessment

Offer emotional support. Obtain baseline SGOT (AST), SGPT (ALT) in pts with a history of hepatitis B or C, cholesterol, triglycerides prior to initiating therapy and at intervals during therapy. Obtain history of all prescription and nonprescription medication (high level of drug interaction).

Intervention/Evaluation

Monitor for CNS psychiatric symptoms: severe acute depression, including suicidal idea-

tion/attempts, dizziness, impaired concentration, somnolence, abnormal dreams, insomnia (begins during first or second day of therapy, generally resolves in 2–4 wks). Assess for evidence of rash (common side effect). Monitor liver enzyme studies for abnormalities. Assess for headache, nausea, diarrhea.

PATIENT/FAMILY TEACHING

Avoid high-fat meals during therapy. If rash appears, contact physician immediately. CNS symptoms occur in over half the pts and may cause dizziness, impaired concentration, delusions, depression. Take medication every day as prescribed. Do not alter dose or discontinue medication w/o informing physician. Avoid tasks that require alertness, motor skills until response to drug is established. Sustiva is not a cure for HIV infection, nor does it reduce risk of transmission to others.

emedastine

em-eh-**das**-teen

(Emadine)

CANADIAN AVAILABILITY

Emadine

PREGNANCY CATEGORY B

CLASSIFICATION

Ophthalmic antihistamine

AVAILABILITY (Rx)

Solution: 0.05%

PHARMACOKINETICS

Absorption: Absorbed into the conjunctiva. **Metabolism:** Converts to two primary metabolites and minor metabolites. **Excretion:** Excreted in the urine as free and conjugated forms. **Half-life:** 3–4 hrs.

ACTION/*THERAPEUTIC EFFECT*

A selective histamine H_1 antagonist, inhibits histamine-stimulated vascular permeability in the conjunctiva, *relieving ocular itching associated with allergic conjunctivitis.*

USES

Temporary relief of signs and symptoms of allergic conjunctivitis.

ADMINISTRATION

OPHTHALMIC:

- Place finger on lower eyelid and pull out until pocket is formed between eye and lower lid. Hold dropper above pocket and place drop into pocket. Close eye gently. Apply digital pressure to lacrimal sac for 1–2 min (minimize drainage into nose and throat, reducing risk of systemic effects). Remove excess solution around eye with tissue.
- Do not apply medication while pt is wearing soft contact lenses (absorbs drug preservative). Lenses may be reinserted 10 min after drug is administered.

INDICATIONS/ROUTES/DOSAGE

Allergic conjunctivitis:

Ophthalmic: Adults, elderly: Apply 1 drop into affected eye(s) up to 4 times/day.

CONTRAINDICATIONS

History of hypersensitivity to medication.

CAUTIONS

None significant.

INTERACTIONS

DRUG: None significant. **HERBAL:** None known. **FOOD:** None significant. **ALTERED LAB VALUES:** None significant.

SIDE EFFECTS

FREQUENT (11%): Headache. **OCCASIONAL (5%):** Abnormal dreams, asthenia (loss of strength, energy), bad taste, blurred vision, burning or stinging, dry eyes, foreign body sensation, tearing.

ADVERSE REACTIONS/TOXIC EFFECTS

Somnolence, malaise occurs rarely.

PATIENT CONSIDERATIONS

INTERVENTIONS/EVALUATION

Monitor for headache, abnormal dreams, loss of strength/energy, bad taste, blurred vision, burning or stinging, dry eyes, foreign body sensation, tearing.

PATIENT/FAMILY TEACHING

Do not touch eyelids or surrounding area with dropper tip of the bottle. Keep bottle tightly closed when not in use. Do not use if the solution has become discolored. Do not apply medication while wearing soft contact lenses (absorbs drug preservative). Reinsert lenses ≥10 min after drug is administered. Vision may be temporarily blurred. Contact physician if any eye symptoms occur.

enalapril maleate

en-**al**-ah-prill

(Vasotec)

FIXED-COMBINATION(S)

W/hydrochlorothiazide, a diuretic **(Vaseretic)**; w/diltrazem, a calcium channel blocker **(Teczem)**; w/felodipine, a calcium channel blocker **(Lexxel)**

CANADIAN AVAILABILITY

Vasotec

PREGNANCY CATEGORY D

CLASSIFICATION

Angiotensin-converting enzyme (ACE) inhibitor, antihypertensive

AVAILABILITY (Rx)

Tablets: 2.5 mg, 5 mg, 10 mg, 20 mg. **Injection:** 1.25 mg/ml.

PHARMACODYNAMICS

	ONSET	PEAK	DURATION
Oral	1 hr	4–6 hrs	24 hrs
IV	15 min	1–4 hrs	6 hrs

PHARMACOKINETICS

Absorption: Readily absorbed from GI tract (not affected by food). **Metabolism:** Converted to active metabolite enalapril. **Excretion:** Primarily excreted in urine. Removed by hemodialysis. **Half-life:** 11 hrs (increased in reduced renal function).

ACTION/*THERAPEUTIC EFFECT*

Suppresses renin-angiotensin-aldosterone system (prevents conversion of angiotensin I to angiotensin II, a potent vasoconstrictor; may inhibit angiotensin II at local vascular, renal sites). Decreases plasma angiotensin II, increases plasma renin activity, decreases aldosterone secretion. *In hypertension, reduces peripheral arterial resistance. In CHF, increases cardiac output, decreases peripheral vascular resistance, B/P, pulmonary capillary wedge pressure, heart size.*

USES/*UNLABELED*

Treatment of hypertension alone or in combination w/other antihypertensives. Adjunctive therapy for CHF (in combination w/cardiac glycosides, diuretics). *Treatment of diabetic nephropathy, hypertension, or renal crisis in scleroderma.*

STORAGE/HANDLING

Store tablets, parenteral form at room temperature. For parenteral form, use only clear, colorless solution. Diluted IV solution is stable for 24 hrs at room temperature.

ADMINISTRATION

ORAL:

- May give w/o regard to food.
- Tablets may be crushed.

IV:

- For direct IV, give undiluted over 5 min.
- May dilute w/5% dextrose or 0.9% NaCl. Infuse over 10–15 min.

INDICATIONS/ROUTES/DOSAGE

Hypertension (used alone):
Oral: Adults, elderly: Initially, 5 mg/day. ***Maintenance:*** 10–40 mg/day as single or in 2 divided doses.

IV: Adults, elderly: 1.25 mg q6h.

Hypertension (w/diuretics):
Note: Discontinue diuretic 2–3 days before initiating enalapril therapy; if unable, initiate w/2.5 mg enalapril (0.625 mg IV).

Dose in renal impairment:
(Based on creatinine clearance.)

Oral: Adults, elderly: Initially, 2.5–5 mg/day. Titrate up to maximum of 40 mg/day.

IV: Adults, elderly (Ccr <30 ml/min): Initially, 0.625 mg. May repeat in 1 hr if no response, then 1.25 mg q6h.

CHF:
Oral: Adults, elderly: Initially, 2.5–5 mg/day. ***Maintenance:*** 5–20 mg/day in 2 divided doses. ***Maximum:*** 40 mg/day in 2 divided doses.

Dosage in renal impairment, hyponatremia (Na <130, Creat >1.6):
Initially, 2.5 mg/day, increase to 2.5 mg 2 times/day, then 5 mg 2 times/day at 4 day intervals (minimum) up to 40 mg/day.

CONTRAINDICATIONS

History of angioedema w/previous treatment w/ACE inhibitors.

CAUTIONS

Renal impairment, those w/sodium depletion or on diuretic therapy, dialysis, hypovolemia, coronary /cerebrovascular insufficiency.

INTERACTIONS

DRUG: ***Alcohol, diuretics, hypotensive agents*** may increase effects. ***NSAIDs*** may decrease effect. ***Potassium-sparing diuretics, potassium supplements*** may cause hyperkalemia. May increase ***lithium*** concentration, toxicity. **HERBAL:** None known. **FOOD:** None significant. **ALTERED LAB VALUES:** May increase potassium, SGOT (AST), SGPT (ALT), alkaline phosphatase, bilirubin, BUN, creatinine. May decrease sodium. May cause positive ANA titer.

SIDE EFFECTS

FREQUENT (5–10%): Hypotension, dizziness. **OCCASIONAL**

(2–5%): Headache, fatigue. **RARE (<2%):** Angina, vertigo, abdominal pain, vomiting, nausea, diarrhea, urinary tract infection, bronchitis, cough, dyspnea, rash asthenia, syncope.

ADVERSE REACTIONS/TOXIC EFFECTS

Excessive hypotension ("first-dose syncope") may occur in those w/CHF, severely salt/volume depleted. Angioedema (swelling of face, lips), hyperkalemia occur rarely. Agranulocytosis, neutropenia may be noted in those w/impaired renal function or collagen vascular disease (systemic lupus erythematosus, scleroderma). Nephrotic syndrome may be noted in those w/history of renal disease.

PATIENT CONSIDERATIONS

Baseline Assessment

Obtain B/P immediately before each dose in addition to regular monitoring (be alert to fluctuations). Renal function tests should be performed before therapy begins. In those w/renal impairment, autoimmune disease, or taking drugs that affect leukocytes or immune response, CBC and differential count should be performed before therapy begins and q2wks for 3 mos, then periodically thereafter.

Intervention/Evaluation

Assist w/ambulation if dizziness occurs. Assess skin for development of rash. Monitor serum potassium, BUN, serum creatinine levels. Monitor pattern of daily bowel activity, stool consistency. Assess for anorexia due to decreased taste sensation. If excessive reduction in B/P occurs, place pt in supine position w/legs elevated.

Patient/Family Teaching

To reduce hypotensive effect, rise slowly from lying to sitting position and permit legs to dangle from bed momentarily before standing. If nausea occurs, noncaffeinated carbonated beverages, unsalted crackers, or dry toast may relieve effect. Report any sign of infection (sore throat, fever). Several wks may be needed for full therapeutic effect of B/P reduction. Skipping doses or voluntarily discontinuing drug may produce severe, rebound hypertension.

enoxacin

en-**ox**-ah-sin
(Penetrex)

PREGNANCY CATEGORY C

CLASSIFICATION

Anti-infective: quinolone

AVAILABILITY (Rx)

Tablets: 200 mg, 400 mg

PHARMACOKINETICS

Absorption: Well absorbed from GI tract. **Metabolism:** Partially metabolized in liver. **Excretion:** Primarily excreted in urine. **Half-life:** 3–6 hrs.

ACTION/*THERAPEUTIC EFFECT*

Inhibits DNA-gyrase in susceptible microorganisms, *interfering w/bacterial DNA replication and repair.*

USES/*UNLABELED*

Treatment of uncomplicated urethral or cervical gonorrhea, uncomplicated (cystitis) or complicated urinary tract infections. *Treatment of chancroid.*

ADMINISTRATION

ORAL:

- Give 1 hr before or 2 hrs after meals.

INDICATIONS/ROUTES/DOSAGE

Uncomplicated (cystitis) urinary tract infection:
Oral: Adults >18 yrs, elderly: 200 mg q12h for 7 days.

Complicated urinary tract infection:
Oral: Adults >18 yrs, elderly: 400 mg q12h for 14 days.

Uncomplicated gonorrhea:
Oral: Adults >18 hrs: 400 mg given as single dose.

Dosage in renal impairment:
The dose and/or frequency is modified based on degree of renal impairment.

CREATININE CLEARANCE	DOSAGE
<30 ml/min	Normal initial dose, then 1/2 regular dose q12h

CONTRAINDICATIONS

Do not use in children <18 years of age.

CAUTIONS

Renal impairment, CNS disorders, seizures, those taking theophylline or caffeine.

INTERACTIONS

DRUG: *Antacids, bismuth subsalicylate, sucralfate* may decrease absorption (give at least 4 hrs before or 2 hrs after enoxacin). Decreases clearance, may increase concentration, toxicity of ***theophylline***. May increase effects of ***oral anticoagulants***. **HERBAL:** None known. **FOOD:** Give 1 hr before or 2 hrs after meals. **ALTERED LAB VALUES:** May increase SGOT (AST), SGPT (ALT), alkaline phosphatase, LDH, bilirubin, BUN, creatinine.

SIDE EFFECTS

FREQUENT (5–10%): Nausea, vomiting. OCCASIONAL (1–5%): Abdominal pain, diarrhea, headache, dizziness. RARE (<1%): Dry mouth, heartburn, constipation, flatulence, fatigue, drowsiness, insomnia, seizures, confusion, photosensitivity reaction.

ADVERSE REACTIONS/TOXIC EFFECTS

Superinfection (particularly enterococcal, fungal). Hypersensitivity reactions, serious and occasionally fatal, have occurred in pts receiving quinolone therapy. Arthropathy may occur if given to children <18 yrs.

PATIENT CONSIDERATIONS

BASELINE ASSESSMENT

Question for history of hypersensitivity to fluoroquinolones, quinolone group of antibacterials (cinoxacin, nalidixic acid).

INTERVENTION/EVALUATION

Monitor stool frequency and consistency. Be alert for superinfection, e.g., genital pruritus, vaginitis, fever, sores, and discomfort in mouth.

PATIENT/FAMILY TEACHING

Drink fluids liberally. Complete full course of therapy. Instruct pt

regarding meals/medications (see Oral Administration). Do not drive or perform activities requiring alertness or dexterity if dizziness occurs. Avoid sunlight/ultraviolet exposure; wear sunscreen and protective clothing.

enoxaparin sodium

en-**ox**-ah-pear-in
(Lovenox)

CANADIAN AVAILABILITY
Lovenox

PREGNANCY CATEGORY B

CLASSIFICATION

Anticoagulant

AVAILABILITY (Rx)

Injection: 30 mg/0.3 ml, 40 mg/0.4 ml, 60 mg/0.6 ml, 80 mg/0.8 ml, 100 mg/1 ml, **prefilled syringes**

PHARMACODYNAMICS

	ONSET	PEAK	DURATION
SubQ	—	3–5 hrs	12 hrs

PHARMACOKINETICS

Absorption: Well absorbed after SubQ administration. **Excretion:** Eliminated primarily in urine. **Half-life:** 4.5 hrs.

ACTION/*THERAPEUTIC EFFECT*

Antithrombin; in presence of low molecular weight heparin, *produces anticoagulation* by inhibition of factor Xa. Enoxaparin causes less inactivation of thrombin, inhibition of platelets, and bleeding than standard heparin. Does not significantly influence bleeding time, prothrombin time (PT), activated partial thromboplastin time (APTT).

USES/*UNLABELED*

Prevention of postop deep vein thrombosis (DVT) following hip or knee replacement surgery, abdominal surgery, nonsurgical acute illness. Long-term DVT prevention following hip replacement surgery. Treatment of unstable angina, non-Q-wave myocardial infarction, acute DVT (w/warfarin). *Prevents DVT following general surgical procedures.*

STORAGE/HANDLING

Parenteral form appears clear and colorless to pale yellow. Store at room temperature.

ADMINISTRATION

Note: Do not mix w/other injections or infusions. Do not give IM.

SUBQ:

- Instruct pt to lie down before administering by deep SubQ injection.
- Inject between left and right anterolateral and left and right posterolateral abdominal wall.
- Introduce entire length of needle ($^1/_2$ inch) into skin fold held between thumb and forefinger, holding skin fold during injection.

INDICATIONS/ROUTES/DOSAGE

Note: Give initial dose as soon as possible after surgery but not more than 24 hrs after surgery.

Prevention of deep vein thrombosis (hip, knee surgery):
SubQ: Adults, elderly: 30 mg twice daily, generally for 7–10 days.

Prevention of DVT abdominal surgery, nonsurgical acute illness:
SubQ: Adults, elderly: 40 mg daily.

E

Angina, myocardial infarction:
SubQ: Adults, elderly: 1 mg/kg q12h.

Acute DVT:
SubQ: Adults, elderly: 1 mg/kg q12h or 1.5 mg/kg once daily.

CONTRAINDICATIONS

Active major bleeding, concurrent heparin therapy, thrombocytopenia associated w/positive in vitro test for antiplatelet antibody, hypersensitivity to heparin or pork products.

CAUTIONS

Conditions w/increased risk of hemorrhage, history of heparin-induced thrombocytopenia, impaired renal function, elderly, uncontrolled arterial hypertension, history of recent GI ulceration and hemorrhage.

INTERACTIONS

DRUG: *Anticoagulants, platelet inhibitors* may increase bleeding (use w/care). **HERBAL:** Feverfew, garlic, ginkgo may increase risk of bleeding. **FOOD:** None significant. **ALTERED LAB VALUES:** Reversible increases in SGOT (AST), SGPT (ALT), alkaline phosphatase, lactic dehydrogenase (LDH).

SIDE EFFECTS

FREQUENT (4–10%): Hemorrhology, fever. **OCCASIONAL (1–4%):** Bleeding, pain/irritation at injection site, nausea, unusually tired/weak, thrombocytopenia, confusion, swelling of ankles.

ADVERSE REACTIONS/TOXIC EFFECTS

Accidental overdosage may lead to bleeding complications ranging from local ecchymoses to major hemorrhage. ***Antidote:*** Dose of protamine sulfate (1% solution) should be equal to the dose of enoxaparin injected. One mg protamine sulfate neutralizes 1 mg enoxaparin. A second dose of 0.5 mg/mg protamine sulfate may be given if APTT tested 2–4 hrs after the first infusion remains prolonged.

PATIENT CONSIDERATIONS

BASELINE ASSESSMENT

Assess complete blood count, including platelet count. Determine initial B/P.

INTERVENTION/EVALUATION

Periodically monitor CBC, platelet count, stool for occult blood (no need for daily monitoring in pts w/normal presurgical coagulation parameters). Assess for any sign of bleeding: bleeding at surgical site, hematuria, blood in stool, bleeding from gums, petechiae, bruising, bleeding from injection sites; monitor B/P for hypotension.

PATIENT/FAMILY TEACHING

Usual length of therapy is 7–10 days. Report any sign of bleeding (as above). Do not take any OTC medication (especially aspirin) w/o consulting physician.

---

entacapone
(Comtan)
See Supplement

---

epinephrine

eh-pih-**nef**-rin
(Adrenalin, Sus-Phrine, Primatene, Bronkaid, AsthmaHaler, Bronitin, MedihalerEpi, EpiPen)

CANADIAN AVAILABILITY
Adrenalin, Bronkaid, Epi-Pen, Vaponefrin

PREGNANCY CATEGORY C

CLASSIFICATION

Sympathomimetic

AVAILABILITY (Rx)

Solution for Inhalation: 2%, 2.25%. **Aerosol:** 0.2 mg/spray, 0.25 mg/spray, 0.3 mg/spray. **Injection:** 1 mg/ml, 0.1 mg/ml, 0.01 mg/ml. **Injection (suspension):** 5 mg/ml. **Ophthalmic Solution:** 0.1%, 0.5%, 1%, 2%.

PHARMACODYNAMICS

	ONSET	PEAK	DURATION
SubQ	5–10 min	20 min	1–4 hrs
IM	5–10 min	20 min	1–4 hrs
Inhalation	3–5 min	20 min	1–3 hrs
Ophthalmic	1 hr	4–8 hrs	12–24 hrs

PHARMACOKINETICS

Absorption: Minimal absorption after inhalation, well absorbed after parenteral administration. **Metabolism:** Metabolized in liver, other tissues, sympathetic nerve endings. **Excretion:** Excreted in urine. ***Ophthalmic:*** May have systemic absorption from drainage into nasal pharyngeal passages. Mydriasis occurs within several min, persists several hours; vasoconstriction occurs within 5 min, lasts <1 hr.

ACTION/*THERAPEUTIC EFFECT*

Stimulates alpha-adrenergic receptors (vasoconstriction, pressor effects), $beta_1$-adrenergic receptors (cardiac stimulation), and $beta_2$-adrenergic receptors (bronchial dilation, vasodilation), *resulting in relaxation of smooth muscle of bronchial tree, peripheral vasculature.* **Ophthalmic:** *Increases outflow of aqueous humor from anterior eye chamber,* dilates pupils (constricts conjunctival blood vessels).

USES/*UNLABELED*

Treatment of acute bronchial asthma attacks, reversible bronchospasm in pts w/chronic bronchitis, emphysema, hypersensitivity reactions. Restores cardiac rhythm in cardiac arrest. ***Ophthalmic:*** Management of chronic open-angle glaucoma alone or in combination w/other agents. ***Systemic:*** *Treatment of gingival/pulpal hemorrhage; priapism.* **Ophthalmic:** *Treatment of conjunctival congestion during surgery; secondary glaucoma.*

STORAGE/HANDLING

Store parenteral forms at room temperature. Do not use if solution appears discolored or contains a precipitate.

ADMINISTRATION

INHALATION:

- Shake container well, exhale completely then holding mouthpiece 1 inch away from lips, inhale and hold breath as long as possible before exhaling.
- Wait 1–10 min before inhaling second dose (allows for deeper bronchial penetration).
- Rinse mouth w/water immediately after inhalation (prevents mouth/throat dryness).

OPHTHALMIC:

- For topical ophthalmic use only.
- Instruct pt to tilt head backward and look up.
- Gently pull lower lid down to form pouch and instill medication.
- Do not touch tip of applicator to lids or any surface.
- When lower lid is released, have pt keep eye open w/o blinking for at least 30 sec.
- Apply gentle finger pressure to lacrimal sac (bridge of the nose, inside corner of the eye) for 1–2 min.

- Remove excess solution around eye w/a tissue. Wash hands immediately to remove medication on hands.

SubQ:
- Shake ampule thoroughly.
- Use tuberculin syringe for SubQ into lateral deltoid region.
- Massage rejection site (minimizes vasoconstriction effect).

IV:
- For injection, dilute each 1 mg of 1:1,000 solution w/10 ml normal saline to provide 1:10,000 solution.
- For infusion, further dilute w/5% dextrose in water.

INDICATIONS/ROUTES/DOSAGE

Cardiac arrest:
IV: Adults, elderly: 0.1–1 mg (1–10 ml of 1:10,000 concentration). May repeat q5min (or may be followed by 0.3 mg SubQ or IV infusion initially at 1 mcg/min up to 4 mcg/min). ***Children:*** 0.01 mg/kg (0.1 ml/kg of 1:10,000 concentration). May repeat q5min (or may give IV infusion initially at 0.1 mcg/kg/min increased at 0.1 mcg/kg/min increments up to maximum of 1 mcg/kg/min). ***Neonates:*** 0.01–0.03 mg/kg (0.1–0.3 ml/kg of 1:10,000 concentration). May repeat q5min.

Intracardiac: Adults, elderly: 0.1–1 mg (1–10 ml of 1:10,000 concentration). ***Children:*** 0.005–0.01 mg/kg (0.05–0.1 ml/kg of 1:10,000 concentration).

Severe anaphylaxis or asthma:
SubQ/IM: Adults, elderly: 0.1–0.5 mg (0.1–0.5 ml of 1:1,000 concentration). May repeat at 10–15 min intervals for anaphylaxis; 20 min-4 hrs for asthma.

SubQ: Children: 0.01 mg/kg (0.01 ml/kg of 1:1,000 concentration). ***Maximum single dose:*** 0.5 mg. May repeat at 20 min-4 hr intervals.

Asthma (prolonged effect):
SubQ: Adults, elderly: Initially, 0.5 mg (0.1 ml of 1:200 concentration). May repeat w/0.5–1.5 mg no sooner than 6 hrs from previous dose. ***Children:*** 0.02–0.025 mg/kg (0.004–0.005 ml/kg of 1:200 concentration). ***Maximum single dose:*** 0.75 mg. May repeat no sooner than 6 hrs from previous dose.

Severe anaphylactic shock:
IV: Adults, elderly: 0.1–0.25 mg (1–2.5 ml of 1:10,000 concentration) over 5–10 min. May repeat q5–15min, or continuous IV infusion initially at 1 mcg/min up to 4 mcg/min. ***Children:*** 0.1 mg (10 ml of 1: 100,000 concentration) over 5–10 min followed w/IV infusion of 0.1 mcg/kg/min up to 1.5 mcg/kg/min.

Usual inhalation dosage:
Inhalation: Adults, elderly, children >4 yrs: 1 inhalation, may repeat in at least 1 min; subsequent doses no sooner than 3 hrs.

Nebulizer: Adults, elderly, children >4 yrs: 1–3 deep inhalations; subsequent doses no sooner than 3 hrs.

Glaucoma:
Ophthalmic: Adults, elderly: 1–2 drops 1–2 times/day.

CONTRAINDICATIONS

Hypertension, hyperthyroidism, ischemic heart disease, cardiac arrhythmias, cerebrovascular insufficiency, narrow-angle glaucoma, shock.

CAUTIONS

Elderly, diabetes mellitus, angina pectoris, tachycardia, myocardial infarction, severe renal/hepatic impairment, psychoneurotic disorders, hypoxia.

INTERACTIONS

DRUG: *Tricyclic antidepressants* may increase cardiovascular effects. May decrease effects of ***beta blockers. Ergonovine, methergine, oxytocin*** may increase vasoconstriction. *Digoxin, sympathomimetics* may increase risk of arrhythmias. **HERBAL:** Ma Huang (Ephedra) may increase effects. **FOOD:** None significant. **ALTERED LAB VALUES:** May decrease serum potassium levels.

SIDE EFFECTS

FREQUENT: *Systemic:* Fast/pounding heartbeat, nervousness. *Ophthalmic:* Headache/brow ache, stinging, burning, other eye irritation, watering of eyes. OCCASIONAL: *Systemic:* Dizziness, lightheadedness, facial flushing, headache, diaphoresis, increased B/P, nausea, trembling, insomnia, vomiting, weakness. *Ophthalmic:* Blurred/decreased vision, eye pain. RARE: *Systemic:* Chest discomfort/pain, irregular heartbeats, bronchospasm, dry mouth/throat.

ADVERSE REACTIONS/TOXIC EFFECTS

Excessive doses may cause acute hypertension, arrhythmias. Prolonged or excessive use may result in metabolic acidosis (due to increased serum lactic acid concentrations). Observe for disorientation, weakness, hyperventilation, headache, nausea, vomiting, diarrhea.

PATIENT CONSIDERATIONS

Baseline Assessment

Offer emotional support (high incidence of anxiety due to difficulty in breathing and sympathomimetic response to drug).

Intervention/Evaluation

Monitor B/P; rate, depth, rhythm, type of respiration; quality and rate of pulse. Assess lung sounds for rhonchi, wheezing, rales. Monitor arterial blood gases. Observe lips, fingernails for blue or dusky color in light-skinned pts; gray in dark-skinned pts. In cardiac arrest, monitor EKG, B/P, pulse. Evaluate for clinical improvement (quieter, slower respirations, relaxed facial expression, cessation of clavicular retractions).

Patient/Family Teaching

Increase fluid intake (decreases lung secretion viscosity). Avoid excessive use of caffeine derivatives (chocolate, coffee, tea, cola, cocoa).

Ophthalmic

Teach proper administration. Slight burning, stinging may occur on initial instillation. Report any new symptoms (rapid pulse, shortness of breath, or dizziness immediately: may be systemic effects).

---

epirubicin

(Ellene)

See Classification section under: Cancer chemotherapy

---

epoetin alfa

eh-po-**ee**-tin

(Epogen, Procrit)

CANADIAN AVAILABILITY

Eprex

PREGNANCY CATEGORY C

CLASSIFICATION

Erythropoietin

AVAILABILITY (Rx)

Injection: 2,000 units, 3,000 units, 4,000 units, 10,000 units, 20,000 units

PHARMACOKINETICS

Absorption: Well absorbed after SubQ administration. After administration, an increase in reticulocyte count seen within 10 days; increases in Hgb, Hct, and RBC count within 2–6 wks. **Half-life:** 4–13 hrs.

ACTION/*THERAPEUTIC EFFECT*

Stimulates division, differentiation of erythroid progenitor cells in bone marrow, *induces erythropoiesis, release of reticulocytes from marrow.*

USES/*UNLABELED*

Treatment of anemia associated w/chronic renal failure or related to zidovudine (AZT) therapy in HIV-infected pts or to chemotherapy in cancer pts, those scheduled for elective nonvascular surgery, reducing need for allogenic blood transfusions. *Prevents anemia in pts donating blood prior to elective surgery, autologous transfusion; treatment of anemia associated w/neoplastic diseases.*

STORAGE/HANDLING

Refrigerate; stable for up to 14 days at room temperature. Use 1 dose/vial; do not reenter vial. Discard unused portion.

INDICATIONS/ROUTES/DOSAGE

Note: May give IV or SubQ.

Chronic renal failure:
IV/SubQ: Adults, elderly: Initially 50–100 units/kg 3 times/wk. Target Hct range: 30–36%. Dosage adjustments not earlier than 1 mo intervals unless clinically indicated. ***Decrease dose:*** Hct increasing and approaching 36% (temporarily hold doses if Hct continues to rise, reinstate lower dose when Hct begins to decrease); Hct increases by >4 points in 2 wk period (monitor Hct 2 times/wk for 2–6 wks). ***Increase dose:*** Hct does not increase 5–6 points after 8 wks (w/iron stores adequate) and Hct below target range. ***Maintenance: (Dialysis):*** 75 units/kg 3 times/wk. ***Range:*** 12.5–525 units/kg. ***(Nondialysis):*** 75–150 units/kg/wk.

AZT-treated, HIV-infected pts:
Note: Pt receiving AZT w/serum erythropoietin levels >500 milliunits likely not to respond to therapy. ***IV/SubQ: Adults:*** Initially, 100 units/kg 3 times/wk for 8 wks; may increase by 50–100 units/kg 3 times/wk. Evaluate response q4–8wks thereafter; adjust dose by 50–100 units/kg 3 times/wk. If doses >300 units/kg 3 times/wk are not eliciting response, unlikely pt will respond. ***Maintenance:*** Titrate to maintain desired Hct.

Chemotherapy pts:
SubQ: Adults, elderly: Initially, 150 units/kg 3 times/wk up to 300 units/kg 3 times/wk.

Reduce allogenic blood transfusions:
SubQ: Adults, elderly: 300 units/kg/day 10 days prior to, on day of, and 4 days after surgery.

CONTRAINDICATIONS

Uncontrolled hypertension, history of sensitivity to mammalian cell-derived products or human albumin.

CAUTIONS

History of seizures, vascular disease, previous controlled hypertension, blood disorders (e.g., sickle-cell anemia).

INTERACTIONS

DRUG: May need to increase heparin (increase in RBC volume may enhance blood clotting). **HERBAL:** None known. **FOOD:** None significant. **ALTERED LAB VALUES:** May decrease bleeding time, iron concentration, serum ferritin. May increase BUN, creatinine, phosphorus, potassium, sodium, uric acid.

SIDE EFFECTS

Note: Generally well tolerated. FREQUENT (10–20%): Hypertension, headache, nausea, arthralgia. OCCASIONAL (5–10%): Fatigue, edema, diarrhea, vomiting, chest pain, reaction at administration site, asthenia, dizziness, clotted access. RARE (<5%): Seizures, stroke, myocardial infarction.

AZT-treated HIV-infected: FREQUENT: Fever, headache, cough, rash, respiratory congestion, nausea, shortness of breath, skin reaction at injection site.

ADVERSE REACTIONS/TOXIC EFFECTS

Hypertensive encephalopathy, thrombosis, cerebrovascular accident, MI, seizures have occurred rarely. Hyperkalemia occurs occasionally, usually in those who do not conform to medication compliance, dietary guidelines, frequency of dialysis.

PATIENT CONSIDERATIONS

Baseline Assessment

Assess B/P before drug initiation (80% of those w/CRF have history of hypertension). B/P often rises during early therapy in those w/history of hypertension. Consider that all pts will eventually need supplemental iron therapy. Assess serum iron (transferrin saturation: should be >20%) and serum ferritin (>100 ng/ml) prior to and during therapy. Establish baseline CBC, differential and platelet counts (especially note hematocrit). Monitor B/P aggressively for increased B/P (25% of those on medication require antihypertension therapy, dietary restrictions).

Intervention/Evaluation

Monitor Hct level diligently (if level increases >4 points in 2 wk period, dosage should be reduced); assess CBC, differential, platelet counts routinely. Monitor temperature, especially in cancer pts on chemotherapy and zidovudine-treated HIV pts, and BUN, uric acid, creatinine, phosphorus, potassium, especially in CRF pts. Evaluate food tolerance and stool frequency, consistency. Provide assistance for dizziness, fatigue, and safety for possible seizures.

Patient/Family Teaching

Compliance w/dietary guidelines and frequency of dialysis is essential (improved sense of well-being may be misleading in CRF pts). Evidence of response to epoetin alfa may be seen in increased reticulocyte count within 10 days; however, Hct changes take 2–6 wks. Does not substitute for emergency transfusions. Avoid tasks that require alertness, motor skills until response to drug is established.

epoprostenol sodium, PG_2, PGX, prostacyclin

ep-oh-**pros**-ten-awl
(Flolan)

CANADIAN AVAILABILITY
Flolan

PREGNANCY CATEGORY B

CLASSIFICATION

Antihypertensive

AVAILABILITY (Rx)

Powder for Injection: 0.5 mg, 1.5 mg

PHARMACOKINETICS

Metabolism: After IV administration, rapidly hydrolyzed, subject to enzymatic degradation. Metabolized to active metabolite. **Half-life:** 6 min.

ACTION/*THERAPEUTIC EFFECT*

Directly vasodilates pulmonary and systemic arterial vascular beds and inhibits platelet aggregation. *Reduces right and left ventricular afterload, increases cardiac output, stroke volume.*

USES/*UNLABELED*

Long-term treatment of primary pulmonary hypertension in class III and class IV pts (New York Heart Association). *Pulmonary hypertension associated w/adult respiratory syndrome, systemic lupus erythematosus, or congenital heart disease; neonatal pulmonary hypertension, cardiopulmonary bypass surgery, hemodialysis, refractory CHF, severe community-acquired pneumonia.*

STORAGE/HANDLING

Store unopened vials at room temperature. Protect both unopened vial and reconstituted solution from light. After reconstitution, refrigerate, protect from light. Do not freeze (discard any frozen solution). Discard any solution refrigerated >48 hrs.

ADMINISTRATION

Note: Refer to manufacturer for concentration and proper dilutions. Give reconstituted solution at room temperature for duration of 8 hrs or may be used w/cold pouch and given ≤24 hrs w/2 frozen 6 oz gel packs. Insulate from temp >77°F or <32°F. Do not expose to direct sunlight.

IV:

Note: Administer through central venous catheter using ambulatory infusion pump. During dose ranging, may administer peripherally. Do not give w/other solutions or medications.

INDICATIONS/ROUTES/DOSAGE

Pulmonary hypertension:

Note: Infused continuously through permanent indwelling central venous catheter using an ambulatory infusion pump. May give through peripheral vein on temporary basis.

IV Infusion: Adults, elderly: (Acute dose-ranging procedure): Initially, 2 ng/kg/min increased in increments of 2 ng/kg/min every 15 min until dose-limiting adverse effects occur. ***(Chronic infusion):*** Start at 4 ng/kg/min less than the maximum dose rate tolerated during acute dose ranging (or ½ maximum rate if rate was below 5 ng/kg/min).

CONTRAINDICATIONS

Chronic use in those w/CHF (severe ventricular systolic dysfunction), hypersensitivity to drug or structurally related compounds.

CAUTIONS

Elderly.

INTERACTIONS

DRUG: Hypotensive effects may be increased by other ***vasodilators*** or using acetate in dialysis fluids. ***Anticoagulants, antiplatelets*** may increase risk of bleeding. ***Vasoconstrictors*** may decrease effect. **HERBAL:** None known. **FOOD:** None significant. **ALTERED LAB VALUES:** None significant.

SIDE EFFECTS

Acute phase: FREQUENT: Flushing (58%), headache (49%), nausea (32%), vomiting (32%), hypotension (16%), anxiety (11%), chest pain (11%), dizziness (8%). OCCASIONAL (2–5%): Bradycardia, abdominal pain, muscle pain, dyspnea, back pain. RARE (<2%): Diaphoresis, dyspepsia, paresthesia, tachycardia. ***Chronic phase:*** FREQUENT (>20%): Dyspnea, asthenia, dizziness, headache, chest pain, nausea, vomiting, palpitations, edema, jaw pain, tachycardia, flushing, myalgia, nonspecific muscle pain, paresthesia, diarrhea, anxiety, chills/fever/flulike symptoms. OCCASIONAL (10–20%): Rash, depression, hypotension, pallor, syncope, bradycardia, ascites.

ADVERSE REACTIONS/TOXIC EFFECTS

Overdose may causes hyperglycemia/ketoacidosis (increased urination, thirst, fruitlike breath). Angina, myocardial infarction, thrombocytopenia occur rarely. Abrupt withdrawal (including large reduction in dosage, interruption in drug delivery) may produce rebound pulmonary hypertension (dyspnea, dizziness, asthenia).

PATIENT CONSIDERATIONS

INTERVENTION/EVALUATION

Monitor functioning of pump devices/catheters. Monitor standing/supine B/P w/any dosage adjustment for several hours after adjustment. Assess for therapeutic response: improvement in pulmonary function, decreased dyspnea on exertion (DOE), fatigue, syncope, chest pain, pulmonary vascular resistance, pulmonary arterial pressure.

PATIENT/FAMILY TEACHING

Instruct pt on drug reconstitution, drug administration, care of the permanent central venous catheter. Brief interruptions in drug delivery may result in rapid, deteriorating symptoms. Drug therapy will be necessary for a prolonged period, possibly years.

eprosartan

eh-pro-**sar**-tan
(Teveten)

PREGNANCY CATEGORY C
First trimester

PREGNANCY CATEGORY D
Second and third trimester.

CLASSIFICATION

Angiotensin II receptor antagonist

AVAILABILITY (Rx)

Tablets: 200 mg

PHARMACOKINETICS

Absorption: Rapidly absorbed following oral administration. **Metabolism:** Undergoes first-pass metabolism in liver to active metabolites. **Excretion:** Excreted in urine and biliary system. **Half-life:** 5–9 hrs.

ACTION/*THERAPEUTIC EFFECT*

Potent vasodilator. Blocks vasoconstrictor and aldosterone-secreting effects of angiotensin II, inhibiting the binding of angiotensin II to the AT1 receptors, *causing vasodilation, decreased peripheral resistance, decrease in B/P.*

USES

Treatment of hypertension.

ADMINISTRATION

ORAL:

- May give w/o regard to food.
- Do not crush or break tablets.

INDICATIONS/DOSAGE/ROUTES

Hypertension:

Oral: Adults, elderly: Initially, 200 mg/day. ***Range:*** 400–600 mg/day.

CONTRAINDICATIONS

None significant.

CAUTIONS

Renal/hepatic function impairment, renal arterial stenosis.

INTERACTIONS

DRUG: None significant. **HERBAL:** None known. **FOOD:** None significant. **ALTERED LAB VALUES:** May increase BUN, serum creatinine, SGOT (AST), SGPT (ALT), alkaline phosphatase, bilirubin. May decrease Hgb, Hct.

SIDE EFFECTS

OCCASIONAL (2–5%): Headache, cough, dizziness. **RARE (<2%):** Muscle pain, fatigue, diarrhea, upper respiratory infection, dyspepsia.

ADVERSE REACTIONS/TOXIC EFFECTS

Overdosage may manifest as hypotension and tachycardia; bradycardia occurs less often.

PATIENT CONSIDERATIONS

BASELINE ASSESSMENT

Obtain B/P and apical pulse immediately before each dose, in addition to regular monitoring (be alert to fluctuations). Question possibility of pregnancy (see Pregnancy Category). Assess medication history (especially diuretic). Question for history of hepatic/renal impairment, renal artery stenosis.

INTERVENTION/EVALUATION

If excessive reduction in B/P occurs, place pt in supine position, feet slightly elevated. Maintain hydration (offer fluids frequently). Assess for evidence of upper respiratory infection, cough. Assist with ambulation if dizziness occurs. Monitor stool frequency and consistency (watery, loose, soft).

PATIENT/FAMILY TEACHING

Inform female pt regarding consequences of second- and third-trimester exposure to medication. Report pregnancy to physician as soon as possible. Avoid tasks that require alertness, motor skills (possible dizziness effect). Report any sign of infection (sore throat, fever). Do not take cold preparations, nasal decongestants. Do not take other medications w/o consulting physician. Restrict sodium and alcohol intake. Follow diet and control weight. Do not stop taking medication. Need for lifelong control. Caution against exercising during hot weather (risk of dehydration, hypotension).

---

eptifibatide

(Integrillin)

See Supplement

---

ergoloid mesylates

ur-go-loyd **mess**-ah-lates

(Gerimal, Hydergine)

CANADIAN AVAILABILITY
Hydergine

CLASSIFICATION

Psychotherapeutic

AVAILABILITY (Rx)

Tablets (sublingual): 0.5 mg, 1 mg. **Tablets:** 0.5 mg, 1 mg. **Capsules:** 1 mg. **Liquid:** 1 mg/ml.

PHARMACOKINETICS

Absorption: Rapidly, incompletely absorbed from GI tract. **Metabolism:** Metabolized in liver. **Excretion:** Eliminated primarily in feces. **Half-life:** 2–5 hrs.

ACTION/*THERAPEUTIC EFFECT*

Central action decreases vascular tone, slows heart rate. Peripheral action blocks alpha adrenergic receptors. *Improves O_2 uptake and improves cerebral metabolism.*

USES

Treatment of age-related (those >60 yrs) mental capacity decline (cognitive and interpersonal skills, mood, self-care, apparent motivation).

ADMINISTRATION

ORAL:

- Instruct pt to allow sublingual tablets to completely dissolve under tongue; do not crush or chew.
- Do not break capsule or tablet form.

INDICATIONS/ROUTES/DOSAGE

Age-related decline in mental capacity:
Oral: Adults, elderly: Initially, 1 mg 3 times/day. ***Range:*** 1.5–12 mg/day.

CONTRAINDICATIONS

Acute or chronic psychosis, regardless of etiology.

CAUTIONS

None significant.

INTERACTIONS

DRUG: None significant. **HERBAL:** None known. **FOOD:** None significant. **ALTERED LAB VALUES:** None significant.

SIDE EFFECTS

OCCASIONAL: GI distress, transient nausea, sublingual irritation, bradycardia, orthostatic hypotension, skin rash.

ADVERSE REACTIONS/TOXIC EFFECTS

Overdose may produce blurred vision, dizziness, syncope, headache, flushed face, nausea, vomiting, decreased appetite, stomach cramps, stuffy nose.

PATIENT CONSIDERATIONS

Baseline Assessment

Exclude possibility that pt's signs and symptoms arise from a possibly reversible and treatable condition secondary to systemic disease, neurologic disease, or primary disturbance of mood before administering medication.

Intervention/Evaluation

Periodically reassess benefit of current therapy.

Patient/Family Teaching

Elimination of symptoms appears gradual. Results may not be noted for 3–4 wks.

ergonovine maleate

er-goe-**noe**-veen
(Ergotrate)

CLASSIFICATION

Uterine stimulant

AVAILABILITY (Rx)

Injection: 0.2 mg/ml

PHARMACODYNAMICS

	ONSET	PEAK	DURATION
IM	3–5 min	—	>3 hrs
IV	40 secs	—	>45 min

PHARMACOKINETICS

Absorption: Rapidly absorbed after IM administration. Distributed to plasma, extracellular fluid. **Metabolism:** Metabolized in liver. **Excretion:** Excreted in urine.

ACTION/*THERAPEUTIC EFFECT*

Directly stimulates uterine muscle *(increases force, frequency of contractions). Induces cervical contractions.* Stimulates alpha adrenergic, serotonin receptors *producing arterial vasoconstriction.* Causes vasospasm of coronary arteries.

USES/*UNLABELED*

To prevent and treat postpartum, postabortion hemorrhage due to atony or involution (not for induction or augmentation of labor). *Treatment of incomplete abortion, diagnosis of angina pectoris.*

STORAGE/HANDLING

Refrigerate parenteral form; protect from light.

ADMINISTRATION

IM/IV:

- IV use in life-threatening emergencies only; may dilute to volume of 5 ml w/0.9% NaCl injection; give over at least 1 min, carefully monitoring B/P.

INDICATIONS/ROUTES/DOSAGE

Oxytocic:

IM/IV: Adults: Initially, 0.2 mg. May repeat no more often than q2–4h for no more than 5 doses total.

CONTRAINDICATIONS

Hypersensitivity to ergot, hypertension, pregnancy, toxemia, untreated hypocalcemia, induction of labor, threatened spontaneous abortions.

CAUTIONS

Renal/hepatic impairment, coronary artery disease, occlusive peripheral vascular disease, sepsis.

INTERACTIONS

DRUG: ***Vasoconstrictors, vasopressors*** may increase effect. **HERBAL:** None known. **FOOD:** None significant. **ALTERED LAB VALUES:** May decrease prolactin concentration.

SIDE EFFECTS

FREQUENT: Nausea, uterine cramping, vomiting. **OCCASIONAL:** Abdominal/stomach pain, diarrhea, headache, dizziness, nasal congestion, sweating, tinnitus, unpleasant taste, bradycardia, chest pain. **RARE:** Pain in arms, legs, or lower back, allergic reaction.

ADVERSE REACTIONS/TOXIC EFFECTS

Severe hypertensive episodes may result in cerebrovascular accident, serious arrhythmias, seizures; hypertensive effects more frequent w/pt susceptibility, rapid IV administration, concurrent regional anesthesia or vasoconstrictors. Peripheral ischemia may lead to gangrene.

PATIENT CONSIDERATIONS

BASELINE ASSESSMENT

Question for hypersensitivity to

any ergot derivatives. Determine calcium, B/P, and pulse baselines. Assess bleeding prior to administration.

INTERVENTION/EVALUATION

Monitor uterine contractions (frequency, strength, duration), bleeding, B/P, and pulse every 15 min until stable (about 1–2 hrs). Assess extremities for color, warmth, movement, pain. Report chest pain promptly. Provide support w/ambulation if dizziness occurs.

PATIENT/FAMILY TEACHING

Avoid smoking because of added vasoconstriction. Report increased cramping, bleeding, or foul-smelling lochia. Pale, cold hands/feet should be reported because may mean decreased circulation.

ergotamine tartrate

er-**got**-a-meen
(Ergostar Medihaler Ergotamine)

dihydroergotamine

(Migranal, D.H.E.)

FIXED-COMBINATION(S)
W/caffeine, a stimulant **(Cafergot, Wigraine)**; w/belladonna, an anticholinergic, and phenobarbital, a sedative-hypnotic **(Bellergal-S)**

CANADIAN AVAILABILITY
Ergomar, Migranal

PREGNANCY CATEGORY D

CLASSIFICATION

Antimigraine

AVAILABILITY (Rx)

Tablets (sublingual): 2 mg. **Aerosol:** 9 mg/ml (0.36 mg/dose). **Injection:** 1 mg/ml. **Nasal Spray.**

PHARMACOKINETICS

Absorption: Slow, incomplete absorption from GI tract, rapid, extensive absorption rectally. **Metabolism:** Undergoes extensive first-pass metabolism in liver. Metabolized to active metabolite. **Excretion:** Eliminated in feces via biliary system. **Half-life:** 21 hrs.

ACTION / *THERAPEUTIC EFFECT*

May have agonist/antagonist actions w/alpha adrenergic, serotonergic, dopaminergic receptors. Directly stimulates vascular smooth muscle, *constricting arteries and veins.* May inhibit reuptake of norepinephrine.

USES

Prevents or aborts vascular headaches (e.g., migraine, cluster headaches).

ADMINISTRATION

SUBLINGUAL:

- Place under tongue; do not swallow.

INHALATION:

- Shake container well; exhale completely; then holding mouthpiece 1 inch away from lips, inhale and hold breath as long as possible before exhaling.
- Wait at least 5 min before inhaling second dose, if needed.
- Rinse mouth w/water immediately after inhalation (prevents mouth/throat dryness).

INDICATIONS/ROUTES/DOSAGE

Note: Initiate therapy as soon as possible after first signs of attack.

Vascular headaches:
Sublingual: Adults, elderly: Initially, 2 mg (1 tablet). May repeat at 30 min intervals. ***Maximum:*** 3 tablets/24 hrs or 5 tablets/wk.

Intranasal: One spray in each nostril; repeat in 15 min.

IM/IV: 1 mg at first sign of headache; repeat in 1 hr. ***Maximum: IM:*** 3 mg; ***IV:*** 2 mg.

Aerosol: Adults, elderly: Initially, 1 inhalation. May repeat in 5 min. *Maximum:* 6 inhalations/24 hrs or 15 inhalations/wk.

CONTRAINDICATIONS

Hypersensitivity to ergot alkaloids, peripheral vascular disease (thromboangitis obliterans, syphilitic arteritis, severe arteriosclerosis, thrombophlebitis, Raynaud's disease), impaired renal/hepatic function, severe pruritus, coronary artery disease, hypertension, sepsis, malnutrition.

CAUTIONS

None significant.

INTERACTIONS

DRUG: *Beta blockers, erythromycin* may increase risk of vasospasm. May decrease effect of ***nitroglycerin. Ergot alkaloids, systemic vasoconstrictors*** may increase pressor effect. HERBAL: None known. FOOD: None significant. ALTERED LAB VALUES: None significant.

SIDE EFFECTS

FREQUENT: Swelling of face, fingers, feet or lower legs, dizziness, drowsiness, diarrhea, nausea, vomiting. OCCASIONAL: Chest pain, change in blood pressure, rapid/weak pulse, confusion, anxiety, pain in arms, legs, numbness of fingers, altered vision.

ADVERSE REACTIONS/TOXIC EFFECTS

Prolonged administration or excessive dosage may produce ergotamine poisoning: nausea, vomiting, weakness of legs, pain in limb muscles, numbness and tingling of fingers/toes, precordial pain, tachycardia or bradycardia, hyper/hypotension. Localized edema, itching due to vasoconstriction of peripheral arteries and arterioles. Feet, hands will become cold, pale, numb. Muscle pain occurs when walking and later, even at rest. Gangrene may occur. Occasionally confusion, depression, drowsiness, convulsions appear.

PATIENT CONSIDERATIONS

BASELINE ASSESSMENT

Question pt regarding history of peripheral vascular disease, renal/hepatic impairment, or possibility of pregnancy. Contact physician w/findings before administering drug. Question pt regarding onset, location, and duration of migraine and possible precipitating symptoms.

INTERVENTION/EVALUATION

Monitor closely for evidence of ergotamine overdosage as result of prolonged administration or excessive dosage (see Adverse Reactions/Toxic Effects). Notify physician of any signs and symptoms of ergotamine poisoning.

PATIENT/FAMILY TEACHING

Initiate therapy at first sign of migraine attack. Report if there is need to progressively increase dose to relieve vascular headaches or if irregular heartbeat, nausea, vomiting, numbness/tingling of fingers/toes, or pain or weakness of extremities is noted.

Discuss contraception w/physician; report suspected pregnancy immediately.

erythrityl

(Cardilate)

See Classification section under: Nitrates

erythromycin base

eh-rith-row-**my**-sin

(E-Mycin, Eryc, Ery-tab, PCE Dispertab, Ilotycin)

erythromycin estolate

(Ilosone)

erythromycin ethylsuccinate

(EES, Pediamycin, EryPed)

erythromycin lactobionate

(Erythrocin)

erythromycin stearate

(Erythrocin, Wyamycin)

erythromycin topical

(Akne-mycin, Eryderm, Erymax)

FIXED-COMBINATION(S)

Erythromycin ethylsuccinate combined w/sulfisoxazole, a sulfonamide **(Pediazole)**

CANADIAN AVAILABILITY

Erybid, Erythrocin, EES

PREGNANCY CATEGORY B

CLASSIFICATION

Antibiotic: Macrolide

AVAILABILITY (Rx)

Powder for Injection: 500 mg, 1 g.

Base: Tablets: 250 mg, 333 mg, 500 mg. **Tablets (delayed-release):** 333 mg. **Capsules (delayed-release):** 250 mg.

Estolate: Tablets: 500 mg. **Capsules:** 250 mg. **Oral Suspension:** 125 mg/5 ml, 250 mg/5 ml.

Ethylsuccinate: Tablets (chewable): 200 mg. **Tablets:** 400 mg. **Oral Suspension:** 200 mg/5 ml, 400 mg/5 ml. **Oral Drops:** 100 mg/2.5 ml.

Stearate: Tablets: 250 mg, 500 mg.

Ophthalmic Ointment: 5 mg/g. **Topical Solution:** 1.5%, 2%. **Topical Gel:** 2%. **Topical Ointment:** 2%.

PHARMACOKINETICS

Absorption: Variably absorbed from GI tract (affected by dosage form used). Widely distributed. **Metabolism:** Metabolized in liver. **Excretion:** Primarily eliminated in feces via bile. Not removed by hemodialysis. **Half-life:** 1.4–2 hrs (increased in reduced renal function).

ACTION / *THERAPEUTIC EFFECT*

Bacteriostatic. Penetrates bacterial cell membrane and reversibly binds to bacterial ribosomes, *inhibiting protein synthesis.*

USES / *UNLABELED*

Respiratory infections, otitis media, pertussis, inflammatory acne vulgaris, diphtheria (adjunctive therapy), Legionnaire's disease, intestinal amebiasis, preop intestinal antisepsis. Prophylaxis for rheumatic fever, bacterial endocarditis, respiratory tract surgery/invasive procedures, gonococcal ophthalmia neonatorum; if penicillin, tetracycline is contraindicated: gonorrheal pelvic inflammatory disease, coexisting chlamydial infections, uncomplicated urogenital infections, Lyme disease (younger than 9 yrs). ***Topical:*** Treatment of acne vulgaris. ***Ophthalmic:*** Treatment of ocular infections, prophylaxis of neonatal conjunctivitis, ophthalmia neonatorium. ***Systemic:*** *Treatment of acne vulgaris, chancroid, Campylobacter enteritis, gastroparesis, Lyme disease.* ***Topical:*** *Treatment of minor skin bacterial infections.* ***Ophthalmic:*** *Treatment of blepharitis, conjunctivitis, chlamydia, keratitis, trachoma.*

STORAGE/HANDLING

Store capsules, tablets at room temperature. Oral suspension stable for 14 days at room temperature. Diluted IV solutions stable for 8 hrs at room temperature, 24 hrs if refrigerated. Discard if precipitate forms.

ADMINISTRATION

ORAL:

- Administer erythromycin base, stearate 1 hr before or 2 hrs after food. Erythromycin estolate, ethylsuccinate may be given w/o regard to meals, but optimal absorption occurs when given on empty stomach.
- Give w/8 oz water.
- If swallowing difficulties exist, sprinkle capsule contents on teaspoon of applesauce, follow w/water.
- Do not swallow chewable tablets whole.

IV:

- For intermittent IV infusion, infuse over 20–60 min.
- Alternating IV sites, use large veins to reduce risk of phlebitis.

OPHTHALMIC:

- Place finger on lower eyelid and pull out until a pocket is formed between eye and lower lid. Place 1/4–1/2 inch ointment into pocket.
- Have pt close eye gently for 1–2 min, rolling eyeball (increases contact area of drug to eye).
- Remove excess ointment around eye w/tissue.

INDICATIONS/ROUTES/DOSAGE

Note: Space doses evenly around the clock: 400 mg erythromycin ethylsuccinate = 250 mg erythromycin base, stearate, or estolate.

Usual parenteral dosage:
IV: Adults, elderly, children: 15–20 mg/kg/day in divided doses. ***Maximum:*** 4 g/day.

Usual oral dosage:
Oral: Adults, elderly: 250 mg q6h; 500 mg q12h; or 333 mg q8h. Increase up to 4 g/day. ***Children:*** 30-50 mg/kg/day in divided doses up to 60–100 mg/kg/day for severe infections.

Preop intestinal antisepsis:
Oral: Adults, elderly: Give 1 g at 1, 2, and 11 PM on day prior to surgery (w/neomycin).

Acne vulgaris:
Topical: Adults: Apply to skin 2 times/day.

Gonococcal ophthalmia neonatorum:
Ophthalmic: Neonates: 0.5–2 cm no later than 1 hr after delivery.

CONTRAINDICATIONS

Hypersensitivity to erythromycins, preexisting liver disease, history of hepatitis due to erythromycins. Do not administer Pediazole to infants <2 mos.

CAUTIONS

Hepatic dysfunction. If combination used (Pediazole), consider precautions of sulfonamides. IV may cause increased HR, prolonged QT interval.

INTERACTIONS

DRUG: May inhibit metabolism of ***carbamazepine***. May decrease effects of ***chloramphenicol, clindamycin***. May increase concentration, toxicity of ***buspirone, cyclosporine, felodipine, lovastatin, simvastatin***. Hepatotoxic medications may increase hepatotoxicity. May increase risk of cardiotoxicity w/***cisapride***. May increase risk of toxicity w/***theophylline***. May increase effect of ***warfarin***. **HERBAL:** None known. **FOOD:** None significant. **ALTERED LAB VALUES:** May increase SGOT (AST), SGPT (ALT), alkaline, phosphatase, bilirubin.

SIDE EFFECTS

FREQUENT: Abdominal discomfort/cramping, phlebitis/thrombophlebitis w/IV administration. ***Topical:*** Dry skin (50%). **OCCASIONAL:** Nausea, vomiting, diarrhea, rash, urticaria. **RARE:** ***Ophthalmic:*** Sensitivity reaction w/increased irritation, burning, itching, inflammation. ***Topical:*** Urticaria.

ADVERSE REACTIONS/TOXIC EFFECTS

Superinfections, especially antibiotic-associated colitis, reversible cholestatic hepatitis may occur. High dosage in renal impairment may lead to reversible hearing loss. Anaphylaxis occurs rarely.

PATIENT CONSIDERATIONS

BASELINE ASSESSMENT

Question pt for history of allergies (particularly erythromycins), hepatitis. Obtain specimens for culture and sensitivity before giving first dose (therapy may begin before results are known).

INTERVENTION/EVALUATION

Check for GI discomfort, nausea, vomiting. Determine pattern of bowel activity, stool consistency. Assess skin for rash. Monitor hepatic function tests, assess for hepatotoxicity: malaise, fever, abdominal pain, GI disturbances. Evaluate for superinfection: genital/anal pruritus, sore mouth or tongue, moderate to severe diarrhea. Check for phlebitis (heat, pain, red streaking over vein).

PATIENT/FAMILY TEACHING

Continue therapy for full length of treatment. Doses should be evenly spaced. Do *not* swallow chewable tablets whole.Take medication w/8 oz water 1 hr before or 2 hrs after food/beverage. Notify physician in event of GI upset, rash, diarrhea, or other new symptom.

Ophthalmic

Report burning, itching, or inflammation: Inquire about use of eye makeup.

Topical

Report excessive dryness, itching, burning. Improvement of acne may not occur for 1–2 mos; maximum benefit may take 3 mos; therapy may last months or years. Use caution in use of other topical acne preparations containing peeling or abrasive agents, medicated or abrasive soaps, cosmetics containing alcohol (e.g., astringents, aftershave lotion).

esmolol hydrochloride

ez-moe-lol
(Brevibloc)

CANADIAN AVAILABILITY
Brevibloc

PREGNANCY CATEGORY C

CLASSIFICATION

Beta$_1$-adrenergic blocker

AVAILABILITY (Rx)

Injection: 10 mg/ml, 250 mg/ml

PHARMACOKINETICS

Widely distributed. **Metabolism:** Rapidly hydrolyzed by esterases in RBCs. **Excretion:** Primarily excreted in urine. **Half-life:** 9 min.

ACTION/*THERAPEUTIC EFFECT*

Selectively blocks beta$_1$-adrenergic receptors, *slowing sinus heart rate, decreasing cardiac output, decreasing B/P* (exact mechanism unknown but may block peripheral adrenergic receptors, decrease sympathetic outflow from CNS or decrease renin release from kidney). Antiarrhythmic activity due to blocking stimulation of cardiac pacemaker potentials.

USES

Rapid, short-term control of ventricular rate in those w/supraventricular arrhythmias, sinus tachycardia. Intra/postop control of tachycardia/hypertension.

STORAGE/HANDLING

Use only clear and colorless to light yellow solution. Alter dilution, solution is stable for 24 hrs. Discard solution if it is discolored or if precipitate forms.

ADMINISTRATION

- **Note:** Give by IV infusion. Avoid butterfly needles, very small veins.
- Must be diluted to concentration of 10 mg/ml (prevents vein irritation).
- For IV infusion, remove 20 ml from 500 ml container of 5% dextrose, 0.9% NaCl, or other compatible IV fluid and dilute 5 g vial esmolol hydrochloride w/remaining 480 ml to provide concentration of 10 mg/ml.
- Administer by controlled infusion device set at rate judged by tolerance and response. Hypotension (systolic B/P below 90 mm Hg) is greatest during first 30 min of IV infusion.

INDICATIONS/ROUTES/DOSAGE

IV: Adults, elderly: Initially, loading dose of 500 mcg/kg/min for 1 min, followed by 50 mcg/kg/min for 4 min. If optimum response is not attained in 5 min, give second loading dose of 500 mcg/kg/min for 1 min, followed by infusion of 100 mcg/kg/min for 4 min. Additional loading doses can be given and infusion increased by 50 mcg/kg/min (up to 200 mcg/kg/min) for 4 min. Once desired response is attained, cease loading dose and increase infusion by no more than 25 mcg/kg/min. Interval between doses may be increased to 10 min. Infusion usually administered over 24–48 hrs in most pts.

CONTRAINDICATIONS

Overt cardiac failure, cardiogenic shock, heart block greater than first degree, sinus bradycardia.

CAUTIONS

History of allergy, bronchial asthma, emphysema, bronchitis, CHF, diabetes, impaired renal function.

INTERACTIONS

DRUG: *Sympathomimetics, xanthines* may mutually inhibit effects. May mask symptoms of hypoglycemia, prolong hypoglycemic effect of ***insulin, oral hypoglycemics. MAO inhibitors*** may cause significant hypertension. **HERBAL:** None known. **FOOD:** None significant. **ALTERED LAB VALUES:** None significant.

SIDE EFFECTS

Generally well tolerated, w/transient and mild side effects. **FREQUENT:** Hypotension (systolic B/P below 90 mm Hg) manifested as dizziness, nausea, diaphoresis, headache, cold extremities, fatigue. **OCCASIONAL:** Anxiety, drowsiness, flushed skin, headache, nausea, vomiting, confusion, cold hands or feet, redness, inflammation at injection site. **RARE:** Bradycardia, breathing difficulties, chest pain, fainting, fever.

ADVERSE REACTIONS/TOXIC EFFECTS

Excessive dosage may produce profound hypotension, bradycardia, dizziness, syncope, drowsiness, breathing difficulty, bluish fingernails/palms of hands, seizures. May potentiate insulin-reduced hypoglycemia in diabetic pts.

PATIENT CONSIDERATIONS

BASELINE ASSESSMENT

Assess B/P, apical pulse immediately before drug is administered (if pulse is 60/min or below, or systolic B/P is below 90 mm Hg, withhold medication, contact physician).

INTERVENTION/EVALUATION

Monitor B/P for hypotension, development of diaphoresis or dizziness (usually first sign of impending hypotension). Assess pulse for strength/weakness, irregular rate, bradycardia. Monitor EKG for cardiac changes, particularly shortening of QT interval, prolongation of PR interval. Assess extremities for coldness. Assist w/ambulation if dizziness occurs. Assess for nausea, diaphoresis, headache, fatigue.

---

estazolam

es-**tay**-zoe-lam

(ProSom)

PREGNANCY CATEGORY X

CLASSIFICATION

Sedative-hypnotic

AVAILABILITY (Rx)

Tablets: 1 mg, 2 mg

PHARMACOKINETICS

Absorption: Well absorbed from GI tract. Crosses blood-brain barrier. **Metabolism:** Metabolized in liver. **Excretion:** Primarily excreted in urine. **Half-life:** 10–24 hrs.

ACTION/*THERAPEUTIC EFFECT*

Enhances action of inhibitory neurotransmitter gamma-aminobutyric acid (GABA). *Depressant effects occur at all levels of CNS.*

USES

Short-term treatment of insomnia (up to 6 wks). Reduces sleep induction time, number of nocturnal awakenings; increases length of sleep.

ADMINISTRATION

ORAL:

- Give w/o regard to meals.
- Tablet may be crushed.

INDICATIONS/ROUTES/DOSAGE

Note: Use smallest effective dose in those w/liver disease, low serum albumin.

Insomnia:

Oral: Adults >18 yrs: 1–2 mg at bedtime. ***Elderly/debilitated:*** 0.5–1 mg at bedtime.

CONTRAINDICATIONS

Sensitivity to other benzodiazepines. Pregnancy.

CAUTIONS

Impaired renal/hepatic function.

INTERACTIONS

DRUG: ***Alcohol, CNS depressants*** may increase CNS depressant effect. **HERBAL:** Kava kava, valerian may have additive effect. **FOOD:** None significant. **ALTERED LAB VALUES:** None significant.

SIDE EFFECTS

FREQUENT: Drowsiness, sedation, rebound insomnia (may occur for 1–2 nights after drug is discontinued), dizziness, confusion, euphoria. **OCCASIONAL:** Weakness, anorexia, diarrhea. **RARE:** Paradoxical CNS excitement, restlessness (particularly noted in elderly/debilitated).

ADVERSE REACTIONS/TOXIC EFFECTS

Abrupt or too rapid withdrawal may result in pronounced restlessness, irritability, insomnia, hand tremors, abdominal/muscle cramps, sweating, vomiting, seizures. Overdosage results in somnolence, confusion, diminished reflexes, coma.

PATIENT CONSIDERATIONS

BASELINE ASSESSMENT

Assess B/P, pulse, respirations immediately before administration. Raise bed rails. Provide environment conductive to sleep (backrub, quiet environment, low lighting).

INTERVENTION/EVALUATION

Assess sleep pattern of pt. Assess elderly/debilitated for paradoxical reaction, particularly during early therapy. Evaluate for therapeutic response: decrease in number of nocturnal awakenings, increase in length of sleep.

PATIENT/FAMILY TEACHING

Smoking reduces drug effectiveness. Do not abruptly withdraw medication following long-term use. Rebound insomnia may occur when drug is discontinued after short-term therapy. Do not use during pregnancy. Avoid alcohol. Use caution while driving or operating machinery.

estradiol

ess-tra-**dye**-ole

(Alora, Climara, Estrace, Esclim, Estring, Estraderm, FemPatch, Vivelle, Vivelle Dot)

estradiol cypionate

(Depo-Estradiol, Depogen)

estradiol valerate

(Delestrogen, Dioval, Valergen 10)

ethinyl estradiol

(Estinyl)

FIXED-COMBINATION(S)

Estradiol w/norethindrone, a pregesterone **(Combipatch);** estradiol cypionate w/testosterone cypionate, an androgen **(DepoTestadiol);** estradiol valerate w/testosterone enanthate, an androgen **(Deladumone, Estra-Testrin);** ethinyl estradiol w/fluoxymesterone, an androgen **(Halodrin);** esterified estrogens w/methyltestosterone, an androgen **(Estratest)**

CANADIAN AVAILABILITY

Climara, Delestrogen, Estrace, Estraderm, Estring, Vivelle

PREGNANCY CATEGORY X

CLASSIFICATION

Antineoplastic, estrogen

AVAILABILITY (Rx)

Injection: (Valerate): 10 mg/ml, 20 mg/ml, 40 mg/ml. **(Cypionate):** 5 mg/ml. **Tablets (ethinyl estradiol):** 0.02 mg, 0.05 mg, 0.5 mg. **Extended-Release Insert (Estring), Vaginal Cream:** 0.1 mg/g. **Topical (transdermal patch):** 0.025 mg, 0.0375 mg, 0.05 mg, 0.075 mg, 0.1 mg.

PHARMACOKINETICS

Absorption: Well absorbed from GI tract. Widely distributed. **Metabolism:** Metabolized in liver. **Excretion:** Primarily excreted in urine. **Half-life:** 50–60 min.

ACTION/*THERAPEUTIC EFFECT*

Increases synthesis of DNA, RNA, and various proteins in responsive tissues. Reduces release of gonadotropin-releasing hormone, reducing follicle-stimulating hormone (FSH) and leuteinizing hormone (LH). *Promotes normal growth, development of female sex organs, maintaining GU function, vasomotor stability. Prevents accelerated bone loss by inhibiting bone resorption, restoring balance of bone resorption and formation.* Inhibits LH, decreases serum concentration of testosterone.

USES/*UNLABELED*

Management of moderate to severe vasomotor symptoms associated w/menopause, female hypogonadism. Palliative treatment of advanced, inoperable metastatic carcinoma of the breast in postmenopausal women (estradiol, ethinyl estradiol), prostate in men (estradiol, estradiol valerate, ethinyl estradiol). Prevention of postpartum breast engorgement (estradiol valerate). Treatment of atrophic vaginitis, kraurosis vulvae (estradiol, estradiol valerate). Treatment of postmenopausal osteoporosis (estradiol transdermal system). Prevention of osteoporosis. *Treatment of Turner's syndrome.*

ADMINISTRATION

ORAL:

- Administer at the same time each day.
- Give w/milk or food if nausea occurs.

IM:

- Rotate vial to disperse drug in solution.
- Inject deep IM in gluteus maximus.

VAGINAL:

- Apply at bedtime for best absorption.
- Assemble and fill applicator per manufacturer's directions.
- Insert end of applicator into vagina, directed slightly toward sacrum; push plunger down completely.
- Avoid skin contact w/cream (prevents skin absorption).

TRANSDERMAL:

- Remove old patch; select new

site (buttocks an alternative application site).
- Peel off protective strip to expose adhesive surface. Apply immediately to clean, dry, intact skin on the trunk of the body (area w/as little hair as possible).
- Press in place for at least 10 sec.
- Do not apply to the breasts or waistline.

INDICATIONS/ROUTES/DOSAGE

ESTRADIOL ORAL, INTRAVAGINAL, TRANSDERMAL:

Vasomotor symptoms, atrophic vaginitis, kraurosis vulvae, female hypogonadism, castration, primary ovarian failure:
Oral: Adults, elderly: Initially, 1–2 mg/day cyclically.

Intravaginal: Adults, elderly: Initially, 2–4 g/day for 12 wks; reduce dose by ½ over 1–2 wks. *Maintenance:* 1 g 1–3 times/wk cyclically.

Topical: Adults, elderly: Initially, 0.05 mg/24 hrs 2 times/wk cyclically; maintenance dose adjusted to pt's needs. *Climara:* Initially, 12.5 cm^2 patch once weekly. *FemPatch:* 0.025 mg once weekly.

Breast cancer:
Oral: Adults, elderly: 10 mg 3 times/day.

Prostate cancer:
Oral: Adults, elderly: 1–2 mg 3 times/day.

Osteoporosis prevention:
Oral: Adults, elderly: 0.5 mg/day (3 wks on, 1 wk off).

Topical (Climara): 0.025–0.1 mg/wk.

ESTRADIOL CYPIONATE:

Vasomotor symptoms:
IM: Adults, elderly: 1–5 mg q3–4 wks.

Female hypogonadism:
IM: Adults, elderly: 1.5–2 mg every month.

ESTRADIOL VALERATE:

Vasomotor symptoms, atrophic vaginitis, kraurosis vulvae, female hypogonadism, castration, primary ovarian failure:
IM: Adults, elderly: 10–20 mg q4wks.

Prevention of postpartum breast engorgement:
IM: Adults, elderly: 10–25 mg as single dose at end of first stage of labor.

Prostate cancer:
IM: Adults, elderly: 30 mg or more q1–2wks.

ETHINYL ESTRADIOL:

Vasomotor symptoms:
Oral: Adults, elderly: 0.02–0.15 mg/day cyclically.

Female hypogonadism:
Oral: Adults, elderly: 0.05 mg 1–3 times/day during first 2 wks menstrual cycle.

Breast cancer:
Oral: Adults, elderly: 1 mg 3 times/day.

Prostate cancer:
Oral: Adults, elderly: 0.15–0.2 mg/day.

Urogenital atrophy:
Vaginal: (Extended-release insert): Once q3mos.

CONTRAINDICATIONS

Known or suspected breast cancer (except select pts w/metastasis), estrogen-dependent neoplasia; undiagnosed abnormal genital bleeding; active thrombophlebitis or thromboembolic disorders; history of thrombophlebitis, thrombosis or thromboembolic disorders w/previous estrogen use, hypersensitivity to estrogen.

CAUTIONS

Conditions that may be aggravated by fluid retention: cardiac, renal/hepatic dysfunction, epilepsy, migraine. Mental depression, metabolic bone disease w/potential hypercalcemia, history of jaundice during pregnancy or strong family history of breast cancer, fibrocystic disease, or breast nodules, children in whom bone growth is not complete.

INTERACTIONS

DRUG: May interfere w/effects of ***bromocriptine.*** May increase concentration of ***cyclosporine,*** increase hepatic, nephrotoxicity. ***Hepatotoxic medications*** may increase hepatotoxicity. **HERBAL:** Increases effects of saw palmetto. **FOOD:** None significant. **ALTERED LAB VALUES:** May affect metapyrone, thyroid function tests. May decrease cholesterol, LDH. May increase calcium, glucose, HDL, triglycerides.

SIDE EFFECTS

FREQUENT: Anorexia, nausea, swelling of breasts, peripheral edema evidenced by swollen ankles, feet. ***Transdermal route:*** Skin irritation, redness. **OCCASIONAL:** Vomiting (especially w/high dosages), headache (may be severe), intolerance to contact lenses, increased B/P, glucose intolerance, brown spots on exposed skin. ***Vaginal route:*** Local irritation, vaginal discharge, changes in vaginal bleeding (spotting, breakthrough or prolonged bleeding). **RARE:** Chorea, cholestatic jaundice, hirsutism, loss of scalp hair, depression.

ADVERSE REACTIONS/TOXIC EFFECTS

Prolonged administration increases risk of gallbladder, thromboembolic disease, and breast, cervical, vaginal, endometrial, and liver carcinoma.

PATIENT CONSIDERATIONS:

BASELINE ASSESSMENT

Question hypersensitivity to estrogen, previous jaundice or thromboembolic disorders associated w/pregnancy or estrogen therapy. Establish baseline B/P, blood glucose.

INTERVENTION/EVALUATION

Assess B/P at least daily. Check for swelling. Weigh daily. Monitor blood glucose 4 times/day for pts w/diabetes. Promptly report signs and symptoms of thromboembolic or thrombotic disorders: sudden severe headache, shortness of breath, vision or speech disturbance, weakness or numbness of an extremity, loss of coordination, pain in chest, groin, or leg. Assess skin for irritation due to transdermal application or brown blotches. Note estrogen therapy on specimens.

PATIENT/FAMILY TEACHING

Importance of medical supervision. Avoid smoking due to increased risk of heart attack or blood clots. Do not take other medications w/o physician approval. Teach how to perform Homan's test, signs and symptoms of blood clots (report these to physician immediately). Notify physician of abnormal vaginal bleeding, depression, other symptoms. Teach female pts to perform breast self-exam. Avoid exposure to sun/ultraviolet light.

Check weight daily; report weekly gain of 5 lbs or more. W/vaginal application: Remain recumbent at least 30 min after application and do not use tampons. Stop taking the medication and contact physician at once if pregnancy is suspected. Give labeling from drug package.

estramustine phosphate sodium

(Emcyt)

See Classification section under: Cancer chemotherapy

estropipate

ess-**troe**-pie-pate

(Ogen)

CANADIAN AVAILABILITY

Ogen

PREGNANCY CATEGORY X

CLASSIFICATION

Estrogen

AVAILABILITY (Rx)

Tablets: 0.625 mg, 1.25 mg, 2.5 mg. **Vaginal Cream:** 1.5 mg/g.

PHARMACOKINETICS

Absorption: Well absorbed from GI tract. Widely distributed. **Metabolism:** Metabolized in liver. **Excretion:** Primarily excreted in urine.

ACTION / *THERAPEUTIC EFFECT*

Increases synthesis of DNA, RNA, and various proteins in responsive tissues. Reduces release of gonadotropin-releasing hormone, reducing follicle-stimulating hormone (FSH) and leuteinizing hormone (LH). *Promotes normal growth, development of female sex organs, maintaining GU function, vasomotor stability. Prevents accelerated bone loss by inhibiting bone resorption, restoring balance of bone resorption and formation.*

USES

Management of moderate to severe vasomotor symptoms associated w/menopause. Treatment of atrophic vaginitis, kraurosis vulvae, female hypogonadism and castration, primary ovarian failure. Prevention of osteoporosis.

ADMINISTRATION

ORAL:

- Administer at the same time each day.

VAGINAL:

- Apply at bedtime for best absorption.
- Assemble and fill applicator per manufacturer's directions.
- Insert end of applicator into vagina, directed slightly toward sacrum; push plunger down completely.
- Avoid skin contact w/cream (prevents skin absorption).

INDICATIONS/ROUTES/DOSAGE

Vasomotor symptoms, atrophic vaginitis, kraurosis vulvae:
Oral: Adults, elderly: 0.625–5 mg/day cyclically.

Atrophic vaginitis, kraurosis vulvae:
Intravaginal: Adults, elderly: 2–4 g/day cyclically.

Female hypogonadism, castration, primary ovarian failure:
Oral: Adults, elderly: 1.25–7.5 mg/day × 21 days; off 8–10 days.

Repeat if bleeding does not occur by end of rest period.

Osteoporosis prevention:
Oral: Adults, elderly: 0.625 mg/day (25 days of 31 day cycle/month).

CONTRAINDICATIONS

Known or suspected breast cancer, estrogen-dependent neoplasia; undiagnosed abnormal genital bleeding; active thrombophlebitis or thromboembolic disorders; history of thrombophlebitis, thrombosis, or thromboembolic disorders w/previous estrogen use, hypersensitivity to estrogen.

CAUTIONS

Conditions that may be aggravated by fluid retention: cardiac, renal, or hepatic dysfunction, epilepsy, migraine. Mental depression, hypercalcemia, history of jaundice during pregnancy or strong family history of breast cancer, fibrocystic disease, or breast nodules, children in whom bone growth is not complete.

INTERACTIONS

DRUG: May interfere w/effects of ***bromocriptine***. May increase concentration of ***cyclosporine***, increase hepatic/nephrotoxicity. ***Hepatotoxic medications*** may increase hepatotoxicity. **HERBAL:** Increases effects of saw palmetto. **FOOD:** None signficant. **ALTERED LAB VALUES:** May affect metapyrone, thyroid function tests. May decrease cholesterol, LDH. May increase calcium, glucose, HDL, triglycerides.

SIDE EFFECTS

FREQUENT: Anorexia, nausea, swelling of breasts, peripheral edema evidenced by swollen ankles, feet. **OCCASIONAL:** Vomiting (especially w/high dosages), headache (may be severe), intolerance to contact lenses, increased B/P, glucose intolerance, brown spots on exposed skin. ***Vaginal route:*** Local irritation, vaginal discharge, changes in vaginal bleeding (spotting, breakthrough or prolonged bleeding). **RARE:** Chorea, cholestatic jaundice, hirsutism, loss of scalp hair, depression.

ADVERSE REACTIONS/TOXIC EFFECTS

Prolonged administration increases risk of gallbladder, thromboembolic disease, and breast, cervical, vaginal, endometrial, and liver carcinoma.

PATIENT CONSIDERATIONS

Baseline Assessment

Question for hypersensitivity to estrogen, previous jaundice, or thromboembolic disorders associated w/pregnancy or estrogen therapy. Establish baseline B/P, blood glucose.

Intervention/Evaluation

Assess B/P at least daily. Check for swelling, weigh daily. Check blood glucose 4 times/day for pts w/diabetes. Promptly report signs and symptoms of thromboembolic or thrombotic disorders: sudden severe headache, shortness of breath, vision or speech disturbance, weakness or numbness of an extremity, loss of coordination, pain in chest, groin, or leg. Note estrogen therapy on specimens.

Patient/Family Teaching

Importance of medical supervision. Avoid smoking because of increased risk of heart attack or blood clots. Do not take other medications w/o physician

approval. Teach how to perform Homan's test, signs and symptoms of blood clots (report these to physician immediately). Also notify physician of abnormal vaginal discharge or bleeding, depression. Teach breast self-exam. Avoid exposure to sun/ultraviolet light. Check weight daily; report weekly gain of 5 lbs or more. W/vaginal application. Remain recumbent at least 30 min after application and do not use tampons. Stop taking estropipate and contact physician if pregnancy suspected. Give labeling from drug package.

etanercept

ee-**tan**-er-cept
(Enbrel)

PREGNANCY CATEGORY B

CLASSIFICATION

Anti-arthritic

AVAILABILITY (Rx)

Powder for Injection: 25 mg

PHARMACOKINETICS

Absorption: Well absorbed following SubQ administration. **Metabolism:** Blocks interactions with cell surface tumor necrosis factor receptors (TNFR). **Half-life:** 115 hrs.

ACTION/*THERAPEUTIC EFFECT*

Binds to tumor necrosis factor (TNF), blocking its interaction with cell surface receptors (TNFR). (TNF is involved in inflammatory and immune responses; elevated TNF is found in synovial fluid of rheumatoid arthritis pts.)

USES

To reduce signs and symptoms of moderately to severely active rheumatoid arthritis (RA). Treatment of active juvenile rheumatoid arthritis.

STORAGE/HANDLING

Refrigerate. Once reconstituted, may be stored under refrigeration for up to 6 hrs.

ADMINISTRATION

SubQ:

- **Note:** Do not add other medications to solution. Do not use filter during reconstitution or administration.
- Reconstitute with 1 ml of sterile bacteriostatic water for injection (0.9% benzyl alcohol). Do not reconstitute with other diluents.
- Slowly inject the diluent into the vial. Some foaming will occur. To avoid excessive foaming, do not shake or agitate vigorously, but slowly swirl contents until powder is dissolved (<5 min).
- Visually inspect solution for particles or discoloration. Reconstituted solution should appear clear and colorless. If discolored, cloudy, or particles remain, discard solution; do not use.
- Withdraw all the solution into syringe. Final volume should be approximately 1 ml.
- May inject into thigh, abdomen, or upper arm. Rotate injection sites.
- Give new injection at least 1 inch from an old site and never into area when skin is tender, bruised, red, or hard.

INDICATIONS/DOSAGE/ROUTES

Rheumatoid arthritis:
SubQ: Adults, elderly: 25 mg twice weekly. ***Children (4–17 yrs):***

0.4 mg/kg (maximum 25 mg dose) twice weekly.

CONTRAINDICATIONS

Sepsis, history of hypersensitivity to etanercept.

CAUTIONS

Avoid use in pts w/infection (may cause serious infection).

INTERACTIONS

DRUG: None significant. **HERBAL:** None known. **FOOD:** None significant. **ALTERED LAB VALUES:** None significant.

SIDE EFFECTS

FREQUENT (37%): Injection site reaction (erythema, itching, pain, swelling). Incidence of abdominal pain, vomiting is higher in children than adults. **OCCASIONAL (4–16%):** Headache, rhinitis, dizziness, pharyngitis, cough, asthenia, abdominal pain, dyspepsia. **RARE (<3%):** Sinusitis, allergic reaction.

ADVERSE REACTIONS/TOXIC EFFECTS

Infection (pyelonephritis, cellulitis, osteomyelitis, wound infection, leg ulcer, septic arthritis, diarrhea), upper respiratory tract infection (bronchitis, pneumonia) occurs frequently **(29–38%)**. Formation of autoimmune antibodies may occur. Serious adverse effects occur rarely (heart failure, hypertension, hypotension, pancreatitis, GI hemorrhage, dyspnea).

PATIENT CONSIDERATIONS

Baseline Assessment

Assess onset, type, location, duration of pain/inflammation. The needle cover of the diluent syringe contains latex and should not be handled by those sensitive to this substance. If pt is to self-administer, instruct in SubQ injection technique, including areas of the body acceptable as injection sites. If a significant exposure to varicella virus has occurred during treatment, therapy should be temporarily discontinued and treatment with varicella zoster immune globulin be considered.

Intervention/Evaluation

Assess for therapeutic response (relief from pain, improved mobility).

Patient/Family Teaching

Injection site reaction generally occurs in first month of treatment and decrease in frequency during continued therapy. Do not receive live vaccines during treatment. In those with juvenile rheumatoid arthritis, immunizations should be brought up to date prior to initiating therapy. Promptly report signs of infection.

---

ethacrynic acid

eth-ah-**krin**-ick

(Edecrin)

ethacrynate sodium

eth-ah-**krin**-ate

(Edecrin Sodium)

CANADIAN AVAILABILITY

Edecrin

PREGNANCY CATEGORY D

CLASSIFICATION

Diuretic: Loop

AVAILABILITY (Rx)

Tablets: 25 mg, 50 mg. **Powder for Injection:** 50 mg.

PHARMACODYNAMICS

	ONSET	PEAK	DURATION
Oral	<30 min	2 hrs	6–8 hrs
IV	<5 min	15–30 min	2 hrs

PHARMACOKINETICS

Absorption: Rapidly absorbed from GI tract. **Metabolism:** Metabolized in liver to active metabolite. **Excretion:** Primarily excreted in urine.

ACTION/*THERAPEUTIC EFFECT*

Enhances excretion of sodium, chloride, potassium at ascending limb of loop of Henle and distal renal tubule *producing diuretic effect.*

USES/*UNLABELED*

Treatment of edema associated w/CHF, severe renal impairment, nephrotic syndrome, hepatic cirrhosis; short-term management of ascites, children w/congenital heart disease. *Treatment of hypertension, hypercalcemia.*

STORAGE/HANDLING

Store oral, parenteral form at room temperature. Discard if parenteral form appears hazy or opalescent. Discard unused reconstituted solution after 24 hrs.

ADMINISTRATION

ORAL:

- Give w/food to avoid GI upset, preferably w/breakfast (may prevent nocturia).

IV:

- For direct IV, administer slowly over several min.
- For IV infusion, reconstitute each 50 mg ethacrynate sodium w/50 ml 5% dextrose injection or NaCl injection.
- Infuse slowly, over 20–30 min, through tubing of running IV infusion.

INDICATIONS/ROUTES/DOSAGE

Edema:

Oral: Adults: 50–100 mg daily. Dosage may be increased in 25–50 mg increments until therapeutic response is achieved. ***Elderly:*** Initially, 25–50 mg/day; increase as needed. ***Children:*** Initially, 25 mg. Dosage may be increased in increments of 25 mg until therapeutic response is achieved. Alternate day scheduling may be used for maintenance therapy.

IV: Adults >18 yrs, elderly: 0.5–1.0 mg/kg or 50 mg for average-sized adult. Single IV dose should not exceed 100 mg.

CONTRAINDICATIONS

Anuria, severe renal impairment.

CAUTIONS

Hepatic cirrhosis, ascites, history of gout, pancreatitis, systemic lupus erythematosus, diabetes mellitus, elderly, debilitated.

INTERACTIONS

DRUG: ***Amphotericin, ototoxic and nephrotoxic agents*** may increase toxicity. May decrease effect of ***anticoagulants, heparin. Hypokalemia-causing agents*** may increase risk of hypokalemia. May increase risk of ***lithium*** toxicity. **HERBAL:** None known. **FOOD:** None significant. **ALTERED LAB VALUES:** May increase glucose, BUN, uric acid, urinary phosphate. May decrease calcium, chloride, magnesium, potassium, sodium.

SIDE EFFECTS

FREQUENT: Diarrhea, decreased appetite, dizziness, lightheadedness. **OCCASIONAL:** Electrolyte imbalance (dry mouth, increased thirst, mental changes, muscle cramps, nausea, vomiting), ringing/buzzing in ears, blurred vision, confusion, headache. **RARE:** Allergic reaction, leukopenia (fever, chills), thrombocytopenia (unusual bruising or bleeding), severe stomach pain, pain at injection site.

ADVERSE REACTIONS/TOXIC EFFECTS

Vigorous diuresis may lead to profound water loss and electrolyte depletion, resulting in hypokalemia, hyponatremia, dehydration, coma, circulatory collapse. Acute hypotensive episodes may also occur, sometimes several days after beginning of therapy. Ototoxicity manifested as deafness, vertigo, tinnitus (ringing/roaring in ears) may occur, especially in those w/severe renal impairment. Can exacerbate diabetes mellitus, systemic lupus erythematosus, gout, pancreatitis. Blood dyscrasias have been reported.

PATIENT CONSIDERATIONS

BASELINE ASSESSMENT

Check vital signs, especially B/P for hypotension prior to administration. Obtain baseline electrolytes. Particularly check for low potassium. Check edema, skin turgor, mucous membranes for hydration status. Assess muscle strength, mental status. Note skin temperature, moisture. Obtain baseline weight. Initiate I&O.

INTERVENTION/EVALUATION

Monitor B/P, vital signs, electrolytes, I&O, weight. Note extent of diuresis. Watch for changes from initial assessment (hypokalemia may result in muscle strength changes, tremor, muscle cramps, change in mental status, cardiac arrhythmias; hyponatremia may result in confusion, thirst, cold/clammy skin).

PATIENT/FAMILY TEACHING

Expect increased frequency and volume of urination. Report irregular heartbeat, signs of electrolyte imbalances (noted above), hearing abnormalities (such as sense of fullness in ears, ringing/roaring in ears). Eat foods high in potassium such as whole grains (cereals), legumes, meat, bananas, apricots, orange juice, potatoes (white, sweet), raisins.

---

ethambutol

eth-**am**-byoo-toll
(Myambutol)

CANADIAN AVAILABILITY
Etibi, Myambutol

PREGNANCY CATEGORY B

CLASSIFICATION

Antitubercular

AVAILABILITY (Rx)

Tablets: 100 mg, 400 mg

PHARMACOKINETICS

Absorption: Rapidly, well absorbed from GI tract. Widely distributed. **Metabolism:** Metabolized in liver. **Excretion:** Primarily excreted in urine. Removed by hemodialysis. **Half-life:** 3–4 hrs (increased in reduced renal function).

ACTION/ *THERAPEUTIC EFFECT*

Interferes w/cell metabolism and multiplication by inhibiting one or more metabolites in susceptible bacteria. Active only during cell division. *Bacteriostatic.*

USES/ *UNLABELED*

In conjunction w/at least one other antitubercular agent for initial treatment and retreatment of clinical tuberculosis. *Treatment of atypical mycobacterial infections.*

ADMINISTRATION

ORAL:

- Give w/food (decreases GI upset).
- Give once q24h.

INDICATIONS/ROUTES/DOSAGE

Tuberculosis:

Oral: Adults, elderly: Initially (no prior anti-TB medication): 15 mg/kg q24h. ***(Prior anti-TB medication):*** 25 mg/kg/day q24h for 60 days, then decrease to 15 mg/kg/day. **Note:** When used in combination therapy and given 2 times/wk, dose is 50 mg/kg. Decrease dose in those w/renal impairment.

CONTRAINDICATIONS

Hypersensitivity to ethambutol, optic neuritis.

CAUTIONS

Renal dysfunction, gout, ocular defects: diabetic retinopathy, cataracts, recurrent ocular inflammatory conditions. Not recommended for children under 13 yrs of age.

INTERACTIONS

DRUG: *Neurotoxic medications* may increase risk of neurotoxicity. **HERBAL:** None known. **FOOD:** Give w/food. **ALTERED LAB VALUES:** May increase uric acid.

SIDE EFFECTS

OCCASIONAL: Acute gouty arthritis (chills, pain, swelling of joints w/hot skin), confusion, abdominal pain, nausea, vomiting, loss of appetite, headache. **RARE:** Rash, fever, blurred vision, eye pain, red-green color blindness, any vision loss.

ADVERSE REACTIONS/TOXIC EFFECTS

Optic neuritis (occurs more often w/high dosage, long-term therapy), peripheral neuritis, thrombocytopenia, anaphylactoid reaction occur rarely.

PATIENT CONSIDERATIONS

BASELINE ASSESSMENT

Question for hypersensitivity to ethambutol. Assure collection of specimens for culture, sensitivity. Evaluate initial CBC, renal and hepatic test results.

INTERVENTION/EVALUATION

Assess for vision changes (altered color perception, decreased visual acuity may be first signs). Discontinue drug and notify physician immediately. Give w/food if GI distress occurs. Monitor uric acid concentrations and assess for hot/painful/swollen joints, especially big toe, ankle, or knee (gout). Check CBC, culture and sensitivity tests, renal and hepatic function results. Monitor I&O in event of renal dysfunction. Report numbness, tingling, burning of extremities (peripheral neuritis). Assess for dizziness and assure assistance w/ambulation. Check mental status. Evaluate skin for rash.

PATIENT/FAMILY TEACHING

Do not skip doses; take for full length of therapy (may take months, years). Office visits, vision and lab tests are essential part of treatment. Do not take any other medication w/o consulting physician. Notify physician immediately of any visual problem (visual effects generally reversible w/discontinuation of ethambutol, but in rare cases may take up to a year to disappear or may be permanent); promptly report rash, swelling and pain of joints, numbness/tingling/burning of hands or feet. Do not drive or use machinery if visual problems or dizziness occurs.

ethosuximide

(Zarontin)

See Classification section under: Anticonvulsants

etidronate disodium

eh-**tye**-droe-nate

(Didronel)

CANADIAN AVAILABILITY

Didronel

PREGNANCY CATEGORY B

(oral)

PREGNANCY CATEGORY C

(parenteral)

CLASSIFICATION

Calcium regulator

AVAILABILITY (Rx)

Tablets: 200 mg, 400 mg. **Injection:** 50 mg/ml.

PHARMACOKINETICS

Absorption: Minimally absorbed from GI tract (1–6%). Chemically adsorbed to bone in areas of elevated osteogenesis. **Excretion:** Absorbed dose excreted in urine; unabsorbed dose eliminated in feces. **Half-life:** 5–7 hrs.

ACTION/*THERAPEUTIC EFFECT*

Binds to calcium phosphate surface of calcium crystals, *retarding bone resorption, bone formation. May also retard accelerated rate of bone turnover in Paget's disease.*

USES

Oral: Treatment of symptomatic Paget's disease of the bone, prevention and treatment of heterotopic ossification following hip replacement or due to spinal injury. ***Parenteral (IV):*** Treatment of hypercalcemia associated w/malignant neoplasms inadequately managed by dietary modification or oral hydration; treatment of hypercalcemia of malignancy persisting after adequate hydration has been restored.

STORAGE/HANDLING

Store tablets at room temperature. After dilution, IV stable for at least 48 hrs.

ADMINISTRATION

ORAL:

- Give on empty stomach, 2 hrs before meals.
- Do not give within 2 hrs of vitamins w/mineral supplements, antacids, or medications high in calcium, magnesium, iron, or aluminum.

IV INFUSION:

- Dilute in at least 250 ml 0.9% NaCl.
- Infuse slowly, over a minimum

of 2 hrs regardless of volume of solution.

INDICATIONS/DOSAGE/ROUTES

Paget's disease:
Oral: Adults, elderly: Initially, 5–10 mg/kg/day not to exceed 6 mos or 11–20 mg/kg/day not to exceed 3 mos. Repeat only after drug-free period of at least 90 days.

Heterotopic ossification (due to spinal cord injury):
Oral: Adults, elderly: 20 mg/kg/day for 2 wks; then 10 mg/kg/day for 10 wks.

Heterotopic ossification (complicating total hip replacement):
Oral: Adults, elderly: 20 mg/kg/day for 1 mo preop; follow w/20 mg/kg/day for 3 mos postop.

Usual parenteral dosage:
IV: Adults, elderly: 7.5 mg/kg/day for 3 days; retreatment no sooner than 7 day intervals between courses. Follow w/oral therapy on day after last infusion (20 mg/kg/day for 30 days; may extend up to 90 days).

CONTRAINDICATIONS

Children, severe renal function.

CAUTIONS

Enterocolitis, renal impairment, pts unable to maintain adequate intake of vitamin D or calcium.

INTERACTIONS

DRUG: *Antacids w/calcium, magnesium, aluminum, foods w/calcium, mineral supplements* may decrease absorption. HERBAL: None known. FOOD: None significant. ALTERED LAB VALUES: None significant.

SIDE EFFECTS

FREQUENT: Nausea, diarrhea increased, continuing or more frequent bone pain in those with Paget's disease. OCCASIONAL: Bone fractures (especially femur). *Parenteral:* Metallic, altered, or loss of taste. RARE: Hypersensitivity reaction (rash, pruritus, urticaria, angioedema).

ADVERSE REACTIONS/TOXIC EFFECTS

Nephrotoxicity (hematuria, dysuria, proteinuria) noted w/parenteral route.

PATIENT CONSIDERATIONS

BASELINE ASSESSMENT

Obtain lab baselines, especially electrolytes, renal function.

INTERVENTION/EVALUATION

Assess food tolerance. Check for diarrhea. Monitor electrolytes. Check I&O, BUN, creatinine in pts w/impaired renal function. Evaluate pain in pts w/Paget's disease. Assess skin for eruptions.

PATIENT/FAMILY TEACHING

May take up to 3 mos for therapeutic response; do not stop taking medication, discuss w/physician. Taste may be altered, usually disappears w/continuation of therapy. Assure milk, dairy products in diet for calcium, vitamin D. Do not take any other medications w/o physician approval. Take medication on empty stomach, 2 hrs from food, vitamins, antacids. Report nausea, diarrhea, rash, or other symptoms.

---

etodolac

eh-**toe**-doe-lack
(Lodine, Lodine XL)

CANADIAN AVAILABILITY
Apo-Etodolac, Ultradol

PREGNANCY CATEGORY C

CLASSIFICATION

Nonsteroidal anti-inflammatory

AVAILABILITY (Rx)

Capsules: 200 mg, 300 mg, 400 mg, 500 mg. **Capsules (extended-release):** 400 mg, 500 mg, 600 mg, 1,200 mg.

PHARMACODYNAMICS

	ONSET	PEAK	DURATION
Oral analgesic			
	30 min	—	4–12 hrs

PHARMACOKINETICS

Absorption: Completely absorbed from GI tract. Widely distributed. **Metabolism:** Metabolized in liver. **Excretion:** Primarily excreted in urine. **Half-life:** 6–7 hrs.

ACTION/*THERAPEUTIC EFFECT*

Produces analgesic and anti-inflammatory effect by inhibiting prostaglandin synthesis, *reducing inflammatory response and intensity of pain stimulus reaching sensory nerve endings.*

USES/*UNLABELED*

Acute and long-term treatment of osteoarthritis, management of pain, treatment of rheumatoid arthritis. *Treatment of acute gouty arthritis, vascular headache.*

ADMINISTRATION

ORAL:

- Do not crush or break capsules, extended-release capsules.
- May give w/food, milk, or antacids if GI distress occurs.

INDICATIONS/ROUTES/DOSAGE

Note: Reduce dosage in elderly; maximum dose for pts weighing <60 kg: 20 mg/kg.

Osteoarthritis:
Oral: Adults, elderly: Initially, 800–1,200 mg/day in 2–4 divided doses. ***Maintenance:*** 600–1,200 mg/day.

Rheumatoid arthritis:
Oral: Adults, elderly: Initially, 300 mg 2–3 times/day or 400–500 mg 2 times/day. ***Maintenance:*** 600–1,200 mg/day.

Analgesia:
Oral: Adults, elderly: 200–400 mg q6–8h as needed. ***Maximum:*** 1,200 mg/day.

CONTRAINDICATIONS

Active peptic ulcer, GI ulceration, chronic inflammation of GI tract, GI bleeding disorders, history of hypersensitivity to aspirin or NSAIDs.

CAUTIONS

Impaired renal/hepatic function, history of GI tract disease, predisposition to fluid retention.

INTERACTIONS

DRUG: May increase effects of ***oral anticoagulants, heparin, thrombolytics.*** May decrease effect of ***antihypertensives, diuretics. Salicylates, aspirin*** may increase risk of GI side effects, bleeding. ***Bone marrow depressants*** may increase risk of hematologic reactions. May increase concentration, toxicity of ***lithium.*** May increase ***methotrexate*** toxicity. ***Probenecid*** may increase concentration. **HERBAL:** Feverfew, ginkgo may increase risk of bleeding. **FOOD:** None significant. **ALTERED LAB VALUES:** May increase bleeding time, creatinine, liver function tests. May decrease uric acid.

SIDE EFFECTS

FREQUENT (3–9%): Dizziness, headache, abdominal pain or cramps, bloated feeling, diarrhea, nausea, indigestion. **OCCASIONAL (1–3%):** Constipation, rash, itching, visual changes, ringing in ears. **RARE (<1%):** Increased blood pressure, anemia, bruising, thrombocytopenia, hepatitis, angioedema.

ADVERSE REACTIONS/TOXIC EFFECTS

Overdosage may result in acute renal failure. In those treated chronically, peptic ulcer, GI bleeding, gastritis, severe hepatic reaction (jaundice), nephrotoxicity (hematuria, dysuria, proteinuria), severe hypersensitivity reaction (bronchospasm, angiofacial edema) occur rarely.

PATIENT CONSIDERATIONS

Baseline Assessment

Assess onset, type, location, duration of pain or inflammation. Inspect appearance of affected joints for immobility, deformities, skin condition.

Intervention/Evaluation

Monitor for headache, dyspepsia. Monitor pattern of daily bowel activity, stool consistency. Evaluate for therapeutic response: relief of pain, stiffness, swelling, increase in joint mobility, reduced joint tenderness, improved grip strength.

Patient/Family Teaching

Swallow capsule whole; do not crush or chew. Avoid aspirin, alcohol during therapy (increases risk of GI bleeding). If GI upset occurs, take w/food, milk. Report GI distress, visual disturbances, rash, edema, headache.

---

etoposide, VP-16

(Etopophos, VePesid)

See Classification section under: Cancer chemotherapy

---

exemestane

(Aromasin)

See Classification section under: Cancer chemotherapy
See Supplement

factor IX complex (human)

(Benefix, Konyne, Profilnine, Heat-treated Propex T)

CANADIAN AVAILABILITY
Immunine VH

PREGNANCY CATEGORY C

CLASSIFICATION

Antihemophilic

AVAILABILITY (Rx)

Injection: Number of units indicated on each vial

ACTION/*THERAPEUTIC EFFECT*

Raises plasma levels of factor IX, restores hemostasis in pts w/factor IX deficiency. *Increases blood clotting factors II, VII, IX, and X.*

USES

Note: Only Propex T controls bleeding in pts w/factor VII deficiency.

Treatment of bleeding caused by hemophilia B (deficiency of factor IX is demonstrated). Treatment of bleeding in pts w/hemophilia A who have factor VIII inhibitors. Reversal of anticoagulant effect of coumarin anticoagulants.

STORAGE/HANDLING

Store in refrigerator. Do not freeze. Reconstituted solutions stable for 12 hrs at room temperature. Begin administration within 3 hrs. Do not refrigerate reconstituted solutions.

ADMINISTRATION

IV:

- Administer by slow IV injection or IV infusion.
- Filter before administration.
- Before reconstitution, warm diluent to room temperature.
- Gently agitate vial until powder is completely dissolved (prevents removal of active components during administration through filter).
- Infuse slowly, not to exceed 3 ml/min. A too rapid IV may produce headache, flushing, change in B/P and pulse rate, tingling sensation. Discontinuing infusion will eliminate effects immediately. Resume IV at slower rate.
- If evidence of disseminated intravascular coagulation (DIC) occurs (change in B/P and pulse rate, respiratory distress, chest pain, cough), stop infusion immediately.

INDICATIONS/ROUTES/DOSAGE

Note: Amount of factor IX required is individualized.

Dosage depends on degree of deficiency, level of each factor desired, weight of pt, severity of bleeding. Give sufficient drug to achieve/maintain plasma level at least 20% of normal until hemostasis achieved.

CONTRAINDICATIONS

Sensitivity to mouse protein.

CAUTIONS

Sensitivity to factor IX, liver impairment, recent surgery.

INTERACTIONS

DRUG: *Aminocaproic acid* may increase risk of thrombosis. **HERBAL:** None known. **FOOD:** None significant. **ALTERED LAB VALUES:** None significant.

SIDE EFFECTS

RARE: Mild hypersensitivity reaction (fever, chills, change in B/P and pulse rate, rash, tingling urticaria [hives]).

ADVERSE REACTIONS/TOXIC EFFECTS

High risk of venous thrombosis during postop period. Acute hypersensitivity reaction, anaphylactoid reaction may occur. ***Antidote:*** Epinephrine 1:1,000. High dosage may produce DIC, MI, thrombosis, pulmonary embolism. There is a risk of transmitting viral hepatitis, other viral diseases.

PATIENT CONSIDERATIONS

BASELINE ASSESSMENT

When monitoring B/P, avoid overinflation of cuff. Remove adhesive tape from any pressure dressing very carefully and slowly. Assess results of coagulation studies and extent of existing bleeding (overt bleeding, bruising, joint pain, and swelling).

INTERVENTION/EVALUATION

Monitor vital signs, I&O. Assess for hypersensitivity reaction (slow infusion and notify physician). Monitor results of coagulation studies closely. Avoid IM or SubQ injections or rectal temperatures. After IV administration, apply direct pressure to venipuncture site for a full 5 min or longer to assure bleeding has stopped. Monitor IV site for oozing q5–15min for 1–2 hrs after administration. Report any evidence of hematuria or change in vital signs immediately. Assess for decrease in B/P, increase in pulse rate, complaint of abdominal/back pain, severe headache (may be evidence of hemorrhage). Question for increase in amount of discharge during menses. Assess peripheral pulses; skin for bruises, petechiae. Check for excessive bleeding from minor cuts, scratches. Assess gums for erythema, gingival bleeding. Evaluate for therapeutic relief of pain, reduction of swelling, and restricted joint movement.

PATIENT/FAMILY TEACHING

Use electric razor, soft toothbrush to prevent bleeding. Report any sign of red/dark urine, black/red stool, coffee-ground vomitus, red-speckled mucus from cough. Do not use OTC medication w/o physician approval (may interfere w/platelet aggregation). Carry identification that indicates disease.

---

famciclovir

fam-**sigh**-klo-vir
(Famvir)

CANADIAN AVAILABILITY
Famvir

PREGNANCY CATEGORY B

CLASSIFICATION

Antiviral

AVAILABILITY (Rx)

Tablets: 125 mg, 250 mg, 500 mg

PHARMACOKINETICS

Absorption: Rapidly, extensively absorbed following oral administration. **Metabolism:** Rapidly metabolized to penciclovir by enzymes in gut wall, plasma, and liver. **Excretion:** Penciclovir eliminated unchanged in urine. **Half-life:** 2 hrs.

ACTION/*THERAPEUTIC EFFECT*

Suppresses herpes simplex virus and varicella zoster virus replication by inhibition of viral DNA synthesis.

USES

Treatment of herpes simplex virus (HSV), acute herpes zoster in immunocompromised pts, recurrent genital herpes, recurrent herpes simplex, prevention of genital herpes.

ADMINISTRATION

ORAL:

- May be given w/o regard to meals.

INDICATIONS/ROUTES/DOSAGE

Herpes zoster:
Oral: Adults: 500 mg q8h for 7 days.

Genital herpes:
Oral: Adults: 125 mg twice daily for 5 days.

Recurrent herpes simplex:
Oral: Adults: 500 mg twice daily for 7 days.

Prevention of genital herpes:
Oral: Adults: 250 mg twice daily.

Dosage in renal impairment:
Dosage based on creatinine clearance (ml/min):

CREATININE CLEARANCE	HERPES ZOSTER	GENITAL HERPES
40–59	500 mg q12h	125 mg q12h
20–39	500 mg q24h	125 mg q24h
<20	250 mg q48h	125 mg q48h

Hemodialysis pts:
Oral: Adults: 250 mg (herpes zoster) or 125 mg (genital herpes) following each dialysis treatment.

CONTRAINDICATIONS

Hypersensitivity to famciclovir.

CAUTIONS

Renal function impairment.

INTERACTIONS

DRUG: None significant. **HERBAL:** None known. **FOOD:** None significant. **ALTERED LAB VALUES:** None significant.

SIDE EFFECTS

FREQUENT: Headache (23%), nausea (12%). **OCCASIONAL (2–10%):** Dizziness, somnolence, numbness of feet, diarrhea, vomiting, constipation, decreased appetite, fatigue, fever, pharyngitis, sinusitis, pruritus. **RARE (<2%):** Inability to sleep, abdominal pain, dyspepsia, flatulence, back pain, arthralgia.

ADVERSE REACTIONS/TOXIC EFFECTS

None significant.

PATIENT CONSIDERATIONS

BASELINE ASSESSMENT

Tissue cultures for herpes simplex virus and varicella zoster virus should be done before giving first dose (therapy may proceed before results are known).

INTERVENTION/EVALUATION

Evaluate cutaneous lesions. Be alert to neurologic effects: headache, dizziness. Provide analgesics and comfort measures; especially exhausting to elderly. Encourage fluids. Keep pt's fingernails short, hands clean.

PATIENT/FAMILY TEACHING

Drink adequate fluids. Notify physician if side effects develop. Do not touch lesions with fingers to avoid spreading infection to new site.

Genital herpes
Continue therapy for full length of treatment. Space doses evenly. Use finger cot or rubber glove to apply topical ointment. Avoid sexual intercourse during duration of lesions to prevent infecting partner. Notify physician if lesions do not improve or recur. Avoid driving or operat-

ing machinery if dizziness is present. Pap smears should be done at least annually.

famotidine

fah-**mow**-tih-deen

(Mylanta AR, Pepcid, Pepcid AC, Pepcid RPD)

CANADIAN AVAILABILITY

Pepcid, Maalox H_2 Acid Controller, Novo-Famotidine, Ulcidine

PREGNANCY CATEGORY B

CLASSIFICATION

H_2 receptor antagonist

AVAILABILITY (Rx)

Chewable Tablets: 10 mg. **Tablets:** 10 mg (OTC), 20 mg, 40 mg. **Powder for Oral Suspension:** 40 mg/5 ml. **Injection:** 10 mg/ml, 20 mg/50 ml NaCl infusion.

PHARMACOKINETICS

Absorption: Rapid, incompletely absorbed from GI tract. **Metabolism:** Partially metabolized in liver. **Excretion:** Primarily excreted in urine. **Half-life:** 2.5–3.5 hrs (increased in reduced renal function).

ACTION / *THERAPEUTIC EFFECT*

Inhibits histamine action at H-2 receptors of parietal cells, *inhibiting gastric acid secretion (fasting, nocturnal, or when stimulated by food, caffeine, insulin).*

USES / *UNLABELED*

Short-term treatment of active duodenal ulcer. Prevention of duodenal ulcer recurrence. Treatment of active benign gastric ulcer, pathologic GI hypersecretory conditions. Short-term treatment of gastroesophageal reflux disease including erosive esophagitis. *Prophylaxis vs. aspiration pneumonitis, autism.*

STORAGE/HANDLING

Store tablets, suspension at room temperature. After reconstitution, suspension is stable for 30 days at room temperature. Refrigerate unreconstituted vials. IV solution appears clear, colorless. After dilution, IV solution is stable for 48 hrs at room temperature.

ADMINISTRATION

ORAL:

- Give w/o regard to meals or antacids. Best given after meals or at bedtime.
- Shake suspension well before use.
- Pepcid RPD dissolves under tongue, does not require water for dosing.

IV:

- For direct IV injection, dilute 20 mg vial w/5–10 ml 0.9% NaCl or other compatible IV solution. Inject over not less than 2 min.
- For intermittent IV infusion (piggyback), dilute w/100 ml 5% dextrose or other compatible IV fluid. Infuse over 15–30 min.

INDICATIONS/ROUTES/DOSAGE

Acute therapy—duodenal ulcer:
Oral: Adults, elderly: 40 mg at bedtime or 20 mg q12h. ***Maintenance:*** 20 mg at bedtime.

Children (1–16 yrs): 0.5 mg/kg/day. ***Maximum:*** 40 mg.

Acute therapy—benign gastric ulcer:
Oral: Adults, elderly: 40 mg at bedtime.

Gastroesophageal reflux disease:
Oral: Adults, elderly: 20 mg 2 times/

day up to 6 wks; 20–40 mg 2 times/day up to 12 wks in pts w/esophagitis (including erosions, ulcerations).

Children (1–16 yrs): 1 mg/kg/day in 2 divided dose. ***Maximum:*** 80 mg/day.

Pathologic hypersecretory conditions:
Oral: Adults, elderly: Initially, 20 mg q6h up to 160 mg q6h.

Usual parenteral dosage:
IV: Adults, elderly: 20 mg q12h.

Children: 0.25 mg/kg q12h. ***Maximum:*** 40 mg/day.

Dosage in renal impairment:
Creatinine clearance equal to or less than 10 ml/min: Decrease dose to 20 mg at bedtime or increase dosage interval to 36–48 hrs.

CONTRAINDICATIONS

None significant.

CAUTIONS

Impaired renal/hepatic function.

INTERACTIONS

DRUG: *Antacids* may decrease absorption (do not give within 1/2–1 hr). May decrease absorption of ***ketoconazole*** (give at least 2 hrs after). **HERBAL:** None known. **FOOD:** None significant. **ALTERED LAB VALUES:** Interferes w/skin tests using allergen extracts. May increase liver function tests.

SIDE EFFECTS

FREQUENT (4–6%): Headache. OCCASIONAL (1–3%): Constipation, diarrhea, dizziness, decreased appetite, joint pain, nausea, vomiting, ringing in ears, skin rash.

ADVERSE REACTIONS/TOXIC EFFECTS

None significant.

PATIENT CONSIDERATIONS

INTERVENTION/EVALUATION

Monitor daily bowel activity and stool consistency. Assess for abdominal pain, GI bleeding signs. Monitor for diarrhea/constipation.

PATIENT/FAMILY TEACHING

IV may produce transient discomfort at injection site. May take w/o regard to meals or antacids. Report headache. Avoid tasks that require alertness, motor skills until drug response is established. Avoid smoking (decreases effectiveness). Do not use OTC medications/alcohol w/o consulting physician.

F

felodipine

feh-**low**-dih-peen
(Plendil)

FIXED-COMBINATIONS
W/enalapril, an ACE inhibitor **(Lexxel)**

CANADIAN AVAILABILITY
Plendil, Renedil

PREGNANCY CATEGORY B

CLASSIFICATION

Calcium channel blocker

AVAILABILITY (Rx)

Tablets (extended-release): 2.5 mg, 5 mg, 10 mg

PHARMACODYNAMICS

	ONSET	PEAK	DURATION
Oral	2–5 hrs	—	—

PHARMACOKINETICS

Absorption: Rapidly, completely absorbed from GI tract. **Metabolism:** Undergoes first-pass metabolism in liver. **Excretion:** Primarily excreted in urine. **Half-life:** 11–16 hrs.

ACTION / *THERAPEUTIC EFFECT*

Inhibits calcium movement across cardiac, vascular smooth muscle. Potent peripheral vasodilator (does not depress SA, AV nodes). *Increases myocardial contractility, heart rate, cardiac output; decreases peripheral vascular resistance.*

USES / *UNLABELED*

Management of hypertension. May be used alone or w/other antihypertensives. *Treatment of chronic angina pectoris, Raynaud's phenomena.*

ADMINISTRATION

ORAL:

- May take w/o regard to food.
- Do not crush or break tablets.

INDICATIONS / ROUTES / DOSAGE

Hypertension:

Oral: Adults: Initially, 5 mg/day as single dose. ***Elderly, pts w/impaired liver function:*** Initially, 2.5 mg/day. Adjust dosage at no less than 2 wk intervals. ***Maintenance:*** 2.5–10 mg/day.

CONTRAINDICATIONS

Sick-sinus syndrome/second- or third-degree AV block (except in presence of pacemaker), severe hypotension, extreme bradycardia, CHF.

CAUTIONS

Impaired renal/hepatic function.

INTERACTIONS

DRUG: ***Beta blockers*** may have additive effect. May increase ***digoxin*** concentration. ***Procainamide, quinidine*** may increase risk of QT interval prolongation. ***Erythromycin*** may increase concentration/toxicity. ***Hypokalemia-producing agents*** may increase risk of arrhythmias. **HERBAL:** DHEA may increase concentration. **FOOD:** Grapefruit juice may increase concentration, hypotensive effect. **ALTERED LAB VALUES:** None significant.

SIDE EFFECTS

FREQUENT (>5%): Dizziness, lightheadedness, headache, peripheral edema, flushed skin, respiratory infection. **OCCASIONAL (2–5%):** Asthenia (loss of strength, weakness), abdominal discomfort, cough. **RARE (<2%):** Nervousness, fainting, inability to sleep, anxiety, nausea, diarrhea, constipation, vomiting, dry mouth, flatulence, hypotension, palpitations, pruritus, rash, nasal congestion, mild gingival hyperplasia.

ADVERSE REACTIONS / TOXIC EFFECTS

Overdosage produces nausea, drowsiness, confusion, slurred speech.

PATIENT CONSIDERATIONS

BASELINE ASSESSMENT

Assess baseline renal/liver function tests. Assess B/P, apical pulse immediately before drug is administered (if pulse is 60/min or below, or systolic B/P is below 90 mm Hg, withhold medication, contact physician).

INTERVENTION / EVALUATION

Assist w/ambulation if lightheadedness, dizziness occur. Assess for peripheral edema behind media/malleolus (sacral area in bedridden pts). Monitor pulse rate for bradycardia. Assess skin for flushing. Monitor liver enzyme tests. Question for headache, asthenia.

PATIENT/FAMILY TEACHING

Do not abruptly discontinue medication. Compliance w/therapy regimen is essential to control hypertension. To avoid hypotensive effect, rise slowly from lying to sitting position. Wait momentarily before standing. Avoid tasks that require alertness, motor skills until response to drug is established. Contact physician/nurse if irregular heartbeat, shortness of breath, pronounced dizziness, or nausea occurs. Swallow whole, do not crush or chew. Maintain good dental hygiene. Avoid grapefruit juice.

fenofibrate

fen-oh-**figh**-brate
(Tricor)

CANADIAN AVAILABILITY
Apo-Fenofibrate

PREGNANCY CATEGORY C

CLASSIFICATION

Antihyperlipidemic

AVAILABILITY (Rx)

Capsules: 67 mg

PHARMACOKINETICS

Absorption: Well absorbed from GI tract. Absorption increased when given with food. **Metabolism:** Rapidly metabolized in liver to active metabolite. Binds to plasma proteins. **Excretion:** Excreted primarily in the urine, lesser amount in feces. **Half-life:** 20 hrs.

ACTION/*THERAPEUTIC EFFECT*

Reduces very low-density lipoprotein (VLDL) and stimulates the catabolism of triglyceride-rich lipoprotein (VLDL), *decreasing plasma triglycerides, cholesterol.* Reduces serum uric acid levels by increasing urinary excretion of uric acid.

F

USES/*UNLABELED*

Adjunct to diet therapy in adult pts with very high elevations of serum triglyceride levels who are at risk of pancreatitis and who do not respond adequately to a determined dietary effort to control triglyceride levels.

ADMINISTRATION

ORAL:
- Give with meals.

INDICATIONS/ROUTES/DOSAGES

Hyperlipidemia:
Oral: Adults, renal function impairment (Ccr <50 ml/min: Initially, 67 mg/day given with meals. ***Maximum:*** 3 capsules/day (201 mg). ***Elderly:*** Limit the dosage to 67 mg/day.

CONTRAINDICATIONS

Hypersensitivity to fenofibrate, severe renal or hepatic dysfunction including primary biliary cirrhosis, unexplained persistent liver function abnormality, preexisting gallbladder disease.

CAUTIONS

Anticoagulant therapy, history of liver disease, substantial alcohol consumption.

INTERACTIONS

DRUG: *Potentiates* effects of ***anticoagulants.*** Concurrent administration with ***cyclosporine*** increases risk of nephrotoxicity. Increased risk of severe myopathy, rhabdomyolysis, acute renal failure may occur with ***HMG-CoA reductase*** *inhibitors. Bile acid sequestrants* impede fenofibrate absorption (give fenofibrate 1 hr before or 4–6 hrs after bile acid sequestrant administration). **HERBAL:** None known. **FOOD:** Food increases drug absorption. **ALTERED LAB VALUES:** May increase serum transaminase (AST, ALT), creatinine kinase (CK), blood urea levels. May decrease Hgb, Hct, WBC, uric acid.

SIDE EFFECTS

FREQUENT (4–8%): Pain, rash, headache, asthenia/fatigue, flu syndrome, dyspepsia, nausea/vomiting, rhinitis. **OCCASIONAL (2–3%):** Diarrhea, abdominal pain, constipation, flatulence, arthralgia, decreased libido, dizziness, pruritus. **RARE (<2%):** Increased appetite, insomnia, polyuria, cough, blurred vision, eye floaters, earache.

ADVERSE REACTIONS/TOXIC EFFECTS

May increase cholesterol excretion into the bile, leading to cholelithiasis. Pancreatitis, hepatitis, thrombocytopenia, agranulocytosis occur rarely.

PATIENT CONSIDERATIONS

BASELINE ASSESSMENT

Obtain lipid cholesterol, triglycerides, liver function tests, including serum ALT, and blood counts during initial therapy and periodically during treatment. Treatment should be discontinued if liver enzyme levels persist > 3 times normal limit.

INTERVENTIONS/EVALUATION

For those on concurrent therapy with HMG-CoA reductase inhibitors, monitor for complaints of myopathy (muscle pain, weakness), including serum creatinine kinase levels. Monitor cholesterol and triglyceride concentrations for therapeutic response.

PATIENT/FAMILY TEACHING

Periodic lab tests are essential part of therapy. Do not take other medications w/o physician's knowledge. Do not stop medication w/o consulting physician.

---

fenoldopam

feh-**noll**-doh-pam
(Corlopam)

PREGNANCY CATEGORY B

CLASSIFICATION

Antihypertensive

AVAILABILITY (Rx)

Injection, Concentrate: 10 mg/ml

PHARMACODYNAMICS

	ONSET	PEAK	DURATION
IV	—	15 min	—

PHARMACOKINETICS

Absorption: Administered as a constant infusion. Binds to alpha$_2$-adrenoceptors. **Excretion:** Eliminated primarily in urine. Clearance is not altered by end-stage renal disease or affected by hepatic failure. **Half-life:** 5 min.

ACTION/*THERAPEUTIC EFFECT*

Rapid-acting vasodilator. An agonist for D$_1$-like dopamine receptors, produces vasodilation in coronary, renal, mesenteric and peripheral arteries, *reducing systolic and diastolic B/P, increase in heart rate.*

USES

Short-term (48 hrs) management of severe hypertension when rapid, but quickly reversible, emergency reduction of B/P is clinically indicated, including malignant hypertension with deteriorating end-organ function.

ADMINISTRATION

IV:

- Dilute each ampoule in 0.9% sodium chloride injection or 5% dextrose injection for final concentration of 40 mcg/ml.
- Add 4 ml of concentrate (40 mg of drug) to 1,000 ml; 2 ml of concentrate (20 mg) to 500 ml; 1 ml of concentrate (10 mg) to 250 ml.
- Infusion can be rapidly discontinued or gradually tapered off to discontinuation.

INDICATIONS/DOSAGE/ROUTES

Hypertension:

Continuous IV infusion: Adults, elderly: 0.01–0.3 mcg/kg/min (do not use bolus dose). Titrate dose upward or downward no more frequently than every 15 min to reach desired therapeutic effect. Avoid rapid decrease in B/P or hypotension. ***Recommended titration increments:*** 0.05–0.1 mcg/kg/min.

CONTRAINDICATIONS

None significant.

CAUTIONS

Glaucoma, intraocular hypertension (increases intraocular pressure), tachycardia, hypotension, hypokalemia, sulfite sensitivity.

INTERACTIONS

DRUG: Concurrent use of ***beta blockers*** may produce excessive hypotension. **HERBAL:** None known. **FOOD:** None significant. **ALTERED LAB VALUES:** May elevate BUN, glucose, transaminase, LDH. May decrease potassium.

SIDE EFFECTS

OCCASIONAL (>5%): Headache, flushing, nausea, hypotension. **RARE (1–4%):** Nervousness/anxiety, vomiting, constipation, nasal congestion, diaphoresis, back pain.

ADVERSE REACTIONS/TOXIC EFFECTS

Excessive hypotension occurs occasionally; B/P must be monitored diligently during infusion. Excessive heart rate may lead to ischemic cardiac events or worsened heart failure. Allergic-type reactions, including anaphylaxis and life-threatening asthmatic attack in those with sulfite sensitivity.

PATIENT CONSIDERATIONS

BASELINE ASSESSMENT

Determine initial B/P and apical pulse. It is essential to monitor B/P diligently during infusion. Assess medication history (especially beta blockers). Obtain baseline serum electrolytes, particularly potassium, and periodically thereafter during infusion. Question asthmatic pts for history of sulfite sensitivity.

INTERVENTION/EVALUATION

Monitor B/P and heart rate at frequent intervals (every 15 min) to avoid hypotension and rapid decrease in B/P. If excessive reduction in B/P occurs, place pt in supine position, feet slightly elevated. Monitor for decrease in serum potassium, particularly <6 hrs of infusion.

fenoprofen calcium

fen-oh-**pro**-fen
(Nalfon)

CANADIAN AVAILABILITY
Nalfon

PREGNANCY CATEGORY B
(D if used in third trimester or near delivery)

CLASSIFICATION

Nonsteroidal anti-inflammatory

AVAILABILITY (Rx)

Capsules: 200 mg, 300 mg. **Tablets:** 600 mg.

PHARMACODYNAMICS

	ONSET	PEAK	DURATION
Oral (antirheumatic)			
	2 days	—	2–3 wks

PHARMACOKINETICS

Absorption: Rapidly absorbed from GI tract. Widely distributed. **Metabolism:** Metabolized in liver. **Excretion:** Primarily excreted in urine. **Half-life:** 3 hrs.

ACTION/*THERAPEUTIC EFFECT*

Produces analgesic and anti-inflammatory effect by inhibiting prostaglandin synthesis, *reducing inflammatory response and intensity of pain stimulus reaching sensory nerve endings.*

USES/*UNLABELED*

Treatment of acute or long-term mild to moderate pain, symptomatic treatment of acute and/or chronic rheumatoid arthritis, osteoarthritis. *Treatment of vascular headaches, ankylosing spondylitis, psoriatic arthritis.*

ADMINISTRATION

ORAL:

- May give w/food, milk, or antacids if GI distress occurs.

INDICATIONS/ROUTES/DOSAGE

Note: Do not exceed 3.2 g/day.

Mild to moderate pain:
Oral: Adults, elderly: 200 mg q4–6h as needed.

Rheumatoid arthritis, osteoarthritis:
Oral: Adults, elderly: 300–600 mg 3–4 times/day.

CONTRAINDICATIONS

Active peptic ulcer, GI ulceration, chronic inflammation of GI tract, GI bleeding disorders, history of hypersensitivity to aspirin/NSAIDs, history of significantly impaired renal function.

CAUTIONS

Impaired renal/hepatic function, history of GI tract diseases, predisposition to fluid retention.

INTERACTIONS

DRUG: May increase effects of ***oral anticoagulants, heparin, thrombolytics.*** May decrease effect of ***antihypertensives, diuretics. Salicylates, aspirin*** may increase risk of GI side effects, bleeding. ***Bone marrow depressants*** may increase risk of hematologic reactions. May increase concentration, toxicity of ***lithium.*** May increase ***methotrexate*** toxicity. ***Probenecid*** may increase concentrations. **HERBAL:** Feverfew, ginkgo may increase risk of bleeding. **FOOD:** None significant. **ALTERED LAB VALUES:** May increase serum transaminase, LDH, alkaline phosphatase, BUN, creatinine, potassium, glucose, protein, bleeding time.

SIDE EFFECTS

FREQUENT (3–9%): Headache, somnolence/drowsiness, dyspepsia (heartburn, indigestion, epigastric pain), nausea, vomiting, constipation. OCCASIONAL (1–3%): Dizziness, pruritus, nervousness, asthenia (loss of strength), diarrhea, abdominal cramps, flatulence, tinnitus, blurred vision, peripheral edema/fluid retention.

ADVERSE REACTIONS/TOXIC EFFECTS

Overdosage may result in acute hypotension, tachycardia. Peptic ulcer, GI bleeding, nephrotoxicity (dysuria, cystitis, hematuria, proteinuria, nephrotic syndrome), gastritis, severe hepatic reaction (cholestasis, jaundice), severe hypersensitivity reaction (bronchospasm, angiofacial edema) occur rarely.

PATIENT CONSIDERATIONS

BASELINE ASSESSMENT

Assess onset, type, location, duration of pain or inflammation. Inspect appearance of affected joints for immobility, deformities, skin condition.

INTERVENTION/EVALUATION

Assist w/ambulation if somnolence/drowsiness/dizziness occurs. Monitor for evidence of dyspepsia. Monitor pattern of daily bowel activity, stool consistency. Check behind medial malleolus for fluid retention (usually first area noted). Evaluate for therapeutic response: relief of pain, stiffness, swelling, increase in joint mobility, reduced joint tenderness, improved grip strength.

PATIENT/FAMILY TEACHING

Swallow capsule whole; do not crush or chew. Avoid tasks that require alertness, motor skills until response to drug is established. If GI upset occurs, take w/food, milk. Avoid aspirin, alcohol during therapy (increases risk of GI bleeding). Report headache, GI distress, visual disturbances, edema, skin rash, itching, black stools.

F

---

fentanyl

fen-tah-nil
(Actig, Duragesic)

fentanyl citrate

(Fentanyl Oralet, Sublimaze)

FIXED-COMBINATION(S)
W/droperidol, an antianxiety, antiemetic **(Innovar)**

CANADIAN AVAILABILITY
Duragesic

PREGNANCY CATEGORY B
(D if used for prolonged periods or at high doses at term)

CLASSIFICATION

Opioid: Analgesic **(Schedule II)**

AVAILABILITY (Rx)

Injection: 0.05 mg/ml. **Transdermal Patch:** 25 mcg/hr, 50 mcg/hr, 75 mcg/hr, 100 mcg/hr. **Lozenges:** 200 mcg, 300 mcg, 400 mcg.

PHARMACODYNAMICS

	ONSET	PEAK	DURATION
IM	7–15 min	20–30 min	1–2 hrs
IV	1–2 min	3–5 min	0.5–1 hr

PHARMACOKINETICS

Absorption: Well absorbed after

topical, IM administration. Transmucosal absorbed through mucosal tissue of mouth, GI tract. **Metabolism:** Metabolized in liver. **Excretion:** Primarily eliminated via biliary system. **Half-life:** 3.6 hrs (increased in elderly).

ACTION / *THERAPEUTIC EFFECT*

Binds at opiate receptor sites within CNS, reducing stimuli from sensory nerve endings, *affecting pain perception, emotional response to pain.*

USES

Analgesic action for short duration surgery, outpt minor surgery, diagnostic procedures requiring pt to be awake or lightly anesthetized; during surgery, immediately after surgery to prevent/relieve tachypnea, postop delirium, adjunct to general/regional anesthesia. Transdermal for management of chronic pain. Transmucosal for anesthetic premedication. ***Actig:*** Treatment breakthrough for pain in chronic cancer or AIDS-related pain.

STORAGE/HANDLING

Store parenteral form at room temperature.

ADMINISTRATION

IV/IM:

- **Note:** Incompatible w/methohexital, pentobarbital, thiopental.
- For initial anesthesia induction dosage, give small amount, via tuberculin syringe.
- Give by slow IV injection (over 1–2 min).
- Too rapid IV increases risk of severe adverse reactions (skeletal and thoracic muscle rigidity resulting in apnea, laryngospasm, bronchospasm, peripheral circulatory collapse, anaphylactoid effects, cardiac arrest).
- Opiate antagonist (naloxone) should be readily available.

TRANSDERMAL:

- Apply to nonhairy area of intact skin of upper torso.
- Use flat, nonirritated site.
- Firmly press evenly for 10–20 sec assuring adhesion is in full contact w/skin and edges are completely sealed.
- Use only water to cleanse site prior to application (soaps, oils, etc., may irritate skin).
- Rotate sites of application.
- Used patches are carefully folded so system adheres to itself; discard in toilet.

TRANSMUCOSAL:

- Suck lozenge vigorously.

INDICATIONS/ROUTES/DOSAGE

Note: Reduce initial dose by 25–33% in those receiving CNS depressants. Reduce dose in elderly, debilitated. Obese (>20% ideal body weight): Adjust dosage based on lean body weight.

Preop:
IM: Adults, elderly: 50–100 mcg (0.05–0.1 mg) 30–60 min before surgery.

Primary agent anesthesia:
IV: Adults, elderly: 50–100 mcg/kg, administered w/oxygen and skeletal muscle relaxant. ***Children 2–12 yrs:*** 1.7–3.3 mcg/kg.

Adjunct to local anesthesia:
IM/IV: Adults, elderly: 50–100 mcg.

Adjunct to general anesthesia:
Total low dose:
IV: Adults, elderly: 2 mcg/kg one time.

Total moderate dose:
IV/IM: Adults, elderly: Initially, 2–20 mcg/kg IV, then 25–100 mcg IM/IV as necessary.

Total high dose:
IV: Adults, elderly: Initially, 20–50 mcg/kg. May give additional doses ranging from 25 mcg up to one-half initial dose.

Postop (recovery room):
IM: Adults, elderly: 50–100 mcg q1–2h, as needed.

Usual transdermal dosage:
Transdermal: Adults, elderly: Individualized. Use lowest effective dose based on previous analgesics given, opioid tolerance, pt condition, medical status.

Usual transmucosal dosage:
Transmucosal: Adults, children: 200–400 mcg.

CONTRAINDICATIONS

Transdermal: Diarrhea, acute respiratory depression.

EXTREME CAUTION

Bradyarrhythmias, severe CNS depression, anoxia, hypercapnia, respiratory depression, seizures, acute alcoholism, shock, untreated myxedema, respiratory dysfunction.

CAUTIONS

Increased intracranial pressure; impaired hepatic, renal function. *Transdermal:* Acute asthma attack, chronic respiratory disease, severe inflammatory bowel disease, impaired liver/renal function, increased intracranial pressure, head injury.

INTERACTIONS

DRUG: *Benzodiazepines* may increase risk of hypotension, respiratory depression. *Buprenorphine* may decrease effect. CNS depressants may increase CNS, respiratory depression, hypotension. **HERBAL:** None known. **FOOD:** None significant. **ALTERED LAB VALUES:** May increase amylase, lipase plasma concentrations.

SIDE EFFECTS

FREQUENT: *Transdermal (3–10%):* Headache, itching skin, nausea, vomiting, sweating, difficulty breathing, confusion, dizziness, drowsiness, diarrhea, constipation, decreased appetite. *IV:* Postop drowsiness, nausea, vomiting. **OCCASIONAL:** *Transdermal (1–3%):* Chest pain, irregular heartbeat, redness, itching, swelling of skin, fainting,agitation, tingling or burning of skin. *IV:* Postop confusion, blurred vision, chills, orthostatic hypotension, constipation, difficulty urinating.

ADVERSE REACTIONS/TOXIC EFFECTS

Overdosage or too rapid IV results in severe respiratory depression, skeletal and thoracic muscle rigidity resulting in apnea, laryngospasm, bronchospasm, cold and clammy skin, cyanosis, coma. Tolerance to analgesic effect may occur w/repeated use.

PATIENT CONSIDERATIONS

BASELINE ASSESSMENT

Resuscitative equipment and opiate antagonist (naloxone, 0.5 mcg/kg) must be available. Establish baseline B/P and respirations. Assess type, location, intensity, and duration of pain.

INTERVENTION/EVALUATION

Monitor B/P and respirations closely. Assist w/ambulation. Encourage pt to turn, cough, and

deep breathe q2h. Check for constipation; increase fluids, bulk, and exercise as appropriate. Assess for relief of pain.

Patient/Family Teaching

Avoid alcohol; do not take other medications w/o consulting physician. Do not drive or perform other activities requiring alertness, coordination. Teach pt proper application of transdermal. Use as directed to avoid overdosage; potential for physical dependence w/prolonged use. After long-term use, must be discontinued slowly.

ferrous fumarate

fair-us **fume**-ah-rate
(Feostat)

ferrous gluconate

fair-us **glue**-kuh-nate
(Fergon, Ferralet, Simron)

ferrous sulfate

fair-us **sul**-fate
(Feosol, Slow-Fe)

FIXED-COMBINATION(S)

W/docusate sodium, a stool softener **(Ferro-Sequels)**; w/aluminum and magnesium hydroxide, antacids **(Fermalox)**

CANADIAN AVAILABILITY

Apo-Ferrous Gluconate, Apo-Ferrous Sulfate, Fer-In-Sol, Slow Fe, Palafer

PREGNANCY CATEGORY A

CLASSIFICATION

Iron preparation

AVAILABILITY (OTC)

Ferrous Fumarate: Tablets: 63 mg, 195 mg, 200 mg, 324 mg, 350 mg. **Tablets (chewable):** 100 mg. **Capsules (controlled-release):** 325 mg. **Suspension:** 100 mg/5 ml. **Oral Drops:** 45 mg/0.6 ml.

Ferrous Gluconate: Tablets: 300 mg, 320 mg. **Tablets (sustained-release):** 320 mg.

Ferrous Sulfate: Tablets: 195 mg, 300 mg, 324 mg. **Capsules:** 250 mg. **Tablets (timed-release):** 525 mg. **Syrup:** 90 mg/5 ml. **Elixir:** 220 mg/5 ml. **Oral Drops:** 125 mg/ml.

Ferrous Sulfate (exsiccated): Tablets: 200 mg. **Capsules:** 190 mg. **Capsules (timed-release):** 159 mg, 250 mg. **Tablets (slow-release):** 160 mg.

PHARMACOKINETICS

Absorption: Absorption increased when iron stores depleted. Primarily absorbed in duodenum, proximal jejunum and stored in hepatocytes and reticuloendothelial system. No physiologic system of elimination (small amounts lost daily in shedding skin, hair, nails). **Half-life:** 6 hrs.

ACTION/*THERAPEUTIC EFFECT*

Essential component in formation of hemoglobin, myoglobin, and enzymes, *necessary for effective erythropoiesis and for transport and utilization of oxygen.*

USES

Prevention and treatment of iron deficiency anemia due to inadequate diet, malabsorption, pregnancy, and/or blood loss.

STORAGE/HANDLING

Store all forms (tablets, capsules, suspension, drops) at room temperature.

ADMINISTRATION

ORAL:

- Ideally, give between meals w/water but may give w/meals if GI discomfort occurs.
- Transient staining of mucous membranes and teeth will occur w/liquid iron preparation. Place liquid on back of tongue w/dropper or straw.
- Avoid simultaneous administration of antacids or tetracycline.
- Do not crush sustained-release preparations.

INDICATIONS/ROUTES/DOSAGE

Note: Dosage expressed in terms of elemental iron. Elemental iron content: ferrous fumarate: 33% (99 mg iron/300 mg tablet); ferrous gluconate: 11.6% (35 mg iron/300 mg tablet); ferrous sulfate: 20% (60 mg iron/300 mg tablet).

Deficiency:

Oral: Adults, elderly: 2–3 mg/kg/day in 3 divided doses. *Children 2–12 yrs:* 3 mg/kg/day in 3–4 divided doses. *Children 6 mos–2 yrs:* Up to 6 mg/kg/day in 3–4 divided doses. *Infants:* 10–25 mg/day in 3–4 divided doses.

CONTRAINDICATIONS

Hemochromatosis, hemosiderosis, hemolytic anemias, those w/peptic ulcer, regional enteritis, or ulcerative colitis.

CAUTIONS

Those w/bronchial asthma, iron hypersensitivity.

INTERACTIONS

DRUG: *Antacids, calcium supplements, pancreatin, pancrelipase* may decrease absorption. May decrease absorption of *quinolones, etidronate, tetracyclines.* HERBAL: None known. FOOD: None significant. **ALTERED LAB VALUES:** May increase bilirubin. May decrease calcium. May obscure occult blood in stools.

SIDE EFFECTS

OCCASIONAL: Mild, transient nausea. **RARE:** Heartburn, anorexia, constipation, or diarrhea.

ADVERSE REACTIONS/TOXIC EFFECTS

Large doses may aggravate existing GI tract disease (peptic ulcer, regional enteritis, ulcerative colitis). Severe iron poisoning occurs mostly in children and is manifested as vomiting, severe abdominal pain, diarrhea, dehydration, followed by hyperventilation, pallor or cyanosis, cardiovascular collapse.

PATIENT CONSIDERATIONS

BASELINE ASSESSMENT

To prevent mucous membrane and teeth staining w/liquid preparation, use dropper or straw and allow solution to drop on back of tongue. Eggs, milk inhibit absorption. Obtain Hgb, Hct results.

INTERVENTION/EVALUATION

Those w/normal iron balance should not take iron preparation routinely. Monitor daily pattern of bowel activity and stool consistency. Assess for clinical improvement and record relief of iron deficiency symptoms (fatigue, irritability, pallor, paresthesia of extremities, headache). Monitor Hgb, Hct results.

PATIENT/FAMILY TEACHING

Expect stools to darken in color. Take on empty stomach. If GI discomfort occurs, take after meals or w/food. Do not take

within 2 hrs of antacids (prevents absorption).

fexofenadine

fecks-**oh**-fen-ah-deen
(Allegra)

FIXED-COMBINATION(S)
W/pseudoephedrine, a sympathomimetic **(Allegra-D)**

CANADIAN AVAILABILITY
Allegra

PREGNANCY CATEGORY C

CLASSIFICATION

Antihistamine

AVAILABILITY (Rx)

Capsules: 60 mg

PHARMACOKINETICS

Absorption: Rapidly absorbed following oral administration. Does not cross blood-brain barrier. **Metabolism:** Minimally metabolized. **Excretion:** Eliminated in feces, excreted in urine. **Half-life:** 14.4 hrs (increased in those w/reduced renal function).

ACTION/*THERAPEUTIC EFFECT*

Prevents, antagonizes most histamine effects (e.g., urticaria, pruritus). *Relieves allergic rhinitis symptoms.*

USES

Relief of symptoms associated w/seasonal allergic rhinitis (sneezing, rhinorrhea, itching of throat/eyes) in adults, children >12 yrs.

ADMINISTRATION

ORAL:

- May take w/o regard to food.

INDICATIONS/ROUTES/DOSAGE

Allergic rhinitis:
Oral: Adults, elderly, children >12 yrs: 60 mg 2 times/day.

Dosage in renal impairment:
Oral: Adults, elderly, children >12 yrs: 60 mg once daily.

CONTRAINDICATIONS

Hypersensitivitiy to fexofenadine or its ingredients.

CAUTIONS

Severe renal impairment.

INTERACTIONS

DRUG: None significant. **HERBAL:** None known. **FOOD:** None significant. **ALTERED LAB VALUES:** May suppress wheal and flare reactions to antigen skin testing. Discontinue at least 4 days before testing.

SIDE EFFECTS

OCCASIONAL (1–3%): Drowsiness, headache, fatigue, nausea, vomiting, abdominal distress, dysmenorrhea.

ADVERSE REACTIONS/TOXIC EFFECTS

None significant.

PATENT CONSIDERATIONS

Baseline Assessment

If pt is undergoing allergic reaction, obtain history of recently ingested foods, drugs, environmental exposure, recent emotional stress. Monitor rate, depth, rhythm, type of respiration; quality and rate of pulse. Assess lung sounds for rhonchi, wheezing, rales.

Intervention/Evaluation

Assess for therapeutic response from allergy: itching, red, watery

eyes, relief from rhinorrhea, sneezing.

PATIENT/FAMILY TEACHING

Avoid tasks that require alertness, motor skills until response to drug is established. Avoid alcoholic beverages during antihistamine therapy. Coffee or tea may help reduce drowsiness.

filgrastim

fill-**grass**-tim
(Neupogen)

CANADIAN AVAILABILITY
Neupogen

PREGNANCY CATEGORY C

CLASSIFICATION

Colony stimulating factor

AVAILABILITY (Rx)

Injection: 300 mcg/ml

PHARMACOKINETICS

Absorption: Readily absorbed after SubQ administration. **Half-life:** 3.5 hrs.

ACTION/*THERAPEUTIC EFFECT*

Regulates production of neutrophils within bone marrow. Primarily affects neutrophil progenitor proliferation, differentiation, and selected end-cell functional activation *(e.g., increased phagocytic ability, antibody-dependent killing)*.

USES/*UNLABELED*

Decrease infection incidence in pt w/nonmyeloid malignancies receiving myelosuppressive therapy associated w/severe neutropenia, fever. Reduce neutropenia duration (and sequelae) in pt w/nonmyeloid malignancies having myeloablative therapy followed by bone marrow transplant (BMT). Mobilization of hematopoietic progenitor cells into peripheral blood for collection by leukapheresis. Improves neutrophoil recovery, reduce fever duration following chemotherapy for acute myeloid leukemia (AML). *Treatment of AIDS-related neutropenia; chronic, severe neutropenia, drug-induced neutropenia; myelodysplastic syndrome.*

STORAGE/HANDLING

Refrigerate. Do not shake vial. Use 1 dose/vial, do not reenter vial. Stable for up to 24 hrs at room temperature (provided vial contents are clear, contain no particulate matter). Remains stable if accidentally exposed to freezing temperature.

ADMINISTRATION

SUBQ/IV:
May be given by SubQ injection or short IV infusion (15–30 min).

INDICATIONS/ROUTES/DOSAGE

Note: Begin at least 24 hrs after last dose of chemotherapy, discontinue at least 24 hrs prior to next dose of chemotherapy.

Myelosuppressive:
SubQ/IV or SubQ Infusion: ***Adults, elderly:*** Initially, 5 mcg/kg/day. May increase by 5 mcg/kg for each chemotherapy cycle based on duration/severity of absolute neutrophil count (ANC) nadir.

Note: Begin at least 24 hrs after last dose of chemotherapy and at least 24 hrs after bone marrow infusion.

BMT:
IV or SubQ Infusion: Adults, elderly: 10 mcg/kg/day. Adjust dose daily during period of neutrophil recovery based on neutrophil response.

Mobilize progenitor cells:
IV/SubQ: Adults: 10 mcg/kg/day beginning at least 4 days before first leukapheresis and continuing until last leukapheresis.

CONTRAINDICATIONS

Hypersensitivity to *Escherichia coli*derived proteins, 24 hrs before or after cytotoxic chemotherapy, use w/other drugs that may result in lowered platelet count.

CAUTIONS

Concurrent use w/mycoloid properties.

INTERACTIONS

DRUG: None significant. **HERBAL:** None known. **FOOD:** None significant. **ALTERED LABVALUES:** May increase alkaline phosphatase, LDH, uric acid, leukocyte (LAP) scores.

SIDE EFFECTS

FREQUENT (>10%): Bone pain, mild to severe (occurs more frequently in those receiving high dose via IV form, less frequently in low dose, SubQ form), nausea, vomiting, alopecia, diarrhea, fever, fatigue. **OCCASIONAL (5–10%):** Anorexia, dyspnea, headache, cough, skin rash. **RARE (<5%):** Psoriasis, hematuria/proteinuria, osteoporosis.

ADVERSE REACTIONS/TOXIC EFFECTS

Chronic administration occasionally produces chronic neutropenia, splenomegaly. Thrombocytopenia, MI arrhythmias occur rarely. Adult respiratory distress syndrome may occur in septic pts.

PATIENT CONSIDERATIONS

BASELINE ASSESSMENT

A CBC, platelet count (differential) should be obtained before initiation of therapy and twice weekly thereafter.

INTERVENTION/EVALUATION

In septic pts, be alert to adult respiratory distress syndrome. Closely monitor those w/preexisting cardiac conditions. Monitor B/P (transient decrease in B/P may occur).

---

finasteride

fin-**ah**-stir-eyd
(Propecia, Proscar)

CANADIAN AVAILABILITY
Proscar, Propecia

PREGNANCY CATEGORY X

CLASSIFICATION

5-alpha reductase inhibitor

AVAILABILITY (Rx)

Tablets: 1 mg, 5 mg

PHARMACODYNAMICS

	ONSET	PEAK	DURATION
Oral	24 hrs	1–2 days	5–7 days

PHARMACOKINETICS

Absorption: Rapidly absorbed from GI tract. Widely distributed. **Metabolism:** Metabolized in liver. **Half-life:** 6–8 hrs.

ACTION/*THERAPEUTIC EFFECT*

Inhibits steroid 5-alpha reductase, an intracellular enzyme that converts testosterone into dihydrotestosterone (DHT) in the prostate gland, providing a reduction in serum DHT, *regressing the enlarged prostate gland.*

USES

Reduce risk of acute urinary retention, need for surgery in symptomatic benign prostatic hyperplasia (BPH). Most improvement noted in hesitancy, feeling of incomplete bladder emptying, interruption of urinary stream, difficulty initiating flow, dysuria, impaired size and force of urinary stream. Treatment for hair loss.

ADMINISTRATION

ORAL:

- Do not break or crush film-coated tablets.
- May take w/o regard to meals.

INDICATIONS/ROUTES/DOSAGE

Benign prostatic hypertrophy:
Oral: Adults, elderly: 5 mg once daily (minimum 6 mos).

Hair loss:
Oral: Adults: 1 mg daily.

CONTRAINDICATIONS

Physical handling of tablet in those who may become, or are, pregnant, exposure to semen in those who may become pregnant.

CAUTIONS

Liver function abnormalities.

INTERACTIONS

DRUG: None significant. **HERBAL:** None known. **FOOD:** None significant. **ALTERED LAB VALUES:** Produces decrease in serum prostate-specific antigen (PSA) levels (even in presence of prostate cancer).

SIDE EFFECTS

OCCASIONAL (2–4%): Impotence, decreased libido, gynecomastia, decreased volume of ejaculate.

ADVERSE REACTIONS/TOXIC EFFECTS

None significant.

PATIENT CONSIDERATIONS

BASELINE ASSESSMENT

Digital rectal exam, serum PSA determination should be performed in those w/benign prostatic hypertrophy before initiating therapy and periodically thereafter.

INTERVENTION/EVALUATION

Diligent monitoring of I&O, especially in those w/large residual urinary volume or severely diminished urinary flow for obstructive uropathy.

PATIENT/FAMILY TEACHING

Pt should be aware of potential impotence. May not notice improved urinary flow even if prostate gland shrinks, need to take medication >6 mos, and it is not known if medication decreases need for surgery. Regular visits to physician and monitoring tests are necessary. Because of potential risk to male fetus, a woman who is or may become pregnant should not handle tablets or be exposed to pt's semen. Volume of ejaculate may be decreased during treatment (decrease does not interfere w/sexual function).

flavoxate

flay-**vocks**-ate
(Urispas)

CANADIAN AVAILABILITY
Urispas

PREGNANCY CATEGORY B

CLASSIFICATION

Antispasmodic

AVAILABILITY (Rx)

Tablets: 100 mg

PHARMACOKINETICS

Absorption: Well absorbed from GI tract. **Excretion:** Primarily excreted in urine.

ACTION/*THERAPEUTIC EFFECT*

Relaxes detrusor and other smooth muscle by cholinergic blockade, counteracting muscle spasm of urinary tract. *Produces anticholinergic, local anesthetic, analgesic effects.*

USES

Symptomatic relief of dysuria, urgency, nocturia, frequency, incontinence associated w/cystitis, prostatitis, urethritis, urethrocystitis, or urethrotrigonitis.

ADMINISTRATION

ORAL:

- May be given w/o regard to food.

INDICATIONS/ROUTES/DOSAGE

Urinary antispasmodic:
Oral: Adults, elderly, adolescent: 100–200 mg 3–4 times/day.

CONTRAINDICATIONS

GI tract obstructive disease, GI hemorrhage, paralytic ileus, obstructive uropathy.

CAUTIONS

None significant.

INTERACTIONS

DRUG: None significant. **HERBAL:** None known. **FOOD:** None significant. **ALTERED LAB VALUES:** None significant.

SIDE EFFECTS

Generally well tolerated. Side effects usually mild and transient. **FREQUENT:** Drowsiness, dry mouth, throat. **OCCASIONAL:** Constipation, difficult urination, blurred vision, dizziness, headache, increased light sensitivity, nausea, vomiting, stomach pain. **RARE:** Confusion (primarily in elderly), hypersensitivity, increased intraocular pressure, leukopenia.

ADVERSE REACTIONS/TOXIC EFFECTS

Anticholinergic effect w/overdose (unsteadiness, severe dizziness, drowsiness, fever, flushed face, shortness of breath, nervousness, irritability).

PATIENT CONSIDERATIONS

BASELINE ASSESSMENT

Assess dysuria, urgency, frequency, incontinence, or suprapubic pain.

INTERVENTION/EVALUATION

Monitor for symptomatic relief. Observe elderly especially for mental confusion.

PATIENT/FAMILY TEACHING

Avoid driving or other tasks requiring alertness, coordination, or manual dexterity (blurred vision, drowsiness). Dry

mouth may be relieved by sips of water, sugarless gum, or hard candy.

flecainide acetate

fleh-kun-eyed
(Tambocor)

CANADIAN AVAILABILITY
Tambocor

PREGNANCY CATEGORY C

CLASSIFICATION

Antiarrhythmic

AVAILABILITY (Rx)

Tablets: 50 mg, 100 mg, 150 mg

PHARMACOKINETICS

Absorption: Completely absorbed from GI tract. Widely distributed. **Metabolism:** Metabolized in liver. **Excretion:** Primarily excreted in urine. Minimal removal by hemodialysis. **Half-life:** 12–27 hrs (increased in decreased renal, liver function, CHF).

ACTION/*THERAPEUTIC EFFECT*

Slows atrial, AV, His-Purkinje, intraventricular conduction *(decreases excitability, conduction velocity, automaticity)*. Greatest effect on His-Purkinje system.

USES

Prevention of documented life-threatening ventricular arrhythmias, paroxysmal supraventricular tachycardias (PSVT) w/o structural heart disease, and paroxysmal atrial fibrillation (PAF).

ADMINISTRATION

ORAL:

- Scored tablets may be crushed.
- Monitor EKG for cardiac changes, particularly widening of QRS, prolongation of PR interval. Notify physician of any significant interval changes.

INDICATIONS/ROUTES/DOSAGE

Life-threatening ventricular arrhythmias, sustained ventricular tachycardia:
Oral: Adults, elderly: Initially, 100 mg q12h, increased by 100 mg (50 mg 2 times/day) every 4 days until effective dose or maximum of 400 mg/day attained.

PSVT, PAF:
Oral: Adults, elderly: Initially, 50 mg q12h, increased by 100 mg (50 mg 2 times/day) every 4 days until effective dose or maximum of 300 mg/day attained. ***Dose in pts w/CHF or myocardial dysfunction:*** Initially, 50–100 mg q12h. Increase by 50 mg 2 times/day every 4 days up to 200 mg q12h (400 mg/day). ***Dose in pts w/renal or hepatic impairment:*** Initially, 100 mg q12h increased at intervals greater than 4 days. Creatinine clearance <35 ml/min/m^2 dose is reduced by 25–50%.

CONTRAINDICATIONS

Cardiogenic shock, preexisting second- or third-degree AV block, right bundle branch block (w/o presence of pacemaker).

CAUTIONS

Impaired myocardial function, second- or third-degree AV block (w/pacemaker), CHF, sick-sinus syndrome.

INTERACTIONS

DRUG: *Urinary acidifiers* may

increase excretion; urinary alkalizers may decrease excretion. Other *antiarrhythmics* may have additive effects. *Beta blockers* may increase negative inotropic effects. May increase *digoxin* concentrations. HERBAL: None known. FOOD: None significant. ALTERED LAB VALUES: None significant.

SIDE EFFECTS

FREQUENT (>10%): Dizziness, dyspnea, visual disturbances. OCCASIONAL (3–10%): Headache, nausea, fatigue, palpitations, chest pain, asthenia (loss of strength), tremor, constipation, abdominal pain. RARE (1–3%): Vomiting, diarrhea, decreased appetite, dry mouth, insomnia, eye pain, fever.

ADVERSE REACTIONS/TOXIC EFFECTS

Has ability to worsen existing arrhythmias or produce new ones. May also produce or worsen CHF. Overdosage may increase QRS duration, QT interval and conduction disturbances, reduce myocardial contractility, conduction disturbances, hypotension.

PATIENT CONSIDERATIONS

BASELINE ASSESSMENT

Obtain medication history (especially other antiarrhythmics), cardiovascular history. Assess liver function studies.

INTERVENTION/EVALUATION

Assess pulse for strength/weakness, irregular rate. Monitor EKG for cardiac changes, particularly widening of QRS, prolongation of PR interval. Notify physician of any significant interval changes. Question for visual disturbances, headache, GI upset. Monitor fluid and electrolyte serum levels. Assess for evidence of CHF: dyspnea (particularly on exertion or lying down), night cough, peripheral edema, distended neck veins. Monitor I&O (increase in weight, decrease in urine output may indicate CHF). Assess hand movement for sign of tremor. Monitor for therapeutic serum level (0.2–1 mcg/ml).

PATIENT/FAMILY TEACHING

Side effects generally disappear w/continued use or decreased dosage. Do not abruptly discontinue medication. Compliance w/therapy regimen is essential to control arrhythmias. Do not use nasal decongestants, OTC cold preparations (stimulants) w/o physician approval. Restrict salt, alcohol intake.

---

floxuridine

(FUDR)

See Classification section under: Cancer chemotherapy

---

fluconazole

flu-**con**-ah-zole
(Diflucan)

CANADIAN AVAILABILITY
Diflucan

PREGNANCY CATEGORY C

CLASSIFICATION

Antifungal

AVAILABILITY (Rx)

Tablets: 50 mg, 100 mg, 150 mg, 200 mg. **Powder for Oral Suspen-**

sion: 10 mg/ml, 40 mg/ml. **Injection:** 2 mg/ml (in 100 or 200 ml containers).

PHARMACOKINETICS

Absorption: Well absorbed from GI tract. Widely distributed (including CSF). **Metabolism:** Partially metabolized in liver. **Excretion:** Primarily excreted unchanged in urine. Partially removed by hemodialysis. **Half-life:** 20–50 hrs (increased in reduced renal function).

ACTION/*THERAPEUTIC EFFECT*

Directly damages fungal membrane, altering membrane function. Interferes w/cytochrome (necessary for ergosterol formation). *Fungistatic.*

USES/*UNLABELED*

Treatment of oropharyngeal, esophageal, vaginal candidiasis, serious systemic candidal infections (e.g., urinary tract infections, peritonitis, pneumonia), *Cryptococcus neoformans* meningitis. Prevent candidiasis in bone marrow transplants. *Treatment of coccidiomycosis, cryptococcosis, onychomycosis, fungal pneumonia/septicemia, ringworm of the hand.*

STORAGE/HANDLING

Store at room temperature. Do not use parenteral form if solution is cloudy, precipitate forms, seal is not intact, or it is discolored.

ADMINISTRATION

ORAL:

- Give w/o regard to meals.
- Not affected by gastric pH.
- Oral and IV therapy equally effective; IV therapy for pt intolerant of the drug or unable to take orally.

IV:

- Do not remove from outer wrap until ready to use.
- Squeeze inner bag to check for minute leaks.
- Discard if solution is cloudy or precipitate is noted.
- Do not add supplementary medication.
- Plastic containers are not to be used in series connections (could cause air embolism).
- Maximum flow rate is 200 mg/hr.

INDICATIONS/ROUTES/DOSAGE

Oropharyngeal candidiasis:
Oral/IV: Adults, elderly: Initially, 200 mg once, then 100 mg/day for at least 14 days. ***Children:*** Initially, 6 mg/kg/day once, then 3 mg/kg/day.

Esophageal candidiasis:
Oral/IV: Adults, elderly: 200 mg once, then 100 mg/day (up to 400 mg/day) for 21 days and at least 14 days following resolution of symptoms. ***Children:*** 6 mg/kg/day once, then 3 mg/kg/day (up to 12 mg/kg/day).

Vaginal candidiasis:
Oral: Adults: 150 mg once.

Candidiasis prevention:
Oral: Adults: 400 mg/day.

Systemic candidiasis:
Oral/IV: Adults, elderly: Initially, 400 mg once, then 200 mg/day (up to 400 mg/day) for at least 28 days and at least 14 days following resolution of symptoms. ***Children:*** 6–12 mg/kg/day.

Cryptococcal meningitis:
Oral/IV: Adults, elderly: Initially, 400 mg once, then 200 mg/day (up to 400 mg/day). Continue for 10–12 wks after CSF becomes negative (200 mg/day for suppression of relapse in pts w/AIDS).

Children: 12 mg/kg/day once, then 6–12 mg/kg/day; 6 mg/kg/day for suppression.

Onychomycosis:
Oral: Adults: 150 mg weekly.

Dosage in renal impairment:

After loading dose of 400 mg, daily dose based on creatinine clearance:

CREATININE CLEARANCE	% OF RECOMMENDED DOSE
>50	100
21–50	50
11–20	25
Dialysis	Dose after dialysis

CONTRAINDICATIONS

Hypersensitivity to fluconazole or any component of preparation.

CAUTIONS

Hepatic impairment. Hypersensitivity to other triazoles (e.g., itraconazole, terconazole) or imidazoles (butoconazole, ketoconazole, etc.).

INTERACTIONS

DRUG: May increase concentration, effects of ***oral hypoglycemics.*** High doses increase ***cyclosporine*** concentration. May decrease metabolism of ***phenytoin, warfarin. Rifampin*** may increase metabolism. May decrease metabolism; increase ***cisapride*** concentration, risk of cardiotoxicity. **HERBAL:** None known. **FOOD:** None significant. **ALTERED LAB VALUES:** May increase SGOT (AST), SGPT (ALT), alkaline phosphatase, bilirubin.

SIDE EFFECTS

OCCASIONAL (1–4%): Hypersensitivity reaction (fever, chills, rash, itching), dizziness, drowsiness, headache, constipation, diarrhea, nausea, vomiting, abdominal pain.

ADVERSE REACTIONS/TOXIC EFFECTS

Exfoliative skin disorders, serious hepatic effects, blood dyscrasias (eosinophilia, thrombocytopenia, anemia, leukopenia) have been reported rarely.

PATIENT CONSIDERATIONS

Baseline Assessment

Question for hypersensitivity to fluconazole or components of preparation. Confirm that a culture or histologic test was done for accurate diagnosis; therapy may begin before results are known. Establish baselines for CBC, potassium.

Intervention/Evaluation

Monitor hepatic function tests; be alert for hepatotoxicity: dark urine, pale stools, anorexia/nausea/vomiting, yellow skin or sclera. Report rash, itching promptly. Check CBC and potassium lab results. Evaluate food tolerance. Monitor temperature at least daily. Determine pattern of bowel activity, stool consistency. Assess for dizziness and provide assistance as needed.

Patient/Family Teaching

Do not drive car, machinery if dizziness, drowsiness occur. Notify physician of dark urine, pale stool, yellow skin/eyes or rash w/or w/o itching. Pts w/oropharyngeal infections should be taught good oral hygiene. Consult physician before taking any other medication.

fludarabine phosphate

(Fludara)

See Classification section under: Cancer chemotherapy

fludrocortisone

floo-droe-**kor**-tih-sone
(Florinef)

CANADIAN AVAILABILITY
Florinef

PREGNANCY CATEGORY C

CLASSIFICATION

Mineralocorticoid

AVAILABILITY (Rx)

Tablets: 0.1 mg

PHARMACOKINETICS

Absorption: Well absorbed from GI tract. Widely distributed. **Metabolism:** Metabolized in liver, kidney. **Excretion:** Primarily excreted in urine. **Half-life:** 3.5 hrs.

ACTION/*THERAPEUTIC EFFECT*

High mineralocorticoid, moderate glucocorticoid activity. Acts at distal tubules to *increase potassium, hydrogen ion excretion, sodium reabsorption, and water retention.*

USES/*UNLABELED*

Partial replacement therapy for primary and secondary adrenocortical insufficiency in Addison's disease. Adjunctive treatment of salt-losing forms of congenital adrenogenital syndrome. *Treatment of idiopathic orthostatic hypotension, acidosis in renal tubular disorders.*

ADMINISTRATION

ORAL:

- Give w/food or milk.
- Administer w/glucocorticoid.

INDICATIONS/ROUTES/DOSAGE

Addison's disease:
Oral: Adults, elderly: 0.05–0.1 mg/day. ***Range:*** 0.1 mg 3 times/wk–0.2 mg/day. Administration w/cortisone/hydrocortisone preferred.

Salt-losing adrenogenital syndrome:
Oral: Adults, elderly: 0.1–0.2 mg/day.

CONTRAINDICATIONS

Hypersensitivity to fludrocortisone, any condition except those requiring high mineralocorticoid activity.

CAUTIONS

CHF, hypertension, renal insufficiency. Prolonged therapy should be discontinued slowly.

INTERACTIONS

DRUG: May increase ***digoxin*** toxicity (hypokalemia). ***Hepatic enzyme inducers (e.g., phenytoin)*** may increase metabolism. ***Hypokalemia-causing medications*** may increase effect. ***Sodium-containing medication*** may increase sodium, edema, B/P. **HERBAL:** None known. **FOOD:** None significant. **ALTERED LAB VALUES:** May increase sodium. May decrease potassium, hematocrit.

SIDE EFFECTS

FREQUENT: Increased appetite, exaggerated sense of well-being, abdominal distension, weight gain, insomnia, mood swings. ***High dose, prolonged therapy, too rapid withdrawal:*** Increased susceptibility to infection (signs/symptoms masked); delayed wound healing, hypokalemia, hypocalcemia, GI distress, diarrhea or constipation, hypertension. **OCCASIONAL:** Headache (frontal or occipital), dizziness, menstrual difficulty or amenorrhea, ulcer development. **RARE:** Hypersensitivity reaction.

ADVERSE REACTIONS/TOXIC EFFECTS

Long-term therapy: muscle wasting (especially arms, legs), osteoporosis, spontaneous fractures, amenorrhea, cataracts, glaucoma, peptic ulcer, CHF. ***Abrupt withdrawal following long-term therapy:*** anorexia, nausea, fever, headache, joint pain, rebound inflammation, fatigue, weakness, lethargy, dizziness, orthostatic hypotension.

PATIENT CONSIDERATIONS

Baseline Assessment

Question for hypersensitivity to any corticosteroids. Obtain baselines for weight, B/P, blood glucose, electrolytes, chest x-ray, EKG.

Intervention/Evaluation

Monitor I&O, daily weight. Check B/P, pulse at least 2 times/day. Assess for signs of edema. Monitor blood glucose and electrolytes. Provide assistance w/ambulation, notify physician of dizziness. Be alert to signs/symptoms of hypokalemia (weakness and muscle cramps, numbness/tingling, especially lower extremities, nausea and vomiting, irritability, EKG changes). Evaluate food tolerance and bowel activity; report hyperacidity promptly. Assess emotional status, ability to sleep. Assess for infection: fever, sore throat, vague symptoms.

Patient/Family Teaching

Take w/food or milk. Usually given in conjunction w/glucocorticoids, electrolytes. Carry identification of drug and dose, physician name and phone number. Do not change dose/schedule or stop taking drug; must taper off gradually under medical supervision. Notify physician of fever, sore throat, muscle aches, sudden weight gain/swelling, continuing headaches. W/dietician give instructions for prescribed diet (usually high potassium). Maintain careful personal hygiene, avoid exposure to disease or trauma. Severe stress (serious infection, surgery, or trauma) may require increased dosage. Do not take aspirin or any other medication w/o consulting physician. Follow-up visits, lab tests are necessary; children must be assessed for growth retardation. Inform dentist or other physicians of fludrocortisone therapy now or within past 12 mos.

---

flumazenil

flew-**maz**-ah-nil
(Romazicon)

CANADIAN AVAILABILITY
Anexate

PREGNANCY CATEGORY C

CLASSIFICATION

Benzodiazepine receptor antagonist

AVAILABILITY (Rx)

Injection: 0.1 mg/ml

PHARMACODYNAMICS

	ONSET	PEAK	DURATION
IV	1–2 min	6–10 min	—

PHARMACOKINETICS

Duration, degree of benzodiazepine reversal related to dosage, plasma concentration. **Metabolism:** Metabolized by liver; excreted in urine.

ACTION/*THERAPEUTIC EFFECT*

Antagonizes sedation, impairment of recall and psychomotor impairment due to benzodiazepine activity on CNS.

USES

Complete or partial reversal of sedative effects of benzodiazepines when general anesthesia has been induced and/or maintained w/benzodiazepines, when sedation has been produced w/benzodiazepines for diagnostic and therapeutic procedures, management of benzodiazepine overdosage.

STORAGE/HANDLING

Store parenteral form at room temperature. Discard after 24 hrs once medication is drawn into syringe, is mixed w/any solutions, or if particulate or discoloration is noted.

ADMINISTRATION

IV:

- **Note:** Compatible w/5% dextrose in water, lactated Ringer's, 0.9% NaCl solutions.
- Rinse spilled medication from skin w/cool water.
- Administer through freely running IV infusion into large vein (local injection produces pain, inflammation at injection site).

INDICATIONS/ROUTES/DOSAGE

Reversal of conscious sedation, in general anesthesia:

*IV: **Adults, elderly:*** Initially, 0.2 mg (2 ml) over 15 sec; may repeat 0.2 mg dose in 45 sec; then at 60 sec intervals. ***Maximum:*** 1 mg (10 ml total dose).

Note: If resedation occurs, repeat dose at 20 min intervals. ***Maximum:*** 1 mg (given as 0.2 mg/min) at any one time, 3 mg in any 1 hr.

Benzodiazepine overdose:

*IV: **Adults, elderly:*** Initially, 0.2 mg (2 ml) over 30 sec; may repeat after 30 sec w/0.3 mg (3 ml) over 30 sec if desired level of consciousness not achieved. Further doses of 0.5 mg (5 ml) over 30 sec may be administered at 60 sec intervals. ***Maximum:*** 3 mg (30 ml) total dose.

Note: If resedation occurs, repeat dose at 20 min intervals. ***Maximum:*** 1 mg (given as 0.5 mg/min) at any one time, 3 mg in any 1 hr.

CONTRAINDICATIONS

History of hypersensitivity to benzodiazepines, in those who have been given a benzodiazepine for control of a potentially life-threatening condition (control of intracranial pressure, status epilepticus), those showing signs of serious cyclic antidepressant overdose manifested by motor abnormalities, dysrhythmias, anticholinergic signs, cardiovascular collapse.

CAUTIONS

Head injury, impaired hepatic function, alcoholism, drug dependency.

INTERACTIONS

DRUG: *Seizure-induced medica-*

tions may increase risk of seizures. **HERBAL:** None known. **FOOD:** None significant. **ALTERED LAB VALUES:** None significant.

SIDE EFFECTS

FREQUENT (3–11%): Agitation, anxiety, dry mouth, dyspnea, insomnia, palpitations, tremors, headache, blurred vision, dizziness, ataxia, nausea, vomiting, pain at injection site, increased sweating. **OCCASIONAL (1–3%):** Fatigue, flushing, hearing disturbances, thrombophlebitis, skin rash. **RARE (<1%):** Hives, itching, hallucinations.

ADVERSE REACTIONS/TOXIC EFFECTS

May produce onset of seizures (particularly those on long-term benzodiazepine use), overdosage, concurrent sedative-hypnotic drug withdrawal, recent therapy w/repeated doses of parenteral benzodiazepine, myoclonic jerking, concurrent cyclic antidepressant poisoning. May provoke panic attack in those w/history of panic disorder.

PATIENT CONSIDERATIONS

BASELINE ASSESSMENT

Arterial blood gases should be obtained before and at 30 min intervals during IV administration. Prepare to intervene in reestablishing airway, assisting ventilation (drug may not fully reverse ventilatory insufficiency induced by benzodiazepines). Note that effects of flumazenil may wear off before effects of benzodiazepines.

INTERVENTION/EVALUATION

Properly manage airway, assisted breathing, circulatory access and support, internal decontamination by lavage and charcoal, adequate clinical evaluation. Monitor for reversal of benzodiazepine effect. Assess for possible resedation, respiratory depression, hypoventilation. Assess closely for return of unconsciousness (narcosis) for at least 1 hr after pt is fully alert.

PATIENT/FAMILY TEACHING

Avoid tasks that require alertness, motor skills, ingestion of alcohol, or taking nonprescription drugs until at least 18–24 hrs after discharge.

flunisolide

flew-**nis**-oh-lide

(AeroBid, Nasalide, Nasarel)

CANADIAN AVAILABILITY

Bronalide aerosol, Rhinalar

PREGNANCY CATEGORY C

CLASSIFICATION

Corticosteroid

AVAILABILITY (Rx)

Aerosol: 250 mcg/activation. **Nasal Spray:** 25 mcg/activation.

PHARMACOKINETICS

Absorption: Minimally absorbed from pulmonary, nasal, and GI tissue. **Metabolism:** Primarily metabolized in liver, lung. **Excretion:** Primarily excreted in urine. **Half-life:** 1–1.5 hrs (nasal: 1–2 hrs).

ACTION/*THERAPEUTIC EFFECT*

Decreases number, activity of anti-inflammatory cells. *Inhibits bronchoconstriction, produces smooth muscle relaxation. Decreases immediate and late-phase allergic reactions.*

USES / *UNLABELED*

Inhalation: Control of bronchial asthma in those requiring chronic steroid therapy. ***Intranasal:*** Relief of symptoms of seasonal/perennial rhinitis. *Prevent recurrence of postsurgical nasal polyps.*

ADMINISTRATION

INHALATION:

- Shake container well; exhale completely; holding mouthpiece 1 inch away from lips, inhale and hold breath as long as possible before exhaling; then exhale slowly.
- Wait 1 min between inhalations when multiple inhalations ordered (allows for deeper bronchial penetration).
- Rinse mouth w/water immediately after inhalation (prevents mouth/throat dryness).

INTRANASAL:

- Clear nasal passages before use (topical nasal decongestants may be needed 5–15 min before use).
- Tilt head slightly forward.
- Insert spray tip up in 1 nostril, pointing toward inflamed nasal turbinates, away from nasal septum.
- Pump medication into 1 nostril while holding other nostril closed and concurrently inspire through nose.
- Discard used nasal solution after 3 mos.

INDICATIONS / ROUTES / DOSAGE

Usual inhalation dosage:

Inhalation: Adults, elderly: 2 inhalations 2 times/day, morning and evening. ***Maximum:*** 4 inhalations 2 times/day. ***Children (6–15 yrs):*** 2 inhalations 2 times/day.

Usual intranasal dosage:

Note: Improvement seen within few days; may take 3 wks. Do not continue beyond 3 wks if no significant improvement occurs.

Intranasal: Adults, elderly: Initially, 2 sprays each nostril 2 times/day, may increase to 2 sprays 3 times/day. ***Maximum:*** 8 sprays each nostril/day. ***Children (6–14 yrs):*** Initially, 1 spray 3 times/day or 2 sprays 2 times/day. ***Maximum:*** 4 sprays each nostril/day. ***Maintenance:*** Smallest amount to control symptoms.

CONTRAINDICATIONS

Hypersensitivity to any corticosteroid or components, primary treatment of status asthmaticus, systemic fungal infections, persistently positive sputum cultures for *Candida albicans.*

CAUTIONS

Adrenal insufficiency.

INTERACTIONS

DRUG: None significant. **HERBAL:** None known. **FOOD:** None significant. **ALTERED LAB VALUES:** None significant.

SIDE EFFECTS

OCCASIONAL: ***Inhalation:*** Throat irritation, hoarseness, dry mouth, coughing, temporary wheezing, localized fungal infection in mouth, pharynx, larynx (particularly if mouth is not rinsed w/water after each administration). ***Intranasal:*** Mild nasopharyngeal irritation; nasal irritation, burning, stinging, dryness, rebound congestion, bronchial asthma, rhinorrhea, loss of sense of taste.

ADVERSE REACTIONS / TOXIC EFFECTS

Acute hypersensitivity reaction (urticaria, angioedema, severe bronchospasm) occurs rarely. Transfer from systemic to local steroid therapy may unmask previously suppressed bronchial asthma condition.

PATIENT CONSIDERATIONS

BASELINE ASSESSMENT

Question for hypersensitivity to any corticosteroids, components. Offer emotional support (high incidence of anxiety due to difficulty in breathing and sympathomimetic response to drug).

INTERVENTION/EVALUATION

In those receiving bronchodilators by inhalation concomitantly w/steroid inhalation therapy, advise pts to use bronchodilator several min before corticosteroid aerosol (enhances penetration of steroid into bronchial tree). Monitor rate, depth, rhythm, type of respiration; quality and rate of pulse. Assess lung sounds for rhonchi, wheezing, rales. Monitor arterial blood gases. Observe lips, fingernails for blue or dusky color in light-skinned pts; gray in dark-skinned pts. Observe for clavicular retractions, hand tremor. Evaluate for clinical improvement (quieter, slower respirations, relaxed facial expression, cessation of clavicular retractions).

PATIENT/FAMILY TEACHING

Do not change dose schedule or stop taking drug; must taper off gradually under medical supervision. Maintain careful mouth hygiene. Rinse mouth w/water immediately after inhalation (prevents mouth/throat dryness, fungal infection of mouth). Contact physician/nurse if sore throat/mouth occurs. Increase fluid intake (decreases lung secretion viscosity). Do not take more than 2 inhalations at any one time (excessive use may produce paradoxical bronchoconstriction or a decreased bronchodilating effect). Avoid excessive use of caffeine derivatives (chocolate, coffee, tea, cola).

---

fluocinolone acetonide

(Flurosyn, Synalar, Synemol)

See Classification section under: Corticosteroids: topical.

---

fluocinonide

(Lidex, Vasoderm)

See Classification section under: Corticosteroids: topical.

---

fluoride

flur-eyd

(Fluoritab, Luride)

CANADIAN AVAILABILITY

Fluor-A-Day, Fluotic

CLASSIFICATION

Dietary supplement

AVAILABILITY (OTC)

Tablets (Chewable): 0.5 mg, 1 mg. **Oral Drops:** 0.125 mg/drop, 0.25 mg/drop.

PHARMACOKINETICS

Absorption: Rapid, completely absorbed from GI tract. Concentrated primarily in bone, developing teeth. **Excretion:** Primarily excreted in urine.

ACTION/*THERAPEUTIC EFFECT*

Increases tooth resistance to acid

dissolution by *promoting remineralization of decalcified enamel, inhibiting dental plaque bacteria, increasing resistance to development of caries.* Maintains bone strength.

USES

Dietary supplement for prevention of dental caries in children. Treatment of osteoporosis.

ADMINISTRATION

ORAL:

- May take w/o regard to food.
- May crush chewable tablets. **Liquid:** Avoid glass (causes etching of glass), may mix w/cereal, juice, food.

INDICATIONS/ROUTES/DOSAGE

Dietary supplement:

WATER FLUORIDE	AGE	MG/DAY
<0.3 ppm	<2 yrs	0.25 mg/day
	2–3 yrs	0.5 mg/day
	3–13 yrs	1 mg/day
0.3–0.7 ppm	<2 yrs	None
	2–3 yrs	0.25 mg/day
	3–13 yrs	0.5 mg/day
>0.7 ppm	None	None

Osteoporosis:

Oral: Adults, elderly: 50–75 mg/day in divided doses.

CONTRAINDICATIONS

Arthralgia, GI ulceration, severe renal insufficiency.

CAUTIONS

None significant.

INTERACTIONS

DRUG: ***Aluminum hydroxide, calcium*** may decrease absorption. **HERBAL:** None known. **FOOD:** None significant. **ALTERED LAB VALUES:** May increase SGOT (AST), alkaline phosphatase.

SIDE EFFECTS

Generally well tolerated. Side effects usually mild and transient. **RARE:** Oral mucous membrane ulceration.

ADVERSE REACTIONS/TOXIC EFFECTS

Hypocalcemia, tetany, bone pain (especially ankles, feet), electrolyte disturbances, arrhythmias, may cause cardiac failure, respiratory arrest. May cause skeletal fluorosis, osteomalacia, osteosclerosis.

PATIENT CONSIDERATIONS

PATIENT/FAMILILY TEACHING

Use only as directed and keep out of reach of children to avoid overdosage. Do not take w/milk or other dairy products (decreases absorption). Rinses and gels should be used at bedtime after brushing or flossing. Expectorate excess—do not swallow. Do not eat, drink, or rinse mouth after application.

fluorouracil

(Adrucil, Efudex, Fluoroplex)

See Classification section under: Cancer chemotherapy

fluoxetine hydrochloride

(Prozac)

CANADIAN AVAILABILITY

Novo-Fluoxetine, Prozac

PREGNANCY CATEGORY B

CLASSIFICATION

Antidepressant

AVAILABILITY (Rx)

Capsules: 10 mg, 20 mg. **Liquid:** 20 mg/5 ml. **Tablets:** 10 mg.

PHARMACOKINETICS

Absorption: Well absorbed from GI tract. Crosses blood-brain barrier. **Metabolism:** Metabolized in liver to active metabolite. **Excretion:** Primarily excreted in urine. **Half-life:** 2–3 days; metabolite: 7–9 days.

ACTION / *THERAPEUTIC EFFECT*

Selectively inhibits serotonin uptake in CNS, enhancing serotonergic function. *Resulting enhancement of synaptic activity produces antidepressant effect.*

USES

Outpt treatment of major depression exhibited as persistent, prominent dysphoria (occurring nearly every day for at least 2 wks) manifested by 4 of 8 symptoms: change in appetite, change in sleep pattern, increased fatigue, impaired concentration, feelings of guilt or worthlessness, loss of interest in usual activities, psychomotor agitation or retardation, or suicidal tendencies. Treatment of obsessive-compulsive disorder (OCD). Treatment of panic disorder, premenstrual disorder, bulimia.

ADMINISTRATION

ORAL:

- Give w/food or milk if GI distress occurs.

INDICATIONS / ROUTES / DOSAGE

Note: Use lower or less frequent doses in those w/renal, hepatic impairment, elderly, those w/concurrent disease or on multiple medications.

Depression, OCD:
Oral: Adults: Initially, 20 mg each morning. If therapeutic improvement does not occur after 2 wks, gradually increase dose to maximum 80 mg/day in 2 equally divided doses in morning, noon. ***Elderly:*** Initially, 10 mg/day. May increase by 10–20 mg q2wks. Avoid administration at night.

Bulimia:
Oral: Adults: 60 mg once daily in morning.

CONTRAINDICATIONS

Within 14 days of MAO inhibitor ingestion.

CAUTIONS

Impaired renal or hepatic function.

INTERACTIONS

DRUG: ***Alcohol, CNS depressants*** antagonize CNS depressant effect. May displace ***highly protein-bound medications*** from protein-binding sites (e.g., oral anticoagulants). ***MAO inhibitors*** may produce serotonin syndrome. May increase ***phenytoin*** concentration, toxicity. **HERBAL:** St. John's wort may have additive effect. **FOOD:** None significant. **ALTERED LAB VALUES:** None significant.

SIDE EFFECTS

FREQUENT (>10%): Headache, asthenia (loss of strength), inability to sleep, anxiety, nervousness, drowsiness, nausea, diarrhea, decreased appetite. **OCCASIONAL (2–10%):** Dizziness, tremor, fatigue, vomiting, constipation, dry mouth, abdominal pain, nasal congestion, increased sweating. **RARE (<2%):** Flushed skin, lightheadedness, decreased ability to concentrate.

ADVERSE REACTIONS / TOXIC EFFECTS

Overdosage may produce seizures, nausea, vomiting, excessive agitation, restlessness.

PATIENT CONSIDERATIONS

BASELINE ASSESSMENT

For those on long-term therapy, liver/renal function tests, blood counts should be performed periodically.

INTERVENTION/EVALUATION

Supervise suicidal risk pt closely during early therapy (as energy level improves, suicide potential increases). Assess appearance, behavior, speech pattern, level of interest, mood. Assist w/ambulation if dizziness occurs. Monitor stool frequency and consistency. Assess skin for appearance of rash.

PATIENT/FAMILY TEACHING

Maximum therapeutic response may require 4 or more wks of therapy. Dry mouth may be relieved by sugarless gum, sips of tepid water. Report visual disturbances. Do not abruptly discontinue medication. Avoid tasks that require alertness, motor skills until response to drug is established. Avoid alcohol.

---

fluoxymesterone

floo-ox-ih-**mes**-teh-rone
(Android-F, Halotestin)

FIXED-COMBINATION(S)
W/ethinyl estradiol, an estrogen **(Halodrin)**

CANADIAN AVAILABILITY
Halotestin

PREGNANCY CATEGORY X

CLASSIFICATION

Androgen

AVAILABILITY (Rx)

Tablets: 2 mg, 5 mg, 10 mg

PHARMACOKINETICS

Metabolism: Metabolized in liver. **Excretion:** Primarily excreted in urine. **Half-life:** 9.2 hrs.

ACTION/*THERAPEUTIC EFFECT*

Suppresses gonadotropin-releasing hormone, LH, and FSH. *Stimulates spermatogenesis, development of male secondary sex characteristics, sexual maturation at puberty.* Stimulates production of RBCs.

USES/*UNLABELED*

Treatment of delayed puberty; testicular failure due to cryptorchidism, bilateral orchism, orchitis, vanishing testis syndrome, or orchidectomy; hypogonadotropic hypogonadism due to pituitary/hypothalamic injury (tumors, trauma, or radiation), idiopathic gonadotropin or LHRH deficiency. Palliative therapy in women 1–5 years past menopause w/advancing, inoperable metastatic breast cancer or premenopausal women who have benefited from oophorectomy and have a hormone-responsive tumor. Prevention of postpartum breast pain and engorgement. In combination w/estrogens for management of moderate to severe vasomotor symptoms associated w/menopause when estrogens alone are not effective. *Treatment of anemia.*

ADMINISTRATION

ORAL:

- May give w/o regard to food.

INDICATIONS/ROUTES/DOSAGE

Males (hypogonadism):
Oral: Adults: 5–20 mg/day.

Males (delayed puberty):
Oral: Adults: 2.5–20 mg/day for 4–6 mos.

Females (inoperable breast cancer):
Oral: Adults: 10–40 mg/day in divided doses for 1–3 mos.

Females (prevent postpartum breast pain/engorgement):
Oral: Adults: Initially, 2.5 mg shortly after delivery, then 5–10 mg/day in divided doses for 4–5 days.

CONTRAINDICATIONS

Hypersensitivity to drug or components of preparation, serious cardiac, renal, or hepatic dysfunction. Do not use for men w/carcinomas of the breast or prostate.

CAUTIONS

Decreased renal or liver function, benign prostate hypertrophy, hypercalcemia (may be aggravated in pts w/metastatic breast cancer), history of myocardial infarction, diabetes mellitus.

INTERACTIONS

DRUG: May increase effect of ***oral anticoagulants. Hepatotoxic medications*** may increase hepatotoxicity. **HERBAL:** None known. **FOOD:** None significant. **ALTERED LAB VALUES:** May increase alkaline phosphatase, SGOT (AST), bilirubin, calcium, potassium, sodium, Hgb, Hct, LDL. May decrease HDL.

SIDE EFFECTS

FREQUENT: *Females:* Amenorrhea, virilism (e.g., acne, decreased breast size, enlarged clitoris, male pattern baldness), deepening voice. *Males:* UTI, breast soreness, gynecomastia, priapism, virilism (e.g., acne, early pubic hair growth). **OCCASIONAL:** Edema, nausea, vomiting, mild acne, diarrhea, stomach pain. *Males*: Impotence, testicular atrophy. **RARE:** Hepatic necrosis, leukopenia.

ADVERSE REACTIONS/TOXIC EFFECTS

Peliosis hepatitis (liver, spleen replaced w/blood-filled cysts), hepatic neoplasms, and hepatocellular carcinoma have been associated w/prolonged high dosage.

PATIENT CONSIDERATIONS

Baseline Assessment

Question for hypersensitivity to drug or components (sensitivity to aspirin may indicate tartrazine sensitivity). Establish baseline weight, B/P, Hgb, Hct. Check liver function test results, electrolytes, and cholesterol if ordered. Wrist x-rays may be ordered to determine bone maturation in children.

Intervention/Evaluation

Weigh daily and report weekly gain of more than 5 lbs; evaluate for edema. Monitor I&O. Check B/P at least 2 times/day. Assess electrolytes, cholesterol, Hgb, Hct (periodically for high dosage), liver function test results. W/breast cancer or immobility, check for hypercalcemia (lethargy, muscle weakness, confusion, irritability). Assure adequate intake of protein, calories. Be alert to signs of virilization. Monitor sleep patterns. Assess for hepatitis: nausea, yellowing of eyes and skin, dark urine, light stools.

Patient/Family Teaching

Regular visits to physician and monitoring tests are necessary.

Do not take any other medications w/o consulting physician. Teach diet high in protein, calories. Food may be tolerated better in small, frequent feedings. Weigh daily, report weekly gain of 5 lbs or more. Teach signs of jaundice; notify physician if these, nausea, vomiting, acne, ankle swelling occur.

Female
Promptly report menstrual irregularities, hoarseness, deepening of voice.

Male
Report frequent erections, difficulty urinating, gynecomastia.

fluphenazine decanoate

flew-**phen**-ah-zeen
(Prolixin)

fluphenazine enanthate

(Prolixin)

fluphenazine hydrochloride

(Prolixin, Permitil)

CANADIAN AVAILABILITY
Apo-Fluphenazine, Moditen

CLASSIFICATION

Antipsychotic

AVAILABILITY (Rx)

Tablets: 1 mg, 2.5 mg, 5 mg, 10 mg. **Elixir:** 2.5 mg/5 ml. **Oral Concentrate:** 5 mg/ml. **Injection:** 2.5 mg/ml.

PHARMACOKINETICS

Absorption: Variably absorbed after oral administration; well absorbed after IM administration. **Metabolism:** Metabolized in liver to active metabolites. **Excretion:** Primarily excreted in urine. **Half-life:** 33 hrs.

ACTION/*THERAPEUTIC EFFECT*

Antagonizes dopamine neurotransmission at synapses by blocking postsynaptic dopaminergic receptors in brain, *decreasing psychotic behavior.* Produces weak anticholinergic, sedative, antiemetic effects, strong extrapyramidal activity.

USES/*UNLABELED*

Management of psychotic disturbances (schizophrenia, delusions, hallucinations). *Treatment of neurogenic pain (adjunct to tricyclic antidepressants).*

STORAGE/HANDLING

Store oral and parenteral form at room temperature. Yellow discoloration of solution does not affect potency, but discard if markedly discolored or if precipitate forms.

ADMINISTRATION

ORAL:

- Mix oral concentrate w/water, carbonated orange or lemon-lime drink, milk, vegetable, pineapple, apricot, prune, orange, tomato, grapefruit juice.
- Do not mix oral concentrate w/caffeine (coffee, cola), tea, apple juice because of physical incompatibility.

IM:

- **Note:** Pt must remain recumbent for 30–60 min in head-low position w/legs raised, to minimize hypotensive effect.

- Use a dry 21 gauge needle, syringe for administering fluphenazine decanoate or enanthate (wet needle and syringe turn solution cloudy).
- Inject slow, deep IM into upper outer quadrant of gluteus maximus. If irritation occurs, further injections may be diluted w/0.9% NaCl or 2% procaine hydrochloride.
- Massage IM injection site to reduce discomfort.

INDICATIONS/ROUTES/DOSAGE

Psychotic disorders:
Oral: Adults: Initially, 0.5–10 mg/day fluphenazine HCl in divided doses q6–8h. Increase gradually until therapeutic response is achieved (usually under 20 mg daily); decrease gradually to maintenance level (1–5 mg/day). ***Elderly:*** Initially, 1–2.5 mg/day.

IM: Adults: Initially, 1.25 mg, followed by 2.5–10 mg/day in divided doses q6–8h.

Chronic schizophrenic disorder:
IM: Adults: Initially, 12.5–25 mg of fluphenazine decanoate q1–6 wks, or 25 mg fluphenazine enanthate q2wks.

Usual elderly dosage (nonpsychotic):
Oral: Initially, 1–2.5 mg/day. May increase by 1–2.5 mg/day q4–7 days. ***Maximum:*** 20 mg/day.

CONTRAINDICATIONS

Severe CNS depression, comatose states, severe cardiovascular disease, bone marrow depression, subcortical brain damage.

CAUTIONS

Impaired respiratory/hepatic/renal/cardiac function, alcohol withdrawal, history of seizures, urinary retention, glaucoma, prostatic hypertrophy, hypocalcemia (increased susceptibility to dystonias).

INTERACTIONS

DRUG: ***Alcohol, CNS depressants*** may increase CNS, respiratory depression, hypotensive effects. ***Tricyclic antidepressants, MAO inhibitors*** may increase sedative, anticholinergic effects. ***Antithyroid agents*** may increase risk of agranulocytosis. Extrapyramidal symptoms (EPS) may increase ***w/EPS-producing medications. Hypotensives*** may increase hypotension. May decrease ***levodopa*** effects. ***Lithium*** may decrease absorption, produce adverse neurologic effects. **HERBAL:** None known. **FOOD:** None significant. **ALTERED LAB VALUES:** May produce false-positive pregnancy test, PKU. EKG changes may occur, including Q and T wave disturbances.

SIDE EFFECTS

FREQUENT: Hypotension, dizziness, and fainting occur frequently after first injection, occasionally after subsequent injections, and rarely w/oral dosage. **OCCASIONAL:** Drowsiness during early therapy, dry mouth, blurred vision, lethargy, constipation or diarrhea, nasal congestion, peripheral edema, urinary retention. **RARE:** Ocular changes, skin pigmentation (those on high doses for prolonged periods).

ADVERSE REACTIONS/TOXIC EFFECTS

Extrapyramidal symptoms appear dose related (particularly high dosage), divided into 3 categories: akathisia (inability to sit still, tapping of feet, urge to move around); parkinsonian symptoms (mask-like face, tremors, shuffling gait, hypersalivation); and acute dystonias: torticollis (neck muscle spasm), opisthotonos (rigidity of back muscles), and oculogyric crisis (rolling back of eyes). Dystonic reaction may also produce profuse sweating, pallor. Tardive dyskinesia (protrusion of tongue, puffing of cheeks, chewing/puckering of the mouth) occurs rarely (may be irreversible). Abrupt withdrawal after long-term therapy may precipitate nausea, vomiting, gastritis, dizziness, tremors. Blood dyscrasias, particularly agranulocytosis, mild leukopenia (sore mouth/gums/throat) may occur. May lower seizure threshold.

PATIENT CONSIDERATIONS

Baseline Assessment

Avoid skin contact w/solution (contact dermatitis). Assess behavior, appearance, emotional status, response to environment, speech pattern, thought content.

Intervention/Evaluation

Monitor B/P for hypotension. Assess for extrapyramidal symptoms. Monitor WBC, differential count for blood dyscrasias. Monitor for fine tongue movement (may be early sign of tardive dyskinesia). Supervise suicidal risk pt closely during early therapy (as depression lessens, energy level improves, increasing suicide potential). Assess for therapeutic response (interest in surroundings, improvement in self-care, increased ability to concentrate, relaxed facial expression).

Patient/Family Teaching

Full therapeutic effect may take up to 6 wks. Urine may darken. Do not abruptly withdraw from long-term drug therapy. Report visual disturbances. Sugarless gum, sips of tepid water may relieve dry mouth. Drowsiness generally subsides during continued therapy. Avoid tasks that require alertness, motor skills until response to drug is established. Avoid alcohol.

flurandrenolide

(Cordran)

See Classification section under: Corticosteroids: topical

flurazepam hydrochloride

(Dalmane)

CANADIAN AVAILABILITY

Apo-Flurazepam, Dalmane

PREGNANCY CATEGORY X

CLASSIFICATION

Sedative-hypnotic **(Schedule IV)**

AVAILABILITY (Rx)

Capsules: 15 mg, 30 mg

PHARMACODYNAMICS

	ONSET	PEAK	DURATION
Oral	15–45 min	—	7–8 hrs

PHARMACOKINETICS

Absorption: Well absorbed from GI tract. Crosses blood-brain barrier. Widely distributed. **Metabo-**

lism: Metabolized in liver to active metabolite. **Excretion:** Primarily excreted in urine. **Half-life:** 2.3 hrs; metabolite: 40–114 hrs.

ACTION/*THERAPEUTIC EFFECT*

Enhances action of inhibitory neurotransmitter gamma-aminobutyric acid (GABA), *producing hypnotic effect due to CNS depression.*

USES

Short-term treatment of insomnia (up to 4 wks). Reduces sleep-induction time, number of nocturnal awakenings; increases length of sleep.

ADMINISTRATION

ORAL:

- Give w/o regard to meals.
- Capsules may be emptied and mixed w/food.

INDICATIONS/ROUTES/DOSAGE

Insomnia:

Oral: Adults: 15–30 mg at bedtime. ***Elderly/debilitated/liver disease/low serum albumin:*** 15 mg at bedtime.

CONTRAINDICATIONS

Acute narrow-angle glaucoma, acute alcohol intoxication.

CAUTIONS

Impaired renal/hepatic function.

INTERACTIONS

DRUG: *Alcohol, CNS depressants* may increase CNS depressant effect. **HERBAL:** Kava kava, valerian may have additive effect. **FOOD:** None significant. **ALTERED LAB VALUES:** None significant.

SIDE EFFECTS

FREQUENT: Drowsiness, dizziness, ataxia, sedation. Morning drowsiness may occur initially. **OCCASIONAL:** Dizziness, GI disturbances, nervousness, blurred vision, dry mouth, headache, confusion, skin rash, irritability, slurred speech. **RARE:** Paradoxical CNS excitement/restlessness (particularly noted in elderly/debilitated).

ADVERSE REACTIONS/TOXIC EFFECTS

Abrupt or too rapid withdrawal may result in pronounced restlessness and irritability, insomnia, hand tremors, abdominal/muscle cramps, sweating, vomiting, seizures. Overdosage results in somnolence, confusion, diminished reflexes, coma.

PATIENT CONSIDERATIONS

BASELINE ASSESSMENT

Assess B/P, pulse, respirations immediately before administration. Raise bed rails. Provide environment conducive to sleep (back rub, quiet environment, low lighting).

INTERVENTION/EVALUATION

Assist w/ambulation. Assess for paradoxical reaction, particularly during early therapy. Evaluate for therapeutic response: decrease in number of nocturnal awakenings, increase in length of sleep duration.

PATIENT/FAMILY TEACHING

Smoking reduces drug effectiveness. Do not abruptly withdraw medication after long-term use. Avoid alcohol. May have disturbed sleep 1–2 nights after discontinuing. Use caution driving, performing other tasks requiring alertness. Notify physician if pregnant or planning to become pregnant.

flurbiprofen

fleur-bih-**pro**-fen
(Ansaid)

flurbiprofen sodium

(Ocufen)

CANADIAN AVAILABILITY
Ansaid, Froben, Ocufen

PREGNANCY CATEGORY B
(D if used in third trimester or near delivery)
Ophthalmic: Pregnancy Category C.

CLASSIFICATION

Nonsteroidal anti-inflammatory

AVAILABILITY (Rx)

Tablets: 50 mg, 100 mg. **Ophthalmic Solution:** 0.03%.

PHARMACOKINETICS

Absorption: Well absorbed from GI tract, penetrates cornea after ophthalmic administration (may be systemically absorbed). Widely distributed. **Metabolism:** Metabolized in liver. **Excretion:** Primarily excreted in urine. **Half-life:** 3–4 hrs.

ACTION/*THERAPEUTIC EFFECT*

Produces analgesic and anti-inflammatory effect by inhibiting prostaglandin synthesis, *reducing inflammatory response and intensity of pain stimulus reaching sensory nerve endings.* Prevents, reduces miosis by relaxing iris sphincter.

USES

Symptomatic treatment of acute and/or chronic rheumatoid arthritis, osteoarthritis; inhibits intraoperative miosis.

ADMINISTRATION

ORAL:
- Do not crush or break enteric-coated form.
- May give w/food, milk, or antacids if GI distress occurs.

OPHTHALMIC:
- Place finger on lower eyelid and pull out until pocket is formed between eye and lower lid.
- Hold dropper above pocket and place prescribed number of drops into pocket. Close eye gently. Apply digital pressure to lacrimal sac for 1–2 min (minimizes drainage into nose and throat, reducing risk of systemic effects). Remove excess solution w/tissue.

INDICATIONS/ROUTES/DOSAGE

Rheumatoid arthritis, osteoarthritis:
Oral: Adults, elderly: 200–300 mg/day in 2–4 divided doses. Do not give >100 mg/dose or 300 mg/day.

Usual ophthalmic dosage:
Ophthalmic: Adults, elderly: Apply 2 drops into conjunctival sac 3, 2, and 1 hr before surgery or 2 drops q4h while pt is awake day before surgery.

CONTRAINDICATIONS

Active peptic ulcer, GI ulceration, chronic inflammation of GI tract, GI bleeding disorders, history of hypersensitivity to aspirin or NSAIDs.

CAUTIONS

Impaired renal/hepatic function, history of GI tract disease, predisposition to fluid retention, those wearing soft contact lenses, surgical pts w/bleeding tendencies.

INTERACTIONS

DRUG: May increase effects of ***oral***

anticoagulants, heparin, thrombolytics. May decrease effect of ***antihypertensives, diuretics. Salicylates, aspirin*** may increase risk of GI side effects, bleeding. ***Bone marrow depressants*** may increase risk of hematologic reactions. May increase concentration, toxicity of ***lithium.*** May increase ***methotrexate*** toxicity. ***Probenecid*** may increase concentration. ***Ophthalmic:*** May decrease effect of ***acetylcholine, carbachol.*** May decrease antiglaucoma effect of ***epinephrine, other antiglaucoma medications.*** **HERBAL:** Feverfew, ginkgo may increase risk of bleeding. **FOOD:** None significant. **ALTERED LAB VALUES:** May increase serum transaminase, alkaline phosphatase, LDH, bleeding time.

SIDE EFFECTS

FREQUENT: *Oral (3–9%):* Headache, abdominal pain, diarrhea, indigestion, nausea, fluid retention. *Ophthalmic:* Burning, stinging on instillation, keratitis, elevated intraocular pressure. OCCASIONAL: *Oral (1–3%):* GI bleeding, blurred vision, palpitations, flushed skin, dizziness, drowsiness, nervousness, insomnia, unusual weakness, constipation, decreased appetite, vomiting. RARE: *Oral (<1%):* Cardiac arrhythmias, increased blood pressure, confusion, hypersensitivity reaction, angioedema, impaired renal function.

ADVERSE REACTIONS/TOXIC EFFECTS

Overdosage may result in acute renal failure. In those treated chronically, peptic ulcer, GI bleeding, gastritis, severe hepatic reaction (jaundice), nephrotoxicity (hematuria, dysuria, proteinuria), severe hypersensitivity reaction (bronchospasm, angiofacial edema) occur rarely.

PATIENT CONSIDERATIONS

BASELINE ASSESSMENT

Anti-inflammatory
Assess onset, type, location, and duration of pain or inflammation. Inspect appearance of affected joints for immobility, deformities, and skin condition.

INTERVENTION/EVALUATION

Monitor for headache, dyspepsia, dizziness. Monitor pattern of daily bowel activity and stool consistency. Evaluate for therapeutic response: relief of pain, stiffness, swelling, increase in joint mobility, reduced joint tenderness, improved grip strength.

PATIENT/FAMILY TEACHING

Swallow tablet whole; do not crush or chew. Avoid aspirin, alcohol during therapy (increases risk of GI bleeding). If GI upset occurs, take w/food, milk. Report GI distress, visual disturbances, rash, edema, headache.

Ophthalmic
Eye burning may occur w/instillation.

flutamide

flew-tah-myd
(Eulexin)

CANADIAN AVAILABILITY
Euflex, Novo-Flutamide

CLASSIFICATION

Antineoplastic

AVAILABILITY (Rx)

Capsules: 125 mg

PHARMACOKINETICS

Absorption: Completely absorbed from GI tract. **Metabolism:** Metabolized in liver to active metabolite. **Excretion:** Primarily excreted in urine. **Half-life:** 6 hrs (increase in elderly).

ACTION/ *THERAPEUTIC EFFECT*

Inhibits androgen uptake and/or binding of androgen in tissues. Interferes w/testosterone at cellular level (complements leuprolide, *suppressing testicular androgen production* by inhibiting LH secretion).

USES

Treatment of metastatic carcinoma of prostate (in combination w/LHRH analogues—i.e., leuprolide). Management of locally confined stage B_2-C and stage D_2.

INDICATIONS/ROUTES/DOSAGE

Prostatic carcinoma:
Oral: Adults, elderly: 250 mg q8h.

CONTRAINDICATIONS

None significant.

CAUTIONS

None significant.

INTERACTIONS

DRUG: None significant. **HERBAL:** None known. **FOOD:** None significant. **ALTERED LAB VALUES:** May increase estradiol, testosterone, SGOT (AST), SGPT (ALT), bilirubin, creatinine.

SIDE EFFECTS

FREQUENT: Hot flashes, loss of libido, impotence, diarrhea, nausea/vomiting, gynecomastia. **OCCASIONAL:** Rash, anorexia. **RARE:** Photosensitivity.

ADVERSE REACTIONS/TOXIC EFFECTS

Hepatitis, hypertension may be noted.

PATIENT CONSIDERATIONS

INTERVENTION/EVALUATION

Monitor B/P periodically and hepatic function tests in long-term therapy. Check for diarrhea, nausea, and vomiting.

PATIENT/FAMILY TEACHING

Do not stop taking medication (both drugs must be continued). Explain side effects and action on carcinoma. Contact physician if nausea/vomiting continues at home.

fluticasone propionate

flew-tih-**cah**-sewn
(Flonase, Cutivate, Flovent)

CANADIAN AVAILABILITY
Flonase, Flovent

PREGNANCY CATEGORY C

CLASSIFICATION

Corticosteroid

AVAILABILITY (Rx)

Cream: 0.05%. **Ointment:** 0.005%. **Intranasal:** 0.05%. **Inhalation:** 44 mcg/actuation, 110 mcg/actuation, 220 mcg/actuation. **Powder for Inhalation:** 50 mcg, 100 mcg, 250 mcg.

PHARMACOKINETICS

Inhalation/intranasal: **Metabolism:** Undergoes extensive first-pass metabolism in liver. **Excretion:** Excreted in urine. **Half-life:** 3–7.8 hrs. ***Topical:*** **Absorption:** Amount absorbed dependent on drug, area, skin condition (absorption increased w/elevated skin temperature, hydration, inflamed/denuded skin).

ACTION/*THERAPEUTIC EFFECT*

Nasal: Inhibits early activation of inflammatory cells, release of inflammatory mediators, generally on late-phase allergic reactions, *decreasing response to seasonal and perennial rhinitis.* ***Topical:*** Stimulates protein synthesis of inhibitory enzymes responsible for anti-inflammatory effects. ***Inhalation:*** Inhibits inflammatory cascade reducing airway hyper-responsiveness. *Decreases bronchial reactivity inhibiting early/late bronchoconstriction* occurring when exposed to inhaled allergens.

USES

Nasal: Relief of seasonal/perennial allergic rhinitis. ***Topical:*** Relief of inflammation/pruritus associated w/steroid-responsive disorders (e.g., contact dermatitis, eczema). ***Inhalation:*** Maintenance treatment of asthma for those requiring oral corticosteroid therapy for asthma. ***Powder:*** Maintenance asthma treatment in children 4 yrs and older.

ADMINISTRATION

INHALATION:

- Shake container well; exhale completely; holding mouthpiece 1 inch away from lips, inhale and hold breath as long as possible before exhaling; then exhale slowly.
- Wait 1 min between inhalations when multiple inhalations ordered (allows for deeper bronchial penetration).
- Rinse mouth w/water immediately after inhalation (prevents mouth/throat dryness).

INTRANASAL:

- Clear nasal passages before use (topical nasal decongestants may be needed 5–15 min before use).
- Tilt head slightly forward.
- Insert spray tip up in 1 nostril, pointing toward inflamed nasal turbinates, away from nasal septum. Pump medication into 1 nostril while holding other nostril closed and concurrently inspire through nose.
- Discard used nasal solution after 3 mos.

INDICATIONS/ROUTES/DOSAGE

Allergic rhinitis:
Intranasal: Adults, elderly: Initially, 200 mcg (2 sprays each nostril once daily or 1 spray each nostril q12h). ***Maintenance:*** 1 spray each nostril once daily. ***Maximum:*** 200 mcg/day. ***Children >4 yrs:*** Initially, 100 mcg (1 spray each nostril once daily). ***Maximum:*** 200 mcg/day.

Usual topical dosage:
Adults, elderly, children >3 mos: Apply sparingly to affected area 1–2 times/day.

Usual inhalation dosage (dry powder formulation):
Children (4–11 yrs): 50–100 mcg twice daily.

Previous treatment: bronchodilators:
Inhalation: Adults, elderly, children >12 yrs: Initially 88 mcg q12h. ***Maximum:*** 440 mcg/day.

Previous treatment: inhaled steroids:
Inhalation: Adults, elderly, children >12 yrs: Initially 88–220 mcg q12h. ***Maximum:*** 440 mcg q12h.

Previous treatment: oral steroids: *Inhalation: Adults, elderly, children >12 yrs:* Initially, 880 mcg q12h.

CONTRAINDICATIONS

Untreated localized infection of nasal mucosa, hypersensitivity of drug or component. ***Inhalation:*** Primary treatment of status asthmaticus or other acute asthma episodes.

CAUTIONS

Active or quiescent tuberculosis, untreated fungal, bacterial, or systemic viral infection of ocular herpes simplex.

INTERACTIONS

DRUG: None significant. **HERBAL:** None known. **FOOD:** None significant. **ALTERED LAB VALUES:** None significant.

SIDE EFFECTS

FREQUENT: ***Inhalation:*** Throat irritation, hoarseness, dry mouth, coughing, temporary wheezing, localized fungal infection in mouth, pharynx, larynx (particularly if mouth is not rinsed w/water after each administration). ***Intranasal:*** Mild nasopharyngeal irritation; nasal irritation, burning, stinging, dryness, rebound congestion, rhinorrhea, loss of sense of taste. **OCCASIONAL:** ***Intranasal:*** Nasal/pharyngeal candidiasis, headache. ***Inhalation:*** Oral candidiasis. ***Topical:*** Burning/itching of skin.

ADVERSE REACTIONS/TOXIC EFFECTS

None significant.

PATIENT CONSIDERATIONS

BASELINE ASSESSMENT

Question for hypersensitivity to any fluticasone. Establish baseline assessment of skin disorder, asthma, or rhinitis.

INTERVENTION/EVALUATION

In those receiving bronchodilators by inhalation concomitantly with inhalation of steroid therapy, advise pt to use bronchodilator several min before corticosteroid aerosol (enhances penetration of steroid into bronchial tree). Monitor rate, depth, rhythm, type of respiration; quality and rate of pulse. Assess lung sounds for rhonchi, wheezing, rales. Monitor arterial blood gases. Observe lips, fingernails for blue or dusky color in light-skinned pts; gray in dark-skinned pts. Observe for clavicular retractions, hand tremor. Evaluate for clinical improvement (quieter, slower respirations, relaxed facial expression, cessation of clavicular retractions).

Topical
Assess involved area for therapeutic response to irritation.

PATIENT/FAMILY TEACHING

Do not change dose schedule or stop taking drug; must taper off gradually under medical supervision.

Inhalation
Teach proper use of inhaler. Maintain careful mouth hygiene. Rinse mouth w/water immediately after inhalation (prevents mouth/throat dryness, fungal infection of mouth). Increase fluid intake (decreases lung secretion viscosity). Contact physician/nurse if sore throat or mouth occurs.

Intranasal
Teach proper use of nasal spray. Clear nasal passages prior to use.

Contact physician if no improvement in symptoms, sneezing or nasal irritation occur. Improvement seen in several days.

Topical
Rub thin film gently into affected area. Use only for prescribed area and no longer than ordered. Report adverse local reaction. Avoid contact w/eyes.

fluvastatin

flu-vah-**stah**-tin
(Lescol)

CANADIAN AVAILABILITY
Lescol

PREGNANCY CATEGORY X

CLASSIFICATION

Antihyperlipoproteinemic

AVAILABILITY (Rx)

Capsules: 20 mg, 40 mg

PHARMACOKINETICS

Absorption: Well absorbed from GI tract (unaffected by food). Does not cross blood-brain barrier. **Excretion:** Primarily eliminated in feces.

ACTION/*THERAPEUTIC EFFECT*

Inhibits HMG-CoA reductase, the enzyme that catalyzes the early step in cholesterol synthesis. *Decreases LDL cholesterol, VLDL, plasma triglycerides.* Increases HDL cholesterol concentration slightly.

USES

Adjunct to diet therapy to decrease elevated total and LDL cholesterol concentrations in those w/primary hypercholesterolemia (types IIa and IIb) and in those w/combined hypercholesterolemia, hypertriglyceridemia. Treatment of elevated triglycerides and apolipoprotein.

ADMINISTRATION

ORAL:
- May give w/o regard to food.

INDICATIONS/ROUTES/DOSAGE

Hyperlipoproteinemia:
Oral: Adults, elderly: Initially, 20 mg/day in the evening. May increase up to 40 mg/day. *Maintenance:* 20–40 mg/day in single or divided doses.

CONTRAINDICATIONS

Hypersensitivity to fluvastatin, active liver disease, unexplained increased serum transaminase.

CAUTIONS

Anticoagulant therapy, history of liver disease, substantial alcohol consumption. Withholding/discontinuing fluvastatin may be necessary when pt at risk for renal failure (secondary to rhabdomyolysis); major surgery, severe acute infection, trauma, hypotension, severe metabolic, endocrine, or electrolyte disorders, or uncontrolled seizures.

INTERACTIONS

DRUG: Increased risk of rhabdomyolysis, acute renal failure w/***cyclosporine, erythromycin, gemfibrozil, niacin, other immunosuppressants.*** **HERBAL:** None known. **FOOD:** None significant. **ALTERED LAB VALUES:** May increase creatinine kinase (CK), serum transaminase concentrations.

SIDE EFFECTS

FREQUENT (>10%): Headache, upper respiratory infection. **OCCASIONAL (2–10%):** Dizziness, inability to sleep, nausea, vomiting, diarrhea, constipation, flatulence, dyspepsia, muscle pain, back pain, rhinitis, cough, rash, flulike symptoms.

ADVERSE REACTIONS/TOXIC EFFECTS

Myositis, w/ or w/o increased CK, muscle weakness. May progress to frank rhabdomyolysis and renal impairment.

PATIENT CONSIDERATIONS

Baseline Assessment

Question for possibility of pregnancy before initiating therapy (Pregnancy Category X). Question history of hypersensitivity to fluvastatin. Assess baseline lab results: cholesterol, triglycerides, liver function tests.

Intervention/Evaluation

Evaluate food tolerance. Determine pattern of bowel activity. Check for headache, dizziness, blurred vision. Assess for rash, pruritus. Monitor cholesterol and triglyceride lab results for therapeutic response. Be alert for malaise, muscle cramping or weakness. Monitor temperature at least twice a day.

Patient/Family Teaching

Follow special diet (important part of treatment). Periodic lab tests are essential part of therapy. Do not take other medications w/o physician knowledge. Do not stop medication w/o consulting physician. Report promptly any muscle pain or weakness, especially if accompanied by fever or malaise. Do not drive or perform activities that require alert response if dizziness occurs.

fluvoxamine maleate

flew-**vox**-ah-meen
(Luvox)

CANADIAN AVAILABILITY
Luvox

PREGNANCY CATEGORY C

CLASSIFICATION

Antidepressant

AVAILABILITY (Rx)

Tablets: 50 mg, 100 mg

PHARMACOKINETICS

Absorption: Well absorbed following oral administration. **Metabolism:** Metabolized in liver (none of metabolites possess actions of parent drug). **Excretion:** Primarily excreted in urine. **Half-life:** 13–15 hrs.

ACTION/*THERAPEUTIC EFFECT*

Selectively inhibits serotonin neuronal uptake in CNS, *producing antidepressant effect.*

USES/*UNLABELED*

Treatment of obsessive-compulsive disorder (OCD). *Treatment of depression.*

ADMINISTRATION

ORAL:

- May give w/o regard to food.

INDICATIONS/ROUTES/DOSAGE

Note: Use lower or less frequent dosing in impaired hepatic function, elderly.

Obsessive-compulsive disorder: *Oral: Adults:* 50 mg at bedtime, increased by 50 mg q4–7days. Doses >100 mg/day in 2 divided doses. *Maximum:* 300 mg/day.

Children 8–17 yrs: 25 mg at bedtime, increased by 25 mg q4–7 days. Doses >50 mg/day in 2 divided doses. *Maximum:* 200 mg/day. .

CONTRAINDICATIONS

Within 14 days of MAO inhibitor ingestion, concurrent astemizole or terfenadine therapy.

CAUTIONS

Impaired renal or hepatic function, elderly.

INTERACTIONS

DRUG: *MAO inhibitors* may produce serious reactions (hyperthermia, rigidity, myoclonus). *Tryptophan, lithium* may enhance serotonergic effects. *Tricyclic antidepressants* may increase concentration. Fluvoxamine may increase concentration/toxicity of *astemizole, benzodiazepines, carbamazepine, clozapine, terfenadine, theophylline.* May increase effects of *warfarin.* HERBAL: St. John's wort may have additive effect. FOOD: None significant. ALTERED LAB VALUES: None significant.

SIDE EFFECTS

FREQUENT (>10%): Nausea (40%), diarrhea, dyspepsia, dry mouth, constipation. OCCASIONAL (2–10%): Vomiting, decreased appetite, upper respiratory infection, increased sweating, altered taste, abnormal ejaculation. RARE (<2%): Cough, dyspnea, bronchitis, arthralgia.

ADVERSE REACTIONS/TOXIC EFFECTS

Overdosage may produce seizures, nausea, vomiting, excessive agitation, restlessness.

PATIENT CONSIDERATIONS

BASELINE ASSESSMENT

For those on long-term therapy, liver/renal function tests, blood counts should be performed periodically.

INTERVENTION/EVALUATION

Supervise suicidal risk pt closely during early therapy (as energy level improves, suicide potential increases). Assess appearance, behavior, speech pattern, level of interest, mood. Assist w/ambulation if dizziness occurs. Monitor stool frequency and consistency. Assess skin for appearance of rash.

PATIENT/FAMILY TEACHING

Change positions slowly to avoid hypotensive effect. Maximum therapeutic response may require 4 or more wks of therapy. Photosensitivity to sun may occur. Dry mouth may be relieved by sugarless gum, sips of tepid water. Report visual disturbances. Do not abruptly discontinue medication. Avoid tasks that require alertness, motor skills until response to drug is established. Avoid alcohol.

---

folic acid (vitamin B_9)

foe-lick
(Folvite)

sodium folate

(Folvite—parenteral)

CANADIAN AVAILABILITY
Apo-Folic

PREGNANCY CATEGORY C

CLASSIFICATION

Coenzyme

AVAILABILITY (Rx)

Tablets: 0.4 mg, 0.8 mg (OTC), 1 mg (Rx). **Injection (Rx):** 5 mg/ml.

PHARMACOKINETICS

Absorption: Almost completely absorbed from GI tract (upper duodenum). **Metabolism:** Metabolized in liver, plasma to active form. **Excretion:** Excreted in urine. Removed by hemodialysis.

ACTION/*THERAPEUTIC EFFECT*

Stimulates production of red and white blood cells and platelets, *essential for nucleoprotein synthesis, maintenance of normal erythropoiesis.*

USES/*UNLABELED*

Treatment of megaloblastic, macrocytic anemia associated w/pregnancy, infancy, childhood, inadequate dietary intake. *Decreases risk of colon cancer.*

ADMINISTRATION

Note: Parenteral form used in acutely ill, parenteral or enteral alimentation, those unresponsive to oral route in GI malabsorption syndrome. Dosage >0.1 mg daily may conceal pernicious anemia.

INDICATIONS/ROUTES/DOSAGE

Deficiency:
Oral/IM/IV: Adults, children: Up to 1 mg/day.

Supplement:
Oral/IM/IV: Adults, elderly, children >4 yrs: 0.4 mg/day. *Children <4 yrs:* 0.3 mg/day. *Children <1 yr:* 0.1 mg/day. *Pregnancy:* 0.8 mg/day.

CONTRAINDICATIONS

Anemias (pernicious, aplastic, normocytic, refractory).

CAUTIONS

None significant.

INTERACTIONS

DRUG: May decrease effects of ***hydantoin anticonvulsants. Analgesics, anticonvulsants, carbamazepine, estrogens*** may increase folic acid requirements. ***Antacids, cholestyramine*** may decrease absorption. ***Methotrexate, triamterene, trimethoprim may antagonize effects.*** **HERBAL:** None known. **FOOD:** None significant. **ALTERED LAB VALUES:** May decrease vitamin B_{12} concentration.

SIDE EFFECTS

None significant.

ADVERSE REACTIONS/TOXIC EFFECTS

Allergic hypersensitivity occurs rarely w/parenteral form. Oral folic acid is nontoxic.

PATIENT CONSIDERATIONS

BASELINE ASSESSMENT

Pernicious anemia should be ruled out by Schilling test and vitamin B_{12} blood level before therapy is initiated (may produce irreversible neurologic damage). Resistance to treatment may occur if decreased hematopoiesis, alcoholism, antimetabolic drugs or deficiency of vitamin B_6, B_{12}, C, or E is evident.

INTERVENTION/EVALUATION

Assess for therapeutic improvement: improved sense of well-being, relief from iron deficiency symptoms (fatigue, shortness of breath, sore tongue, headache, pallor).

PATIENT/FAMILY TEACHING

Take only under medical supervision. Follow diet as ordered. Eat foods rich in folic acid including fruits, vegetables, and

organ meats. Report rash or hives promptly.

follitropin alpha

fole-eh-**trow**-pin al-pha
(Gonal-F)

CANADIAN AVAILABILITY
Gonal F

PREGNANCY CATEGORY X

CLASSIFICATION

Gonadotropin

AVAILABILITY (Rx)

Powder for Injection: 75 IU, 150 IU

PHARMACOKINETICS

Absorption: Absorption following SubQ is slower than elimination rate. Body weight decreases absorption rate. **Half-life:** 30 hrs.

ACTION/*THERAPEUTIC EFFECT*

A human follicle-stimulating hormone (FSH), stimulates ovarian follicular growth, *inducing ovulation.*

USES

For induction of ovulation and pregnancy in anovulatory infertile pts in whom the cause of infertility is functional and not caused by primary ovarian failure. Stimulates production of multiple follicles in ovulatory pts undergoing in vitro fertilization.

ADMINISTRATION

SubQ:

- Dissolve contents of ampoule(s) in 0.5–1 ml sterile water for injection.
- Concentration should not exceed 225 IU/0.5 ml.

INDICATIONS/DOSAGE/ROUTES

Ovulation induction:
SubQ: Adults: 75 IU day. Incremental dosage adjustment up to 37.5 IU/day may be considered after 14 days; similar adjustments, if needed, every 7 days thereafter.

Follicle stimulation:
SubQ: Adults: 150 IU/day until sufficient follicular development is attained, usually not to exceed 10 days.

CONTRAINDICATIONS

High levels of FSH indicating primary ovarian failure, uncontrolled thyroid or adrenal dysfunction, presence of any cause of infertility other than anovulation, tumor of ovary, breast, uterus, hypothalamus or pituitary gland, abnormal vaginal bleeding of undetermined origin, ovarian cysts or enlargement not due to polycystic ovary syndrome, hypersensitivity to drug, pregnancy.

CAUTIONS

None significant.

INTERACTIONS

DRUG: None significant. **HERBAL:** None known. **FOOD:** None significant. **ALTERED LAB VALUES:** None significant.

SIDE EFFECTS

FREQUENT (20%): Mild to moderate ovarian enlargement accompanied by abdominal distension/pain (generally regresses within 2–3 weeks). **OCCASIONAL (4–10%):** Flulike symptoms (fever, chills, musculoskeletal aches, joint pain, headache, malaise), GI disturbances (nausea, vomiting, diarrhea, abdominal cramps), breast tenderness, headache, dermatologic symptoms (dry skin, body rash, hair loss, hives). **RARE (1–4%):** Dizziness, dysmenorrhea, redness, pain at injection site, somnolence, dyspepsia, decreased appetite, palpitations, itching.

ADVERSE REACTIONS/TOXIC EFFECTS

Ovarian hyperstimulation syndrome (OHSS) is characterized by severe ovarian enlargement, abdominal pain/distension, nausea, vomiting, diarrhea, dyspnea, oliguria, and may be accompanied by ascites, pleural effusion, hypovolemia, electrolyte imbalance, hemoperitoneum and thromboembolic events. Syndrome occurs 7–10 days immediately following treatment. Hospitalization is necessary. Pulmonary complications may occur (atelectasis, acute respiratory distress syndrome, exacerbation of asthma).

PATIENT CONSIDERATIONS

BASELINE ASSESSMENT

Inform pts of duration of treatment and monitoring required, possible adverse reactions, risk of multiple births (12%). Rule out possibility of early pregnancy before initiating therapy (Pregnancy Category X). Exclude primary ovarian failure by determination of gonadotropin levels.

INTERVENTION/EVALUATION

Monitor ovarian response with serum estradiol and vaginal ultrasound periodically. Monitor hospitalized OHSS pts for fluid I&O, weight, Hct, serum and urinary electrolytes, urine specific gravity, BUN, creatinine, abdominal girth. Monitor follicular maturation by sonographic visualization of ovaries and endometrial lining or measuring serum estradiol levels. Clinical confirmation of ovulation indicated by rise in basal body temperature, increase in serum progesterone, menstruation following shift in basal body temperature.

fomivirsen sodium

foam-ih-**vir**-sen
(Vitravene)

PREGNANCY CATEGORY C

CLASSIFICATION

Antiviral

AVAILABILITY (Rx)

Injection (as sodium): 6.6 mg/ml

PHARMACOKINETICS

Absorption: Absorbed through vitreous humor; 40% bound to proteins. **Metabolism:** Cleared from vitreous by combination of tissue distribution and metabolism. Metabolized by enzymes yielding metabolites that are further catabolized to nucleotides. **Excretion:** Metabolism is primary route of elimination from the eye. Excreted as low molecular weight metabolites. A small amount is eliminated in urine and feces.

ACTION/*THERAPEUTIC EFFECT*

Inhibits protein synthesis, *preventing human cytomegalovirus (CMV) replication.*

USES

Treatment of cytomegalovirus (CMV) retinitis in those with acquired immunodeficiency syndrome (AIDS).

ADMINISTRATION

INTRAVITREAL (OPHTHALMIC) INJECTION:

- Apply topical or local anesthetics and antimicrobials using 30 gauge needle on a tuberculin syringe.
- Attach a 5 micron filter needle to injection syringe for solution withdrawal and withdraw 0.15 ml through filter needle.
- Remove filter needle and attach a 30 gauge needle to syringe containing fomivirsen sodium.
- Physician to deliver injection volume.
- Roll cotton tip applicator over injection site as needle is withdrawn to reduce loss of eye fluid.

INDICATIONS/ROUTES/DOSAGES

Cytomegalovirus (CMV) retinitis:

Intravitreal (ophthalmic) injection: Adults, elderly: 330 mcg (0.05 ml/eye) as a single intravitreal injection every other week for 2 doses. *Maintenance:* 330 mg (0.05 ml/eye) once every 4 weeks.

CONTRAINDICATIONS

History of hypersensitivity to medication, those who have recently (2–4 weeks) been treated with either IV or intravitreal cidofovir (increased risk of exaggerated ocular inflammation).

CAUTIONS

Impaired liver function.

INTERACTIONS

DRUG: None significant. **HERBAL:** None known. **FOOD:** None significant. **ALTERED LAB VALUES:** None significant.

SIDE EFFECTS

FREQUENT (25%): Ocular inflammation (uveitis), including iritis and vitritis. **OCCASIONAL (5–20%):** Abnormal vision, blurred vision, cataract, decreased visual acuity, eye pain, floaters, photophobia, abdominal pain, asthenia, diarrhea, fever, headache, nausea, rash, sinusitis, vomiting. **RARE (2–5%):** Conjunctivitis, decreased peripheral vision, eye irritation, application site reaction.

ADVERSE REACTIONS/TOXIC EFFECTS

Increased intraocular pressure (IOP), conjunctival bleeding, retinal detachment, retinal edema, retinal pigment changes, abnormal liver function occur occasionally.

PATIENT CONSIDERATIONS

Baseline Assessment

Periodic ophthalmologic follow-up examination should be performed. Monitor IOP at each visit; manage IOP elevations with medications to lower IOP.

Interventions/Evaluation

Monitor for lid reaction (redness, swelling, and discharge), conjunctivitis. Monitor for extraocular CMV infections (pneumonitis, colitis) or retinitis in untreated eye.

Patient/Family Teaching

Medication is not a cure for CMV retinitis and some pts may continue to experience progression of retinitis during and following treatment. Regular follow-up examination must be diligently followed. Medication treats only the eye(s) in which it has been injected and does not treat systemic CMV disease. Continue all other antiretroviral

medication presently being taken by HIV-infected pts.

foscarnet sodium

fos-**car**-net
(Foscavir)

PREGNANCY CATEGORY C

CLASSIFICATION

Antiviral

AVAILABILITY (Rx)

Injection: 24 mg/ml

PHARMACOKINETICS

Sequestered into bone, cartilage. **Excretion:** Primarily excreted unchanged in urine. Removed by hemodialysis. **Half-life:** 3.3–6.8 hrs (increased in decreased renal function).

ACTION/*THERAPEUTIC EFFECT*

Provides selective inhibition at binding site on virus-specific DNA polymerases and reverse transcriptases, *inhibiting replication of herpes virus.*

USES/*UNLABELED*

Treatment of CMV retinitis in pts w/AIDS; in combination w/ganciclovir for relapsed AIDS-related CMV retinitis; acyclovir-resistant herpes simplex virus (HSV) in immunocompromised pts. *Treatment of CMV disease, herpes simplex, varicella zoster.*

STORAGE/HANDLING

Store parenteral vials at room temperature. After dilution, stable for 24 hrs at room temperature.

ADMINISTRATION

IV:

- Do not give IV injection or rapid infusion (increases toxicity).
- Administer only by IV infusion over a minimum of 1 hr (no more than 1 mg/kg/min).
- To minimize toxicity and phlebitis, use central venous lines or veins w/adequate blood to permit rapid dilution and dissemination of foscarnet.
- Use IV infusion pump to prevent accidental overdose.
- The standard 24 mg/ml solution may be used w/o dilution when central venous catheter is used for infusion; 24 mg/ml solution *must* be diluted to 12 mg/ml when peripheral vein catheter is being used. Only 5% dextrose in water or normal saline solution for injection should be used for dilution.
- Because dosage is calculated on body weight, unneeded quantity may be removed before start of infusion to avoid overdosage. Aseptic technique must be used and solution administered within 24 hrs of first entry into sealed bottle.
- Do not use if solution is discolored or contains particulate material.

INDICATIONS/ROUTES/DOSAGE

CMV retinitis:
*IV: **Adults:*** Initially, 60 mg/kg q8h for 2–3 wks. ***Maintenance:*** 90 mg/kg/day; may increase up to 120 mg/kg/day if retinitis progresses.

Herpes simplex:
*IV: **Adults:*** 40 mg/kg q8–12h for 2–3 wks or until healed.

Dosage in renal impairment:
Dosage individualized according

to pt's creatinine clearance. Refer to dosing guide provided by manufacturer.

CONTRAINDICATIONS

Hypersensitivity to foscarnet sodium.

CAUTIONS

Neurologic or cardiac abnormalities, history of renal impairment, altered calcium or other electrolyte levels.

INTERACTIONS

DRUG: ***Nephrotoxic medications*** may increase risk of renal toxicity. ***Pentamidine (IV)*** may cause reversible hypocalcemia, hypomagnesemia, nephrotoxicity. ***Zidovudine*** may increase anemia. **HERBAL:** None known. **FOOD:** None significant. **ALTERED LAB VALUES:** May increase SGOT (AST), SGPT (ALT), alkaline phosphatase, bilirubin, creatinine. May decrease magnesium, potassium. May alter calcium, phosphate concentrations.

SIDE EFFECTS

FREQUENT: Fever (65%), nausea (47%), vomiting, diarrhea (30%), abnormal renal functioning, anemia (33%), bone marrow suppression, headache, seizures (10%), mineral and electrolyte imbalances. **OCCASIONAL:** Pain and inflammation at injection site, back and chest pain, hyper/hypotension, tachycardia, ulcerative stomatitis, rash or urticaria, taste perversions, insomnia, bronchospasm, pneumonia, urinary retention or polyuria. **RARE:** Ascites, hemoptysis, hypothermia, abnormal crying, earache, deafness, retinal detachment, photophobia, alopecia, abnormal gait, speech disorders, cholestatic hepatitis, cholecystitis.

ADVERSE REACTIONS/TOXIC EFFECTS

Renal impairment is a major toxicity that occurs to some extent in most pts. Seizures and mineral/electrolyte imbalances may be life threatening.

PATIENT CONSIDERATIONS

BASELINE ASSESSMENT

Question for hypersensitivity to foscarnet. Obtain baseline mineral and electrolyte levels, vital signs, CBC values, renal functioning.

INTERVENTION/EVALUATION

Monitor electrolyte results closely; assess for signs of electrolyte imbalance, especially hypocalcemia (perioral tingling, numbness/paresthesia of extremities) or hypokalemia (weakness, muscle cramps, numbness/tingling of extremities, irritability). Maintain accurate I&O, provide adequate hydration to assure diuresis before and during dosing, and monitor renal function tests to avoid or identify promptly renal impairment. Assess for tremors; provide safety measures for potential seizures. Evaluate vital signs at least 2 times/day. Provide small, attractive meals; avoid unattractive sights, smells, especially at mealtimes, and administer ordered antiemetics to support nutrition. Monitor number, consistency of stools. Assess for bleeding, anemia, or developing superinfections.

PATIENT/FAMILY TEACHING

Foscarnet is not a cure for CMV retinitis; regular ophthalmologic examinations are part of therapy. Dose modifications may be necessary, especially w/regard to controlling side effects; close medical supervision is essential. Infusion rate must be controlled to prevent overdosage (no more than 1 mg/kg/min). Important to report perioral tingling, numbness in the extremities, or paresthesias during or after infusion (may indicate electrolyte abnormalities). Risk of renal impairment can be reduced by sufficient fluid intake to assure diuresis before and during dosing. Tremors should be reported promptly because of potential for seizures.

fosfomycin

fos-foe-**my**-sin
(Monurol)

PREGNANCY CATEGORY B

CLASSIFICATION

Antibiotic: Broad-spectrum

AVAILABILITY (Rx)

Granules: 3 g

PHARMACODYNAMICS

	ONSET	PEAK	DURATION
Oral	2–3 days	—	—

PHARMACOKINETICS

Absorption: Rapidly absorbed following oral administration. Distributed to kidneys, bladder wall, prostate, seminal vesicles. **Excretion:** Excreted unchanged in urine and feces. **Half-life:** 4–8 hrs.

ACTION/*THERAPEUTIC EFFECT*

Inhibits bacterial cell wall synthesis, reduces adherence of bacteria to uroepithelial cells, *producing bactericidal activity in gram-positive and gram-negative aerobic microorganisms.*

USES

Treatment of uncomplicated urinary tract infection (acute cystitis) in women.

ADMINISTRATION

ORAL:

- Give w/o regard to meals.
- Do not give in dry form; to be mixed with water before ingestion.
- Pour entire contents of single-dose packet into 90–120 ml (3–4 oz) water; stir to dissolve.
- Give immediately after dissolved in water (do not use hot water).

INDICATIONS/ROUTES/DOSAGES

Urinary tract infection:
Oral: Adults ≥18 yrs, elderly: One packet (3 g) mixed in water as a single dose.

CONTRAINDICATIONS

History of hypersensitivity to medication.

CAUTIONS

None significant.

INTERACTIONS

DRUG: *Metoclopramide* lowers serum concentration and urinary excretion of fosfomycin. **HERBAL:** None known. **FOOD:** None significant. **ALTERED LAB VALUES:** May increase SGOT (AST), SGOT (ALT), alkaline phosphatase, bilirubin, eosinophil count; may decrease Hct, Hgb. May either increase or decrease WBC count, platelet count.

F

SIDE EFFECTS

OCCASIONAL (3–9%): Diarrhea, vaginitis, rhinitis, nausea, headache, back pain. RARE (1–2%): Dysmenorrhea, pharyngitis, abdominal pain, rash, dizziness, dyspepsia, asthenia.

ADVERSE REACTIONS/TOXIC EFFECTS

None significant.

PATIENT CONSIDERATIONS

Baseline Assessment

Question for hypersensitivity to fosfomycin. Do not use more than one single dose of medication to treat a single episode of acute cystitis.

Intervention/Evaluation

Monitor bowel activity and stool consistency. Provide symptomatic relief for nausea, headache. Monitor hematology reports.

Patient/Family Teaching

May be taken w/ or w/o food. Do not take in dry form; always mix fosfomycin with water before ingesting. Symptoms should improve within 2–3 days. If not improved, contact physician.

fosinopril

foh-**sin**-oh-prill
(Monopril)

CANADIAN AVAILABILITY
Monopril

PREGNANCY CATEGORY D

CLASSIFICATION

Angiotensin-converting enzyme (ACE) inhibitor

AVAILABILITY (Rx)

Tablets: 10 mg, 20 mg

PHARMACODYNAMICS

	ONSET	PEAK	DURATION
Oral	1 hr	2–6 hrs	24 hrs

PHARMACOKINETICS

Absorption: Slowly absorbed from GI tract. **Metabolism:** Metabolized in liver, GI mucosa to active metabolite. **Excretion:** Primarily excreted in urine. Minimal removal by hemodialysis. **Half-life:** 11.5 hrs.

ACTION/*THERAPEUTIC EFFECT*

Suppresses renin-angiotensin-aldosterone system (prevents conversion of angiotensin I to angiotensin II, a potent vasoconstrictor; may also inhibit angiotensin II at local vascular and renal sites). Decreases plasma angiotensin II, increases plasma renin activity, decreases aldosterone secretion. *Reduces peripheral arterial resistance, pulmonary capillary wedge pressure, improves cardiac output, exercise tolerance.*

USES/*UNLABELED*

Treatment of hypertension. Used alone or in combination w/other antihypertensives. Treatment of heart failure. *Treatment of renal crisis in scleroderma.*

ADMINISTRATION

ORAL:

- May give w/o regard to food.
- Tablets may be crushed.

INDICATIONS/ROUTES/DOSAGE

Hypertension (used alone):
Oral: Adults, elderly: Initially, 10 mg/day. ***Maintenance:*** 20–40 mg/day. ***Maximum:*** 80 mg/day.

Hypertension (w/diuretic):
Note: Discontinue diuretic 2–3

days before initiation of fosinopril therapy.

Oral: Adults, elderly: Initially, 10 mg/day titrated to pt's needs.

Heart failure:
Oral: Adults, elderly: Initially, 5–10 mg. *Maintenance:* 20–40 mg/day.

CONTRAINDICATIONS

History of angioedema w/previous treatment w/ACE inhibitors.

CAUTIONS

Renal impairment, those w/sodium depletion or on diuretic therapy, dialysis, hypovolemia, coronary or cerebrovascular insufficiency.

INTERACTIONS

DRUG: *Alcohol, diuretics, hypotensive agents* may increase effects. *NSAIDs* may decrease effect. *Potassium-sparing diuretics, potassium supplements* may cause hyperkalemia. May increase *lithium* concentration, toxicity. **HERBAL:** None known. **FOOD:** None significant. **ALTERED LAB VALUES:** May increase potassium, SGOT (AST), SGPT (ALT), alkaline phosphatase, bilirubin, BUN, creatinine. May decrease sodium. May cause positive ANA titer.

SIDE EFFECTS

FREQUENT (4–10%): Hypotension, dizziness, cough. **OCCASIONAL (1–4%):** Orthostatic hypotension, fatigue, vomiting, nausea, diarrhea, upper respiratory infection, chest pain. **RARE (<1%):** Palpitations, inability to sleep, confusion, abdominal pain, rash, constipation, dry mouth, photosensitivity reaction.

ADVERSE REACTIONS/TOXIC EFFECTS

Excessive hypotension ("first-dose syncope") may occur in pts w/CHF, severely salt/volume depleted. Angioedema (swelling of face/lips), hyperkalemia occur rarely. Agranulocytosis, neutropenia may be noted in those w/impaired renal function or collagen vascular disease (systemic lupus erythematosus, scleroderma). Nephrotic syndrome may be noted in those w/history of renal disease.

PATIENT CONSIDERATIONS

BASELINE ASSESSMENT

Obtain B/P immediately before each dose, in addition to regular monitoring (be alert to fluctuations). Renal function tests should be performed before therapy begins. In pts w/renal impairment, autoimmune disease, or taking drugs that affect leukocytes or immune response, CBC and differential count should be performed before therapy begins and q2wks for 3 mos, then periodically thereafter.

INTERVENTION/EVALUATION

If excessive reduction in B/P occurs, place pt in supine position w/legs elevated. Assist w/ambulation if dizziness occurs. Assess for urinary frequency. Auscultate lung sounds for rales, wheezing in those w/CHF. Monitor urinalysis for proteinuria. Monitor serum potassium levels in those on concurrent diuretic therapy. Monitor pattern of daily bowel activity and stool consistency.

PATIENT/FAMILY TEACHING

Report any sign of infection (sore throat, fever). Several weeks may be needed for full therapeutic effect of B/P reduction. Skipping doses or voluntarily discontinuing drug may pro-

duce severe, rebound hypertension. To reduce hypotensive effect, rise slowly from lying to sitting position and permit legs to dangle from bed momentarily before standing.

fosphenytoin

fos-**phen**-ih-twon
(Cerebyx)

CANADIAN AVAILABILITY
Cerebyx

PREGNANCY CATEGORY D

CLASSIFICATION

Anticonvulsant

AVAILABILITY (Rx)

Injection: 75 mg/ml (50 mg phenytoin sodium)

PHARMACOKINETICS

Absorption: Completely absorbed following IM administration. **Metabolism:** After IM or IV administration, rapidly/completely hydrolyzed to phenytoin. **Half-life:** Half-life for conversion to phenytoin: 8–15 min.

ACTION/*THERAPEUTIC EFFECT*

Stabilizes neuronal membranes, limits spread of seizure activity. Decreases sodium, calcium, ion influx in neurons. Decreases post-tetanic potentiation and repetitive afterdischarge. *Decreases seizure activity.*

USES

Acute treatment, control of generalized convulsive status epilepticus, prevention, treatment of seizures occurring during neurosurgery, short-term substitution of oral phenytoin.

STORAGE/HANDLING

Refrigerate. Do not store at room temperature >48 hrs. After dilution, solution stable for 8 hrs at room temperature or 24 hrs if refrigerated.

ADMINISTRATION

IV:

- Dilute in 5% dextrose or 0.9% NaCl to a concentration ranging from 1.5 to 25 mg PE/ml (PE: phenytoin equivalent).
- Administer at rate of ≤150 mg PE/min (decreases risk of hypotension).

INDICATIONS/ROUTES/DOSAGE

Note: 150 mg fosphenytoin yields 100 mg phenytoin. Dose, concentration solution, infusion rate of fosphenytoin expressed in terms of phenytoin equivalents (PE). Lower, less frequent dosing in elderly may be required. Not approved for pediatric use.

Status epilepticus:
IV: Adults: Loading dose: 15–20 mg PE/kg infused at rate of 100–150 mg PE/min.

Nonemergent seizures:
IV: Adults: Loading dose: 10–20 mg PE/kg. ***Maintenance:*** 4–6 mg PE/kg/day.

CONTRAINDICATIONS

Hypersensitivity to fosphenytoin, phenytoin, or any of its ingredients, severe bradycardia, SA block, second- or third-degree AV block, Adams-Stokes syndrome.

CAUTIONS

Porphyria, hypotension, severe myocardial insufficiency, renal/hepatic disease, hypoalbuminemia.

INTERACTIONS

DRUG: May decrease effect of *glucocorticoids. Alcohol, CNS depressants* may increase CNS depression. *Antacids* may decrease absorption. *Amiodarone, anticoagulants, cimetidine, disulfiram, fluoxetine, isoniazid, sulfonamides* may increase fosphenytoin concentration, effects, toxicity. *Fluconazole, ketoconazole, miconazole* may increase concentration. *Lidocaine, propranolol* may increase cardiac depressant effects. *Valproic acid* may increase concentration, decrease metabolism. May increase *xanthine* metabolism. **HERBAL:** None known. **FOOD:** None significant. **ALTERED LAB VALUES:** May increase alkaline phosphatase, GGT, glucose.

SIDE EFFECTS

FREQUENT: Dizziness, paresthesia, tinnitus, pruritus, headache, somnolence. **OCCASIONAL:** Morbilliform rash.

ADVERSE REACTIONS/TOXIC EFFECTS

A too high fosphenytoin blood concentration may produce ataxia (muscular incoordination), nystagmus (rhythmic oscillation of eyes), double vision, lethargy, slurred speech, nausea, vomiting, hypotension. As level increases, extreme lethargy to comatose states occur.

PATIENT CONSIDERATIONS

Baseline Assessment

Review history of seizure disorder (intensity, frequency, duration, level of consciousness). Initiate seizure precautions. Obtain vital signs, medication history (especially use of phenytoin or other anticonvulsants). Observe clinically.

Intervention/Evaluation

Measure cardiac function, EKG, determination of respiratory function, B/P during and immediately after infusion (10–20 min). Discontinue if skin rash appears. Interrupt or decrease rate if hypotension or arrhythmias are detected. Assess pt postinfusion (may feel dizzy, ataxic, or drowsy). Assess blood levels of fosphenytoin (2 hrs post IV infusion or 4 hrs post IM injection).

Patient/Family Teaching

Teach pts about their seizure condition and role in its management. If noncompliance is an issue in causing acute seizures, discuss reasons for noncompliance and address them.

furosemide

feur-**oh**-sah-mide
(Lasix)

CANADIAN AVAILABILITY
Apo-Furosemide, Lasix

PREGNANCY CATEGORY C

CLASSIFICATION

Diuretic: Loop

AVAILABILITY (Rx)

Tablets: 20 mg, 40 mg, 80 mg. **Oral Solution:** 10 mg/ml, 40 mg/5 ml. **Injection:** 10 mg/ml.

PHARMACODYNAMICS

	ONSET	PEAK	DURATION

Oral	30–60 min	1–2 hrs	6–8 hrs
IM	—	30 min	—
IV	5 min	20–60 min	2 hrs

PHARMACOKINETICS

Absorption: Well absorbed from GI tract. **Metabolism:** Partially metabolized in liver. **Excretion:** Primarily excreted in urine (in severe renal impairment, nonrenal clearance increases). **Half-life:** 30–90 min (increased in decreased renal, liver function and in neonates).

ACTION/*THERAPEUTIC EFFECT*

Enhances excretion of sodium, chloride, potassium by direct action at ascending limb of loop of Henle, *producing diuretic effect.*

USES/*UNLABELED*

Treatment of edema associated w/CHF, chronic renal failure including nephrotic syndrome, hepatic cirrhosis, acute pulmonary edema. Treats hypertension, either alone or in combination w/other antihypertensives. *Treatment of hypercalcemia.*

STORAGE/HANDLING

Solution appears clear, colorless. Discard yellow injections or discolored tablet.

ADMINISTRATION

ORAL:

- Give w/food to avoid GI upset, preferably w/breakfast (may prevent nocturia).

IM:

- Temporary pain at injection site may be noted.

IV:

- May give undiluted but is compatible w/5% dextrose in water, 0.9% sodium chloride, or lactated Ringer's solutions.
- Administer direct IV over 1–2 min, preferably through Y tube or 3-way stopcock.
- Do not exceed administration rate of 4 mg/min in those w/renal impairment.

INDICATIONS/ROUTES/DOSAGE

Edema:
Oral: Adults: 20–80 mg daily given as single dose in morning. May increase in 20–40 mg increments q6–8h. Give effective dose 1–2 times/day. ***Maximum:*** 600 mg.

IM/IV: Adults: 20–40 mg given as single injection. May increase in 20 mg increments no sooner than 2 hrs after previous dose. May give effective dose 1–2 times/day.

Acute pulmonary edema:
IV: Adults: 40 mg slow IV, given over 1–2 min. If satisfactory response is not reached in 1 hr, may increase to 80 mg slow IV, given over 1–2 min.

Hypertension:
Oral: Adults: Initially 40 mg 2 times/day based on pt response.

Usual elderly dosage:
Oral/IM/IV: Initially, 20 mg/day. May increase slowly to desired response.

Usual dosage for children:
Oral: 2 mg/kg given as single dose. May be increased in 1–2 mg/kg increments q6–8h. ***Maximum:*** 6 mg/kg/day.

IV/IM: 1 mg/kg given as single dose. May increase by 1 mg/kg no sooner than 2 hrs after previous dose. ***Maximum:*** 6 mg/kg/day.

CONTRAINDICATIONS

Anuria, hepatic coma, severe electrolyte depletion.

CAUTIONS

Acute MI, oliguria, hepatic cirrhosis, history of gout, diabetes, systemic lupus erythematosus, pancreatitis.

INTERACTIONS

DRUG: *Amphotericin, ototoxic, nephrotoxic agents* may increase toxicity. May decrease effect of ***anticoagulants, heparin. Hypokalemia-causing agents*** may increase risk of hypokalemia. May increase risk of ***lithium*** toxicity. ***Probenecid*** may increase concentrations. **HERBAL:** None known. **FOOD:** None significant. **ALTERED LAB VALUES:** May increase glucose, BUN, uric acid. May decrease calcium, chloride, magnesium, potassium, sodium.

SIDE EFFECTS

EXPECTED: Increase in urinary frequency/volume. **FREQUENT:** Nausea, gastric upset w/cramping, diarrhea, or constipation, electrolyte disturbances. **OCCASIONAL:** Dizziness, lightheadedness, headache, blurred vision, paresthesia, photosensitivity, rash, weakness, urinary frequency/bladder spasm, restlessness, diaphoresis. **RARE:** Flank pain, loin pain.

ADVERSE REACTIONS/TOXIC EFFECTS

Vigorous diuresis may lead to profound water loss and electrolyte depletion, resulting in hypokalemia, hyponatremia, dehydration. Sudden volume depletion may result in increased risk of thrombosis, circulatory collapse, sudden death. Acute hypotensive episodes may also occur, sometimes several days after beginning of therapy. Ototoxicity manifested as deafness, vertigo, tinnitus (ringing/roaring in ears) may occur, especially in those w/severe renal impairment. Can exacerbate diabetes mellitus, systemic lupus erythematosus, gout, pancreatitis. Blood dyscrasias have been reported.

PATIENT CONSIDERATIONS

BASELINE ASSESSMENT

Check vital signs, especially B/P for hypotension before administration. Assess baseline electrolytes, particularly check for low potassium. Assess edema, skin turgor, mucous membranes for hydration status. Assess muscle strength, mental status. Note skin temperature, moisture. Obtain baseline weight. Initiate I&O monitoring.

INTERVENTION/EVALUATION

Monitor B/P, vital signs, electrolytes, I&O, weight. Note extent of diuresis. Watch for changes from initial assessment (hypokalemia may result in changes in muscle strength, tremor, muscle cramps, change in mental status, cardiac arrhythmias). Hyponatremia may result in confusion, thirst, cold/clammy skin.

PATIENT/FAMILY TEACHING

Expect increased frequency and volume of urination. Report irregular heartbeat, signs of electrolyte imbalances (noted above), hearing abnormalities (such as sense of fullness in ears, ringing/roaring in ears). Eat foods high in potassium such as whole grains (cereals), legumes, meat, bananas, apricots, orange juice, potatoes (white, sweet), raisins. Avoid sun/sunlamps.

gabapentin

gah-bah-**pen**-tin
(Neurontin)

CANADIAN AVAILABILITY
Neurontin

PREGNANCY CATEGORY C

CLASSIFICATION

Anticonvulsant

AVAILABILITY (Rx)

Capsules: 100 mg, 300 mg, 400 mg
Tablets: 600 mg, 800 mg

PHARMACOKINETICS

Absorption: Well absorbed from GI tract (not affected by food). Widely distributed. Crosses blood-brain barrier. **Excretion:** Primarily excreted unchanged in urine. Removed by hemodialysis. **Half-life:** 5–7 hrs (increased in decreased renal function, elderly).

ACTION/*THERAPEUTIC EFFECT*

Exact mechanism unknown. May be due to increased gamma-aminobutyric acid (GABA) synthesis rate, increased GABA accumulation, or binding to as yet undefined receptor sites in brain tissue *to produce anticonvulsant activity.*

USES/*UNLABELED*

Adjunctive therapy in treatment of partial seizures and partial seizures w/secondary generalization in adults. *Neuropathic pain, psychiatric disorders, hot flashes, essential tremor, muscle cramps.*

ADMINISTRATION

ORAL:

- May be given w/o regard to meals; may give w/food to avoid or reduce GI upset.
- If treatment is discontinued or anticonvulsant therapy is added, do so gradually over at least 1 wk (reduces risk of loss of seizure control).

INDICATIONS/ROUTES/DOSAGE

Seizure control:
Note: Maximum time between doses should not exceed 12 hrs.
Oral: Adults, elderly: 900–1,800 mg/day given in divided doses q8h. May titrate to effective dose rapidly: ***Day 1:*** 300 mg (give at bedtime). ***Day 2:*** 300 mg q12h. ***Day 3:*** 300 mg q8h.

Renal function impairment:
Based on creatinine clearance:

CREATININE CLEARANCE	DOSAGE
>60 ml/min	400 mg q8h
30–60 ml/min	300 mg q12h
15–30 ml/min	300 mg daily
<15 ml/min	300 mg every other day
Hemodialysis	200–300 mg after each 4 hr hemodialysis

CONTRAINDICATIONS

None significant.

CAUTIONS

Renal impairment. Discontinue/add anticonvulsant therapy gradually (reduces loss of seizure control).

INTERACTIONS

DRUG: None significant. **HERBAL:** None known. **FOOD:** None significant. **ALTERED LAB VALUES:** May decrease WBCs.

SIDE EFFECTS

FREQUENT (>10%): Fatigue, somnolence, dizziness, ataxia. **OCCASIONAL (2–10%):** Increase in weight, dyspepsia, muscle pain, rhinitis, double vision, tremor, nystagmus (rolling eye movements), loss of memory. **RARE (<2%):** Back pain, peripheral edema, dry mouth, constipation, increased appetite, cough, altered thinking/coordination, itching, impotence.

ADVERSE REACTIONS/TOXIC EFFECTS

Abrupt withdrawal may increase seizure frequency. Overdosage may result in double vision, slurred speech, drowsiness, lethargy, diarrhea.

PATIENT CONSIDERATIONS

Baseline Assessment

Review history of seizure disorder (type, onset, intensity, frequency, duration, level of consciousness). Routine laboratory monitoring of blood serum levels unnecessary for safe use. Obtain vital signs, medication history.

Intervention/Evaluation

Provide safety measures as needed. Assess for seizure activity.

Patient/Family Teaching

Take gabapentin only as prescribed; do not abruptly stop taking drug because seizure frequency may be increased. Do not drive, operate machinery, or perform activities requiring mental acuity due to potential dizziness, somnolence. Avoid alcohol. Carry identification card/bracelet to note anticonvulsant therapy. Teach pt about his or her seizure condition and role in its management. If noncompliance is an issue in causing acute seizures, discuss reasons for noncompliance and address them.

gallium nitrate

gal-lee-um
(Ganite)

PREGNANCY CATEGORY C

G

CLASSIFICATION

Antihypercalcemic

AVAILABILITY (Rx)

Injection: 25 mg/ml

PHARMACOKINETICS

Excretion: Primarily excreted in urine. **Half-life:** 24 hrs.

ACTION/*THERAPEUTIC EFFECT*

Inhibits abnormal bone resorption, reduces flow of calcium from resorbing bone into blood, *decreasing calcium serum levels.*

USES

Treatment of hypercalcemia or malignancy that is inadequately managed by oral hydration alone. Use concomitantly w/saline (increases urine output) and diuretics (increases rate of calcium excretion).

STORAGE/HANDLING

Store undiluted vials at room temperature. After dilution, stable for 48 hrs at room temperature or up to 7 days refrigerated.

ADMINISTRATION

IV:

- Must dilute daily dose in 1,000 ml 0.9% NaCl or 5% dextrose.

INDICATIONS/ROUTES/DOSAGE

Hypercalcemia:

IV Infusion: Adults, elderly: 100–200 mg/m^2/day over 24 hrs for 5 days. May repeat after waiting 3–4 wks.

CONTRAINDICATIONS

Decreases renal function when serum creatinine >2.5 mg/dl.

CAUTIONS

Renal function when serum creatinine 2–2.5 mg/dl.

INTERACTIONS

DRUG: *Calcium-containing medications, products, vitamin D* may decrease effect. *Nephrotoxic medications* may increase nephrotoxicity. HERBAL: None known. FOOD: None significant. ALTERED LAB VALUES: None significant.

SIDE EFFECTS

FREQUENT: Hypophosphatemia (e.g., bone pain, muscle weakness, anorexia), nephrotoxicity (blood in urine, nausea, vomiting), diarrhea, metallic taste. OCCASIONAL: Hypocalcemia (abnormal cramps, confusion, muscle spasms). RARE: Anemia.

ADVERSE REACTIONS/TOXIC EFFECTS

None significant.

PATIENT CONSIDERATIONS

Baseline Assessment

Assure no other nephrotoxic drugs are being given concurrently. Determine initial serum calcium and creatinine levels. Establish adequate hydration w/oral or IV fluids, preferably saline, to counteract dehydration (caused by hypercalcemia) and increase excretion of calcium. Assure satisfactory urine output (2 L/day recommended) before starting gallium therapy.

Intervention/Evaluation

Throughout therapy maintain adequate hydration w/o overhydrating pt w/compromised cardiovascular status. Monitor urinary output. Assess serum calcium, phosphorus, creatinine, and BUN frequently (therapy should be discontinued if serum creatinine level exceeds 2.5 mg/dl).

Patient/Family Teaching

Explain rationale of therapy and importance of fluids, I&O.

ganciclovir sodium

gan-**sye**-klo-vir
(Cytovene, Vitrasert)

CANADIAN AVAILABILITY
Cytovene

PREGNANCY CATEGORY C

CLASSIFICATION

Antiviral

AVAILABILITY (Rx)

Capsules: 250 mg, 500 mg. **Powder for Injection:** 500 mg. **Implant.**

PHARMACOKINETICS

Widely distributed. **Metabolism:** Undergoes minimal metabolism. **Excretion:** Primarily excreted unchanged in urine. Removed by hemodialysis. **Half-life:** 2.5–3.6 hrs (increased in decreased renal function).

ACTION/*THERAPEUTIC EFFECT*

Converted intracellularly, competes w/viral DNA polymerases and direct incorporation into growing viral DNA chains, *interfering w/DNA synthesis and viral replication.* Congener of acyclovir.

USES/*UNLABELED*

Treatment of cytomegalovirus (CMV) retinitis in immunocompromised pts (e.g., AIDS, bone marrow recipients); in combination w/foscarnet for relapsed AIDS-related CMV retinitis; prevention of CMV in transplant pts. ***Oral:*** Maintenance treatment of CMV. **Vitrasert: intraocular implant:** Treatment of CMV in pts w/AIDS. *IV: Treatment of other CMV infections (e.g., pneumonitis, gastroenteritis, hepatitis).*

STORAGE/HANDLING

Store vials at room temperature. Reconstituted solution in vial stable for 12 hrs at room temperature. Do not refrigerate. After dilution, refrigerate, use within 24 hrs. Discard if precipitate forms, discoloration occurs. Avoid exposure to skin, eyes, mucous membranes. Wear latex gloves.

ADMINISTRATION

ORAL:

- Take w/food.

IV:

- Latex gloves and safety glasses should be used during preparation and handling of solution. Avoid inhalation. (If solution contacts skin, mucous membrane wash carefully w/soap and water; rinse eyes thoroughly w/plain water.)
- Reconstitute 500 mg vial w/10 ml sterile water for injection to provide a concentration of 50 mg/ml; do *not* use bacteriostatic water (contains parabens, which is incompatible w/ganciclovir).
- Further dilute w/100 ml D_5W, 0.9% NaCl, or other compatible fluid to provide a concentration of 5 mg/ml.
- Administer only by IV infusion over 1 hr.
- Do not give IV injection or rapid infusion (increases toxicity).
- Do not give IM or SubQ; protect from infiltration (high pH causes severe tissue irritation).
- Use veins w/adequate blood to permit rapid dilution and dissemination of ganciclovir (minimize phlebitis); central venous catheters tunneled under subcutaneous tissue may reduce catheter-associated infection.

INDICATIONS/ROUTES/DOSAGE

Note: Do not give if neutrophil count <500 cells/mm^3 or platelets <25,000/mm^3.

CMV retinitis treatment:
IV: Adults: Initially, 5 mg/kg q12h for 14–21 days.

CMV disease prevention:
IV: Adults: Initially, 5 mg/kg q12h for 7–14 days.

Maintenance:
***IV:* Adults:** 5 mg/kg/day for 7 days or 6 mg/kg for 5 days.
Oral: Adults: 1,000 mg 3 times/day or 500 mg 6 times/day q3h given w/food.

Dosage in renal impairment:

CREATININE CLEARANCE	DOSAGE	DOSING INTERVAL
≥80 ml/min	5 mg/kg	12 hrs
50–79 ml/min	2.5 mg/kg	12 hrs
25–49 ml/min	2.5 mg/kg	24 hrs
<25 ml/min	1.25 mg/kg	24 hrs

CONTRAINDICATIONS

Hypersensitivity to ganciclovir or acyclovir. Not for use in immunocompetent persons or those w/congenital or neonatal CMV disease.

CAUTIONS

Extreme caution in children because of long-term carcinogenicity, reproductive toxicity. Renal impairment, preexisting cytopenias or history of cytopenic reactions to other drugs, elderly (at greater risk of renal impairment).

INTERACTIONS

DRUG: *Bone marrow depressants* may increase bone marrow depression. May increase risk of seizures w/***imipenem-cilastatin.*** May increase hematologic toxicity w/***zidovudine.*** **HERBAL:** None known. **FOOD:** None significant. **ALTERED LAB VALUES:** May increase SGOT (AST), SGPT (ALT), alkaline phosphatase, bilirubin.

SIDE EFFECTS

FREQUENT (>10%): Fever **(40%)**, diarrhea **(41%)**, nausea **(25%)**, abdominal pain, vomiting, decreased appetite, anemia, leukopenia. ***Intraocular insert:*** Visual acuity loss, vitreous hemorrhage, retinal detachment. **OCCASIONAL (1–10%):** Infection, chills, flatulence, numbness in hands, feet, itching, pneumonia, neutropenia. ***Intraocular insert:*** Cataracts, macular abnormalities, increased IOP, optic disk/nerve changes, uveitis. **RARE (<1%):** Headache, dizziness, thought disorders, behavioral changes, psychosis, coma, seizures, abnormal dreams, intention tremor, chills, malaise, cardiac arrhythmias, hyper/hypotension, pruritus, hematuria, diarrhea, paresthesia, ataxia, edema, alopecia.

ADVERSE REACTIONS/TOXIC EFFECTS

Hematologic toxicity, GI hemorrhage occur rarely.

PATIENT CONSIDERATIONS

Baseline Assessment

Question for hypersensitivity to ganciclovir or acyclovir. Evaluate hematologic baseline. Obtain specimens for support of differential diagnosis (urine, feces, blood, throat) because usually retinal infection due to hematogenous dissemination.

Intervention/Evaluation

Monitor I&O and assure adequate hydration (minimum 1,500 ml/24 hrs). Check IV site, rate of infusion q15min during dosage administration. Diligently evaluate hematology reports for potentially life-threatening neutropenia, thrombocytopenia, decreased platelets (hold ganciclovir and notify physician immediately of neutrophil count less than 500/mm^3, platelet count less than 25,000/mm^3). Monitor B/P at least 2 times/day for hyper/hypotension. Check temperature at least 2 times/day for onset or increase in fever. Assess pt carefully for change (i.e., increased bleeding tendency, signs of infection). Question pt regarding vision, therapeutic improvement, or complications. Be alert for behavior changes, thought disorders, confusion, or other nervous system effects and report promptly. Assess for rash, pruritus.

Patient/Family Teaching

Ganciclovir provides suppression, not cure of CMV retinitis. Frequent blood tests and eye exams are necessary during therapy because of toxic nature of drug. It is essential to report any new symptom promptly. May temporarily or permanently inhibit sperm production in men, suppress fertility in women. Barrier contraception should be used during and for 90 days after therapy because of mutagenic potential.

gatifloxacin
(Tequin)
See Supplement

gemfibrozil
gem-**fie**-bro-zill
(Lopid)

CANADIAN AVAILABILITY
Lopid

PREGNANCY CATEGORY C

CLASSIFICATION

Antihyperlipoproteinemic

AVAILABILITY (Rx)

Tablets: 600 mg

PHARMACOKINETICS

Absorption: Well absorbed from GI tract. **Metabolism:** Metabolized in liver. **Excretion:** Primarily excreted in urine. **Half-life:** 1.5 hrs.

ACTION/*THERAPEUTIC EFFECT*

Inhibits lipolysis of fat in adipose tissue; decreases liver uptake of free fatty acids (reduces hepatic triglyceride production). Inhibits synthesis of VLDL carrier apolipoprotein B. *Lowers serum cholesterol and triglycerides (decreases VLDL, LDL, increases HDL).*

USES

Treatment of hyperlipidemia, decreases risk of coronary heart disease in pts w/type IIB hyperlipidemia. Treatment of severe primary hyperlipidemia (types IV, V).

ADMINISTRATION

ORAL:

- Give 30 min before morning and evening meals.

INDICATIONS/ROUTES/DOSAGE

Hyperlipidemia:
Oral: Adults, elderly: 900 mg to 1.5 g/day in 2 divided doses.

CONTRAINDICATIONS

Hypersensitivity to gemfibrozil, hepatic dysfunction (including primary biliary cirrhosis), severe renal dysfunction, preexisting gallbladder disease.

CAUTIONS

Hypothyroidism, diabetes mellitus, estrogen or anticoagulant therapy.

INTERACTIONS

DRUG: May increase effect of ***warfarin.*** May cause rhabdomyolysis, leading to acute renal failure w/***lovastatin.*** **HERBAL:** None known. **FOOD:** None significant. **ALTERED LAB VALUES:** May increase SGOT (AST), SGPT (ALT), alkaline phosphatase, bilirubin, creatinine kinase, LDH. May decrease Hgb, Hct, potassium, leukocyte counts.

SIDE EFFECTS

FREQUENT (20%): Dyspepsia. **OCCASIONAL (2–10%):** Abdominal pain, diarrhea, nausea, vomiting, fatigue. **RARE (<2%):** Constipation, acute appendicitis, vertigo, headache, rash, altered taste.

ADVERSE REACTIONS/TOXIC EFFECTS

Cholelithiasis, cholecystitis, acute appendicitis, pancreatitis, malignancy occur rarely.

PATIENT CONSIDERATIONS

BASELINE ASSESSMENT

Question for history of hypersensitivity to gemfibrozil. Assess baseline lab results: serum glucose, triglyceride, cholesterol levels, liver function tests, CBC.

INTERVENTION/EVALUATION

Evaluate food tolerance. Determine pattern of bowel activity. Monitor LDL, VLDL, serum triglyceride, and cholesterol lab results for therapeutic response. Assess for rash, pruritus. Check for headache and dizziness, blurred vision. Monitor liver function and hematology tests. Assess for pain, especially right upper quadrant/epigastric pain suggestive of adverse gallbladder effects. Monitor serum glucose for those receiving insulin or oral antihyperglycemics.

PATIENT/FAMILY TEACHING

Follow special diet (important part of treatment). Do not take other medication w/o checking w/physician. Do not stop medication w/o physician's knowledge. Periodic lab tests are essential part of therapy. Notify physician in event of new symptoms, particularly abdominal/epigastric pain. Do not drive or perform other activities that require alert response if dizziness occurs.

---

gemtuzumab

(Mylotarg)

See Classification section under: Cancer chemotherapy

---

gentamicin sulfate

jen-tah-**my**-sin

(Garamycin, Genoptic, Gentacidin, Jenamicin)

CANADIAN AVAILABILITY

Alcomicin, Cidomycin, Garamycin

PREGNANCY CATEGORY C

CLASSIFICATION

Antibiotic: Aminoglycoside

AVAILABILITY (Rx)

Injection: 10 mg/ml, 40 mg/ml, 2 mg/ml (Intrathecal). **Ophthalmic Solution:** 3 mg/ml. **Ophthalmic Ointment:** 3 mg/g. **Cream:** 0.5%. **Ointment:** 0.1%.

PHARMACOKINETICS

Absorption: Rapid, complete absorption after IM administration. Widely distributed (does not cross blood-brain barrier, low concentrations in CSF). **Excretion:** Excreted unchanged in urine. Removed by hemodialysis. **Half-life:** 2–4 hrs (increased in decreased renal function, neonates; decreased in cystic fibrosis, burn or febrile pts).

ACTION / *THERAPEUTIC EFFECT*

Bactericidal. Irreversibly binds to protein of bacterial ribosomes, *interfering in protein synthesis of susceptible microorganisms.*

USES / *UNLABELED*

Parenteral: Treatment of skin/skin structure, bone, joint, respiratory tract, intra-abdominal, complicated urinary tract, and acute pelvic infections; postop, burns, septicemia, meningitis. ***Ophthalmic:*** Ointment/solution for superficial eye infections. ***Topical:*** Cream/ointment for superficial skin infections. Ophthalmic or topical applications may be combined w/systemic administration for serious, extensive infections. ***Topical:*** *Prophylaxis of minor bacterial skin infections, treatment of dermal ulcer.*

STORAGE/HANDLING

Store vials, ophthalmic, topical preparations at room temperature. Solutions appear clear or slightly yellow. Intermittent IV infusion (piggyback) stable for 24 hrs at room temperature. Discard if precipitate forms. Use intrathecal forms immediately after preparation. Discard unused portion.

ADMINISTRATION

Note: Coordinate peak and trough lab draws w/administration times.

IM:

- To minimize discomfort, give deep IM slowly. Less painful if injected into gluteus maximus rather than lateral aspect of thigh.

IV:

- Dilute w/50–200 ml 5% dextrose, 0.9% NaCl, or other compatible fluid. Amount of diluent for infants, children depends on individual needs.
- Infuse over 30–60 min for adults, older children, and over 60–120 min for infants, young children.
- Alternating IV sites, use large veins to reduce risk of phlebitis.

INTRATHECAL:

- Use only 2 mg/ml intrathecal preparation w/o preservative.
- Mix w/10% estimated CSF volume or sodium chloride.
- Give over 3–5 min.

OPHTHALMIC:

- Place finger on lower eyelid and pull out until a pocket is formed between eye and lower lid.
- Hold dropper above pocket and place correct number of drops (1/4–1/2 inch ointment) into pocket. Close eye gently.
- ***Solution:*** Apply digital pressure to lacrimal sac for 1–2 min (minimizes drainage into nose and throat, reducing risk of systemic effects). ***Ointment:*** Close eye for 1–2 min, rolling eyeball (increases contact area of drug to eye).
- Remove excess solution or ointment around eye w/tissue.

INDICATIONS/ROUTES/DOSAGE

Note: Space parenteral doses evenly around the clock. Dosage based on ideal body weight. Peak, trough level determined periodically to maintain desired serum concentrations (minimizes risk of toxicity). ***Recommended peak level:*** 4–10 mcg/ml; ***trough level:*** 1–2 mcg/ml.

Moderate to severe infections:
IM/IV: Adults, elderly: 3 mg/kg/day in divided doses q8h. ***Children:*** 6–7.5 mg/kg/day in divided doses q8h. ***Infants, neonates:*** 7.5 mg/kg/day in divided doses q8h. ***Premature or full-term neonates <7 days:*** 5/mg/kg/day in divided doses q12h.

Life-threatening infections:
IM/IV: Adults, elderly: Up to 5 mg/kg/day in divided doses 3–4 times/day.

Intrathecal: Adults, elderly: 4–8 mg as single daily dose (w/IM/IV doses). ***Children >3 mos:*** 1–2 mg as single daily dose (w/IM/IV doses).

Dosage in renal impairment:
Dose and/or frequency is modified according to degree of renal impairment, serum concentration of drug. After loading dose of 1–2 mg/kg, maintenance dose/frequency based on serum creatinine or creatinine clearance.

Usual ophthalmic dosage:
Adults, elderly: Ointment: Thin strip to conjunctiva q6–12h. ***Solution:*** 1 drop q4–8h to conjunctiva.

Usual topical dosage:
Adults, elderly: Apply 3–4 times/day.

CONTRAINDICATIONS

Hypersensitivity to gentamicin, other aminoglycosides (cross-sensitivity). Sulfite sensitivity may result in anaphylaxis, especially in asthmatics.

CAUTIONS

Elderly, neonates because of renal insufficiency or immaturity; neuromuscular disorders (potential for respiratory depression), prior hearing loss, vertigo, renal impairment. Cumulative effects may occur w/concurrent systemic administration and topical application to large areas.

INTERACTIONS

DRUG: Other ***aminoglycosides, nephrotoxic, ototoxic-producing medications*** may increase toxicity. May increase effects of ***neuromuscular blocking agents.*** **HERBAL:** None known. **FOOD:** None significant. **ALTERED LAB VALUES:** May increase BUN, SGPT (ALT), SGOT (AST), bilirubin, creatinine, LDH concentrations; may decrease serum calcium, magnesium, potassium, sodium concentrations.

SIDE EFFECTS

OCCASIONAL: Pain, induration at IM injection site; phlebitis, thrombophlebitis w/IV administration; hypersensitivity reactions: rash, fever, urticaria, pruritus. ***Ophthalmic:*** Burning, tearing, itching, blurred vision. ***Topical:*** Redness, itching. **RARE:** Alopecia, hypertension, weakness.

ADVERSE REACTIONS/TOXIC EFFECTS

Nephrotoxicity (evidenced by increased BUN and serum creatinine, decreased creatinine clearance) may be reversible if drug stopped at first sign of symptoms; irreversible ototoxicity (tinnitus, dizziness, ringing/roaring in ears, reduced hearing) and neurotoxicity (headache, dizziness, lethargy, tremors, visual disturbances) occur occasionally. Risk is greater w/higher dosages, prolonged therapy, or if solution is applied directly to mucosa. Superinfections, particularly w/fungi, may result from bacterial imbalance via any route of administration. Ophthalmic application may cause paresthesia of conjunctiva, mydriasis.

PATIENT CONSIDERATIONS

BASELINE ASSESSMENT

Dehydration must be treated before parenteral therapy is begun. Establish baseline hearing acuity. Question for history of allergies, especially to aminoglycosides and sulfite (and parabens for topical/ophthalmic routes). Obtain specimens for culture, sensitivity before giving first dose (therapy may begin before results are known).

INTERVENTION/EVALUATION

Monitor I&O (maintain hydration), urinalysis (casts, RBCs, WBCs, decrease in specific gravity). Monitor results of peak/trough blood tests. Be alert to ototoxic and neurotoxic symptoms (see Adverse Reactions/Toxic Effects). Check IM injection site for pain, induration. Evaluate IV site for phlebitis (heat, pain, red streaking over vein). Assess for rash (*ophthalmic:* assess for redness, burning, itching, tearing; *topical:* assess for redness, itching). Be alert for superinfection, particularly genital/anal pruritus, changes in oral mucosa, diarrhea.

When treating those w/neuromuscular disorders, assess respiratory response carefully.

Patient/Family Teaching

Continue antibiotic for full length of treatment. Space doses evenly. Discomfort may occur w/IM injection. Blurred vision or tearing may occur briefly after each ophthalmic dose. Notify physician in event of any hearing, visual, balance, urinary problems, even after therapy is completed.

Ophthalmic
Contact physician if tearing, redness, or irritation continues.

Topical
Cleanse area gently before applying; notify physician if redness, itching occurs. Do not take other medication w/o consulting physician. Lab tests are an essential part of therapy.

glatiramer acetate

glah-**tie**-rah-mir
(Copaxone)

PREGNANCY CATEGORY B

CLASSIFICATION

Neurologic agent

AVAILABILITY (Rx)

Injection: 20 mg/ml

PHARMACOKINETICS

Absorption: A substantial amount of SubQ injection is hydrolyzed locally. **Metabolism:** A fraction of injection enters lymphatic circulation, reaching regional lymph nodes; some may enter systemic circulation.

ACTION/*THERAPEUTIC EFFECT*

Exact mechanism unknown but is thought to act by modifying immune response to myelin, thought to be responsible for the pathogenesis of multiple sclerosis (MS), *relieving symptoms of MS.*

USES/*UNLABELED*

For reduction of the frequency of relapses in pts with relapsing-remitting multiple sclerosis.

ADMINISTRATION

SubQ:

- Reconstitute with the diluent supplied, sterile bacteriostatic water for injection.
- Gently swirl the glatiramer acetate vial and let stand at room temperature until the solid material is completely dissolved.
- May inject into thigh, abdomen, or upper arms.
- Rotate injection sites.
- Give new injection at least 1 inch from an old site and never into area when skin is tender, bruised, red, or hard.

INDICATIONS/DOSAGE/ROUTES

Muscular dystrophy:
SubQ: Adults, elderly: 20 mg/day.

CONTRAINDICATIONS

History of hypersensitivity to glatiramer acetate or mannitol.

CAUTIONS

None significant.

INTERACTIONS

DRUG: None significant. **HERBAL:** None known. **FOOD:** None signifi-

cant. **ALTERED LAB VALUES:** None significant.

SIDE EFFECTS

Note: Effects are generally self-limiting and transient. **FREQUENT (40–73%):** Injection site reaction (pain, erythema, inflammation, itching, mass), infection, asthenia (loss of strength, energy), chest pain, generalized pain, vasodilation, arthralgia, anxiety, hypertonia, nausea. **OCCASIONAL (10–19%):** Flu syndrome, dyspnea, rash, pruritus, palpitations, back pain, sweating, rhinitis, diarrhea, lymphadenopathy, induration/welt at injection site, urinary urgency. **RARE (4–9%):** Bronchitis, fever, neck pain, anorexia, ecchymosis, tremor, peripheral edema, ear pain, facial edema, vertigo, vomiting, dysmenorrhea, tachycardia, migraine, syncope, GI disturbance, urticaria.

ADVERSE REACTIONS/TOXIC EFFECTS

Blood dyscrasias (leukopenia, anemia, pancytopenia) and cardiovascular disturbances (atrial fibrillation, bradycardia, hypotension, systolic murmur) occur in ≤1%.

PATIENT CONSIDERATIONS

BASELINE ASSESSMENT

Provide supportive measures, (e.g., bed rest, positioning, exercise, moist heat as indicated). Determine degree of immobility.

INTERVENTION/EVALUATION

Assess for therapeutic response from signs/symptoms of MS.

PATIENT/FAMILY TEACHING

Inform physician if you are pregnant or are planning to get pregnant while on medication. Do not stop taking this medication w/o consulting your doctor.

glimepiride

glim-**eh**-purr-eyd
(Amaryl)

PREGNANCY CATEGORY C

CLASSIFICATION

Hypoglycemic: Oral

AVAILABILITY (Rx)

Tablets: 1 mg, 2 mg, 4 mg

PHARMACODYNAMICS

	ONSET	PEAK	DURATION
Oral	—	2–3 hrs	24 hrs

PHARMACOKINETICS

Absorption: Completely absorbed from GI tract. **Metabolism:** Metabolized in liver. **Excretion:** Excreted in urine and eliminated in feces. **Half-life:** 5–9.2 hrs.

ACTION/*THERAPEUTIC EFFECT*

Promotes release of insulin from beta cells of pancreas, increases insulin sensitivity at peripheral sites, *lowering blood glucose concentration.*

USES

Adjunct to diet/exercise in management of noninsulin-dependent diabetes mellitus (type II, NIDDM). Use in combination w/insulin or metformin in pts not controlled by diet/exercise in conjunction w/oral hypoglycemic agent.

ADMINISTRATION

ORAL:

- Take w/breakfast or first main meal.

INDICATIONS/ROUTES/DOSAGE

Diabetes mellitus:
Oral: Adults: Initially, 1–2 mg once daily, w/breakfast or first main meal. *Maintenance:* 1–4 mg once daily. After dose of 2 mg is reached, dosage should be increased in increments of up to 2 mg every 1–2 wks, based on blood glucose response. *Maximum:* 8 mg/day.

Combination therapy w/insulin:
Oral: Adults: 8 mg once daily w/breakfast or first main meal w/low-dose insulin.

Renal function impairment:
Oral: Adults: 1 mg once/day.

CONTRAINDICATIONS

Sole therapy for type I diabetes mellitus, diabetic complications (ketosis, acidosis, diabetic coma), stress situations (severe infection, trauma, surgery), hypersensitivity to drug, severe renal or hepatic impairment.

CAUTIONS

Severe diarrhea, intestinal obstruction, prolonged vomiting, liver disease, hyperthyroidism (not controlled), impaired renal function, adrenal insufficiency, debilitated, malnourished, pituitary insufficiency.

INTERACTIONS

DRUG: May increase effect of ***oral anticoagulants. Fluconazole, cimetidine, ranitidine, ciprofloxacin, MAO inhibitors, quinidine, salicylates*** (large doses) may increase effect. ***Beta blockers*** may increase hypoglycemic effect, mask signs of hypoglycemia. ***Corticosteroids, thiazide diuretics, lithium*** may decrease effect. **HERBAL:** None known. **FOOD:** None significant. **ALTERED LAB VALUES:** May increase alkaline phosphatase, SGOT (AST), LDH, creatinine, BUN.

SIDE EFFECTS

FREQUENT: Altered taste sensation, dizziness, drowsiness, weight gain, constipation, diarrhea, heartburn, nausea, vomiting, stomach fullness, headache. **OCCASIONAL:** Increased skin sensitivity to sunlight, peeling of skin, itching, rash.

ADVERSE REACTIONS/TOXIC EFFECTS

Hypoglycemia may occur due to overdosage, insufficient food intake especially w/increased glucose demands. GI hemorrhage, cholestatic hepatic jaundice, leukopenia, thrombocytopenia, pancytopenia, agranulocytosis, aplastic or hemolytic anemia occurs rarely.

PATIENT CONSIDERATIONS

Baseline Assessment

Question for hypersensitivity to glimepiride. Check blood glucose level. Discuss lifestyle to determine extent of learning, emotional needs. Assure follow-up instruction if pt/family do not thoroughly understand diabetes management or glucose-testing technique.

Intervention/Evaluation

Monitor blood glucose and food intake. Assess for hypoglycemia (cool wet skin, tremors, dizziness, anxiety, headache, tachycardia, numbness in mouth, hunger, diplopia) or hyperglycemia

(polyuria, polyphagia, polydipsia, nausea, vomiting, dim vision, fatigue, deep rapid breathing). Check for adverse skin reactions, jaundice. Monitor hematology reports. Assess for bleeding or bruising. Be alert to conditions that alter glucose requirements: fever, increased activity or stress, surgical procedure.

PATIENT/FAMILY TEACHING

Prescribed diet is principal part of treatment; do not skip or delay meals. Diabetes mellitus requires lifelong control. Check blood glucose/urine as ordered. Carry candy, sugar packets, or other sugar supplements for immediate response to hypoglycemia. Wear medical alert identification. Check w/physician when glucose demands are altered (e.g., fever, infection, trauma, stress, heavy physical activity). Avoid alcoholic beverages. Do not take other medication w/o consulting physician. Weight control, exercise, hygiene (including foot care), and nonsmoking are essential part of therapy. Notify physician promptly of skin eruptions, itching, bleeding, yellow skin, dark urine. Inform dentist, physician, or surgeon of this medication before any treatment.

glipizide

glip-ih-zide
(Glucotrol, Glucotrol XL)

PREGNANCY CATEGORY C

CLASSIFICATION

Hypoglycemic: Oral

AVAILABILITY (Rx)

Tablets: 5 mg, 10 mg. **Tablets (extended-release):** 2.5 mg, 5 mg, 10 mg.

PHARMACODYNAMICS

	ONSET	PEAK	DURATION
Oral	10–30 min	0.5–2 hrs	24 hrs

PHARMACOKINETICS

Absorption: Well absorbed from GI tract. **Metabolism:** Metabolized in liver. **Excretion:** Excreted in urine. **Half-life:** 2–4 hrs.

ACTION/*THERAPEUTIC EFFECT*

Promotes release of insulin from beta cells of pancreas, increases insulin sensitivity at peripheral sites, *lowering blood glucose concentration.*

USES

Adjunct to diet/exercise in management of stable, mild to moderately severe noninsulin-dependent diabetes mellitus (type II, NIDDM). May be used to supplement insulin in those w/type I diabetes mellitus.

ADMINISTRATION

ORAL:

- May take w/food (response better if taken 15–30 min before meals).
- Do not crush extended-release tablets.

INDICATIONS/ROUTES/DOSAGE

Diabetes mellitus:

Oral: Adults: Initially, 5 mg/day (2.5 mg in geriatric or those w/liver disease). Adjust dosage in 2.5–5 mg increments at intervals of several days. ***Maximum single dose:*** 15 mg. ***Maximum dose/day:*** 40 mg. ***Maintenance:*** 10 mg/day.

Usual elderly dosage:
Oral: Initially, 2.5–5 mg/day. May increase by 2.5–5 mg/day q1–2wks.

CONTRAINDICATIONS

Sole therapy for type I diabetes mellitus, diabetic complications (ketosis, acidosis, diabetic coma), stress situations (severe infection, trauma, surgery), hypersensitivity to drug, severe renal or hepatic impairment.

CAUTIONS

Severe diarrhea, intestinal obstruction, prolonged vomiting, liver disease, hyperthyroidism (not controlled), impaired renal function, adrenal insufficiency, debilitated, malnourished, pituitary insufficiency.

INTERACTIONS

DRUG: May increase effect of ***oral anticoagulants. Fluconazole, cimetidine, ranitidine, ciprofloxacin, MAO inhibitors, quinidine, salicylates*** (large doses) may increase effect. ***Beta blockers*** may increase hypoglycemic effect, mask signs of hypoglycemia. ***Corticosteroids, thiazide diuretics, lithium*** may decrease effect. **HERBAL:** None known. **FOOD:** None significant. **ALTERED LAB VALUES:** May increase alkaline phosphatase, SGOT (AST), LDH, creatinine, BUN.

SIDE EFFECTS

FREQUENT: Altered taste sensation, dizziness, drowsiness, weight gain, constipation, diarrhea, heartburn, nausea, vomiting, stomach fullness, headache. **OCCASIONAL:** Increased skin sensitivity to sunlight, peeling of skin, itching, rash.

ADVERSE REACTIONS/TOXIC EFFECTS

Hypoglycemia may occur because of overdosage, insufficient food intake especially w/increased glucose demands. GI hemorrhage, cholestatic hepatic jaundice, leukopenia, thrombocytopenia, pancytopenia, agranulocytosis, aplastic or hemolytic anemia occurs rarely.

G

PATIENT CONSIDERATIONS

BASELINE ASSESSMENT

Question for hypersensitivity to glipizide. Check blood glucose level. Discuss lifestyle to determine extent of learning, emotional needs. Assure follow-up instruction if pt/family do not thoroughly understand diabetes management or glucose-testing technique.

INTERVENTION/EVALUATION

Monitor blood glucose and food intake. Assess for hypoglycemia (cool wet skin, tremors, dizziness, anxiety, headache, tachycardia, numbness in mouth, hunger, diplopia) or hyperglycemia (polyuria, polyphagia, polydipsia, nausea, vomiting, dim vision, fatigue, deep rapid breathing). Check for adverse skin reactions, jaundice. Monitor hematology reports. Assess for bleeding or bruising. Be alert to conditions that alter glucose requirements: fever, increased activity or stress, surgical procedure.

PATIENT/FAMILY TEACHING

Prescribed diet is principal part of treatment; do not skip or delay meals. Diabetes mellitus requires lifelong control. Check blood glucose/urine as ordered. Carry candy, sugar packets, or other sugar supplements for immediate response to hypoglycemia. Wear medical alert identification. Check w/physician when glucose demands are altered (e.g., fever, infection, trauma, stress, heavy

physical activity). Avoid alcoholic beverages. Do not take other medication w/o consulting physician. Weight control, exercise, hygiene (including foot care), and nonsmoking are essential part of therapy. Inform dentist, physician, or surgeon of this medication before any treatment.

glucagon hydrochloride

glue-ka-gon
(Glucagon Emergency Kit)

CANADIAN AVAILABILITY
Glucagon Emergency Kit

PREGNANCY CATEGORY B

CLASSIFICATION

Antihypoglycemic

AVAILABILITY (Rx)

Powder for Injection: 1 mg, 10 mg

PHARMACOKINETICS

Absorption: Well absorbed after IM, SubQ administration. **Metabolism:** Undergoes enzymatic proteolysis in liver/kidney. **Half-life:** 10 min. Peak hyperglycemia occurs within 30 min, lasting 1–2 hrs. Return to consciousness in 5–20 min.

ACTION/*THERAPEUTIC EFFECT*

Promotes hepatic glycogenolysis, gluconeogenesis. Stimulates enzyme to increase production of cAMP, *resulting in increased plasma glucose concentration, relaxant effect on smooth muscle, and inotropic myocardial effect.*

USES/*UNLABELED*

Treatment of severe hypoglycemia in diabetic pts. Not for use in chronic hypoglycemia or hypoglycemia due to starvation, adrenal insufficiency because liver glycogen unavailable. Diagnostic aid in radiographic examination of GI tract. *Treatment of toxicity associated w/beta blockers, calcium channel blockers; esophageal obstruction due to foreign bodies.*

STORAGE/HANDLING

Store vial at room temperature. After reconstitution, stable for 48 hrs if refrigerated. If reconstituted w/sterile water for injection, use immediately. Do not use glucagon solution unless clear.

ADMINISTRATION

- **Note:** Place pt on side to avoid potential aspiration (glucagon, as well as hypoglycemia, may produce nausea and vomiting).
- Reconstitute powder w/manufacturer's diluent when preparing 2 mg doses or less. For doses exceeding 2 mg, dilute w/sterile water for injection.
- To provide 1 mg glucagon/ml, use 1 ml diluent. For 1 mg vial of glucagon, use 10 ml diluent for 10 mg vial.
- Pt will usually awaken in 5–20 min. Although 1–2 additional doses may be administered, the concern for effects of continuing cerebral hypoglycemia requires consideration of parenteral glucose.
- When pt awakens, give supplemental carbohydrate to restore liver glycogen and prevent secondary hypoglycemia. If pt fails to respond to glucagon, IV glucose is necessary.

INDICATIONS/ROUTES/DOSAGE

Note: Administer IV dextrose if pt fails to respond to glucagon.

Hypoglycemia:
SubQ/IM/IV: Adults, elderly: 0.5–1 mg (0.5–1 unit). May repeat 1–2 additional doses if response is delayed.

Diagnostic aid:
IM: Adults, elderly: 1–2 mg (1–2 units).

IV: Adults, elderly: 0.25–2 mg (0.25–2 units).

CONTRAINDICATIONS

Pheochromocytoma, hypersensitivity to glucagon (protein).

CAUTIONS

History of insulinoma or pheochromocytoma.

INTERACTIONS

DRUG: May increase ***anticoagulant*** effect. HERBAL: None known. FOOD: None significant. ALTERED LAB VALUES: May decrease potassium.

SIDE EFFECTS

OCCASIONAL: Nausea, vomiting. RARE: Allergic reaction (urticaria, respiratory distress, hypotension).

ADVERSE REACTIONS/TOXIC EFFECTS

Overdose may produce continuing nausea, vomiting, hypokalemia (severe weakness, decreased appetite, irregular heartbeat, muscle cramps).

PATIENT CONSIDERATIONS

Baseline Assessment

Obtain immediate assessment, including history, clinical signs, and symptoms. If hypoglycemic coma is established, give glucagon promptly as described above.

Intervention/Evaluation

Monitor response time carefully. Have IV dextrose readily available in event pt does not awaken within 5–20 min. Assess for possible allergic reaction (urticaria, respiratory difficulty, hypotension). When pt is conscious, give carbohydrate and review insulin/diet needs w/physician.

Patient/Family Teaching

Recognize significance of recognizing symptoms of hypoglycemia: pale cool skin, anxiety, difficulty concentrating, headache, hunger, nausea, nervousness, shakiness, sweating, unusual tiredness, weakness, unconsciousness. Instruct pt, family, or friend to give sugar form first (orange juice, honey, hard candy, sugar cubes, or table sugar dissolved in water or juice) if symptoms of hypoglycemia develop, followed by cheese and crackers or half a sandwich or glass of milk. Inform physician of hypoglycemic episode and use of glucagon so that regimen can be regulated appropriately. Replace glucagon as soon as possible.

---

glyburide

glye-byoo-ride
(Diabeta, Micronase)

FIXED-COMBINATION(S)
W/metformin, an antidiabetic (Glucovance)

CANADIAN AVAILABILITY
Diabeta, Euglucon

PREGNANCY CATEGORY C

CLASSIFICATION

Hypoglycemic: Oral

AVAILABILITY (Rx)

Tablets: 1.25 mg, 2.5 mg, 5 mg

PHARMACODYNAMICS

	ONSET	PEAK	DURATION
Oral	0.25–1 hr	1–2 hrs	24 hrs

PHARMACOKINETICS

Absorption: Well absorbed from GI tract. **Metabolism:** Metabolized in liver to weakly active metabolite. **Excretion:** Primarily excreted in urine. **Half-life:** 10 hrs.

ACTION/*THERAPEUTIC EFFECT*

Promotes release of insulin from beta cells of pancreas, increases insulin sensitivity at peripheral sites, *lowering blood glucose concentration.*

USES

Adjunct to diet/exercise in management of stable, mild to moderately severe noninsulin-dependent diabetes mellitus (type II, NIDDM). May be used to supplement insulin in those w/type I diabetes mellitus.

ADMINISTRATION

ORAL:

- May take w/food (response better if taken 15–30 min before meals).

INDICATIONS/ROUTES/DOSAGE

Diabetes mellitus:
Oral: Adults: Initially, 2.5 mg up to 20 mg/day. ***Range:*** 1.25–20 mg/day as a single or in divided doses. ***Maintenance:*** 7.5 mg/day.

Usual elderly dosage:
Oral: Initially, 1.25–2.5 mg/day. May increase by 1.25–2.5 mg/day q1–3wks.

CONTRAINDICATIONS

Sole therapy for type I diabetes mellitus, diabetic complications (ketosis, acidosis, diabetic coma), stress situations (severe infection, trauma, surgery), hypersensitivity to drug, severe renal or hepatic impairment.

CAUTIONS

Severe diarrhea, intestinal obstruction, prolonged vomiting, liver disease, hyperthyroidism (not controlled), impaired renal function, adrenal insufficiency, debilitated, malnourished, pituitary insufficiency.

INTERACTIONS

DRUG: May increase effect of ***oral anticoagulants. Fluconazole, cimetidine, ranitidine, ciprofloxacin, MAO inhibitors, quinidine, salicylates*** (large doses) may increase effect. ***Beta blockers*** may increase hypoglycemic effect, mask signs of hypoglycemia. ***Corticosteroids, thiazide diuretics, lithium*** may decrease effect. **HERBAL:** None known. **FOOD:** None significant. **ALTERED LAB VALUES:** May increase alkaline phosphatase, SGOT (AST), LDH, creatinine, BUN.

SIDE EFFECTS

FREQUENT: Altered taste sensation, dizziness, drowsiness, weight gain, constipation, diarrhea, heartburn, nausea, vomiting, stomach fullness, headache. **OCCASIONAL:** Increased skin sensitivity to sunlight, peeling of skin, itching, rash.

ADVERSE REACTIONS/TOXIC EFFECTS

Overdosage, insufficient food intake may produce hypoglycemia, especially w/increased glucose demands. Cholestatic jaundice, leukopenia, thrombocytopenia, pancytopenia, agranulocytosis, aplastic or hemolytic anemia occurs rarely.

PATIENT CONSIDERATIONS

Baseline Assessment

Question for hypersensitivity to glyburide. Check blood glucose level. Discuss lifestyle to determine extent of learning, emotional needs. Assure follow-up instruction if pt/family does not thoroughly understand diabetes management or glucose-testing techniques.

Intervention/Evaluation

Monitor blood glucose and food intake. Assess for hypoglycemia (cool wet skin, tremors, dizziness, anxiety, headache, tachycardia, numbness in mouth, hunger, diplopia) or hyperglycemia (polyuria, polyphagia, polydipsia, nausea and vomiting, dim vision, fatigue, deep rapid breathing). Be alert to conditions altering glucose requirements: fever, increased activity or stress, surgical procedure. Check for adverse skin reactions, jaundice. Monitor hematology reports. Assess for bleeding or bruising.

Patient/Family Teaching

Prescribed diet is principal part of treatment; do not skip or delay meals. Diabetes mellitus requires lifelong control. Check blood glucose/urine as ordered. Signs and symptoms, treatment of hypo/hyperglycemia. Carry candy, sugar packets, or other sugar supplements for immediate response to hypoglycemia; wear medical alert identification. Check w/physician when glucose demands change (e.g., fever, infection, trauma, stress, heavy physical activity). Avoid alcoholic beverages. Do not take other medication w/o consulting physician. Weight control, exercise, hygiene (including foot care), and nonsmoking are essential part of therapy. Inform dentist, physician, or surgeon of this medication before any treatment.

glycopyrrolate

gly-ko-**pie**-roll-ate
(Robinul)

CANADIAN AVAILABILITY
Robinul

PREGNANCY CATEGORY B

CLASSIFICATION

Anticholinergic

AVAILABILITY (Rx)

Tablets: 1 mg, 2 mg. **Injection:** 0.2 mg/ml.

PHARMACOKINETICS

Absorption: Incompletely absorbed from GI tract. Well absorbed after IM administration. **Metabolism:** Metabolized in liver. **Excretion:** Primarily excreted in urine. **Half-life:** 1.7 hrs.

ACTION/*THERAPEUTIC EFFECT*

Inhibits action of acetylcholine on structures innervated by postganglionic sites: smooth, cardiac muscle, SA, AV nodes, exocrine glands. Larger doses may decrease motility, secretory activity of GI system, tone of ureter, urinary bladder. *Reduces salivation and excessive secretions of respiratory tract; reduces gastric secretions, acidity.*

USES

Treatment of peptic ulcer disease. Preop medication to prevent cholinergic effect during surgery (i.e., arrhythmias; reduces salivation, secretions). Given concurrently w/anticholinesterase agents to block adverse muscarinic effects. Blocks vagal inhibitory reflexes during anesthesia induction and intubation. Used intraoperatively to counter vagal reflexes w/arrhythmias. Protects against peripheral muscarinic effects (bradycardia, secretions) of cholinergic agents.

ADMINISTRATION

ORAL:

- Administer before meals (food decreases absorption) and bedtime.

IM:

- For preop, may be given in same syringe w/other compatible preop medication.

IV:

- Give by direct IV injection.
- May be given via tubing or running IV infusion of compatible solution.
- When used concurrently w/neostigmine or physostigmine, may be administered via same syringe.

INDICATIONS/ROUTES/DOSAGE

Peptic ulcer disease:
Oral: Adults, elderly: Initially, 1 mg 3 times/day. *Maintenance:* 1 mg 2 times/day. *Maximum:* 8 mg/day.
IM/IV: Adults, elderly: 0.1–0.2 mg q4h (3–4 times/day). *Maximum:* 4 doses/day.

Preop:
IM: Adults, elderly, children >2 yrs: 0.004 mg/kg 30–60 min before anesthesia. *Children <2 yrs:* Up to 0.004 mg/lb.

Intraoperative (prevent cholinergic effects):
IV: Adults, elderly, children: 0.1 mg (0.5 ml). May repeat at 2–3 min intervals.

Block effects of anticholinesterase agents:
IV: Adults, elderly: 0.2 mg for each 1 mg neostigmine or 5 mg pyridostigmine.

CONTRAINDICATIONS

Narrow-angle glaucoma, severe ulcerative colitis, toxic megacolon, obstructive disease of GI tract, paralytic ileus, intestinal atony, bladder neck obstruction due to prostatic hypertrophy, myasthenia gravis in those not treated w/neostigmine, tachycardia secondary to cardiac insufficiency or thyrotoxicosis, cardiospasm, unstable cardiovascular status in acute hemorrhage.

EXTREME CAUTION

Autonomic neuropathy, known or suspected GI infections, diarrhea, mild to moderate ulcerative colitis.

CAUTIONS

Hyperthyroidism, hepatic or renal disease, hypertension, tachyarrhythmias, CHF, coronary artery disease, gastric ulcer, esophageal reflux or hiatal hernia associated w/reflux esophagitis, infants, elderly, those w/COPD.

INTERACTIONS

DRUG: *Antacids, antidiarrheals* may decrease absorption. *Anticholinergics* may increase effects.

May decrease absorption of ***ketoconazole.*** May increase severity of GI lesions with ***potassium chloride*** (wax matrix). **HERBAL:** None known. **FOOD:** None significant. **ALTERED LAB VALUES:** May decrease uric acid.

SIDE EFFECTS

FREQUENT: Dry mouth (sometimes severe), decreased sweating, constipation. **OCCASIONAL:** Blurred vision, bloated feeling, urinary hesitancy, drowsiness (w/high dosage), headache, intolerance to light, loss of taste, nervousness, flushing, insomnia, impotence, mental confusion/excitement (particularly in elderly, children). Parenteral form may produce temporary lightheadedness, local irritation. **RARE:** Dizziness, faintness.

ADVERSE REACTIONS/TOXIC EFFECTS

Overdosage may produce temporary paralysis of ciliary muscle, pupillary dilation, tachycardia, palpitation, hot/dry/flushed skin, absence of bowel sounds, hyperthermia, increased respiratory rate, EKG abnormalities, nausea, vomiting, rash over face/upper trunk, CNS stimulation, psychosis (agitation, restlessness, rambling speech, visual hallucination, paranoid behavior, delusions), followed by depression.

PATIENT CONSIDERATIONS

Baseline Assessment

Before giving medication, instruct pt to void (reduces risk of urinary retention).

Intervention/Evaluation

Monitor daily bowel activity and stool consistency. Palpate bladder for urinary retention. Monitor changes in B/P, temperature. Assess skin turgor, mucous membranes to evaluate hydration status (encourage adequate fluid intake), bowel sounds for peristalsis. Be alert for fever (increased risk of hyperthermia).

G

Patient/Family Teaching

Take 30 min before meals (food decreases absorption of medication). Use care not to become overheated during exercise in hot weather (may result in heat stroke). Avoid hot baths, saunas. Avoid tasks that require alertness, motor skills until response to drug is established. Sugarless gum, sips of tepid water may relieve dry mouth. Do not take antacids or medicine for diarrhea within 1 hr of taking this medication (decreased effectiveness).

gold sodium thiomalate

gold sodium thigh-oh-**mal**-ate
(Myochrysine)

CANADIAN AVAILABILITY
Myochrysine

PREGNANCY CATEGORY C

CLASSIFICATION

Antirheumatic, anti-inflammatory

AVAILABILITY (Rx)

Injection: 25 mg/ml, 50 mg/ml

PHARMACOKINETICS

Absorption: Rapidly absorbed after IM administration. Widely distributed. **Metabolism:** Metabolic fate unknown. **Excretion:**

Primarily excreted in urine. **Half-life:** 3–27 days after single dose up to 168 days w/multiple doses. Contains approximately 50% gold.

ACTION/*THERAPEUTIC EFFECT*

Inhibits phagocytosis, lysomal enzyme activity, decreasing concentration of rheumatoid factor, immunoglobulins. *Decreases synovial inflammation, retards cartilage and bone destruction (suppresses or prevents, but does not cure, arthritis, synovitis).*

USES/*UNLABELED*

Management of rheumatoid arthritis in those w/insufficient therapeutic response to nonsteroidal anti-inflammatory agents. *Treatment of psoriatic arthritis.*

ADMINISTRATION

IM:

- Give in upper outer quadrant of gluteus maximus.
- Pt to be lying down when administered.

INDICATIONS/ROUTES/DOSAGE

Rheumatoid arthritis:
Note: Give as weekly injections.

IM: Adults, elderly: Initially, 10 mg, then 25 mg for second dose. Follow w/25 mg/wk until improvement noted or total of 1 g administered. ***Maintenance:*** 25–50 mg q2wks for 2–20 wks; if stable, may increase to q3–4wk intervals. ***Children:*** Initially, 10 mg, then 1 mg/kg/wk. ***Maximum single dose:*** 50 mg.

CONTRAINDICATIONS

History of gold-induced pathoses (necrotizing enterocolitis, exfoliative dermatitis, pulmonary fibrosis, blood dyscrasias), hepatic dysfunction or history of hepatitis, uncontrolled diabetes or CHF, urticaria, eczema, colitis, hemorrhagic conditions, systemic lupus erythematosus, recent radiation therapy.

CAUTIONS

Renal/hepatic disease, inflammatory bowel disease.

INTERACTIONS

DRUG: ***Bone marrow depressants, hepatotoxic, nephrotoxic medications*** may increase toxicity. ***Penicillamine*** may increase risk of hematologic or renal adverse effects. **HERBAL:** None known. **FOOD:** None significant. **ALTERED LAB VALUES:** May decrease Hgb, Hct, platelets, WBCs. May alter liver function tests. May increase urine protein.

SIDE EFFECTS

FREQUENT: Diarrhea/loose stools, rash, pruritus, abdominal pain, nausea. **OCCASIONAL:** Vomiting, anorexia, flatulence, dyspepsia, conjunctivitis, photosensitivity. **RARE:** Constipation, urticaria, rash.

ADVERSE REACTIONS/TOXIC EFFECTS

Signs of gold toxicity: decreased hemoglobin, leukopenia (WBC below 4,000 mm^3), reduced granulocyte counts (below 150,000/mm^3), proteinuria, hematuria, stomatitis, blood dyscrasias (anemia, leukopenia, thrombocytopenia, eosinophilia), glomerulonephritis, nephrotic syndrome, cholestatic jaundice.

PATIENT CONSIDERATIONS

BASELINE ASSESSMENT

Rule out pregnancy before beginning treatment; CBC, urinalysis, platelet and differential, renal and

liver function tests should be performed before therapy begins.

INTERVENTION/EVALUATION

Monitor daily bowel activity and stool consistency. Assess urine tests for proteinuria or hematuria. Monitor WBC, hemoglobin, differential, platelet count, renal and hepatic function studies. Question for skin pruritus (may be first sign of impending rash). Assess skin daily for rash, purpura, or ecchymoses. Assess oral mucous membranes, borders of tongue, palate, pharynx for ulceration, complaint of metallic taste sensation (signs of stomatitis). Evaluate for therapeutic response: relief of pain, stiffness, swelling, increase in joint mobility, reduced joint tenderness, improved grip strength.

PATIENT/FAMILY TEACHING

Therapeutic response may take 6 mos or longer. Avoid exposure to sunlight (gray to blue pigment may appear). Contact physician/nurse if pruritus, rash, sore mouth, indigestion, or metallic taste occurs. Maintain diligent oral hygiene.

gonadorelin acetate

go-nad-oh-**rell**-in

(Lutrepulse)

gonadorelin hydrochloride

(Factrel)

CANADIAN AVAILABILITY

Factrel, Lutrepulse

PREGNANCY CATEGORY B

CLASSIFICATION

Gonadotropin-releasing hormone

AVAILABILITY (Rx)

Powder for Injection: (acetate): 0.8 mg, 3.2 mg; **(hydrochloride):** 100 mcg, 500 mcg

G

PHARMACOKINETICS

Metabolism: Rapidly metabolized. **Excretion:** Primarily excreted in urine. **Half-life:** 10–40 min.

ACTION/*THERAPEUTIC EFFECT*

Diagnostic aid. *Stimulates synthesis, release of luteinizing hormone (LH), follicle-stimulating hormone (FSH)* from anterior pituitary. *Stimulates release of gonadotropin-releasing hormone* from hypothalamus.

USES/*UNLABELED*

As a single dose, to evaluate the functional capacity and response of gonadotropes of anterior pituitary in suspected gonadotropic deficiency (does not differentiate between hypothalamus or pituitary disorders). Multiple injection testing is used to evaluate residual gonadotropic function of pituitary after removal of a pituitary tumor by surgery and/or irradiation. Induction of ovulation in women w/primary hypothalamic amenorrhea. *Acetate: Treatment of delayed puberty, infertility.*

STORAGE/HANDLING

Solution should appear clear, colorless, free of particulate matter. Do not use if discolored/precipitate formed. Discard unused portion.

ADMINISTRATION

GONADORELIN ACETATE:

- Reconstitute vial w/8 ml diluent

immediately before use. Inject diluent onto dry product cake.

- Shake a few seconds.
- Transfer solution to plastic reservoir.
- Set Lutrepulse pump to deliver appropriate volume/pulse over 1 min q90min.
- Solution will supply doses for approximately 7 days.

Gonadorelin Hydrochloride:

- Reconstitute 100 mcg w/1 ml of sterile diluent supplied.
- Reconstitute 500 mcg w/2 ml of sterile diluent supplied.
- Prepare solution immediately before use.

INDICATIONS/ROUTES/DOSAGE

Note: Test should be conducted in the absence of other drugs that affect pituitary secretion of gonadotropins.

Gonadorelin Acetate:

Primary hypothalamic amenorrhea:
IV Pump: Adults: 5 mcg q90min (range 1–20 mcg); treatment interval 21 days. Refer to manufacturer's manual for proper dilutions/settings on pump. Response usually occurs 2–3 wks after initiation. Continue additional 2 wks after ovulation occurs (maintains corpus luteum).

Gonadorelin Hydrochloride:

Diagnostic agent:
IV/SubQ: Adults: 100 mcg. In females, perform test in early follicular phase of menstrual cycle.

CONTRAINDICATIONS

Hypersensitivity to gonadorelin, components. *Gonadorelin acetate:* Women w/any condition exacerbated by pregnancy, ovarian cysts, or causes of anovulation other than hypothalamic in origin.

CAUTIONS

None significant.

INTERACTIONS

DRUG: None significant. **HERBAL:** None known. **FOOD:** None significant. **ALTERED LAB VALUES:** None significant.

SIDE EFFECTS

OCCASIONAL: *Gonadorelin acetate:* Multiple pregnancy, inflammation, infection, mild phlebitis, hematoma at catheter site. *Gonadorelin hydrochloride:* Swelling, pain, or itching at injection site w/SubQ administration. Local or generalized skin rash w/chronic SubQ administration. **RARE:** *Gonadorelin acetate:* Ovarian hyperstimulation. *Gonadorelin hydrochloride:* Headache, nausea, lightheadedness, abdominal discomfort, hypersensitivity reactions (bronchospasm, tachycardia, flushing, urticaria), induration at injection site.

ADVERSE REACTIONS/TOXIC EFFECTS

Anaphylactic reaction occurs rarely.

PATIENT CONSIDERATIONS

Baseline Assessment

Before test is started, assure that pt understands procedure. Question for hypersensitivity to gonadorelin or components.

Gonadorelin acetate
Pt instructions included w/kit from manufacturer.

Gonadorelin hydrochloride
Venous blood sample (for LH) to be drawn immediately before gonadorelin hydrochloride administration.

INTERVENTION/EVALUATION

Gonadorelin acetate
W/baseline pelvic ultrasound, follow-up studies.

Gonadorelin hydrochloride
At 7 and 14 days of therapy, change cannula and IV site at 48 hr intervals. Assure protocol for test is maintained: usually venous blood samples (for LH) drawn after administration at intervals of 15, 30, 45, 60, and 120 min.

goserelin acetate

(Zoladex)
See Classification section under: Cancer chemotherapy

granisetron

gran-**is**-eh-tron
(Kytril)

CANADIAN AVAILABILITY
Kytril

PREGNANCY CATEGORY B

CLASSIFICATION

Antiemetic

AVAILABILITY (Rx)

Tablets: 1 mg, 2 mg. **Injection:** 1 mg/ml.

PHARMACOKINETICS

Rapid, widely distributed to tissues. **Metabolism:** Metabolized in liver to active metabolite. **Excretion:** Excreted in urine, eliminated in feces. **Half-life:** 10–12 hrs (increased in elderly).

ACTION/*THERAPEUTIC EFFECT*

Selectively blocks serotonin stimulation at receptor sites on abdominal vagal afferent nerve and chemoreceptor trigger zone, *preventing nausea, vomiting.*

USES/*UNLABELED*

Prevents nausea, vomiting associated w/emetogenic cancer therapy (includes high-dose cisplatin). *Oral:* Prevention of nausea/vomiting associated w/radiation therapy. *Prophylaxis of nausea/vomiting associated w/cancer radiotherapy.*

STORAGE/HANDLING

Clear, colorless solution. Store at room temperature. After dilution, stable for at least 24 hrs at room temperature. Inspect for particulates, discoloration.

ADMINISTRATION

IV:
- Dilute calculated dose w/20–50 ml 0.9% NaCl or 5% dextrose. Do not mix w/other medications.
- Infuse IV over 5 min.
- May give undiluted over 30 sec.

INDICATIONS/ROUTES/DOSAGE

Antiemetic:
IV: Adults, elderly, children >2 yrs: 10 mcg/kg beginning within 30 min before initiating chemotherapy.

Oral: Adults, elderly: 1 mg up to 1 hr before chemotherapy and 12 hrs after first dose or 2 mg once 1 hr prior to chemotherapy.

Give only on days that chemotherapy is administered.

CONTRAINDICATIONS

None significant.

CAUTIONS

Safety in children <2 yrs of age not established.

INTERACTIONS

DRUG: *Hepatic enzyme inducers* may decrease effect. **HERBAL:** None known. **FOOD:** None significant. **ALTERED LAB VALUES:** May increase SGOT (AST), SGPT (ALT).

SIDE EFFECTS

FREQUENT (10–20%): Headache, constipation, asthenia (loss of strength), nausea, leukopenia. **OCCASIONAL (2–10%):** Abdominal pain, diarrhea, vomiting, decreased appetite, chills, hair loss. **RARE (<2%):** Chest pain, angina, hypertension, altered taste, hypersensitivity reaction.

ADVERSE REACTIONS/TOXIC EFFECTS

None significant.

PATIENT CONSIDERATIONS

Baseline Assessment

Assure granisetron is given within 30 min before start of chemotherapy.

Intervention/Evaluation

Monitor for therapeutic effect. Assess for headache. Monitor frequency and consistency of stools.

Patient/Family Teaching

Granisetron is effective shortly after administration; prevents nausea, vomiting. Explain that transitory taste disorder may occur.

---

grepafloxacin

grep-ah-**flocks**-ah-sin
(Raxar)

CANADIAN AVAILABILITY
Raxar

PREGNANCY CATEGORY C

CLASSIFICATION

Antibiotic: Fluoroquinolone

AVAILABILITY (Rx)

Tablets: 200 mg

PHARMACOKINETICS

Absorption: Well absorbed from GI tract. Widely distributed. **Metabolism:** Metabolized in liver. **Excretion:** Primarily excreted in urine. **Half-life:** 12–20 hrs.

ACTION/*THERAPEUTIC EFFECT*

Inhibits the DNA enzyme, gyrase, in susceptible microorganisms, interfering with bacterial DNA replication and repair, *producing bactericidal activity.*

USES/*UNLABELED*

Treatment of mild to moderate acute bacterial exacerbation of chronic bronchitis, community-acquired pneumonia, uncomplicated gonorrhea, nongonococcal urethritis/cervicitis.

ADMINISTRATION

ORAL:

- Give w/o regard to meals.
- Do not administer antacids (aluminum, magnesium) within 2 hrs of grepafloxacin dosage.
- Encourage cranberry juice, citrus fruits (acidifies urine).

INDICATIONS/ROUTES/DOSAGES

Bronchitis:
Oral: Adults, elderly: 400–600 mg once daily for 10 days.

Pneumonia:
Oral: Adults, elderly: 600 mg once daily for 10 days.

Nongonococcal urethritis or cervicitis:
Oral: Adults, elderly: 400 mg once daily for 7 days.

Uncomplicated gonorrhea:
Oral: Adults, elderly: 400 mg given as a single dose.

CONTRAINDICATIONS

Hepatic failure, pts with known QT prolongation, those concurrently taking medications known to produce an increase in QT interval or torsade de pointes (e.g., terfenadine) unless appropriate cardiac monitoring can be ensured.

CAUTIONS

Hypersensitivity to fluoroquinolones, impaired hepatic function, severe cerebral arterosclerosis, epilepsy.

INTERACTIONS

DRUG: ***Antacids, sucralfate, didanosine, iron preparations*** decreases grepafloxacin serum levels. May increase effect of ***anticoagulants.*** May increase concentration, toxicity of ***theophylline.*** Nephrotoxic effects may be increased with ***cyclosporine.*** ***NSAIDs*** may increase risk CNS toxicity. ***Medication prolonging QT interval (e.g., amiodarone, cisapride, procainamide, quinidine)*** may increase risk of cardiac arrhythmias. **HERBAL:** None known. **FOOD:** None significant. **ALTERED LAB VALUES:** May increase SGOT (AST), SGOT (ALT), alkaline phosphatase, bilirubin, LDH, BUN, creatinine.

SIDE EFFECTS

FREQUENT: Altered taste, mild diarrhea, dizziness, lightheadedness, headache, nausea, vomiting, vaginal pain/discharge. **OCCASIONAL:** Increased sensitivity of skin to sunlight. **RARE:** CNS stimulation (e.g., confusion, hallucinations, acute psychosis), pain in calves, swelling of calves or lower legs.

ADVERSE REACTIONS/TOXIC EFFECTS

Superinfection (particularly enterococcal or fungal overgrowth of nonsusceptible organisms) may occur. Hypersensitivity reactions have occurred in those receiving fluoroquinolone therapy. QT interval prolongation (irregular/slow heartbeat, recurrent fainting). Pseudomembranous colitis (fever, severe diarrhea, abdominal cramps/pain).

PATIENT CONSIDERATIONS

BASELINE ASSESSMENT

Question for hypersensitivity to grepafloxacin or other fluoroquinolones. Obtain specimens for culture and sensitivity test (therapy may begin before results are known).

INTERVENTION/EVALUATION

Report hypersensitivity reaction: skin rash, urticaria, pruritus, fever promptly. Be alert for superinfection (e.g., genital-anal pruritus, ulceration or changes in oral mucosa, moderate to severe diarrhea, new or increased fever). Provide symptomatic relief for nausea, vomiting. Evaluate food tolerance, change in taste sensation. Question for headache, dizziness; provide ambulation assistance if needed.

PATIENT/FAMILY TEACHING

Do not take antacids 2 hrs before or after taking medication (reduces/destroys effectiveness). Continue medication for full length of treatment. Sugarless gum, hard candy may relieve altered taste. Avoid prolonged exposure to sun. Use caution operating machinery, driving (may cause dizziness).

griseofulvin

griz-ee-oh-**full**-vin
(Fulvicin, Grisactin, GrisPEG)

CANADIAN AVAILABILITY
Fulvicin, Grisovin-FP

PREGNANCY CATEGORY C

CLASSIFICATION

Antifungal

AVAILABILITY (Rx)

Microsize: **Tablets:** 250 mg, 500 mg. **Capsules:** 125 mg, 250 mg. **Oral Suspension:** 125 mg/5 ml.

Ultra Microsize: **Tablets:** 125 mg, 165 mg, 250 mg, 330 mg.

PHARMACOKINETICS

Absorption: *Microsize:* Variably absorbed from GI tract. *Ultra microsize:* Completely absorbed from GI tract. Primarily deposited in keratin layer of skin, hair, nails. **Metabolism:** Metabolized in liver. **Excretion:** Primarily excreted in urine. **Half-life:** 24 hrs.

ACTION/*THERAPEUTIC EFFECT*

Inhibits fungal cell mitosis by disrupting mitotic spindle structure. *Fungistatic.*

USES

Treatment of tineas (ringworm): t. capitis, t. corporis, t. cruris, t. pedis, t. unguium.

ADMINISTRATION

ORAL:

- Take w/or after meals (decreases GI irritation, increases absorption).
- Shake suspension well before administration.
- Distinguish carefully between microsize and ultra microsize doses.

INDICATIONS/ROUTES/DOSAGE

Note: Give orally as a single dose or in 2–4 divided doses. Dosage is individualized.

Tinea corporis, tinea cruris, tinea capitis:
Oral: Adults, elderly: **Ultra microsize:** 330–375 mg/day. **Microsize:** 500 mg/day.

Tinea pedis, tinea unguium:
Oral: Adults, elderly: Ultra microsize: 660–750 mg/day. **Microsize:** 750 mg to 1 g/day. ***Children >2 yrs:*** Ultra microsize: 7.3 mg/kg/day. **Microsize:** 10–11 mg/kg/day.

CONTRAINDICATIONS

Hypersensitivity to griseofulvin, porphyria, hepatocellular failure.

CAUTIONS

Exposure to sun or ultraviolet light (photosensitivity), hypersensitivity to penicillins.

INTERACTIONS

DRUG: May decrease effects of ***warfarin, oral contraceptives.*** **HERBAL:** None known. **FOOD:** None significant. **ALTERED LAB VALUES:** None significant.

SIDE EFFECTS

OCCASIONAL: Hypersensitivity reaction (rash, pruritus, urticaria), headache, nausea, diarrhea, excessive thirst, flatulence, oral thrush, dizziness, insomnia. **RARE:** Paresthesia of hands/feet, proteinuria.

ADVERSE REACTIONS/TOXIC EFFECTS

Granulocytopenia should cause discontinuation of drug.

PATIENT CONSIDERATIONS

Baseline Assessment

Question for history of allergies, especially to griseofulvin, penicillins. Confirm that a culture/histologic test was done for accurate diagnosis.

Intervention/Evaluation

Assess skin for rash and response to therapy. Evaluate food intake, tolerance. Determine pattern of bowel activity and stool consistency. Question presence of headache: onset, location, type of discomfort. Assess mental status for dizziness and provide ambulation assistance when necessary.

Patient/Family Teaching

Prolonged therapy (weeks or months) is usually necessary. Do not miss a dose; continue therapy as long as ordered. Avoid alcohol (may produce tachycardia, flushing). Maintain good hygiene (prevents superinfection). Separate personal items in direct contact w/affected areas. Do not apply other preparations or take other medications w/o consulting physician. Avoid exposure to sunlight. Keep areas dry; wear light clothing for ventilation. Take w/foods high in fat such as milk, ice cream (reduces GI upset and assists absorption).

---

guaifenesin (glyceryl guaiacolate)

guay-**fen**-ah-sin
(Glycotuss, Humibid, Robitussin)

FIXED-COMBINATION(S)
W/phenylephrine and phenylpropanolamine, sympathomimetics **(Entex)**.

CANADIAN AVAILABILITY
Balminil, Benylin E, Robitussin

G

PREGNANCY CATEGORY C

CLASSIFICATION

Expectorant

AVAILABILITY (OTC)

Tablets: 100 mg, 200 mg. **Tablets (sustained-release):** 600 mg. **Capsules:** 200 mg. **Capsules (sustained-release):** 300 mg. **Syrup:** 100 mg/5 ml. **Liquid:** 200 mg/5 ml.

PHARMACOKINETICS

Absorption: Well absorbed from GI tract. **Metabolism:** Metabolized in liver. **Excretion:** Excreted in urine.

ACTION/*THERAPEUTIC EFFECT*

Enhances fluid output of respiratory tract by decreasing adhesiveness and surface tension, *promoting removal of viscous mucus.*

USES

Symptomatic relief of cough in presence of mucus in respiratory tract. Not for use w/persistent cough due to smoking, asthma, emphysema or cough accompanied by excessive secretions.

STORAGE/HANDLING

Store syrup, liquid, capsules at room temperature.

ADMINISTRATION

ORAL:

- Give w/o regard to meals.
- Do not crush or break sustained-

release capsule. May sprinkle contents on soft food, then swallow w/o crushing/chewing.

INDICATIONS/ROUTES/DOSAGE

Note: Give extended-release at 12 hr intervals.

Expectorant:
Oral: Adults, elderly, children >12 yrs: 200–400 mg q4h. *Maximum:* 2.4 g/day. *Children 6–12 yrs:* 100–200 mg q4h. *Maximum:* 1.2 g/day. *Children 2–6 yrs:* 50–100 mg q4h. *Maximum:* 600 mg/day.

CONTRAINDICATIONS

None significant.

CAUTIONS

None significant.

INTERACTIONS

DRUG: None significant. **HERBAL:** None known. **FOOD:** None significant. **ALTERED LAB VALUES:** None significant.

SIDE EFFECTS

RARE: Dizziness, headache, rash, diarrhea, nausea, vomiting, stomach pain.

ADVERSE REACTIONS/TOXIC EFFECTS

Excessive dosage may produce nausea, vomiting.

PATIENT CONSIDERATIONS

Baseline Assessment

Assess type, severity, frequency of cough and productions. Increase fluid intake and environmental humidity to lower viscosity of lung secretions.

Intervention/Evaluation

Initiate deep breathing and coughing exercises, particularly in those w/impaired pulmonary function. Assess for clinical improvement and record onset of relief of cough.

Patient/Family Teaching

Avoid tasks that require alertness, motor skills until response to drug is established. Do not take for chronic cough. Inform physician if cough persists or if fever, rash, headache, or sore throat is present w/cough. Maintain adequate hydration.

guanabenz acetate

gwan-ah-benz
(Wytensin)

PREGNANCY CATEGORY C

CLASSIFICATION

Antihypertensive

AVAILABILITY (Rx)

Tablets: 4 mg, 8 mg

PHARMACODYNAMICS

	ONSET	PEAK	DURATION
Oral	1 hr	2–4 hrs	6–8 hrs

PHARMACOKINETICS

Absorption: Well absorbed from GI tract. Widely distributed. **Metabolism:** Metabolized in liver. **Excretion:** Primarily excreted in urine. **Half-life:** 7–10 hrs.

ACTION/*THERAPEUTIC EFFECT*

Stimulates alpha$_2$-adrenergic receptors. Inhibits sympathetic cardioaccelerator and vasoconstrictor center to heart, kidneys, peripheral vasculature. *Decreases systolic, diastolic B/P.* Chronic use *decreases peripheral vascular resistance.*

USES

Treatment of hypertension. Used alone or in combination w/thiazide-type diuretics.

ADMINISTRATION

ORAL:

- May give w/food if GI distress occurs.
- Tablets may be crushed.
- Give last dose at bedtime (ensures control of B/P at night, minimizing daytime drowsiness).

INDICATIONS/ROUTES/DOSAGE

Hypertension:

Oral: Adults: Initially, 4 mg 2 times/day. Increase by 4–8 mg at 1–2 wk intervals. ***Elderly:*** Initially, 4 mg/day. May increase q1–2wks. ***Maintenance:*** 8–16 mg/day. ***Maximum:*** 32 mg/day.

CONTRAINDICATIONS

None significant.

CAUTIONS

Severe coronary insufficiency, recent MI, cerebrovascular disease, severe hepatic, renal failure.

INTERACTIONS

DRUG: *Beta-adrenergic blockers, hypotension-producing medications* may increase antihypertensive effect. **HERBAL:** None known. **FOOD:** None significant. **ALTERED LAB VALUES:** May decrease cholesterol, total triglyceride concentrations.

SIDE EFFECTS

FREQUENT (>10%): Dizziness, drowsiness (20–39%), dry mouth (28–38%), weakness. **OCCASIONAL (3–10%):** Headache, nausea, decreased sexual ability. **RARE (<3%):** Chest pain, palpitations, anxiety, ataxia, sleep disturbances, rash, itching, diarrhea, constipation, altered taste, muscle aches.

ADVERSE REACTIONS/TOXIC EFFECTS

Abrupt withdrawal may result in rebound hypertension manifested as nervousness, agitation, anxiety, insomnia, hand tingling, tremor, flushing, sweating. Overdosage produces hypotension, somnolence, lethargy, irritability, bradycardia, miosis (pupillary constriction).

PATIENT CONSIDERATIONS

BASELINE ASSESSMENT

Obtain B/P immediately before each dose administration, in addition to regular monitoring (be alert to B/P fluctuations).

INTERVENTION/EVALUATION

Sedative effect, drowsiness may require assistance w/ambulation, especially during early therapy. Assess for peripheral edema of hands, feet (usually, first area of low extremity swelling is behind medial malleolus). Assess skin for development of rash. If excessive reduction in B/P occurs, place pt in supine position w/legs elevated. Assess for anorexia secondary to decreased taste perception. Monitor pattern of daily bowel activity and stool consistency.

PATIENT/FAMILY TEACHING

Side effects may occur during first 2 wks of therapy but generally diminish or disappear during continued therapy. Sugarless gum, sips of tepid water may relieve dry mouth. Skipping

G

doses or voluntarily discontinuing drug may produce severe, rebound hypertension. Avoid alcohol. Use caution driving or operating machinery until tolerance to medication established.

guanadrel sulfate

gwan-ah-drel
(Hylorel)

PREGNANCY CATEGORY B

CLASSIFICATION

Antihypertensive

AVAILABILITY (Rx)

Tablets: 10 mg, 25 mg

PHARMACODYNAMICS

	ONSET	PEAK	DURATION
Oral	2 hrs	4–6 hrs	—

PHARMACOKINETICS

Absorption: Rapidly, completely absorbed from GI tract. Widely distributed. **Metabolism:** Metabolized in liver. **Excretion:** Primarily excreted in urine. **Half-life:** 10 hrs.

ACTION/*THERAPEUTIC EFFECT*

Depletes norepinephrine from adrenergic nerve endings, *reducing B/P.* Prevents release of norepinephrine normally produced by nerve stimulation.

USES

Treatment of hypertension in those not controlled w/thiazide-type diuretic. Combine w/diuretic therapy for optimum control of B/P.

ADMINISTRATION

ORAL:

- May give w/o regard to food.
- Tablets may be crushed.

INDICATIONS/ROUTES/DOSAGE

Hypertension:
Oral: Adults: Initially, 5 mg 2 times/day. Increase at 1–4 wk intervals. ***Elderly:*** Initially, 5 mg/day. May gradually increase at 1–4 wk intervals. ***Maintenance:*** 20–75 mg/day in 2 divided doses.

CONTRAINDICATIONS

Frank CHF, pheochromocytoma.

EXTREME CAUTION

CHF, regional vascular disease.

CAUTIONS

Elderly, bronchial asthma, peptic ulcer.

INTERACTIONS

DRUG: *Tricyclic antidepressants, MAO inhibitors, phenothiazines, sympathomimetics* may decrease antihypertensive effect. **HERBAL:** None known. **FOOD:** None significant. **ALTERED LAB VALUES:** None significant.

SIDE EFFECTS

FREQUENT (30–65%): Fatigue, headache, faintness, drowsiness, nocturia, urinary frequency, change in weight, aching limbs. OCCASIONAL (10–30%): Cough, shortness of breath (resting), Change in vision, confusion, constipation, decreased appetite, peripheral edema, leg cramps. RARE (<10%): Depression, altered sleep, nausea, vomiting, dry mouth, throat, impotence, backache, joint pain.

ADVERSE REACTIONS/TOXIC EFFECTS

Overdose may produce blurred vision, severe dizziness/faintness.

PATIENT CONSIDERATIONS

Baseline Assessment

Obtain B/P immediately before each dose, in addition to regular monitoring (be alert to B/P fluctuations). Therapy should be discontinued 2–3 days before elective surgery. Advise anesthesiologist of drug therapy if emergency surgery is necessary.

Intervention/Evaluation

Monitor pattern of daily bowel activity and stool consistency. If excessive reduction in B/P occurs, place pt in supine position w/legs elevated. Assess for peripheral edema of hands, feet (usually, first area of low extremity swelling is behind medial malleolus in ambulatory, sacral area in bedridden). Monitor both erect and supine B/P.

Patient/Family Teaching

To reduce hypotensive effect, rise slowly from lying to sitting position and permit legs to dangle from bed momentarily before standing. Avoid sudden or prolonged standing, exercise, hot environment or hot shower, alcohol ingestion, particularly in morning (may aggravate orthostatic hypotension). If dizziness or weakness occurs, sit or lie down immediately. If nausea occurs, cola, unsalted crackers, or dry toast may relieve effect. Sugarless gum, sips of tepid water may relieve dry mouth.

guanfacine

gwan-**fah**-seen
(Tenex)

PREGNANCY CATEGORY B

CLASSIFICATION

Antihypertensive

AVAILABILITY (Rx)

Tablets: 1 mg, 2 mg

PHARMACODYNAMICS

	ONSET	PEAK	DURATION
Oral	—	1–4 hrs	—

PHARMACOKINETICS

Absorption: Rapidly, completely absorbed from GI tract. Widely distributed. **Metabolism:** Metabolized in liver. **Excretion:** Primarily excreted in urine. **Half-life:** 10–30 hrs.

ACTION/*THERAPEUTIC EFFECT*

Stimulates alpha$_2$-adrenergic receptors. Inhibits sympathetic cardioaccelerator and vasoconstrictor center to heart, kidneys, peripheral vasculature. *Decreases systolic, diastolic B/P.* Chronic use *decreases peripheral vascular resistance.*

USES/*UNLABELED*

Management of hypertension alone or in combination w/other antihypertensives, especially thiazide-type diuretics. *Attention deficit hyperactivity disorder (ADHD), tic disorders.*

ADMINISTRATION

ORAL:

- Give w/o regard to food.
- Tablets may be crushed.
- Administer at bedtime (minimizes daytime drowsiness).

INDICATIONS/ROUTES/DOSAGE

Hypertension:

Oral: Adults, elderly: Initially, 1 mg/day. Increase by 1 mg/day at intervals of 3–4 wks up to 3 mg/day in single or divided doses.

CONTRAINDICATIONS

None significant.

CAUTIONS

Impaired renal function.

INTERACTIONS

DRUG: *Beta-$_1$ adrenergic blockers, hypotension-producing medications* may increase antihypertensive effect. HERBAL: None known. FOOD: None significant. ALTERED LAB VALUES: May increase growth hormone concentration. May decrease urinary catecholamine, VMA excretion.

SIDE EFFECTS

FREQUENT (>10%): Constipation, dizziness, drowsiness, dry mouth. OCCASIONAL (2–10%): Confusion, depression, conjunctivitis (dry, itching, burning eyes), decreased sexual ability, headache, nausea, vomiting, inability to sleep, unusually tired.

ADVERSE REACTIONS/TOXIC EFFECTS

Overdosage may produce difficult breathing, dizziness, faintness, severe drowsiness, bradycardia.

PATIENT CONSIDERATIONS

Baseline Assessment

Obtain B/P and pulse immediately before each dose. Withhold medication and notify physician if systolic B/P <90 mm Hg and/or pulse rate <60/min.

Intervention/Evaluation

Monitor B/P, pulse. Sedative effect, drowsiness may require assistance w/ambulation, especially during early therapy. If excessive B/P reduction occurs, place pt in supine position w/legs elevated.

Patient/Family Teaching

Sugarless gum or sips of tepid water may help relieve dry mouth. Avoid tasks that require alertness, motor skills until drug response is established. Side effects usually diminish w/continued therapy. Tolerance to alcohol or other CNS depressants may be reduced. Do not abruptly withdraw medication after long-term use. Therapeutic effect may take 1 wk; peak effect noted in 1–3 mos. Best taken at bedtime.

halcinonide

(Halog)
See Classification section under: Corticosteroids: topical

halobetasol

(Ultravate)
See Classification section under: Corticosteroids: topical

haloperidol

hal-oh-**pear**-ih-dawl
(Haldol)

CANADIAN AVAILABILITY

Apo-Haloperidol, Haldol, Novo-peridol, Peridol

PREGNANCY CATEGORY C

CLASSIFICATION

Antipsychotic

AVAILABILITY (Rx)

Tablets: 0.5 mg, 1 mg, 2 mg, 5 mg, 10 mg, 20 mg. **Oral Concentrate:** 2 mg/ml. **Injection:** 5 mg/ml. **Injection (Decanoate):** 50 mg/ml, 100 mg/ml.

PHARMACOKINETICS

Absorption: Readily absorbed from GI tract. **Metabolism:** Extensively metabolized in liver. **Excretion:** Primarily excreted in urine. **Half-life:** *Oral:* 12–37 hrs; *IM:* 17–25 hrs, *IV:* 10–19 hrs.

ACTION/ *THERAPEUTIC EFFECT*

Competitively blocks postsynaptic dopamine receptors, increases turnover of brain dopamine, *producing tranquilizing effect.* Has anticholinergic, alpha-adrenergic blocking activity.

USES/ *UNLABELED*

Management of psychotic disorders, control of tics, vocal utterances in Tourette's syndrome. Used in management of severe behavioral problems in children, short-term treatment of hyperactivity in children. *Treatment of infantile autism, Huntington's chorea, nausea/vomiting associated w/cancer chemotherapy.*

STORAGE/HANDLING

Store all preparations at room temperature. Discard if precipitate forms, discoloration occurs.

ADMINISTRATION

ORAL:

- Give w/o regard to meals.
- Scored tablets may be crushed.

IM:

- Pt must remain recumbent for 30–60 min in head-low position w/legs raised to minimize hypotensive effect.
- Prepare Decanoate IM injection using 21 gauge needle.
- Do not exceed maximum volume of 3 ml per IM injection site.
- Inject slow, deep IM into upper outer quadrant of gluteus maximus.

INDICATIONS/ROUTES/DOSAGE

Note: Increase dosage gradually to optimum response, then decrease to lowest effective level for maintenance. Replace parenteral therapy w/oral therapy as soon as possible.

Moderate symptoms:

Oral: Adults, elderly: Initially, 0.5–2 mg 2–3 times/day; may titrate up to 100 mg/day. *Maintenance:* Lowest effective dose.

Severe symptoms:
Oral: Adults, elderly: Initially, 3–5 mg 2–3 times/day; may titrate up to 100 mg/day. *Maintenance:* Lowest effective dose.

Usual parenteral dosage:
IM: Adults, elderly: 2–5 mg; may repeat at 1–8 hr intervals. Give oral dose 12–24 hrs after last parenteral dose administered.

Usual elderly dosage: (Nonpsychotic):
Oral: Initially, 0.25–0.5 mg 1–2 times/day. May increase by 0.25–0.5 mg q4–7days. *Maximum:* 50 mg/day.

Usual pediatric dosage:
Oral: Children (3–12 yrs): Initially, 0.5 mg/day. May increase by 0.5 mg q5–7days. Total daily dose given in 2–3 doses/day. *Psychotic disorders:* 0.05–0.15 mg/kg/day. *Nonpsychiatric disorders, Tourette's disorder:* 0.05–0.075 mg/kg/day.

CONTRAINDICATIONS

Coma, alcohol ingestion, Parkinson's disease, thyrotoxicosis.

CAUTIONS

Impaired respiratory/hepatic/cardiovascular function, alcohol withdrawal, history of seizures, urinary retention, glaucoma, prostatic hypertrophy, elderly.

INTERACTIONS

DRUG: *Alcohol, CNS depressants* may increase CNS depression. *Epinephrine* may block alpha-adrenergic effects. *Extrapyramidal symptom (EPS)-producing medications* may increase EPS. *Lithium* may increase neurologic toxicity. HERBAL: None known. FOOD: None significant. **ALTERED LAB VALUES:** None significant.

SIDE EFFECTS

FREQUENT: Blurred vision, constipation, dry mouth, swelling or soreness of female breasts, increased weight. OCCASIONAL: Allergic reaction, difficulty urinating, decreased thirst, dizziness, lightheadedness, decreased sexual ability, drowsiness, nausea, vomiting, increased skin sensitivity to sunlight, lethargy, transient leukopenia.

ADVERSE REACTIONS/TOXIC EFFECTS

Extrapyramidal symptoms appear to be dose related and may be noted in first few days of therapy. Marked drowsiness and lethargy, excessive salivation, fixed stare may be mild to severe in intensity. Less frequently seen are severe akathisia (motor restlessness) and acute dystonias: torticollis (neck muscle spasm), opisthotonos (rigidity of back muscles), and oculogyric crisis (rolling back of eyes). Tardive dyskinesia (protrusion of tongue, puffing of cheeks, chewing/puckering of the mouth) may occur during long-term administration or following drug discontinuance, and may be irreversible. Risk is greater in female geriatric pts. Abrupt withdrawal following long-term therapy may provoke transient dyskinesia signs.

PATIENT CONSIDERATIONS

BASELINE ASSESSMENT

Assess behavior, appearance, emotional status, response to environment, speech pattern, thought content.

INTERVENTION/EVALUATION

Supervise suicidal risk pt close-

ly during early therapy (as depression lessens, energy level improves, causing increased suicide potential). Monitor B/P for hypotension. Assess for peripheral edema behind medial malleolus (sacral area in bedridden pts). Assess stool consistency and frequency. Monitor for rigidity, tremor, mask-like facial expression, fine tongue movement. Assess for therapeutic response (interest in surroundings, improvement in self-care, increased ability to concentrate, relaxed facial expression).

PATIENT/FAMILY TEACHING

Full therapeutic effect may take up to 6 wks. Do not abruptly withdraw from long-term drug therapy. Report visual disturbances. Sugarless gum, sips of tepid water may relieve dry mouth. Drowsiness generally subsides during continued therapy. Avoid tasks that require alertness, motor skills until response to drug is established. Avoid alcohol. Report sore throat, fever, rash, change in vision, involuntary muscle twitching, muscle stiffness. Avoid exposure to sunlight, overheating, and dehydration (increased risk heat stroke).

haloprogin

(Halotex)

See Classification section under: Antifungals: topical

heparin sodium

hep-ah-rin

(Liquaemin)

CANADIAN AVAILABILITY

Hepalean

PREGNANCY CATEGORY B

CLASSIFICATION

Anticoagulant

AVAILABILITY (Rx)

Injection: 10 units/ml, 100 units/ml, 1,000 units/ml, 2,500 units/ml, 5,000 units/ml, 7,500 units/ml, 10,000 units/ml, 20,000 units/ml, 40,000 units/ml, 25,000 units/500 ml infusion

PHARMACOKINETICS

Absorption: Well absorbed after SubQ administration. **Metabolism:** Metabolized in liver, removed from circulation by uptake by reticuloendothelial system. **Excretion:** Primarily excreted in urine. **Half-life:** 1–6 hrs.

ACTION/*THERAPEUTIC EFFECT*

Blocks conversion of prothrombin to thrombin and fibrinogen to fibrin. *Prevents further extension of existing thrombi or new clot formation.* No effect on existing clots.

USES

Prophylaxis, treatment of venous thrombosis, pulmonary embolism, peripheral arterial embolism, atrial fibrillation w/embolism. Prevention of thromboembolus in cardiac and vascular surgery, dialysis procedures, blood transfusions, and blood sampling for laboratory purposes. Adjunct in treatment of coronary occlusion w/acute MI. Maintains patency of indwelling intravascular devices. Diagnosis and treatment of acute/chronic consumptive coagulation pathology (e.g., DIC). Prevents cerebral thrombosis in progressive strokes.

H

STORAGE/HANDLING

Store parenteral form at room temperature.

ADMINISTRATION

Note: Do *not* give by IM injection (pain, hematoma, ulceration, erythema).

SubQ:

- **Note:** Used in low-dose therapy.
- After withdrawal of heparin from vial, change needle before injection (prevents leakage along needle track).
- Inject above iliac crest or in abdominal fat layer. Do not inject within 2 inches of umbilicus, or any scar tissue.
- Withdraw needle rapidly, apply prolonged pressure at injection site. Do not massage.
- Rotate injection sites.

IV:

- **Note:** Used in full-dose therapy. Intermittent IV produces higher incidence of bleeding abnormalities. Continuous IV preferred.
- Dilute IV infusion in isotonic sterile saline, 5% dextrose in water, or lactated Ringer's.
- Invert container at least 6 times (ensures mixing, prevents pooling of medication).
- Use constant-rate IV infusion pump or microdrip.

INDICATIONS/ROUTES/DOSAGE

Note: Dosage expressed in USP units. Dosage requirements highly individualized.

SubQ: Adults, elderly: 5,000 units IV injection and 10,000–20,000 units SubQ, followed by 8,000–10,000 units q8h or 15,000–20,000 units q12h.

Prophylaxis of postop thrombosis:
SubQ: Adults, elderly: 5,000 units given 2 hrs before surgery, then q8–12h after surgery for 5–7 days or when pt is ambulatory.

Full-dose therapy:
Continuous IV: Adults, elderly: 5,000 units IV injection to start, followed by 20,000–40,000 units IV infusion given over 24 hrs. ***Children:*** 50 units/kg IV to start, followed by 20,000 units/m^2 continuous IV infusion per 24 hrs.
Intermittent IV: Adults, elderly: 10,000 units to start, followed by 5,000–10,000 units q4–6h. ***Children:*** 100 units/kg to start, followed by 50–100 units/kg q4h.

Maintaining patency of indwelling intravascular devices:
IV: Adults, elderly: 10–100 units injected into diaphragm of device after each use, designated interval, or as necessary.

CONTRAINDICATIONS

Bleeding abnormalities, vitamin K insufficiency, chronic alcoholism, severe hepatic/renal disease, salicylate therapy, severe hypertension, pregnancy, hypersensitivity to heparin, ergot alkaloids, lidocaine; peripheral artery disease, coronary insufficiency, angina, sepsis, thrombocytopenia, brain/spinal cord surgery, spinal anesthesia, eye surgery, oral anticoagulants.

CAUTIONS

Severe hypertension, peripheral vascular disease, indwelling catheters, those >60 yrs, factors increasing risk of hemorrhage, diabetes, mild hepatic/renal disease.

INTERACTIONS

DRUG: ***Anticoagulants, platelet aggregation inhibitors, thrombolytics*** may increase risk of bleeding. ***Antithyroid medications, cef-***

operazone, cefotetan, valproic acid may cause hypoprothrombinemia. *Probenecid* may increase effect. **HERBAL:** Feverfew effect may be decreased. Ginkgo may increase risk of bleeding. **FOOD:** None significant. **ALTERED LAB VALUES:** May increase free fatty acids, SGOT (AST), SGPT (ALT). May decrease triglycerides, cholesterol.

SIDE EFFECTS

OCCASIONAL: Itching, burning, particularly on soles of feet (due to vasospastic reaction). **RARE:** Pain, cyanosis of extremity 6–10 days after initial therapy, lasts 4–6 hrs; hypersensitivity reaction (chills, fever, pruritus, urticaria, asthma, rhinitis, lacrimation, headache).

ADVERSE REACTIONS/TOXIC EFFECTS

Bleeding complications ranging from local ecchymoses to major hemorrhage occur more frequently in high-dose therapy, intermittent IV infusion, and in women >60 yrs. ***Antidote:*** Protamine sulfate 1–1.5 mg for q 100 units heparin SubQ if overdosage occurred before 30 min, 0.5–0.75 mg for q 100 units heparin SubQ if overdosage occurred within 30–60 min, 0.25–0.375 mg for q 100 units heparin SubQ if 2 hrs have elapsed since overdosage, 25–50 mg if heparin given by IV infusion.

PATIENT CONSIDERATIONS

BASELINE ASSESSMENT

Cross-check dose w/co-worker. Determine activated partial thromboplastin time (APTT) before administration and 24 hrs after initiation of therapy, then 24–48 hrs for first week of therapy or until maintenance dose is established. Follow with APTT determinations 1–2 times weekly for 3–4 wks. Long-term therapy: 1–2 times/month.

INTERVENTION/EVALUATION

Monitor APTT (therapeutic dosage at 1.5–2.5 times normal) diligently. Assess hematocrit, platelet count, urine/stool culture for occult blood, SGOT (AST), SGPT (ALT), regardless of route of administration. Assess for decrease in B/P, increase in pulse rate, complaint of abdominal or back pain, severe headache (may be evidence of hemorrhage). Question for increase in amount of discharge during menses. Check peripheral pulses; skin for bruises, petechiae. Check for excessive bleeding from minor cuts, scratches. Assess gums for erythema, gingival bleeding. Assess urine output for hematuria. Avoid IM injections of other medications because of potential for hematomas. When converting to warfarin therapy, monitor PT results (will be 10–20% higher while heparin is given concurrently).

PATIENT/FAMILY TEACHING

Use electric razor, soft toothbrush to prevent bleeding. Report any sign of red or dark urine, black or red stool, coffee-ground vomitus, red-speckled mucus from cough. Do not use any OTC medication w/o physician approval (may interfere w/platelet aggregation). Wear/carry identification that notes anticoagulant therapy. Inform dentist, other physicians of heparin therapy.

---

hepatitis A

(Havrix, Vaqta)

See Supplement

hetastarch

het-ah-starch
(Hespan, Hextend)

PREGNANCY CATEGORY C

CLASSIFICATION

Plasma volume expander

AVAILABILITY (Rx)

Injection: 6 g/100 ml 0.9% NaCl (500 ml infusion container)

PHARMACOKINETICS

Excretion: Smaller molecules (<50,000 molecular weight) rapidly excreted by kidneys; larger molecules (>50,000 molecular weight) slowly degraded to smaller sized molecules, then excreted. **Half-life:** 17 days.

ACTION/*THERAPEUTIC EFFECT*

Exerts osmotic pull on tissue fluids; *reducing hemoconcentration and blood viscosity, increasing circulating blood volume.*

USES

Fluid replacement and plasma volume expansion in treatment of shock due to hemorrhage, burns, surgery, sepsis, trauma, leukapheresis.

STORAGE/HANDLING

Store solutions at room temperature. Solution should appear clear, pale yellow to amber. Do not use if discolored (deep turbid brown) or if precipitate forms.

ADMINISTRATION

IV:

- Administer only by IV infusion.
- Do not add drugs or mix w/other IV fluids.
- In acute hemorrhagic shock, administer at rate approaching 1.2 g/kg (20 ml/kg) per hour. Use slower rates for burns, septic shock.
- Monitor central venous pressure (CVP) when given by rapid infusion. If there is a precipitous rise in CVP, immediately discontinue drug (overexpansion of blood volume).

INDICATIONS/ROUTES/DOSAGE

Plasma volume expansion:
IV: Adults, elderly: 500–1,000 ml/day up to 1,500 ml/day (20 mg/kg) at a rate up to 20 ml/kg/hr in hemorrhagic shock (slower rates for burns or septic shock).

Leukapheresis:
IV: Adults, elderly: 250–700 ml infused at constant rate, usually 1:8 to venous whole blood.

CONTRAINDICATIONS

Severe bleeding disorders, severe CHF, oliguria, anuria.

CAUTIONS

Thrombocytopenia, elderly or very young, pulmonary edema, CHF, impaired renal function, hepatic disease, those on sodium restriction.

INTERACTIONS

DRUG: None significant. **HERBAL:** None known. **FOOD:** None significant. **ALTERED LAB VALUES:** May prolong prothrombin time (PT), partial thromboplastin time (PTT), bleeding, and clotting times; decrease hematocrit.

SIDE EFFECTS

RARE: Allergic reaction resulting in vomiting, mild temperature elevation, chills, itching; submaxillary and parotid gland enlargement, peripheral edema of lower extremities, mild flulike symptoms: headache, muscle aches.

ADVERSE REACTIONS/TOXIC EFFECTS

Fluid overload (headache, weakness, blurred vision, behavioral changes, incoordination, isolated muscle twitching) and pulmonary edema (rapid breathing, rales, wheezing, coughing, increased B/P, distended neck veins) may occur. Anaphylactoid reaction may be observed as periorbital edema, urticaria, wheezing.

PATIENT CONSIDERATIONS

INTERVENTION/EVALUATION

Monitor for fluid overload (peripheral and/or pulmonary edema, impending CHF symptoms). Assess lung sounds for wheezing, rales. During leukapheresis, monitor CBC, leukocyte and platelet counts, differential, hemoglobin, hematocrit, PT, PTT, I&O. Monitor central venous B/P (detects overexpansion of blood volume). Monitor urine output closely (increase in output generally occurs in oliguric pts after administration). Assess for periorbital edema, itching, wheezing, urticaria (allergic reaction). Monitor for oliguria, anuria, any change in output ratio. Monitor for bleeding from surgical or trauma sites.

hyaluronate sodium

hi-al-**your**-on-ate
(Hyalgan, Synvisc)
Hyalgan, Synvisc

PREGNANCY CATEGORY C

CLASSIFICATION

Anti-arthritic

AVAILABILITY (Rx)

Solution: 20 mg/2 ml, 16 mg/2 ml

PHARMACOKINETICS

Absorption: Widely distributed in synovial and capsular tissues and intracellular fluids. Permeates articular cartilage, through joint tissues and passes through the lymph system into systemic circulation. **Metabolism:** Metabolized in the liver, yielding carbon dioxide and water in 7 days. **Excretion:** Once yielding CO_2 and H_20, it immediately clears the joint and does not accumulate in any body tissues.

ACTION/*THERAPEUTIC EFFECT*

Naturally occurring; supports the lubricating and shock-absorbing properties of auricular cartilage, *improving elasticity and viscosity of synovial fluid.*

USES

For the treatment of osteoarthritis of the knee in those who have failed to respond adequately to conservative nonpharmacologic therapy and simple analgesics.

ADMINISTRATION

INTRA-ARTICULAR:

- Do not prepare injection site with skin disinfectants containing quaternary ammonium salts (precipitate of drug can occur).
- Do not give other intra-articular injections concurrently.
- If treatment is bilateral, use a separate 2 ml vial/syringe for each knee.
- Remove effusion, if present, before drug administration.

- Do not use same syringe for removing effusion fluid and injecting hyaluronate.

INDICATIONS/DOSAGE/ROUTES

Osteoarthritis:
Intra-articular: Adults, elderly: **Hyalgan:** 5 injections per treatment cycle. **Synvisc:** 3 injections per treatment cycle.

CONTRAINDICATIONS

History of hypersensitivity to hyaluronate; infections or skin diseases in area of injection site; concurrent skin disinfectants containing quaternary ammonium salts (may cause drug precipitate).

CAUTIONS

Severely inflamed knee joints, evidence of lymphatic or venous stasis in treatment leg, allergy to avian proteins, feathers, egg products.

INTERACTIONS

DRUG: None significant. **HERBAL:** None known. **FOOD:** None significant. **ALTERED LAB VALUES:** None significant.

SIDE EFFECTS

Hyalgan:
FREQUENT (14–23%): Injection site pain, headache, skin reaction (ecchymosis, rash). **OCCASIONAL (7%):** Pruritus.

Synvisc:
OCCASIONAL (7%): Knee pain or swelling. **RARE (1–2%):** Rash on thorax and back, pruritus, calf cramps, ankle edema, muscle pain.

ADVERSE REACTIONS/TOXIC EFFECTS

Tachyarrhythmia, phlebitis with varicosity. Hypersensitivity reaction occurs rarely but does not recur following subsequent administration.

PATIENT CONSIDERATIONS

Baseline Assessment

Assess knee joint for swelling, tenderness, pain as baseline to monitor for therapeutic effect. If effusion is present, must be removed before therapy begins.

Intervention/Evaluation

Assess for therapeutic response (relief from pain, improved mobility, decreased swelling, reduced tenderness).

Patient/Family Teaching

Transient pain/swelling of the treated joint may occur, especially in those with rheumatoid or gouty arthritis. Avoid strenuous or prolonged (>1 hr) weight-bearing activities (e.g., jogging, tennis) within 48 hrs after treatment. Pain relief may not be noted until after the last injection.

hydralazine hydrochloride

hy-**dral**-ah-zeen
(Apresoline)

FIXED-COMBINATION(S)
W/hydrochlorothiazide, a diuretic **(Apresodex, Apresoline-Esidrex, Apresazide, Hydralazine PLUS, Hydrazide)**; w/reserpine, an antihypertensive **(Serpasil-Apresoline)**; w/hydrochlorothiazide and reserpine **(Cherapas, Ser-Ap-Es, Serathide)**.

CANADIAN AVAILABILITY
Apresoline, Novohylazin

PREGNANCY CATEGORY C

CLASSIFICATION

Antihypertensive

AVAILABILITY (Rx)

Tablets: 10 mg, 25 mg, 50 mg, 100 mg. **Injection:** 20 mg/ml.

PHARMACODYNAMICS

	ONSET	PEAK	DURATION
Oral	10–20 min	0.5–2 hrs	2–4 hrs

PHARMACOKINETICS

Absorption: Well absorbed from GI tract. Widely distributed. **Metabolism:** Metabolized in liver to active metabolite. **Excretion:** Primarily excreted in urine. **Half-life:** 3–7 hrs (increased in decreased renal function).

ACTION/*THERAPEUTIC EFFECT*

Directly relaxes vascular smooth muscle (greater effect on arterioles), *reducing B/P.* Produces decreased peripheral vascular resistance, increased heart rate, cardiac output. Decreases afterload (increases CO, decreases systemic resistance).

USES/*UNLABELED*

Management of moderate/severe hypertension. *Treatment of congestive heart failure.*

STORAGE/HANDLING

Store oral form at room temperature.

ADMINISTRATION

ORAL:

- Best given w/food or regularly spaced meals.
- Tablets may be crushed.

INDICATIONS/ROUTES/DOSAGE

Hypertension:

Oral: Adults: Initially, 10 mg 4 times/day for 2–4 days. Increase to 25 mg 4 times/day for remainder of first week. Increase second week and subsequent weeks to 50 mg 4 times/day. *Elderly:* Initially, 10 mg 2–3 times/day. May increase by 10–25 mg/day q2–5days. *Children:* Initially, 0.75 mg/kg in 4 divided doses (maximum 25 mg). May be increased over 1–4 wks up to 7.5 mg/kg/day or 200 mg/day.

IM/IV: Adults, elderly: 20–40 mg. Children: 0.1–0.2 mg/kg/dose.

CONTRAINDICATIONS

Coronary artery disease, rheumatic heart disease, lupus erythematosus.

CAUTIONS

Impaired renal function, cerebrovascular disease.

INTERACTIONS

DRUG: *Diuretics, other hypotensives* may increase hypotensive effect. **HERBAL:** None known. **FOOD:** None significant. **ALTERED LAB VALUES:** May produce positive direct Coombs' test.

SIDE EFFECTS

FREQUENT: Diarrhea, palpitations, tachycardia, headache, decreased appetite, nausea, vomiting. **OCCASIONAL:** Angina, numbness of hands/feet, fluid retention, edema, lupus erythematosis–like reaction (fever, facial rash, muscle and joint aches, splenomegaly), dizziness, flushed face, shortness of breath, nasal congestion.

H

ADVERSE REACTIONS/TOXIC EFFECTS

Severe orthostatic hypotension, generalized skin flushing, severe headache, myocardial ischemia, cardiac arrhythmias may develop. Profound shock may occur in cases of severe overdosage.

PATIENT CONSIDERATIONS

Baseline Assessment

Obtain B/P, pulse immediately before each dose administration, in addition to regular monitoring (be alert to fluctuations). Keep tissues readily available at pt's bedside for lacrimation, nasal congestion.

Intervention/Evaluation

Assess for peripheral edema of hands, feet (usually, first area of low extremity swelling is behind medial malleolus in ambulatory, sacral area in bedridden). Monitor temperature for fever (lupus-like reaction). Monitor pattern of daily bowel activity and stool consistency.

Patient/Family Teaching

To reduce hypotensive effect, rise slowly from lying to sitting position and permit legs to dangle from bed momentarily before standing. Unsalted crackers, dry toast may relieve nausea. Report muscle and joint aches, fever (lupus-like reaction).

hydrochlorothiazide

high-drow-chlor-oh-**thigh**-ah-zide
(HydroDIURIL, Esidrix, Microzide, Oretic)

FIXED-COMBINATION(S)

W/methyldopa, an antihypertensive **(Aldoril)**; w/propranolol, a beta blocker **(Inderide)**; w/hydralazine, a vasodilator **(Apresazide)**; w/candesartan, an angiotensin II inhibitor **(Atacand HCT)**; w/captopril, an ACE inhibitor **(Capozide)**; w/enalapril, an ACE inhibitor **(Vaseretic)**; w/irbesartan, an angiotensin II inhibitor **(Avalide)**; w/losartan, an angiotensin II inhibitor **(Hyzaar)**; w/metoprolol, a beta blocker **(Lopressor HCT)**; w/moexipril, an ACE inhibitor **(Uniretic)**; w/timolol, a beta blocker **(Timolide)**; w/labetolol, an alpha-beta blocker **(Normozide)**; w/potassium-sparing diuretics (amiloride) **[Moduretic]** (spironolactone) **[Aldactazide]** (triamterene) **[Dyazide, Maxzide]**; w/quinapril, an ACE inhibitor **(Accuretic)**; w/telmisartan, an angiotensin II inhibitor **(Micardis HCT)**; w/valsartan, an angiotensin II inhibitor **(Diovan HCT)**.

CANADIAN AVAILABILITY

Apo-Hydro, Hydrodiuril

PREGNANCY CATEGORY D

CLASSIFICATION

Diuretic: Thiazide

AVAILABILITY (Rx)

Capsules: 12.5 mg. **Tablets:** 25 mg, 50 mg, 100 mg. **Oral Solution:** 50 mg/5 ml, 100 mg/ml.

PHARMACODYNAMICS

	ONSET	PEAK	DURATION
Oral (diuretic)			
	2 hrs	4–6 hrs	6–12 hrs

PHARMACOKINETICS

Absorption: Variably absorbed from GI tract. **Excretion:** Primarily excreted unchanged in liver. **Half-life:** 5.6–14.8 hrs.

ACTION/*THERAPEUTIC EFFECT*

Diuretic: Blocks reabsorption of

water, electrolytes (sodium, potassium) at cortical diluting segment of distal tubule, *promoting renal excretion.* ***Antihypertensive:*** Reduces plasma, extracellular fluid volume, decreases peripheral vascular resistance (PVR) by direct effect on blood vessels, *reducing B/P.*

USES / *UNLABELED*

Adjunctive therapy in edema associated w/CHF, hepatic cirrhosis, corticoid or estrogen therapy, renal impairment. In treatment of hypertension, may be used alone or w/other antihypertensive agents. *Treatment of diabetes insipidus; prevents calcium-containing renal stones.*

ADMINISTRATION

ORAL:

- May give w/food or milk if GI upset occurs, preferably w/breakfast (may prevent nocturia).

INDICATIONS / ROUTES / DOSAGE

Edema:
Oral: Adults: Initially, 25–200 mg in 1–3 divided doses. ***Maintenance:*** 25–100 mg/day. ***Maximum:*** 200 mg/day.

Hypertension:
Oral: Adults: Initially, 12.5–25 mg/day. Gradually increase up to 50 mg/day. ***Maintenance:*** 25–50 mg/day.

Usual elderly dosage:
Oral: 12.5–25 mg/day.

Usual dosage for children:
Oral: Children 2–12 yrs: 37.5–100 mg/day. ***Children <2 yrs:*** 12.5–37.5 mg/day.

CONTRAINDICATIONS

History of hypersensitivity to sulfonamides or thiazide diuretics, renal decompensation, anuria.

CAUTIONS

Severe renal disease, impaired hepatic function, diabetes mellitus, elderly/debilitated, thyroid disorders.

INTERACTIONS

DRUG: ***Cholestyramine, colestipol*** may decrease absorption, effects. May increase ***digoxin*** toxicity (due to hypokalemia). May increase ***lithium*** toxicity. **HERBAL:** None known. **FOOD:** None significant. **ALTERED LAB VALUES:** May increase bilirubin, serum calcium, LDL, cholesterol, triglycerides, creatinine, glucose, uric acid. May decrease urinary calcium, magnesium, potassium, sodium.

SIDE EFFECTS

EXPECTED: Increase in urine frequency/volume. **FREQUENT:** Potassium depletion. **OCCASIONAL:** Postural hypotension, headache, GI disturbances, photosensitivity reaction.

ADVERSE REACTIONS / TOXIC EFFECTS

Vigorous diuresis may lead to profound water loss and electrolyte depletion, resulting in hypokalemia, hyponatremia, dehydration. Acute hypotensive episodes may occur. Hyperglycemia may be noted during prolonged therapy. GI upset, pancreatitis, dizziness, paresthesias, headache, blood dyscrasias, pulmonary edema, allergic pneumonitis, dermatologic reactions occur rarely. Overdosage can lead to lethargy, coma w/o changes in electrolytes or hydration.

PATIENT CONSIDERATIONS

BASELINE ASSESSMENT

Check vital signs, especially B/P for hypotension prior to adminis-

tration. Assess baseline electrolytes; particularly check for low potassium. Evaluate edema, skin turgor, mucous membranes for hydration status. Assess muscle strength, mental status. Note skin temperature, moisture. Obtain baseline weight. Initiate I&O.

INTERVENTION/EVALUATION

Continue to monitor B/P, vital signs, electrolytes, I&O, weight. Note extent of diuresis. Watch for changes from initial assessment (hypokalemia may result in weakness, tremor, muscle cramps, nausea, vomiting, change in mental status, tachycardia; hyponatremia may result in confusion, thirst, cold/clammy skin). Be especially alert for potassium depletion in pts taking digoxin (cardiac arrhythmias). Potassium supplements are frequently ordered. Check for constipation (may occur w/exercise diuresis).

PATIENT/FAMILY TEACHING

Expect increased frequency and volume of urination. To reduce hypotensive effect, rise slowly from lying to sitting position and permit legs to dangle momentarily before standing. Eat foods high in potassium such as whole grains (cereals), legumes, meat, bananas, apricots, orange juice, potatoes (white, sweet), raisins. Protect skin from sun/ultraviolet rays (photosensitivity may occur).

hydrocodone bitartrate

high-drough-**koe**-doan

FIXED-COMBINATION(S)

W/acetaminophen **(Anexsia, Lortab, Vicodin, Vicodin HP, Zydone)**; w/aspirin **(Lortab ASA)**; w/chlorpheniramine, an antihistamine **(Tussionex)**; w/ibuprofen, a NSAID **(Vicoprofen)**; w/phenypropanolamine, a sympathomimetic **(Hycomine)**.

CANADIAN AVAILABILITY

Hycodan, Robidone

PREGNANCY CATEGORY C

(D if used for prolonged periods or at high doses at term)

CLASSIFICATION

Opioid: Analgesic **(Schedule III)**

PHARMACODYNAMICS

	ONSET	PEAK	DURATION
Oral	—	—	4–6 hrs

PHARMACOKINETICS

Absorption: Well absorbed from GI tract. **Metabolism:** Metabolized in liver. **Excretion:** Primarily excreted in urine. **Half-life:** 3.8 hrs (increased in elderly).

ACTION / *THERAPEUTIC EFFECT*

Binds at opiate receptor sites in CNS. *Reduces intensity of pain stimuli incoming from sensory nerve endings, altering pain perception and emotional response to pain; suppresses cough reflex.*

USES

Relief of moderate to moderately severe pain, nonproductive cough.

ADMINISTRATION

ORAL:

- Give w/o regard to meals.
- Tablets may be crushed.

INDICATIONS/ROUTES/DOSAGE

Analgesia:
Oral: Adults, children >12 yrs: 5–10 mg q4–6h. *Elderly:* 2.5–5 mg q4–6h.

Antitussive:
Oral: Adults: 5–10 mg q4–6h as needed. ***Maximum:*** 15 mg/dose. ***Children:*** 0.6 mg/kg/day in 3–4 divided doses at intervals of no less than 4 hrs. ***Maximum single dose in children 2–12 yrs:*** 5 mg. ***Maximum single dose in children <2 yrs:*** 1.25 mg.

Extended-release:
Oral: Adults: 10 mg q12h. ***Children 6–12 yrs:*** 5 mg q12h.

CONTRAINDICATIONS

None significant.

EXTREME CAUTION

CNS depression, anoxia, hypercapnia, respiratory depression, seizures, acute alcoholism, shock, untreated myxedema, respiratory dysfunction.

CAUTIONS

Increased intracranial pressure, impaired hepatic function, acute abdominal conditions, hypothyroidism, prostatic hypertrophy, Addison's disease, urethral stricture, COPD.

INTERACTIONS

DRUG: ***Alcohol, CNS depressants*** may increase CNS or respiratory depression, hypotension. ***MAO inhibitors*** may produce severe, fatal reaction (reduce dose to 1/4 usual dose). **HERBAL:** None known. **FOOD:** None significant. **ALTERED LAB VALUES:** May increase amylase, lipase plasma concentrations.

SIDE EFFECTS

Note: Effects are dependent on dosage amount but occur infrequently w/oral antitussives. Ambulatory pts and those not in severe pain may experience dizziness, nausea, vomiting, hypotension more frequently than those who are in supine position or having severe pain. **FREQUENT:** Histamine release reaction (decreased blood pressure, increased sweating, flushed face, wheezing), dizziness, drowsiness, hypotension, unusually tired. **OCCASIONAL:** Trouble breathing, decreased urination, blurred vision, constipation, dry mouth, euphoria, headache, nausea, vomiting, difficult/painful urination.

ADVERSE REACTIONS/TOXIC EFFECTS

Overdosage results in respiratory depression, skeletal muscle flaccidity, cold clammy skin, cyanosis, extreme somnolence progressing to convulsions, stupor, coma. Tolerance to analgesic effect, physical dependence may occur w/repeated use. Prolonged duration of action, cumulative effect may occur in those w/impaired hepatic, renal function.

PATIENT CONSIDERATIONS

Baseline Assessment

Obtain vital signs before giving medication. If respirations are 12/min or lower (20/min or lower in children), w/hold medication, contact physician.

Analgesic
Assess onset, type, location, and duration of pain. Effect of medication is reduced if full pain recurs before next dose.

Antitussive
Assess type, severity, frequency of cough, and productions.

Intervention/Evaluation

Increase fluid intake and environmental humidity to improve viscosity of lung secretions. Palpate bladder for urinary retention. Monitor pattern of daily bowel activity and stool consistency. Initiate deep breathing and coughing exercises, particularly in those w/impaired pulmonary function. Assess for clinical improvement and record onset of relief of pain or cough.

Patient/Family Teaching

Change positions slowly to avoid orthostatic hypotension. Avoid tasks that require alertness, motor skills until response to drug is established. Tolerance/dependence may occur w/prolonged use of high doses. Avoid alcohol. Report nausea, vomiting, constipation, shortness of breath, difficulty breathing. May take w/food.

---

hydrocortisone

high-droe-**core**-tah-sewn
(Cortef, Cort-Dome, Cortenema, Hydrocortone, Hytone, Locoid, Pandel)

hydrocortisone acetate

(Cortaid, Corticaine, Proctocort)

hydrocortisone cypionate

(Cortef Suspension)

hydrocortisone sodium phosphate

(Hydrocortone Phosphate)

hydrocortisone sodium succinate

(A-hydroCort, Solu-Cortef)

hydrocortisone valerate

(WestCort)

FIXED-COMBINATION(S)

W/Neomycin, an antibiotic **(Neo-Cort-Dome)**; w/Bacitracin, Neomycin, Polymyxin B, anti-infectives **(Cortisporin)**; w/ciprofloxacin, an antibiotic **(Cipro HC Otic)**; hydrocortisone acetate w/Neomycin, an antibiotic **(Neo-Cortef)**, w/ciprofloxacin, an antibiotic **(Cipro HC Otic)**.

CANADIAN AVAILABILITY

Cortamed, Cortef, Cortenema, Corticreme, Westcort

CLASSIFICATION

Corticosteroid

AVAILABILITY (Rx)

Hydrocortisone: Tablets: 5 mg, 10 mg, 20 mg. **Gel:** 0.5%, 1% (OTC). **Lotion:** 0.25%, 0.5%, 1%, 2%, 2.5%. **Cream:** 0.5%, 1% (OTC), 2.5%. **Ointment:** 0.5%, 1% (OTC), 2.5%. **Topical Solution:** 1%.

Cypionate: Oral Suspension: 10 mg/5 ml.

Sodium phosphate: Injection: 50 mg/ml.

Sodium succinate: Injection: 100 mg, 250 mg, 500 mg, 1,000 mg.

Acetate: Injection: 25 mg/ml, 50 mg/ml. **Suppository:** 10 mg, 25 mg, 30 mg. **Cream:** 0.5%, 1%. **Ointment:** 0.5%, 1%.

Valerate: Cream: 0.2%.

PHARMACOKINETICS

Absorption: Well absorbed from GI tract, after IM administration. Widely distributed. **Metabolism:** Metabolized in liver. **Half-life:** *plasma:* 1.5–2 hrs; *biologic:* 8–12 hrs.

ACTION/*THERAPEUTIC EFFECT*

Inhibits accumulation of inflammatory cells at inflammation sites, phagocytosis, lysosomal enzyme release and synthesis and/or release of mediators of inflammation. *Prevents/suppresses cell-mediated immune reactions. Decreases/prevents tissue response to inflammatory process.*

USES

Substitution therapy in deficiency states (acute/chronic adrenal insufficiency, congenital adrenal hyperplasia, adrenal insufficiency secondary to pituitary insufficiency); nonendocrine disorders (arthritis, rheumatic carditis, allergic, collagen, intestinal tract, liver, ocular, renal, skin diseases, bronchial asthma, cerebral edema, malignancies). ***Rectal:*** Adjunctive therapy in treatment of ulcerative colitis.

STORAGE/HANDLING

Store parenteral forms at room temperature. ***Hydrocortisone sodium succinate:*** After reconstitution, use solution within 72 hrs. Use immediately if further diluted w/5% dextrose, 0.9% NaCl, or other compatible diluent.

ADMINISTRATION

ORAL:

- Give w/milk or food (decreases GI upset).
- Give single dose before 9 AM; give multiple doses at evenly spaced intervals.

IM/IV:

- Once reconstituted, solution stable for 72 hrs at room temperature.
- May further dilute w/5% dextrose or 0.9% NaCl.

TOPICAL:

- Gently cleanse area prior to application.
- Use occlusive dressings only as ordered.
- Apply sparingly and rub into area thoroughly.

RECTAL:

- Shake homogeneous suspension well.
- Instruct pt to lie on left side w/left leg extended, right leg flexed.
- Gently insert applicator tip into rectum, pointed slightly toward navel (umbilicus).
- Aim nozzle to back, then slowly instill medication.

INDICATIONS/ROUTES/DOSAGE

Hydrocortisone:
Oral: Adults, elderly: 20–240 mg/day.
IM: Adults, elderly: 1/3–1/2 oral dose q12h.

Hydrocortisone sodium phosphate:
IM/IV/SubQ: Adults, elderly: 15–240 mg/day, usually 1/3–1/2 oral dose q12h.

Hydrocortisone sodium succinate:
IM/IV: Adults, elderly: Initially, 100–500 mg/day.

Hydrocortisone acetate:
Intra-articular, intralesional, soft tissue: Adults, elderly: 5–50 mg.

Usual rectal dosage:
Rectal: Adults, elderly: 100 mg at bedtime for 21 nights or until clinical and proctologic remission occurs (may require 2–3 mos therapy).

Cortifoam: Adults, elderly: 1 applicator 1–2 times/day for 2–3 wks, then every second day thereafter.

Usual topical dosage:
Adults, elderly: Apply sparingly 2–4 times/day.

CONTRAINDICATIONS

Hypersensitivity to any corticosteroid or sulfite, systemic fungal infection, peptic ulcers (except life-threatening situations). Avoid live virus vaccine such as smallpox. ***Topical:*** Marked circulation impairment. Do not instill ocular solution when topical corticosteroids are being used on eyelids or surrounding skin.

CAUTIONS

Thromboembolic disorders, history of tuberculosis (may reactivate disease), hypothyroidism, cirrhosis, nonspecific ulcerative colitis, CHF, hypertension, psychosis, renal insufficiency, seizure disorders. Prolonged therapy should be discontinued slowly. ***Topical:*** Do not apply to extensive areas.

INTERACTIONS

DRUG: *Amphotericin* may increase hypokalemia. May decrease effect of ***oral hypoglycemics, insulin, diuretics, potassium supplements.*** May increase ***digoxin*** toxicity (due to hypokalemia). ***Hepatic enzyme inducers*** may decrease effect. ***Live virus vaccines*** may potentiate virus replication, increase vaccine side effects, decrease pt's antibody response to vaccine. HERBAL: None known. FOOD: None significant. ALTERED LAB VALUES: May decrease calcium, potassium, thyroxine. May increase cholesterol, lipids, glucose, sodium, amylase.

SIDE EFFECTS

FREQUENT: Insomnia, heartburn, nervousness, abdominal distension, increased sweating, acne, mood swings, increased appetite, facial flushing, delayed wound healing, increased susceptibility to infection, diarrhea/constipation. OCCASIONAL: Headache, edema, change in skin color, frequent urination. ***Topical:*** Itching, redness, irritation. RARE: Tachycardia, allergic reaction (rash, hives), psychic changes, hallucinations, depression. ***Topical:*** Allergic contact dermatitis, purpura. Systemic absorption more likely w/occlusive dressings or extensive application in young children.

ADVERSE REACTIONS/TOXIC EFFECTS

Long-term therapy: Hypocalcemia, hypokalemia, muscle wasting (especially arms, legs), osteoporosis, spontaneous fractures, amenorrhea, cataracts, glaucoma, peptic ulcer, CHF. *Abrupt withdrawal following long-term therapy:* Anorexia, nausea, fever, headache, sudden severe joint pain, rebound inflammation, fatigue, weakness, lethargy, dizziness, orthostatic hypertension.

PATIENT CONSIDERATIONS

BASELINE ASSESSMENT

Question for hypersensitivity to any of the corticosteroids. Obtain baseline values for weight, B/P, glucose, cholesterol, electrolytes. Check results of initial tests (e.g., TB skin test, x-rays, EKG).

INTERVENTION/EVALUATION

Monitor I&O, daily weight; assess

for edema. Check B/P, vital signs at least 2 times/day. Be alert to infection (reduced immune response): sore throat, fever, or vague symptoms. Evaluate bowel activity. Monitor electrolytes. Watch for hypocalcemia (muscle twitching, cramps, positive Trousseau's or Chvostek's signs) or hypokalemia (weakness and muscle cramps, numbness/tingling especially lower extremities, nausea and vomiting, irritability, EKG changes). Assess emotional status, ability to sleep.

Patient/Family Teaching

Take oral dose w/food or milk. Carry identification of drug and dose, physician's name and phone number. Do not change dose/schedule or stop taking drug; *must* taper off under medical supervision. Notify physician of fever, sore throat, muscle aches, sudden weight gain/swelling. W/dietician, give instructions for prescribed diet (usually sodium restricted w/high vitamin D, protein, and potassium). Maintain fastidious oral hygiene. Severe stress (serious infection, surgery, or trauma) may require increased dosage. Do not take aspirin or any other medication w/o consulting physician. Follow-up visits, lab tests are necessary; children must be assessed for growth retardation. Inform dentist or other physicians of cortisone therapy now or within past 12 mos. Caution against overuse of joints injected for symptomatic relief.

Topical

Apply after shower or bath for best absorption. Do not cover unless physician orders; do not use tight diapers, plastic pants, or coverings. Avoid contact w/eyes.

hydromorphone hydrochloride

high-dro-**more**-phone
(Dilaudid, Dilaudid HP)

H

FIXED-COMBINATION(S)
W/guaifenesin, an expectorant **(Dilaudid Cough Syrup).**

CANADIAN AVAILABILITY
Dilaudid, Hydromorph Contin

PREGNANCY CATEGORY B
(D if used for prolonged periods or at high doses at term)

CLASSIFICATION

Opioid: Analgesic **(Schedule II)**

AVAILABILITY (Rx)

Tablets: 1 mg, 2 mg, 3 mg, 4 mg. **Injection:** 1 mg/ml, 2 mg/ml, 3 mg/ml, 4 mg/ml, 10 mg/ml. **Suppository:** 3 mg.

PHARMACODYNAMICS

	ONSET	PEAK	DURATION
Oral	30 min	90–120 min	4 hrs
SubQ	15 min	30–90 min	4 hrs
IM	15 min	30–60 min	4–5 hrs
IV	10–15 min	15–30 min	2–3 hrs
Rectal	15–30 min	—	—

PHARMACOKINETICS

Absorption: Well absorbed from GI tract, after IM administration. Widely distributed. **Metabolism:** Metabolized in liver. **Excretion:** Excreted in urine. **Half-life:** 1–3 hrs.

ACTION/*THERAPEUTIC EFFECT*

Binds at opiate receptor sites in CNS. *Reduces intensity of pain stimuli incoming from sensory nerve endings, altering pain per-*

ception and emotional response to pain; suppresses cough reflex.

USES

Relief of moderate to severe pain, persistent nonproductive cough.

STORAGE/HANDLING

Store oral/parenteral form at room temperature. Slight yellow discoloration of parenteral form does not indicate loss of potency. Refrigerate suppositories.

ADMINISTRATION

ORAL:

- Give w/o regard to meals.
- Tablets may be crushed.

SubQ/IM:

- Use short 30 gauge needle for SubQ injection.
- Administer slowly, rotating injection sites.
- Pts w/circulatory impairment experience higher risk of overdosage because of delayed absorption of repeated administration.

IV:

- **Note:** High concentration injection (10 mg/ml) should only be used in those tolerant to opiate agonists, currently receiving high doses of another opiate agonist for severe, chronic pain due to cancer.
- Administer very slowly (over 2–3 min).
- Rapid IV increases risk of severe adverse reactions (chest wall rigidity, apnea, peripheral circulatory collapse, anaphylactoid effects, cardiac arrest).

RECTAL:

- Moisten suppository w/cold water before inserting well up into rectum.

INDICATIONS/ROUTES/DOSAGE

Analgesia:

Oral/SubQ/IM/IV: Adults, elderly: 2 mg q4–6h, as needed. Severe pain may require up to 4 mg q4–6h.

Rectal: Adults, elderly: 3 mg q6–8h.

Antitussive:

Oral: Adults, children >12 yrs, elderly: 1 mg q3–4h. ***Children 6–12 yrs:*** 0.5 mg q3–4h.

CONTRAINDICATIONS

None significant.

EXTREME CAUTION

CNS depression, anoxia, hypercapnia, respiratory depression, seizures, acute alcoholism, shock, untreated myxedema, respiratory dysfunction.

CAUTIONS

Increased intracranial pressure, impaired hepatic function, acute abdominal conditions, hypothyroidism, prostatic hypertrophy, Addison's disease, urethral stricture, COPD.

INTERACTIONS

DRUG: ***Alcohol, CNS depressants*** may increase CNS or respiratory depression, hypotension. ***MAO inhibitors*** may produce severe, fatal reaction (reduce dose to 1/4 usual dose). **HERBAL:** None known. **FOOD:** None significant. **ALTERED LAB VALUES:** May increase amylase, lipase plasma concentrations.

SIDE EFFECTS

Note: Effects are dependent on dosage amount, route of administration but occur infrequently w/oral antitussives. Ambulatory pts and those not in severe pain may experience dizziness, nausea, vomiting, hypotension more frequently than those in supine position or having severe pain. **FREQUENT:** Dizziness, drowsiness, hypotension, decreased appetite, unusually tired. **OCCASIONAL:** Confusion, pounding heartbeat, histamine reaction (decreased blood pressure, increased sweating, flushed face, trouble breathing), decreased urination, constipation, dry mouth, nausea, vomiting, headache, pain at injection site, confusion.

ADVERSE REACTIONS/TOXIC EFFECTS

Overdosage results in respiratory depression, skeletal muscle flaccidity, cold clammy skin, cyanosis, extreme somnolence progressing to convulsions, stupor, coma. Tolerance to analgesic effect, physical dependence may occur w/repeated use. Prolonged duration of action, cumulative effect may occur in those w/impaired hepatic, renal function.

PATIENT CONSIDERATIONS

BASELINE ASSESSMENT

Obtain vital signs before giving medication. If respirations are 12/min or lower (20/min or lower in children), withhold medication, contact physician.

Analgesic

Assess onset, type, location, and duration of pain. Effect of medication is reduced if full pain recurs before next dose.

Antitussive

Assess type, severity, frequency of cough and productions.

INTERVENTION/EVALUATION

Monitor B/P, pulse, respirations. Assess cough, lung sounds. Increase fluid intake and environmental humidity to improve viscosity of lung secretions. To prevent pain cycles, instruct pt to request pain medication as soon as discomfort begins. Check for constipation (especially in long-term use) and increase fiber, fluids, and exercise as appropriate. Initiate deep breathing and coughing exercises, particularly in those w/impaired pulmonary function. Assess for clinical improvement and record onset of relief of pain or cough.

PATIENT/FAMILY TEACHING

Discomfort may occur w/injection. Change positions slowly to avoid orthostatic hypotension. Avoid tasks that require alertness, motor skills until response to drug is established. Tolerance/dependence may occur w/prolonged use of high doses. Avoid alcohol. Report nausea, vomiting, constipation, shortness of breath, difficulty breathing.

H

hydroxychloroquine sulfate

hi-drocks-ee-**klor**-oh-kwin
(Plaquenil Sulfate)

CANADIAN AVAILABILITY
Plaquenil

PREGNANCY CATEGORY C

CLASSIFICATION

Antimalarial, antirheumatic

AVAILABILITY (Rx)

Tablets: 200 mg

PHARMACOKINETICS

Absorption: Variably absorbed from GI tract. Widely distributed. **Excretion:** Slowly excreted in urine. Minimal removal by hemodialysis. **Half-life:** 1.9–5.5 hrs.

ACTION / *THERAPEUTIC EFFECT*

Concentrates in parasite acid vesicles, interfering w/parasite protein synthesis, increasing pH *(inhibits parasite growth)*. Antirheumatic action unknown, but may involve suppressing formation of antigens responsible for hypersensitivity reactions.

USES / *UNLABELED*

Treatment of falciparum malaria (terminates acute attacks and cures nonresistant strains), suppression of acute attacks and prolongation of interval between treatment/relapse in vivax, ovale, malariae malaria. Treatment of discoid or systematic lupus erythematosus, acute and chronic rheumatoid arthritis. *Treatment of juvenile arthritis, sarcoid-associated hypercalcemia.*

ADMINISTRATION

ORAL:

- Administer w/meals to reduce GI upset.

INDICATIONS / ROUTES / DOSAGE

Note: 200 mg hydroxychloroquine = 155 mg base.

Suppression of malaria:
Oral: Adults: 310 mg base weekly on same day each week. ***Children:*** 5 mg base/kg/wk. Begin 2 wks prior to exposure; continue 6–8 wks after leaving endemic area or if therapy is not begun prior to exposure.

Oral: Adults: 620 mg base. ***Children:*** 10 mg base/kg given in 2 divided doses 6 hrs apart.

Treatment of malaria (acute attack): Dose (mg base)

DOSE	TIMES	ADULTS	CHILDREN
Initial	Day 1	620 mg	10 mg/kg
2nd	6 hrs later	310 mg	5 mg/kg
3rd	Day 2	310 mg	5 mg/kg
4th	Day 3	310 mg	5 mg/kg

Rheumatoid arthritis:
Oral: Adults: Initially, 400–600 mg (310–465 mg base) daily for 5–10 days; gradually increase dose to optimum response level. ***Maintenance (usually within 4–12 wks):*** Decrease dose by 50%, continue at level of 200–400 mg/day. Maximum effect may not be seen for several months.

Lupus erythematosus:
Oral: Adults: Initially, 400 mg 1–2 times/day for several weeks or months. ***Maintenance:*** 200–400 mg/day.

CONTRAINDICATIONS

Hypersensitivity to 4-aminoquinolones, retinal or visual field changes, long-term therapy for children, psoriasis, porphyria. After weighing risk/benefit ratio, physician may still elect to use drug, especially w/plasmodial forms.

CAUTIONS

Alcoholism, hepatic disease, G-6-PD deficiency. Children are especially susceptible to hydroxychloroquine fatalities.

INTERACTIONS

DRUG: May increase concentration of ***penicillamine,*** increase risk of hematologic/renal or severe skin reaction. **HERBAL:** None known. **FOOD:** None significant. **ALTERED LAB VALUES:** None significant.

SIDE EFFECTS

FREQUENT: Mild transient headache, anorexia, nausea, vomiting. OCCASIONAL: Visual disturbances (blurring and difficulty focusing); nervousness; fatigue; pruritus (especially of palms, soles, scalp); bleaching of hair; irritability, personality changes, diarrhea, skin eruptions. RARE: Stomatitis, exfoliative dermatitis, reduced hearing (nerve deafness).

ADVERSE REACTIONS/TOXIC EFFECTS

Ocular toxicity (especially retinopathy, which may progress even after drug is discontinued). *Prolonged therapy:* peripheral neuritis, neuromyopathy, hypotension, EKG changes, agranulocytosis, aplastic anemia, thrombocytopenia, convulsions, psychosis. *Overdosage:* headache, vomiting, visual disturbance, drowsiness, convulsions, hypokalemia followed by cardiovascular collapse, death.

PATIENT CONSIDERATIONS

BASELINE ASSESSMENT

Question for hypersensitivity to hydroxychloroquine sulfate or chloroquine. Evaluate CBC, hepatic function results.

INTERVENTION/EVALUATION

Monitor and report any visual disturbances promptly. Evaluate for GI distress. Give dose w/food (for malaria); discuss w/physician dividing the dose into separate days during week. Monitor hepatic function tests and check for fatigue, jaundice, other signs of hepatic effects. Assess skin and buccal mucosa; inquire about pruritus. Check vital signs. Be alert to signs/symptoms of overdosage (especially w/children). Monitor CBC results for adverse hematologic effects. Report reduced hearing immediately. W/prolonged therapy, test for muscle weakness.

PATIENT/FAMILY TEACHING

Continue drug for full length of treatment. In long-term therapy therapeutic response may not be evident for up to 6 mos. Immediately notify physician of *any* new symptom of visual difficulties, muscular weakness, decreased hearing, tinnitus. Do not take any other medication w/o consulting physician. Periodic lab and visual tests are important part of therapy. Keep out of reach of children (small amount can cause serious effects, death).

---

hydroxyurea
(Droxia, Hydrea)
See Classification section under: Cancer chemotherapy

---

hydroxyzine hydrochloride

high-**drox**-ih-zeen
(Atarax, Vistaril)

hydroxyzine pamoate

(Vistaril)

CANADIAN AVAILABILITY
Apo-Hydroxyzine, Atarax, Novohydroxyzin

PREGNANCY CATEGORY C

CLASSIFICATION

Antihistamine

AVAILABILITY (Rx)

Tablets: 10 mg, 25 mg, 50 mg, 100 mg. **Capsules:** 25 mg, 50 mg, 100 mg. **Syrup:** 10 mg/5 ml. **Oral Suspension:** 25 mg/5 ml. **Injection:** 25 mg/ml, 50 mg/ml.

PHARMACODYNAMICS

	ONSET	PEAK	DURATION
Oral			
	15–30 min	—	—

PHARMACOKINETICS

Absorption: Well absorbed from GI tract, parenteral administration. **Metabolism:** Metabolized in liver. **Excretion:** Primarily excreted in urine. **Half-life:** 20–25 hrs (increased in elderly).

ACTION / *THERAPEUTIC EFFECT*

Suppresses activity at subcortical levels of CNS, *producing anticholinergic, antihistaminic, analgesic effects, skeletal muscle relaxation.* Diminishes vestibular stimulation and depresses labyrinthine function, *controlling nausea, vomiting.*

USES

Relief of anxiety, tension; pruritus caused by allergic conditions, preop and postop sedation, control of muscle spasm, nausea, and vomiting.

STORAGE/HANDLING

Store oral solution/suspension, parenteral form at room temperature.

ADMINISTRATION

ORAL:

- Shake oral suspension well.
- Scored tablets may be crushed.
- Do not crush or break capsule.

IM:

- **Note:** Significant tissue damage, thrombosis, gangrene may occur if injection is given SubQ, intra-arterial, or IV injection.
- IM may be given undiluted.
- Use Z-track technique of injection to prevent SubQ infiltration.
- Inject deep IM into gluteus maximus or midlateral thigh in adults, midlateral thigh in children.

INDICATIONS/ROUTES/DOSAGE

Anxiety, tension:
Oral: Adults, elderly: 25-100 mg 3–4 times/day. ***Children >6 yrs:*** 50–100 mg/day in divided doses. ***Children <6 yrs:*** 50 mg/day in divided doses.

IM: Adults, elderly: 25–100 mg q4–6h, as needed. ***Children:*** 0.5 mg/kg.

Nausea, vomiting:
IM: Adults, elderly: 25–100 mg. ***Children:*** 1.1 mg/kg.

Pruritus:
Oral: Adults, elderly: 25 mg 3–4 times/day. ***Children >6 yrs:*** 50–100/day in divided doses. ***Children <6 yrs:*** 50 mg/day in divided doses.

Agitation due to alcohol withdrawal:
IM: Adults, elderly: 50–100 mg. May be repeated q4–6h, as needed.

CONTRAINDICATIONS

None significant.

CAUTIONS

None significant.

INTERACTIONS

DRUG: *Alcohol, CNS depressants* may increase CNS depressant effects. ***MAO inhibitors*** may increase anticholinergic, CNS depressant effects. **HERBAL:** None known. **FOOD:** None significant. **ALTERED LAB VALUES:** May cause false positives w/17-hydroxy corticosteroid determinations.

SIDE EFFECTS

Side effects are generally mild and transient. **FREQUENT:** Drowsiness, dry mouth, marked discomfort w/IM injection. **OCCASIONAL:** Dizziness, ataxia (muscular incoordination), weakness, slurred speech, headache, agitation, increased anxiety. **RARE:** Paradoxical CNS hyperactivity/nervousness in children, excitement/restlessness in elderly/debilitated pts (generally noted during first 2 wks of therapy, particularly noted in presence of uncontrolled pain).

ADVERSE REACTIONS/TOXIC EFFECTS

Hypersensitivity reaction (wheezing, dyspnea, tightness of chest).

PATIENT CONSIDERATIONS

BASELINE ASSESSMENT

Anxiety

Offer emotional support to anxious pt. Assess motor responses (agitation, trembling, tension) and autonomic responses (cold, clammy hands, sweating).

Antiemetic

Assess for dehydration (poor skin turgor, dry mucous membranes, longitudinal furrows in tongue).

INTERVENTION/EVALUATION

For those on long-term therapy, liver/renal function tests, blood counts should be performed periodically. Monitor lung sounds for signs of hypersensitivity reaction. Monitor serum electrolytes in those w/severe vomiting. Assess for paradoxical reaction, particularly during early therapy. Assist w/ambulation if drowsiness, lightheadedness occurs.

PATIENT/FAMILY TEACHING

Marked discomfort may occur w/IM injection. Sugarless gum, sips of tepid water may relieve dry mouth. Drowsiness usually diminishes w/continued therapy. Avoid tasks that require alertness, motor skills until response to drug is established.

hyoscyamine hydrobromide

high-oh-**sigh**-ah-meen

hyoscyamine sulfate

(Anaspaz, Levsin, Levsinex, Neoquess, Cystospaz)

FIXED-COMBINATION(S)
W/phenobarbital, a sedative-hypnotic **(Levsinex w/PB, Anaspaz PB)**

CANADIAN AVAILABILITY
Buscopan, Levsin

PREGNANCY CATEGORY C

CLASSIFICATION

Anticholinergic

AVAILABILITY (Rx)

Tablets: 0.125 mg, 0.15 mg. **Capsules (timed-release):** 0.375 mg. **Oral Solution:** 0.125 mg/ml. **Elixir:** 0.125 mg/5 ml. **Injection:** 0.5 mg/ml. **Ophthalmic Solution:** 0.25%.

PHARMACOKINETICS

Absorption: Well absorbed from GI tract. Widely distributed. **Metabolism:** Metabolized in liver. **Excretion:** Primarily excreted in urine. **Half-life:** 3.5 hrs.

ACTION/*THERAPEUTIC EFFECT*

Inhibits action of acetylcholine at postganglionic (muscarinic) receptor sites, *decreasing secretions (bronchial, salivary, sweat glands, gastric juices). Reduces motility of GI and urinary tract.*

USES

Adjunct in treatment of peptic ulcer disease; GI hypermotility (i.e., irritable bowel syndrome). Treatment of neurogenic bowel syndrome. Drying agent in acute rhinitis. Aid in controlling gastric secretion, visceral spasm, hypermotility in spastic colitis, spastic bladder, pylorospasm, associated abdominal cramps. Reduces duodenal motility to facilitate diagnostic radiologic procedure. Preop to reduce salivary, tracheobronchial, pharyngeal secretions. Reduces volume, acidity of gastric secretions.

ADMINISTRATION

ORAL:

- May give w/o regard to meals.
- Tablets may be crushed, chewed.
- Extended-release capsule should be swallowed whole.

INDICATIONS/ROUTES/DOSAGE

Usual oral dose:
Oral: Adults, elderly: 0.125–0.25 mg 3–4 times/day. ***(Extended-release):*** 0.375–0.750 mg q12h. ***Children:*** Based on weight q4h as needed.

Usual parenteral dosage:
IM/IV/SubQ: Adults, elderly: 0.25–0.5 mg 2–4 times/day.

Duodenography:
IV: Adults, elderly: 0.25–0.5 mg 10 min prior to procedure.

Preop:
IM: Adults, elderly: 0.5 mg (0.005 mg/kg) 30–60 min prior to induction of anesthesia or administration of preop medications.

CONTRAINDICATIONS

Narrow-angle glaucoma, severe ulcerative colitis, toxic megacolon, obstructive disease of GI tract, paralytic ileus, intestinal atony, bladder neck obstruction due to prostatic hypertrophy, myasthenia gravis in those not treated w/neostigmine, tachycardia secondary to cardiac insufficiency or thyrotoxicosis, cardiospasm, unstable cardiovascular status in acute hemorrhage.

EXTREME CAUTION

Autonomic neuropathy, known or suspected GI infections, diarrhea, mild to moderate ulcerative colitis, bronchial asthma.

CAUTIONS

Hyperthyroidism, hepatic or renal disease, hypertension, tachyarrhythmias, CHF, coronary artery disease, gastric ulcer, esophageal reflux or hiatal hernia associated w/reflux esophagitis, infants, elderly, those w/COPD.

INTERACTIONS

DRUG: ***Antacids, antidiarrheals*** may decrease absorption. ***Anticholinergics*** may increase effects. May decrease absorption of ***ketoconazole.*** May increase severity of GI lesions with ***potassium chloride (wax matrix).*** HERBAL: None known. **FOOD:** None significant. **ALTERED LAB VALUES:** None significant.

SIDE EFFECTS

FREQUENT: Dry mouth (sometimes severe), decreased sweating, constipation. **OCCASIONAL:** Blurred vision, bloated feeling, urinary hesitancy, drowsiness (w/high dosage), headache, intolerance to light, loss of taste, nervousness, flushing, insomnia, impotence, mental confusion/excitement (particularly in elderly, children). Parenteral form may produce temporary lightheadedness, local irritation. **RARE:** Dizziness, faintness.

ADVERSE REACTIONS/TOXIC EFFECTS

Overdosage may produce temporary paralysis of ciliary muscle, pupillary dilation, tachycardia, palpitation, hot/dry/flushed skin, absence of bowel sounds, hyperthermia, increased respiratory rate, EKG abnormalities, nausea, vomiting, rash over face/upper trunk, CNS stimulation, psychosis (agitation, restlessness, rambling speech, visual hallucination, paranoid behavior, delusions), followed by depression.

PATIENT CONSIDERATIONS

BASELINE ASSESSMENT

Before giving medication, instruct pt to void (reduces risk of urinary retention).

INTERVENTION/EVALUATION

Monitor daily bowel activity and stool consistency. Palpate bladder for urinary retention. Monitor changes in B/P, temperature. Assess skin turgor, mucous membranes to evaluate hydration status (encourage adequate fluid intake), bowel sounds for peristalsis. Be alert for fever (increased risk of hyperthermia).

PATIENT/FAMILY TEACHING

Do not become overheated during exercise in hot weather (may result in heat stroke). Avoid hot baths, saunas. Avoid tasks that require alertness, motor skills until response to drug is established. Sugarless gum, sips of tepid water may relieve dry mouth. Do not take antacids or medicine for diarrhea within 1 hr of taking this medication (decreased effectiveness).

ibuprofen

eye-byew-**pro**-fen
(Advil, Motrin, Nuprin, Rufen, Trendar)

FIXED-COMBINATION(S)
W/hydrocodone, an opioid analgesic **(Vicoprofen)**

CANADIAN AVAILABILITY
Advil, Motrin, Novoprofen

PREGNANCY CATEGORY B
(D if used in third trimester or near delivery)

CLASSIFICATION

Nonsteroidal anti-inflammatory

AVAILABILITY (Rx)

Tablets: 100 mg, 200 mg (OTC), 400 mg, 600 mg, 800 mg. **Tablets (chewable):** 50 mg (OTC), 100 mg (OTC). **Oral Suspension:** 100 mg/5 ml (OTC). **Oral Drops:** 40 mg/ml.

PHARMACODYNAMICS

	ONSET	PEAK	DURATION
Oral (analgesic)			
	0.5 hrs	—	4–6 hrs
Oral (antirheumatic)			
	2 days	1–2 wks	—

PHARMACOKINETICS

Absorption: Rapidly absorbed from GI tract. **Metabolism:** Metabolized in liver. **Excretion:** Primarily excreted in urine. **Half-life:** 2–4 hrs.

ACTION / *THERAPEUTIC EFFECT*

Produces analgesic and anti-inflammatory effect by inhibiting prostaglandin synthesis, *reducing inflammatory response and intensity of pain stimulus reaching sensory nerve endings.* Antipyresis produced by effect on hypothalamus, producing vasodilation, *thereby decreasing elevated body temperature.*

USES / *UNLABELED*

Symptomatic treatment of acute/chronic rheumatoid arthritis and osteoarthritis; reduces fever. Relief of mild to moderate pain, primary dysmenorrhea. Temporary relief of minor aches/pain associated w/common cold, headache, toothache, muscular aches, backaches, menstrual cramps. Treatment of migraines. *Treatment of psoriatic arthritis, vascular headaches.*

ADMINISTRATION

ORAL:
- Do not crush or break enteric-coated form.
- May give w/food, milk, or antacids if GI distress occurs.

INDICATIONS / ROUTES / DOSAGE

Note: Do not exceed 3.2 g/day.

Acute/chronic rheumatoid arthritis, osteoarthritis:
Oral: Adults, elderly: 300–800 mg 3–4 times/day.

Mild to moderate pain, primary dysmenorrhea:
Oral: Adults, elderly: 400 mg q4–6h.

Fever, minor aches/pain:
Oral: Adults, elderly: 200–400 mg q4–6h. ***Maximum:*** 1.2 g/day. ***Children:*** 5–10 mg/kg/dose. ***Maximum:*** 40 mg/kg/day.

Juvenile arthritis:
Oral: Children: 30–70 mg/kg/day in 3–4 divided doses.

CONTRAINDICATIONS

Active peptic ulcer, GI ulceration, chronic inflammation of GI tract, GI bleeding disorders, history of hypersensitivity to aspirin or NSAIDs.

CAUTIONS

Impaired renal/hepatic function,

history of GI tract disease, predisposition to fluid retention.

INTERACTIONS

DRUG: May increase effects of ***oral anticoagulants, heparin, thrombolytics.*** May decrease effect of ***antihypertensives, diuretics. Salicylates, aspirin*** may increase risk of GI side effects, bleeding. ***Bone marrow depressants*** may increase risk of hematologic reactions. May increase concentration, toxicity of ***lithium.*** May increase ***methotrexate*** toxicity. ***Probenecid*** may increase concentration. **HERBAL:** Ginkgo may increase risk of bleeding. May decrease effect of feverfew. **FOOD:** None significant. **ALTERED LAB VALUES:** May prolong bleeding time. May alter blood glucose. May increase BUN, creatinine, potassium, liver function tests. May decrease Hgb, Hct.

SIDE EFFECTS

FREQUENT (3–9%): Skin rash, dizziness, abdominal cramps, epigastric pain, heartburn, nausea. OCCASIONAL (1–3%): Itching, ringing in ears, fluid retention/edema, headache, constipation, diarrhea, indigestion, vomiting, decreased appetite. RARE (<1%): Confusion, increased blood pressure, blurred vision, dry swollen eyes, renal impairment.

ADVERSE REACTIONS/TOXIC EFFECTS

Acute overdosage may result in metabolic acidosis. Peptic ulcer, GI bleeding, gastritis, severe hepatic reaction (cholestasis, jaundice) occur rarely. Nephrotoxicity (dysuria, hematuria, proteinuria, nephrotic syndrome) and severe hypersensitivity reaction (particularly those w/systemic lupus erythematosus, other collagen diseases) occur rarely.

PATIENT CONSIDERATIONS

BASELINE ASSESSMENT

Assess onset, type, location, and duration of pain or inflammation. Inspect appearance of affected joints for immobility, deformities, and skin condition.

INTERVENTION/EVALUATION

Monitor for evidence of nausea, dyspepsia. Monitor pattern of daily bowel activity and stool consistency. Check behind medial malleolus for fluid retention (usually first area noted). Assess skin for evidence of rash. Assist w/ambulation if dizziness occurs. Evaluate for therapeutic response: relief of pain, stiffness, swelling, increase in joint mobility, reduced joint tenderness, improved grip strength.

PATIENT/FAMILY TEACHING

Avoid aspirin, alcohol during therapy (increases risk of GI bleeding). If GI upset occurs, take w/food, milk, or antacids. Report blurred vision, ringing/roaring in ears. Avoid tasks that require alertness until response to drug is established. Do not crush or chew enteric-coated tablet.

ibutilide fumarate

eye-**byewt**-ih-lied
(Corvert)

PREGNANCY CATEGORY C

CLASSIFICATION

Antiarrhythmic

AVAILABILITY (Rx)

Injection: 0.1 mg/ml solution

PHARMACOKINETICS

After IV administration, highly distributed, rapidly cleared. **Excretion:** Primarily excreted in urine as metabolite. **Half-life:** 2–12 hrs (avg: 6 hrs).

ACTION/ *THERAPEUTIC EFFECT*

Prolongs both atrial and ventricular action potential duration and increases atrial and ventricular refractory period. Activates slow, inward current (sodium), produces mild slowing of sinus rate and AV conduction, dose-related prolongation of QT interval. Converts arrhythmias to sinus rhythm.

USES

Rapid conversion of atrial fibrillation or flutter of recent onset to sinus rhythm (arrhythmias of longer duration less likely to respond to therapy).

STORAGE/HANDLING

Admixtures w/diluent stable at room temperature for 24 hrs, 48 hrs if refrigerated.

ADMINISTRATION

IV:

- **Note:** Compatible w/5% dextrose injection, 0.9% NaCl diluents. Compatible w/polyvinyl chloride plastic and polyolefin bag admixtures.
- Give undiluted or diluted in 50 ml diluent.
- Give infusion over 10 min.
- Monitor pt w/continuous EKG reading for at least 4 hrs following infusion or until QT interval has returned to baseline.

INDICATIONS/ROUTES/DOSAGE

Atrial arrhythmias:

IV Infusion: Adults, elderly ≥60 kg (132 lbs): One vial (1 mg) given over 10 min. If arrhythmia does not stop within 10 min after end of initial infusion, a second 10 min infusion may be given 10 min after completion of first infusion. ***Adults, elderly <60 kg (132 lbs):*** 0.1 ml/kg (0.01 mg/kg) given over 10 min. If arrhythmia does not stop within 10 min after end of initial infusion, a second 10 min infusion may be given 10 min after completion of first infusion.

CONTRAINDICATIONS

Hypersensitivity to ibutilide.

CAUTIONS

Abnormal liver function, heart block.

INTERACTIONS

DRUG: Do not give concurrently w/***class Ia (disopyramide, quinidine, procainamide, moricizine) or class III (amiodarone, sotalol, bretylium) antiarrhythmics*** or within 4 hrs postinfusion of ibutilide. ***Phenothiazines, tricyclic and tetracyclic antidepressants, H-1 receptor antagonists*** may prolong QT interval. **HERBAL:** None known. **FOOD:** None significant. **ALTERED LAB VALUES:** None significant.

SIDE EFFECTS

Generally well tolerated. **OCCASIONAL:** Ventricular extrasystoles (5.1%), ventricular tachycardia (4.9%), headache (3.6%), hypotension, postural hypotension (2%). **RARE:** Bundle-branch block, AV block, bradycardia, hypertension.

ADVERSE REACTIONS/TOXIC EFFECTS

Sustained polymorphic ventricular tachycardia, occasionally w/QT prolongation (torsades de pointes) occurs rarely. Overdosage results in CNS toxicity (CNS depression, rapid gasping breathing, seizures). May exaggerate expected prolongation of repolarization. May worsen existing arrhythmias or produce new arrhythmias.

PATIENT CONSIDERATIONS

BASELINE ASSESSMENT

Those w/atrial fibrillation of >2–3 days duration must be treated w/anticoagulants generally for at least 2 wks prior to ibutilide therapy. Cardiac monitoring equipment, intracardiac pacing facility, cardioverter/defibrillator, medications for treatment of sustained ventricular tachycardia (VT), including polymorphic VT, must be available during and after administration. Anticipate proarrhythmic events.

INTERVENTION/EVALUATION

Observe pt w/continuous EKG monitoring for at least 4 hrs following infusion or until QT interval has returned to baseline. If any arrhythmic activity is noted, continue EKG monitoring. Monitor for symptoms of electrolyte abnormalities, especially magnesium and potassium, and overdrive cardiac pacing, electrical cardioversion, or defibrillation.

idarubicin hydrochloride

(Idamycin)

See Classification section under: Cancer chemotherapy

ifosfamide

(Ifex)

See Classification section under: Cancer chemotherapy

imiglucerase

(Cerezyme)

See Supplement

imipenem/cilastatin sodium

im-ih-**peh**-nem/sill-as-**tah**-tin
(Primaxin)

CANADIAN AVAILABILITY
Primaxin

PREGNANCY CATEGORY C

CLASSIFICATION

Antibiotic

AVAILABILITY (Rx)

Injection for IM: 500 mg, 750 mg.
Injection for IV: 250 mg, 500 mg.

PHARMACOKINETICS

Absorption: Readily absorbed after IM administration. Widely distributed. **Metabolism:** Metabolized in kidney. **Excretion:** Primarily excreted in urine. Removed by hemodialysis. **Half-life:** 1 hr (increased in decreased renal function).

ACTION/*THERAPEUTIC EFFECT*

Imipenem: Bactericidal. Binds to bacterial membranes, *inhibiting bacterial cell wall synthesis. Cilastatin:* Prevents renal metabolism of imipenem.

USES

Treatment of respiratory tract, skin/skin structure, gynecologic, bone/joint, intra-abdominal, complicated/uncomplicated urinary tract infections, endocarditis, polymicrobic infections, septicemia; serious nosocomial infections.

STORAGE/HANDLING

Solution appears colorless to yellow; discard if solution turns brown. IV infusion (piggyback) stable for 4 hrs at room temperature, 24 hrs if refrigerated. Discard if precipitate forms.

ADMINISTRATION

IM:

- Prepare w/1% lidocaine 500 mg vial w/2 ml, 750 mg vial w/3 ml lidocaine HCl.
- Administer suspension within 1 hr of preparation.
- Do not mix w/any other medications.
- Inject deep in large muscle; aspirate to decrease risk of injection into a blood vessel.

IV:

- Give by intermittent IV infusion (piggyback). Do not give IV push.
- Dilute each 250 mg or 500 mg vial w/100 ml 5% dextrose; 0.9% NaCl, or other compatible IV fluid. Infuse >20–30 min (1 g dose >40–60 min).
- Use large veins to reduce risk of phlebitis; alternate sites.
- Observe pt during first 30 min of infusion to observe for possible hypersensitivity reaction.

INDICATIONS/ROUTES/DOSAGE

Note: Space doses evenly around the clock.

Uncomplicated urinary tract infections:
IV: Adults, elderly: 250 mg q6h.

Complicated urinary tract infections:
IV: Adults, elderly: 500 mg q6h.

Mild infections:
IV: Adults, elderly: 250–500 mg q6h.

Moderate infections:
IV: Adults, elderly: 500 mg q6–8h.

Severe, life-threatening infections:
IV: Adults, elderly: 500 mg q6h.

Usual pediatric dosage:
IV: Children (>3 mos): 10–25 mg/kg/dose q6h.

Dosage in renal impairment:
Dose and/or frequency is modified based on creatinine clearance and/or severity of infection.

CREATININE CLEARANCE	DOSAGE
31–70 ml/min	500 mg q8h
21–30 ml/min	500 mg q12h
0–20 ml/min	250 mg q12h

USUAL INTRAMUSCULAR DOSAGE:

Note: Do not use for severe or life-threatening infections.

Mild to moderate lower respiratory tract, skin/skin structure, gynecologic infections:
IM: Adults, elderly: 500–750 mg q12h.

Mild to moderate intra-abdominal infections:
IM: Adults, elderly: 750 mg q12h.

CONTRAINDICATIONS

Hypersensitivity to imipenem/cilastatin sodium, other beta lactams. *IM:* Hypersensitivity to any local anesthetics of amide type; pts w/severe shock or heart block (due to use of lidocaine diluent).

CAUTIONS

Hypersensitivity to penicillins, cephalosporins, other allergens;

renal dysfunction, CNS disorders, particularly w/history of seizures.

INTERACTIONS

DRUG: None significant. **HERBAL:** None known. **FOOD:** None significant. **ALTERED LAB VALUES:** May increase SGOT (AST), SGPT (ALT), alkaline phosphatase, LDH, bilirubin, BUN, creatinine. May decrease Hgb, Hct.

SIDE EFFECTS

OCCASIONAL (1–3%): Allergic reaction (rash, itching, fever), confusion, dizziness, seizures, tremors, pain at injection site, diarrhea, nausea, vomiting. RARE (<1%): Infusion rate reaction (dizziness, sweating, nausea, vomiting, unusual tiredness).

ADVERSE REACTIONS/TOXIC EFFECTS

Antibiotic-associated colitis, other superinfections may occur. Anaphylactic reactions in those receiving beta lactams have occurred.

PATIENT CONSIDERATIONS

BASELINE ASSESSMENT

Question pt for history of allergies, particularly to imipenem/cilastatin sodium, other beta lactams, penicillins, cephalosporins. Inquire about history of seizures. Obtain culture and sensitivity tests before giving first dose (therapy may begin before results are known).

INTERVENTION/EVALUATION

Evaluate for phlebitis (heat, pain, red streaking over vein), pain at IV injection site. Assess for GI discomfort, nausea, vomiting. Determine pattern of bowel activity and stool consistency. Assess skin for rash. Monitor I&O, renal function tests. Check mental status, be alert to tremors and possible seizures. Assess temperature, B/P twice daily, more often if necessary. Assess for hearing loss, tinnitus. Monitor electrolytes, especially potassium.

PATIENT/FAMILY TEACHING

Continue therapy for full length of treatment. Doses should be evenly spaced. Do not take any other medication unless approved by physician. Notify physician in event of tremors, seizures, rash, diarrhea, or other new symptom.

imipramine hydrochloride

ih-**mih**-prah-meen
(Janimine, Tofranil)

imipramine pamoate

(Tofranil-PM)

CANADIAN AVAILABILITY
Api-Imipramine, Tofranil

PREGNANCY CATEGORY D

CLASSIFICATION

Antidepressant: Tricyclic

AVAILABILITY (Rx)

Hydrochloride: Tablets: 10 mg, 25 mg, 50 mg. **Injection:** 25 mg/ml.

Pamoate: Capsules: 75 mg, 100 mg, 125 mg, 150 mg.

PHARMACOKINETICS

Absorption: Rapidly, well absorbed from GI tract. Widely distributed. **Metabolism:** Metabolized in liver, undergoing first-pass effect. **Excretion:** Primarily excreted in urine. **Half-life:** 11–25 hrs.

ACTION/ *THERAPEUTIC EFFECT*

Blocks reuptake of neurotransmitters (norepinephrine, serotonin) at presynaptic membranes, increasing concentration at postsynaptic receptor sites, *resulting in antidepressant effect.* Anticholinergic effect *controls nocturnal enuresis.*

USES/ *UNLABELED*

Treatment of various forms of depression, often in conjunction w/psychotherapy. Treatment of nocturnal enuresis in children >6 yrs. *Treatment of panic disorder, neurogenic pain, attention deficit hyperactivity disorder (ADHD), cataplexy associated w/narcolepsy.*

STORAGE/HANDLING

Parenteral form takes on yellow or reddish hue when exposed to light. Slight discoloration does not affect potency but marked discoloration is associated w/potency loss.

ADMINISTRATION

ORAL:

- Give w/food or milk if GI distress occurs.
- Do not crush or break film-coated tablets.

IM:

- Give by IM only if oral administration is not feasible.
- Crystals may form in injection. Redissolve by immersing ampule in hot water for 1 min.
- Give deep IM slowly.

INDICATIONS/ROUTES/DOSAGE

Depression:
Oral: Adults: Initially, 75–100 mg daily. Dosage may be gradually increased to 300 mg daily for hospitalized pts, 200 mg for outpts, then reduce dosage to effective maintenance level (50–150 mg daily). ***Elderly:*** Initially, 10–25 mg/day at bedtime. May increase by 10–25 mg q3–7days. ***Range:*** 50–150 mg. ***Adolescents:*** 30–40 mg daily in divided doses to maximum of 100 mg/day.

IM: Adults: Do not exceed 100 mg/day, administered in divided doses.

Childhood enuresis:
Oral: Children >6 yrs: 25 mg 1 hr before bedtime.

CONTRAINDICATIONS

Acute recovery period following MI, within 14 days of MAO inhibitor ingestion.

CAUTIONS

Prostatic hypertrophy, history of urinary retention or obstruction, glaucoma, diabetes mellitus, history of seizures, hyperthyroidism, cardiac/hepatic/renal disease, schizophrenia, increased intraocular pressure, hiatal hernia.

INTERACTIONS

DRUG: ***Alcohol, CNS depressants*** may increase CNS, respiratory depression, hypotensive effects. ***Antithyroid agents*** may increase risk of agranulocytosis. ***Phenothiazines*** may increase sedative, anticholinergic effects. ***Cimetidine*** may increase concentration, toxicity. May decrease effects of ***clonidine, guanadrel.*** May increase cardiac effects w/***sympathomimetics.*** May increase risk of hypertensive crisis, hyperpyretic, convulsions w/***MAO inhibitors. Phenytoin*** may decrease concentrations. HERBAL: None known. FOOD:

None significant. **ALTERED LAB VALUES:** May alter EKG readings, glucose.

SIDE EFFECTS

FREQUENT: Drowsiness, fatigue, dry mouth, blurred vision, constipation, delayed micturition, postural hypotension, excessive sweating, disturbed concentration, increased appetite, urinary retention. **OCCASIONAL:** GI disturbances (nausea, metallic taste sensation). **RARE:** Paradoxical reaction (agitation, restlessness, nightmares, insomnia), extrapyramidal symptoms (particularly fine hand tremor).

ADVERSE REACTIONS/TOXIC EFFECTS

High dosage may produce cardiovascular effects (severe postural hypotension, dizziness, tachycardia, palpitations, arrhythmias) and seizures. May also result in altered temperature regulation (hyperpyrexia or hypothermia). Abrupt withdrawal from prolonged therapy may produce headache, malaise, nausea, vomiting, vivid dreams.

PATIENT CONSIDERATIONS

BASELINE ASSESSMENT

For those on long-term therapy, liver/renal function tests, blood counts should be performed periodically.

INTERVENTION/EVALUATION

Supervise suicidal risk pt closely during early therapy (as depression lessens, energy level improves, causing increased suicide potential). Assess appearance, behavior, speech pattern, level of interest, mood. Monitor pattern of daily bowel activity and stool consistency. Monitor B/P, pulse for hypotension, arrhythmias. Assess for urinary retention by bladder palpation.

PATIENT/FAMILY TEACHING

Change positions slowly to avoid hypotensive effect. Tolerance to postural hypotension, sedative, and anticholinergic effects usually develops during early therapy. Therapeutic effect may be noted within 2–5 days, maximum effect within 2–3 wks. Photosensitivity to sun may occur. Dry mouth may be relieved by sugarless gum, sips of tepid water. Report visual disturbances. Do not abruptly discontinue medication. Avoid tasks that require alertness, motor skills until response to drug is established. Avoid alcohol.

---

imiquimod

(Aldara)

See Supplement

---

immune globulin IM (IGIM, gamma globulin, ISG)

(Gamastan, Gammar)

immune globulin IV (IGIV)

(Gamimune N, Gammagard, Gammar-IV, Iveegam, Sandoglobulin, Venoglobulin-I)

CANADIAN AVAILABILITY

Gamimune N, Iveegam

PREGNANCY CATEGORY C

CLASSIFICATION

Immune serum

AVAILABILITY (Rx)

Injection: 5%, 10%. **Powder for Injection:** 50 mg/ml, 1 g, 3 g, 6 g, 12 g.

PHARMACOKINETICS

Evenly distributed between intravascular and extravascular space. **Half-life:** 21–23 days.

ACTION/*THERAPEUTIC EFFECT*

Increases antibody titer and antigen-antibody reaction, *providing passive immunity against infection.* Induces rapid increase in platelet counts. Produces anti-inflammatory effect.

USES/*UNLABELED*

IGIM: Provides passive immunity to those exposed to hepatitis A virus, hepatitis B virus, or hepatitis B surface antigen (HBsAg); prevents or modifies symptoms of measles (rubeola) in susceptible individuals exposed <6 days previously; provides replacement therapy in prophylactic management of infections with those with IgG or other antibody deficiency diseases. *IGIV:* Maintenance treatment in those unable to produce sufficient amounts of IgG antibodies; treatment of idiopathic thrombocytopenic purpura (ITP); prevents bacterial infections in those with hypogammaglobulinemia and/or recurrent bacterial infections associated with B-cell chronic lymphocytic leukemia (CLL). Treatment of Kawasaki disease, *prevents acute infections in immunosuppressed pts, controls/prevents infections in infants/children immunosuppressed in association w/AIDs or ARC. Prophylaxis/treatment of infections in high-risk, preterm, low birth weight neonates, treatment of chronic inflammatory demyelinating polyneuropathies.*

STORAGE/HANDLING

Refrigerate IM vials; refer to individual IV preparations for storage requirements, stability after reconstitution. Reconstitute only with diluent provided by manufacturer. Discard partially used or turbid preparations.

ADMINISTRATION

Note: Do not mix with other medications. Do not perform skin testing prior to administration.

IM:

- Inject into deltoid muscle or anterolateral aspect of thigh.
- Use upper outer quadrant of gluteal muscle only for large volumes or multiple injections (when dose >10 ml).

IV:

- Give by infusion only.
- After reconstituted, administer via separate tubing.
- Avoid mixing with other medication/IV infusion fluids.
- Rate of infusion varies with product used.
- Monitor vital signs and B/P diligently during and immediately following IV administration (precipitous fall in B/P may produce picture of anaphylactic reaction). Stop infusion immediately. Epinephrine should be readily available.

INDICATIONS/ROUTES/DOSAGE

Hepatitis A infection:
IM: Adults, elderly, children: (after exposure): 0.02 ml/kg as single dose as soon as possible after exposure; (before exposure): 0.02

ml/kg as single dose; 0.06 ml/kg if exposure >3 mos, repeat q4–6mos.

Non-A, non-B hepatitis:
IM: Adults, elderly, children: 0.06 ml/kg as single dose as soon as possible after exposure.

Measles (after exposure):
IM: Adults, children: 0.25 ml/kg as single dose within 6 days of exposure; 0.5 ml/kg if pt suspected of having leukemia, lymphoma, generalized malignancy, or immunodeficiency disorder, receiving steroids, or other immunosuppression therapy.

Immunodeficiency diseases:
IM: Adults, elderly, children: Initially, 1.2 ml/kg. ***Maintenance:*** 0.6 ml/kg (at least 100 mg/kg) q2–4wks. ***Maximum single dose:*** 30–50 ml (adults); 20–30 ml (infants, small children).

Primary immunodeficiency diseases:
IV Infusion: Adults, elderly, children: (Gamimune N): 100–200 mg/kg or 2–4 ml/kg once monthly; may increase to 400 mg/kg or 8 ml/kg once monthly or more frequently. ***(Gammagard):*** 200–400 mg/kg once monthly. Minimum: 100 mg/kg once monthly. ***(Gammar-IV):*** 100–200 mg/kg q3–4wks. Loading dose 200 mg/kg may be given at more frequent intervals until therapeutic concentration attained. ***(Iveegam):*** 200 mg/kg once monthly. ***(Sandoglobulin):*** 200 mg/kg once monthly, may increase to 300 mg/kg once monthly or at more frequent intervals. ***(Venoglobulin-I):*** 200 mg/kg once monthly, may increase to 300–400 mg/kg once monthly or at more frequent intervals.

Idiopathic thrombocytopenic purpura (ITP):
IV Infusion: Adults, elderly, children: (Gamimune-N, Sandoglobulin): Initially, 400 mg/kg/day for 2–5 days depending on platelet count/clinical response. ***(Gammagard):*** 1 g/kg as single dose; may give up to 3 doses on alternate days. ***(Venoglobulin-I):*** Initially, 500 mg/kg/day for 2–7 days; then, if necessary, 500–2,000 mg/kg q2wks or less to maintain platelets >30,000/m^3 in children or >20,000/m^3 in adults.

Kawasaki syndrome:
IV: Adults: 80–100 mg/kg/day.

Hypogammaglobulinemia and/or recurrent bacterial infections in B-cell CLL:
IV Infusion: Adults, elderly, children: (Gammagard): 400 mg/kg q3–4wks.

CONTRAINDICATIONS

History of allergic response to gamma globulin or anti-immunoglobulin A (IgA) antibodies, allergic response to thimerosal, those with isolated immunoglobulin A (IgA) deficiency. IM also contraindicated in those who have severe thrombocytopenia and any coagulation disorder.

CAUTIONS

Prior systemic allergic reactions following administration of human immunoglobulin preparations. Preexisting renal dysfunction, diabetes; those >65 yrs are at high risk of acute renal failure.

INTERACTIONS

DRUG: *Live virus vaccines* may potentiate virus replication, increase vaccine side effects, decrease pt's antibody response to vaccine. **HERBAL:** None known. **FOOD:** None significant. **ALTERED LAB VALUES:** None significant.

SIDE EFFECTS

FREQUENT: Dyspnea, tachycardia, backache or pain, headache, joint or muscle pain. **OCCASIONAL:** Fatigue, wheezing, rash or pain at injection site, leg cramps, hives, bluish color of lips, nailbeds, lightheadedness.

ADVERSE REACTIONS/TOXIC EFFECTS

Anaphylactic reactions occur rarely but increased incidence when given large IM doses or in those receiving repeated injections of immune globulin. Epinephrine should be readily available. Overdose may produce chest tightness, chills, diaphoresis, dizziness, flushed face, nausea, vomiting, fever, hypotension.

PATIENT CONSIDERATIONS

Baseline Assessment

Inquire about history of exposure to disease for both pt and family as appropriate. Have epinephrine readily available. Pt should be well hydrated prior to infusion.

Intervention/Evaluation

Control rate of IV infusion carefully; too rapid infusion increases risk of precipitous fall in B/P and signs of anaphylaxis (facial flushing, chest tightness, chills, fever, nausea, vomiting, diaphoresis). Assess pt closely during infusion, especially 1st hour; monitor vital signs continuously. Stop infusion temporarily if above signs noted. For treatment of ITP, monitor platelets.

Patient/Family Teaching

Explain rationale for therapy. Rapid response, lasts 1–3 mos. Local pain or muscle tenderness may occur at IM injection site.

indapamide

in-**dap**-ah-myd
(Lozol)

CANADIAN AVAILABILITY
Lozide

PREGNANCY CATEGORY D

CLASSIFICATION

Diuretic: Thiazide

AVAILABILITY (Rx)

Tablets: 1.25 mg, 2.5 mg

PHARMACODYNAMICS

	ONSET	PEAK	DURATION
Oral (diuretic)	1–2 hrs	<2 hrs	Up to 36 hrs

PHARMACOKINETICS

Absorption: Completely absorbed from GI tract. **Metabolism:** Metabolized in liver. **Excretion:** Primarily excreted in urine. **Half-life:** 14–18 hrs.

ACTION/*THERAPEUTIC EFFECT*

Diuretic: Blocks reabsorption of water, electrolytes (sodium, potassium) at cortical diluting segment of distal tubule, *promoting renal excretion.* ***Antihypertensive:*** Reduces plasma, extracellular fluid volume, decreases peripheral vascular resistance (PVR) by direct effect on blood vessels, *reducing B/P.*

USES

Treatment of hypertension and edema associated w/CHF. May be used alone or w/antihypertensive agents.

ADMINISTRATION

ORAL:

- Give w/food or milk if GI upset occurs, preferably w/breakfast (may prevent nocturia).
- Do not crush or break tablets.

INDICATIONS/ROUTES/DOSAGE

Edema:
Oral: Adults: Initially, 2.5 mg/day, may increase to 5 mg/day in 1 wk.

Hypertension:
Oral: Adults: Initially, 1.25 mg, may increase to 2.5 mg/day in 4 wks or 5 mg/day after additional 4 wks.

Usual elderly dosage:
Oral: Initially, 1.25 mg/day or every other day. May increase up to 5 mg/day.

CONTRAINDICATIONS

None significant.

CAUTIONS

History of hypersensitivity to sulfonamides or thiazide diuretics, renal decompensation, anuria, severe renal disease, impaired hepatic function, diabetes mellitus, elderly/debilitated, thyroid disorders.

INTERACTIONS

DRUG: May increase risk of ***digoxin*** toxicity (due to hypokalemia). May decrease clearance, increase toxicity of ***lithium.*** **HERBAL:** None known. **FOOD:** None significant. **ALTERED LAB VALUES:** May increase plasma renin activity. May decrease calcium, protein-bound iodine, potassium, sodium.

SIDE EFFECTS

OCCASIONAL: Headache, dizziness, lightheadedness, upset stomach, decreased appetite, diarrhea. **RARE:** Allergic reaction (rash, itching), electrolyte imbalance (especially decreased sodium, potassium).

ADVERSE REACTIONS/TOXIC EFFECTS

Vigorous diuresis may lead to profound water loss and electrolyte depletion, resulting in hypokalemia, hyponatremia, dehydration. Acute hypotensive episodes may occur. Hyperglycemia may be noted during prolonged therapy. GI upset, pancreatitis, dizziness, paresthesias, headache, blood dyscrasias, pulmonary edema, allergic pneumonitis, dermatologic reactions occur rarely. Overdosage can lead to lethargy, coma w/o changes in electrolytes or hydration.

PATIENT CONSIDERATIONS

BASELINE ASSESSMENT

Check vital signs, especially B/P for hypotension prior to administration. Assess baseline electrolytes, particularly check for low potassium. Assess edema, skin turgor, mucous membranes for hydration status. Assess muscle strength, mental status. Note skin temperature, moisture. Obtain baseline weight. Initiate I&O.

INTERVENTION/EVALUATION

Continue to monitor B/P, vital signs, electrolytes, I&O, weight. Note extent of diuresis. Watch for electrolyte disturbances (hypokalemia may result in weakness, tremor, muscle cramps, nausea, vomiting, change in mental status, tachycardia; hyponatremia may result in confusion, thirst, cold/clammy skin).

PATIENT/FAMILY TEACHING

Expect increased frequency and volume of urination. To reduce hypotensive effect, rise slowly

from lying to sitting position and permit legs to dangle momentarily before standing. Eat foods high in potassium such as whole grains (cereals), legumes, meat, bananas, apricots, orange juice, potatoes (white, sweet), raisins.

indinavir

in-**din**-oh-vir
(Crixivan)

CANADIAN AVAILABILITY
Crixivan

PREGNANCY CATEGORY C

CLASSIFICATION

Antiviral

AVAILABILITY (Rx)

Capsules: 200 mg, 333 mg, 400 mg

PHARMACOKINETICS

Absorption: Rapidly absorbed following oral administration. **Metabolism:** Metabolized in liver. **Excretion:** Primarily excreted in urine. **Half-life:** 1.8 hrs (increased in pts w/impaired liver function).

ACTION / *THERAPEUTIC EFFECT*

Suppresses human immunodeficiency virus (HIV) protease, an enzyme necessary for splitting viral polyprotein precursors into mature and infectious virus particles. *Resultant effect interrupts HIV replication, forms immature noninfectious viral particles.*

USES

Treatment of human immunodeficiency virus (HIV) when antiretroviral therapy is warranted.

STORAGE/HANDLING

Store at room temperature. Protect from moisture (capsules sensitive to moisture; keep in original bottle).

ADMINISTRATION

ORAL:

- Best given w/o food but w/water only (optimal absorption) 1 hr before or 2 hrs after a meal but may give w/water, skim milk, juice, coffee or tea, or w/light meal (e.g., dry toast w/jelly, juice and coffee w/skim milk and sugar; or cornflakes, skim milk and sugar). Do not give w/meal high in fat, calories, and protein.
- If indinavir and didanosine are given concurrently, give at least 1 hr apart on an empty stomach.

INDICATIONS/ROUTES/DOSAGE

HIV infection:
Oral: Adults: 800 mg (two 400 mg capsules) q8h.

Dosage w/hepatic insufficiency:
Oral: Adults: 600 mg q8h.

CONTRAINDICATIONS

Hypersensitivity to indinavir; nephrolithiasis.

CAUTIONS

Renal, hepatic function impairment.

INTERACTIONS

DRUG: Avoid concurrent administration of indinavir w/***terfenadine, triazolam, midazolam*** (potential for arrhythmias, prolonged sedation). **HERBAL:** St. John's wort may decrease concentration, effect. **FOOD:** None significant. **ALTERED LAB VALUES:** May increase bilirubin (occurs in 10% of pts), SGOT (AST), SGPT (ALT).

SIDE EFFECTS

FREQUENT: Nausea (12%), abdominal pain (9%), headache (6%), diarrhea (5%). OCCASIONAL: Vomiting, asthenia, fatigue (4%), insomnia, accumulation of fat in waist, stomach, or back of neck. RARE: Abnormal taste sensation, heartburn, symptomatic urinary tract disease, transient kidney dysfunction.

ADVERSE REACTIONS/TOXIC EFFECTS

Nephrolithiasis (flank pain with or w/o hematuria) occurs in 4% of pts.

PATIENT CONSIDERATIONS

Baseline Assessment

Offer emotional support. Establish baseline lab values. Emphasize need for close monitoring of renal function (urinalysis, serum creatinine) during therapy.

Intervention/Evaluation

Encourage adequate hydration. Pt should drink 48 oz (1.5 L) of liquid for each 24 hrs during therapy. Monitor for evidence of nephrolithiasis (flank pain, hematuria) and contact physician if symptoms occur (therapy should be interrupted for 1–3 days). Monitor stool frequency and consistency (watery, loose, soft). Assess for abdominal discomfort, headache.

Patient/Family Teaching

Advise that indinavir is not cure for HIV, and condition may progress in spite of treatment. Do not modify or discontinue treatment w/o physician approval. If dose is missed, take next dose at regularly scheduled time (do *not* double the dose). Best taken w/o food but water only (optimal absorption) 1 hr before or 2 hrs after a meal but may take with water, skim milk, juice, coffee or tea, or w/light meal (e.g., dry toast w/jelly, juice and coffee w/skim milk and sugar; or cornflakes, skim milk and sugar).

indomethacin

in-doe-**meth**-ah-sin
(Indocin, Indocin-SR)

indomethacin sodium trihydrate

(Indocin IV)

CANADIAN AVAILABILITY
Apo-Indomethacin, Indocid, Indotec, Novomethacin

PREGNANCY CATEGORY B
(D if used more than 48 hrs, after 34 wks gestation, or close to delivery)

CLASSIFICATION

Nonsteroidal anti-inflammatory

AVAILABILITY (Rx)

Capsules: 25 mg, 50 mg. **Capsules (sustained-release):** 75 mg. **Oral Suspension:** 25 mg/5 ml. **Suppository:** 50 mg. **Powder for Injection:** 1 mg.

PHARMACODYNAMICS

	ONSET	PEAK	DURATION
Oral (analgesic)			
	0.5 hr	—	4–6 hrs
Oral (antirheumatic)			
	7 days	1–2 wks	—

PHARMACOKINETICS

Absorption: Well absorbed from GI tract. **Metabolism:** Metabolized in liver. **Excretion:** Primarily excreted in urine. **Half-life:** 4–6 hrs (increased in neonates: 2–60 hrs).

ACTION/*THERAPEUTIC EFFECT*

Produces analgesic and anti-inflammatory effect by inhibiting prostaglandin synthesis, *reducing inflammatory response and intensity of pain stimulus reaching sensory nerve endings.* ***Patent ductus:*** Inhibits prostaglandin synthesis, increases sensitivity of premature ductus to dilating effects of prostaglandins, *causing closure of patent ductus arteriosus.*

USES/*UNLABELED*

Treatment of active stages of rheumatoid arthritis, osteoarthritis, ankylosing spondylitis, acute gouty arthritis, acute painful shoulder. Relief of acute bursitis and/or tendinitis of shoulder. For closure of hemodynamically significant patent ductus arteriosus of premature infants weighing 500–1,750 g. *Treatment of psoriatic arthritis, rheumatic complications associated w/Paget's disease of bone, fever due to malignancy, vascular headache, pericarditis.*

STORAGE/HANDLING

Store capsules, suppositories, oral suspension at room temperature. IV solutions made w/o preservatives should be used immediately. Use IV immediately after reconstitution. IV solution appears clear; discard if cloudy or if precipitate forms. Discard unused portion.

ADMINISTRATION

ORAL:

- Give after meals or w/food or antacids.
- Do not crush sustained-release capsules.

RECTAL:

- If suppository is too soft, chill for 30 min in refrigerator or run cold water over foil wrapper.
- Moisten suppository w/cold water before inserting well up into rectum.

IV:

- **Note:** IV injection preferred for patent ductus arteriosus in neonate (may give dose orally via NG tube or rectally).
- To 1 mg vial, add 1–2 ml preservative-free sterile water for injection or 0.9% NaCl injection to provide concentration of 1 mg or 0.5 mg/ml, respectively. Do not further dilute.
- Administer over 5–10 sec.
- Restrict fluid intake.

INDICATIONS/ROUTES/DOSAGE

Moderate to severe rheumatoid arthritis, osteoarthritis, ankylosing spondylitis:
Oral: Adults, elderly: Initially, 25 mg 2–3 times/day. Increase by 25–50 mg/wk up to 150–200 mg/day. ***Extended-release: Adults, elderly:*** Initially, 75 mg/day up to 75 mg two times/day.

Acute gouty arthritis:
Oral: Adults, elderly: Initially, 100 mg, then 50 mg three times/day.

Acute painful shoulder:
Oral: Adults, elderly: 75–150 mg/day in 3–4 divided doses.

Usual rectal dosage:
Adults, elderly: 50 mg four times/day. ***Children:*** Initially, 1.5–2.5 mg/kg/day, up to 4 mg/kg/day. Do not exceed 150–200 mg/day.

Patent ductus arteriosus:
Note: May give up to 3 doses at 12–24 hr intervals.

IV: Neonates: Initially, 0.2 mg/kg. ***<48 hrs old:*** 0.1 mg/kg for 2nd and

3rd doses. ***Age 2–7 days:*** 0.2 mg/kg for 2nd and 3rd doses. ***>7 days old:*** 0.25 mg/kg for 2nd and 3rd doses.

CONTRAINDICATIONS

History of allergic reaction to aspirin or other NSAIDs, history of recurrent or active GI lesions. *Suppositories:* History of proctitis or recent rectal bleeding.

CAUTIONS

Impaired renal/hepatic function, elderly, volume depletion, CHF, sepsis, epilepsy, parkinsonism, psychiatric disturbances, coagulation defects.

INTERACTIONS

DRUG: May increase effects of ***oral anticoagulants, heparin, thrombolytics.*** May decrease effect of ***antihypertensives, diuretics. Salicylates, aspirin*** may increase risk of GI side effects, bleeding. ***Bone marrow depressants*** may increase risk of hematologic reactions. May increase concentration, toxicity of ***lithium.*** May increase ***methotrexate*** toxicity. ***Probenecid*** may increase concentration. May increase concentration of ***aminoglycosides*** in neonates. HERBAL: Feverfew, ginkgo may increase risk of bleeding. FOOD: None significant. ALTERED LAB VALUES: May prolong bleeding time. May alter blood glucose. May increase BUN, creatinine, potassium, liver function tests. May decrease sodium, platelet count.

SIDE EFFECTS

FREQUENT: *Oral (3–9%):* Fluid retention, edema, dizziness, headache, abdominal cramps, nausea, indigestion. *Patent ductus arteriosus:* Impaired renal function, vomiting. OCCASIONAL: *Oral (1–3%):* Depression, ringing in ears, increased sweating, drowsiness, constipation, diarrhea, vomiting. *Patent ductus arteriosus:* Bleeding disturbances. RARE: *Oral (<1%):* Increased blood pressure, confusion, hives, itching, skin rash, blurred vision. *Patent ductus arteriosus:* Acidosis, apnea, bradycardia, alkalosis.

ADVERSE REACTIONS/TOXIC EFFECTS

Ulceration of esophagus, stomach, duodenum, or small intestine, paralytic ileus may occur. In those w/impaired renal function, hyperkalemia along w/worsening of impairment may occur. May aggravate depression or psychiatric disturbances, epilepsy, parkinsonism. Nephrotoxicity (dysuria, hematuria, proteinuria, nephrotic syndrome) occurs rarely.

PATIENT CONSIDERATIONS

BASELINE ASSESSMENT

May mask signs of infection. Do not give concurrently w/triamterene (may potentiate acute renal failure). Assess onset, type, location, and duration of pain, fever, or inflammation. Inspect appearance of affected joints for immobility, deformities, and skin condition.

INTERVENTION/EVALUATION

Monitor for evidence of nausea, dyspepsia. Assist w/ambulation if dizziness occurs. Evaluate for therapeutic response: relief of pain, stiffness, swelling, increase in joint mobility, reduced joint tenderness, improved grip strength.

PATIENT/FAMILY TEACHING

Avoid aspirin, alcohol during therapy (increases risk of GI bleeding). If GI upset occurs, take w/food, milk. Report headache. Avoid tasks that require alertness, motor skills until response to drug is established.

Swallow capsule whole; do not crush or chew.

infliximab

in-**flicks**-ih-mab
(Remicade)

PREGNANCY CATEGORY C

CLASSIFICATION

Monoclonal antibody

AVAILABILITY (Rx)

Powder for injection: 100 mg

PHARMACOKINETICS

Absorption: Absorbed into GI tissue; primarily distributed in the vascular compartment. **Half-life:** 9.5 days.

ACTION/*THERAPEUTIC EFFECT*

Binds to soluble and transmembrane cytokines, inhibiting receptor binding and functional activity, *reducing infiltration of inflammatory cells, decreasing inflamed areas of the intestine.*

USES

Treatment of moderate-to-severe Crohn's disease, treatment of those with fistulizing Crohn's disease for the reduction in number of draining enterocutaneous fistula(s). Treatment of rheumatoid arthritis.

ADMINISTRATION

Note: Do not infuse infliximab concurrently in the same IV line with other agents.

IV INFUSION:

- Reconstitute each vial with 10 ml sterile water for injection, using 21 gauge or smaller needle. Direct the stream of sterile water to the glass wall of the vial.
- Swirl the vial gently by rotating the vial to dissolve the contents. Do not shake.
- Allow the solution to stand for 5 min.
- As infliximab is a protein, the solution may develop a few translucent particles; do not use if particles are opaque or foreign particles are present.
- Solution should appear colorless to light yellow and opalescent; do not use if discolored.
- Withdraw a volume of 0.9% sodium chloride injection from a 250 ml bag to equal the volume of reconstituted solution to be injected into the 250 ml bag (approximately 10 ml). Total dose to be infused should equal 250 ml.
- Slowly add the reconstituted infliximab solution to the 250 ml infusion bag. Gently mix. Infusion concentration should range between 0.4 and 4 mg/ml.
- Begin infusion within 3 hrs after reconstitution.
- Administer the IV infusion 2≥ hrs, using set with a low-protein-binding filter.

INDICATIONS/ROUTES/DOSAGES

Moderate-to-severe Crohn's disease:
IV infusion: Adults, elderly: 5 mg/kg as a single IV infusion.

Fistulizing Crohn's disease:
IV infusion: Adults, elderly: Initially, 5 mg/kg followed with additional 5mg/kg doses at 2 and 6 wks after the first infusion.

CONTRAINDICATIONS

Hypersensitivity to murine proteins or other components of the product.

CAUTIONS

Elderly, those on immunosuppressive therapy.

INTERACTIONS

DRUG: None significant. **HERBAL:** None known. **FOOD:** None significant. **ALTERED LAB VALUES:** None significant.

SIDE EFFECTS

FREQUENT (10–22%): Headache, nausea, fatigue, fever. **OCCASIONAL (5–9%):** Fever/chills during infusion, pharyngitis, vomiting, pain, dizziness, bronchitis, rash, rhinitis, coughing, pruritus, sinusitis, myalgia, back pain. **RARE (1–4%):** Hypo/hypertension, paresthesia, anxiety, depression, insomnia, diarrhea, urinary tract infection.

ADVERSE REACTIONS/TOXIC EFFECTS

Potential for hypersensitivity reaction, lupus-like syndrome.

PATIENT CONSIDERATIONS

BASELINE ASSESSMENT

Determine pattern of bowel activity. Check baseline hydration status: skin turgor, mucous membranes for dryness, urinary status.

INTERVENTIONS/EVALUATION

Monitor stool frequency and consistency (watery, loose, soft, semisolid, solid). Assess bowel sounds for peristaltic activity. Encourage adequate fluid intake.

---

insulin

in-sull-in

Rapid acting:

INSULIN LISPRO

(Humalog)

INSULIN INJECTION

(Humulin R, Novolin R, Regular, Velosulin)

PROMPT INSULIN ZINC SUSPENSION

(Semilente)

Intermediate acting:

ISOPHANE INSULIN SUSPENSION

(Humulin N, Insulatard, Novolin N, NPH)

INSULIN ZINC SUSPENSION

(Humulin L, Lente, Novolin L)

Long acting:

EXTENDED INSULIN ZINC SUSPENSION

(Humulin U, Ultralente)

FIXED-COMBINATION(S)
Isophane Insulin Suspension w/insulin injection: **Humulin 70/30, Mixtard, Novolin 70/30, Humulin 50/50.**

CANADIAN AVAILABILITY
See above.

PREGNANCY CATEGORY B

CLASSIFICATION

Hypoglycemic

AVAILABILITY (OTC)

Regular, NPH, 70/30, 50/50, Lente, Ultralente: all 100 units/ml

PHARMACODYNAMICS

	ONSET (HRS)	PEAK (HRS)	DURATION (HRS)
Regular	0.5–1	—	6–8
Semilente	1–1.5	5–10	12–16
NPH	1–1.5	4–12	24
Lente	1–2.5	7–15	24
Ultralente	4–8	10–30	>36

ACTION/*THERAPEUTIC EFFECT*

Facilitates passage of glucose, K, Mg across cellular membranes of skeletal and cardiac muscle, adipose tissue; controls storage and metabolism of carbohydrates, protein, fats. Promotes conversion of glucose to glycogen in liver.

USES

Treatment of insulin-dependent type I diabetes mellitus; noninsulin-dependent type 2 diabetes mellitus when diet/weight control therapy has failed to maintain satisfactory blood glucose levels or in event of pregnancy, surgery, trauma, infection, fever, severe renal, hepatic, or endocrine dysfunction. Regular insulin used in emergency treatment of ketoacidosis, to promote passage of glucose across cell membrane in hyperalimentation, to facilitate intracellular shift of K+ in hyperkalemia.

STORAGE/HANDLING

Store currently used insulin at room temperature (avoid extreme temperatures, direct sunlight). Store extra vials in refrigerator. Discard unused vials if not used for several weeks. No insulin should have precipitate or discoloration.

ADMINISTRATION

SubQ:

- Give SubQ only. (Regular insulin is the *only* insulin that may be given IV, IM for ketoacidosis or other specific situations.)
- Do not give cold insulin; warm to room temperature.
- Rotate vial gently between hands; do not shake. Regular insulin should be clear; no insulin should have precipitate or discoloration.
- Usually administered approximately 30 min before a meal (Insulin lispro given up to 15 min before meals). Check blood glucose concentration before administration; dosage highly individualized.
- When insulin is mixed, regular insulin is always drawn up first. Mixtures should be administered at once (binding can occur within 5 min). Humalog may be mixed w/Humulin-N, -L.
- SubQ injections may be given in thigh, abdomen, upper arm, buttocks, or upper back if there is adequate adipose tissue.
- Rotation of injection sites is essential; maintain careful record.
- For home situations, prefilled syringes are stable for 1 wk under refrigeration (this includes mixtures once they have stabilized, (e.g., 15 min for NPH/Regular, 24 hrs for Lente/Regular). Prefilled syringes should be stored in vertical or oblique position to avoid plugging; plunger should be pulled back slightly and the syringe rocked to remix the solution before injection.

INDICATIONS/ROUTES/DOSAGE

Dosage for insulin is individualized/monitored.

Usual dosage guidelines:
Note: Adjust dosage to achieve premeal and bedtime glucose level of 80–140 mg/dl (children <5 yrs: 100–200 mg/dl).

SubQ: Adults, elderly, children: 0.5–1 unit/kg/day. ***Adolescents (during growth spurt):*** 0.8–1.2 units/kg/day.

CONTRAINDICATIONS

Hypersensitivity or insulin resistance may require change of type or species source of insulin.

INTERACTIONS

DRUG: ***Glucocorticoids, thiazide diuretics*** may increase blood glucose. ***Alcohol*** may increase insulin effect. ***Beta-adrenergic blockers*** may increase risk of hypo/hyperglycemia, mask signs of hypoglycemia, prolong period of hypoglycemia. **HERBAL:** None known. **FOOD:** None significant. **ALTERED LAB VALUES:** May decrease potassium, magnesium, phosphate concentrations.

SIDE EFFECTS

OCCASIONAL: Local redness, swelling, itching (due to improper injection technique or allergy to cleansing solution or insulin). **INFREQUENT:** Somogyi effect (rebound hyperglycemia) w/chronically excessive insulin doses. Systemic allergic reaction (rash, angioedema, anaphylaxis), lipodystrophy (depression at injection site due to breakdown of adipose tissue), lipohypertrophy (accumulation of SubQ tissue at injection site due to lack of adequate site rotation). **RARE:** Insulin resistance.

ADVERSE REACTIONS/TOXIC EFFECTS

Severe hypoglycemia (due to hyperinsulinism) may occur in overdose of insulin, decrease or delay of food intake, excessive exercise, or those w/brittle diabetes. Diabetic ketoacidosis may result from stress, illness, omission of insulin dose, or long-term poor insulin control.

PATIENT CONSIDERATIONS

BASELINE ASSESSMENT

Question for allergies. Check blood glucose level. Discuss lifestyle to determine extent of learning, emotional needs.

INTERVENTION/EVALUATION

Monitor blood glucose and food intake; assure between meal/bedtime nourishments. Assess for hypoglycemia (refer to pharmacokinetics table for peak times/duration): cool wet skin, tremors, dizziness, headache, anxiety, tachycardia, numbness in mouth, hunger, diplopia. Check sleeping pt for restlessness or diaphoresis. Check for hyperglycemia: polyuria (excessive urine output), polyphagia (excessive food intake), polydipsia (excessive thirst), nausea and vomiting, dim vision, fatigue, deep rapid breathing. Be alert to conditions altering glucose requirements: fever, increased activity or stress, surgical procedure.

PATIENT/FAMILY TEACHING

Prescribed diet is essential part of treatment; do not skip or delay meals. Diabetes mellitus requires lifelong control. Check blood glucose/urine as ordered. Instruct signs and symptoms, treatment of hypo/hyperglycemia, proper handling, and administration of medication. Carry candy, sugar packets, other sugar supplements for immediate response to hypoglycemia. Wear/carry medical alert identification. Check w/physician when insulin demands are altered (e.g., fever, infection, trauma, stress, heavy physical activity). Avoid alcoholic beverages. Do not take other medication w/o consulting physician. Weight con-

trol, exercise, hygiene (including foot care), and not smoking are integral part of therapy. Protect skin, limit sun exposure. Avoid exposure to infections. Important to keep follow-up appointments. Select clothing, positions that do not restrict blood flow. Inform dentist, physician, or surgeon of medication before any treatment is given. Assure follow-up instruction if pt/family does not thoroughly understand diabetes management or administration techniques.

interferon alfacon-1

inn-ter-**fear**-on
(Infergen)

CANADIAN AVAILABILITY
Infergen

PREGNANCY CATEGORY C

CLASSIFICATION

Antiviral

AVAILABILITY (Rx)

Injection: 9 mcg, 15 mcg

PHARMACOKINETICS

Absorption: Plasma concentration following SubQ administration is undetectable.

ACTION/*THERAPEUTIC EFFECT*

Inhibits viral replication in virus-infected cells, suppresses cell proliferation, *increases phagocytic action of macrophages, augments specific cytotoxicity of lymphocytes.*

USES/*UNLABELED*

Treatment of chronic hepatitis C virus (HCV) infections in pts ≥ 18 yrs with compensated liver disease who have anti-HCV serum antibodies or the presence of HCV RNA. *Treatment of hairy-cell leukemia.*

INDICATIONS/ROUTES/DOSAGE

Hepatitis C infection:
SubQ: Adults, elderly: 9 mcg as a single injection 3 times/wk for 24 wks. At least 48 hrs should elapse between doses. Those who did not respond to previous interferon therapy or relapsed following its discontinuation may be treated with 15 mcg 3 times/wk for 6 mos.

CONTRAINDICATIONS

Sensitivity to alpha interferon alfacon-1, decompensated hepatic disease (jaundice, ascites, coagulopathy, decreased serum albumin), history severe psychiatric disorders.

CAUTIONS

History of depression, preexisting cardiac disease, those concurrently receiving myelosuppressive medication, autoimmune disorders, bone marrow depression, history endocrine disorders.

INTERACTIONS

DRUG: *Bone marrow depressants* may have additive effect. **HERBAL:** None known. **FOOD:** None significant. **ALTERED LAB VALUES:** May increase SGOT (AST), SGPT (ALT), alkaline phosphatase, bilirubin, serum creatinine, creatinine clearance, LDH, thyroid (TSH and T_4), serum triglycerides. May decrease Hgb, Hct, platelet count, WBC count.

SIDE EFFECTS

FREQUENT (39–82%): Flulike symptoms (headache, fatigue, fever, chills, myalgia, arthralgia), abdominal pain, nausea, insomnia, back pain. **OCCASIONAL (12–34%):** Upper respiratory tract infection (pharyngitis, cough, sinusitis, rhinitis), nervousness, diarrhea, musculoskeletal pain, mild-to-moderate depression, anorexia, injection site erythema, dizziness, dyspepsia, pruritus, anxiety, hot flashes, paresthesia, vomiting, rash. **RARE (9%):** Injection site pain, peripheral edema, constipation.

ADVERSE REACTIONS/TOXIC EFFECTS

Potential for blood dyscrasias (granulocytopenia, thrombocytopenia, leukopenia). May exacerbate preexisting cardiac abnormalities. Hypothyroidism occurs occasionally. Hypersensitivity reaction, ophthalmologic abnormalities occur rarely.

PATIENT CONSIDERATIONS

Baseline Assessment

CBC, blood chemistry, urinalysis, renal and liver function tests, thyroid function tests should be performed prior to initial therapy and routinely thereafter.

Intervention/Evaluation

Monitor all levels of clinical function (numerous side effects). Monitor all lab results; assess ANC (therapy should be withheld if ANC <500). Assess for depression and suicidal ideation.

Patient/Family Teaching

Flulike symptoms tend to diminish with continued therapy. Do not have immunizations w/o physician's approval (drug lowers body's resistance). Avoid contact with those who have recently received live virus vaccine. Report if signs of depression, blurred vision or loss of visual field occur.

---

interferon alfa-2a

(Roferon-A)

See Classification section under: Cancer chemotherapy

---

interferon alfa-2b

(Intron-A)

See Classification section under: Cancer chemotherapy

---

interferon alfa-n3

(Alferon N)

See Classification section under: Cancer chemotherapy

---

interferon beta 1a

inn-ter-**fear**-on
(Avonex)

CANADIAN AVAILABILITY
Rebif

PREGNANCY CATEGORY C

CLASSIFICATION

Interferon

AVAILABILITY (Rx)

Powder for Injection: 33 mcg (6.6 million units)

PHARMACOKINETICS

Following IM administration, peak serum levels attained in 3–15 hrs. Biologic markers increase within 12 hrs and remain elevated for 4 days. **Half-life:** 10 hrs (IM).

ACTION/*THERAPEUTIC EFFECT*

Interacts w/specific cell receptors found on surface of human cells. *Possesses antiviral and immunoregulatory activities.*

USES/*UNLABELED*

Treatment of relapsing multiple sclerosis to slow progression of physical disability, decrease frequency of clinical exacerbations. *Treatment of AIDS, AIDS-related Kaposi's sarcoma, renal cell carcinoma, malignant melanoma, acute non-A, non-B hepatitis.*

STORAGE/HANDLING

Refrigerate vials. Following reconstitution, use within 6 hrs if refrigerated. Discard if discolored, contains a precipitate.

ADMINISTRATION

IM:

- Reconstitute 33 mcg (6.6 million IU) vial w/1.1 ml diluent (supplied by manufacturer).
- Gently swirl to dissolve medication; do not shake.
- Discard if discolored, contains particulate matter.
- Discard unused portion (contains no preservative).

INDICATIONS/ROUTES/DOSAGE

Relapsing-remitting multiple sclerosis:
IM: Adults: 30 mcg once weekly.

CONTRAINDICATIONS

Hypersensitivity to interferon, albumin.

CAUTIONS

Chronic progressive multiple sclerosis, children <18 yrs.

INTERACTIONS

DRUG: None significant. **HERBAL:** None known. **FOOD:** None significant. **ALTERED LAB VALUES:** May increase SGOT (AST), SGPT (ALT), bilirubin, alkaline phosphatase, BUN, calcium, glucose. May decrease Hgb, platelets, WBCs, neutrophils.

SIDE EFFECTS

FREQUENT: Headache (67%), flu-like symptoms (61%), myalgia (34%), upper respiratory infection (31%), pain (24%), asthenia, chills (21%), sinusitis (18%), infection (11%). **OCCASIONAL:** Abdominal pain, arthralgia (9%), chest pain, dyspnea (6%), malaise, syncope (4%). **RARE:** Injection site reaction, hypersensitivity reaction (3%).

ADVERSE REACTIONS/TOXIC EFFECTS

Anemia occurs in 8% of pts.

PATIENT CONSIDERATIONS

BASELINE ASSESSMENT

Obtain Hgb, CBC and differential, platelet count, blood chemistries including liver function tests. Assess home situation for support of therapy.

INTERVENTION/EVALUATION

Assess for headache, flulike symptoms, muscle ache (see Side Effects). Periodically monitor lab results and reevaluate injection technique. Assess for depression and suicidal ideation.

PATIENT/FAMILY TEACHING

Do not change schedule or dosage w/o consultation w/physician. Instruct on correct reconstitution of product and administration, including aseptic technique. Provide puncture-resistant container for used needles, syringes, and explain proper disposal. Explain that injection site reactions may occur. These do not require discontinuation of therapy, but note type and extent carefully.

Depression or suicidal ideation must be reported immediately.

interferon beta 1b

inn-ter-**fear**-on
(Betaseron)

CANADIAN AVAILABILITY
Betaseron

PREGNANCY CATEGORY C

CLASSIFICATION

Interferon

AVAILABILITY (Rx)

Powder for Injection: 0.3 mg (9.6 million units)

PHARMACOKINETICS

Half-life: 8 min–4.3 hrs.

ACTION/*THERAPEUTIC EFFECT*

Interacts w/specific cell receptors found on surface of human cells. *Possesses antiviral and immunoregulatory activities.*

USES/*UNLABELED*

Reduces frequency of clinical exacerbations w/pts w/relapsing-remitting multiple sclerosis (recurrent attacks of neurologic dysfunction). *Treatment of AIDS, AIDS-related Kaposi's sarcoma, renal cell carcinoma, malignant melanoma, acute non-A, non-B hepatitis.*

STORAGE/HANDLING

Refrigerate vials. After reconstitution, stable for 3 hrs if refrigerated. Use within 3 hrs of reconstitution. Discard if discolored, contains a precipitate.

ADMINISTRATION

SubQ:

- Reconstitute 0.3 mg (9.6 million IU) vial w/1.2 ml diluent (supplied by manufacturer) to provide concentration of 0.25 mg/ml (8 million U/ml).
- Gently swirl to dissolve medication; do not shake.
- Discard if discolored, contains particulate matter.
- Withdraw 1 ml solution and inject SubQ into arms, abdomen, hips, or thighs using 27 gauge needle.
- Discard unused portion (contains no preservative).

INDICATIONS/ROUTES/DOSAGE

Relapsing-remitting multiple sclerosis:
SubQ: Adults: 0.25 mg (8 million IU) every other day.

CONTRAINDICATIONS

Hypersensitivity to interferon, albumin.

CAUTIONS

Chronic progressive multiple sclerosis, children <18 yrs of age.

INTERACTIONS

DRUG: None significant. **HERBAL:** None known. **FOOD:** None significant. **ALTERED LAB VALUES:** May increase SGOT (AST), SGPT (ALT), bilirubin, alkaline phosphatase, BUN, calcium, glucose, WBCs. May decrease Hgb, platelets, WBCs, neutrophils.

SIDE EFFECTS

FREQUENT: Injection site reaction (85%), headache (84%), flulike symptoms (76%), fever (59%), pain (52%), asthenia (49%), myalgia (44%), sinusitis (36%), diarrhea, dizziness (35%), mental symptoms (29%), constipation (24%), diaphoresis (23%), vomiting (21%). **OCCASIONAL:** Malaise (15%), somnolence (6%), alopecia (4%).

ADVERSE REACTIONS/TOXIC EFFECTS

Seizures occur rarely.

PATIENT CONSIDERATIONS

Baseline Assessment

Obtain Hgb, CBC and differential, platelet count, blood chemistries including liver function tests. Assess home situation for support of therapy.

Intervention/Evaluation

Periodically monitor lab results and reevaluate injection technique. Assess for nausea (high incidence). Monitor sleep pattern. Monitor stool frequency and consistency (watery, loose, soft). Assist w/ambulation if dizziness occurs. Question for evidence of heartburn, epigastric discomfort. Monitor food intake. Assess for depression and suicidal ideation.

Patient/Family Teaching

Do not change schedule or dosage w/o consultation w/physician. Instruct on correct reconstitution of product and administration, including aseptic technique. Provide puncture-resistant container for used needles, syringes, and explain proper disposal. Explain that injection site reactions may occur. These do not require discontinuation of therapy, but note type and extent carefully. Depression or suicidal ideation must be reported immediately. Inform physician of flulike symptoms (occur commonly but decrease over time). Wear sunscreens, protective clothing if exposed to ultraviolet light or sunlight until tolerance known. Interferon beta 1b has abortifacient potential.

interferon gamma-1b

inn-ter-**fear**-on
(Actimmune)

PREGNANCY CATEGORY C

CLASSIFICATION

Biologic response modifier

AVAILABILITY (Rx)

Injection: 100 mcg (3 million units)

PHARMACOKINETICS

Absorption: Slowly absorbed following SubQ administration. **Metabolism:** Metabolic fate unknown.

ACTION/*THERAPEUTIC EFFECT*

Induces activation of macrophages in blood monocytes to phagocytes (necessary in cellular immune response to intracellular and extracellular pathogens). *Enhances phagocytic function, antimicrobial activity of monocytes.*

USES

Reduces frequency, severity of serious infections due to chronic granulomatous disease. Treatment of osteoporosis.

STORAGE/HANDLING

Refrigerate vials. Do not freeze. Do not keep at room temperature >12 hrs; discard if left out longer. Vials are single dose; discard unused portion. Clear, colorless solution. Do not use if discolored, precipitate formed.

ADMINISTRATION

- **Note:** Avoid excessive agitation of vial; do not shake.

SubQ:

- When given 3 times/week, give in left deltoid, right deltoid, and anterior thigh.

INDICATIONS/ROUTES/DOSAGE

Chronic granulomatous disease: *SubQ: Adults, children >1 yr:* 50 mcg/m^2 (1.5 million units/m^2) in pts with body surface area (BSA) >0.5 m^2; 1.5 mcg/kg/dose in pts with ≤BSA 0.5 m^2. Give 3 times/wk.

CONTRAINDICATIONS

Hypersensitivity to *Escherichia coli* products.

CAUTIONS

Seizure disorders, compromised CNS function, preexisting cardiac disease (including ischemia, CHF, arrhythmia), myelosuppression.

INTERACTIONS

DRUG: *Bone marrow depressants* may increase bone marrow depression. **HERBAL:** None known. **FOOD:** None significant. **ALTERED LAB VALUES:** None significant.

SIDE EFFECTS

FREQUENT (>15%): Fever, headache, rash, chills, fatigue, diarrhea. **OCCASIONAL (4–14%):** Nausea, vomiting, muscle aches. **RARE (1–3%):** Anorexia, hypersensitivity reaction.

ADVERSE REACTIONS/TOXIC EFFECTS

May exacerbate preexisting CNS, cardiac abnormalities demonstrated as decreased mental status, gait disturbance, dizziness.

PATIENT CONSIDERATIONS

BASELINE ASSESSMENT

CBC, differential and platelet counts, blood chemistries, urinalysis, renal and liver function tests should be performed prior to initial therapy and at 3 mo intervals during course of treatment.

INTERVENTION/EVALUATION

Monitor for flulike symptoms (fever, chills, fatigue, muscle aches). Assess for evidence of hypersensitivity reaction. Check for gait disturbance, dizziness. Assist with walking if these symptoms appear.

PATIENT/FAMILY TEACHING

Flulike symptoms (fever, chills, fatigue, muscle aches) are generally mild and tend to disappear as treatment continues. Symptoms may be minimized by bedtime administration. Avoid tasks that require alertness, motor skills until response to drug is established. If home use prescribed, instruct in proper technique of administration, care in proper disposal of needles, syringes. Vial should remain refrigerated.

ipecac syrup

ip-eh-kak

CANADIAN AVAILABILITY
PMS Ipecac Syrup

PREGNANCY CATEGORY C

CLASSIFICATION

Antidote

AVAILABILITY (OTC)

Syrup: 15 ml, 30 ml

PHARMACODYNAMICS

	ONSET	PEAK	DURATION
Oral	<30 min	—	—

PHARMACOKINETICS

After administration, vomiting occurs within 20–30 min.

ACTION/*THERAPEUTIC EFFECT*

Acts centrally by stimulating medullary chemoreceptor trigger zone and locally by irritating gastric mucosa, *producing emesis.*

USES

Induces vomiting in early treatment of unabsorbed oral poisons, drug overdosage.

STORAGE/HANDLING

Store syrup at room temperature.

ADMINISTRATION

ORAL:

- Before administering, instruct pt to sit upright before drinking syrup (enhances emetic effect).
- Do not confuse ipecac fluid extract w/ipecac syrup (fluid extract is 14 times more potent and may cause death if given inadvertently at syrup dosage).
- Emetic action may be facilitated if 200–300 ml water or clear liquid is given immediately following ipecac.

INDICATIONS/ROUTES/DOSAGE

Note: If vomiting has not occurred within 20 min after first dose, repeat w/15 ml. If vomiting has not occurred within 30 min after last dose, initiate gastric lavage, activated charcoal.

Emetic:

Oral: Adults, elderly, children >12 yrs: 15–30 ml; give w/3–4 glasses water immediately following administration. *Children 1–12 yrs:* 15 ml; follow w/1–2 glasses water. *Children 6 mos–1 yr:* 5–10 ml; follow w/1 glass water. If vomiting has not occurred within 30 min, repeat initial dosage.

CONTRAINDICATIONS

Ingestion of petroleum distillates (paint thinner, gasoline, kerosene), alkali (lye), acids, strychnine.

CAUTIONS

Impaired cardiac function, pathologic blood vessel disease.

INTERACTIONS

DRUG: *Antiemetics* may decrease effect. **HERBAL:** None known. **FOOD:** Avoid carbonated beverages (causes stomach distension), milk or milk products (decreases effectiveness). **ALTERED LAB VALUES:** None significant.

SIDE EFFECTS

FREQUENT: Nausea, vomiting. After vomiting, diarrhea and CNS symptoms (drowsiness, mild CNS depression) commonly occur.

ADVERSE REACTIONS/TOXIC EFFECTS

Cardiotoxicity may occur if ipecac syrup is not vomited (noted as hypotension, tachycardia, precordial chest pain, pulmonary congestion, dyspnea, ventricular tachycardia and fibrillation, cardiac arrest). Overdose may produce diarrhea, fast/irregular heartbeat, nausea continuing >30 min, stomach pain, respiratory difficulty, unusually tired, aching/stiff muscles.

PATIENT CONSIDERATIONS

BASELINE ASSESSMENT

Do not administer to semiconscious, unconscious, or convuls-

ing pt. Gastric lavage, activated charcoal is necessary if vomiting does not occur within 30 min of second dosage to avoid drug toxicity (bloody stools, vomitus, abdominal pain, hypotension, dyspnea, shock, cardiac disturbances, seizures, coma). Maintain pt in upright position to enhance emetic effect.

INTERVENTION/EVALUATION

Closely monitor vital signs, EKG during and after drug is administered. Watch for changes from initial assessment. Check for reversal of poisoning or overdosage symptoms. Monitor daily bowel activity and stool consistency (watery, loose, soft, semisolid, solid) and record time of evacuation. Assess for dehydration in excessive vomiting: poor skin turgor, dry mucous membranes, longitudinal furrows in tongue.

ipratropium bromide

ih-prah-**trow**-pea-um
(Atrovent)

FIXED-COMBINATION(S)
W/albuterol, a bronchodilator (Combivent)

CANADIAN AVAILABILITY
Atrovent

PREGNANCY CATEGORY B

CLASSIFICATION

Bronchodilator

AVAILABILITY (Rx)

Aerosol Solution for Inhalation: 0.02% (500 mcg). **Nasal Spray:** 0.03%, 0.06%

PHARMACODYNAMICS

	ONSET	PEAK	DURATION
Inhalation			
	<15 min	1–2 hrs	3–4 hrs

PHARMACOKINETICS

Absorption: Minimal systemic absorption. **Metabolism:** Metabolized in liver (systemic absorption). **Excretion:** Primarily eliminated in feces. **Half-life:** 1.5–4 hrs.

ACTION/ *THERAPEUTIC EFFECT*

Inhibits vagal mediated response by reversing action of acetylcholine, *producing smooth muscle relaxation, bronchodilating response.* Produces significant increase in forced vital lung capacity.

USES

Maintenance treatment of bronchospasm due to chronic obstructive airway disease, including bronchitis, emphysema. Adjunct to bronchodilators for maintenance treatment of bronchial asthma. Not to be used for immediate bronchospasm relief. ***Nasal spray:*** Rhinorrhea (0.03% associated w/perineal rhinitis, 0.06% associated w/common cold).

ADMINISTRATION

INHALATION:

- Shake container well, exhale completely, then holding mouthpiece 1 inch away from lips, inhale and hold breath as long as possible before exhaling.
- Wait 1–10 min before inhaling second dose (allows for deeper bronchial penetration).
- Rinse mouth w/water immediately after inhalation (prevents mouth/throat dryness).

INDICATIONS/ROUTES/DOSAGE

Bronchospasm:
Inhalation: Adults, elderly: 2 inhalations 4 times/day. Wait 1–10 min before administering second inhalation. *Maximum:* 12 inhalations/24 hrs.

Nebulization: Adults, elderly: 500 mcg 3–4 times/day.

Rhinorrhea:
Intranasal: Adults, children >6 yrs: 0.03%: 2 sprays 2–3 times/day. *Adults, children >12 yrs: 0.06%:* 2 sprays 3–4 times/day.

CONTRAINDICATIONS

History of hypersensitivity to atropine.

CAUTIONS

Narrow-angle glaucoma, prostatic hypertrophy, bladder neck obstruction.

INTERACTIONS

DRUG: Avoid mixing w/*cromolyn inhalation solution* (forms precipitate). HERBAL: None known. FOOD: None significant. ALTERED LAB VALUES: None significant.

SIDE EFFECTS

FREQUENT: *Inhalation (3–10%):* Cough, dry mouth, headache, dizziness, nervousness, upset stomach, nausea. *Nasal:* Dry nose/mouth, headache, nasal irritation. OCCASIONAL: *Inhalation (1–3%):* Increased bronchospasm, visual changes, hypotension, insomnia, metallic/unpleasant taste, palpitations, urinary retention. *Nasal:* Diarrhea/constipation, dry throat, stomach pain, stuffy nose.

ADVERSE REACTIONS/TOXIC EFFECTS

Worsening of narrow-angle glaucoma, acute eye pain, hypotension occur rarely.

PATIENT CONSIDERATIONS

BASELINE ASSESSMENT

Offer emotional support (high incidence of anxiety due to difficulty in breathing and sympathomimetic response to drug).

INTERVENTION/EVALUATION

Monitor rate, depth, rhythm, type of respiration; quality and rate of pulse. Assess lung sounds for rhonchi, wheezing, rales. Monitor arterial blood gases. Observe lips, fingernails for blue or dusky color in light-skinned pts; gray in dark-skinned pts. Observe for clavicular retractions, hand tremor. Evaluate for clinical improvement (quieter, slower respirations, relaxed facial expression, cessation of clavicular retractions).

PATIENT/FAMILY TEACHING

Increase fluid intake (decreases lung secretion viscosity). Do not take more than 2 inhalations at any one time (excessive use may produce paradoxical bronchoconstriction or a decreased bronchodilating effect). Rinsing mouth with water immediately after inhalation may prevent mouth/throat dryness. Avoid excessive use of caffeine derivatives (chocolate, coffee, tea, cola, cocoa).

irbesartan

ir-beh-**sar**-tan
(Avapro)

FIXED-COMBINATION(S)
W/hydrochlorothiazide, a diuretic (**Avalide**)

CANADIAN AVAILABILITY
Avapro

PREGNANCY CATEGORY C
(first trimester)

PREGNANCY CATEGORY D
(second and third trimester)

CLASSIFICATION

Angiotensin II receptor antagonist

AVAILABILITY (Rx)

Tablets: 75 mg, 150 mg, 300 mg

PHARMACOKINETICS

Absorption: Rapidly and completely absorbed following oral administration. **Metabolism:** Undergoes hepatic metabolism to inactive metabolite. **Excretion:** Recovered primarily in feces and to a lesser extent, in urine. Not removed by hemodialysis. **Half-life:** 11–15 hrs.

ACTION/*THERAPEUTIC EFFECT*

Potent vasodilator. An angiotensin II receptor (type AT_1) antagonist; blocks vasoconstrictor and aldosterone-secreting effects of angiotensin II, inhibiting the binding of angiotensin II to the AT_1 receptors, *producing vasodilation, decreased peripheral resistance, decrease in B/P.*

USES/*UNLABELED*

Treatment of hypertension alone or in combination with other antihypertensives. *Treatment of heart failure.*

ADMINISTRATION

ORAL:

- Give w/o regard to meals.

INDICATIONS/ROUTES/DOSAGES

Note: May be given concurrently w/other antihypertensives. If B/P is not controlled by irbesartan alone, a diuretic may be added.

Hypertension:
Oral: Adults, elderly, mildly impaired renal or hepatic function: 150 mg once daily in pts who are not volume depleted. May be titrated to 300 mg once daily.

CONTRAINDICATIONS

None significant.

CAUTIONS

Renal/hepatic function impairment, renal arterial stenosis.

INTERACTIONS

DRUG: *Hydrochlorothiazide* produces further dose reduction in B/P. **HERBAL:** None known. **FOOD:** None significant. **ALTERED LAB VALUES:** Minor increase in BUN, serum creatinine. May decrease Hgb.

SIDE EFFECTS

OCCASIONAL (3–9%): Upper respiratory infection, fatigue, diarrhea, cough. **RARE (1–2%):** Heartburn, dizziness, headache, nausea, rash.

ADVERSE REACTIONS/TOXIC EFFECTS

Overdosage may manifest as hypotension and tachycardia; bradycardia occurs less often. Institute supportive measures.

PATIENT CONSIDERATIONS

BASELINE ASSESSMENT

Obtain B/P and apical pulse immediately before each dose, in addition to regular monitoring (be alert to fluctuations). If excessive reduction in B/P occurs, place pt in supine position, feet slightly elevated. Question possibility of preg-

nancy (see Pregnancy Category). Assess medication history (especially diuretic). Question for history of hepatic/renal impairment, renal artery stenosis. Obtain BUN, serum creatinine, Hgb, and vital signs, particularly B/P, pulse rate.

INTERVENTION/EVALUATION

Maintain hydration (offer fluids frequently). Assess for evidence of upper respiratory infection. Assist with ambulation if dizziness occurs. Monitor all blood serum levels. Assess B/P for hypertension/hypotension.

PATIENT/FAMILY TEACHING

Inform female pt regarding consequences of second- and third-trimester exposure to irbesartan. Report pregnancy to physician as soon as possible. Avoid tasks that require alertness, motor skills (possible dizziness effect). Report any sign of infection (sore throat, fever). Do not stop taking medication. Need for lifelong control. Caution against exercising during hot weather (risk of dehydration, hypotension).

---

irinotecan

(Camptsar)

See Classification section under: Cancer chemotherapy

---

iron dextran

iron **dex**-tran

(Infed)

CANADIAN AVAILABILITY

Dexiron, Infufer

PREGNANCY CATEGORY C

CLASSIFICATION

Hematinic

AVAILABILITY (Rx)

Injection: 50 mg/ml

PHARMACOKINETICS

Absorption: Readily absorbed after IM administration. Major portion of absorption occurs within 72 hrs; remainder within 3–4 wks. Iron is bound to protein to form hemosiderin, ferritin, or transferrin. **Excretion:** No physiologic system of elimination. Small amounts lost daily in shedding of skin, hair, and nails, and in feces, urine, and perspiration. **Half-life:** 5–20 hrs.

ACTION/*THERAPEUTIC EFFECT*

Essential component of formation of hemoglobin, *replenishes hemoglobin and depleted iron stores.* Necessary for effective erythropoiesis and oxygen transport capacity of blood. Serves as cofactor of several essential enzymes.

USES

Treatment of established iron deficiency anemia. Use only when oral administration is not feasible or when rapid replenishment of iron is warranted.

STORAGE/HANDLING

Store at room temperature. Dark brown, slightly viscous liquid.

ADMINISTRATION

- **Note:** Test doses are generally given before the full dosage; stay w/pt for several min after injection due to potential for anaphylactic reaction and keep epinephrine and resuscitative equipment available.

IM:

- Draw up medication w/one needle, use new needle for injection (minimizes skin staining).
- Administer deep IM in upper outer quadrant of buttock only.
- Use Z-tract technique (displacement of SubQ tissue lateral to injection site before inserting needle) to minimize skin staining.

IV:

- **Note:** A too rapid IV rate may produce flushing, chest pain, shock, hypotension, tachycardia.
- May give undiluted or diluted in normal saline for infusion.
- Do not exceed IV administration rate of 50 mg/min (1 ml/min).
- Pt must remain recumbent 30–45 min following IV administration (avoid postural hypotension).

INDICATIONS/ROUTES/DOSAGE

Note: Discontinue oral iron form before administering iron dextran. Dosage expressed in terms of milligrams of elemental iron. Dosage individualized based on degree of anemia, pt weight, presence of any bleeding. Use periodic hematologic determinations as guide to therapy.

Iron deficiency anemia (no blood loss):
IM/IV: Adults, elderly: Mg iron = 0.66 × weight (kg) × (100–Hgb <g/dl>/14.8).

Replacement secondary to blood loss:
IM/IV: Adults, elderly: Replacement iron (mg) = blood loss (ml) × hematocrit.

CONTRAINDICATIONS

All anemias except iron deficiency anemia (eliminates pernicious, aplastic, normocytic, refractory).

EXTREME CAUTION

Serious liver impairment.

CAUTIONS

History of allergies, bronchial asthma, rheumatoid arthritis.

I

INTERACTIONS

DRUG: None significant. **HERBAL:** None known. **FOOD:** None significant. **ALTERED LAB VALUES:** None significant.

SIDE EFFECTS

FREQUENT: Allergic reaction (rash, itching), backache, muscle pain, chills, dizziness, headache, fever, nausea, vomiting, flushed skin, pain or redness at injection site. Brown discoloration of skin, metallic taste.

ADVERSE REACTIONS/TOXIC EFFECTS

Anaphylaxis has occurred during the first few min after injection, causing death on rare occasions. Leukocytosis, lymphadenopathy occur rarely.

PATIENT CONSIDERATIONS

Baseline Assessment

Do not give concurrently w/oral iron form (excessive iron may produce excessive iron storage [hemosiderosis]). Be alert to those w/rheumatoid arthritis or iron deficiency anemia (acute exacerbation of joint pain and swelling may occur). Inguinal lymphadenopathy may occur w/IM injection. Assess for adequate muscle mass before injecting medication.

INTERVENTION/EVALUATION

Monitor IM site for abscess formation, necrosis, atrophy, swelling, brownish color to skin. Question pt regarding soreness, pain, inflammation at or near IM injection site. Check IV site for phlebitis. Monitor serum ferritin levels.

PATIENT/FAMILY TEACHING

Pain and brown staining may occur at injection site. Oral iron should not be taken when receiving iron injections. Stools frequently become black w/iron therapy; this is harmless unless accompanied by red streaking, sticky consistency of stool, abdominal pain or cramping, which should be reported to physician. Oral hygiene, hard candy, or gum may reduce metallic taste. Notify physician immediately if fever, back pain, headache occur.

isoetharine hydrochloride

eye-sew-**eth**-ah-reen
(Bronkosol, Dey-Dose)

isoetharine mesylate

(Bronkometer)

PREGNANCY CATEGORY C

CLASSIFICATION

Bronchodilator

AVAILABILITY (Rx)

Aerosol Solution for Inhalation: 0.062%, 0.08%, 0.1%, 0.125%, 0.167%, 0.17%, 0.2%, 0.25%, 1%

PHARMACODYNAMICS

	ONSET	PEAK	DURATION
Aerosol	1–6 min	5–15 min	1–4 hrs
Nebulization	1–6 min	5–15 min	1–4 hrs
IPPB	1–6 min	5–15 min	1–4 hrs

PHARMACOKINETICS

Absorption: Inhaled medication rapidly absorbed from respiratory tract. **Metabolism:** Metabolized in GI tract, lungs, liver. **Excretion:** Excreted in urine.

ACTION/*THERAPEUTIC EFFECT*

Stimulates $beta_2$-adrenergic receptors in lungs, resulting in relaxation of bronchial smooth muscle, *relieving bronchospasm; reduces airway resistance.*

USES

Relief of acute bronchial asthma, bronchospasm associated w/chronic bronchitis, emphysema.

STORAGE/HANDLING

Store at room temperature. Do not use if solution is pink to brown, contains a precipitate, or becomes cloudy.

ADMINISTRATION

METERED DOSE INHALER (I. Mesylate):

- Shake container well, exhale completely, then holding mouthpiece 1 inch away from lips, inhale and hold breath as long as possible before exhaling.
- Wait 1–10 min before inhaling 2nd dose (allows for deeper bronchial penetration).
- Rinse mouth w/water immediately after inhalation (prevents mouth/throat dryness).

NEBULIZATION, IPPB
(I. Hydrochloride):

- Dilute 0.5 or 1% solution with sterile water, sterile purified water, or 0.45 or 0.9% NaCl solution at 1:3 ratio (0.125, 0.2, or 0.25% may be given undiluted).
- Adjust oxygen flow rate at 4–6 L/min over 120 min.
- For IPPB, adjust at 15 L/min at cycling pressure of 15 cm water (allowing for adjustment of flow rate, cycling pressure, further dilution).

INDICATIONS/ROUTES/DOSAGE

Bronchospasm:
Hand-bulb Nebulizer: Adults, elderly: 4 inhalations (*range:* 3–7 inhalations) undiluted. May be repeated up to 5 times/day.

Metered Dose Inhalation: Adults, elderly: 1–2 inhalations q4h. Wait 1 min before administering 2nd inhalation.

IPPB, Oxygen Aerolization: Adults, elderly: 0.5–1 ml of a 0.5% or 0.5 ml of a 1% solution diluted 1:3.

CONTRAINDICATIONS

History of hypersensitivity to sympathomimetics.

CAUTIONS

Hypertension, cardiovascular disease, hyperthyroidism, diabetes mellitus.

INTERACTIONS

DRUG: May decrease effects of ***beta blockers. Digoxin*** may increase risk of arrhythmias. **HERBAL:** None known. **FOOD:** None significant. **ALTERED LAB VALUES:** May decrease serum potassium levels.

SIDE EFFECTS

OCCASIONAL: Tremor, nausea, nervousness, palpitations, tachycardia, peripheral vasodilation, dryness of mouth, throat, diziness, vomiting, weakness, headache, increased blood pressure, insomnia.

ADVERSE REACTIONS/TOXIC EFFECTS

Excessive sympathomimetic stimulation may cause palpitations, extrasystoles, tachycardia, chest pain, slight increase in B/P followed by a substantial decrease, chills, sweating, and blanching of skin. Too frequent or excessive use may lead to loss of bronchodilating effectiveness and/or severe, paradoxical bronchoconstriction.

PATIENT CONSIDERATIONS

BASELINE ASSESSMENT

Offer emotional support (high incidence of anxiety due to difficulty in breathing and sympathomimetic response to drug).

INTERVENTION/EVALUATION

Monitor rate, depth, rhythm, type of respiration; quality and rate of pulse. Assess lung sounds for rhonchi, wheezing, rales. Monitor arterial blood gases. Observe lips, fingernails for blue or dusky color in light-skinned pts; gray in dark-skinned pts. Observe for clavicular retractions, hand tremor. Evaluate for clinical improvement (quieter, slower respirations, relaxed facial expression, cessation of clavicular retractions).

PATIENT/FAMILY TEACHING

Increase fluid intake (decreases lung secretion viscosity). Do not take more than 2 inhalations at any one time (excessive use may produce paradoxical bronchoconstriction or a decreased bronchodilating effect). Rinsing mouth with water immediately after inhalation may prevent mouth/

throat dryness. Avoid excessive use of caffeine derivatives (chocolate, coffee, tea, cola, cocoa).

isoflurophate

(Floropryl)

See Classification section under: Antiglaucoma

isoniazid

eye-sew-**nye**-ah-zid

(INH, Laniazid, Nydrazid)

FIXED-COMBINATION(S)

W/rifampin, an antitubercular **(Rifamate)**; w/pyrazinamide and rifampin, antituberculars **(Rifater)**.

CANADIAN AVAILABILITY

Isotamine, PMS Isoniazid

PREGNANCY CATEGORY C

CLASSIFICATION

Antitubercular

AVAILABILITY (Rx)

Tablets: 50 mg, 100 mg, 300 mg. **Syrup:** 50 mg/5 ml. **Injection:** 100 mg/ml.

PHARMACOKINETICS

Absorption: Readily absorbed from GI tract. Widely distributed (including CSF). **Metabolism:** Metabolized in liver. **Excretion:** Primarily excreted in urine. Removed by hemodialysis. **Half-life:** 0.5–5 hrs.

ACTION/*THERAPEUTIC EFFECT*

Inhibits mycolic acid synthesis that causes disruption of bacterial cell wall and loss of acid-fast properties in susceptible mycobacteria. Active only during cell division. *Bactericidal.*

USES

Drug of choice in tuberculosis prophylaxis. Used in combination w/one or more other antitubercular agents for treatment of all forms of active tuberculosis.

ADMINISTRATION

ORAL:

- Give 1 hr before or 2 hrs after meals (may give w/food to decrease GI upset, but will delay absorption).
- Administer at least 1 hr before antacids, especially those containing aluminum.

INDICATIONS/ROUTES/DOSAGE

Tuberculosis (treatment):

Oral/IM: Adults, elderly: 5 mg/kg/day (maximum 300 mg/day) as single dose. ***Children:*** 10–20 mg/kg/day (maximum 300 mg/day) as single dose.

Tuberculosis (prevention):

Oral/IM: Adults, elderly: 300 mg/day as single dose. ***Children:*** 10 mg/kg/day (maximum 300 mg/day) as single dose.

CONTRAINDICATIONS

Acute liver disease, history of hypersensitivity reactions or hepatic injury w/previous isoniazid therapy.

CAUTIONS

Chronic liver disease or alcoholism, severe renal impairment. May be cross sensitive w/nicotinic acid or other chemically related medications.

INTERACTIONS

DRUG: *Alcohol* may increase hepatotoxicity, metabolism. May increase toxicity of ***carbamazepine, phenytoin.*** May decrease ***ketoconazole*** concentrations. ***Disulfiram*** may increase CNS effects. ***Hepatotoxic medications*** may increase hepatotoxicity. **HERBAL:** None known. **FOOD:** Tuna, sauerkraut, aged cheeses, smoked fish may cause reaction such as red/itching skin, pounding heartbeat, lightheadedness, hot or clammy feeling, headache. **ALTERED LAB VALUES:** May increase SGOT (AST), SGPT (ALT), bilirubin.

SIDE EFFECTS

FREQUENT: Hepatitis (dark urine, yellow eyes or skin, loss of appetite, unusually tired or weak), peripheral neuritis (clumsy or unsteadiness, numbness, tingling, burning or pain in hands or feet), nausea, vomiting, diarrhea, stomach pain. **RARE:** Pain at injection site, hypersensitivity reaction, optic neuritis.

ADVERSE REACTIONS/TOXIC EFFECTS

Neurotoxicity, hepatotoxicity occur rarely.

PATIENT CONSIDERATIONS

Baseline Assessment

Question for history of hypersensitivity reactions or hepatic injury from isoniazid, sensitivity to nicotinic acid or chemically related medications. Assure collection of specimens for culture, sensitivity. Evaluate initial hepatic function results.

Intervention/Evaluation

Monitor hepatic function test results and assess for hepatitis: anorexia, nausea, vomiting, weakness, fatigue, dark urine, jaundice (hold INH and inform physician promptly). Check for tingling, numbness, or burning of extremities (those especially at risk for neuropathy may be given pyridoxine prophylactically: malnourished, elderly, diabetics, those w/chronic liver disease, including alcoholics). Be alert for fever, skin eruptions (hypersensitivity reaction). Report vision difficulties at once. Evaluate mental status. Check for dizziness; assist w/ambulation as needed. Monitor CBC results and blood sugar.

Patient/Family Teaching

Do not skip doses; continue taking isoniazid for full length of therapy (6–24 mos). Office visits, vision and lab tests are important part of treatment. Take preferably 1 hr before or 2 hrs after meals (w/food if GI upset). Avoid alcohol during treatment. Do not take any other medications w/o consulting physician, including antacids; must take isoniazid at least 1 hr before antacid. Avoid tuna, sauerkraut, aged cheeses, smoked fish (provide list of tyramine-containing foods) that may cause reaction such as red/itching skin, pounding heartbeat, lightheadedness, hot or clammy feeling, headache; contact physician. Be certain pt not experiencing vision difficulty, dizziness, or other impairment before driving, using machinery. Notify physician of any new symptom immediately for vision difficulties, nausea/vomiting, dark urine, yellowing of skin/eyes, fatigue, numbness or tingling of hands or feet.

isoproterenol hydrochloride

eye-sew-pro-**tear**-en-all
(Isuprel, Dey-Dose)

isoproterenol sulfate

(Medihaler-Iso)

FIXED-COMBINATION(S)
W/phenylephrine, a vasoconstrictor **(Duo-Medihaler)**

CANADIAN AVAILABILITY
Isuprel

PREGNANCY CATEGORY C

CLASSIFICATION

Cardiac stimulant, bronchodilator

AVAILABILITY (Rx)

Injection: 1:5,000 (0.2 mg/ml). **Tablets (sublingual):** 10 mg, 15 mg. **Solution for Inhalation:** 0.25%, 0.5%, 1%. **Aerosol.**

PHARMACODYNAMICS

	ONSET	PEAK	DURATION
Inhalation	2–5 min	—	0.5–2 hrs
Sublingual	15–30 min	—	1–2 hrs
SubQ, IM	Prompt	—	1–2 hrs
IV	Immediate	—	Length of infusion

PHARMACOKINETICS

Absorption: Rapidly absorbed after inhalation/parenteral administration. **Metabolism:** Metabolized in liver. **Excretion:** Primarily excreted in urine. **Half-life:** 2.5–5 min.

ACTION/*THERAPEUTIC EFFECT*

Stimulates $beta_1$-adrenergic receptors, *increasing myocardial contractility, stroke volume, cardiac output.* Also stimulates $beta_2$-adrenergic receptors, resulting in relaxation of bronchial smooth muscle, *relieving bronchospasm; reduces airway resistance.*

USES

Treatment of carotid sinus hypersensitivity, Adams-Stokes syndrome, ventricular arrhythmias due to AV nodal block, reversible bronchospasm, diagnosis of coronary artery disease; adjunct in treatment of shock. Treatment of bronchospasm due to bronchial asthma, emphysema, bronchitis, bronchiectasis.

STORAGE/HANDLING

Do not use if solution is pink to brown, contains a precipitate, or appears cloudy.

ADMINISTRATION

SUBLINGUAL:

- Dissolve sublingual tablet under tongue (do not chew or swallow tablet).
- Do not swallow saliva until tablet is dissolved.

INHALATION:

- Shake container well, exhale completely, then holding mouthpiece 1 inch away from lips, inhale and hold breath as long as possible before exhaling.
- Wait 1–10 min before inhaling second dose (allows for deeper bronchial penetration).
- Rinse mouth w/water immediately after inhalation (prevents mouth/throat dryness).

IV:

- **Note:** May also be given SubQ, IM, intracardiac.
- For IV injection, dilute 0.2 mg (1 ml) of 1:5,000 solution to a vol-

ume of 10 ml 0.9% NaCl injection or 5% dextrose injection.

- Administer IV injection at rate of 1 ml/min, regulated by EKG monitoring.
- For IV infusion, dilute 0.2–2 mg (1–10 ml) of 1:5,000 solution in 500 ml of 5% dextrose in water to provide a solution of 0.4–4 mcg/ml.
- Rate of IV infusion determined by pt's heart rate, central venous pressure, systemic B/P, and urine flow measurements.
- Use microdrip (60 drops/ml) or infusion pump to administer drug.
- If EKG changes occur, heart rate exceeds 110 beats/min, or premature beats occur, consider reducing rate of infusion or temporarily stopping infusion.

INDICATIONS/ROUTES/DOSAGE

Arrhythmias:
IV Bolus: Adults, elderly: Initially, 0.02–0.06 mg (1–3 ml of diluted solution). Subsequent dose range: 0.01–0.2 mg (0.5–10 ml of diluted solution).

IV Infusion: Adults, elderly: Initially, 5 mcg/min (1.25 ml/min of diluted solution). Subsequent dose range: 2–20 mcg/min. ***Children:*** 2.5 mcg/min or 0.1 mcg/kg per min.

IM/SubQ: Adults, elderly: 0.2 mg, then 0.02–1 mg, as needed.

Mild arrhythmias:
Sublingual: Adults, elderly: 10–30 mg 4–6 times/day.

Complete heart block following closure of ventricular septal defects:
IV: Adults, elderly: 0.04–0.06 mg (2–3 ml of diluted solution). ***Infants:*** 0.01–0.03 (0.5–1.5 ml of diluted solution).

Shock:
IV Infusion: Adults, elderly: Rate of 0.5–5 mcg/min (0.25–2.5 ml of 1:500,000 dilution); rate of infusion based on clinical response (heart rate, central venous pressure, systemic B/P, urine flow measurements).

Bronchospasm:
Metered Dose Inhalation: Adults, elderly, children >6 yrs: 1–2 inhalations 4–6 times/day at no less than 3–4 hr intervals. Wait 1–5 min before administering second inhalation.

IPPB: Adults, elderly: 2 ml (0.125%) or 2.5 ml (0.1%) up to 5 times/day. Flow rate adjusted to administer dose over 15–20 min IPPB: 10–20 min via nebulization. ***Children:*** 2 ml (0.0625%) or 2.5 ml (0.05%) up to 5 times/day.

Nebulization Solution: Adults, elderly, children: 6–12 inhalations (0.025%). Repeat at 5–15 min intervals (maximum 3 treatments). ***Maximum:*** 8 treatments/24 hrs.

Sublingual: Adults, elderly: 10–20 mg q6–8h. ***Children >6 yrs:*** 5–10 mg q6–8h.

IV Infusion: Adults, elderly: 0.01–0.02 mg (0.5–1 ml of a diluted solution). ***Children:*** $^{1}/_{10}$–$^{1}/_{12}$ adult dose.

CONTRAINDICATIONS

Tachycardia due to digitalis toxicity, preexisting arrhythmias, angina, precordial distress.

CAUTIONS

Hypersensitivity to sulfite, elderly/debilitated, hypertension, cardiovascular disease, impaired renal function, hyperthyroidism, diabetes mellitus, prostatic hypertrophy, glaucoma. Safety and efficacy in children not established.

INTERACTIONS

DRUG: *Tricyclic antidepressants* may increase cardiovascular effects. May decrease effects of *beta blockers. Digoxin* may increase risk of arrhythmias. HERBAL: None known. FOOD: None significant. ALTERED LAB VALUES: May decrease serum potassium levels.

SIDE EFFECTS

FREQUENT: Dry, irritated mouth, nervousness, inability to sleep. OCCASIONAL: Coughing, dizziness, flushed skin, headache, increased sweating, nausea, pounding heartbeat, tremors, vomiting.

ADVERSE REACTIONS/TOXIC EFFECTS

Excessive sympathomimetic stimulation may cause palpitations, extrasystoles, tachycardia, chest pain, slight increase in B/P followed by a substantial decrease, chills, sweating, and blanching of skin. Ventricular arrhythmias may occur if heart rate is above 130 beats/min. When used for bronchospasm, too frequent or excessive use may lead to loss of bronchodilating effectiveness and/or severe, paradoxical bronchoconstriction. Parotid gland swelling may occur w/prolonged use.

PATIENT CONSIDERATIONS

BASELINE ASSESSMENT

Be alert to anginal pain or precordial distress, pulse rate exceeding 110 beats/min.

INTERVENTION/EVALUATION

Cardiac stimulant
Monitor EKG, blood P_{CO_2} or bicarbonate and blood pH, central venous pressure, pulse, systemic B/P, urine output.

Bronchospasm
Monitor rate, depth, rhythm, type of respiration; quality and rate of pulse. Assess lung sounds for rhonchi, wheezing, rales. Monitor arterial blood gases. Observe lips, fingernails for blue or dusky color in light-skinned pts; gray in dark-skinned pts. Observe for clavicular retractions, hand tremor. Evaluate for clinical improvement (quieter, slower respirations, relaxed facial expression, cessation of clavicular retractions).

PATIENT/FAMILY TEACHING

Bronchospasm
Increase fluid intake (decreases lung secretion viscosity). Do not take more than 2 inhalations at any one time (excessive use may produce paradoxical bronchoconstriction or a decreased bronchodilating effect). Rinsing mouth with water immediately after inhalation may prevent mouth/throat dryness. Saliva may turn pink after sublingual administration. Due to acidity of drug, frequent sublingual use may damage teeth. Avoid excessive use of caffeine derivatives (chocolate, coffee, tea, cola, cocoa).

---

isosorbide dinitrate

eye-sew-**sore**-bide
(Dilatrate, Isordil, Sorbitrate)

isosorbide mononitrate

(Imdur, ISMO, Monoket)

CANADIAN AVAILABILITY
Apo-ISDN, Cedocard, Imdur, Ismo, Isordil

PREGNANCY CATEGORY C

CLASSIFICATION

Nitrate

AVAILABILITY (Rx)

Dinitrate: Tablets: 5 mg, 10 mg, 20 mg, 30 mg, 40 mg. **Tablets (sublingual):** 2.5 mg, 5 mg, 10 mg. **Tablets (chewable):** 5 mg, 10 mg. **Tablets (sustained-release):** 40 mg. **Capsules (sustained-release):** 40 mg.

Mononitrate: Tablets: 10 mg, 20 mg. **Tablets (extended-release):** 60 mg.

PHARMACODYNAMICS

	ONSET	PEAK	DURATION
Chewable			
	5–20 min	15–60 min	1–4 hrs
Sublingual			
	5–20 min	15–60 min	1–4 hrs
Extended-release			
	up to 4 hrs	—	6–8 hrs
Tablets, capsules			
	20–40 min	45–120 min	4–6 hrs
Mononitrate			
	30–60 min	—	—

PHARMACOKINETICS

Absorption: Poorly absorbed from GI tract; well absorbed after sublingual administration. **Metabolism:** Metabolized in liver (undergoes first-pass effect). **Excretion:** Primarily excreted in urine. **Half-life:** ***oral:*** 4 hrs, ***sublingual:*** 1 hr. ***Mononitrate:*** Not subjected to first-pass metabolism in liver.

ACTION/*THERAPEUTIC EFFECT*

Decreases myocardial O_2 demand, increases myocardial O_2 supply, reducing wall tension by venous dilation (preload) and arterial dilation (afterload). *Dilates coronary arteries; improves collateral blood flow to ischemic areas within myocardium.*

USES

Treatment and prevention of angina pectoris. Chronic prophylaxis of angina. *Mononitrate:* Prevention of angina pectoris due to coronary artery disease.

ADMINISTRATION

ORAL:

- Best if taken on an empty stomach.
- Oral tablets may be crushed.
- Do not crush or break sublingual or extended-release form.
- Do not crush chewable form before administering.

SUBLINGUAL:

- Do not crush/chew sublingual tablets.
- Dissolve tablets under tongue; do not swallow.

INDICATIONS/ROUTES/DOSAGE

Note: Drug-free interval at least 14 hrs. Patch: Allow 10–12 hr drug-free interval.

Acute angina, prophylactic management in situations likely to provoke attack:
Sublingual/Chewable: Adults, elderly: Initially, 2.5–5 mg. Repeat at 5–10 min intervals. No more than 3 doses in 15–30 min period.

Acute prophylactic management of angina:
Sublingual/Chewable: Adults, elderly: 5–10 mg q2–3h.

Long-term prophylaxis of angina:
Oral: Adults, elderly: Initially, 5–20 mg 3–4 times/day. ***Maintenance:*** 10–40 mg q6h. Consider 2–3 times/day, last dose no later than 7 PM to minimize intolerance.

Mononitrate: Adults, elderly: 20 mg 2 times/day, 7 hrs apart. First dose upon awakening in morning.

Extended-Release: Adults, elderly: Initially, 40 mg. *Maintenance:* 40–80 mg 2–3 times/day. Consider 1–2 times/day, last dose at 2 PM to minimize intolerance.

Imdur: 60–120 mg/day as single dose.

CONTRAINDICATIONS

Hypersensitivity to nitrates, severe anemia, closed-angle glaucoma, postural hypotension, head trauma, increased intracranial pressure. *Extended-release:* GI hypermotility/malabsorption, severe anemia.

CAUTIONS

Acute MI, hepatic/renal disease, glaucoma (contraindicated in closed-angle glaucoma), blood volume depletion from diuretic therapy, systolic B/P below 90 mm Hg.

INTERACTIONS

DRUG: *Alcohol, antihypertensives, vasodilators* may increase risk of orthostatic hypotension. HERBAL: None known. FOOD: None significant. ALTERED LAB VALUES: May increase urine catecholamines, urine VMA (vanilmandelic acid).

SIDE EFFECTS

FREQUENT: Headache (may be severe) occurs mostly in early therapy, diminishes rapidly in intensity, usually disappears during continued treatment; transient flushing of face and neck, dizziness (especially if pt is standing immobile or is in a warm environment), weakness, postural hypotension, nausea, vomiting, restlessness. *Sublingual:* Burning, tingling sensation at oral point of dissolution. OCCASIONAL: GI upset, blurred vision, dry mouth.

ADVERSE REACTIONS/TOXIC EFFECTS

Drug should be discontinued if blurred vision, dry mouth occurs. Severe postural hypotension manifested by fainting, pulselessness, cold/clammy skin, profuse sweating. Tolerance may occur w/repeated, prolonged therapy (minor tolerance w/intermittent use of sublingual tablets). Tolerance may not occur w/extended-release form. High dose tends to produce severe headache.

PATIENT CONSIDERATIONS

BASELINE ASSESSMENT

Record onset, type (sharp, dull, squeezing), radiation, location, intensity, and duration of anginal pain, and precipitating factors (exertion, emotional stress). If headache occurs during management therapy, administer medication w/meals.

INTERVENTION/EVALUATION

Assist w/ambulation if lightheadedness, dizziness occurs. Assess for facial/neck flushing. Monitor B/P for hypotension.

PATIENT/FAMILY TEACHING

Rise slowly from lying to sitting position and dangle legs momentarily before standing. Take oral form on empty stomach (however, if headache occurs during management therapy, take medication w/meals). Dissolve sublingual tablet under tongue; do not swallow. Take at first signal of angina. If not relieved within 5 min, dissolve second tablet under tongue. Repeat if no relief in another 5 min. If pain continues,

contact physician. Expel from mouth any remaining sublingual tablet after pain is completely relieved. Do not change from one brand of drug to another. Avoid alcohol (intensifies hypotensive effect). If alcohol is ingested soon after taking nitroglycerin, possible acute hypotensive episode (marked drop in B/P, vertigo, pallor) may occur.

isotretinoin

eye-sew-**tret**-ih-noyn
(Accutane)

CANADIAN AVAILABILITY
Accutane, Isotrex

PREGNANCY CATEGORY X

CLASSIFICATION

Acne aid

AVAILABILITY (Rx)

Capsules: 10 mg, 20 mg, 40 mg

PHARMACOKINETICS

Absorption: Rapidly absorbed from GI tract. **Metabolism:** Metabolized in liver. **Excretion:** Excreted in urine via biliary system. **Half-life:** 10–20 hrs.

ACTION/*THERAPEUTIC EFFECT*

Reduces sebaceous gland size, inhibiting its activity. *Produces antikeratinizing, anti-inflammatory effects.*

USES/*UNLABELED*

Treatment of severe, recalcitrant cystic acne that is unresponsive to conventional acne therapies. *Treatment of gram-negative folliculitis, severe rosacea; correcting severe keratinization disorders.*

ADMINISTRATION

ORAL:

- Administer whole; do not crush.
- Give w/food to facilitate absorption.

INDICATIONS/ROUTES/DOSAGE

Recalcitrant cystic acne:
Oral: Adults: Initially, 0.5–2 mg/kg/day divided in 2 doses for 15–20 wks. May repeat after at least 2 mos of therapy.

CONTRAINDICATIONS

Hypersensitivity to isotretinoin or parabens (component of capsules).

CAUTIONS

Renal, hepatic dysfunction. Safety in children not established.

INTERACTIONS

DRUG: ***Etretinate, tretinoin, vitamin A*** may increase toxic effects. ***Tetracycline*** may increase potential of pseudotumor cerebri. **HERBAL:** None known. **FOOD:** None significant. **ALTERED LAB VALUES:** May increase triglycerides, cholesterol, SGPT (ALT), SGOT (AST), alkaline phosphatase, LDH, sedimentation rate, fasting blood glucose, uric acid; may decrease HDL.

SIDE EFFECTS

FREQUENT: Cheilitis (inflammation of lips) (90%); skin/mucous membrane dryness (80%); skin fragility, pruritus, epistaxis, dry nose/mouth; conjunctivitis (40%); hypertriglyceridemia (25%); nausea, vomiting, abdominal pain (20%). **OCCASIONAL:** Musculoskeletal symptoms (16%) including bone or joint pain, arthralgia, generalized muscle aches; photosensitivity (5–10%). RARE: Decreased night vision, depression.

ADVERSE REACTIONS/TOXIC EFFECTS

Inflammatory bowel disease and pseudotumor cerebri (benign intracranial hypertension) have been temporarily associated w/isotretinoin therapy.

PATIENT CONSIDERATIONS

Baseline Assessment

Question for hypersensitivity to isotretinoin or parabens. Assess baselines for blood lipids and glucose.

Intervention/Evaluation

Assess acne for decreased cysts. Evaluate skin and mucous membranes for excessive dryness. Monitor blood glucose, lipids.

Patient/Family Teaching

A transient exacerbation of acne may occur during initial period. May have decreased tolerance to contact lenses during and after therapy. Topical acne agents should not be used w/o physician approval. Do not take vitamin supplements w/vitamin A because of additive effects. Notify physician immediately of onset of abdominal pain, severe diarrhea, rectal bleeding (possible inflammatory bowel disease), or headache, nausea and vomiting, visual disturbances (possible pseudotumor cerebri). Decreased night vision may occur suddenly; take caution w/night driving. Minimize or eliminate alcohol consumption (may potentiate serum triglyceride elevation), prolonged exposure to sunlight; use sunscreens, protective clothing until sunlight or ultraviolet light tolerance established. Do not donate blood during or for 1 mo after treatment.

Women

Explain the serious risk to fetus if pregnancy occurs (both oral and written warnings are given, w/pt acknowledging in writing that she understands the warnings and consents to treatment). Must have a negative serum pregnancy test within 2 wks prior to starting therapy; therapy will begin on the second or third day of the next normal menstrual period. Effective contraception (using 2 reliable forms of contraception simultaneously) must be used for at least 1 mo before, during, and for at least 1 mo after therapy w/isotretinoin.

isradipine

iss-**ray**-dih-peen
(DynaCirc, DynaCirc CR)

PREGNANCY CATEGORY C

CLASSIFICATION

Calcium channel blocker

AVAILABILITY (Rx)

Capsules: 2.5 mg, 5 mg. **Extended-Release Capsules:** 5 mg, 10 mg.

PHARMACODYNAMICS

	ONSET	PEAK	DURATION
Oral	2–3 hrs	—	—

PHARMACOKINETICS

Absorption: Well absorbed from

GI tract. **Metabolism:** Metabolized in liver (undergoes first-pass effect). **Excretion:** Primarily excreted in urine. **Half-life:** 8 hrs.

ACTION / *THERAPEUTIC EFFECT*

Inhibits calcium movement across cardiac, vascular smooth muscle. Potent peripheral vasodilator (does not depress SA, AV nodes). *Increases myocardial contractility, heart rate, cardiac output; decreases peripheral vascular resistance.*

USES / *UNLABELED*

Management of hypertension. May be used alone or w/thiazide-type diuretics. *Treatment of chronic angina pectoris, Raynaud's phenomena.*

ADMINISTRATION

ORAL:

- Do not crush or break capsule.

INDICATIONS / ROUTES / DOSAGE

Hypertension:

Oral: Adults, elderly: Initially, 2.5 mg 2 times/day. May increase by 5 mg q2–4wks. ***Maximum:*** 20 mg/day.

CONTRAINDICATIONS

Sick-sinus syndrome/second- or third-degree AV block (except in presence of pacemaker).

CAUTIONS

Impaired renal/hepatic function, CHF.

INTERACTIONS

DRUG: ***Beta blockers*** may have additive effect. **HERBAL:** None known. **FOOD:** None significant. **ALTERED LAB VALUES:** None significant.

SIDE EFFECTS

FREQUENT: Headache, peripheral edema, dizziness/lightheadedness. **OCCASIONAL:** Palpitations, facial flushing. **RARE:** Nausea, vomiting, diarrhea, rash, dyspepsia, cough.

ADVERSE REACTIONS / TOXIC EFFECTS

CHF occurs rarely. Overdosage produces nausea, drowsiness, confusion, slurred speech.

PATIENT CONSIDERATIONS

BASELINE ASSESSMENT

Assess baseline renal/liver function tests. Assess B/P, apical pulse immediately before drug is administered (if pulse is 60/min or below, or systolic B/P is below 90 mm Hg, withhold medication, contact physician).

INTERVENTION/EVALUATION

Assist w/ambulation if lightheadedness, dizziness occurs. Assess for peripheral edema behind medial malleolus (sacral area in bedridden pts). Monitor pulse rate for bradycardia. Assess skin for flushing. Monitor liver enzyme tests.

PATIENT/FAMILY TEACHING

Do not abruptly discontinue medication. Compliance w/therapy regimen is essential to control hypertension. To avoid hypotensive effect, rise slowly from lying to sitting position, wait momentarily before standing. Avoid tasks that require alertness, motor skills until response to drug is established. Contact physician/nurse if irregular heartbeat, shortness of breath, pronounced dizziness, or nausea occurs.

itraconazole

eye-tra-**con**-ah-zoll
(Sporanox)

CANADIAN AVAILABILITY
Sporanox

PREGNANCY CATEGORY C

CLASSIFICATION

Antifungal

AVAILABILITY (Rx)

Capsules: 100 mg. **Oral Solution:** 10 mg/ml. **Injection.**

PHARMACOKINETICS

Absorption: Moderately absorbed from GI tract (increased w/food). Widely distributed (primarily in liver, kidney, fatty tissue). **Metabolism:** Metabolized in liver to active metabolite. **Excretion:** Primarily excreted in urine. Not removed by hemodialysis. **Half-life:** 21 hrs; metabolite: 12 hrs.

ACTION/*THERAPEUTIC EFFECT*

Inhibits synthesis of ergosterol (vital component of fungal cell formation), damaging fungal cell membrane. *Fungistatic.*

USES/*UNLABELED*

Treatment of blastomycosis (pulmonary, extrapulmonary), histoplasmosis, aspergillosis, onychomycosis, dermatophyte skin infections, tinea pedis in pts unable to take topical therapy. Solution: Oral, esophageal candidiasis. *Suppresses histoplasmosis; treatment of fungal pneumonia/septicemia, disseminated sporotrichosis, ringworm of hand.*

ADMINISTRATION

ORAL:

- Take w/food (increases absorption).

IV:

- Infuse over 1 hr.

INDICATIONS/ROUTES/DOSAGE

Note: Doses >200 mg given in 2 divided doses.

Blastomycosis, histoplasmosis:
Oral: Adults, elderly: Initially, 200 mg/day w/food. May increase in 100 mg increments. ***Maximum:*** 400 mg/day.

Aspergillosis:
Oral: Adults, elderly: 200–400 mg/day.

Onychomycosis:
Oral: Adults, elderly: 200 mg/day for 12 consecutive wks or 200 mg twice daily for 1 wk; 3 wk rest period; repeat.

Life-threatening infection:
Oral: Adults, elderly: Initially, 200 mg 3 times/day for 3 days as loading dose.

Oral candidiasis:
Oral: Adults: 200 mg daily for 1–2 wks.

Esophageal candidiasis:
Oral: Adults: 100–200 mg daily for 3 wks.

Usual IV dosage:
IV: Adults: 200 mg 2 times/day × 4 doses; then, 4 times/day.

CONTRAINDICATIONS

Coadministration of terfenadine. Hypersensitivity to itraconazole, fluconazole, ketoconazole, miconazole.

CAUTIONS

Hepatitis, HIV-infected pts, pts w/achlorhydria, hypochlorhydria (decreases absorption), impaired liver function.

INTERACTIONS

DRUG: May increase ***buspirone, cyclosporine, digoxin, lovastatin, simvastatin*** concentrations. May increase effect of ***oral anticoagulants. Phenytoin, rifampin*** may decrease concentrations. ***Antacids, H-2 antagonists, didanosine*** may decrease absorption. **HERBAL:** None known. **FOOD:** None significant. **ALTERED LAB VALUES:** May increase SGOT (AST), SGPT (ALT), alkaline phosphatase, LDH, bilirubin. May decrease potassium.

SIDE EFFECTS

FREQUENT: Nausea (11%), rash (9%), abdominal pain, nausea, vomiting, constipation, headache. **OCCASIONAL:** Vomiting (5%), headache, peripheral edema (4%), diarrhea, hypertension (3%). **RARE:** Fatigue, fever, pruritus (2%).

ADVERSE REACTIONS/TOXIC EFFECTS

Hepatitis (anorexia, abdominal pain, unusual tiredness/weakness, jaundice, dark urine) occurs rarely.

PATIENT CONSIDERATIONS

BASELINE ASSESSMENT

Obtain specimens for fungal cultures and other lab studies before first dose. Therapy may begin before results are known. Determine baseline temperature, liver function tests. Assess allergies.

INTERVENTION/EVALUATION

Assess for signs and symptoms of liver dysfunction and monitor hepatic enzyme test results in pts w/preexisting liver dysfunction. Check temperature.

PATIENT/FAMILY TEACHING

Take w/food. Therapy will continue for at least 3 mos and until lab tests and clinical presentation indicate infection is controlled. Report the following at once: unusual fatigue, yellow skin, dark urine, pale stool, anorexia/nausea/vomiting.

---

ivermectin

(Stromectol)

See Supplement

I

kanamycin sulfate

can-ah-**my**-sin
(Kantrex)

PREGNANCY CATEGORY D

CLASSIFICATION

Antibiotic: Aminoglycoside

AVAILABILITY (Rx)

Injection: 75 mg/2 ml, 500 mg/2 ml, 1 g/3 ml. **Capsules:** 500 mg.

PHARMACOKINETICS

Absorption: Rapid, complete absorption after IM administration. Widely distributed (does not cross blood-brain barrier; low concentrations in CSF). **Excretion:** Excreted unchanged in urine. Removed by hemodialysis. **Half-life:** 2–4 hrs (increased in decreased renal function, neonates; decreased in cystic fibrosis, burn or febrile pts).

ACTION/*THERAPEUTIC EFFECT*

Irreversibly binds to protein on bacterial ribosome, *interfering in protein synthesis of susceptible microorganisms.*

USES

Treatment of skin/skin structure, bone, joint, respiratory tract, intra-abdominal and complicated urinary tract infections; wound and surgical site irrigation, burns, septicemia, hepatic encephalopathy. Adjunctive therapy for tuberculosis; before operation for intestinal antisepsis.

STORAGE/HANDLING

Store parenteral form, capsules at room temperature. Solutions appear clear, colorless to pale yellow. Darkening of solution does not indicate loss of potency. Intermittent IV infusion (piggyback) stable for 24 hrs at room temperature. Discard if precipitate forms.

ADMINISTRATION

Note: Coordinate peak and trough lab draws w/administration times.

ORAL:
- Give w/o regard to meals.
- If GI upset occurs, give w/food or milk.

IM:
- To minimize discomfort, give deep IM slowly.
- Less painful to inject into gluteus maximus rather than lateral aspect of thigh.

IV:
- Dilute each 500 mg w/100–200 ml 5% dextrose, 0.9% NaCl, or other compatible IV fluid. Amount of diluent for infants, children depends on individual needs.
- Administer IV infusion (piggyback) over 30–60 min.
- Alternating IV sites, use large veins to reduce risk of phlebitis.

INDICATIONS/ROUTES/DOSAGE

Space doses evenly around the clock.

Mild to moderate infections:
IM/IV: Adults, children: 15 mg/kg/day in divided doses q8–12h (IM doses may be given q6h). *Elderly:* 5–7.5 mg/kg/dose q12–24h.

Hepatic encephalopathy (adjunctive treatment):
Oral: Adults, elderly: 8–12 g/day in 4 divided doses.

Preop intestinal antisepsis:
Oral: Adults, elderly: 1 g every

hour for 4 doses, then 1 g q6h for up to 3 days.

Intraperitoneal instillation:
Adults: 500 mg dissolved in 20 ml sterile water, instilled via catheter into wound.

Irrigation:
Adults: 0.25% solution to irrigate pleural space, ventricular or abscess cavities, wounds, or surgical sites.

Inhalation:
Adults: 250 mg diluted w/3 ml 0.9% NaCl and nebulized 2–4 times/day.

Dosage in renal impairment:
Dose and/or frequency is modified based on degree of renal impairment, serum concentration of drug.

CONTRAINDICATIONS

Hypersensitivity to kanamycin, other aminoglycosides (cross-sensitivity). Oral administration contraindicated in intestinal obstruction.

CAUTIONS

Elderly, neonates (due to renal insufficiency or immaturity); neuromuscular disorders (potential for respiratory depression), prior hearing loss, vertigo, renal impairment. Not for long-term therapy due to associated toxicities. Cumulative effects may occur when given via more than one route.

INTERACTIONS

DRUG: Other *aminoglycosides, nephrotoxic, ototoxic medications* may increase toxicity. May increase effects of *neuromuscular blocking agents.* HERBAL: None known. FOOD: None significant. ALTERED LAB VALUES: May increase BUN, SGPT (ALT), SGOT (AST), bilirubin, creatinine, LDH concentrations; may decrease serum calcium, magnesium, potassium, sodium concentrations.

SIDE EFFECTS

FREQUENT: *Oral:* Nausea, vomiting, diarrhea. OCCASIONAL: *IM:* Pain, irritation at injection site. *IV:* Phlebitis; hypersensitivity reactions: rash, fever, urticaria, pruritus. RARE: Headache.

ADVERSE REACTIONS/TOXIC EFFECTS

Nephrotoxicity (evidenced by increased BUN and serum creatinine, decreased creatinine clearance) may be reversible if drug stopped at first sign of symptoms; irreversible ototoxicity (tinnitus, dizziness, ringing/roaring in ears, reduced hearing) and neurotoxicity (headache, dizziness, lethargy, tremors, visual disturbances) occur occasionally. Risk is greater w/higher dosages, prolonged therapy. Superinfections, particularly w/fungi, may result from bacterial imbalance. Severe respiratory depression, anaphylaxis occur rarely.

PATIENT CONSIDERATIONS

Baseline Assessment

Dehydration must be treated before aminoglycoside therapy. Establish pt's baseline hearing acuity before beginning therapy. Question for history of allergies, especially to aminoglycosides. Obtain specimens for culture, sensitivity before giving first dose (therapy may begin before results are known). Maintain adequate hydration.

Intervention/Evaluation

Monitor I&O (maintain hydration),

K

urinalysis (casts, RBCs, WBCs, decrease in specific gravity). Monitor results of peak/trough blood tests. Be alert to ototoxic and neurotoxic symptoms (see Adverse Reactions/Toxic Effects). Check IM injection site for pain, induration. Evaluate IV site for phlebitis (heat, pain, red streaking over vein). Assess for rash. Be alert to respiratory depression. Assess for superinfection, particularly genital/anal pruritus, changes of oral mucosa, diarrhea.

PATIENT/FAMILY TEACHING

Continue antibiotic for full length of treatment. Space doses evenly. Discomfort may occur w/IM injection. Notify physician in event of headache, shortness of breath, dizziness, hearing or urinary problem even after therapy is completed. Do not take other medication w/o consulting physician. Lab tests are an essential part of therapy.

kaolin/pectin

kay-oh-lyn
(Kaopectate, Kapectolin)

FIXED-COMBINATION(S)
W/atropine, hyoscyamine, scopolamine, belladonna alkaloids, opium **(Donnagel PG, Kapectolin PG)**; w/opium **(Parepectolin)**

CANADIAN AVAILABILITY
Kaopectate

PREGNANCY CATEGORY C

CLASSIFICATION

Antidiarrheal

AVAILABILITY (OTC)

Suspension

PHARMACOKINETICS

Absorption: Not absorbed orally. **Metabolism:** Up to 90% of pectin decomposed in GI tract.

ACTION/*THERAPEUTIC EFFECT*

Adsorbent, protectant *(adsorbs bacteria, toxins, reduces water loss)*.

USES

Symptomatic treatment of mild to moderate acute diarrhea.

ADMINISTRATION

ORAL:
- Shake suspension well before administration.

INDICATIONS/ROUTES/DOSAGE

Antidiarrheal:
Oral: Adults, elderly: 60–120 ml after each loose bowel movement (LBM). ***Children >12 yrs:*** 60 ml after each LBM; ***6–12 yrs:*** 30–60 ml after each LBM; ***3–6 yrs:*** 15–30 ml after each LBM.

CONTRAINDICATIONS

None significant.

CAUTIONS

None significant.

INTERACTIONS

DRUG: May decrease absorption of ***digoxin.*** **HERBAL:** None known. **FOOD:** None significant. **ALTERED LAB VALUES:** None significant.

SIDE EFFECTS

RARE: Constipation.

ADVERSE REACTIONS/TOXIC EFFECTS

None significant.

PATIENT CONSIDERATIONS

Intervention/Evaluation

Encourage adequate fluid intake. Assess bowel sounds for peristalsis. Assess stools for frequency and consistency (watery, loose, soft, semisolid, solid).

Patient/Family Teaching

Do not use for more than 2 days or w/high fever. Not for children under 3 yrs of age w/o physician direction.

---

ketamine hydrochloride

(Ketalar)

See Classification section under: Anesthetics: general

---

ketoconazole

keet-oh-**con**-ah-zol

(Nizoral, Nizoral AD)

CANADIAN AVAILABILITY

Apo-Ketoconazole, Nizoral

PREGNANCY CATEGORY C

CLASSIFICATION

Antifungal

AVAILABILITY (Rx)

Tablets: 200 mg. **Cream:** 2%. **Shampoo:** 2%, 1% **(OTC)**.

PHARMACOKINETICS

Oral: **Absorption:** Readily absorbed from GI tract. Widely distributed. **Metabolism:** Metabolized in liver. Primarily excreted via biliary elimination. **Half-life:** 8 hrs. ***Topical:*** **Absorption:** Minimal systemic absorption.

ACTION/*THERAPEUTIC EFFECT*

Inhibits synthesis of ergosterol (vital component of fungal cell formation), damaging fungal cell membrane. ***Fungistatic.***

USES/*UNLABELED*

Treatment of histoplasmosis, blastomycosis, candidiasis, chronic mucocutaneous candidiasis, coccidioidomycosis, paracoccidioidomycosis, chromomycosis, seborrheic dermatitis, tineas (ringworm): corporis, capitis, manus, cruris, pedis, unguium (onychomycosis), oral thrush, candiduria. ***Shampoo:*** Reduces scaling due to dandruff. Treatment tinea versicolor. ***Topical:*** Treatment of tineas, pityriasis versicolor, cutaneous candidiasis, seborrhea dermatitis, dandruff. ***Systemic:*** *Treatment of fungal pneumonia, septicemia, prostate cancer.*

ADMINISTRATION

ORAL:

- Give w/food to minimize GI irritation.
- Tablets may be crushed.
- Ketoconazole requires acidity; give antacids, anticholinergics, H-2 blockers *at least* 2 hrs after dosing.

INDICATIONS/ROUTES/DOSAGE

Mild to moderate infections:
Oral: Adults, elderly: 200 mg/day. ***Children >2 yrs:*** 3.3–6.6 mg/kg/day as single dose.

Severe infections:
Oral: Adults, elderly: 400 mg/day.

Cutaneous fungal infections:
Topical: Adults, elderly: Apply 1–2 times/day for 2–4 wks.

Tinea versicolor:
Shampoo: Adults: Apply to damp

skin w/wide margin around it, lather, leave 5 min, rinse.

Dandruff:
Shampoo: Adults, elderly: 2 times/wk for 4 wks, allowing at least 3 days between shampooing. Intermittent use to maintain control.

CONTRAINDICATIONS

Hypersensitivity to ketoconazole, children <2 yrs.

CAUTIONS

Hepatic impairment.

INTERACTIONS

DRUG: *Alcohol, hepatotoxic medications* may increase hepatotoxicity. *Antacids, anticholinergics, H-2 antagonists, omeprazole* may decrease absorption (allow 2 hr interval). May increase concentration, toxicity of *cyclosporine, lovastatin, simvastatin. Isoniazid, rifampin* may decrease concentration. May increase concentration of *cisapride, terfenadine* causing cardiotoxicity. HERBAL: None known. FOOD: None significant. ALTERED LAB VALUES: May increase SGOT (AST), SGPT (ALT), alkaline phosphatase, bilirubin. May decrease corticosteroid, testosterone concentrations.

SIDE EFFECTS

FREQUENT (3–10%): Nausea, vomiting, pruritus. OCCASIONAL (1–3%): Abdominal pain, diarrhea or constipation, GI bleeding, rash, urticaria, photophobia, headache, dizziness, gynecomastia, fever, chills, abnormal dreams, somnolence, impotence, arthralgia, adrenocortical insufficiency. RARE (<1%): Topical application may cause itching, burning, irritation.

ADVERSE REACTIONS/TOXIC EFFECTS

Hematologic toxicity occurs occasionally (thrombocytopenia, hemolytic anemia, leukopenia). Hepatotoxicity may occur within first week to several months of therapy. Anaphylaxis occurs rarely.

PATIENT CONSIDERATIONS

BASELINE ASSESSMENT

Question for history of allergies, especially to ketoconazole (sulfite when using topical cream). Confirm that a culture or histologic test was done for accurate diagnosis; therapy may begin before results known.

INTERVENTION/EVALUATION

Monitor hepatic function tests; be alert for hepatotoxicity: dark urine, pale stools, fatigue, anorexia/nausea/vomiting (unrelieved by giving medication w/food). Determine pattern of bowel activity, stool consistency, check for blood in stool. Assess mental status (dizziness, somnolence) and provide assistance as needed. Evaluate skin for rash, urticaria, itching. Check sleep pattern.

Topical
Check for local burning, itching, irritation.

PATIENT/FAMILY TEACHING

Prolonged therapy (weeks or months) is usually necessary. Do not miss a dose; continue therapy as long as directed. Avoid alcohol (due to potential liver problem). Wear sunglasses and avoid bright light in event of photophobia. Do not drive car, machinery if dizziness occurs. Take any antacids/antiulcer medications at least 2 hrs after ketoconazole. Notify physician of dark urine, pale stool, yellow skin/eyes, increased irritation in topical use, or onset of other new symp-

tom. Consult physician before taking any other medication.

Topical
Rub well into affected areas. Avoid contact w/eyes. Keep skin clean, dry; wear light clothing for ventilation. Separate personal items in direct contact w/affected area. Do not use other preparations or occlusive covering w/o consulting physician.

Shampoo
Apply shampoo to wet hair to produce enough lather to wash hair and scalp. Leave in place about 1 min, then rinse. Apply shampoo and lather a second time, leaving on scalp 3 min, then rinse again thoroughly. Initially use twice weekly for 4 wks w/at least 3 days between shampooing; frequency then will be determined by response.

ketoprofen

key-**toe**-pro-fen

(Actron, Orudis, Orudis KT, Oruvail)

CANADIAN AVAILABILITY
Apo-Keto, Orafen, Orudis, Rhodis

PREGNANCY CATEGORY B
(D if used in third trimester or near delivery)

CLASSIFICATION

Nonsteroidal anti-inflammatory

AVAILABILITY (Rx)

Tablets: (OTC) 12.5 mg. **Capsules:** 25 mg, 50 mg, 75 mg. **Capsules (extended-release):** 100 mg, 150 mg, 200 mg.

PHARMACOKINETICS

Absorption: Rapid, complete absorption from GI tract. **Metabolism:** Primarily metabolized in liver. **Excretion:** Excreted in urine. Removed by hemodialysis. **Half-life:** 1.5–4 hrs.

ACTION / *THERAPEUTIC EFFECT*

Produces analgesic and anti-inflammatory effect by inhibiting prostaglandin synthesis, *reducing inflammatory response and intensity of pain stimulus reaching sensory nerve endings.*

K

USES / *UNLABELED*

Symptomatic treatment of acute and chronic rheumatoid arthritis and osteoarthritis. Relief of mild to moderate pain, primary dysmenorrhea. *Treatment of ankylosing spondylitis, psoriatic arthritis, acute gouty arthritis, vascular headache.*

ADMINISTRATION

ORAL:

- May give w/food, milk, or full glass (8 oz) water (minimizes potential GI distress).
- Do not break, chew extended-release capsules.

INDICATIONS / ROUTES / DOSAGE

Note: Do not exceed 300 mg/day. Oruvail not recommended as initial therapy in pts who are small, >75 yrs of age, or renally impaired.

Acute and chronic rheumatoid arthritis, osteoarthritis:
Oral: Adults: Initially, 75 mg three times/day or 50 mg four times/day. ***Elderly:*** Initially, 25–50 mg 3–4 times/day. ***Maintenance:*** 150–300 mg/day in 3–4 divided doses. ***Extended-release:*** 100–200 mg/day as single dose.

Mild to moderate pain, dysmenorrhea:
Oral: Adults: 25–50 mg q6–8h.

CONTRAINDICATIONS

Active peptic ulcer, GI ulceration, chronic inflammation of GI tract, GI bleeding disorders, history of hypersensitivity to aspirin or NSAIDs.

CAUTIONS

Impaired renal/hepatic function, history of GI tract disease, predisposition to fluid retention.

INTERACTIONS

DRUG: May increase effects of ***oral anticoagulants, heparin, thrombolytics.*** May decrease effect of ***antihypertensives, diuretics. Salicylates, aspirin*** may increase risk of GI side effects, bleeding. ***Bone marrow depressants*** may increase risk of hematologic reactions. May increase concentration, toxicity of ***lithium.*** May increase ***methotrexate*** toxicity. ***Probenecid*** may increase concentration. HERBAL: May decrease effect of feverfew. Ginkgo may increase risk of bleeding. FOOD: None significant. ALTERED LAB VALUES: May prolong bleeding time. May increase alkaline phosphatase, LDH, liver function tests. May decrease sodium, Hgb, Hct.

SIDE EFFECTS

FREQUENT (3–9%): Dyspepsia (heartburn, indigestion, epigastric pain). OCCASIONAL (1–3%): Nausea, diarrhea/constipation, flatulence, headache, dizziness, peripheral edema/fluid retention. RARE (<1%): Anorexia, vomiting, visual disturbances.

ADVERSE REACTIONS/TOXIC EFFECTS

Peptic ulcer, GI bleeding, gastritis, severe hepatic reaction (cholestasis, jaundice) occur rarely. Nephrotoxicity (dysuria, hematuria, proteinuria, nephrotic syndrome) and severe hypersensitivity reaction (bronchospasm, angiofacial edema) occur rarely.

PATIENT CONSIDERATIONS

Baseline Assessment

Assess onset, type, location, and duration of pain or inflammation. Inspect appearance of affected joints for immobility, deformities, skin condition.

Intervention/Evaluation

Monitor for evidence of nausea, dyspepsia. Monitor pattern of daily bowel activity and stool consistency. Assist w/ambulation if dizziness occurs. Check behind medial malleolus for fluid retention (usually first area noted). Evaluate for therapeutic response: relief of pain, stiffness, swelling, increase in joint mobility, reduced joint tenderness, improved grip strength.

Patient/Family Teaching

Avoid aspirin, alcohol during therapy (increases risk of GI bleeding). If GI upset occurs, take w/food, milk. Avoid tasks that require alertness, motor skills until response to drug is established. Swallow capsule whole; do not crush or chew.

ketorolac tromethamine

key-**tore**-oh-lack
(Toradol, Acular, Acular PF)

CANADIAN AVAILABILITY
Acular, Toradol

PREGNANCY CATEGORY C
(D if used in third trimester)

CLASSIFICATION

Nonsteroidal anti-inflammatory

AVAILABILITY (Rx)

Tablets: 10 mg. **Injection:** 15 mg/ml, 30 mg/ml. **Ophthalmic Solution:** 0.5%.

PHARMACODYNAMICS

	ONSET	PEAK	DURATION
IM	10 min	1–2 hrs	4–6 hrs
IV	10 min	1–2 hrs	4–6 hrs

PHARMACOKINETICS

Absorption: Readily absorbed from GI tract, after IM administration. **Metabolism:** Partially metabolized primarily in kidneys. **Excretion:** Primarily excreted in urine. **Half-life:** 3.8–6.3 hrs (increased in decreased renal function, elderly).

ACTION/*THERAPEUTIC EFFECT*

Produces analgesic effect by inhibiting prostaglandin synthesis, *reducing intensity of pain stimulus reaching sensory nerve endings.* Reduces prostaglandin levels in aqueous humor, *reducing intraocular inflammation.*

USES/*UNLABELED*

Short-term relief of mild to moderate pain. ***Ophthalmic:*** Relief of ocular itching due to seasonal allergic conjunctivitis. Treatment postop for inflammation following cataract extraction, pain following incisional refractive surgery. ***Ophthalmic:*** *Prophylaxis/treatment of ocular inflammation.*

STORAGE/HANDLING

Store oral, parenteral form at room temperature.

ADMINISTRATION

ORAL:

- May give w/food, milk, or antacids if GI distress occurs.

IM:

- Give slowly, deeply into muscle.

IV:

- Give over at least 15 sec.

OPHTHALMIC:

- Place finger on lower eyelid and pull out until pocket is formed between eye and lower lid. Hold dropper above pocket and place prescribed number of drops in pocket.
- Close eye gently. Apply digital pressure to lacrimal sac for 1–2 min (minimized drainage into nose and throat, reducing risk of systemic effects).
- Remove excess solution w/tissue.

INDICATIONS/ROUTES/DOSAGE

Note: Combined duration of IM/IV and oral not to exceed 5 days. May give as single dose, regular, or as needed schedule.

Analgesic (multiple dosing):
Oral: Adults, elderly: 10 mg q4–6h. ***Maximum:*** 40 mg/24 hrs.

IV/IM: Adults <65 yrs: 30 mg q6h. ***Maximum:*** 120 mg/24 hrs. ***>65 yrs, renally impaired, <50 kg:*** 15 mg q6h. ***Maximum:*** 60 mg/24 hrs.

Analgesic (single dose):
IM: Adults <65 yrs: 60 mg; ***>65 yrs, renally impaired, <50 kg:*** 30 mg.

IV: Adults <65 yrs: 30 mg; ***>65 yrs, renally impaired, <50 kg:*** 15 mg.

Usual ophthalmic dosage:
Adults, elderly: 1 drop 4 times/day.

CONTRAINDICATIONS

Active peptic ulcer, GI ulceration, chronic inflammation of GI tract,

K

GI bleeding disorders, history of hypersensitivity to aspirin or NSAIDs.

CAUTIONS

Renal/hepatic function, history of GI tract disease, predisposition to fluid retention.

INTERACTIONS

DRUG: May increase effects of ***oral anticoagulants, heparin, thrombolytics. Salicylates, aspirin*** may increase risk of GI side effects, bleeding. May increase concentration, toxicity of ***lithium.*** May increase ***methotrexate*** toxicity. ***Probenecid*** may increase concentration. **HERBAL:** May decrease effect of feverfew. Ginkgo may increase risk of bleeding. **FOOD:** None significant. **ALTERED LAB VALUES:** May prolong bleeding time. May increase liver function tests.

SIDE EFFECTS

Note: Age increases possibility of side effects. **FREQUENT (3–9%):** Diarrhea/constipation, indigestion, nausea, maculopapular rash, dermatitis, dizziness, headache. *Ophthalmic:* Transient stinging and burning. **OCCASIONAL (1–3%):** Anorexia, GI cramps, flatulence. *Ophthalmic:* Ocular irritation, allergic reactions, superficial ocular infection, keratitis.

ADVERSE REACTIONS/TOXIC EFFECTS

GI bleeding, peptic ulcer occur infrequently. Nephrotoxicity (glomerular nephritis, interstitial nephritis, and nephrotic syndrome) may occur in those with preexisting impaired renal function. Acute hypersensitivity reaction (fever, chills, joint pain) occurs rarely.

PATIENT CONSIDERATIONS

Baseline Assessment

Assess onset, type, location, and duration of pain.

Intervention/Evaluation

Assist with ambulation if dizziness occurs. Monitor stool frequency, consistency. Assess for evidence of rash. Evaluate for therapeutic response: relief of pain, stiffness, swelling, increase in joint mobility, reduced joint tenderness, improved grip strength. Be alert to signs of bleeding (may also occur w/ophthalmic due to systemic absorption).

Patient/Family Teaching

Avoid aspirin, alcohol during therapy w/oral or ophthalmic ketorolac (increases tendency to bleed). If GI upset occurs, take with food, milk. Avoid tasks that require alertness, motor skills until response to drug is established.

Ophthalmic

Transient stinging and burning may occur upon instillation. Do not administer while wearing soft contact lenses.

---

ketotifen

(Zaditor)

See Supplement

labetolol hydrochloride

lah-**bet**-ah-lol
(Normodyne, Trandate)

FIXED-COMBINATION(S)
W/hydrochlorothiazide, a diuretic **(Normozide)**

CANADIAN AVAILABILITY
Trandate

PREGNANCY CATEGORY C
(D if used in second or third trimester)

CLASSIFICATION

Beta-adrenergic blocker

AVAILABILITY (Rx)

Tablets: 100 mg, 200 mg, 300 mg. **Injection:** 5 mg/ml.

PHARMACODYNAMICS

	ONSET	PEAK	DURATION
Oral	0.5–2 hrs	2–4 hrs	8–12 hrs
IV	2–5 min	5–15 min	2–4 hrs

PHARMACOKINETICS

Absorption: Completely absorbed from GI tract. **Metabolism:** Undergoes first-pass metabolism. Metabolized in liver. **Excretion:** Primarily excreted in urine. **Half-life:** oral: 6–8 hrs; IV: 5.5 hrs.

ACTION/*THERAPEUTIC EFFECT*

Selectively blocks $beta_1$-adrenergic receptors, *slowing sinus heart rate, decreasing cardiac output, decreasing B/P* (exact mechanism unknown but may block peripheral adrenergic receptors, decrease sympathetic outflow from CNS or decrease renin release from kidney). Large dose may block $beta_2$-adrenergic receptors, *increasing airway resistance.* Alpha blockage *causes vasodilation, decreased peripheral vascular resistance.*

USES/*UNLABELED*

Management of mild, moderate, severe hypertension. May be used alone or in combination w/other antihypertensives. *Treatment of chronic angina pectoris; produces controlled hypotension during surgery.*

STORAGE/HANDLING

Store oral, parenteral form at room temperature. After dilution, IV solution is stable for 24 hrs. Solution appears clear, colorless to light yellow. Discard if precipitate forms or discoloration occurs.

ADMINISTRATION

ORAL:

- May give w/o regard to food.
- Tablets may be crushed.

IV:

- **Note:** Pt must be in supine position for IV administration and for 3 hrs after receiving medication (substantial drop in B/P on standing should be expected).
- For IV injection, give over 2 min at 10 min intervals.
- For IV infusion, dilute 200 mg in 160 ml 5% dextrose, 0.9% NaCl, or other compatible IV fluid to provide concentration of 1 mg/ml.
- Administer at rate of 2 mg/min (2 ml/min) initially. Rate is adjusted according to B/P.
- Monitor B/P immediately before, and every 5–10 min during IV administration (maximum effect occurs within 5 min).

INDICATIONS/ROUTES/DOSAGE

Hypertension:
Oral: Adults: Initially, 100 mg 2 times/day adjusted in increments

L

of 100 mg 2 times/day every 2–3 days. *Maintenance:* 200–400 mg 2 times/day. *Maximum:* 2.4 g/day.

Usual elderly dosage:
Oral: Initially, 100 mg 1–2 times/day. May increase as needed.

Severe hypertension, hypertensive emergency:
IV: Adults: Initially, 20 mg. Additional doses of 20–80 mg may be given at 10 min intervals, up to total dose of 300 mg.

IV Infusion: Adults: Initially, 2 mg/min up to total dose of 300 mg.

Oral: Adults: (After IV therapy): Initially, 200 mg; then, 200–400 mg in 6–12 hrs. Increase dose at 1 day intervals to desired level.

CONTRAINDICATIONS

Bronchial asthma, uncontrolled CHF, second- or third-degree heart block, severe bradycardia, cardiogenic shock.

CAUTIONS

Drug-controlled CHF, nonallergic bronchospastic disease (chronic bronchitis, emphysema), impaired hepatic, cardiac function, pheochromocytoma, diabetes mellitus.

INTERACTIONS

DRUG: *Diuretics, other hypotensives* may increase hypotensive effect; *sympathomimetics, xanthines* may mutually inhibit effects; may mask symptoms of hypoglycemia, prolong hypoglycemic effect of *insulin, oral hypoglycemics. MAO inhibitors* may produce hypertension. **HERBAL:** None known. **FOOD:** None significant. **ALTERED LAB VALUES:** May increase ANA titer, SGOT (AST), SGPT (ALT), alkaline phosphatase, LDH, bilirubin, BUN, creatinine, potassium uric acid, lipoproteins, triglycerides.

SIDE EFFECTS

FREQUENT: Drowsiness, trouble sleeping, unusually tired or weak, decreased sexual ability. **OCCASIONAL:** Dizziness, difficulty breathing, swelling of hands, feet, depression, anxiety, constipation, diarrhea, nasal congestion, nausea, vomiting, stomach discomfort. **RARE:** Altered taste, dry eyes, increased urination, numbness or tingling in fingers, toes, or scalp.

ADVERSE REACTIONS/TOXIC EFFECTS

May precipitate or aggravate CHF (due to decreased myocardial stimulation). Abrupt withdrawal may precipitate ischemic heart disease, producing sweating, palpitations, headache, tremulousness. Beta blockers may mask signs, symptoms of acute hypoglycemia (tachycardia, B/P changes) in diabetic pts.

PATIENT CONSIDERATIONS

BASELINE ASSESSMENT

Assess baseline renal/liver function tests. Assess B/P, apical pulse immediately before drug is administered (if pulse is 60/min or below, or systolic B/P is below 90 mm Hg, withhold medication, contact physician).

INTERVENTION/EVALUATION

Monitor B/P for hypotension, respiration for shortness of breath. Assess pulse for strength/weakness, irregular rate, bradycardia. Monitor EKG for cardiac arrhythmias. Monitor stool frequency and consistency. Assist w/ambulation if dizziness occurs. Assess for evidence of CHF: dyspnea (particularly on exertion or lying down), night cough, peripheral edema, distended neck veins. Monitor I&O (increase in weight,

decrease in urine output may indicate CHF). Assess for nausea, diaphoresis, headache, fatigue.

PATIENT/FAMILY TEACHING

Do not discontinue drug except upon advice of physician (abrupt discontinuation may precipitate heart failure). Transient scalp tingling may occur, especially when drug is initiated. Compliance w/therapy regimen is essential to control hypertension, arrhythmias. Avoid tasks that require alertness, motor skills until response to drug is established. Report shortness of breath, excessive fatigue, weight gain, prolonged dizziness or headache. Do not use nasal decongestants, OTC cold preparations (stimulants) w/o physician approval. Outpatients should monitor B/P, pulse before taking medication. Restrict salt, alcohol intake.

lactulose

lack-tyoo-lows
(Chronulac, Evalose, Heptalac)

CANADIAN AVAILABILITY
Acilac, Duphalac, Laxilose

PREGNANCY CATEGORY B

CLASSIFICATION

Laxative: Osmotic

AVAILABILITY (Rx)

Syrup: 10 g/15 ml

PHARMACODYNAMICS

	ONSET	PEAK	DURATION
Oral	24–48 hrs	—	—
Rectal	30–60 min	—	—

PHARMACOKINETICS

Absorption: Poorly absorbed from GI tract. Acts in colon.

ACTION / *THERAPEUTIC EFFECT*

Retains ammonia in colon (decreases blood ammonia concentration), producing osmotic effect. *Promotes increased peristalsis, bowel evacuation (expelling ammonia from colon).*

USES

Prevention/treatment of portal systemic encephalopathy (including hepatic precoma, coma); treatment of constipation.

STORAGE/HANDLING

Store solution at room temperature. Solution appears pale yellow to yellow, sweet, viscous liquid. Cloudiness, darkened solutions do not indicate potency loss.

ADMINISTRATION

ORAL:
- Drink water, juice, or milk w/each dose (aids stool softening, increases palatability).

RECTAL:
- Lubricate anus w/petroleum jelly before enema insertion.
- Insert carefully (prevents damage to rectal wall) w/nozzle toward navel.
- Squeeze container until entire dose expelled.
- Retain until definite lower abdominal cramping felt.

INDICATIONS/ROUTES/DOSAGE

Constipation:
Oral: Adults, elderly: 15–30 ml/day up to 60 ml/day.

Portal-systemic encephalopathy:
Oral: Adults, elderly: Initially, 30–45 ml every hour. Then, 30–45

ml 3–4 times/day. Adjust dose every 1–2 days to produce 2–3 soft stools/day. ***Children:*** 40–90 ml/day in divided doses. ***Infants:*** 2.5–10 ml/day in divided doses.

Usual rectal dosage (as retention enema):
Adults, elderly: 300 ml w/700 ml water or saline; retain 30–60 min; repeat every 4–6 hrs. (If evacuation occurs too promptly, repeat immediately.)

CONTRAINDICATIONS

Those on galactose-free diet, abdominal pain, nausea, vomiting, appendicitis.

CAUTIONS

Diabetes mellitus.

INTERACTIONS

DRUG: May decrease transit time of concurrently administered ***oral medication,*** decreasing absorption. **HERBAL:** None known. **FOOD:** None significant. **ALTERED LAB VALUES:** May decrease potassium concentration.

SIDE EFFECTS

OCCASIONAL: Cramping, diarrhea, flatulence, increased thirst, abdominal discomfort. **RARE:** Electrolyte imbalance, nausea, vomiting, magnesium accumulation in pts w/renal impairment.

ADVERSE REACTIONS/TOXIC EFFECTS

Diarrhea indicates overdosage. Long-term use may result in laxative dependence, chronic constipation, loss of normal bowel function.

PATIENT CONSIDERATIONS

INTERVENTION/EVALUATION

Encourage adequate fluid intake. Assess bowel sounds for peristalsis. Monitor daily bowel activity and stool consistency (watery, loose, soft, semisolid, solid) and record time of evacuation. Assess for abdominal disturbances. Monitor serum electrolytes in those exposed to prolonged, frequent, or excessive use of medication.

PATIENT/FAMILY TEACHING

Evacuation occurs in 24–48 hrs of initial dose. Institute measures to promote defecation. Increase fluid intake, exercise, high-fiber diet. Cola, unsalted crackers, dry toast may relieve nausea.

lamivudine

lah-mih-**view**-deen
(Epivir)

FIXED-COMBINATION(S)
w/zidovudine, an antiviral **(Combivir);** w/abacavir and zidovudine, antivirals **(Trizivir)**

CANADIAN AVAILABILITY
3TC

PREGNANCY CATEGORY C

CLASSIFICATION

Antiviral

AVAILABILITY (Rx)

Tablets: 100 mg, 150 mg. **Oral Solution:** 5 mg/ml, 10 mg/ml

PHARMACOKINETICS

Absorption: Rapidly, completely absorbed from GI tract. Widely distributed (crosses blood-brain barrier). **Excretion:** Primarily excreted unchanged in urine. Unknown if removed by hemo/peritoneal dialysis. **Half-life:** 11–15 hrs (intracellular); serum (adults) 2–11 hrs, (children) 1.7–2 hrs. Half-life increases w/diminished renal function.

ACTION / *THERAPEUTIC EFFECT*

Inhibits HIV reverse transcriptase via viral DNA chain termination. Also inhibits RNA- and DNA-dependent DNA polymerase, an enzyme necessary for viral HIV replication, *slowing HIV replication, reducing progression of HIV infection.*

USES / *UNLABELED*

Used in combination w/zidovudine for treatment of HIV infection when therapy is necessary based on clinical or immunologic evidence of disease. Treatment chronic hepatitis B. *Prophylaxis in health-care workers at risk of acquiring HIV after occupational exposure to virus.*

ADMINISTRATION

ORAL:

- May give w/o regard to meals.

INDICATIONS/ROUTES/DOSAGE

Note: Complete prescribing information for zidovudine should be consulted before concurrent therapy w/lamivudine and zidovudine is begun.

HIV infection:
Oral: Adults, children 12–16 yrs, >50 kg (>100 lbs): 150 mg twice daily in combination w/zidovudine. *Adults <50 kg:* 2 mg/kg twice daily in combination w/zidovudine. *Children 3 mos–12 yrs:* 4 mg/kg twice daily (up to 150 mg) in combination w/zidovudine.

Chronic hepatitis B:
Oral: Adults: 100 mg daily.

Dosage in renal impairment:
Dose and/or frequency is modified based on creatinine clearance.

CREATININE CLEARANCE	DOSAGE
≤ 50	150 mg twice daily
30–49	150 mg once daily
15–29	150 mg first dose, then 100 mg once daily
5–14	150 mg first dose, then 50 mg once daily
< 5	50 mg first dose, then 25 mg once daily

CONTRAINDICATIONS

None significant.

CAUTIONS

Peripheral neuropathy or history of peripheral neuropathy, history of pancreatitis in children, impaired renal function.

INTERACTIONS

DRUG: *Trimethoprim-sulfamethoxazole* increases lamivudine concentration. **HERBAL:** St. John's wort may decrease concentration, effect. **FOOD:** None significant. **ALTERED LAB VALUES:** May increase neutrophil count, SGOT (AST), SGPT (ALT), amylase serum level, Hgb.

SIDE EFFECTS

FREQUENT: Headache (35%), nausea (33%), malaise/fatigue (27%), nasal disturbances (20%), diarrhea, cough (18%), musculoskeletal pain, neuropathy (12%), insomnia (11%), anorexia, dizziness, fever/chills (10%). **OCCASIONAL:** Depression, (9%), myalgia (8%), abdominal cramps (6%), dyspepsia, arthralgia (5%).

ADVERSE REACTIONS/TOXIC EFFECTS

Pancreatitis occurs in 13% of pediatric pts. Anemia, neutropenia, thrombocytopenia occur rarely.

PATIENT CONSIDERATIONS

BASELINE ASSESSMENTS

Offer emotional support. Establish baseline lab values, especially renal function. Advise parents to closely monitor pediatric pts for symptoms of pancreatitis (severe, steady abdominal pain often radiating to the back, clammy skin, reduced B/P; nausea and vomiting may accompany abdominal pain). Question for hypersensitivity to lamivudine, pregnancy.

INTERVENTION/EVALUATION

Monitor amylase, lipase, BUN, serum creatinine. Assess for headache, nausea, cough. Determine pattern of bowel activity and stool consistency. Modify diet, or administer laxative as needed. Assess for dizziness, sleep pattern. If pancreatitis in children occurs, movement aggravates abdominal pain; sitting up or flexion at the waist relieves the pain.

PATIENT/FAMILY TEACHING

Continue therapy for full length of treatment. Doses should be evenly spaced. Do not take any medications w/o consulting physician. Inform pt lamivudine is not a cure and pt may continue to experience illnesses, including opportunistic infections. Do not drive, use machinery, or engage in other activities that require mental acuity if experiencing dizziness.

---

lamotrigine

lam-**oh**-trih-geen
(Lamictal)

CANADIAN AVAILABILITY
Lamictal

PREGNANCY CATEGORY C

CLASSIFICATION

Anticonvulsant

AVAILABILITY (Rx)

Tablets: 25 mg, 100 mg, 150 mg, 200 mg. **Chewable Tablets:** 5 mg, 25 mg.

PHARMACOKINETICS

Absorption: Rapidly, completely absorbed following oral administration (not affected by food). Binds to melanin-containing tissue (e.g., eye, pigmented skin). **Metabolism:** Metabolized in liver. **Excretion:** Primarily excreted unchanged in urine. Partially removed by hemodialysis. **Half-life:** 7.5–12.5 hrs (increased in pts receiving other anticonvulsants).

ACTION/*THERAPEUTIC EFFECT*

Exact mechanism unknown. May be due to inhibition of voltage-sensitive sodium channels, stabilizing neuronal membranes and regulating presynaptic transmitter release of excitatory amino acids, *producing anticonvulsant activity.*

USES/*UNLABELED*

Adjunctive therapy in adults w/partial seizures, adults and children in treatment of generalized seizures of Lennox-Gastaut syndrome. Conversion to monotherapy in adults treated w/another enzyme-inducing anti-epileptic drug (EIAED).

INDICATIONS/ROUTES/DOSAGE

Note: If pt currently on valproic acid, reduce lamotrigine dosage to less than half the normal dosage.

Seizure control in pts receiving enzyme-inducing antiepileptic drugs (AEDs), but not valproate:
Oral: Adults, elderly, children >12 yrs: Recommended as add-on therapy: 50 mg once/day for 2 wks,

followed by 100 mg/day in 2 divided doses for 2 wks. *Maintenance:* Dose may be increased by 100 mg/day every week, up to 300–500 mg/day in 2 divided doses.

Children (2–12 yrs): 0.6 mg/kg/day in 2 divided doses for 2 wks; then, 1.2 mg/kg/day in 2 divided doses for wks 3 and 4. *Maintenance:* 5–15 mg/kg/day. *Maximum:* 400 mg/day.

Seizure control in pts receiving combination therapy of valproic acid and enzyme-inducing antiepileptic drugs (AEDs): *Oral: Adults, elderly, children >12 yrs:* 25 mg every other day for 2 wks, followed by 25 mg once/day for 2 wks. *Maintenance:* Dose may be increased by 25–50 mg/day every 1–2 wks, up to 150 mg/day in 2 divided doses.

Children (2–12 yrs): 0.15 mg/kg/day in 2 divided doses for 2 wks; then, 0.3 mg/kg/day in 2 divided doses for wks 3 and 4. *Maintenance:* 1–5 mg/kg/day in 2 divided doses. *Maximum:* 200 mg/day.

Conversion to monotherapy: *Oral: Adults, children >12 yrs:* Add lamotrigine 50 mg/day for 2 wks; then, 100 mg/day during wks 3 and 4; then, increase by 100 mg/day q1–2wks until maintenance dosage achieved (300–500 mg/day in 2 divided doses/day). Gradually discontinue other EIAED over 4 wks once maintenance dose achieved.

Renal function impairment: **Note:** Same dosage as combination therapy (see above).

Discontinuation therapy: **Note:** A reduction in dosage over at least 2 wks (approx. 50% per week) is recommended.

CONTRAINDICATIONS

None significant.

CAUTIONS

Renal/hepatic function impairment, cardiac function impairment.

INTERACTIONS

DRUG: Lamotrigine may increase ***carbamazepine, valproic acid*** serum levels. ***Phenobarbital, primidone, phenytoin, carbamazepine, valproic acid*** decreases lamotrigine concentration. **HERBAL:** None known. **FOOD:** None significant. **ALTERED LAB VALUES:** None significant.

SIDE EFFECTS

FREQUENT: Dizziness (38%), double vision (28%), headache (29%), ataxia [muscular incoordination] (22%), nausea (19%), blurred vision (16%), somnolence, rhinitis (14%). **OCCASIONAL:** Rash (10%), pharyngitis, vomiting (9%), cough (8%), flu syndrome (7%), diarrhea, dysmenorrhea, fever, insomnia (6%), dyspepsia (5%). **RARE:** Constipation, tremor, anxiety, pruritus, vaginitis.

ADVERSE REACTIONS/TOXIC EFFECTS

Abrupt withdrawal may increase seizure frequency. Severe, potentially life-threatening rash.

PATIENT CONSIDERATIONS

BASELINE ASSESSMENT

Review history of seizure disorder (type, onset, intensity, frequency, duration, level of consciousness), drug history (especially other anticonvulsants), other medical conditions (e.g., renal function impairment). Provide safety precautions, quiet, dark environment. Obtain vital signs.

INTERVENTION/EVALUATION

Report to physician promptly if evidence of rash occurs (drug discontinuation may be necessary). Assist w/ambulation if dizziness, ataxia occurs. Observe frequently for recurrence of seizure activity. Assess for clinical improvement (decrease in intensity/frequency of seizures). Assess for visual abnormalities, headache.

PATIENT/FAMILY TEACHING

Take lamotrigine only as prescribed; do not abruptly withdraw medication after long-term therapy. Avoid tasks that require alertness, motor skills until response to drug is established. Avoid alcohol. Carry identification card/bracelet to note anticonvulsant therapy. Strict maintenance of drug therapy is essential for seizure control. If noncompliance is an issue in causing acute seizures, discuss reasons for noncompliance and address it. Report first sign of rash to physician.

lansoprazole

lan-sew-**prah**-zoll
(Prevacid)

CANADIAN AVAILABILITY
Prevacid

PREGNANCY CATEGORY B

CLASSIFICATION

Gastric acid pump inhibitor

AVAILABILITY (Rx)

Capsules (extended-release): 15 mg, 30 mg

PHARMACODYNAMICS

	ONSET	PEAK	DURATION
15 mg	2–3 hrs	—	24 hrs
30 mg	1–2 hrs	—	>24 hrs

PHARMACOKINETICS

Absorption: Once leaving stomach, rapid and complete absorption (food may decrease absorption). Distributed primarily to gastric parietal cells, converted to two active metabolites. **Metabolism:** Extensively metabolized in liver. Eliminated from body in bile and urine. **Half-life:** 1.5 hrs (increased in elderly, pts w/liver impairment).

ACTION/*THERAPEUTIC EFFECT*

Converted to active metabolites that irreversibly bind to and inhibit H+/K+ ATPase (an enzyme on surface of gastric parietal cells). Inhibits hydrogen ion transport into gastric lumen, *increasing gastric pH, reducing gastric acid production.*

USES/*UNLABELED*

Short-term treatment (up to 4 wks) for healing and symptomatic relief of active duodenal ulcer, short-term treatment (up to 8 wks) for healing and symptomatic relief of erosive esophagitis. Long-term treatment of pathologic hypersecretory conditions including Zollinger-Ellison syndrome. Short-term treatment (up to 8 wks) of active gastric ulcer. *H. pylori*–associated duodenal ulcer, maintenance treatment for healed duodenal ulcer. Treatment of gastroesophageal reflux disease (GERD).

ADMINISTRATION

ORAL:

- Give while fasting or before meals (food diminishes absorption).
- Do not chew or crush delayed-release capsules.

- If pt has difficulty swallowing capsules, open capsules and sprinkle granules on 1 tablespoon of applesauce and swallow immediately.

INDICATIONS/ROUTES/DOSAGE

Duodenal ulcer:
Oral: Adults, elderly: 15–30 mg/day, before eating, preferably in AM, for up to 4 wks.

Erosive esophagitis:
Oral: Adults, elderly: 30 mg/day, before eating, for up to 8 wks. If healing does not occur within 8 wks (5–10%), may give for additional 8 wks.

Gastric ulcer:
Oral: Adults: 30 mg/day for up to 8 wks.

Healed duodenal ulcer, GERD:
Oral: Adults: 15 mg/day

H. pylori:
Oral: Adults: 30 mg 2 times/day for 10 days (w/amoxicillin, clarithromycin).

Pathologic hypersecretory conditions (including Zollinger-Ellison syndrome):
Oral: Adults, elderly: 60 mg/day. Individualize dosage according to pt needs and for as long as clinically indicated. May increase to >120 mg/day in divided doses.

CONTRAINDICATIONS

None significant.

CAUTIONS

Impaired hepatic function.

INTERACTIONS

DRUG: May interfere with ***ketoconazole, ampicillin, iron salts, digoxin*** absorption. ***Sucralfate*** may delay lansoprazole absorption (give lansoprazole 30 min before sucralfate). **HERBAL:** None known. **FOOD:** Diminishes absorption. **ALTERED LAB VALUES:** May increase SGOT (AST), SGPT (ALT), serum creatinine, alkaline phosphatase, bilirubin, triglycerides, uric acid, LDH, cholesterol. May produce abnormal WBC, RBC and platelet counts, albumin/globulin ratio, electrolyte balance. May increase Hct, Hgb.

SIDE EFFECTS

OCCASIONAL (3–10%): Diarrhea, abdominal pain, rash, pruritus, altered appetite. **RARE (1–3%):** Nausea, headache.

ADVERSE REACTIONS/TOXIC EFFECTS

Bilirubinemia, eosinophilia, hyperlipemia occur rarely.

PATIENT CONSIDERATIONS

BASELINE ASSESSMENT

Obtain baseline lab values. Assess drug history, especially use of sucralfate.

INTERVENTION/EVALUATION

Monitor ongoing laboratory results. Assess for therapeutic response (i.e., relief of GI symptoms). Question if diarrhea, abdominal pain, nausea occur.

PATIENT/FAMILY TEACHING

Do not chew or crush delayed-release capsules. For those who have difficulty swallowing capsules, open capsules and sprinkle granules on 1 tablespoon of applesauce and swallow immediately. Report any adverse reactions.

latanoprost

lah-**tan**-oh-prost
(Xalatan)

CANADIAN AVAILABILITY
Xalatan

PREGNANCY CATEGORY C

CLASSIFICATION

Anti-glaucoma (prostaglandin)

AVAILABILITY (Rx)

Solution: 0.005% (50 mcg/ml)

PHARMACODYNAMICS

	ONSET	PEAK	DURATION
Ophthalmic			
	3–4 hrs	8–12 hrs	24 hrs

PHARMACOKINETICS

Absorption: A prodrug, rapidly hydrolyzed to active latanoprost acid in the cornea/plasma. Only minimal amount penetrates the eye (balance absorbed into systemic circulation). **Metabolism:** Metabolized in liver. **Excretion:** Primarily excreted in urine). **Half-life:** 17 min.

ACTION/*THERAPEUTIC EFFECT*

Increases uveoscleral (iris, ciliary body, choroid, sclera) outflow of aqueous humor, *decreasing intraocular pressure (IOP), ocular hypertension.*

USES

Reduces intraocular pressure (IOP) in management of chronic open-angle glaucoma, ocular hypertension in pts intolerant of other IOP-lowering medications or insufficiently responsive to another IOP-lowering medication.

STORAGE/HANDLING

Refrigerate unopened bottle. Once opened, may store container at room temperature for up to 6 wks.

ADMINISTRATION

OPHTHALMIC:

- Instruct pt to lie down or tilt head backward and look up.
- Gently pull lower eyelid down to form pocket between eye and lower lid. Hold dropper above pocket and place prescribed number of drops in pocket (do not touch tip of applicator to any surface).
- Close eye gently. Apply gentle finger pressure to lacrimal sac (bridge of nose, inside corner of eye) for 1–2 min (minimizes drainage into nose and throat, reducing risk of systemic effects).
- Remove excess solution around eye w/tissue.
- Tell pt not to close eyes tightly or blink more often than necessary.
- Never rinse dropper.

INDICATIONS/ROUTES/DOSAGE

Note: May be used concurrently w/other topical ophthalmics to lower IOP, but administer the medications at least 5 min apart (may cause precipitate).

Glaucoma:

Ophthalmic: Adults, elderly: One drop (1.5 mcg) in affected eye(s) once daily in the evening.

CONTRAINDICATIONS

Hypersensitivity to latanoprost or any component of medication.

CAUTIONS

None significant.

INTERACTIONS

DRUG: None significant. **HERBAL:** None known. **FOOD:** None signifi-

cant. **ALTERED LAB VALUES:** None significant.

SIDE EFFECTS

FREQUENT (5–15%): Transient blurred vision, burning/stinging, foreign body sensation, conjunctival hyperemia (excess blood), change in eye color (increase in amount of brown pigment), itching. **OCCASIONAL (1–4%):** Dry eye, eye pain, lid crusting, excessive tearing, lid edema, lid erythema, lid discomfort/pain, photophobia. **RARE (<1%):** Conjunctivitis, blurred vision, eye discharge, darkened eyelids/eyelashes; increased growth of eyelashes.

ADVERSE REACTIONS/TOXIC EFFECTS

Systemic events produce upper respiratory tract infection/cold/flu (4%), and rarely, musculoskeletal pain, chest pain, angina pectoris, allergic skin reaction (1–2%).

PATIENT CONSIDERATIONS

Baseline Assessment

Question for hypersensitivity to latanoprost or any component of medication. Assess physical appearance of eye and pt's perception of vision.

Intervention/Evaluation

Monitor for potential systemic reaction.

Patient/Family Teaching

Inform pt of possibility of iris color change, darkened eyelids, eyelashes, longer eyelashes, increased amount of brown pigment (more noticeable w/green-brown, blue/gray-brown or yellow-brown iris). Change may be permanent. Remove contact lenses prior to administration. Lenses may be inserted 15 min following administration. Instruct pt on proper administration of drops, particularly to avoid allowing tip of container to contact eye or surrounding area (increased risk of ocular infections due to contamination). If more than one ophthalmic drug is being used, administer drugs at least 5 min apart. Transient stinging, transient blurred vision, or foreign body sensation is common; notify physician if conjunctivitis or lid reaction occurs.

L

leflunomide

lee-**flew**-no-mide
(Arava)

PREGNANCY CATEGORY X

CLASSIFICATION

Immunomodulatory agent

AVAILABILITY (Rx)

Tablets: 10 mg, 20 mg.

PHARMACOKINETICS

Absorption: Well absorbed following oral administration. **Metabolism:** Metabolized to active metabolite in gastrointestinal wall and liver. **Excretion:** Mechanisms of excretion include both renal and biliary systems. **Half-life:** 16 days.

ACTION/*THERAPEUTIC EFFECT*

Attenuates the immune response exhibited in rheumatoid synovium, hinders proliferation of lymphocytes, possesses anti-inflammatory action. *Reduces signs and symptoms of rheumatoid arthritis and retards structural damage.*

USES

Treatment of active rheumatoid arthritis.

ADMINISTRATION

ORAL:

- May take w/o regard to food.

INDICATIONS/ROUTES/DOSAGES

Rheumatoid arthritis:
Oral: Adults, elderly: Initially, 100 mg daily for 3 days, then 10–20 mg daily.

CONTRAINDICATIONS

History of hypersensitivity to leflunomide, pregnancy or planning to become pregnant (Pregnancy Category X).

CAUTIONS

Impaired hepatic/renal function, positive hepatitis B or C serology, pts w/immunodeficiency or bone marrow dysplasias, nursing mothers.

INTERACTIONS

DRUG: *Rifampin* increases concentration of leflunomide. **HERBAL:** None known. **FOOD:** None significant. **ALTERED LAB VALUES:** May increase liver enzymes (especially ALT, AST).

SIDE EFFECTS

FREQUENT (10–20%): Diarrhea, respiratory tract infections, hair loss, rash, nausea.

ADVERSE REACTIONS/TOXIC EFFECTS

Transient thrombocytopenia and leukopenia occur rarely.

PATIENT CONSIDERATIONS

BASELINE ASSESSMENT

Question for hypersensitivity to leflunomide, pregnancy. Assess limitations in activities of daily living due to rheumatoid arthritis.

INTERVENTION/EVALUATION

Monitor tolerance to medication. Assess symptomatic relief of rheumatoid arthritis.

PATIENT/FAMILY TEACHING

May take w/o regard to food. Improvement may take >8 wks. Caution when driving or anything requiring alertness (possible dizziness, lightheadedness) until effects of medication known. Report if pain, inflammation, or rupture of a tendon is experienced.

lepirudin

leh-**pier**-ruh-din
(Refludan)

PREGNANCY CATEGORY B

CLASSIFICATION

Anticoagulant

AVAILABILITY (Rx)

Powder for Injection: 50 mg

PHARMACOKINETICS

Distributed primarily in extracellular fluid. **Excretion:** Eliminated primarily by kidneys. **Half-life:** 1.3 hrs. Half-life prolonged in those with severely impaired renal function.

ACTION/*THERAPEUTIC EFFECT*

Inhibits thrombogenic action of thrombin *producing increase in activated partial thromboplasitn time (APTT)*. Action independent of antithrombin II and not inhibited by platelet factor 4.

USES

Anticoagulant in pts w/heparin-induced thrombocytopenia and associated thromboembolic disease to prevent further thromboembolic complications.

ADMINISTRATION

IV:

- Reconstitute by adding 1 ml of water for injection or 0.9% NaCl to 50 mg vial.
- For administration by IV injection, further dilute w/sterile water for injection, 0.9% NaCl or 5% dextrose to volume of 10 ml (5 mg/ml).
- For continuous IV infusion, contents of 2 vials (100 mg) are transferred into 500 ml or 250 ml of 0.9% NaCl or 5% dextrose (0.2 or 0.4 mg/ml, respectively).

INDICATIONS/ROUTES/DOSAGE

Note: Give initial dose as soon as possible after surgery but not more than 24 hrs after surgery.

Anticoagulant:
IV injection/IV infusion: Adults, elderly: 0.2–0.4 mg/kg, IV slowly over 15–20 sec followed by IV infusion of 0.15 mg/kg/hr for 2–10 hrs or longer.

CONTRAINDICATIONS

None significant.

CAUTIONS

Conditions w/increased risk of hemorrhage, acute bacterial endocarditis, congenital or acquired bleeding disorders, active ulcerative and angiodysplastic GI disease, nonhemorrhagic stroke, shortly after brain, spinal, or ophthalmologic surgery, postoperative indwelling epidural catheter use, severe uncontrolled hypertension, renal/hepatic function impairment.

INTERACTIONS

DRUG: *Anticoagulants, platelet inhibitors, thrombolytics* may increase risk of bleeding complications (use w/care). **HERBAL:** Ginkgo may increase risk of bleeding. **FOOD:** None significant.

ALTERED LAB VALUES: Increased APTT, thrombin time.

SIDE EFFECTS

FREQUENT (>10%): Bleeding complications (e.g., bleeding from puncture sites/wound), hematoma. **OCCASIONAL (1–10%):** Allergic reaction (rash, itching), unusually tired, blood in urine, GI and rectal bleeding, nosebleed, vaginal bleeding, fever, swelling of feet or lower legs, pneumonia.

ADVERSE REACTIONS/TOXIC EFFECTS

Accidental overdosage may lead to bleeding complications ranging from minor ecchymosis to major hemorrhage.

PATIENT CONSIDERATIONS

BASELINE ASSESSMENT

Assess APTT.

INTERVENTION/EVALUATION

Periodically monitor APTT, stool for occult blood. Assess for any sign of bleeding: bleeding at surgical site, hematuria, and blood in stool, bleeding from gums, petechiae, bruising, bleeding from injection sites.

---

letrozole

(Femara)
See Supplement

---

leucovorin calcium (folinic acid, citrovorum factor)

lou-**koe**-vor-in
(Wellcovorin)

CANADIAN AVAILABILITY

Lederle, Leucovorin

PREGNANCY CATEGORY C

CLASSIFICATION

Folic acid antagonist

AVAILABILITY (Rx)

Tablets: 5 mg, 15 mg, 25 mg. **Injection:** 3 mg/ml. **Powder for Injection:** 50 mg, 100 mg, 350 mg.

PHARMACOKINETICS

Absorption: Readily absorbed from GI tract. Widely distributed. Primarily concentrated in liver. **Metabolism:** Metabolized in liver, intestinal mucosa to active metabolite. **Excretion:** Primarily excreted in urine. **Half-life:** 6.2 hrs.

ACTION/*THERAPEUTIC EFFECT*

Competes w/methotrexate for same transport processes into cells (limits methotrexate action on normal cells). *Allows purine, DNA, RNA, protein synthesis.*

USES

Antidote (diminishes toxicity, counteracts effect of unintentional overdose of folic acid antagonists [e.g., methotrexate]); prevention/treatment of undesired hematopoietic effects of folic acid antagonists (e.g., rescue w/high-dose methotrexate therapy); treatment of megaloblastic anemias due to folic acid deficiency. Palliative treatment of advanced colorectal cancer (in combination w/5-fluorouracil).

STORAGE/HANDLING

Store tablets/vials for parenteral use at room temperature. Injection is clear, yellowish solution.

ADMINISTRATION

ORAL:

- Scored tablets may be crushed.

IV:

- Reconstitute each 50 mg vial w/5 ml sterile water for injection or bacteriostatic water for injection containing benzyl alcohol to provide concentration of 10 mg/ml. Due to benzyl alcohol in 1 mg ampule and in bacteriostatic water, reconstitute doses >10 mg/m^2 w/sterile water.
- Use immediately if reconstituted w/sterile water; stable for 7 days if reconstituted w/bacteriostatic water for injection.
- Further dilute w/5% dextrose or 0.9% NaCl.
- Do not exceed 160 mg/min if given by IV infusion (because of calcium content).

INDICATIONS/ROUTES/DOSAGE

Antidote, prevention/treatment of hematopoietic effects of folic acid antagonists:

Note: For rescue therapy in cancer chemotherapy, refer to specific protocol being used for optimal dosage and sequence of leucovorin administration.

Conventional rescue dosage:
10 mg/m^2 parenterally one time then q6h orally until serum methotrexate <10^{-8}M. If 24 hr serum creatinine increased by 50% or more over baseline or methotrexate >5×10^{-6}M or 48 hr level >9×10^{-7}M, increase to 100 mg/m^2 IV q3h until methotrexate level <10^{-8}M.

Megaloblastic anemia:
IM: Adults: Up to 1 mg/day.

Advanced colorectal cancer:
IV: Adults: 200 mg/m^2 over minimum of 3 min (follow w/5-fluorouracil 370 mg/m^2 by IV injection) or 20 mg/m^2 (follow w/5-fluorouracil 425 mg/m^2). Repeat daily for 5 days; repeat cycle at 4 wk intervals for 2 cycles; then, at 4–5 wk intervals. **Note:** Do not start

next cycle until pt recovered from prior treatment course (until WBC is 4,000/mm^3 and platelets are 130,000/mm^3).

CONTRAINDICATIONS

Pernicious anemia, other megaloblastic anemias secondary to vitamin B_{12} deficiency.

CAUTIONS

History of allergies, bronchial asthma. ***W/5-fluorouracil:*** Pts w/GI toxicities (more common/severe).

INTERACTIONS

DRUG: May decrease effect of ***anticonvulsants***. May increase effect, toxicity of ***5-fluorouracil.*** **HERBAL:** None known. **FOOD:** None significant. **ALTERED LAB VALUES:** None significant.

SIDE EFFECTS

FREQUENT: ***W/5-fluorouracil:*** Diarrhea, stomatitis, nausea, vomiting, lethargy/malaise/fatigue, alopecia, anorexia. **OCCASIONAL:** Urticaria, dermatitis.

ADVERSE REACTIONS/TOXIC EFFECTS

Excessive dosage may negate chemotherapeutic effect of folic acid antagonists. Anaphylaxis occurs rarely. Diarrhea may cause rapid clinical deterioration and death.

PATIENT CONSIDERATIONS

Baseline Assessment

Give as soon as possible, preferably within 1 hr, for treatment of accidental overdosage of folic acid antagonists.

Intervention/Evaluation

Monitor for vomiting—may need to change from oral to parenteral therapy. Observe elderly and debilitated closely because of risk of severe toxicities. Assess CBC, differential, platelet count (also electrolytes and liver function tests for combination w/5-fluorouracil).

Patient/Family Teaching

Explain purpose of medication in treatment of cancer. Report allergic reaction, vomiting.

L

leuprolide acetate

leu-pro-lied
(Lupron, Lupron Depot Ped)

CANADIAN AVAILABILITY
Lupron

PREGNANCY CATEGORY X

CLASSIFICATION

Antineoplastic

AVAILABILITY (Rx)

Injection: 5 mg/ml. **Lypholized Microspheres for Injection:** 3.75 mg, 7.5 mg, 11.25 mg, 15 mg, 22.5 mg, 30 mg.

PHARMACOKINETICS

Absorption: Rapid, well absorbed after SubQ administration. Slow absorption after IM administration. **Half-life:** 3–4 hrs.

ACTION/*THERAPEUTIC EFFECT*

Initial or intermittent administration stimulates release of luteinizing hormone (LH) and follicle-stimulating hormone (FSH) from anterior pituitary, increasing (within 1 wk) testosterone level in males, estradiol in premenopausal women. Continuous daily administration suppresses secretion of gonadotropin-releasing hormone, *producing fall (within 2–4 wks) in testosterone levels to castrate level in males, estrogen level in premenopausal women to postmenopausal levels. In central precocious puberty, gonadotropins reduced to prepubertal levels.*

USES

Treatment of advanced prostatic carcinoma, endometriosis, central precocious puberty, uterine fibroid tumors, anemia caused by uterine leiomyomata.

STORAGE/HANDLING

Note: May be carcinogenic, mutagenic, or teratogenic. Handle w/extreme care during preparation/administration.

Injection appears clear, colorless. Refrigerate. Store opened vial at room temperature. Discard if precipitate forms or solution appears discolored. ***Depot vials:*** Store at room temperature. Reconstitute only w/diluent provided; use immediately. Do not use needles <22 gauge.

ADMINISTRATION

SubQ:

- Use syringes provided by manufacturer (0.5 ml low-dose insulin syringe may be used as alternative).

INDICATIONS/ROUTES/DOSAGE

Prostatic carcinoma:
SubQ: Adults, elderly: 1 mg daily.

IM: Adults, elderly: Depot: 7.5 mg q28–33days or 22.5 mg q3mos or 30 mg q4mos.

Endometriosis, uterine leiomyomata:
IM: Adults: Depot: 3.75 mg monthly or 11.25 mg as single injection.

Central precocious puberty:
SubQ: Children: Initially, 50 mcg/kg/day; if down regulation not achieved, titrate upward by 10 mcg/kg/day.

IM: Children: Initially, 0.3 mg/kg 4 wks (minimum: 7.5 mg); if down regulation not achieved, titrate upward in 3.75 mg increments q4wks.

CONTRAINDICATIONS

None significant.

EXTREME CAUTION

Pts w/life-threatening disease when rapid symptomatic relief is necessary.

CAUTIONS

Hypersensitivity to benzyl alcohol.

INTERACTIONS

DRUG: None significant. **HERBAL:** None known. **FOOD:** None significant. **ALTERED LAB VALUES:** May increase serum acid phosphatase. Initially increases testosterone, then decreases testosterone concentration.

SIDE EFFECTS

FREQUENT: Hot flashes (ranging from mild flushing to sweating). ***Females:*** Amenorrhea, spotting. **OCCASIONAL:** Arrhythmias/palpitations, blurred vision, dizziness, edema, headache, burning/itching, swelling at injection site, nausea, insomnia, increased weight. ***Females:*** Deepening voice, increased hair growth, decreased libido, increased breast tenderness, vaginitis, altered mood. ***Males:*** Constipation, decreased testicle size, gynecomastia, impotence, decreased appetite, angina. **RARE:** ***Males:*** Thrombophlebitis.

ADVERSE REACTIONS/TOXIC EFFECTS

Occasionally, a worsening of signs/symptoms of prostatic carcinoma occurs 1–2 wks after initial dosing (subsides during continued therapy). Increased bone pain and less frequently dysuria or hematuria, weakness or paresthesia of lower extremities may be noted. Myocardial infarction, pulmonary embolism occur rarely.

PATIENT CONSIDERATIONS

BASELINE ASSESSMENT

Question for possibility of pregnancy before initiating therapy (Pregnancy Category X). Obtain serum testosterone, prostatic acid phosphatase (PAP) levels periodically during therapy. Serum testosterone and PAP levels should increase during first week of therapy. Testosterone level then should decrease to baseline level or less within 2 wks, PAP level within 4 wks.

INTERVENTION/EVALUATION

Monitor closely for signs/symptoms of worsening of disease.

PATIENT/FAMILY TEACHING

Hot flashes tend to decrease during continued therapy. A temporary exacerbation of signs/symptoms of disease may occur during first few weeks of therapy.

levalbuterol

(Xopenex)

See Classification section under: Bronchodilators

levamisole hydrochloride

(Ergamisol)

See Classification section under: Cancer chemotherapy

levetiracetam

(Keppra)

See Supplement

levobunolol hydrochloride

(Betagan Liquifilm)

See Classification section under: Antiglaucoma agents

levobupivacaine

(Chirocaine)

See Classification section under: Local anesthetics

levocabastine hydrochloride

lev-oh-cah-**bass**-teen

(Livostin)

CANADIAN AVAILABILITY

Livostin

PREGNANCY CATEGORY C

CLASSIFICATION

Antiallergic

AVAILABILITY (Rx)

Ophthalmic Suspension: 0.05%

PHARMACODYNAMICS

	ONSET	PEAK	DURATION
Ophthalmic	—	—	2 hrs

PHARMACOKINETICS

Absorption: Minimal systemic absorption.

ACTION/*THERAPEUTIC EFFECT*

Selective H-1 receptor antagonist. *Blocks histamine-associated symptoms of allergic conjunctivitis.*

USES

Temporary relief of signs and symptoms of seasonal allergic conjunctivitis.

STORAGE/HANDLING

Store at room temperature, protect from freezing. Discard if suspension is discolored. Keep tightly closed.

ADMINISTRATION

OPHTHALMIC:

- Instruct pt to lie down or tilt head backward and look up.
- Shake suspension well.
- Gently pull lower lid down to form pouch and instill medication.
- Do not touch tip of applicator to any surface.
- When lower lid is released, have pt keep eye open w/o blinking for at least 30 sec.
- Apply gentle finger pressure to lacrimal sac (bridge of the nose, inside corner of the eye) for 1–2 min.
- Remove excess solution around eye w/tissue.
- Tell pt not to close eyes tightly or blink more often than necessary.
- Never rinse dropper.

INDICATIONS/ROUTES/DOSAGE

Allergic conjunctivitis:
Ophthalmic: Adults, elderly, children >12 yrs: 1 drop 4 times/day, for up to 2 wks.

CONTRAINDICATIONS

Hypersensitivity. Wearing soft contact lenses (product contains benzalkonium chloride).

CAUTIONS

For ophthalmic use only. Not for injection. Safety in children <12 years not known.

INTERACTIONS

DRUG: None significant. **HERBAL:** None known. **FOOD:** None significant. **ALTERED LAB VALUES:** None significant.

SIDE EFFECTS

FREQUENT (5–15%): Transient stinging, burning, discomfort, headache. **OCCASIONAL (3–5%):** Dry mouth, fatigue, eye dryness, lacrimation/discharge, eyelid edema. **RARE (1–3%):** Rash, erythema, nausea, dyspnea.

ADVERSE REACTIONS/TOXIC EFFECTS

None significant.

PATIENT CONSIDERATIONS

Baseline Assessment

Assess for hypersensitivity to any component of suspension. Evaluate ocular signs and symptoms.

Patient/Family Teaching

Shake well before using. Do not use if suspension is discolored. Teach correct procedure for administration of drops. Do not wear soft contact lenses during therapy. For ophthalmic use only. May experience mild transitory burning, stinging upon instillation. Therapy may last up to 2 wks. If disorder does not improve or new symptoms develop, notify physician.

levofloxacin

leave-oh-**flocks**-ah-sin
(Levaquin, Quixin)

CANADIAN AVAILABILITY
Levaquin

PREGNANCY CATEGORY C

CLASSIFICATION

Antibiotic: Fluoroquinolone

AVAILABILITY (Rx)

Tablets: 250 mg, 500 mg, 750 mg. **Injection:** 500 mg/20 ml vials. **Premix:** 250 mg/50 ml, 500 mg/100 ml, 750 mg/100 ml. **Ophthalmic Solution:** 0.5%.

PHARMACOKINETICS

Absorption: Well absorbed following both oral and IV administration. Penetrates rapidly and extensively into leukocytes, epithelial cells and macrophages. Lung concentrations are 2–5 times higher than those of plasma. **Excretion:** Eliminated unchanged in the urine. **Half-life:** 8 hrs.

ACTION/*THERAPEUTIC EFFECT*

Inhibits the DNA enzyme, gyrase, in susceptible microorganisms, interfering with bacterial DNA replication and repair, *producing bactericidal activity.*

USES

Treatment of acute bacterial exacerbation of chronic bronchitis, community-acquired pneumonia, acute maxillary sinusitis, mild-moderate complicated urinary tract infections, acute pyelonephritis, uncomplicated mild to moderate skin and skin-structure infections.

ADMINISTRATION

ORAL:

- Do not administer antacids (aluminum, magnesium), sucralfate, iron and multivitamin preparations with zinc within 2 hrs of levofloxacin administration (significantly reduces levofloxacin absorption).
- Encourage cranberry juice, citrus fruits (acidifies urine).
- May take w/o regard to food.

IV:

- Compatible with 0.9% sodium chloride, 5% dextrose, 5% dextrose in lactated Ringer's, plasma-lyte 56/5% dextrose, 5% dextrose/0.45% sodium chloride, 0.15% potassium chloride, sodium lactate.
- Administer slowly, over a period of not less than 60 min.

INDICATIONS/ROUTES/DOSAGES

Bronchitis:
Oral/IV: Adults, elderly: 500 mg q24h for 7 days.

Pneumonia:
Oral/IV: Adults, elderly: 500 mg q24h for 7–14 days.

Acute maxillary sinusitis:
Oral/IV: Adults, elderly: 500 mg q24h for 10–14 days.

Skin, skin-structure:
Oral/IV: Adults, elderly: 500 mg q24h for 7–10 days.

Urinary tract infection, acute pyelonephritis:
Oral/IV: Adults, elderly: 250 mg q24h for 10 days.

Dosage in renal impairment:
Bronchitis, pneumonia, sinusitis, skin, skin-structure infections:

CREATININE CLEARANCE	DOSAGE
50–80 ml/min	No change
20–49 ml/min	500 mg initially, then 250 mg q24h
10–19 ml/min, dialysis	500 mg initially, then 250 mg q48h

Urinary tract infection, pyelonephritis:

CREATININE CLEARANCE	DOSAGE
≥20 ml/min	No change
10–19 ml/min	250 mg initially, then 250 mg q48h

CONTRAINDICATIONS

History of hypersensitivity to fluoroquinolone antibiotics, cinoxacin, nalidixic acid.

CAUTIONS

Impaired renal/hepatic function, diabetes mellitus.

INTERACTIONS

DRUG: *Antacids, sucralfate, iron preparations* decreases levofloxacin absorption. *NSAIDs* may increase risk of CNS stimulation/seizures. **HERBAL:** None known. **FOOD:** None significant. **ALTERED LAB VALUES:** May alter blood glucose concentrations.

SIDE EFFECTS

OCCASIONAL (1–3%): Diarrhea, nausea, stomach pain, dizziness, drowsiness, headache, lightheadedness. **RARE (<1%):** Vaginitis, flatulence, rash with pruritus, abdominal pain, taste perversion, phototoxicity (rash, itching, blister, swelling, sensation of skin burning), pain, inflammation or swelling in calves, hands or shoulder.

ADVERSE REACTIONS/TOXIC EFFECTS

Superinfection may occur. Hypersensitivity reactions have occurred in those receiving fluoroquinolone therapy. Pseudomembranous colitis (severe abdominal pain/cramps, severe watery diarrhea, fever).

PATIENT CONSIDERATIONS

BASELINE ASSESSMENT

Question for hypersensitivity to levofloxacin or other fluoroquinolones. Obtain specimens for culture and sensitivity test (therapy may begin before results are known).

INTERVENTION/EVALUATION

Report hypersensitivity reaction: skin rash, urticaria, pruritus, photosensitivity promptly. Be alert for superinfection (e.g., genital-anal pruritus, ulceration or changes in oral mucosa, moderate to severe diarrhea, new or increased fever). Provide symptomatic relief for nausea. Evaluate food tolerance, change in taste sensation.

PATIENT/FAMILY TEACHING

Do not take antacids 2 hrs before or after taking medication (reduces/destroys effectiveness). Possible photoxic reaction. Continue medication for full length of treatment. Check w/physician if no improvement within a few days. Discontinue at first sign of skin rash or other allergic reaction. Caution when driving or anything requiring alertness (possible dizziness, lightheadedness) until effects of medication known. Report if pain, inflammation, or rupture of a tendon is experienced.

levorphanol tartrate

leh-**vor**-phan-ole

(Levo-Dromoran)

PREGNANCY CATEGORY B
(D if used for prolonged periods or at high doses at term)

CLASSIFICATION

Opioid: Analgesic **(Schedule II)**

AVAILABILITY (Rx)

Tablets: 2 mg. **Injection:** 2 mg/ml.

PHARMACODYNAMICS

	ONSET	PEAK	DURATION
Oral	30–45 min	60–120 min	4 hrs (analgesic) 4–6 hrs (antitussive)
IM	10–30 min	30–60 min	4 hrs
SubQ	10–30 min	—	2.5–4 hrs

PHARMACOKINETICS

Absorption: Well absorbed from GI tract, after IM, SubQ administration. **Metabolism:** Metabolized in liver. **Excretion:** Primarily excreted in urine. **Half-life:** 11 hrs.

ACTION/*THERAPEUTIC EFFECT*

Binds w/opioid receptors within CNS, *altering processes affecting pain perception, emotional response to pain.*

USES

Relief of moderate to severe pain. Used preoperatively to produce sedation, and as adjunct w/nitrous oxide/oxygen anesthesia.

STORAGE/HANDLING

Store oral, parenteral forms at room temperature.

ADMINISTRATION

ORAL:

- May be given w/o regard to meals.
- Tablets may be crushed.

SUBQ:

- Pt should be in recumbent position before administering.
- Those w/circulatory impairment may experience overdosage due to delayed absorption of repeated SubQ administration.

IV:

- Always administer very slowly (over 2–3 min).
- Rapid IV increases risk of severe adverse reactions (chest wall rigidity, apnea, peripheral circulatory collapse, anaphylactoid effect, cardiac arrest).

INDICATIONS/ROUTES/DOSAGE

Note: Reduce initial dosage in those w/hypothyroidism, Addison's disease, renal insufficiency, elderly/debilitated, those on concurrent CNS depressants.

Oral/SubQ: Adults, elderly: 2 mg. May be increased to 3 mg, if needed.

IV: Adults: Optimum dosage not established.

CONTRAINDICATIONS

None significant.

EXTREME CAUTION

CNS depression, anoxia, hypercapnia, respiratory depression, seizures, acute alcoholism, shock, untreated myxedema, respiratory dysfunction.

CAUTIONS

Increased intracranial pressure, impaired hepatic function, acute abdominal conditions, hypothyroidism, prostatic hypertrophy, Addison's disease, urethral stricture, COPD.

INTERACTIONS

DRUG: *Alcohol, CNS depressants* may increase CNS or respiratory depression, hypotension. ***MAO inhibitors*** may produce severe, fatal reaction (reduce dose to usual 1/4 dose). **HERBAL:** None known. **FOOD:** None significant. **ALTERED LAB VALUES:** May increase amylase, lipase plasma concentrations.

SIDE EFFECTS

Note: Effects are dependent on dosage amount, route of administration. Ambulatory pts and those not in severe pain may experience dizziness, nausea, vomiting, hypotension more frequently than those in supine position or having severe pain. **FREQUENT:** Dizziness, drowsiness, hypotension, nausea, vomiting, unusually tired. **OCCASIONAL:** Shortness of breath, trouble breathing, confusion, decreased urination, stomach cramps, altered vision, constipation, dry mouth, headache, redness, pain, swelling at injection site, difficult or painful urination. **RARE:** Allergic reaction (rash, itching), histamine reaction (decreased blood pressure, increased sweating, flushed face, wheezing), paralytic ileus, inability to sleep.

ADVERSE REACTIONS/TOXIC EFFECTS

Overdosage results in respiratory depression, skeletal muscle flaccidity, cold clammy skin, cyanosis, extreme somnolence progressing to convulsions, stupor, coma. Tolerance to analgesic effect, physical dependence may occur w/repeated use.

PATIENT CONSIDERATIONS

BASELINE ASSESSMENT

Pt should be in a recumbent position before drug is administered by parenteral route. Assess onset, type, location, and duration of pain. Obtain vital signs before giving medication. If respirations are 12/min or lower (20/min or lower in children), withhold medication, contact physician.

INTERVENTION/EVALUATION

Monitor vital signs after parenteral administration for decreased B/P, a change in rate or quality of pulse, decreased respirations. Assess for adequate voiding, possible constipation. Initiate deep breathing and coughing exercises, particularly in those w/impaired pulmonary function. Assess therapeutic response and contact physician if pain relief is inadequate.

PATIENT/FAMILY TEACHING

Promptly report recurrence of pain (effect of medication is reduced if full pain recurs before next dose). Discomfort may occur w/injection. Change positions slowly to avoid orthostatic hypotension. Avoid tasks that require alertness, motor skills until response to drug is established. Tolerance/dependence may occur w/prolonged use of high doses. Avoid alcohol. Report nausea, vomiting, constipation, shortness of breath, difficulty breathing.

levothyroxine

lee-voe-thye-**rox**-een
(Eltroxin, Levothroid, Levoxyl, Synthroid)

FIXED-COMBINATION(S)
W/liothyronine, T_3 **(Thyrolar)**

CANADIAN AVAILABILITY

Eltroxin, Levotec, Synthroid

PREGNANCY CATEGORY A

CLASSIFICATION

Thyroid

AVAILABILITY (Rx)

Tablets: 0.025 mg, 0.05 mg, 0.075 mg, 0.088 mg, 0.1 mg, 0.112 mg, 0.125 mg, 0.137 mg, 0.15 mg, 0.175 mg, 0.2 mg, 0.3 mg. **Injection:** 200 mcg, 500 mcg.

PHARMACOKINETICS

Absorption: Variable, incomplete absorption from GI tract. Widely distributed. **Metabolism:** Deiodinated in peripheral tissues, minimal metabolism in liver. **Excretion:** Eliminated by biliary excretion. **Half-life:** 6–7 days.

ACTION / *THERAPEUTIC EFFECT*

Involved in normal metabolism, growth and development (especially CNS of infants). Possesses catabolic and anabolic effects. *Increases basal metabolic rate, enhances gluconeogenesis, stimulates protein synthesis.*

USES

Replacement in decreased or absent thyroid function (partial or complete absence of gland, primary atrophy, functional deficiency, effects of surgery, radiation or antithyroid agents, pituitary or hypothalamic hypothyroidism); management of simple (nontoxic) goiter and chronic lymphocytic thyroiditis; treatment of thyrotoxicosis (w/antithyroid drugs) to prevent goitrogenesis and hypothyroidism. Management of thyroid cancer. Diagnostic in thyroid suppression tests.

ADMINISTRATION

Do not interchange brands because there have been problems w/bioequivalence between manufacturers.

ORAL:

- Give at same time each day to maintain hormone levels.
- Administer before breakfast to prevent insomnia.
- Tablets may be crushed.

IV:

- Reconstitute 200 mcg or 500 mcg vial w/5ml 0.9% NaCl to provide a concentration of 40 or 100 mcg/ml, respectively; shake until clear.
- Do not use or mix w/other IV solutions.
- Use immediately and discard unused portions.

INDICATIONS / ROUTES / DOSAGE

Note: Begin therapy w/small doses; gradually increase.

Hypothyroidism:
Oral: Adults, elderly: Initially, 0.05 mg/day. Increase by 0.025 mg q2–3 wks. *Maintenance:* 0.1–0.2 mg/day.

Myxedema coma or stupor (medical emergency):
IV: Adults, elderly: Initially, 0.4 mg. Follow w/daily supplements of 0.1–0.2 mg. *Maintenance:* 0.05–0.1 mg/day.

Thyroid suppression therapy:
Oral: Adults, elderly: 2.6 mcg/kg/day for 7–10 days.

TSH suppression in thyroid cancer, nodules, euthyroid goiters:
Oral: Adults, elderly: Use larger doses than that used for replacement therapy.

Congenital hypothyroidism:
Oral: Children >12 yrs: >0.15 mg/day; *Children 6–12 yrs:* 0.1–0.15 mg/day; *Children 1–5 yrs:* 0.075–0.1 mg/day; *Children 6–12 mos:* 0.05–0.075 mg/day; *Infants 0–6 mos:* 0.025–0.05 mg/day.

Usual parenteral dosage:
IV: Adults, elderly: Initial dosage approximately one-half the previously established oral dosage.

CONTRAINDICATIONS

Thyrotoxicosis and myocardial infarction uncomplicated by hypothyroidism, hypersensitivity to any component (w/tablets: tartrazine, allergy to aspirin, lactose intolerance), treatment of obesity.

CAUTIONS

Elderly, angina pectoris, hypertension or other cardiovascular disease.

INTERACTIONS

DRUG: May alter effect of *oral anticoagulants. Cholestyramine, colestipol* may decrease absorption. *Sympathomimetics* may increase effects, coronary insufficiency. HERBAL: None known. FOOD: None significant. ALTERED LAB VALUES: None significant.

SIDE EFFECTS

OCCASIONAL: Children may have reversible hair loss upon initiation. RARE: Dry skin, GI intolerance, skin rash, hives, pseudotumor cerebri (severe headache in children).

ADVERSE REACTIONS/TOXIC EFFECTS

Excessive dosage produces signs/symptoms of hyperthyroidism: weight loss, palpitations, increased appetite, tremors, nervousness, tachycardia, increased B/P, headache, insomnia, menstrual irregularities. Cardiac arrhythmias occur rarely.

PATIENT CONSIDERATIONS

BASELINE ASSESSMENT

Question for hypersensitivity to tartrazine, aspirin, lactose. Obtain baseline weight, vital signs. Check results of thyroid function tests. Signs and symptoms of diabetes mellitus, diabetes insipidus, adrenal insufficiency, hypopituitarism may become intensified. Treat w/adrenocortical steroids prior to thyroid therapy in coexisting hypothyroidism and hypoadrenalism.

INTERVENTION/EVALUATION

Monitor pulse for rate, rhythm (report pulse of 100 or marked increase). Assess for tremors, nervousness. Check appetite and sleep pattern.

PATIENT/FAMILY TEACHING

Do not discontinue; replacement for hypothyroidism is lifelong. Follow-up office visits and thyroid function tests are essential. Take medication at the same time each day, preferably in morning. Monitor pulse, report marked increase, pulse of 100 or above, change of rhythm. Do not change brands. Take other medications only on advice of physician. Notify physician promptly of chest pain, weight loss, nervousness or tremors, insomnia. Children may have reversible hair loss or increased aggressiveness during the first few months of therapy. Full therapeutic effect may take 1–3 wks.

lidocaine hydrochloride

lie-doe-cane
(LidoPen, Xylocaine)

FIXED-COMBINATION(S)

W/epinephrine, a sympathomimetic (**Lidocaine with Epinephrine, Xylocaine with Epinephrine**)

CANADIAN AVAILABILITY

Xylocaine, Xylocard, Zilactin-L

PREGNANCY CATEGORY C

CLASSIFICATION

Antiarrhythmic, anesthetic

AVAILABILITY (Rx)

Injection: IM: 300 mg/3 ml. **Direct IV:** 10 mg/ml, 20 mg/ml. **IV Admixture:** 40 mg/ml, 100 mg/ml, 200 mg/ml. **IV Infusion:** 2 mg/ml, 4 mg/ml, 8 mg/ml. **Injection (anesthesia):** 0.5%, 1%, 1.5%, 2%, 4%. **Topical: Liquid:** 2.5%, 5%. **Ointment:** 2.5%, 5%. **Cream:** 0.5%. **Gel:** 0.5%, 2.5%. **Spray:** 0.5%. **Solution:** 2%, 4%. **Jelly:** 2%. **Dermal Patch:** 5%.

PHARMACODYNAMICS

	ONSET	PEAK	DURATION
IV			
	30–90 sec	—	10–20 min
Local anesthetic			
	2.5 min	—	30–60 min

PHARMACOKINETICS

Absorption: Completely absorbed after IM administration. Widely distributed. **Metabolism:** Metabolized in liver. **Excretion:** Primarily excreted in urine. **Half-life:** 1–2 hrs.

ACTION / *THERAPEUTIC EFFECT*

Anesthetic: Inhibits conduction of nerve impulses, *causing temporary loss of feeling and sensation.* ***Antiarrhythmic:*** Decreases depolarization, automaticity, excitability of ventricle during diastole by direct action, *reversing ventricular arrhythmias.*

USES

Antiarrhythmic: Rapid control of acute ventricular arrhythmias following myocardial infarction, cardiac catheterization, cardiac surgery, digitalis-induced ventricular arrhythmias. ***Local anesthetic:*** Infiltration or nerve block for dental or surgical procedures, childbirth. ***Topical anesthetic:*** Local skin disorders (minor burns, insect bites, prickly heat, skin manifestations of chicken pox, abrasions). Mucous membranes (local anesthesia of oral, nasal, and laryngeal mucous membranes, respiratory or urinary tracts; relieve discomfort of pruritus ani, hemorrhoids, pruritus vulvae). ***Dermal patch:*** Treatment of shingles-related skin pain.

ADMINISTRATION

Note: Resuscitative equipment and drugs (including oxygen) must always be readily available when administering lidocaine by any route.

IM:

- Use 10% (100 mg/ml); clearly identify lidocaine that is *for IM use.*
- Give in deltoid muscle (blood level is significantly higher than if injection is given in gluteus muscle or lateral thigh).

IV:

- **Note:** Use only lidocaine w/o preservative, clearly marked *for IV use.*
- For direct IV, use 1% (10 mg/ml) or 2% (20 mg/ml).
- Administer for direct IV at rate of 25–50 mg/min.
- For IV infusion, prepare solution by adding 1 g to 1 L 5% dextrose to provide concentration of 1 mg/ml (0.1%).
- Commercially available preparations of 0.2%, 0.4%, and 0.8% may be used for IV infusion.
- Administer for IV infusion at rate of 1–4 mg/min (1–4 ml); use volume control IV set.

- Monitor EKG constantly during infusion.
- Terminate IV infusion when cardiac rhythm is stable or toxic effects occur.
- Monitor pt response during IV administration.
- If excessive cardiac depression (arrhythmias; prolongation of PR interval, QRS complex) occurs, discontinue medication immediately, institute supportive measures.
- Unused lidocaine w/o preservative must be discarded.

INFILTRATION/NERVE BLOCK:

- **Note:** Only clinicians skilled in administration of anesthetics may give lidocaine for local anesthesia.
- For spinal or epidural anesthesia, use only preservative-free solutions.
- Monitor B/P, pulse, respirations, and pt's state of consciousness throughout regional anesthesia due to potential for cardiovascular or CNS toxicity.
- Consult standard textbooks for positioning and general care of pts undergoing regional anesthesia.

TOPICAL:

- Not for ophthalmic use.
- For skin disorders, apply directly to affected area or put on gauze or bandage, which is then applied to the skin.
- For mucous membrane use, apply to desired area using manufacturer's insert.
- Administer the lowest dose possible that still provides anesthesia.

INDICATIONS/ROUTES/DOSAGE

Ventricular arrhythmias:
IM: Adults, elderly: 300 mg (or 4.3 mg/kg). May repeat in 60–90 min.

IV: Adults, elderly: Initially, 50–100 mg (1 mg/kg) IV bolus at rate of 25–50 mg/min. May repeat in 5 min. Give no more than 200–300 mg in 1 hr. ***Maintenance:*** 20–50 mcg/kg/min (1–4 mg/min) as IV infusion. ***Children, infants:*** Initially, 0.5–1 mg/kg IV bolus; may repeat but total dose not to exceed 3–5 mg/kg. ***Maintenance:*** 10–50 mcg/kg/min as IV infusion.

Usual local anesthetic dosage:
Note: Do not use any preparation containing preservatives for spinal or epidural anesthesia.

Infiltration: 0.5 or 1% solution.

Epidural (Including Caudal): 1 or 2% solution.

Peripheral Nerve Block: 1 or 1.5% solution.

Sympathetic Nerve Block: 1% solution.

Spinal Anesthesia: 1.5 or 5% solution (with dextrose).

Usual topical dosage:
Topical: Adults, elderly: Apply to affected areas as needed.

Dermal Patch: Apply to intact skin over most painful area. (Up to 3 patches once for up to 12 hrs in 24-hr period.)

CONTRAINDICATIONS

Hypersensitivity to amide-type local anesthetics, Adams-Stokes syndrome, supraventricular arrhythmias, Wolff-Parkinson-White syndrome. Spinal anesthesia contraindicated in septicemia.

CAUTIONS

Dosage should be reduced for elderly, debilitated, acutely ill; safety in children not established. Severe renal/hepatic disease, hypovolemia, CHF, shock, heart block, marked hypoxia, severe respiratory depression, bradycardia, incomplete heart block. Anesthetic solutions containing epinephrine should be used with caution in peripheral or hypertensive vascular disease, and during or following potent general anesthesia. Sulfite sensitivity or asthma for some local and topical anesthetic preparations. Tartrazine or aspirin sensitivity with some topical preparations.

INTERACTIONS

DRUG: May increase cardiac effects w/other ***antiarrhythmics. Anticonvulsants*** may increase cardiac depressant effects. ***Beta-adrenergic blockers*** may increase risk of toxicity. **HERBAL:** None known. **FOOD:** None significant. **ALTERED LAB VALUES:** IM lidocaine may increase CPK level (used in diagnostic test for presence of acute MI).

SIDE EFFECTS

CNS effects generally dose related and of short duration. **OCCASIONAL:** *IM:* Pain at injection site. ***Topical:*** Burning, stinging, tenderness. **RARE:** Generally with high dose: drowsiness, dizziness, disorientation, lightheadedness, tremors, apprehension, euphoria, sensation of heat/cold/numbness, blurred/double vision, ringing/roaring in ears (tinnitus), nausea.

ADVERSE REACTIONS/TOXIC EFFECTS

Although serious adverse reactions to lidocaine are uncommon, high dosage by any route may produce cardiovascular depression: bradycardia, somnolence, hypotension, arrhythmias, heart block, cardiovascular collapse, cardiac arrest. Potential for malignant hyperthermia. CNS toxicity may occur, especially with regional anesthesia use, progressing rapidly from mild side effects to tremors, convulsions, vomiting, respiratory depression, arrest. Methemoglobinemia (evidenced by cyanosis) has occurred following topical application of lidocaine for teething discomfort and laryngeal anesthetic spray. Overuse of oral lidocaine has caused seizures in children. Allergic reactions are rare.

PATIENT CONSIDERATIONS

Baseline Assessment

Question for hypersensitivity to lidocaine, amide anesthetics, or components of preparation. Obtain baseline B/P, pulse, respirations, EKG, and electrolytes.

Intervention/Evaluation

Monitor EKG, vital signs closely during and after drug is administered for cardiac performance. If EKG shows arrhythmias, prolongation of PR interval or QRS complex, inform physician immediately. Assess pulse for irregularity, strength/weakness, bradycardia. Assess B/P for evidence of hypotension. Monitor I&O, electrolyte serum level. Monitor for therapeutic serum level (1.5–6 mcg/ml). For lidocaine given by all routes, monitor vital signs and pt's state of consciousness. Drowsiness should be considered a warning sign of high blood levels of lidocaine.

Patient/Family Teaching

Explain action of lidocaine. Report drowsiness or CNS effects promptly (see Adverse Reactions/Toxic Effects).

Local anesthesia
Assure that pt understands loss of feeling, sensation and need for protection until anesthetic wears off (e.g., no ambulation, including special positions for some regional anesthesia; not chewing gum, eating, or drinking following administration to oral area, etc.).

L

Topical anesthesia
Use only as directed; too frequent use may cause overdosage. Do not eat, drink, or chew gum for 1 hr following application (swallowing reflex may be impaired increasing risk of aspiration; numbness of tongue or buccal mucosa may lead to biting trauma).

linezolid

(Zyvox)
See Supplement

liothyronine

lye-oh-**thigh**-roe-neen
(Cytomel)

FIXED-COMBINATION(S)
W/levothyroxine, T_4 **(Thyrolar)**

PREGNANCY CATEGORY A

CLASSIFICATION

Thyroid

AVAILABILITY (Rx)

Tablets: 5 mcg, 25 mcg, 50 mcg. **Injection:** 10 mcg/ml.

PHARMACOKINETICS

Absorption: Almost complete absorption from GI tract. Widely distributed. **Metabolism:** Deiodinated in peripheral tissues, minimal metabolism in liver. **Excretion:** Eliminated by biliary excretion. **Half-life:** 1 day.

ACTION/*THERAPEUTIC EFFECT*

Involved in normal metabolism, growth and development (especially CNS of infants). Possesses catabolic and anabolic effects. *Increases basal metabolic rate, enhances gluconeogenesis, stimulates protein synthesis.*

USES

Oral: Replacement in decreased or absent thyroid function (partial or complete absence of gland, primary atrophy, functional deficiency, effects of surgery, radiation or antithyroid agents, pituitary or hypothalamic hypothyroidism). Management of simple (nontoxic) goiter; diagnostically in T_3 suppression test (differentiates hyperthyroidism from euthyroidism). *IV:* Myxedema coma, precoma.

STORAGE/HANDLING

Refrigerate parenteral dosage form; store oral tablets at room temperature.

ADMINISTRATION

ORAL:

- Give at the same time each day to maintain hormone levels.
- Administer before breakfast to prevent insomnia.
- When transferred *from* another thyroid preparation, the other thyroid agent should be discontinued first; begin liothyronine at low dose.
- When transferring *to* another thyroid preparation, continue liothyronine for several days to prevent relapse (rapid action, short duration).

IV:

- Do not administer IM or SubQ.
- Switch to oral as soon as pt stabilized clinically. Initiate oral therapy at low dose, increasing gradually according to pt response.

INDICATIONS/ROUTES/DOSAGE

Hypothyroidism:
Oral: Adults: Initially, 25 mcg/day.

Increase by 12.5–25 mcg q1–2 wks. *Elderly:* Initially, 5 mcg/day. May increase by 5 mcg/day q1–2 wks. *Maintenance:* 25–75 mcg/day.

Myxedema:
Oral: Adults, elderly: Initially, 5 mcg/day. Increase by 5–10 mcg q1–2wks (after 25 mcg/day reached, may increase by 12.5 mcg increments). *Maintenance:* 50–100 mcg/day.

Nontoxic goiter:
Oral: Adults, elderly: Initially, 5 mcg/day. Increase by 5–10 mcg/day q1–2 wks. When 25 mcg/day obtained, may increase by 12.5–25 mcg/day q1–2 wks. *Maintenance:* 75 mcg/day.

Congenital hypothyroidism:
Oral: Children: Initially, 5 mcg/day. Increase by 5 mcg/day q3–4days. *Maintenance: (Infants):* 20 mcg /day. *(1 yr):* 50 mcg/day. *(>3 yrs):* Full adult dosage.

T_3 suppression test:
Oral: Adults, elderly: 75–100 mcg/day for 7 days, then repeat I^{131} thyroid uptake test.

Myxedema coma, precoma:
Note: Initial and subsequent dosage based on pt's clinical status, response. Administer IV dose at least 4 hrs but no longer than 12 hrs apart.

IV: Adults, elderly: Initially, 25–50 mcg (10–20 mcg in pts w/cardiovascular disease). Total dose at least 65 mcg/day.

CONTRAINDICATIONS

Thyrotoxicosis and MI uncomplicated by hypothyroidism, treatment of obesity.

CAUTIONS

Elderly, angina pectoris, hypertension, or other cardiovascular disease.

INTERACTIONS

DRUG: May alter effect of ***oral anticoagulants. Cholestyramine, colestipol*** may decrease absorption. ***Sympathomimetics*** may increase effects, coronary insufficiency. **HERBAL:** None known. **FOOD:** None significant. **ALTERED LAB VALUES:** None significant.

SIDE EFFECTS

OCCASIONAL: Children may have reversible hair loss upon initiation. **RARE:** Dry skin, GI intolerance, skin rash, hives, pseudotumor cerebri (severe headache in children).

ADVERSE REACTIONS/TOXIC EFFECTS

Excessive dosage produces signs/symptoms of hyperthyroidism: weight loss, palpitations, increased appetite, tremors, nervousness, tachycardia, increased B/P, headache, insomnia, menstrual irregularities. Cardiac arrhythmias occur rarely.

PATIENT CONSIDERATIONS

BASELINE ASSESSMENT

Question for hypersensitivity to tartrazine, aspirin. Obtain baseline weight, vital signs. Check results of thyroid function tests. Signs and symptoms of diabetes mellitus, diabetes insipidus, adrenal insufficiency, hypopituitarism may become intensified. Treat w/adrenocortical steroids prior to thyroid therapy in coexisting hypothyroidism and hypoadrenalism.

INTERVENTION/EVALUATION

Monitor pulse for rate, rhythm (report pulse ≥100 or marked increase). Assess for tremors, nervousness. Check appetite and sleep pattern.

PATIENT/FAMILY TEACHING

Do not discontinue; replacement for hypothyroidism is lifelong. Follow-up office visits and thyroid function tests are essential. Take medication at the same time each day, preferably in morning. Teach pt or family to take pulse correctly, report marked increase, pulse of 100 or above, change of rhythm. Do not change brands (not equivalent). Take other medications only on advice of physician. Notify physician promptly of chest pain, weight loss, nervousness or tremors, insomnia. Children may have reversible hair loss or increased aggressiveness during first few months of therapy.

lisinopril

lih-**sin**-oh-prill
(Prinivil, Zestril)

FIXED-COMBINATION(S)
W/hydrochlorothiazide, a diuretic **(Prinzide, Zestoretic)**

CANADIAN AVAILABILITY
Prinivil, Zestril

PREGNANCY CATEGORY D

CLASSIFICATION

Angiotensin-converting enzyme (ACE) inhibitor

AVAILABILITY (Rx)

Tablets: 2.5 mg, 5 mg, 10 mg, 20 mg, 40 mg

PHARMACODYNAMICS

	ONSET	PEAK	DURATION
Oral	1 hr	6 hrs	24 hrs

PHARMACOKINETICS

Absorption: Incompletely absorbed from GI tract. **Excretion:** Primarily excreted unchanged in urine. Removed by hemodialysis. **Half-life:** 12 hrs (prolonged in decreased renal function).

ACTION/*THERAPEUTIC EFFECT*

Suppresses renin-angiotensin-aldosterone system (prevents conversion of angiotensin I to angiotensin II, a potent vasoconstrictor; may also inhibit angiotensin II at local vascular and renal sites). Decreases plasma angiotensin II, increases plasma renin activity, decreases aldosterone secretion. *Reduces peripheral arterial resistance, B/P (afterload), pulmonary capillary wedge pressure (preload), pulmonary vascular resistance.* In those w/heart failure, *also decreases heart size, increases cardiac output, exercise tolerance time.*

USES/*UNLABELED*

Treatment of hypertension. Used alone or in combination w/other antihypertensives. Adjunctive therapy in management of heart failure. Improves survival in pts who had myocardial infarction. *Treatment of hypertension/renal crises w/scleroderma.*

ADMINISTRATION

ORAL:

- May give w/o regard to food.
- Tablets may be crushed.

INDICATIONS/ROUTES/DOSAGE

Hypertension (used alone):
Oral: Adults: Initially, 10 mg/day. ***Maintenance:*** 20–40 mg/day as single dose.

Hypertension (combination therapy):
Note: Discontinue diuretic 2–3 days prior to initiating lisinopril therapy.

Oral: Adults: Initially, 5 mg/day titrated to pt's needs.

Heart failure:
Oral: Adults: Initially, 5 mg/day (2.5 mg/day in pts w/hyponatremia). *Range:* 5–20 mg/day.

Myocardial infarction:
Oral: Adults, elderly: Initially, 5 mg, then 5 mg after 24 hrs, 10 mg after 48 hrs, then 10 mg/day × 6 wks. (Pts w/low systolic B/P: 2.5 mg/day for 3 days, then 2.5–5 mg/day).

Usual elderly dosage:
Oral: Initially, 2.5–5 mg/day. May increase by 2.5–5 mg/day at 1–2 wk intervals. *Maximum:* 40 mg/day.

Dosage in renal impairment:
Titrate to pt's needs after giving the following initial dose:

CREATININE CLEARANCE	INITIAL DOSE
>30 ml/min	10 mg
10–30 ml/min	5 mg
<10 ml/min	2.5 mg

CONTRAINDICATIONS

MI, coronary insufficiency, angina, evidence of coronary artery disease, hypersensitivity to phentolamine, history of angioedema w/previous treatment w/ACEIs.

CAUTIONS

Renal impairment, those w/sodium depletion or on diuretic therapy, dialysis, hypovolemia, coronary or cerebrovascular insufficiency.

INTERACTIONS

DRUG: *Alcohol, diuretics, hypotensive agents* may increase effects. ***NSAIDs*** may decrease effect. ***Potassium-sparing diuretics, potassium supplements*** may cause hyperkalemia. May increase ***lithium*** concentration, toxicity. **HERBAL:** None known. **FOOD:** None significant. **ALTERED LAB VALUES:** May increase potassium, SGOT (AST), SGPT (ALT), alkaline phosphatase, bilirubin, BUN, creatinine. May decrease sodium. May cause positive ANA titer.

SIDE EFFECTS

FREQUENT (5–10%): Headache, dizziness. **OCCASIONAL (1–5%):** Chest pain, lightheadedness, fatigue, rash, abdominal pain, nausea, diarrhea, upper respiratory infection. **RARE (<1%):** Palpitations, tachycardia, peripheral edema (swelling of feet), inability to sleep, numbness in hands, feet, confusion, constipation, dry mouth, muscle cramps.

ADVERSE REACTIONS/TOXIC EFFECTS

Excessive hypotension ("first-dose syncope") may occur in those w/CHF, severely salt/volume depleted. Angioedema (swelling of face/lips), hyperkalemia occurs rarely. Agranulocytosis, neutropenia may be noted in those w/impaired renal function or collagen vascular disease (systemic lupus erythematosus, scleroderma). Nephrotic syndrome may be noted in those w/history of renal disease.

PATIENT CONSIDERATIONS

BASELINE ASSESSMENT

Obtain B/P and apical pulse immediately before each dose, in addition to regular monitoring (be alert to fluctuations). If excessive reduction in B/P

occurs, place pt in supine position, feet slightly elevated. Renal function tests should be performed before therapy begins. In those w/renal impairment, autoimmune disease, or taking drugs that affect leukocytes or immune response, CBC and differential count should be performed before therapy begins and q2wks for 3 mos, then periodically thereafter.

Intervention/Evaluation

Assess for edema; check lungs for rales. Monitor I&O; weigh daily. Assess stools for frequency and consistency; prevent constipation. Assist w/ambulation if dizziness occurs.

Patient/Family Teaching

To reduce hypotensive effect, rise slowly from lying to sitting position and permit legs to dangle from bed momentarily before standing. Full therapeutic effect may take 2–4 wks. Report any sign of infection (sore throat, fever), swelling of hands or feet or face, chest pain, difficulty breathing or swallowing. Skipping doses or voluntarily discontinuing drug may produce severe, rebound hypertension. Do not take cold preparations, nasal decongestants. Restrict sodium and alcohol as ordered.

lithium carbonate

lith-ee-um
(Eskalith, Lithane, Lithobid)

lithium citrate

(Cibalith-S)

CANADIAN AVAILABILITY
Carbolith, Duralith, Lithane

PREGNANCY CATEGORY D

CLASSIFICATION

Antimanic

AVAILABILITY (Rx)

Capsules: 150 mg, 300 mg, 600 mg. **Tablets:** 300 mg. **Tablets (slow-release):** 300 mg, 450 mg. **Syrup:** 300 mg/5 ml.

PHARMACOKINETICS

Absorption: Rapid, complete absorption from GI tract. **Excretion:** Primarily excreted unchanged in urine. **Half-life:** 18–24 hrs (increased in elderly).

ACTION/*THERAPEUTIC EFFECT*

Alters ion transport at cellular sites in body tissue. Cations necessary in synthesis, storage, release, reuptake of neurotransmitters involved in *producing antimanic, antidepressant effects.*

USES/*UNLABELED*

Prophylaxis, treatment of acute mania, manic phase of bipolar disorder (manic-depressive illness). *Treatment of mental depression, prophylaxis of vascular headache, treatment of neutropenia.*

STORAGE/HANDLING

Store all forms at room temperature.

ADMINISTRATION

ORAL:

- Preferable to administer w/meals or milk.
- Do not crush, chew, or break extended-release or film-coated tablets.

INDICATIONS/ROUTES/DOSAGE

Note: During acute phase, therapeutic serum lithium concentration of 1–1.4 mEq/L is required. Desired level during long-term control: 0.5–1.3 mEq/L.

Acute manic phase:
Oral: Adults: Initially, 1.8 g (or 20–30 mg/kg) lithium carbonate or 30 ml lithium citrate/day, in 2–3 divided doses. ***Elderly:*** 600–900 mg/day.

Long-term control:
Oral: Adults: 900 mg-1.2 g lithium carbonate or 15–20 ml lithium citrate, daily, in 2–4 divided doses.

Usual elderly dosage:
Oral: Initially, 300 mg 2 times/day. May increase by 300 mg/day at weekly intervals. ***Maintenance:*** 900–1,200 mg/day.

CONTRAINDICATIONS

Severe cardiovascular disease, severe renal disease, severe dehydration/sodium depletion, debilitated patients.

CAUTIONS

Cardiovascular disease, thyroid disease, elderly.

INTERACTIONS

DRUG: May increase effects of ***antithyroid medication, iodinated glycerol, potassium iodide. NSAIDs*** may increase concentration, toxicity. May decrease absorption of ***phenothiazines. Phenothiazines*** may increase intracellular concentration, increase renal excretion, extrapyramidal symptoms (EPS), delirium, mask early signs of lithium toxicity. ***Diuretics*** may increase concentration, toxicity. ***Haloperidol*** may increase EPS, neurologic toxicity. ***Molindone*** may increase risk of neurotoxic symptoms. **HERBAL:** None known. **FOOD:** None significant. **ALTERED LAB VALUES:** May increase blood glucose, calcium, immunoreactive parathyroid hormone.

SIDE EFFECTS

FREQUENT: Diarrhea, polydipsia (excessive thirst), polyuria (increased urination). Loss of bladder control, fine hand tremor. **OCCASIONAL:** Leukocytosis, increased weight, fast or slow heartbeat, dyspnea, irregular pulse, acne, skin rash, muscle twitching, bloated, pressure in stomach. **RARE:** Blue color or pain in fingers, toes, coldness in arms or legs, pseudotumor cerebri (eye pain, headache, vision problems, noises in ears).

ADVERSE REACTIONS/TOXIC EFFECTS

Serum lithium concentration of 1.5–2.0 mEq/L may produce vomiting, diarrhea, drowsiness, incoordination, coarse hand tremor, muscle twitching, EKG T-wave depression, mental confusion. Serum lithium concentration of 2.0–2.5 mEq/L may result in ataxia, giddiness, tinnitus, blurred vision, clonic movements, severe hypotension. Acute toxicity characterized by seizures, oliguria, circulatory failure, coma, death.

PATIENT CONSIDERATIONS

Baseline Assessment

Serum lithium levels should be tested every 3–4 days during initial phase of therapy, every 1–2 mos thereafter, and weekly if there is no improvement of disorder or adverse effects occur.

Intervention/Evaluation

Lithium serum testing should be performed as close as possible to 12th hour after last dose. Besides serum lithium concentra-

tion levels, clinical assessment of therapeutic effect or tolerance to drug effect is necessary for correct dosing-level management. Assess behavior, appearance, emotional status, response to environment, speech pattern, thought content. Monitor serum lithium concentrations, differential count, urinalysis, creatinine clearance. Assess for increased urine output, persistent thirst. Report polyuria, prolonged vomiting, diarrhea, fever to physician (may need to reduce or discontinue dosage temporarily). Monitor for signs of lithium toxicity. Supervise suicidal risk pt closely during early therapy (as depression lessens, energy level improves, and suicide potential increases). Assess for therapeutic response (interest in surroundings, improvement in self-care, increased ability to concentrate, relaxed facial expression).

Patient/Family Teaching

Take as directed; do not discontinue except on physician's advice. Do not engage in activities requiring alert response until effects of drug are known. Thirst, frequent urination may occur. A fluid intake of 2–3 quarts liquid per day and maintenance of a normal salt intake are necessary during initial phase of treatment to avoid dehydration. Thereafter, 1–1.5 L fluid intake daily is necessary. GI disturbances generally disappear during continued therapy. Thyroid function tests should be performed q6–12mos in elderly pts (increased incidence of goiter, hypothyroidism). Therapeutic improvement noted in 1–3 wks. Avoid alcohol and OTC drugs. Consult physician regarding contraception.

Iodoxamide tromethamine

low-**dox**-ah-myd
(Alomide)

CANADIAN AVAILABILITY
Alomide

PREGNANCY CATEGORY B

CLASSIFICATION

Antiallergic

AVAILABILITY (Rx)

Ophthalmic Solution: 0.1%

PHARMACOKINETICS

Absorption: Minimal systemic absorption. **Excretion:** Primarily excreted in urine. **Half-life:** 8.5 hrs.

ACTION/*THERAPEUTIC EFFECT*

Mast cell stabilizer. Prevents increase in cutaneous vascular permeability, antigen-stimulated histamine release and may prevent calcium influx into mast cells, *inhibiting hypersensitivity reaction.*

USES

Treatment of vernal keratoconjunctivitis, conjunctivitis, and keratitis.

STORAGE/HANDLING

Keep at room temperature; protect from freezing. Do not use if discolored. Keep tightly closed.

ADMINISTRATION

OPHTHALMIC:

- Instruct pt to lie down or tilt head backward and look up.
- Gently pull lower lid down to form pouch and instill medication.

- Do not touch tip of applicator to any surface.
- When lower lid is released, have pt keep eye open w/o blinking for at least 30 sec.
- Apply gentle finger pressure to lacrimal sac (bridge of the nose, inside corner of the eye) for 1–2 min.
- Remove excess solution around eye w/tissue.
- Tell pt not to close eyes tightly or blink more often than necessary.
- Never rinse dropper.

INDICATIONS/ROUTES/DOSAGE

Usual ophthalmic dosage:
Adults, elderly, children >2 yrs: 1–2 drops 4 times/day, for up to 3 mos.

CONTRAINDICATIONS

Hypersensitivity. Wearing soft contact lenses (product contains benzalkonium chloride).

CAUTIONS

For ophthalmic use only. Not for injection. Safety in children <2 yrs not known.

INTERACTIONS

DRUG: None significant. **HERBAL:** None known. **FOOD:** None significant. **ALTERED LAB VALUES:** None significant.

SIDE EFFECTS

FREQUENT: Transient stinging, burning, instillation discomfort. **OCCASIONAL:** Ocular itching, blurred vision, dry eye, tearing/discharge/foreign body sensation, headache. **RARE:** Scales on lid/lash, ocular swelling, sticky sensation, dizziness, somnolence, nausea, sneezing, dry nose, rash.

ADVERSE REACTIONS/TOXIC EFFECTS

None significant.

PATIENT CONSIDERATIONS

BASELINE ASSESSMENT

Assess for hypersensitivity to any component of suspension. Evaluate ocular signs and symptoms.

PATIENT/FAMILY TEACHING

Teach correct procedure for administration of drops. Do not wear soft contact lenses during therapy. For ophthalmic use only. May experience mild transitory burning, stinging upon instillation; inform physician if continues. Therapy may last up to 3 mos. If disorder does not improve or new symptoms develop, notify physician.

lomefloxacin hydrochloride

low-meh-**flocks**-ah-sin
(Maxaquin)

PREGNANCY CATEGORY C

CLASSIFICATION

Anti-infective: Quinolone

AVAILABILITY (Rx)

Tablets: 400 mg

PHARMACOKINETICS

Absorption: Well absorbed from GI tract. Widely distributed. **Metabolism:** Metabolized in liver. **Excretion:** Primarily excreted in urine. Minimal removal by hemodialysis. **Half-life:** 4–6 hrs (increased in decreased renal function, elderly).

ACTION/*THERAPEUTIC EFFECT*

Inhibits the enzyme DNA-gyrase in susceptible microorganisms, *interfering w/bacterial DNA replication and repair. Bactericidal.*

USES

Treatment of infections of urinary tract, lower respiratory tract, postop prophylaxis in pts undergoing transurethral procedures.

ADMINISTRATION

ORAL:

- May be given w/o regard to meals (preferred dosing time: 2 hrs after meals).
- Do not administer antacids (aluminum, magnesium) within 2 hrs of lomefloxacin.
- Encourage cranberry juice, citrus fruits (to acidify urine).

INDICATIONS/ROUTES/DOSAGE

Urinary tract infections:
Oral: Adults, elderly: 400 mg/day for 10–14 days.

Uncomplicated UTI:
Oral: Adults (females): 400 mg/day for 3 days.

Lower respiratory tract infections:
Oral: Adults, elderly: 400 mg/day for 10 days.

Postop prophylaxis:
Oral: Adults, elderly: 400 mg 2–6 hrs prior to surgery.

Dosage in renal impairment:
The dose and/or frequency is modified in pts based on severity of renal impairment.

CREATININE CLEARANCE	DOSAGE
>40 ml/min	No change
10–40 ml/min	400 mg initially, then 200 mg/day for 10–14 days

CONTRAINDICATIONS

Hypersensitivity to lomefloxacin, quinolones, any component of the preparation.

CAUTIONS

Renal impairment, CNS disorders, seizures, those taking theophylline or caffeine.

INTERACTIONS

DRUG: ***Antacids, iron prep, sucralfate*** may decrease absorption. Decreases clearance, may increase concentration, toxicity of ***theophylline.*** May increase effects of ***oral anticoagulants.*** **HERBAL:** None known. **FOOD:** None significant. **ALTERED LAB VALUES:** May increase SGOT (AST), SGPT (ALT), alkaline phosphatase, LDH, serum bilirubin, BUN, serum creatinine concentration.

SIDE EFFECTS

FREQUENT: Nausea, diarrhea, headache, dizziness, photosensitivity.

ADVERSE REACTIONS/TOXIC EFFECTS

Superinfection (bacterial or fungal overgrowth of nonsusceptible organisms), photosensitivity reaction.

PATIENT CONSIDERATIONS

BASELINE ASSESSMENT

Question for history of hypersensitivity to lomefloxacin, quinolones, any component of preparation. Obtain specimen for diagnostic tests before giving first dose (therapy may begin before results are known).

INTERVENTION/EVALUATION

Evaluate food tolerance. Determine pattern of bowel activity; be alert to blood in feces. Check for dizziness, headache. Monitor

B/P at least twice daily. Assess for chest, joint pain.

Patient/Family Teaching

Do not skip dose; take full course of therapy. Take w/8 oz water; drink several glasses of water between meals. Eat/drink high sources of ascorbic acid to prevent crystalluria (cranberry juice, citrus fruits). Do not take antacids (reduces/destroys effectiveness). Avoid sunlight/ultraviolet exposure; wear sunscreen, protective clothing if photosensitivity develops. Notify nurse/physician if new symptoms occur. Report inflammation or tendon pain.

lomustine

(CeeNU)
See Classification section under: Cancer chemotherapy

loperamide hydrochloride

low-**pear**-ah-myd
(Imodium, Imodium A-D)

FIXED-COMBINATION(S)
W/simethicone, an antiflatulent (Imodium Advanced)

CANADIAN AVAILABILITY
Apo-Loperamide, Imodium, Loperacap, Novo-Loperamide

PREGNANCY CATEGORY B

CLASSIFICATION

Antidiarrheal

AVAILABILITY (OTC)

Tablets: 2 mg. **Capsules (Rx):** 2 mg. **Liquid:** 1 mg/5 ml.

PHARMACOKINETICS

Absorption: Poorly absorbed from GI tract. **Metabolism:** Metabolized in liver. **Excretion:** Eliminated in feces, excreted in urine. **Half-life:** 9.1–14.4 hrs.

ACTION/*THERAPEUTIC EFFECT*

Direct effect on intestinal wall muscles; *slows intestinal motility, prolongs transit time of intestinal contents (reduces fecal volume, diminishes loss of fluid/electrolytes, increases viscosity, bulk).*

USES

Controls, provides symptomatic relief of acute nonspecific diarrhea; chronic diarrhea associated w/inflammatory bowel disease; traveler's diarrhea. Reduces volume of discharge from ileostomy.

INDICATIONS/ROUTES/DOSAGE

Acute diarrhea (capsules):
Oral: Adults, elderly: Initially, 4 mg, then 2 mg after each unformed stool. *Maximum:* 16 mg/day. ***Children, 8–12 yrs, >30 kg:*** Initially, 2 mg 3 times/day for 24 hrs; ***5–8 yrs, 20–30 kg:*** Initially, 2 mg 2 times/day for 24 hrs; ***2–5 yrs, 13–20 kg:*** Initially, 1 mg 3 times/day for 24 hrs. ***Maintenance:*** 1 mg/10 kg only after loose stool.

Chronic diarrhea:
Oral: Adults, elderly: Initially 4 mg, then 2 mg after each unformed stool until diarrhea is controlled.

Traveler's diarrhea:
Oral: Adults, elderly: Initially, 4 mg, then 2 mg after each loose bowel movement (LBM). ***Maximum:*** 8 mg/day for 2 days. ***Children 9–11 yrs:*** Initially 2 mg, then 1 mg after each LBM. ***Maximum:*** 6 mg/day for 2 days. ***Children 6–8 yrs:*** Initially, 1 mg, then 1 mg after each LBM. ***Maximum:*** 4 mg/day for 2 days.

CONTRAINDICATIONS

Those who must avoid constipation, diarrhea associated w/pseudomembranous enterocolitis due to broad-spectrum antibiotics or w/organisms that invade intestinal mucosa (*Escherichia coli*, shigella, salmonella), acute ulcerative colitis (may produce toxic megacolon).

CAUTIONS

Those w/fluid/electrolyte depletion, hepatic impairment.

INTERACTIONS

DRUG: *Opioid (narcotic) analgesics* may increase risk of constipation. HERBAL: None known. FOOD: None significant. ALTERED LAB VALUES: None significant.

SIDE EFFECTS

RARE: Allergic reaction (rash, itching,), toxic megacolon (constipation, decreased appetite, severe stomach pain w/nausea, vomiting), dry mouth, dizziness, drowsiness.

ADVERSE REACTIONS/TOXIC EFFECTS

Toxicity results in constipation, GI irritation including nausea, vomiting, CNS depression. Treatment: Activated charcoal.

PATIENT CONSIDERATIONS

Baseline Assessment

Do not administer in presence of bloody diarrhea or temperature >101°F.

Intervention/Evaluation

Encourage adequate fluid intake. Assess bowel sounds for peristalsis. Monitor stool frequency and consistency (watery, loose, soft, semisolid, solid). Withhold drug and notify physician promptly in event of abdominal pain, distension, or fever.

Patient/Family Teaching

Do not exceed prescribed dose. Avoid tasks that require alertness, motor skills until response to drug is established. Notify physician if diarrhea does not stop within 3 days, if abdominal distension or pain occurs, or if fever develops.

---

lopinavir/ritonavir

(Kaletra)

See Supplement

---

loracarbef

laur-ah-**car**-bef

(Lorabid)

PREGNANCY CATEGORY B

CLASSIFICATION

Antibiotic: Cephalosporin

AVAILABILITY (Rx)

Capsules: 200 mg. **Powder for Oral Suspension:** 100 mg/5 ml.

PHARMACOKINETICS

Absorption: Well absorbed from GI tract. Widely distributed. **Excretion:** Primarily excreted unchanged in urine. Removed by hemodialysis. **Half-life:** 1 hr (increased in decreased renal function).

ACTION/*THERAPEUTIC EFFECT*

Bactericidal. Binds to bacterial membranes, *inhibiting bacterial cell wall synthesis.*

USES

Treatment of bronchitis, otitis media, pharyngitis, pneumonia, sinusitis, skin and soft tissue infections, urinary tract infections (uncomplicated cystitis, pyelonephritis).

STORAGE/HANDLING

After reconstitution, powder for suspension may be kept at room temperature for 14 days. Discard unused portion after 14 days.

ADMINISTRATION

ORAL:

- Give 1 hr before or 2 hrs after meal.
- Shake oral suspension well before using.

INDICATIONS/ROUTES/DOSAGE

Bronchitis:
Oral: Adults, elderly, children >12 yrs: 200–400 mg q12h for 7 days.

Pharyngitis:
Oral: Adults, elderly, children >12 yrs: 200 mg q12h for 10 days. *Children 6 mos–12 yrs:* 7.5 mg/kg q12h for 10 days.

Pneumonia:
Oral: Adults, elderly, children >12 yrs: 400 mg q12h for 14 days.

Sinusitis:
Oral: Adults, elderly, children >12 yrs: 400 mg q12h for 10 days. *Children 6 mos–12 yrs:* 15 mg/kg q12h for 10 days.

Skin, soft tissue infections:
Oral: Adults, elderly, children >12 yrs: 200 mg q12h for 7 days. *Children 6 mos–12 yrs:* 7.5 mg/kg q12h for 7 days.

Urinary tract infections:
Oral: Adults, elderly, children >12 yrs: 200–400 mg q12h for 7–14 days.

Otitis media:
Oral: Children (6 mos–12 yrs): 15 mg/kg q12h for 10 days.

CONTRAINDICATIONS

History of hypersensitivity to cephalosporins, anaphylactic reaction to penicillins.

CAUTIONS

Renal impairment.

INTERACTIONS

DRUG: *Probenecid* increases serum concentrations, half-life of loracarbef. **HERBAL:** None known. **FOOD:** None significant. **ALTERED LAB VALUES:** May increase SGOT (AST), SGPT (ALT), alkaline phosphatase, BUN, creatinine. May decrease leukocytes, platelets.

SIDE EFFECTS

FREQUENT: Abdominal pain, anorexia, nausea, vomiting, diarrhea. **OCCASIONAL:** Skin rash, itching. **RARE:** Dizziness, headache, vaginitis.

ADVERSE REACTIONS/TOXIC EFFECTS

Antibiotic-associated colitis, other superinfections may result from altered bacterial balance. Hypersensitivity reactions (ranging from rash, urticaria, fever to anaphylaxis) occur in less than 5%, generally those w/history of allergies, especially penicillin.

PATIENT CONSIDERATIONS

BASELINE ASSESSMENT

Question history of allergies, particularly cephalosporins, penicillins. Obtain culture and sensitivity test before giving first dose (therapy may begin before results are known).

INTERVENTION/EVALUATION

Assess for nausea, vomiting. Check stool frequency and consistency. Assess skin for rash (dia-

per area in children). Monitor I&O, urinalysis, renal function reports for nephrotoxicity. Be alert for superinfection: genital/anal pruritus, moniliasis, abdominal pain, sore mouth or tongue, moderate to severe diarrhea.

PATIENT/FAMILY TEACHING

Continue antibiotic therapy for full length of treatment. Doses should be evenly spaced, given at least 1 hr before or 2 hrs after a meal. Notify physician in event of diarrhea, rash, or onset of other new symptoms.

loratadine

low-**rah**-tah-deen
(Claritin, Claritin Reditabs)

FIXED-COMBINATION(S)
W/pseudoephedrine, a sympathomimetic **(Claritin-D)**

CANADIAN AVAILABILITY
Claritin

PREGNANCY CATEGORY B

CLASSIFICATION

Antihistamine

AVAILABILITY (Rx)

Tablets: 10 mg. **Syrup:** 10 mg/10 ml.

PHARMACODYNAMICS

	ONSET	PEAK	DURATION
Oral	1–3 hrs	8–12 hrs	24 hrs

PHARMACOKINETICS

Absorption: Rapidly, almost completely absorbed from GI tract. Distributed mainly in liver, lungs, GI tract, bile. **Metabolism:** Metabolized in liver to active metabolite (undergoes extensive first-pass metabolism). **Excretion:** Excreted in urine, eliminated in feces. **Half-life:** 3–20 hrs; metabolite: 28 hrs (increased in elderly, liver disease).

ACTION/*THERAPEUTIC EFFECT*

Long-acting w/selective peripheral histamine H-1 receptor antagonist action. Competes w/histamine for receptor site *to prevent allergic responses mediated by histamine (urticaria, pruritus)*. Has no significant anticholinergic effects.

USES/*UNLABELED*

Relief of nasal and non-nasal symptoms of seasonal allergic rhinitis (hay fever). Treatment of idiopathic chronic urticaria (hives). *Adjunct treatment of bronchial asthma.*

ADMINISTRATION

ORAL:

- Preferably give on an empty stomach (food delays absorption).

INDICATIONS/ROUTES/DOSAGE

Allergic rhinitis, hives:
Oral: Adults, elderly, children >6 yrs: 10 mg once daily. *Hepatic function impairment:* 10 mg every other day.

CONTRAINDICATIONS

Hypersensitivity to loratadine or any ingredient.

CAUTIONS

Pts w/liver impairment. Safety in children <6 yrs not known.

INTERACTIONS

DRUG: *Ketoconazole, erythromycin* may increase concentrations.

HERBAL: None known. **FOOD:** None significant. **ALTERED LAB VALUES:** May suppress wheal and flare reactions to antigen skin testing, unless antihistamines are discontinued 4 days before testing.

SIDE EFFECTS

OCCASIONAL: Altered salivation/lacrimation, increased sweating, flushing, blurred vision, dry skin.

ADVERSE REACTIONS/TOXIC EFFECTS

None significant.

PATIENT CONSIDERATIONS

BASELINE ASSESSMENT

Assess lung sounds, rhinitis, urticaria, or other symptoms.

INTERVENTION/EVALUATION

For upper respiratory allergies, increase fluids to maintain thin secretions and offset thirst, loss of fluids from increased sweating. Monitor symptoms for therapeutic response.

PATIENT/FAMILY TEACHING

Take loratadine on an empty stomach. Does not cause drowsiness; however, if blurred vision or eye pain occurs, do not drive or perform activities requiring visual acuity. Avoid alcohol during antihistamine therapy.

lorazepam

low-**raz**-ah-pam
(Alzapam, Ativan)

CANADIAN AVAILABILITY
Apo-Lorazepam, Ativan, Novolorazepam

PREGNANCY CATEGORY D

CLASSIFICATION

Antianxiety

AVAILABILITY (Rx)

Tablets: 0.5 mg, 1 mg, 2 mg. **Injection:** 2 mg/ml, 4 mg/ml.

PHARMACODYNAMICS

	ONSET	PEAK	DURATION
IM	15–30 min	—	12–24 hrs
IV	1–5 min	—	12–24 hrs

PHARMACOKINETICS

Absorption: Well absorbed after oral, IM administration. Widely distributed. **Metabolism:** Metabolized in liver. **Excretion:** Primarily excreted in urine. **Half-life:** 10–20 hrs.

ACTION/*THERAPEUTIC EFFECT*

Enhances inhibitory neurotransmitter gamma-aminobutyric acid (GABA) neurotransmission at CNS, *producing anxiolytic effect.* Inhibits spinal afferent pathways, *producing skeletal muscle relaxation.* Depressant effects occur at all levels of CNS. Directly depresses motor nerve, muscle function.

USES/*UNLABELED*

Management of anxiety disorders associated w/depressive symptoms. Parenteral form used preoperatively to provide sedation, relieve anxiety, and produce anterograde amnesia. Treatment of status epilepticus. *Treatment of alcohol withdrawal, adjunct to endoscopic procedures (diminishes pt recall), panic disorders, skeletal muscle spasms, cancer chemotherapy–induced nausea/vomiting, tension headache, tremors.*

STORAGE/HANDLING

Refrigerate parenteral form. Do not use if precipitate forms or solution appears discolored. Avoid freezing.

ADMINISTRATION

ORAL:

- Give w/food.
- Tablets may be crushed.

IM:

- Give deep IM into large muscle mass.

IV:

- Dilute w/equal volume of sterile water for injection, 0.9% NaCl injection, or 5% dextrose injection.
- To dilute prefilled syringe, remove air from half-filled syringe, aspirate equal volume of diluent, pull plunger back slightly to allow for mixing, and gently invert syringe several times (do not shake vigorously).
- Give by direct IV injection or into tubing of free-flowing IV infusion (0.9% NaCl, 5% dextrose) at rate of infusion not to exceed 2 mg/min.
- Direct IV injection should be made w/repeated aspiration to ensure prevention of intra-arterial administration (produces arteriospasm; may result in gangrene).

INDICATIONS/ROUTES/DOSAGE

Anxiety:
Oral: Adults: 1–2 mg daily in 2–3 evenly divided doses. ***Elderly:*** Initially, 0.5–1 mg/day. May increase gradually.

Insomnia due to anxiety:
Oral: Adults: 2–4 mg at bedtime. ***Elderly:*** 0.5–1 mg at bedtime.

Preop:
IM: Adults, elderly: 0.05 mg/kg given 2 hrs before procedure. Do not exceed 4 mg.
IV: Adults, elderly: 0.044 mg/kg (up to 2 mg total) 15–20 min before surgery.

Status epilepticus:
IV: Adults: 4 mg, may repeat in 10–15 min. Give slowly 2 mg/min.

CONTRAINDICATIONS

Acute narrow-angle glaucoma, acute alcohol intoxication.

CAUTIONS

Impaired kidney/liver function.

INTERACTIONS

DRUG: ***Alcohol, CNS depressants*** may increase CNS depressant effect. **HERBAL:** Kava kava, valerian may increase CNS depression. **FOOD:** None significant. **ALTERED LAB VALUES:** None significant.

SIDE EFFECTS

FREQUENT: Drowsiness, dizziness, incoordination. Morning drowsiness may occur initially. **OCCASIONAL:** Blurred vision, slurred speech, hypotension, headache. **RARE:** Paradoxical CNS restlessness, excitement in elderly/debilitated (generally noted during first 2 wks of therapy, particularly noted in presence of uncontrolled pain).

ADVERSE REACTIONS/TOXIC EFFECTS

Abrupt or too rapid withdrawal may result in pronounced restlessness, irritability, insomnia, hand tremors, abdominal/muscle cramps, sweating, vomiting, seizures. Overdosage results in somnolence, confusion, diminished reflexes, coma.

PATIENT CONSIDERATIONS

BASELINE ASSESSMENT

Offer emotional support to anxious pt. Pt must remain recum-

bent for up to 8 hrs (individualized) after parenteral administration to reduce hypotensive effect. Assess motor responses (agitation, trembling, tension) and autonomic responses (cold, clammy hands, sweating).

INTERVENTION/EVALUATION

For those on long-term therapy, liver/renal function tests, blood counts should be performed periodically. Assess for paradoxical reaction, particularly during early therapy. Assist w/ambulation if drowsiness, lightheadedness occurs. Evaluate for therapeutic response: a calm facial expression, decreased restlessness and/or insomnia.

PATIENT/FAMILY TEACHING

Drowsiness usually disappears during continued therapy. If dizziness occurs, change positions slowly from recumbent to sitting position before standing. Avoid tasks that require alertness, motor skills until response to drug is established. Smoking reduces drug effectiveness. Do not abruptly withdraw medication after long-term therapy. Do not use alcohol or CNS depressants. Contraception is recommended for long-term therapy. Notify physician at once if pregnancy is suspected.

losartan

loh-**sar**-tan
(Cozaar)

FIXED-COMBINATION(S)
W/hydrochlorothiazide, a thiazide diuretic **(Hyzaar)**

CANADIAN AVAILABILITY
Cozaar

PREGNANCY CATEGORY C
First trimester.

PREGNANCY CATEGORY D
Second and third trimesters (fetal/neonatal morbidity/mortality).

CLASSIFICATION

Angiotensin II receptor antagonist

AVAILABILITY (Rx)

Tablets: 25 mg, 50 mg

PHARMACODYNAMICS

	ONSET	PEAK	DURATION
Oral	—	6 hrs	24 hrs

PHARMACOKINETICS

Absorption: Well absorbed following oral administration. **Metabolism:** Undergoes first-pass metabolism in liver to active metabolites. **Excretion:** Excreted in urine and via biliary system. Not removed by hemodialysis. **Half-life:** 2 hrs.

ACTION/*THERAPEUTIC EFFECT*

Potent vasodilator. An angiotensin II receptor (type AT_1) antagonist; blocks vasoconstrictor and aldosterone-secreting effects of angiotensin II, inhibiting the binding of angiotensin II to the AT_1 receptors, *causing vasodilation, decreased peripheral resistance, decrease in B/P.*

USES

Treatment of hypertension. Used alone or in combination w/other antihypertensives.

ADMINISTRATION

ORAL:
- May give w/o regard to food.
- Do not crush or break tablets.

INDICATIONS/ROUTES/DOSAGE

Note: If antihypertensive effect using once-daily dosing is inadequate, twice-daily regimen at same total daily dose or an increase in dose may provide therapeutic response. May be given concurrently w/other antihypertensives. If B/P not controlled by losartan alone, a low-dose diuretic may be added.

Hypertension:
Oral: Adults, elderly: Initially, 50 mg once daily. ***Maximum:*** May be given once or twice daily w/total daily doses ranging from 25 to 100 mg.

Hypertension (pts treated w/potassium-depleting diuretics, history of hepatic impairment):
Oral: Adults, elderly: Initially, 25 mg once daily. ***Maximum:*** May be given once or twice daily w/total daily doses ranging from 25 to 100 mg.

CONTRAINDICATIONS

None significant.

CAUTIONS

Renal/hepatic function impairment, renal arterial stenosis.

INTERACTIONS

DRUG: ***Cimetidine*** may increase effects. ***Phenobarbital, rifampin*** may decrease effects. May inhibit effects of ***ketoconazole, troleandomycin, sulfaphenazole.*** May increase concentration of ***lithium.*** **HERBAL:** None known. **FOOD:** None significant. **ALTERED LAB VALUES:** May increase BUN, serum creatinine, SGOT (AST), SGPT (ALT), alkaline phosphatase, bilirubin. May decrease Hgb, Hct.

SIDE EFFECTS

FREQUENT (5–10%): Upper respiratory infection, headache. **OCCASIONAL (1–5%):** Dizziness, inability to sleep, diarrhea, dyspepsia, heartburn, pain, muscle cramps, nasal congestion , back pain, fatigue. **RARE (<1%):** Anxiety, muscle pain, sinusitis, cough, insomnia.

ADVERSE REACTIONS/TOXIC EFFECTS

Overdosage may manifest as hypotension and tachycardia; bradycardia occurs less often. Institute supportive measurement.

PATIENT CONSIDERATIONS

Baseline Assessment

Obtain B/P and apical pulse immediately before each dose, in addition to regular monitoring (be alert to fluctuations). If excessive reduction in B/P occurs, place pt in supine position, feet slightly elevated. Question possibility of pregnancy (see Pregnancy/Lactation). Assess medication history (especially diuretic). Question for history of hepatic/renal impairment, renal artery stenosis.

Intervention/Evaluation

Maintain hydration (offer fluids frequently). Assess for evidence of upper respiratory infection, cough. Assist w/ambulation if dizziness occurs. Monitor stool frequency and consistency (watery, loose, soft).

Patient/Family Teaching

Inform female pt regarding consequences of second- and third-trimester exposure to losartan. Report pregnancy to physician as soon as possible. Avoid tasks that require alertness, motor skills (possible dizziness effect). Report any sign of infection

(sore throat, fever), chest pain. Do not take cold preparations, nasal decongestants. Restrict sodium and alcohol as indicated. Follow diet and control weight. Do not take other medications w/o consulting physician. Do not stop taking medication. Need for lifelong control. Caution against exercising during hot weather (risk of dehydration, hypotension).

loteprednol

low-teh-**pred**-noll
(Lotemax, Alrex)

PREGNANCY CATEGORY C

CLASSIFICATION

Ophthalmic corticosteroid

AVAILABILITY (Rx)

Suspension: 0.2% **(Altrex),** 0.5% **(Lotemax)**

PHARMACOKINETICS

Metabolism: Metabolized by enzymes in the eye, minimizing systemic effects.

ACTION/*THERAPEUTIC EFFECT*

Suppresses eye inflammation and edema, fibrin deposit, capillary dilation, scar formation, collagen deposit and capillary and fibroblastic proliferation by *exerting anti-inflammatory effect on conjunctiva, sclera, cornea, lids, iris, and anterior segment of the globe.*

USES

0.2% suspension: Temporary relief of signs and symptoms of seasonal allergic conjunctivitis. ***0.5% suspension:*** Treatment of ocular inflammatory conditions including acne rosacea, superficial or herpes zoster keratitis, allergic conjunctivitis, iritis, cyclitis, infective conjunctivitis. Treatment of postop inflammation following ocular surgery.

ADMINISTRATION

OPHTHALMIC:

- Shake well before using.
- Instruct patient to lie down or tilt head backward and look up.
- Gently pull lower eyelid down until a pocket (pouch) is formed between eye and lower lid (conjunctival sac).
- Hold dropper above pocket and place drop into pocket w/o touching tip of eye dropper to eyelid or conjunctival sac (placing drops directly onto eye may cause a sudden squeezing of eyelid, with subsequent loss of solution).
- Continue to hold eyelid for a moment (allows medication to distribute along entire conjunctival sac) before closing eye gently.
- Apply digital pressure to lacrimal sac at inner canthus (bridge of nose, inside corner of eye) for 1–2 min (minimizes drainage into nose and throat, reducing risk of systemic effects).
- Do not apply medication while pt is wearing soft contact lenses (absorbs drug preservative). Lenses may be reinserted ≥15 min after drug is administered.

INDICATIONS/ROUTES/DOSAGE

Seasonal allergic conjunctivitis (0.2% suspension):
Ophthalmic: Adults, elderly: Apply 1 drop into affected eye(s) up to 4 times/day.

Ocular inflammatory conditions (0.5% suspension):
Ophthalmic: Adults, elderly: Initially, apply 1–2 drops into conjunctival sac up to 4 times/day. During the first week, may increase dosage up to 1 drop every hour.

Postop inflammation (0.5% suspension):
Ophthalmic: Adults, elderly: Apply 1–2 drops into conjunctival sac of operated eye(s) 4 times/day beginning 14 hrs after surgery and continuing through first 2 wks post surgery.

CONTRAINDICATIONS

Acute epithelial herpes simplex keratitis, fungal diseases of ocular structures, vaccinia, varicella and other viral disease of cornea and conjunctive, ocular tuberculosis, hypersensitivity, after uncomplicated removal of superficial corneal foreign body, mycobacterial eye infection, acute purulent untreated eye infections that may be masked or enhanced by presence of steroids.

CAUTIONS

Stromal herpes simplex keratitis, sulfite sensitivity.

INTERACTIONS

DRUG: None significant. **HERBAL:** None known. **FOOD:** None significant. **ALTERED LAB VALUES:** None significant.

SIDE EFFECTS

FREQUENT (5–15%): Blurred vision, swelling of membrane covering white part of eye, redness or swelling of eye, burning when applied, dry eye, watery eye, headache, itching, sore throat, increased sensitivity of eye to light, rhinitis. **OCCASIONAL (1–5%):** Redness of eye, eyelid, or inner lining of eyelid, eye discomfort or irritation, increased intraocular pressure, uveitis (eye pain, tearing, sensitivity of eye to light, blurred vision).

ADVERSE REACTIONS/TOXIC EFFECTS

Prolonged use may result in glaucoma, optic nerve damage, loss of visual acuity and field of vision, cataracts, secondary ocular fungal infection. In diseases that cause thinning of cornea or sclera, perforation may occur.

PATIENT CONSIDERATIONS

INTERVENTIONS/EVALUATION

Do not touch applicator tip to any surface of lid (contaminated ocular solutions can produce ocular infection, eye damage). Monitor for dry eyes, photophobia, blurred vision, foreign body sensation.

PATIENT/FAMILY TEACHING

Do not touch eyelids or surrounding area with dropper tip of the bottle. Keep bottle tightly closed when not in use. Do not apply medication while wearing soft contact lenses (absorbs drug preservative). Reinsert lenses ≥15 min after drug is administered. Vision may be temporarily blurred. Check w/physician if symptoms do not improve or condition worsens.

lovastatin

low-vah-**stah**-tin
(Mevacor)

CANADIAN AVAILABILITY
Mevacor

PREGNANCY CATEGORY X

CLASSIFICATION

Antihyperlipoproteinemic

AVAILABILITY (Rx)

Tablets: 10 mg, 20 mg, 40 mg

PHARMACOKINETICS

Absorption: Incompletely absorbed from GI tract (increased on empty stomach). **Metabolism:** Hydrolyzed in liver to active metabolite. **Excretion:** Primarily eliminated in feces. **Half-life:** 3 hrs.

ACTION/*THERAPEUTIC EFFECT*

Inhibits HMG-CoA reductase, the enzyme that catalyzes the early step in cholesterol synthesis. *Decreases LDL cholesterol, VLDL cholesterol, plasma triglycerides; increases HDL cholesterol.*

USES

Treatment of hypercholesterolemia and coronary atherosclerosis. Reduces risk of myocardial infarction, unstable angina, need for revascularization procedures in pts w/o symptomatic cardiovascular disease, w/average to moderately elevated total cholesterol and LDL cholesterol levels and below average HDL cholesterol levels.

ADMINISTRATION

ORAL:

- Give w/meals.

INDICATIONS/ROUTES/DOSAGE

Hyperlipoproteinemia:

Oral: Adults, elderly: Initially: 20–40 mg/day w/evening meal. Increase at 4 wk intervals up to maximum of 80 mg/day. ***Maintenance:*** 20–80 mg/day in single or divided doses.

CONTRAINDICATIONS

Hypersensitivity to lovastatin, active liver disease, unexplained elevated liver function tests.

CAUTIONS

Anticoagulant therapy, history of liver disease, substantial alcohol consumption.
Withholding/discontinuing lovastatin may be necessary when pt is at risk for renal failure (secondary to rhabdomyolysis); major surgery, severe acute infection, trauma, hypotension, severe metabolic, endocrine or electrolyte disorders, or uncontrolled seizures.

INTERACTIONS

DRUG: Increased risk of rhabdomyolysis, acute renal failure ***w/cyclosporine, erythromycin, gemfibrozil, niacin, other immunosuppressants. Erythromycin, itraconazole, ketoconazole*** may increase concentration causing severe muscle pain, inflammation, weakness. **HERBAL:** None known. **FOOD:** Large amounts of grapefruit juce may increase risk of side effects (e.g., muscle pain, weakness). **ALTERED LAB VALUES:** May increase creatinine kinase, serum transaminase concentrations.

SIDE EFFECTS

FREQUENT (5–10%): Flatulence, headache. **OCCASIONAL (1–5%):** Nausea, diarrhea, vomiting, abdominal pain or cramps, constipation, heartburn, dyspepsia, muscle pain, dizziness, rash. **RARE (<1%):** Altered taste, dry mouth, pain, arthralgia, inability to sleep, chest pain, blurred vision, hair loss.

ADVERSE REACTIONS/TOXIC EFFECTS

Potential for malignancy, cataracts.

PATIENT CONSIDERATIONS

BASELINE ASSESSMENT

Question for possibility of pregnancy before initiating therapy (Pregnancy Category X). Question history of hypersensitivity to lovastatin. Assess baseline lab results: cholesterol, triglycerides, liver function tests.

INTERVENTION/EVALUATION

Evaluate food tolerance. Determine pattern of bowel activity. Check for headache, dizziness, blurred vision. Assess for rash, pruritus. Monitor cholesterol and triglyceride lab results for therapeutic response. Be alert for malaise, muscle cramping or weakness. Monitor temperature at least twice a day.

PATIENT/FAMILY TEACHING

Take w/meals. Follow special diet (important part of treatment). Avoid large amounts of grapefruit juice. Periodic lab tests are essential part of therapy. Do not take other medications w/o physician's knowledge. Do not stop medication w/o consulting physician. Report promptly any muscle pain or weakness, especially if accompanied by fever or malaise. Do not drive or perform activities that require alert response if dizziness occurs.

loxapine hydrochloride

lox-ah-peen

(Loxitane)

loxapine succinate

(Loxitane)

CANADIAN AVAILABILITY

Apo-Loxapine, Loxapac

PREGNANCY CATEGORY C

CLASSIFICATION

Antipsychotic

AVAILABILITY (Rx)

Capsules: 5 mg, 10 mg, 25 mg, 50 mg. **Oral Concentrate:** 25 mg/ml. **Injection:** 50 mg/ml.

PHARMACODYNAMICS

	ONSET	PEAK	DURATION
PO (sedation)			
	20–30 min	1.5–3 hrs	12 hrs
IM (sedation)			
	15–30 min	—	12 hrs

PHARMACOKINETICS

Absorption: Well absorbed after oral, IM administration. **Metabolism:** Metabolized in liver to active metabolite. **Excretion:** Primarily excreted in urine. **Half-life:** 12–19 hrs.

ACTION/*THERAPEUTIC EFFECT*

Blocks dopamine at postsynaptic receptor sites in brain. *Suppresses locomotor activity, produces tranquilization.* Strong anticholinergic effects.

USES/*UNLABELED*

Symptomatic management of psychotic disorders. *Management of anxiety associated w/mental depression.*

STORAGE/HANDLING

Store oral, parenteral form at room temperature. Yellow discoloration of solutions does not affect potency, but discard if markedly discolored.

ADMINISTRATION

Note: Give by oral or IM route.

ORAL:

- Give w/o regard to meals.
- Dilute oral concentrate w/orange or grapefruit juice.

IM:

- Inject slow, deep IM into upper outer quadrant of gluteus maximus.

INDICATIONS/ROUTES/DOSAGE

Psychotic disorders:
Oral: Adults: 10 mg 2 times/day. Increase dosage rapidly during first week to 50 mg, if needed. ***Usual therapeutic, maintenance range:*** 60–100 mg daily in 2–4 divided doses. ***Maximum:*** 250 mg/day.

IM: Adults: 12.5–50 mg q4–6h.

Usual elderly dosage:
Oral: Initially, 5–10 mg 1–2 times/day. May increase by 5–10 mg q4–7days.

IM: 12.5–25 mg q48h. May increase by 12.5 mg up to 50 mg.

CONTRAINDICATIONS

Severe CNS depression, comatose states.

EXTREME CAUTION

History of seizures.

CAUTION

Cardiovascular disorders, glaucoma, history of urinary retention, prostatic hypertrophy.

INTERACTIONS

DRUG: *Alcohol, CNS depressants* may increase CNS depression. *Antacids, antidiarrheals* may decrease absorption. *Extrapyramidal symptom (EPS)–producing medications* may increase risk of EPS. HERBAL: None known. FOOD: None significant. ALTERED LAB VALUES: None significant.

SIDE EFFECTS

FREQUENT: Blurred vision, confusion, drowsiness, dry mouth, dizziness, lightheadedness. OCCASIONAL: Allergic reaction (rash, itching), decreased urination, constipation, decreased sexual ability, enlarged breasts. Headache, increased skin sensitivity to sunlight, nausea, vomiting, inability to sleep, increased weight.

ADVERSE REACTIONS/TOXIC EFFECTS

Extrapyramidal symptoms frequently noted are akathisia (motor restlessness, anxiety). Less frequently noted are akinesia (rigidity, tremor, salivation, mask-like facial expression, reduced voluntary movements). Infrequently noted dystonias: torticollis (neck muscle spasm), opisthotonos (rigidity of back muscles), and oculogyric crisis (rolling back of eyes). Tardive dyskinesia (protrusion of tongue, puffing of cheeks, chewing/puckering of mouth) occurs rarely but may be irreversible. Risk is greater in female elderly pts. Grand mal seizures may occur in epileptic pts (risk higher w/IM administration).

PATIENT CONSIDERATIONS

Baseline Assessment

Assess behavior, appearance, emotional status, response to environment, speech pattern, thought content.

Intervention/Evaluation

Supervise suicidal risk pt closely during early therapy (as depression lessens, energy level improves, and suicide potential increases). Monitor B/P for hypotension. Assess for peripheral edema behind medial malleo-

lus (sacral area in bedridden pts). Assess stool consistency and frequency. Monitor for rigidity, tremor, mask-like facial expression (especially in those receiving IM injection). Assess for therapeutic response (interest in surroundings, improvement in self-care, increased ability to concentrate, relaxed facial expression).

PATIENT/FAMILY TEACHING

Full therapeutic effect may take up to 6 wks. Report visual disturbances. Sugarless gum, sips of tepid water may relieve dry mouth. Drowsiness generally subsides during continued therapy. Avoid tasks that require alertness, motor skills until response to drug is established. Avoid alcohol, CNS depressants, OTC medications. Describe signs and symptoms of extrapyramidal involvement and tardive dyskinesia for pt to report immediately.

mafenide acetate

ma-fe-nide
(Sulfamylon)

PREGNANCY CATEGORY C

CLASSIFICATION

Burn preparation

AVAILABILITY (Rx)

Cream: 85 mg/g. **Topical Solution:** 5%

PHARMACOKINETICS

Absorption: Absorbed through devascularized areas into systemic circulation. **Metabolism:** Rapidly metabolized. **Excretion:** Primarily excreted in urine.

ACTION/*THERAPEUTIC EFFECT*

Decreases number of bacteria in avascular tissue of second- and third-degree burns. *Bacteriostatic. Promotes spontaneous healing of deep partial-thickness burns.*

USES

Adjunctive therapy for second- and third-degree burns to prevent infection, septicemia; protection against conversion from partial- to full-thickness wounds (infection causes extended tissue destruction). ***Solution:*** Adjunct to control bacterial infection when used under moist dressing over meshed autografts on excised burn wounds.

ADMINISTRATION

TOPICAL:

- Apply to cleansed, debrided burns using sterile glove.
- Keep burn areas covered w/mafenide cream at all times; reapply to any areas where removed (e.g., w/pt activity).
- Dressings usually not required; if ordered (e.g., when eschar begins to separate), apply thin layer.

INDICATIONS/ROUTES/DOSAGE

Usual topical dosage:
Adults, elderly: Apply 1–2 times/day.

CONTRAINDICATIONS

Hypersensitivity to mafenide or sulfite.

CAUTIONS

Impaired renal function that increases risk of metabolic acidosis. Cross-sensitivity to sulfonamides not certain.

INTERACTIONS

DRUG: None significant. **HERBAL:** None known. **FOOD:** None significant. **ALTERED LAB VALUES:** None significant.

SIDE EFFECTS

Difficult to distinguish side effects and effects of severe burn. **FREQUENT:** Pain, burning upon application. **OCCASIONAL:** Allergic reaction (usually 10–14 days after initiation of mafenide): itching, rash, facial edema, swelling; unexplained syndrome of marked hyperventilation w/respiratory alkalosis. **RARE:** Delay in eschar separation, excoriation of new skin.

ADVERSE REACTIONS/TOXIC EFFECTS

Hemolytic anemia, porphyria, bone marrow depression, superinfections (especially w/fungi), metabolic acidosis occurs rarely.

PATIENT CONSIDERATIONS

BASELINE ASSESSMENT

Question for hypersensitivity to mafenide, sulfite (more frequent

in asthmatics). Evaluate arterial blood gases (ABGs) for acid-base balance, renal function tests and CBCs for baseline.

INTERVENTION/EVALUATION

Be alert to fluid balance and renal function: Monitor I&O, renal function tests, urinary pH, and promptly report changes. Watch for signs/symptoms of metabolic acidosis: Kussmaul's respirations, nausea, vomiting, diarrhea, headache, tremors, weakness and cardiac arrhythmias (due to associated hyperkalemia), sensorium changes, decreased PCO_2, blood pH, and HCO_3. Monitor vital signs, evaluate ABG results. Assess burns, surrounding skin areas for allergic reaction or superinfection: rash, excoriation, swelling, itching, increased pain, purulent exudate. Monitor hematologic tests.

PATIENT/FAMILY TEACHING

Application may cause temporary pain or burning; burn areas must be completely covered by cream. Therapy must not be interrupted (attempts will be made to reduce adverse reaction before considering discontinuance of drug). Inform physician if condition worsens, irritation occurs or hyperventilation occurs. Bathe burn area daily.

---

magnesium

magnesium chloride

(Slow-Mag)

magnesium citrate

(Citrate of Magnesia, Citroma, Citro-Nesia)

magnesium hydroxide

(MOM)

magnesium oxide

(Mag-Ox 400, Maox)

magnesium protein complex

(Mg-PLUS)

magnesium sulfate

(Epsom salt, Magnesium Sulfate injection)

FIXED-COMBINATION(S)

W/aluminum, an antacid (**Aludrox, Delcid, Gaviscon, Maalox**); w/aluminum and simethicone, an antiflatulent (**Di-Gel, Gelusil, Maalox Plus, Mylanta, Silain-Gel**); w/aluminum and calcium, an antacid (**Camalox**); w/mineral oil, a lubricant laxative (**Haley's MO**); w/magnesium oxide and aluminum oxide, antacids (**Riopan**).

CANADIAN AVAILABILITY

Citro-Mag, Phillips' Magnesia Tablets, Slow-Mag

PREGNANCY CATEGORY B

(anticonvulsant/laxative)

CLASSIFICATION

Antacid, anticonvulsant, electrolyte, laxative

AVAILABILITY (OTC)

Tablets: 400 mg, 500 mg. **Tablets (chewable):** 311 mg. **Tablets (sustained-release):** 535 mg. **Capsules:** 140 mg. **Liquid:** 54 mg/5 ml, 400 mg/5 ml, 800 mg/5 ml. **MOM:** 30 ml, 60 ml. **Injection (Rx):** 10%, 12.5%, 20%, 50%.

PHARMACOKINETICS

Antacid, laxative: **Absorption:** Minimal absorption through intestine. **Excretion:** Absorbed dose primarily excreted in urine. ***Systemic:*** Widely distributed. **Excretion:** Primarily excreted in urine.

ACTION/*THERAPEUTIC EFFECT*

Antacid: Acts in stomach to neutralize *gastric acid, increase pH.* Laxative: Osmotic effect primarily in small intestine. Draws water into intestinal lumen, produces *distension, promotes peristalsis, bowel evacuation.* ***Systemic (dietary supplement, replacement):*** Found primarily in intracellular fluids. Essential *for enzyme activity, nerve conduction, and muscle contraction.* ***Anticonvulsant:*** Blocks neuromuscular transmission, amount of acetylcholine released at motor end plate, *producing seizure control.*

USES

Antacid: Symptomatic relief of upset stomach associated w/hyperacidity (heartburn, acid indigestion, sour stomach), gastric, duodenal ulcers. Symptomatic treatment of GERD. Prophylactic treatment of GI bleeding secondary to gastritis and stress ulceration. ***Laxative:*** Evacuation of colon for rectal and bowel examination, elective colon surgery. Accelerates excretion of various parasites, poisonous substances (except acid or alkali) from GI tract. ***Systemic:*** Dietary supplement, replacement therapy. Nutritional adjunct in hyperalimentation. ***Anticonvulsant:*** Immediate control of life-threatening seizures in treatment of severe toxemia of pregnancy, seizures associated w/acute nephritis in children.

STORAGE/HANDLING

Store oral, parenteral forms at room temperature. Refrigerate citrate of magnesia (retains potency, palatability).

ADMINISTRATION

ORAL (ANTACID):

- Suspensions to be shaken well before use.
- Chew chewable tablets thoroughly before swallowing and follow w/full glass of water.

ORAL (LAXATIVE):

- Drink full glass of liquid (8 oz) w/each dose (prevents dehydration).
- Flavor improved by following w/fruit juice or citrus carbonated beverage.

IM:

- For adults, elderly, use 250 mg/ml (25%) or 500 mg/ml (50%) magnesium sulfate concentration.
- For infants, children, do not exceed 200 mg/ml (20%).

IV:

- For IV infusion, do not exceed magnesium sulfate concentration 200 mg/ml (20%).
- Do not exceed IV infusion rate of 150 mg/min.

INDICATIONS/ROUTES/DOSAGE

Note: 1 g = 8.12 mEq as magnesium sulfate.

ANTACID:

Magnesium hydroxide:
Oral: Adults, elderly, children >12 yrs: 5–15 ml or 0.65–1.3 g 4 times/day.

Magnesium oxide:
Oral: Adults, elderly: 400–840 mg/day.

M

LAXATIVE:

Citrate of magnesia:
Oral: Adults, elderly: 240 ml as needed. *Children:* 1/2 adult dose, repeat as needed.

Magnesium hydroxide:
Oral: Adults, elderly: 30–60 ml/day w/liquids. *Children ≥2 yrs:* 5–30 ml (dependent on age).

Magnesium sulfate:
Oral: Adults, elderly: 10–15 g in glass of water. *Children:* 5–10 g in glass of water.

DIETARY SUPPLEMENT:

Oral: Adults, elderly: 54–483 mg/day (refer to individual products).

MILD DEFICIENCY:

IM: Adults, elderly: 1 g q6h for 4 doses.

SEVERE DEFICIENCY:

IM/IV Infusion: Adults, elderly: 0.5–1 mEq/kg/day (lean body weight) in divided doses.

HYPERALIMENTATION:

IV: Adults, elderly: 1–3 g (8–24 mEq)/day. *Children:* 0.25–1.25 g (2–10 mEq)/day.

ANTICONVULSANT:

IM: Adults: 4–5 g (32–40 mEq) of 50% solution q4h as needed. *Children:* 20–40 mg/kg of 20% solution, may repeat as needed.

IV: Adults: 4 g (32 mEq) of 10–20% solution (do not exceed rate of 1.5 ml/min of 10% solution).

IV Infusion: Adults: 4–5 g (32–40 mEq)/250 ml 5% dextrose or 0.9% NaCl (do not exceed rate of 3 ml/min).

CONTRAINDICATIONS

Antacids: Severe renal impairment, appendicitis or symptoms of appendicitis, ileostomy, intestinal obstruction. *Laxative:* Appendicitis, undiagnosed rectal bleeding, CHF, intestinal obstruction, hypersensitivity, colostomy, ileostomy. *Systemic:* Heart block, myocardial damage, renal failure.

CAUTIONS

Safety in children <6 yrs not known. *Antacids:* Undiagnosed gastrointestinal or rectal bleeding, ulcerative colitis, colostomy, diverticulitis, chronic diarrhea. *Laxative:* Diabetes mellitus or pts on low-salt diet (some products contain sugar, sodium). *Systemic:* Severe renal impairment

INTERACTIONS

DRUG: *Antacids:* May decrease absorption of ***ketoconazole, tetracyclines.*** May decrease effect of ***methenamine.*** *Antacids, laxatives:* May decrease effects of ***oral anticoagulants, digoxin, phenothiazines.*** May form nonabsorbable complex w/***tetracyclines.*** *Systemic:* ***Calcium*** may neutralize effects. ***CNS depression–producing medications*** may increase CNS depression. May cause changes in cardiac conduction/heart block w/***digoxin.*** HERBAL: None known. FOOD: None significant. ALTERED LAB VALUES: *Antacid:* May increase gastrin, pH. *Laxative:* May decrease potassium. *Systemic:* None significant.

SIDE EFFECTS

FREQUENT: *Antacid:* Chalky taste, diarrhea, laxative effect. OCCASIONAL: *Antacid:* Nausea, vomiting, stomach cramps. *Antacid, laxative:* Prolonged use or large dose w/renal impairment may cause increased magnesium (dizziness, irregular heartbeat, mental changes, tiredness, weakness). *Laxative:* Cramping, diarrhea, increased thirst, gas. *Systemic:* Reduced respiratory rate, decreased reflexes, flushing, hypotension, decreased heart rate.

ADVERSE REACTIONS/TOXIC EFFECTS

Antacid, laxative: None significant. *Systemic:* May produce prolonged PQ interval, widening of QRS intervals. May cause loss of deep tendon reflexes, heart block, respiratory paralysis, and cardiac arrest. *Antidote:* 10–20 ml 10% calcium gluconate (5–10 mEq of calcium).

PATIENT CONSIDERATIONS

BASELINE ASSESSMENT

Assess if pt is sensitive to magnesium.

Antacid
Assess gastrointestinal pain (duration, location, time of occurrence, relief w/food or caused by food or alcohol, constant or sporadic, worsened when lying down or bending over).

Laxative
Assess color, amount, consistency of stool. Assess bowel habits (usual pattern), bowel sound for peristalsis. Assess pt for any abdominal pain, weight loss, nausea, vomiting, history of recent abdominal surgery

Systemic
Assess renal function, magnesium level.

INTERVENTION/EVALUATION

Antacid
Assess for relief of gastric distress. Monitor renal function (especially if dosing is long term or frequent).

Laxative
Monitor stools for diarrhea or constipation. Maintain adequate fluid intake.

Systemic
Monitor renal function, magnesium levels, EKG for cardiac function. Test patellar reflex or knee jerk reflexes before giving repeat parenteral doses (used as indication of CNS depression; suppressed reflex may be sign of impending respiratory arrest). Patellar reflex must be present, respiratory rate >16/min before each parenteral dose. Provide seizure precautions.

PATIENT/FAMILY TEACHING

Antacid
Give at least 2 hrs apart from other medication. Do not take >2 wks unless directed by physician. For peptic ulcer take 1 and 3 hrs after meals and at bedtime for 4–6 wks. Chew tablets thoroughly followed w/glass of water; shake suspensions well. Repeat dosing/large doses may have laxative effect.

Laxative
Drink full glass (8 oz) liquid to aid stool softening. Use only for short term. Teach other methods of bowel regulation (diet, exercise, increased fluid intake). Do not use if abdominal pain, vomiting, nausea are present. Inform pt of normal bowel movement range: 3 per day to 3 per week.

Systemic
Inform physician of any signs of hypermagnesemia (confusion, irregular heartbeat, cramping,

unusual tiredness or weakness, lightheadedness, or dizziness).

mannitol

man-ih-toll
(Osmitrol)

CANADIAN AVAILABILITY
Osmitrol

PREGNANCY CATEGORY C

CLASSIFICATION

Osmotic diuretic

AVAILABILITY (Rx)

Injection: 5%, 10%, 15%, 20%, 25%

PHARMACOKINETICS

Remains in extracellular fluid. **Excretion:** Primarily excreted in urine. **Half-life:** 100 min. Onset diuresis occurs in 1–3 hrs, decreases intraocular pressure in 0.5–1 hr, duration 4–6 hrs. Decreases cerebral spinal fluid pressure in 15 min, duration 3–8 hrs.

ACTION/*THERAPEUTIC EFFECT*

Elevates osmotic pressure of glomerular filtrate, increases flow of water into interstitial fluid and plasma, inhibiting renal tubular reabsorption of sodium, chloride, *producing diuresis.* Enhances flow of water from eye into plasma, *reducing intraocular pressure (IOP).*

USES

Prevention, treatment of oliguric phase of acute renal failure (before evidence of permanent renal failure). Reduces increased intracranial pressure due to cerebral edema, edema of injured spinal cord, intraocular pressure due to acute glaucoma. Promotes urinary excretion of toxic substances (aspirin, bromides, imipramine, barbiturates).

STORAGE/HANDLING

Store at room temperature. Crystallization can occur. Do not use if crystals remain after warming procedure (see IV Administration).

ADMINISTRATION

IV:

- **Note:** Assess IV site for patency before each dose. Extravasation noted w/pain, thrombosis.
- Rate of administration should be titrated to promote urinary output of 30–50 ml/hr.
- If crystals are noted in solution, warm bottle in hot water and shake vigorously at intervals. Cool to body temperature before administration.
- Use filter for infusion of 20% or more concentration.
- Do not add KCl or NaCl to mannitol 20% or greater. Do not add to whole blood for transfusion.

INDICATIONS/ROUTES/DOSAGE

Note: Dosage based on pt's condition/fluid requirements, urinary output, concentration and rate of administration.

Test dose for marked oliguria/suspected inadequate renal function:
IV: Adults, elderly: 0.2 g/kg or 12.5 g w/15–20% solution. Infuse over 3–5 min to produce urinary output of 30–50 ml in 2–3 hrs. Test dose may be repeated once.

Oliguria/acute renal failure prevention:
IV: Adults, elderly: 50–100 g of a

concentrated solution followed by 5–10% solution.

Treatment of oliguria:
IV: Adults, elderly: 100 g w/15–20% solution infused over 90 min to a few hours.

Intracranial/intraocular pressure:
IV: Adults, elderly: 1.5–2 g/kg administered as a 15-20-25% solution, infused over 30–60 min. Rebound increase of intracranial pressure may occur 12 hrs after use. For preop use, administer 1–1½ hrs before surgery.

Treatment of drug intoxications:
IV: Adults, elderly: Loading dose of 25 g followed by dosage titrated to maintain urinary output of 100–500 ml/hr. For barbiturates, 0.5 g/kg w/5–10% solutions titrated to urine output. Dosage and treatment based on fluid balance, urine pH, urine volume.

CONTRAINDICATIONS

Increasing oliguria or anuria, CHF, pulmonary edema, organic CNS disease, severe dehydration, fluid overload, active intracranial bleeding (except during craniotomy), severe electrolyte depletion.

CAUTIONS

Impaired renal, hepatic function.

INTERACTIONS

DRUG: May increase ***digoxin*** toxicity (due to hypokalemia). **HERBAL:** None known. **FOOD:** None significant. **ALTERED LAB VALUES:** May decrease phosphate, potassium, sodium.

SIDE EFFECTS

FREQUENT: Dry mouth, thirst. **OCCASIONAL:** Blurred vision, increased urination, headache, arm pain, backache, nausea, vomiting, urticaria (hives), dizziness, hypotension, hypertension, tachycardia, fever, anginalike chest pain.

ADVERSE REACTIONS/TOXIC EFFECTS

Fluid and electrolyte imbalance may occur because of rapid administration of large doses or inadequate urinary output resulting in overexpansion of extracellular fluid. Circulatory overload may produce pulmonary edema, CHF. Excessive diuresis may produce hypokalemia, hyponatremia. Fluid loss in excess of electrolyte excretion may produce hypernatremia, hyperkalemia.

M

PATIENT CONSIDERATIONS

Baseline Assessment

Check B/P, pulse before giving medication. Baseline electrolyte, renal and hepatic function, BUN may be ordered. Assess skin turgor, mucous membranes, mental status, muscle strength. Obtain baseline weight. I&O. For acute situations, a Foley catheter may assist in measuring hourly outputs.

Intervention/Evaluation

Monitor urinary output to ascertain therapeutic response. Monitor electrolyte, BUN, renal, hepatic reports. Assess vital signs, skin turgor, mucous membranes. Weigh daily. Signs of hyponatremia include confusion, drowsiness, thirst or dry mouth, cold/clammy skin. Signs of hypokalemia include changes in muscle strength, tremors, muscle cramps, changes in mental status, cardiac arrhythmias. Signs of hyperkalemia include colic, diarrhea, muscle twitching followed by weakness or paralysis, arrhythmias.

PATIENT/FAMILY TEACHING

Expect increased frequency and volume of urination.

maprotiline hydrochloride

mah-**pro**-tih-leen
(Ludiomil)

CANADIAN AVAILABILITY
Ludiomil

PREGNANCY CATEGORY B

CLASSIFICATION

Antidepressant

AVAILABILITY (Rx)

Tablets: 25 mg, 50 mg, 75 mg

PHARMACOKINETICS

Absorption: Slowly, completely absorbed from GI tract. Widely distributed. **Metabolism:** Metabolized in liver to active metabolites. **Excretion:** Primarily excreted in urine. **Half-life:** 27–58 hrs; metabolite: 60–90 hrs.

ACTION/*THERAPEUTIC EFFECT*

Blocks reuptake of norepinephrine by CNS presynaptic neuronal membranes, increasing availability at postsynaptic neuronal receptor sites. Resulting enhancement of synaptic activity *produces antidepressant effect.* Moderate anticholinergic activity.

USES/*UNLABELED*

Relief of depressive-affective (mood) disorders, including depressive neurosis, major depression. Also used for depression phase of bipolar disorder (manic-depressive illness). *Treatment of neurogenic pain.*

ADMINISTRATION

ORAL:

- Give w/food or milk if GI distress occurs.
- Do not crush or break enteric-coated tablets.
- Scored tablets may be crushed.

INDICATIONS/ROUTES/DOSAGE

Mild to moderate depression:
Oral: Adults: 75 mg/day to start, in 1–4 divided doses. ***Elderly:*** 50–75 mg/day. In 2 wks, increase dosage gradually in 25 mg increments until therapeutic response is achieved. Reduce to lowest effective maintenance level.

Severe depression:
Oral: Adults: 100–150 mg/day in 1–4 divided doses. May increase gradually to maximum 225 mg/day.

Usual elderly dosage:
Oral: Initially, 25 mg at bedtime. May increase by 25 mg q3–7days. ***Maintenance:*** 50–75 mg/day.

CONTRAINDICATIONS

Acute recovery period following MI, within 14 days of MAO inhibitor ingestion, known or suspected seizure disorders.

CAUTIONS

Prostatic hypertrophy, history of urinary retention or obstruction, glaucoma, diabetes mellitus, history of seizures, hyperthyroidism, cardiac/hepatic/renal disease, schizophrenia, increased intraocular pressure, hiatal hernia.

INTERACTIONS

DRUG: *Alcohol, CNS depressants* may increase effect. *MAO inhibitors* may increase risk of hypertensive crisis, severe convulsions. *Sympathomimetics* may increase cardiovascular effects (arrhythmias, tachycardia, severe hypertension). **HERBAL:** None known. **FOOD:** None significant. **ALTERED LAB VALUES:** None significant.

SIDE EFFECTS

FREQUENT: Drowsiness, fatigue, dry mouth, blurred vision, constipation, delayed micturition, postural hypotension, excessive sweating, disturbed concentration, increased appetite, urinary retention. **OCCASIONAL:** GI disturbances (nausea, GI distress, metallic taste sensation), increased sensitivity of skin to sunlight. **RARE:** Paradoxical reaction (agitation, restlessness, nightmares, insomnia), extrapyramidal symptoms (particularly fine hand tremor).

ADVERSE REACTIONS/TOXIC EFFECTS

Higher incidence of seizures than w/tricyclic antidepressants (especially in those w/no previous history of seizures). High dosage may produce cardiovascular effects (severe postural hypotension, dizziness, tachycardia, palpitations, arrhythmias) and seizures. May also result in altered temperature regulation (hyperpyrexia or hypothermia). Abrupt withdrawal from prolonged therapy may produce headache, malaise, nausea, vomiting, vivid dreams.

PATIENT CONSIDERATIONS

Baseline Assessment

For those on long-term therapy, liver/renal function tests, blood counts should be performed periodically.

Intervention/Evaluation

Supervise suicidal risk pt closely during early therapy (as depression lessens, energy level improves, increasing suicide potential). Assess appearance, behavior, speech pattern, level of interest, mood. Monitor bowel activity; avoid constipation. Monitor B/P, pulse for hypotension, arrhythmias. Assess for urinary retention.

Patient/Family Teaching

Change positions slowly to avoid hypotensive effect. Tolerance to postural hypotension, sedative and anticholinergic effects usually develops during early therapy. Therapeutic effect may be noted within 3–7 days, maximum effect within 2–3 wks. Wear protective clothing, use sunscreen to protect skin from ultraviolet light or sunlight. Dry mouth may be relieved by sugarless gum, sips of tepid water. Report visual disturbances. Do not abruptly discontinue medication. Avoid tasks that require alertness, motor skills until response to drug is established.

---

masoprocol

mass-oh-**pro**-call
(Actinex)

PREGNANCY CATEGORY B

CLASSIFICATION

Topical

AVAILABILITY (Rx)

Cream: 10%

PHARMACOKINETICS

Absorption: Minimal absorption systemically (<2%).

ACTION/*THERAPEUTIC EFFECT*

Produces antiproliferative activity against keratinocytes.

USES

Topical treatment for actinic (solar) keratoses.

ADMINISTRATION

TOPICAL:

- Wash and dry affected area before application.
- Apply directly to desired area, massaging gently (avoid eyes and mucous membranes of nose/mouth).
- Avoid occlusive dressing.
- If applied w/fingers, wash hands immediately w/soap and water after use.

INDICATIONS/ROUTES/DOSAGE

Actinic (solar) keratoses:
Topical: Adults, elderly: Apply to area topically as needed. Do not cover surface (minimizes irritation). Repeat each morning and evening for 28 days.

CONTRAINDICATIONS

Hypersensitivity to masoprocol or other components of preparation.

CAUTIONS

Sulfite sensitivity. For external use only. Avoid occlusive dressings. Safety in children not established.

INTERACTIONS

DRUG: None significant. **HERBAL:** None known. **FOOD:** None significant. **ALTERED LAB VALUES:** None significant.

SIDE EFFECTS

FREQUENT (>5%): Erythema, flaking (46%), itching (32%), edema (14%), burning (12%), soreness. **OCCASIONAL (1–5%):** Bleeding, crusting, eye irritation, rash, skin irritation, stinging, tightness, tingling. **RARE (<1%):** Blistering, excoriation, fissuring, skin roughness, wrinkling.

ADVERSE REACTIONS/TOXIC EFFECTS

Allergic contact dermatitis represents sensitization. Discontinue medication, contact physician.

PATIENT CONSIDERATIONS

BASELINE ASSESSMENT

Question for hypersensitivity to masoprocol or other components of preparation.

INTERVENTION/EVALUATION

Assess for irritation.

PATIENT/FAMILY TEACHING

Use only as directed. For external use only. Take special care to avoid eyes, nose, mouth. If contact w/eyes occurs, rinse promptly and thoroughly w/water. If applied w/fingers, wash hands immediately after application. Do not use occlusive coverings. Do not use other skin products or makeup during therapy w/o advice of physician. May stain clothing, fabrics. Does not cause photosensitivity, but avoid undue sun exposure because of keratoses. May have transient local burning after application. Contact physician if oozing, blistering, or other severe reaction occurs.

mebendazole

meh-**ben**-dah-zole
(Vermox)

CANADIAN AVAILABILITY
Vermox

PREGNANCY CATEGORY C

CLASSIFICATION

Anhelminthic

AVAILABILITY (Rx)

Tablets (chewable): 100 mg

PHARMACOKINETICS

Absorption: Poorly absorbed from GI tract (absorption increases w/food). Highest concentration in liver. **Metabolism:** Metabolized in liver. **Excretion:** Primarily eliminated in feces. **Half-life:** 2.5–9 hrs (increased in decreased renal function).

ACTION/*THERAPEUTIC EFFECT*

Vermicidal. Degrades parasite cytoplasmic microtubules, irreversibly blocks glucose uptake in helminths and larvae *(depletes glycogen, decreases ATP, causes helminth death).*

USES

Treatment of trichuriasis (whipworm), enterobiasis (pinworm), ascariasis (roundworm), hookworm caused by *Ancylostoma duodenale* or *Necator americanus.* Effective in mixed helminthic infections due to broad spectrum of activity.

ADMINISTRATION

ORAL:

- No special fasting is required.
- Tablet may be crushed, chewed, swallowed, or mixed w/food.
- For high dosage, best if taken w/food.

INDICATIONS/ROUTES/DOSAGE

Trichuriasis, ascariasis, hookworm:
Oral: Adults, elderly, children >2 yrs: 1 tablet in morning and at bedtime for 3 days.

Enterobiasis:
Oral: Adults, elderly, children >2 yrs: 1 tablet one time.

CONTRAINDICATIONS

None significant.

CAUTIONS

None significant.

INTERACTIONS

DRUG: *Carbamazepine* may decrease concentrations. **HERBAL:** None known. **FOOD:** None significant. **ALTERED LAB VALUES:** May increase SGOT (AST), SGPT (ALT), alkaline phosphatase, BUN. May decrease Hgb.

SIDE EFFECTS

OCCASIONAL: Nausea, vomiting, headache, dizziness. Transient abdominal pain, diarrhea w/massive infection and expulsion of helminths. **RARE:** Fever.

ADVERSE REACTIONS/TOXIC EFFECTS

High dosage may produce reversible myelosuppression (granulocytopenia, leukopenia, neutropenia).

PATIENT CONSIDERATIONS

BASELINE ASSESSMENT

Question for history of hypersensitivity to mebendazole. Obtain

M

specimens to confirm diagnosis: (1) Stool must be collected in clean, dry bedpan or container (parasites may be destroyed by urine, water, or medications). (2) Obtain pinworm specimens early in morning by applying transparent tape to tongue blade and pressing sticky side of tape to perianal area (female pinworms usually deposit eggs in this area during night).

INTERVENTION/EVALUATION

Encourage intake of fruits, vegetables, fluids to avoid constipation (parasites expelled by normal peristalsis). Collect stool or perianal specimens as required to confirm cure. Monitor CBC w/high dosage. Assess food tolerance. Provide assistance w/ambulation if dizzy.

PATIENT/FAMILY TEACHING

Complete full course of therapy; may need to repeat. Wash hands thoroughly after toileting, before eating. Keep hands away from mouth, fingernails short. Disinfect toilet facilities daily. Due to high transmission of pinworm infections, all family members should be treated simultaneously; infected person should sleep alone, shower frequently. Do not shake bedding; change and launder underclothing, pajamas, bedding, towels, and washcloths daily. W/hookworm, avoid walking barefoot (larval entry into system). Continue iron supplements as long as ordered (may be 6 mos after treatment) for anemia associated w/whipworm, hookworm. Notify physician if symptoms do not improve in a few days or if they become worse. Follow-up w/office visits, stool collection are important parts of therapy. Don't drive, use machinery if dizzy.

mechlorethamine hydrochloride

(Mustargen)

See Classification section under: Cancer chemotherapy

meclizine

mek-lih-zeen

(Antivert, Bonine)

CANADIAN AVAILABILITY

Bonamine

PREGNANCY CATEGORY B

CLASSIFICATION

Antiemetic, antivertigo

AVAILABILITY (Rx)

Tablets: 12.5 mg, 25 mg, 50 mg. **Tablets (chewable):** 25 mg. **Capsules:** 25 mg.

PHARMACODYNAMICS

	ONSET	PEAK	DURATION
Oral	30–60 min	—	12–24 hrs

PHARMACOKINETICS

Absorption: Well absorbed from GI tract. Widely distributed. **Metabolism:** Metabolized in liver. **Excretion:** Primarily excreted in urine. **Half-life:** 6 hrs.

ACTION/*THERAPEUTIC EFFECT*

Reduces labyrinth excitability, diminishes vestibular stimulation of labyrinth, affecting chemoreceptor trigger zone (CTZ), *reduc-*

ing nausea, vomiting, vertigo. Anticholinergic activity.

USES

Prevention and treatment of nausea, vomiting, vertigo due to motion sickness. Treatment of vertigo associated with diseases affecting vestibular system.

ADMINISTRATION

ORAL:

- Give w/o regard to meals.
- Scored tablets may be crushed.
- Do not crush or break capsule form.

INDICATIONS/ROUTES/DOSAGE

Motion sickness:
Oral: Adults, elderly, children >12 yrs: 25–50 mg 1 hr before exposure to motion. Repeat q24h as needed.

Vertigo:
Oral: Adults, elderly, children >12 yrs: 25–100 mg/day in divided doses as needed.

CONTRAINDICATIONS

None significant.

CAUTIONS

Narrow-angle glaucoma, prostatic hypertrophy, pyloroduodenal or bladder neck obstruction, asthma, COPD, increased intraocular pressure, cardiovascular disease, hyperthyroidism, hypertension, seizure disorders.

INTERACTIONS

DRUG: *Alcohol, CNS depression–producing medications* may increase CNS depressant effect. **HERBAL:** None known. **FOOD:** None significant. **ALTERED LAB VALUES:** May suppress wheal, flare reactions to antigen skin testing, unless meclizine discontinued 4 days before testing.

SIDE EFFECTS

Note: Elderly (>60 yrs) tend to develop sedation, dizziness, hypotension, mental confusion, disorientation, agitation, psychotic-like symptoms. **FREQUENT:** Drowsiness. **OCCASIONAL:** Blurred vision, dry mouth, nose, or throat.

ADVERSE REACTIONS/TOXIC EFFECTS

Children may experience dominant paradoxical reaction (restlessness, insomnia, euphoria, nervousness, tremors). Overdosage in children may result in hallucinations, convulsions, death. Hypersensitivity reaction (eczema, pruritus, rash, cardiac disturbances, photosensitivity) may occur. Overdosage may vary from CNS depression (sedation, apnea, cardiovascular collapse, death) to severe paradoxical reaction (hallucinations, tremor, seizures).

PATIENT CONSIDERATIONS

INTERVENTION/EVALUATION

Monitor B/P, especially in elderly (increased risk of hypotension). Monitor children closely for paradoxical reaction. Monitor serum electrolytes in those with severe vomiting. Assess skin turgor, mucous membranes to evaluate hydration status.

PATIENT/FAMILY TEACHING

Tolerance to sedative effect may occur. Avoid tasks that require alertness, motor skills until response to drug is established. Dry mouth, drowsiness, dizziness may be an expected response of drug. Avoid alcoholic beverages during therapy.

Sugarless gum, sips of tepid water may relieve dry mouth. Coffee or tea may help reduce drowsiness.

meclofenamate sodium

(Meclodium, Meclomen)
See Classification section under: Nonsteroidal anti-inflammatory drugs (NSAIDs)

medroxyprogesterone acetate

meh-drocks-ee-pro-**jes**-ter-own
(Amen, Curretab, Depo-Provera, Provera)

FIXED-COMBINATION(S)
W/conjugated estrogens **(Lunelle, Premphase, Prempro)**

CANADIAN AVAILABILITY
Novo-Medrone, Depo-Provera, Provera

PREGNANCY CATEGORY D

CLASSIFICATION

Progestin, antineoplastic

AVAILABILITY (Rx)

Tablets: 2.5 mg, 5 mg, 10 mg. **Injection:** 100 mg/ml, 150 mg/ml, 400 mg/ml.

PHARMACOKINETICS

Absorption: Slow absorption after IM administration. **Metabolism:** Metabolized in liver. **Excretion:** Primarily excreted in urine.

ACTION/*THERAPEUTIC EFFECT*

Transforms endometrium from proliferative to secretory (in an estrogen-primed endometrium); inhibits secretion of pituitary gonadotropins, *preventing follicular maturation and ovulation.* Stimulates growth of mammary alveolar tissue; relaxes uterine smooth muscle. *Restores hormonal imbalance.*

USES/*UNLABELED*

Oral: Prevention of endometrial hyperplasia (concurrently given w/estrogen to women with intact uterus), treatment of secondary amenorrhea, abnormal uterine bleeding. ***IM:*** Adjunctive therapy, palliative treatment of inoperable, recurrent, metastatic endometrial carcinoma, renal carcinoma; prevention of pregnancy. *Treatment of endometriosis, hormonal replacement therapy in estrogen-treated menopausal women.*

ADMINISTRATION

ORAL:

- Give w/o regard to meals.

IM:

- Shake vial immediately before administering (ensures complete suspension).
- Rarely, a residual lump, change in skin color, or sterile abscess occurs at injection site.

INDICATIONS/ROUTES/DOSAGE

Endometrial hyperplasia:
Oral: Adults: 2–10 mg/day for 14 days.

Secondary amenorrhea:
Oral: Adults: 5–10 mg/day for 5–10 days (begin at any time during menstrual cycle).

Abnormal uterine bleeding:
Oral: Adults: 5–10 mg/day for 5–10 days (begin on calculated day 16 or day 21 of menstrual cycle).

Endometrial, renal carcinoma:
IM: Adults, elderly: Initially, 400–1,000 mg, repeat at 1 wk intervals. If improvement occurs, disease stabilized, begin maintenance w/as little as 400 mg/mo.

Pregnancy prevention:
IM: Adults: 150 mg q3mos.

CONTRAINDICATIONS

History of or active thrombotic disorders (cerebral apoplexy, thrombophlebitis, thromboembolic disorders), hypersensitivity to progestins, severe liver dysfunction, estrogen-dependent neoplasia, undiagnosed abnormal genital bleeding, missed abortion, use as pregnancy test, undiagnosed vaginal bleeding, carcinoma of breast, known or suspected pregnancy.

CAUTIONS

Those w/conditions aggravated by fluid retention (asthma, seizures, migraine, cardiac or renal dysfunction), diabetes, history of mental depression.

INTERACTIONS

DRUG: May interfere w/effects of ***bromocriptine.*** **HERBAL:** None known. **FOOD:** None significant. **ALTERED LAB VALUES:** May increase alkaline phosphatase, LDL. May decrease HDL cholesterol.

SIDE EFFECTS

FREQUENT: Transient menstrual abnormalities (spotting, change in menstrual flow or cervical secretions, amenorrhea) at initiation of therapy. **OCCASIONAL:** Edema, weight change, breast tenderness, nervousness, insomnia, fatigue, dizziness. **RARE:** Alopecia, mental depression, dermatologic changes, headache, fever, nausea.

ADVERSE REACTIONS/TOXIC EFFECTS

Thrombophlebitis, pulmonary or cerebral embolism, retinal thrombosis occurs rarely.

PATIENT CONSIDERATIONS

Baseline Assessment

Question for hypersensitivity to progestins, possibility of pregnancy before initiating therapy (Pregnancy Category X). Obtain baseline weight, blood glucose, B/P.

Intervention/Evaluation

Check weight daily; report weekly gain of 5 lbs or more. Check B/P periodically. Assess skin for rash, hives. Report immediately the development of chest pain, sudden shortness of breath, sudden decrease in vision, migraine headache, pain (especially w/swelling, warmth, and redness) in calves, numbness of an arm or leg (thrombotic disorders). Monitor I&O in those with renal carcinoma or those experiencing weight gain. Note medroxyprogesterone therapy on pathology specimens.

Patient/Family Teaching

Importance of medical supervision. Do not take other medications w/o physician approval. Use sunscreens, protective clothing to protect from sunlight or ultraviolet light until tolerance determined. Notify physician of abnormal vaginal bleeding or other symptoms. Teach how to perform Homans' test and the signs and symptoms of blood clots (report these to physician immediately). Teach breast self-exam. Stop taking medication and contact physician at once if pregnancy is suspected.

medrysone

med-rih-sohn
(HMS Liquifilm)

PREGNANCY CATEGORY C

CLASSIFICATION

Corticosteroid, ophthalmic

AVAILABILITY (Rx)

Ophthalmic Suspension: 1%

PHARMACOKINETICS

Absorption: Absorbed into conjunctival sac, systemically absorbed.

ACTION/*THERAPEUTIC EFFECT*

Produces vasoconstriction, inhibits edema, fibrin deposition, and migration of leukocytes and phagocytes due to inflammatory response to mechanical, chemical, or immunologic agents.

USES

Symptomatic relief of inflammatory conditions of the conjunctiva, cornea, lid, and anterior segment of the globe (e.g., allergic conjunctivitis, superficial punctate keratitis, herpes zoster keratitis and cyclitis). Also used to help prevent fibrosis, scarring and potential visual impairment caused by chemical, radiation, or thermal burns or penetration of foreign bodies.

ADMINISTRATION

OPHTHALMIC:

- For topical ophthalmic use only.
- Position pt w/head tilted back, looking up.
- Gently pull lower lid down to form pouch and instill drops.
- Do not touch tip of applicator to lids or any surface.
- When lower lid is released, have pt keep eye open w/o blinking for at least 30 sec.
- Apply gentle finger pressure to lacrimal sac (bridge of the nose, inside corner of the eye) for 1–2 min after administration of solution.
- Remove excess solution around eye with a tissue. Wash hands immediately to remove medication.

INDICATIONS/ROUTES/DOSAGE

Usual ophthalmic dosage:
Adults, elderly: Instill 1 drop into conjunctival sac q4h; may increase to 1 drop q1–2h for severe cases. Gradually taper dosage when discontinuing medication.

CONTRAINDICATIONS

Hypersensitivity to any component of preparation, acute superficial herpes simplex keratitis, fungal diseases of ocular structure. In pts w/vaccinia, varicella, or most other viral diseases of the cornea and conjunctiva; ocular tuberculosis. Not for use in iritis or uveitis.

CAUTIONS

Safety and efficacy in children not established.

INTERACTIONS

DRUG: None significant. **HERBAL:** None known. **FOOD:** None significant. **ALTERED LAB VALUES:** None significant.

SIDE EFFECTS

OCCASIONAL: Transient stinging, burning on instillation. High doses may slow corneal healing. **RARE:** Filtering blebs after cataract surgery; hypersensitivity.

ADVERSE REACTIONS/TOXIC EFFECTS

Systemic reactions occur rarely with extensive use.

PATIENT CONSIDERATIONS

Baseline Assessment

Question for hypersensitivity to any components of preparation.

Intervention/Evaluation

Assess for therapeutic response, superinfection, delayed healing or irritation.

Patient/Family Teaching

Explain possible burning or stinging upon application. Visual acuity may be decreased after administration; avoid driving or operating machinery if vision decreases. Do not discontinue use w/o consulting physician. Notify physician if no improvement in 7–8 days, if condition worsens, or if pain, itching, or swelling of eye occurs. Sensitivity to bright light may occur; wear sunglasses to minimize discomfort.

megestrol acetate

meh-**jes**-troll
(Megace)

CANADIAN AVAILABILITY
Megace

PREGNANCY CATEGORY X
(Not recommended in first 4 mos of pregnancy)

CLASSIFICATION

Antineoplastic

AVAILABILITY (Rx)

Tablets: 20 mg, 40 mg. **Suspension:** 40 mg/ml.

PHARMACOKINETICS

Absorption: Well absorbed from GI tract. **Metabolism:** Metabolized in liver. **Excretion:** Excreted in urine.

ACTION/*THERAPEUTIC EFFECT*

Suppresses release of luteinizing hormone from anterior pituitary by inhibiting pituitary function, *regressing tumor size. Increases appetite* (mechanism unknown).

USES/*UNLABELED*

Palliative management of recurrent, inoperable, or metastatic endometrial or breast carcinoma. Treatment of anorexia, cachexia, or unexplained significant weight loss in pts w/AIDS. *Treatment of hormonally dependent/advanced prostate carcinoma.*

INDICATIONS/ROUTES/DOSAGE

Palliative treatment of advanced breast cancer:
Oral: Adults, elderly: 160 mg/day in 4 equally divided doses.

Palliative treatment of advanced endometrial carcinoma:
Oral: Adults, elderly: 40–320 mg/day in divided doses. *Maximum:* 800 mg/day.

Anorexia, cachexia, weight loss:
Oral: Adults, elderly: 800 mg (20 ml)/day.

CONTRAINDICATIONS

Known or suspected pregnancy.

CAUTIONS

History of thrombophlebitis.

INTERACTIONS

DRUG: None significant. **HERBAL:** None known. **FOOD:** None significant. **ALTERED LAB VALUES:** May increase serum glucose levels.

SIDE EFFECTS

FREQUENT: Weight gain sec-

M

ondary to increased appetite. **OCCASIONAL:** Nausea, breakthrough bleeding, backache, headache, breast tenderness, carpal tunnel syndrome. **RARE:** Feeling of coldness.

ADVERSE REACTIONS/TOXIC EFFECTS

Thrombophlebitis, pulmonary embolism occurs rarely.

PATIENT CONSIDERATIONS

BASELINE ASSESSMENT

Question for possibility of pregnancy before initiating therapy (Pregnancy Category X). Provide support to pt, family, recognizing this drug is palliative, not curative.

PATIENT/FAMILY TEACHING

Importance of contraception. Notify physician if headache, nausea, breast tenderness, or other symptom persists.

---

meloxicam
(Mobic)
See Supplement

---

melphalan
(Alkeran)
See Classification section under: Cancer chemotherapy

---

menotropins

men-oh-**troe**-pins
(Humegon, Pergonal, Repronex)

CANADIAN AVAILABILITY
Pergonal

PREGNANCY CATEGORY X

CLASSIFICATION

Gonadotropin

AVAILABILITY (Rx)

Powder for Injection: 75 IU FSH/LH, 150 IU FSH/LH activity

PHARMACOKINETICS

Absorption: Well absorbed after IM administration. **Excretion:** Excreted in urine. **Half-life:** ***FSH:*** *70 hrs;* ***LH:*** *4 hrs.*

ACTION/ *THERAPEUTIC EFFECT*

Gonadotropic agent w/follicle-stimulating hormone (FSH) and luteinizing hormone (LH) actions. *Promotes ovarian follicular growth and maturation in women; stimulates spermatogenesis in men.*

USES

Treatment of infertility in conjunction w/chorionic gonadotropin (HCG) to stimulate ovulation and pregnancy in women w/secondary ovarian dysfunction and to stimulate spermatogenesis in men w/primary or secondary hypogonadotropic hypogonadism.

STORAGE/HANDLING

Powder for reconstitution may be refrigerated or kept at room temperature.

ADMINISTRATION

IM:

- Reconstitute w/1–2 ml 0.9% NaCl injection.
- Administer immediately after reconstitution; discard unused portion.
- Give IM only.

INDICATIONS/ROUTES/DOSAGE

Induction ovulation/pregnancy: *IM: Adults:* Initially, 75 IU FSH/75 IU LH per day for 9–12 days. Follow w/10,000 IU HCG 1 day after last dose menotropin. May repeat at least 2 courses before increasing dose to 150 IU FSH/150 IU LH if evidence of ovulation, but no pregnancy.

Note: Omit HCG if hyperstimulation syndrome likely to occur (total estrogen excretion >100 mcg/24 hrs or estradiol excretion >50 mcg/24 hrs) or ovaries abnormally enlarged on last day of menotropin therapy.

Stimulation of spermatogenesis: **Note:** Pretreat w/HCG alone (5,000 IU 3 times/wk) until normal serum testosterone level and masculinization. May take 4–6 mos.

IM: Adults: Initially, 75 IU FSH/75 IU LH 3 times/wk and HCG 2,000 IU 2 times/wk for at least 4 mos. If no response, may increase dose to 150 IU FSH/150 IU LH w/same HCG dose.

CONTRAINDICATIONS

Prior hypersensitivity to menotropins; primary ovarian failure; thyroid or adrenal dysfunction; organic intracranial lesion (e.g., pituitary tumor); ovarian cysts or enlargement not due to polycystic ovary syndrome; abnormal vaginal bleeding of undetermined origin; men w/normal urinary gonadotropin concentrations, primary testicular failure or infertility problems other than hypogonadotropic hypogonadism.

INTERACTIONS

DRUG: None significant. **HERBAL:** None known. **FOOD:** None significant. **ALTERED LAB VALUES:** None significant.

SIDE EFFECTS

FREQUENT: Irritation, pain, swelling at injection site, rash. ***Females:*** Ovarian enlargement/ovarian cysts w/abdominal distension. **OCCASIONAL:** *Males:* Erythrocytosis (shortness of breath, irregular heartbeat, dizziness, anorexia, headache, fainting), gynecomastia.

ADVERSE REACTIONS/TOXIC EFFECTS

Risk of atelectasis and acute respiratory distress syndrome, intravascular thrombosis and embolism, ovarian hyperstimulation syndrome (OHSS), high incidence (20%) of multiple births (premature deliveries and neonatal prematurity), ruptured ovarian cysts.

PATIENT CONSIDERATIONS

Baseline Assessment

Question for prior allergic reaction to drug.

Intervention/Evaluation

Monitor carefully for OHSS; early signs include weight gain, severe pelvic pain, nausea, vomiting progressing to ascites, dyspnea; report immediately. (Ascitic, pleural, or pericardial fluids should not be removed unless absolutely necessary because of potential injury to the ovary.) Pelvic examination should be avoided due to potential rupture of an ovarian cyst.

Patient/Family Teaching

Importance of close physician supervision during treatment. Promptly report abdominal pain/distension, vaginal bleeding or signs of edema (weigh 2–3 times/week; report >5 lbs/wk gain or swelling of fingers or feet). In anovulation

treatment, teach proper method of taking/recording daily basal temperature; advise intercourse daily beginning the day preceding HCG treatment. Intercourse should be discontinued w/significant ovarian enlargement. Possibility of multiple births.

meperidine hydrochloride

meh-**pear**-ih-deen
(Demerol)

CANADIAN AVAILABILITY
Demerol

PREGNANCY CATEGORY B
(D if used for prolonged periods or at high doses at term)

CLASSIFICATION

Opiate analgesic **(Schedule II)**

AVAILABILITY (Rx)

Tablets: 50 mg, 100 mg. **Syrup:** 50 mg/5 ml. **Injection:** 10 mg/ml, 25 mg/ml, 50 mg/ml, 75 mg/ml, 100 mg/ml.

PHARMACODYNAMICS

	ONSET	PEAK	DURATION
Oral			
	15 min	60 min	2–4 hrs
SubQ			
	10–15 min	30–50 min	2–4 hrs
IM			
	10–15 min	30–50 min	2–4 hrs
IV			
	1 min	5–7 min	2–4 hrs

PHARMACOKINETICS

Absorption: Variably absorbed from GI tract, well absorbed after IM administration. Widely distributed. **Metabolism:** Metabolized in liver to active metabolite. **Excretion:** Primarily excreted in urine. **Half-life:** 2.4–4 hrs (increased in elderly).

ACTION / *THERAPEUTIC EFFECT*

Binds w/opioid receptors within CNS, *altering processes affecting pain perception, emotional response to pain.*

USES

Relief of moderate to severe pain, preop sedation, obstetrical support, anesthesia adjunct.

STORAGE/HANDLING

Store oral, parenteral form at room temperature. Do not use if solution appears cloudy or contains a precipitate.

ADMINISTRATION

ORAL:

- May give w/o regard to meals.
- Dilute syrup in glass H_2O (prevents anesthetic effect on mucous membranes).

SUBQ/IM:

- **Note:** IM preferred over SubQ route (SubQ produces pain, local irritation, induration).
- Administer slowly.
- Those with circulatory impairment experience higher risk of overdosage due to delayed absorption of repeated administration.

IV:

- **Note:** Give by slow IV injection or IV infusion. Physically incompatible with amobarbital, aminophylline, ephedrine, heparin, hydrocortisone, methicillin, methylprednisolone, morphine, nitrofurantoin, oxytetracycline, pentobarbital, phenobarbital, secobarbital, sodium bicarbonate, sodium iodide, tetracycline, thiamylal, thiopental, solutions containing potassium iodide, aminosalicylic acid, salicylamide.

- Dilute in 5% dextrose and lactated Ringer's, dextrose-saline combination, 2.5%, 5%, or 10% dextrose in water, Ringer's, lactated Ringer's, 0.45% or 0.9% NaCl, or molar sodium lactate diluent for IV injection or infusion.
- IV dosage must always be administered very slowly, over 2–3 min.
- Rapid IV increases risk of severe adverse reactions (chest wall rigidity, apnea, peripheral circulatory collapse, anaphylactoid effects, cardiac arrest).

INDICATIONS/ROUTES/DOSAGE

Pain:
Oral/IM/SubQ: Adults: 50–150 mg q3–4h. ***Children:*** 1.1–1.8 mg/kg q3–4h. Do not exceed single pediatric dose 100 mg.

IV: Adults: 15–35 mg/hr.

Usual elderly dosage:
Oral: 50 mg q4h as needed.

IM: 25 mg q4h as needed.

Preop:
IM/SubQ: Adults: 50–100 mg given as single dose 30–90 min before induction of anesthesia. ***Children:*** 1–2 mg/kg 30–90 min before anesthesia.

Labor:
IM: Adults: 50–100 mg when labor pains are regular. Repeat at 1–3 hr intervals.

CONTRAINDICATIONS

Those receiving MAO inhibitors in past 14 days, diarrhea due to poisoning, delivery of premature infant.

CAUTIONS

Impaired renal, hepatic function, elderly/debilitated, supraventricular tachycardia, cor pulmonale, history of seizures, acute abdominal conditions, increased intracranial pressure, respiratory abnormalities.

INTERACTIONS

DRUG: ***Alcohol, CNS depressants*** may increase CNS or respiratory depression, hypotension. ***MAO inhibitors*** may produce severe, fatal reaction (reduce dose to 1/4 usual dose). **HERBAL:** None known. **FOOD:** None significant. **ALTERED LAB VALUES:** May increase amylase, lipase.

SIDE EFFECTS

Note: Effects are dependent on dosage amount, route of administration. Ambulatory pts and those not in severe pain may experience dizziness, nausea, vomiting more frequently than those in supine position or having severe pain. **FREQUENT:** Histamine reaction (decreased blood pressure, increased sweating, flushed face, wheezing), constipation, dizziness, drowsiness, hypotension, nausea, vomiting, unusually tired. **OCCASIONAL:** Shortness of breath, trouble breathing, confusion, irregular heartbeat, tremors, decreased urination, stomach pain, dry mouth, headache, redness, pain, swelling at injection site. **RARE:** Allergic reaction (rash, itching), paralytic ileus, inability to sleep.

ADVERSE REACTIONS/TOXIC EFFECTS

Overdosage results in respiratory

M

depression, skeletal muscle flaccidity, cold clammy skin, cyanosis, extreme somnolence progressing to convulsions, stupor, coma. Antidote: 0.4 mg naloxone (Narcan). Tolerance to analgesic effect, physical dependence may occur with repeated use.

PATIENT CONSIDERATIONS

Baseline Assessment

Pt should be in recumbent position before drug is administered by parenteral route. Assess onset, type, location, duration of pain. Obtain vital signs before giving medication. If respirations are 12/min or lower (20/min or lower in children), withhold medication, contact physician. Effect of medication is reduced if full pain recurs before next dose.

Intervention/Evaluation

Monitor vital signs 15–30 min after SubQ/IM dose, 5–10 min after IV dose (monitor for decreased B/P, change in rate/quality of pulse). Monitor stools; avoid constipation. Check for adequate voiding. Initiate deep breathing and coughing exercises, particularly in those with impaired pulmonary function.

Patient/Family Teaching

Medication should be taken before pain fully returns, within ordered intervals. Discomfort may occur with injection. Change positions slowly to avoid orthostatic hypotension. Avoid tasks that require alertness, motor skills until response to drug is established. Increase fluids, bulk to prevent constipation. Tolerance/dependence may occur with prolonged use of high doses. Avoid alcohol and other CNS depressants.

---

mepivacaine hydrochloride

(Carbocaine, Polocaine)

FIXED-COMBINATION(S)
W/levonordefrin, a vasoconstrictor (Isocaine)

See Classification section under: Anesthetics: local

---

mercaptopurine

(Purinethol)
See Classification section under: Cancer chemotherapy

---

meropenem

murr-oh-**pen**-em
(Merrem IV)

CANADIAN AVAILABILITY
Merrem IV

PREGNANCY CATEGORY B

CLASSIFICATION

Antibiotic

AVAILABILITY (Rx)

Powder for Injection: 500 mg, 1 g

PHARMACOKINETICS

Following IV administration, widely distributed into tissues/fluid including cerebrospinal fluid. **Excretion:** Primarily excreted unchanged in urine. Removed by hemodialysis. **Half-life:** 1 hr.

ACTION/*THERAPEUTIC EFFECT*

Penetrates most gram-positive and gram-negative cell walls, *inhibiting bacterial cell wall synthesis. Bactericidal.*

USES / *UNLABELED*

Treatment of intra-abdominal infections, bacterial meningitis (pediatric pts ≤3 mos only), cystic fibrosis. *Lowers respiratory infections, febrile neutropenia, obstetric/gynecologic infections, sepsis.*

STORAGE/HANDLING

Store vials at room temperature. After reconstitution w/0.9% NaCl, stable for 4 hrs at room temperature, 24 hrs if refrigerated (w/5% dextrose, stable for 1 hr at room temperature, 4 hrs if refrigerated).

ADMINISTRATION

IV:

- May give by IV bolus injection or IV intermittent infusion (piggyback).
- If administering as IV intermittent infusion (piggyback), give over 15–30 min; if administered by IV bolus injection (5–20 ml), give over 3–5 min.

INDICATIONS/ROUTES/DOSAGE

Note: Space doses evenly around the clock.

Usual parenteral dosage:
IV: Adults, elderly: 1 g q8h.

Intra-abdominal (pediatric):
IV: Children ≥3 mos: 20 mg/kg q8h. *Children >50 kg:* 1 g q8h. *Maximum:* 2 g q8h.

Meningitis (pediatric):
IV: Children ≥3 mos: 40 mg/kg q8h. *Children >50 kg:* 2 g q8h. *Maximum:* 2 g q8h.

Dosage in renal impairment:
Reduce dosage in pts w/creatinine clearance <50 ml/min.

CREATININE CLEARANCE	DOSAGE	DOSING INTERVAL
26–50 ml/min	Recommended dose (1,000 mg)	q12h
10–25 ml/min	½ recommended dose	q12h
<10 ml/min	½ recommended dose	q24h

CONTRAINDICATIONS

Hypersensitivity to meropenem, other beta lactams.

CAUTIONS

Hypersensitivity to penicillins, cephalosporins, other allergens; renal function impairment, CNS disorders, particularly w/history of seizures.

INTERACTIONS

DRUG: *Probenecid* inhibits renal excretion of meropenem (do not use concurrently). **HERBAL:** None known. **FOOD:** None significant. **ALTERED LAB VALUES:** May increase SGOT (AST), SGPT (ALT), alkaline phosphatase, LDH, bilirubin, BUN, creatinine. May decrease Hgb, Hct, potassium.

SIDE EFFECTS

FREQUENT: Diarrhea (5%), nausea, vomiting (4%), headache, inflammation at injection site (3%). **OCCASIONAL:** Oral moniliasis, rash, pruritus (2%). **RARE:** Constipation, glossitis.

ADVERSE REACTIONS/TOXIC EFFECTS

Antibiotic-associated colitis, other superinfections may occur. Anaphylactic reactions in those receiving beta lactams have occurred. Seizures may occur in those w/CNS disorders (brain lesions, history of seizures) or w/bacterial meningitis or impaired renal function.

M

PATIENT CONSIDERATIONS

BASELINE ASSESSMENT

Question pt for history of allergies, particularly to meropenem, other beta lactams, penicillins, cephalosporins. Inquire about history of seizures. Obtain culture and sensitivity tests before giving first dose (therapy may begin before results are known).

INTERVENTION/EVALUATION

Monitor daily bowel activity and stool consistency (watery, loose, soft). Monitor for nausea, vomiting. Evaluate hydration status. Evaluate for inflammation at IV injection site. Assess skin for rash. Monitor I&O, renal function tests. Check mental status; be alert to tremors and possible seizures. Assess temperature, B/P twice daily, more often if necessary. Monitor electrolytes, especially potassium.

PATIENT/FAMILY TEACHING

Continue therapy for full length of treatment. Doses should be evenly spaced. Do not take any other medication unless approved by physician. Notify physician in event of tremors, seizures, rash, diarrhea, or other new symptom.

---

mesalamine (5-aminosalicylic acid, 5-ASA)

mess-**al**-ah-meen

(Asacol, Fiv-ASA, Pentasa, Rowasa)

CANADIAN AVAILABILITY

Asacol, Mesasal, Pentasa, Quintasa, Salofalk

PREGNANCY CATEGORY B

CLASSIFICATION

Anti-inflammatory agent

AVAILABILITY (Rx)

Tablets (delayed-release): 400 mg. **Capsules (control-release):** 250 mg. **Suppository:** 500 mg. **Rectal Suspension:** 4 g/60 ml.

PHARMACOKINETICS

Absorption: Poorly absorbed from colon. Moderately absorbed from GI tract. **Metabolism:** Metabolized in liver to active metabolite. **Excretion:** Unabsorbed portion eliminated in feces; absorbed portion excreted in urine. **Half-life:** 0.5–1.5 hrs; metabolite: 5–10 hrs.

ACTION/*THERAPEUTIC EFFECT*

Produces local inhibitory effect on arachidonic acid metabolite production (increased in pts w/chronic inflammatory bowel disease). *Blocks prostaglandin production, diminishes inflammation in colon.*

USES

Treatment of active mild to moderate distal ulcerative colitis, proctosigmoiditis, or proctitis. Asacol: Maintenance of remission of ulcerative colitis.

STORAGE/HANDLING

Store rectal suspension, suppository, oral forms at room temperature.

ADMINISTRATION

ORAL:

- Have pt swallow whole; do not break outer coating of tablet.
- May take w/o regard to food.

RECTAL:

- Shake bottle well.
- Instruct pt to lie on left side with

lower leg extended, upper leg flexed forward.

- Knee-chest position may also be used.
- Insert applicator tip into rectum, pointing toward umbilicus.
- Squeeze bottle steadily until contents are emptied.

INDICATIONS/ROUTES/DOSAGE

Ulcerative colitis, proctosigmoiditis, proctitis:
Oral: Adults, elderly: (Asacol): 800 mg 3 times/day for 6 wks; *(Pentasa):* 1 g 4 times/day for 8 wks.

Rectal: Adults, elderly: (suppository): 500 mg 2 times/day. Retain 1–3 hrs (suspension) 4 g (60 ml) daily, preferably at bedtime.

Maintenance of remission ulcerative colitis:
Oral: Adults, elderly: 1.6 g/day in divided doses.

CONTRAINDICATIONS

None significant.

CAUTIONS

Preexisting renal disease, sulfasalazine sensitivity.

INTERACTIONS

DRUG: None significant. **HERBAL:** None known. **FOOD:** None significant. **ALTERED LAB VALUES:** May increase SGOT (AST), SGPT (ALT), alkaline phosphatase, BUN, serum creatinine.

SIDE EFFECTS

Note: Generally well tolerated, with only mild and transient effects. **FREQUENT (>6%):** *Oral:* Abdominal cramps, pain, diarrhea, dizziness, headache, nausea, vomiting, rhinitis, unusually tired. *Rectal:* Abdominal or stomach cramps, flatulence, headache, nausea. **OCCASIONAL (2–6%):** *Oral:* Mild hair loss, flatulence, decreased appetite, back or joint pain, acne. *Rectal:* Alopecia. **RARE (<2%):** *Oral:* Hepatitis, pancreatitis, pericarditis. *Rectal:* Anal irritation, hepatitis, pancreatitis, pericarditis.

ADVERSE REACTIONS/TOXIC EFFECTS

Sulfite sensitivity in susceptible pts noted as cramping, headache, diarrhea, fever, rash, hives, itching, wheezing. Discontinue drug immediately. Hepatitis, pancreatitis, pericarditis occur rarely w/oral dosage.

PATIENT CONSIDERATIONS

INTERVENTION/EVALUATION

Encourage adequate fluid intake. Assess bowel sounds for peristalsis. Monitor daily bowel activity and stool consistency (watery, loose, soft, semisolid, solid) and record time of evacuation. Assess for abdominal disturbances. Assess skin for rash, hives. Discontinue medication if rash, fever, cramping, or diarrhea occurs.

PATIENT/FAMILY TEACHING

Avoid tasks that require alertness, motor skills until response to drug is established.

mesna

mess-nah
(Mesnex)

CANADIAN AVAILABILITY
Uromitexan

PREGNANCY CATEGORY B

M

CLASSIFICATION

Antidote

AVAILABILITY (Rx)

Injection: 100 mg/ml

PHARMACOKINETICS

Metabolism: Rapidly metabolized after IV administration to mesna disulfide, which is reduced to mesna in kidney. **Excretion:** Excreted in urine. **Half-life:** 0.36 hrs.

ACTION/*THERAPEUTIC EFFECT*

Reduced to free thiol compound, mesna, which reacts with urotoxic ifosfamide metabolites (detoxification). *Inhibits ifosfamide-induced hemorrhagic cystitis.*

USES

Decreased incidence of ifosfamide-induced hemorrhagic cystitis.

STORAGE/HANDLING

Store parenteral form at room temperature. After dilution, stable for 24 hrs at room temperature (recommended use within 6 hrs). Discard unused medication.

ADMINISTRATION

IV:

- Dilute each 100 mg with 5% dextrose or 0.9% NaCl to provide concentration of 20 mg/ml.
- Administer direct IV injection.

INDICATIONS/ROUTES/DOSAGE

Hemorrhagic cystitis:
IV: Adults, elderly: 20% of ifosfamide dose at time of ifosfamide administration and 4 and 8 hrs after each dose of ifosfamide. Total dose: 60% of ifosfamide dosage.

CONTRAINDICATIONS

None significant.

CAUTIONS

None significant.

INTERACTIONS

DRUG: None significant. **HERBAL:** None known. **FOOD:** None significant. **ALTERED LAB VALUES:** May produce false-positive test for urinary ketones.

SIDE EFFECTS

FREQUENT (>17%): Bad taste in mouth, soft stools. ***Large doses:*** Diarrhea, limb pain, headache, fatigue, nausea, hypotension, allergic reaction.

ADVERSE REACTIONS/TOXIC EFFECTS

Hematuria occurs occasionally.

PATIENT CONSIDERATIONS

BASELINE ASSESSMENT

Each dose must be administered with ifosfamide.

INTERVENTION/EVALUATION

Assess morning urine specimen for hematuria. If such occurs, dosage reduction or discontinuation may be necessary. Monitor daily bowel activity and stool consistency (watery, loose, soft, semisolid, solid) and record time of evacuation. Monitor B/P for hypotension.

PATIENT/FAMILY TEACHING

Inform physician/nurse if headache, limb pain, or nausea occurs.

mesoridazine besylate

mess-oh-**rid**-ah-zeen
(Serentil)

CANADIAN AVAILABILITY
Serentil

PREGNANCY CATEGORY C

CLASSIFICATION

Antipsychotic

AVAILABILITY (Rx)

Tablets: 10 mg, 25 mg, 50 mg, 100 mg. **Oral Concentrate:** 25 mg/ml. **Injection:** 25 mg/ml.

PHARMACOKINETICS

Absorption: Variably absorbed from GI tract. **Metabolism:** Metabolized in liver to some active metabolites. **Excretion:** Primarily excreted in urine. **Half-life:** 20–40 hrs.

ACTION/*THERAPEUTIC EFFECT*

Blocks dopamine at postsynaptic receptor sites in brain. *Suppresses behavioral response in psychosis.* Strong anticholinergic, sedative effects.

USES

Symptomatic management of psychotic disorders, treatment of hyperactivity, uncooperativeness associated w/mental deficiency, chronic brain syndrome; as adjunctive treatment of alcohol dependence, management of anxiety/tension associated w/neurosis.

STORAGE/HANDLING

Store oral, parenteral form at room temperature. Yellow discoloration of solution does not affect potency, but discard if markedly discolored or if precipitate forms.

ADMINISTRATION

ORAL:

- Dilute oral solution w/water, orange or grape juice.

IM:

- **Note:** Pt must remain recumbent for 30–60 min in head-low position w/legs raised, to minimize hypotensive effect.
- Inject slow, deep IM into upper outer quadrant of gluteus maximus. If irritation occurs, further injections may be diluted w/0.9% NaCl or 2% procaine hydrochloride.
- Massage IM injection site to reduce discomfort.

INDICATIONS/ROUTES/DOSAGE

Note: Increase dosage gradually to optimum response, then decrease to lowest effective level for maintenance. Replace parenteral therapy w/oral therapy as soon as possible.

Usual parenteral dosage:
IM: Adults, children >12 yrs: 25 mg given as single dose. May repeat in 30–60 min, if needed. ***Maximum dose:*** 200 mg/day.

Psychotic disorders:
Oral: Adults, children >12 yrs: Initially, 50 mg 3 times/day. ***Maintenance:*** 100–400 mg/day.

Hyperactivity:
Oral: Adults, children >12 yrs: 25 mg 3 times/day. ***Maintenance:*** 75–300 mg/day.

Alcohol dependence:
Oral: Adults, children >12 yrs: 25 mg twice/day. ***Maintenance:*** 50–200 mg/day.

Anxiety/tension:
Oral: Adults, children >12 yrs: 10 mg 3 times/day. ***Maintenance:*** 30–150 mg/day.

Usual elderly dosage (nonpsychotic):
Oral: Initially, 10 mg 1–2 times/day. May increase by 10–25 mg/day every 7–10 days. ***Maximum:*** 250 mg/day.

CONTRAINDICATIONS

Severe CNS depression, comatose states, severe cardiovascular disease, bone marrow depression, subcortical brain damage.

CAUTIONS

Impaired respiratory/hepatic/renal/cardiac function, alcohol withdrawal, history of seizures, urinary retention, glaucoma, prostatic hypertrophy.

INTERACTIONS

DRUG: ***Alcohol, CNS depressants*** may increase CNS, respiratory depression, hypotensive effects. ***Tricyclic antidepressants, MAO inhibitors*** may increase sedative, anticholinergic effects. ***Antithyroid agents*** may increase risk of agranulocytosis. Extrapyramidal symptoms (EPS) may increase ***w/EPS-producing medications. Hypotensives*** may increase hypotension. May decrease ***levodopa*** effects. ***Lithium*** may decrease absorption, produce adverse neurologic effects. **HERBAL:** None known. **FOOD:** None significant. **ALTERED LAB VALUES:** May produce false-positive pregnancy test, PKU. EKG changes may occur, including Q and T wave disturbances.

SIDE EFFECTS

FREQUENT: Orthostatic hypotension, dizziness, and fainting occur frequently after first injection, occasionally after subsequent injections, and rarely w/oral dosage. **OCCASIONAL:** Drowsiness during early therapy, dry mouth, blurred vision, lethargy, constipation or diarrhea, nasal congestion, peripheral edema, urinary retention. **RARE:** Ocular changes, skin pigmentation (those on high doses for prolonged periods).

ADVERSE REACTIONS/TOXIC EFFECTS

Abrupt withdrawal following long-term therapy may precipitate nausea, vomiting, gastritis, dizziness, tremors. Blood dyscrasias, particularly agranulocytosis, mild leukopenia (sore mouth/gums/throat) may occur. May lower seizure threshold.

PATIENT CONSIDERATIONS

BASELINE ASSESSMENT

Avoid skin contact w/solution (contact dermatitis). Assess behavior, appearance, emotional status, response to environment, speech pattern, thought content.

INTERVENTION/EVALUATION

Assess for orthostatic hypotension. Monitor stool frequency and consistency (watery, loose, soft, semisolid, solid). Monitor WBC, differential count for blood dyscrasias. Supervise suicidal risk pt closely during early therapy (as depression lessens, energy level improves, increasing suicide potential). Assess for therapeutic response (interest in surroundings, improvement in self-care, increased ability to concentrate, relaxed facial expression).

PATIENT/FAMILY TEACHING

Full therapeutic effect may take up to 6 wks. Urine may become pink, reddish brown. Do not abruptly withdraw from long-term drug therapy. Report visual disturbances. Sugarless gum, sips of tepid water may relieve dry mouth. Drowsiness generally subsides during continued therapy. Avoid tasks that require alertness, motor skills until response to drug is established. Do not use alcohol or other CNS depressants. Use sunscreen, protective clothing for possible photosensitivity.

metaproterenol sulfate

met-ah-pro-**tair**-in-all
(Alupent, Metaprel)

CANADIAN AVAILABILITY
Alupent

PREGNANCY CATEGORY C

CLASSIFICATION

Bronchodilator

AVAILABILITY (Rx)

Tablets: 10 mg, 20 mg. **Syrup:** 10 mg/5 ml. **Aerosol Solution for Inhalation:** 0.4%, 0.6%, 5%.

PHARMACODYNAMICS

	ONSET	PEAK	DURATION
Aerosol			
	1 min	1 hr	4 hrs
Oral	15 min	1 hr	4 hrs
Nebulization			
	5–30 min	1 hr	3–4 hrs

PHARMACOKINETICS

Absorption: Partially absorbed from GI tract, minimal after inhalation. **Metabolism:** Metabolized in liver. **Excretion:** Primarily excreted in urine.

ACTION/*THERAPEUTIC EFFECT*

Stimulates $beta_2$-adrenergic receptors resulting in relaxation of bronchial smooth muscle, *relieving bronchospasm; reduces airway resistance.*

USES

Relief of reversible bronchospasm due to bronchial asthma, bronchitis, emphysema.

STORAGE/HANDLING

Do not use solution for nebulization if brown in color or contains a precipitate.

ADMINISTRATION

AEROSOL:

- Shake container well, exhale completely, then holding mouthpiece 1 inch away from lips, inhale and hold breath as long as possible before exhaling.
- Wait 1–10 min before inhaling second dose (allows for deeper bronchial penetration).
- Rinse mouth w/water immediately after inhalation (prevents mouth/throat dryness).

ORAL:

- Give w/o regard to meals.
- Tablets may be crushed.

NEBULIZATION:

- Administer undiluted solution in hand nebulizer.

IPPB:

- Dilute in 2.5 ml saline solution.

INDICATIONS/ROUTES/DOSAGE

Bronchospasm:
Metered-Dose Inhalation: Adults, elderly, children >12 yrs: 2–3 inhalations as single dose. Wait 2 min before administering second dose. Do not repeat for 3–4 hrs. ***Maximum:*** 12 inhalations/day.

Oral: Adults, children >9 yrs or weigh >60 lbs: 20 mg 3–4 times/day. ***Children 6–9 yrs or weigh <60 lbs:*** 10 mg 3–4 times/day.

Nebulization: Adults, elderly, children >12 yrs: 10 inhalations (range 5–15 inhalations) of undiluted 5% solution, up to 3–4 times/day.

IPPB: Adults, elderly: 0.3 ml 3–4 times/day. May repeat no more often than q4h.

Usual elderly dosage:
Oral: Initially, 10 mg 3–4 times/day. May increase up to 20 mg 3–4 times/day.

CONTRAINDICATIONS

Preexisting arrhythmias.

CAUTIONS

Impaired cardiac function, diabetes mellitus, hypertension, hyperthyroidism.

INTERACTIONS

DRUG: *Tricyclic antidepressants* may increase cardiovascular effects. *MAO inhibitors* may increase risk of hypertensive crises. May decrease effects of *beta blockers. Digoxin, sympathomimetics* may increase risk of arrhythmias. **HERBAL:** Ma Huang (Ephedra) may increase CNS stimulation. **FOOD:** None significant. ALTERED LAB VALUES: May decrease serum potassium levels.

SIDE EFFECTS

FREQUENT (>10%): Tremors, tachycardia, shakiness, nervousness, nausea, vomiting, dry mouth. OCCASIONAL (1–10%): Palpitations, dizziness, vertigo,weakness, headache, GI distress, cough, dry throat. **RARE (<1%):** Changes in blood pressure, drowsiness, diarrhea, unusual taste.

ADVERSE REACTIONS/TOXIC EFFECTS

Excessive sympathomimetic stimulation may cause palpitations, extrasystoles, tachycardia, chest pain, slight increase in B/P followed by a substantial decrease, chills, sweating, and blanching of skin. Too frequent or excessive use may lead to loss of bronchodilating effectiveness and/or severe, paradoxical bronchoconstriction.

PATIENT CONSIDERATIONS

BASELINE ASSESSMENT

Offer emotional support (high incidence of anxiety because of difficulty in breathing and sympathomimetic response to drug).

INTERVENTION/EVALUATION

Monitor rate, depth, rhythm, type of respiration; quality and rate of pulse. Assess lung sounds for rhonchi, wheezing, rales. Monitor arterial blood gases. Observe lips, fingernails for blue or dusky color in light-skinned pts; gray in dark-skinned pts. Observe for clavicular retractions, hand tremor. Evaluate for clinical improvement (quieter, slower respirations, relaxed facial expression, cessation of clavicular retractions).

PATIENT/FAMILY TEACHING

Increase fluid intake (decreases lung secretion viscosity). Do not take more than 2 inhalations at any one time (excessive use may produce paradoxical bronchoconstriction or a decreased bronchodilating effect). Rinsing mouth w/water immediately after inhalation may prevent mouth/throat dryness. Avoid excessive use of caffeine derivatives (chocolate, coffee, tea, cola, cocoa).

---

metaraminol bitartrate

(Aramine)

See Classification section under: Sympathomimetics

metformin

met-**for**-min
(Glucophage)

FIXED-COMBINATION(S)
W/glyburide, an antidiabetic **(Glucovance)**

CANADIAN AVAILABILITY
Glucophage, Novo-Metformin

PREGNANCY CATEGORY B

CLASSIFICATION

Antidiabetic (antihyperglycemic)

AVAILABILITY (Rx)

Tablets: 500 mg, 850 mg. **Extended-Release Tablet.**

PHARMACOKINETICS

Absorption: Slowly, incompletely absorbed following oral administration (food delays/decreases extent of absorption). Primarily distributed to intestinal mucosa, salivary glands. **Excretion:** Primarily excreted unchanged in urine. Removed by hemodialysis. **Half-life:** 8.9–19 hrs.

ACTION/*THERAPEUTIC EFFECT*

Lowers both basal and postprandial plasma glucose by decreasing hepatic glucose production, intestinal absorption of glucose and improves insulin sensitivity. *Provides improvement in glycemic control, stabilizes or decreases body weight, improves lipid profile.*

USES/*UNLABELED*

Adjunct to diet in management of noninsulin-dependent diabetes mellitus (type 2, NIDDM) whose hyperglycemia cannot be managed by diet alone. May be used concurrently with a sulfonylurea antidiabetic agent or insulin when diet and metformin or a sulfonylurea alone do not result in adequate glycemic control. *Treatment of metabolic complications of AIDS, weight loss.*

ADMINISTRATION

ORAL:

- When transferring pts from oral hypoglycemic agents other than chlorpropamide, no transition period necessary. When transferring from chlorpropamide, exercise care during first 2 wks (prolonged retention of chlorpropamide) as overlapping drug effects, possible hypoglycemia may occur.
- If no adequate response to maximum dose of metformin within 4 wks, gradually add oral sulfonylurea antidiabetic agent while continuing metformin at maximum dose.
- Do not crush film-coated tablets.
- Give w/meals.

INDICATIONS/ROUTES/DOSAGE

Diabetes mellitus (500 mg tablet):

Oral: Adults, elderly: Initially, 500 mg twice daily (w/morning and evening meals). May increase dosage in 500 mg increments every week, in divided doses. Can be given twice daily up to 2,000 mg/day (e.g., 1,000 mg twice daily w/morning and evening meals). If 2,500 mg/day dose is required, give 3 times/day w/meals. ***Maximum dose/day:*** 2,500 mg/day.

Diabetes mellitus (850 mg tablet):

Oral: Adults, elderly: Initially, 850 mg/day, w/morning meal. May increase dosage in 850 mg increments every *other* week, in divided doses. ***Maintenance:*** 850 mg twice daily (w/morning and evening meals). ***Maximum dose/day:*** 2,550 mg (850 mg 3 times/day).

CONTRAINDICATIONS

History of lactic acidosis, conditions associated w/hypoxemia (e.g., CHF), hypersensitivity to metformin, renal disease or dysfunction (serum creatinine >1.5 mg/dl [males], >1.4 mg/dl [females]) or abnormal creatinine clearance (Ccr), acute or chronic metabolic acidosis, including diabetic ketoacidosis, with or w/o coma.

CAUTIONS

Conditions delaying food absorption (e.g., diarrhea, gastroparesis, vomiting), causing hyperglycemia (e.g., high fever) or hypoglycemia (e.g., malnutrition), uncontrolled hypo/hyperthyroidism, cardiovascular pts, concurrent drugs that effect renal function, hepatic impairment, elderly, malnourished, or debilitated. Pts w/decreased renal function, CHF, excessive alcohol intake, chronic respiratory difficulty.

INTERACTIONS

DRUG: ***Alcohol, amiloride, digoxin, morphine, procainamide, quinidine, quinine, ranitidine, triamterene, trimethoprim, vancomycin, cimetidine, furosemide, nifedipine*** increases metformin concentration. ***Furosemide, hypoglycemia-causing medication*** may decrease dosage of metformin needed. ***Iodinated contrast studies*** may produce acute renal failure (increases risk of lactic acidosis). **HERBAL:** None known. **FOOD:** None significant. **ALTERED LAB VALUES:** None significant.

SIDE EFFECTS

FREQUENT (>3%): GI disturbances are transient and resolve spontaneously during therapy (diarrhea, nausea, vomiting, abdominal bloating, flatulence, anorexia). **OCCASIONAL (1–3%):** Unpleasant or metallic taste (resolves spontaneously during therapy).

ADVERSE REACTIONS/TOXIC EFFECTS

Lactic acidosis occurs rarely (0.03 cases/1,000 pts) but is a serious, often fatal (50%) complication. Characterized by increase in blood lactate levels (>5 mmol/L), decrease in blood pH, electrolyte disturbances. Symptoms include unexplained hyperventilation, myalgia, malaise, somnolence. May advance to cardiovascular collapse (shock), acute CHF, acute MI, prerenal azotemia.

PATIENT CONSIDERATIONS

BASELINE ASSESSMENT

Inform pt of potential risks and advantages of therapy (see Adverse Reactions/Toxic Effects) and of alternative modes of therapy. Before initiation of therapy and annually thereafter, assess Hgb, Hct, RBC, and renal function (serum creatinine) tests. Discuss lifestyle to determine extent of learning, emotional needs. Assure follow-up instruction if pt/family do not thoroughly understand diabetes management or glucose-testing technique.

INTERVENTION/EVALUATION

Encourage adequate hydration, particularly if diarrhea or vomiting occurs. Monitor folic acid, renal function tests for evidence of early lactic acidosis. Monitor serum B_{12} levels. If low, encourage parenteral B_{12} supplementation. Monitor blood glucose and

glycosylated hemoglobin. If pt is on concurrent oral sulfonylureas, assess for hypoglycemia (cool wet skin, tremors, dizziness, anxiety, headache, tachycardia, numbness in mouth, hunger, diplopia). Monitor serum electrolytes, ketones, blood glucose, blood pH, lactate, pyruvate and metformin levels. Fasting glucose should be obtained to assess therapeutic response. Be alert to conditions altering glucose requirements: fever, increased activity/ stress, surgery. Withhold medication, contact physician in presence of hypoxemia or dehydration (may potentiate acute renal impairment).

Patient/Family Teaching

Discontinue metformin and contact physician immediately if evidence of lactic acidosis appears (unexplained hyperventilation, muscle aches, extreme tiredness, unusual sleepiness). Contact physician if significant diarrhea and vomiting continue. Prescribed diet is principal part of treatment; do not skip or delay meals. Diabetes mellitus requires lifelong control. Check blood glucose/urine as ordered. Wear medical alert identification. Check w/physician when glucose demands are altered (e.g., fever, infection, trauma, stress, heavy physical activity). Avoid excessive alcoholic beverages. Do not take other medication w/o consulting physician. Weight control, exercise, hygiene (including foot care) and nonsmoking are essential part of therapy. Inform dentist, physician, or surgeon of this medication before any treatment.

methadone hydrochloride

meth-ah-doan
(Dolophine)

PREGNANCY CATEGORY B
(D if used for prolonged periods or at high doses at term)

CLASSIFICATION

Opioid analgesic **(Schedule II)**

AVAILABILITY (Rx)

Tablets: 5 mg, 10 mg. **Tablets (dispersable):** 40 mg. **Oral Solution:** 5 mg/5 ml, 10 mg/5 ml. **Oral Concentrate:** 10 mg/ml. **Injection:** 10 mg/ml.

PHARMACODYNAMICS

	ONSET	PEAK	DURATION
Oral	30–60 min	0.5–1 hr	4–6 hrs
SubQ	10–15 min	—	4–6 hrs
IM	10–15 min	—	4–6 hrs

PHARMACOKINETICS

Absorption: Well absorbed after IM injection. **Metabolism:** Metabolized in liver. **Excretion:** Primarily excreted in urine. **Half-life:** 15–25 hrs.

ACTION/*THERAPEUTIC EFFECT*

Binds w/opioid receptors within CNS, *altering processes affecting analgesia, emotional response to acute withdrawal syndrome.*

USES

Relief of severe pain, detoxification, and temporary maintenance treatment of narcotic abstinence syndrome.

STORAGE/HANDLING

Store oral, parenteral form at room temperature. Do not use if solution appears cloudy or contains a precipitate.

ADMINISTRATION

ORAL:
- May give w/o regard to meals.
- Dilute syrup in glass of H_2O (prevents anesthetic effect on mucous membranes).

SUBQ/IM:
- **Note:** IM preferred over SubQ route (SubQ produces pain, local irritation, induration).
- Administer slowly.
- Those w/circulating impairment experience higher risk of overdosage because of delayed absorption of repeated administration.

INDICATIONS/ROUTES/DOSAGE

Pain:
Oral/SubQ/IM: Adults: 2.5–10 mg q3–4h as necessary. ***Elderly:*** 2.5 mg q8–12h.

Detoxification:
Note: Refer to local FDA-approved methadone programs.

Oral: Adults: 15–40 mg/day until suppression of withdrawal symptoms. ***Maintenance:*** 20–100 mg/day.

CONTRAINDICATIONS

Hypersensitivity to narcotics, diarrhea due to poisoning, delivery of premature infant, during labor.

CAUTIONS

Impaired renal, hepatic function, elderly/debilitated, supraventricular tachycardia, cor pulmonale, history of seizures, acute abdominal conditions, increased intracranial pressure, respiratory abnormalities.

INTERACTIONS

DRUG: ***Alcohol, CNS depressants*** may increase CNS, respiratory depression, hypotension. ***MAO inhibitors*** may produce severe, fatal reaction (reduce dose to 1/4 usual dose). Effects may be decreased w/***buprenorphine.*** **HERBAL:** None known. **FOOD:** None significant. **ALTERED LAB VALUES:** May increase amylase, lipase.

SIDE EFFECTS

Note: Effects are dependent on dosage amount, route of administration. Ambulatory pts and those not in severe pain may experience dizziness, nausea, vomiting more frequently than those in supine position or having severe pain. **FREQUENT:** Histamine reaction (decreased blood pressure, increased sweating, flushed face, wheezing), constipation, dizziness, drowsiness, hypotension, nausea, vomiting, unusually tired. **OCCASIONAL:** Shortness of breath, trouble breathing, confusion, decreased urination, pounding heartbeat, stomach cramps, visual changes, dry mouth, headache, decreased appetite, nervousness, inability to sleep. **RARE:** Allergic reaction (rash, itching,), paralytic ileus.

ADVERSE REACTIONS/TOXIC EFFECTS

Overdosage results in respiratory depression, skeletal muscle flaccidity, cold clammy skin, cyanosis, extreme somnolence progressing to convulsions, stupor, coma. ***Antidote:*** 0.4 mg naloxone (Narcan). Tolerance to analgesic effect, physical dependence may occur w/repeated use.

PATIENT CONSIDERATIONS

Baseline Assessment

Pt should be in recumbent position before drug is administered by parenteral route. Assess onset, type, location, duration of pain. Obtain vital signs before giving medication. If respirations are 12/min or lower (20/min or lower in children), withhold medication, contact physician. Effect of medication is reduced if full pain recurs before next dose.

Intervention/Evaluation

Monitor vital signs 15–30 min after SubQ/IM dose, 5–10 min after IV dose (monitor for decreased B/P and/or respirations, change in rate or quality of pulse). Oral medication is one-half as potent as parenteral. Assess for adequate voiding. Monitor stools; avoid constipation with increased fluids, bulky foods, and exercise. Initiate deep breathing and coughing exercises, particularly in those w/impaired pulmonary function. Assess for clinical improvement and record onset of relief of pain. Provide support to pt in detoxification program; monitor for withdrawal symptoms.

Patient/Family Teaching

Discomfort may occur with injection. Change positions slowly to avoid orthostatic hypotension. Avoid tasks that require alertness, motor skills until response to drug is established. Tolerance/dependence may occur w/prolonged use of high doses. Do not take alcohol or other CNS depressants.

methicillin sodium

meth-ih-**sill**-in
(Staphcillin)

PREGNANCY CATEGORY B

M

CLASSIFICATION

Antibiotic: Penicillin

AVAILABILITY (Rx)

Powder for Injection: 1 g, 4 g, 6 g, 10 g

PHARMACOKINETICS

Widely distributed. **Metabolism:** Partially metabolized in liver. **Excretion:** Primarily excreted in urine. **Half-life:** 0.4–0.8 hrs (increased in decreased renal function).

ACTION/*THERAPEUTIC EFFECT*

Binds to bacterial membranes, *inhibiting cell wall synthesis. Bactericidal.*

USES

Treatment of respiratory tract, skin/skin structure infections, osteomyelitis, meningitis, endocarditis, perioperatively, especially cardiovascular, orthopedic procedures. Predominantly treatment of infections caused by penicillinase-producing staphylococci.

STORAGE/HANDLING

Solution for IM injection is stable for 24 hrs at room temperature, 96 hrs if refrigerated; IV infusion (piggyback) is stable for 8 hrs at room temperature. Discard if precipitate forms.

ADMINISTRATION

- **Note:** Space doses evenly around the clock for full effectiveness.

IM:

- Reconstitute 500 mg vial w/1.5 ml sterile water for injection or 0.9% NaCl injection to provide concentration of 500 mg/ml.
- Inject IM deeply into gluteus maximus.
- Administer IM injection slowly.

IV:

- For IV injection, further dilute w/20–25 ml sterile water for injection or 0.9% NaCl injection; administer at rate of 10 ml/min.
- For intermittent IV infusion (piggyback), infuse over 20–30 min.
- Alternating IV sites, use large veins to reduce risk of phlebitis.
- Because of potential for hypersensitivity/anaphylaxis, start initial dose at few drops per minute, increase slowly to ordered rate; stay w/pt first 10–15 min, then check q10min.

INDICATIONS/ROUTES/DOSAGE

Usual adult dosage:
IM/IV: Adults, elderly: 1–2 g q4–6h.

Usual pediatric dosage:
IM/IV: Children >1 mo: 100–300 mg/kg/day in divided doses q4–6h.

Usual dosage (neonates):
IM/IV: Neonates 0–7 days, <2 kg: 50–100 mg/kg/day in divided doses q12h. *Neonates 7–28 days, <2 kg or 0–7 days, >2 kg:* 75–150 mg/kg/day in divided doses q8h. *Neonates 7–28 days, >2 kg:* 100–200 mg/kg/day in divided doses q6h.

CONTRAINDICATIONS

Hypersensitivity to any penicillin.

CAUTIONS

Renal impairment, history of allergies, particularly cephalosporins.

INTERACTIONS

DRUG: ***Probenecid*** may increase concentration, toxicity risk. **HERBAL:** None known. **FOOD:** None significant. **ALTERED LAB VALUES:** May increase SGOT (AST). May cause positive Coombs' test.

SIDE EFFECTS

FREQUENT: Mild hypersensitivity reaction (fever, rash, pruritus), nausea, vomiting, diarrhea more common w/oral therapy. **OCCASIONAL:** Phlebitis, thrombophlebitis (more common in elderly). **RARE:** Sterile abscess at IM injection site.

ADVERSE REACTIONS/TOXIC EFFECTS

Superinfections, potentially fatal antibiotic-associated colitis may result from bacterial imbalance. Neurotoxicity w/IV methicillin. Adverse hematologic effects, severe hypersensitivity reactions, rarely anaphylaxis. Acute interstitial nephritis occurs occasionally.

PATIENT CONSIDERATIONS

Baseline Assessment

Question history of allergies, especially penicillins, cephalosporins. Obtain specimen for culture and sensitivity before giving first dose (therapy may begin before results are known).

Intervention/Evaluation

Hold medication and promptly report rash (possible hypersensitivity) or diarrhea (w/fever, abdominal pain, mucus and

blood in stool may indicate antibiotic-associated colitis). Assess food tolerance. Evaluate IV site for phlebitis (heat, pain, red streaking over vein). Monitor I&O; check for hematuria. Assess IM injection sites for pain, induration. Be alert for superinfection: increased fever, onset sore throat, nausea, vomiting, diarrhea, ulceration or changes of oral mucosa, anal/genital pruritus. Check hematology reports (especially WBCs), periodic renal or hepatic reports in prolonged therapy.

PATIENT/FAMILY TEACHING

Space doses evenly. Continue antibiotic for full length of treatment. Discomfort may occur w/IM injection. Notify physician in event of diarrhea, rash, blood in urine, or other new symptom.

methimazole

meth-im-**ah**-zole
(Tapazole)

CANADIAN AVAILABILITY
Tapazole

PREGNANCY CATEGORY D

CLASSIFICATION

Antithyroid

AVAILABILITY (Rx)

Tablets: 5 mg, 10 mg

PHARMACOKINETICS

Absorption: Readily absorbed from GI tract (food may alter absorption). Primarily concentrated in thyroid gland. **Metabolism:** Metabolized in liver. **Excretion:** Primarily excreted in urine. Minimally removed by hemodialysis. **Half-life:** 5–6 hrs.

ACTION/*THERAPEUTIC EFFECT*

Inhibits thyroid hormone synthesis, *effective in treatment of hyperthyroidism.*

USES

Palliative treatment of hyperthyroidism; adjunct to relieve hyperthyroidism in preparation for surgical treatment or radioactive iodine therapy.

M

ADMINISTRATION

ORAL:

- Space doses evenly, usually at 8 hr intervals.

INDICATIONS/ROUTES/DOSAGE

Hyperthyroidism:
Oral: Adults, elderly: Initially, 15–60 mg/day. *Maintenance:* 5–15 mg/day. *Children:* Initially, 0.4 mg/kg/day. *Maintenance:* One-half the initial dose.

CONTRAINDICATIONS

Hypersensitivity to the drug.

CAUTIONS

Pts >40 yrs or in combination w/other agranulocytosis-inducing drugs.

INTERACTIONS

DRUG: *Amiodarone, iodinated glycerol, iodine, potassium iodide* may decrease response. May decrease effect of ***oral anticoagulants.*** May increase concentration of ***digoxin*** (as pt becomes euthyroid). May decrease thyroid uptake of I^{131}. **HERBAL:** None known. **FOOD:** None significant. **ALTERED LAB VALUES:** May increase SGOT (AST), SGPT (ALT), alkaline phosphatase, LDH, bilirubin, prothrombin time. May decrease prothrombin level.

SIDE EFFECTS

FREQUENT (3–5%): Fever, rash, itching. **OCCASIONAL (1–3%):** Dizziness, loss of taste, nausea, vomiting, stomach pain, peripheral neuropathy (numbness in fingers, toes, face). **RARE (<1%):** Swollen lymph nodes, salivary glands.

ADVERSE REACTIONS/TOXIC EFFECTS

Agranulocytosis (which may occur as long as 4 mos after therapy); pancytopenia and fatal hepatitis have occurred.

PATIENT CONSIDERATIONS

BASELINE ASSESSMENT

Question for hypersensitivity. Obtain baseline weight, pulse.

INTERVENTION/EVALUATION

Monitor pulse and weight daily. Assess food tolerance. Check for skin eruptions, itching, swollen lymph glands. Be alert to hepatitis: nausea, vomiting, drowsiness, jaundice. Monitor hematology results for bone marrow suppression; check for signs of infection or bleeding.

PATIENT/FAMILY TEACHING

Do not exceed ordered dose; follow-up w/physician is essential. Space evenly around the clock. Take resting pulse (teach pt/family) daily to monitor therapeutic results and report as directed. Do not take other medications w/o approval of physician. Seafood and iodine products may be restricted. Report illness, unusual bleeding, or bruising immediately. Inform physician of sudden or continuous weight gain, cold intolerance or depression.

---

methocarbamol

(Robaxin)

FIXED-COMBINATION(S):
W/aspirin, a salicylate **(Robaxisal)**

See Classification section under: Skeletal muscle relaxants

---

methohexital sodium

(Brevital)

See Classification section under: Anesthetics: general

---

methotrexate sodium

(Folex, Mexate, Rheumatrex)

See Classification section under: Cancer chemotherapy

---

methylcellulose

meth-ill-**cell**-you-los
(Citrucel, Cologel)

PREGNANCY CATEGORY C

CLASSIFICATION

Laxative: Bulk-forming

AVAILABILITY (OTC)

Powder

PHARMACODYNAMICS

	ONSET	PEAK	DURATION
Oral	12–24 hrs	—	—

PHARMACOKINETICS

Full effect may not be evident for 2–3 days. Acts in small/large intestine.

ACTION/THERAPEUTIC EFFECT

Dissolves and expands in water, *providing increased bulk, moisture content in stool, increasing peristalsis, bowel motility.*

USES

Prophylaxis in those who should not strain during defecation. Facilitates defecation in those w/diminished colonic motor response.

ADMINISTRATION

ORAL:

- Instruct pt to drink 6–8 glasses of water/day (aids stool softening).
- Not to be swallowed in dry form; mix w/at least 1 full glass (8 oz) liquid.

INDICATIONS/ROUTES/DOSAGE

Laxative:

Oral: Adults, elderly: 1 tbsp (15 ml) in 8 oz water 1–3 times/day. ***Children 6–12 yrs:*** 1 tsp (5 ml) in 4 oz water 3–4 times/day.

CONTRAINDICATIONS

Abdominal pain, nausea, vomiting, symptoms of appendicitis, partial bowel obstruction, dysphagia.

CAUTIONS

None significant.

INTERACTIONS

DRUG: May interfere w/effects of ***potassium-sparing diuretics, potassium supplements.*** May decrease effect of ***oral anticoagulants, digoxin, salicylates*** by decreasing absorption. **HERBAL:** None known. **FOOD:** None significant. **ALTERED LAB VALUES:** May increase glucose. May decrease potassium.

SIDE EFFECTS

RARE: Some degree of abdominal discomfort, nausea, mild cramps, griping, faintness.

ADVERSE REACTIONS/TOXIC EFFECTS

Esophageal or bowel obstruction may occur if administered with insufficient liquid (less than 250 ml or 1 full glass).

PATIENT CONSIDERATIONS

INTERVENTION/EVALUATION

Encourage adequate fluid intake. Assess bowel sounds for peristalsis. Monitor daily bowel activity and stool consistency (watery, loose, soft, semisolid, solid) and record time of evacuation. Monitor serum electrolytes in those exposed to prolonged, frequent, or excessive use of medication.

PATIENT/FAMILY TEACHING

Institute measures to promote defecation: increase fluid intake, exercise, high-fiber diet.

M

---

methyldopa

meth-ill-**doe**-pah
(Aldomet)

methyldopate hydrochloride

FIXED-COMBINATION(S)
W/hydrochlorothiazide, a diuretic **(Aldoril)**; w/chlorothiazide, a diuretic **(Aldoclor)**.

CANADIAN AVAILABILITY
Aldomet, Apo-Methyldopa, Novomedopa

PREGNANCY CATEGORY C

CLASSIFICATION

Antihypertensive

AVAILABILITY (Rx)

Tablets: 125 mg, 250 mg, 500 mg. **Oral Suspension:** 250 mg/5 ml. **Injection:** 250 mg/5 ml.

PHARMACODYNAMICS

	ONSET	PEAK	DURATION
Oral	—	4–6 hrs	—
IV	—	4–6 hrs	10–16 hrs

PHARMACOKINETICS

Absorption: Variably absorbed from GI tract. **Metabolism:** Metabolized in liver. **Excretion:** Primarily excreted in urine. Removed by hemodialysis. **Half-life:** 1.7 hrs (increased in decreased renal function).

ACTION / *THERAPEUTIC EFFECT*

Stimulates central inhibitory alpha-adrenergic receptors (lowers arterial pressure, reduces plasma renin activity). *Reduces standing and supine B/P.*

USES

Management of moderate to severe hypertension.

STORAGE/HANDLING

Store tablets at room temperature. IV solution is stable for 24 hrs at room temperature.

ADMINISTRATION

ORAL:

- May give w/o regard to food. If GI upset occurs, give w/food.
- Tablets may be crushed.

IV:

- Give by IV infusion (piggyback). Avoid SubQ, IM (unpredictable absorption).
- For IV infusion, dilute 250 or 500 mg vial w/50 or 100 ml 5% dextrose.
- Infuse slowly over 30–60 min.

INDICATIONS/ROUTES/DOSAGE

Hypertension:
Oral: Adults: Initially, 250 mg 2–3 times/day for 2 days. Adjust dosage at intervals of 2 days (minimum). ***Elderly:*** Initially, 125 mg 1–2 times/day. May increase by 125 mg q2–3days. ***Maintenance:*** 500 mg to 2 g/day in 2–4 divided doses. ***Children:*** Initially, 10 mg/kg/day in 2–4 divided doses. Adjust dose at intervals of 2 days (minimum). ***Maximum:*** 65 mg/kg/day or 3 g/day, whichever is less.

IV: ***Adults:*** 250–500 mg q6h up to 1 g q6h. ***Children:*** 20–40 mg/kg/day in divided doses q6h. ***Maximum:*** 65 mg/kg/day or 3 g/day, whichever is less.

CONTRAINDICATIONS

Acute hepatitis, active cirrhosis.

CAUTIONS

Impaired hepatic function.

INTERACTIONS

DRUG: ***Tricyclic antidepressants, NSAIDs*** may decrease effect. ***Hypotensive-producing medications*** may increase effect. May increase risk of toxicity of ***lithium***. May cause hyperexcitability ***w/MAO inhibitors. Sympathomimetics*** may decrease effects. **HERBAL:** None known. **FOOD:** None significant. **ALTERED LAB VALUES:** May increase SGOT (AST), SGPT (ALT), alkaline phosphatase, bilirubin, BUN, creatinine, potassium, sodium, prolactin, uric acid. May produce false-positive Coombs' test, prolong prothrombin time.

SIDE EFFECTS

FREQUENT: Peripheral edema (swelling in feet), drowsiness, headache, dry mouth. **OCCASIONAL:** Mental changes (e.g., anxiety depression), decreased sexual ability or interest, diarrhea, swelling of breasts, nausea, vomiting, lightheadedness, numbness in hands, feet, rhinitis.

ADVERSE REACTIONS/TOXIC EFFECTS

Hepatotoxicity (abnormal liver function tests, jaundice, hepatitis), hemolytic anemia, unexplained fever and flulike symptoms: Discontinue medication, contact physician.

PATIENT CONSIDERATIONS

Baseline Assessment

Obtain baseline B/P, pulse, weight.

Intervention/Evaluation

Monitor B/P, pulse closely q30min until stabilized. Monitor weight daily during initial therapy. Monitor liver function tests. Assess for peripheral edema of hands, feet (usually, first area of low extremity swelling is behind medial malleolus in ambulatory, sacral area in bedridden).

Patient/Family Teaching

Urine may darken in color. To reduce hypotensive effect, rise slowly from lying to sitting position and permit legs to dangle from bed momentarily before standing. Avoid sudden or prolonged standing, exercise, hot environment or hot shower, alcohol ingestion, particularly in morning (may aggravate orthostatic hypotension). Full therapeutic effect of oral administration may take 2–3 days. Drowsiness usually disappears during continued therapy. Sugarless gum, sips of tepid water may relieve dry mouth.

methylergonovine

meth-ill-er-go-**noe**-veen
(Methergine)

PREGNANCY CATEGORY C

CLASSIFICATION

Oxytocic

AVAILABILITY (Rx)

Tablets: 0.2 mg. **Injection:** 0.2 mg/ml.

PHARMACODYNAMICS

	ONSET	PEAK	DURATION
Oral	5–10 min	—	—
IM	2–5 min	—	—
IV	Immediate	—	3 hrs

PHARMACOKINETICS

Absorption: Rapidly absorbed from GI tract, after IM administration. Distributed rapidly to plasma, extracellular fluid, tissues. **Metabolism:** Metabolized in liver (undergoes first-pass effect). **Excretion:** Primarily excreted in urine.

ACTION/*THERAPEUTIC EFFECT*

Stimulates alpha-adrenergic, serotonin receptors, producing arterial vasoconstriction. Causes vasospasm of coronary arteries. Directly stimulates uterine muscle *(increases strength, frequency of contractions, decreases uterine bleeding).*

USES/*UNLABELED*

To prevent and treat postpartum,

postabortion hemorrhage due to atony or involution (not for induction or augmentation of labor). *Treatment of incomplete abortion.*

ADMINISTRATION

- Initial dose may be given parenterally, followed by oral regimen.
- IV use in life-threatening emergencies only; dilute to volume of 5 ml w/0.9% NaCl injection and give over at least 1 min, carefully monitoring B/P.

INDICATIONS/ROUTES/DOSAGE

Usual oral dosage:
Oral: Adults: 0.2 mg 3–4 times/day for maximum of 7 days.

Usual parenteral dosage:
IM/IV: Adults: Initially, 0.2 mg. May repeat no more often than q2–4h for no more than 5 doses total.

CONTRAINDICATIONS

Hypersensitivity to ergot, hypertension, pregnancy, toxemia, untreated hypocalcemia.

CAUTIONS

Renal or hepatic impairment, coronary artery disease, occlusive peripheral vascular disease, sepsis.

INTERACTIONS

DRUG: ***Vasoconstrictors, vasopressors*** may increase effect. **HERBAL:** None known. **FOOD:** None significant. **ALTERED LAB VALUES:** May decrease prolactin concentration.

SIDE EFFECTS

FREQUENT: Nausea, uterine cramping, vomiting. **OCCASIONAL:** Abdominal or stomach pain, diarrhea, dizziness, sweating, ringing in ears, bradycardia, chest pain. **RARE:** Allergic reaction (rash, itching), dyspnea, sudden severe hypertension.

ADVERSE REACTIONS/TOXIC EFFECTS

Severe hypertensive episodes may result in cerebrovascular accident, serious arrhythmias, seizures; hypertensive effects more frequent w/pt susceptibility, rapid IV administration, concurrent regional anesthesia or vasoconstrictors. Peripheral ischemia may lead to gangrene.

PATIENT CONSIDERATIONS

BASELINE ASSESSMENT

Question for hypersensitivity to any ergot derivatives. Determine calcium, B/P, and pulse baselines. Assess bleeding prior to administration.

INTERVENTION/EVALUATION

Monitor uterine tone, bleeding, B/P, and pulse q15min until stable (about 1–2 hrs). Assess extremities for color, warmth, movement, pain. Report chest pain promptly. Provide support w/ambulation if dizziness occurs.

PATIENT/FAMILY TEACHING

Avoid smoking because of added vasoconstriction. Report increased cramping, bleeding, or foul-smelling lochia. Pale, cold hands or feet should be reported because may mean decreased circulation.

methylphenidate hydrochloride

meh-thyl-**fen**-ih-date
(Concerta, Methylin, Ritalin)

CANADIAN AVAILABILITY
Ritalin

PREGNANCY CATEGORY C

CLASSIFICATION

CNS stimulant

AVAILABILITY (Rx)

Tablets: 5 mg, 10 mg, 20 mg. **Tablets (sustained-release):** 20 mg. **Concerta:** 18 mg, 36 mg, 54 mg.

PHARMACODYNAMICS

	ONSET	PEAK	DURATION
Oral (tablets)			
	—	—	3–6 hrs
Oral (extended-release)			
	—	—	8 hrs

PHARMACOKINETICS

Absorption: Slowly, incompletely absorbed from GI tract. **Metabolism:** Metabolized in liver. **Excretion:** Excreted in urine, eliminated in feces via biliary system. **Half-life:** 2–4 hrs.

ACTION / *THERAPEUTIC EFFECT*

Blocks reuptake mechanisms of dopaminergic neurons. *Decreases motor restlessness, enhances ability to pay attention. Increases motor activity, mental alertness; diminishes sense of fatigue, enhances spirit, produces mild euphoria.*

USES / *UNLABELED*

Adjunct to treatment of attention deficit disorder with moderate to severe distractability, short attention spans, hyperactivity, emotional impulsivity in children >6 yrs. Management of narcolepsy in adults. *Treatment of secondary mental depression.*

ADMINISTRATION

ORAL:

- Do not give drug in afternoon or evening (drug causes insomnia).
- Do not crush or break sustained-release capsules.
- Tablets may be crushed.
- Give dose 30–45 min before meals.

INDICATIONS / ROUTES / DOSAGE

Note: Do not use extended release for initial therapy.

Attention deficit disorder:
Oral: Children >6 yrs: Initially, 5 mg before breakfast and lunch. May increase dosage by 5–10 mg/day at weekly intervals. ***Maximum:*** 60 mg/day. Therapy usually discontinued when adolescence reached.

Narcolepsy:
Oral: Adults, elderly: 10 mg 2–3 times/day. ***Range:*** 10–60 mg/day.

CONTRAINDICATIONS

History of marked anxiety, tension, agitation; glaucoma, those with motor tics, family history of Tourette's disorder.

CAUTIONS

History of seizures, hypertension, history of drug dependence.

INTERACTIONS

DRUG: ***CNS stimulants*** may have additive effect. ***MAO inhibitors*** may increase effects. **HERBAL:** None known. **FOOD:** None significant. **ALTERED LAB VALUES:** None significant.

SIDE EFFECTS

FREQUENT: Loss of appetite, nervousness, insomnia, increased blood pressure, tachycardia. **OCCASIONAL:** Dizziness, drowsiness, headache, nausea, stomach pain, fever, rash, angina, joint pain, uncontrolled body movements. **RARE:** Blurred vision, Tourette's

M

syndrome (uncontrolled vocal outbursts, repeated body movements).

ADVERSE REACTIONS/TOXIC EFFECTS

Prolonged administration to children w/attention deficit disorder may produce a temporary suppression of normal weight gain pattern. Overdose may produce tachycardia, palpitations, cardiac irregularities, chest pain, psychotic episode, seizures, coma. Hypersensitivity reactions, blood dyscrasias occur rarely.

PATIENT CONSIDERATIONS

INTERVENTION/EVALUATION

CBC, differential, and platelet count should be performed routinely during therapy. If paradoxical return of attention deficit occurs, dosage should be reduced or discontinued.

PATIENT/FAMILY TEACHING

Avoid tasks that require alertness, motor skills until response to drug is established. Dry mouth may be relieved by sugarless gum, sips of tepid water. Report any increase in seizures. Take last dose early in evening to avoid insomnia. Report nervousness, palpitations, fever, vomiting, skin rash.

---

methylprednisolone

meth-ill-pred-**niss**-oh-lone

(Medrol)

methylprednisolone sodium succinate

(Solu-Medrol, A-Methapred)

methylprednisolone acetate

(Depo-Medrol, Duralone)

FIXED-COMBINATIONS

Methylprednisolone acetate w/Neomycin, an anti-infective **(Neo-Medrol)**

CANADIAN AVAILABILITY

Medrol, Depo-Medrol, Solu-Medrol

PREGNANCY CATEGORY C

CLASSIFICATION

Corticosteroid

AVAILABILITY (Rx)

Tablets: 2 mg, 4 mg, 8 mg, 16 mg, 24 mg, 32 mg

Succinate: Powder for Injection: 40 mg, 125 mg, 500 mg, 1 g, 2 g

Acetate: Injection: 20 mg/ml, 40 mg/ml, 80 mg/ml

PHARMACOKINETICS

Absorption: Well absorbed from GI tract, after IM administration. Widely distributed. **Metabolism:** Metabolized in liver. **Excretion:** Excreted in urine. **Half-life:** >3.5 hrs.

ACTION/*THERAPEUTIC EFFECT*

Inhibits accumulation of inflammatory cells at inflammation sites, phagocytosis, lysosomal enzyme release and synthesis and/or release of mediators of inflammation. *Prevents/suppresses cell-mediated immune reactions. Decreases/prevents tissue response to inflammatory process.*

USES

Substitution therapy of deficiency states: acute/chronic adrenal insufficiency, congenital adrenal hyperplasia, adrenal insufficiency secondary to pituitary insufficiency. Nonendocrine disorders: arthritis, rheumatic carditis, allergic, collagen, intestinal tract, liver, ocular, renal, and skin diseases, bronchial asthma, cerebral edema, malignancies.

ADMINISTRATION

ORAL:

- Give w/food or milk.
- Give single doses before 9 AM; give multiple doses at evenly spaced intervals.

IM:

- Methylprednisolone acetate should not be further diluted.
- Methylprednisolone sodium succinate should be reconstituted w/bacteriostatic water.
- Give deep IM in gluteus maximus.

IV:

- For infusion, add to 5% dextrose, 0.9% NaCl, or 5% dextrose in 0.9% NaCl.
- Do *not* give methylprednisolone acetate IV.

INDICATIONS/ROUTES/DOSAGE

Note: Individualize dose based on disease, pt, and response.

Oral Methylprednisolone:

Oral: Adults, elderly: Initially, 4–48 mg/day.

Methylprednisolone Sodium Succinate:

IV: Adults, elderly: (High dose): 30 mg/kg over at least 30 min. Repeat q4–6h for 48–72 hrs.

IV: Adults, elderly: Initially, 10–40 mg q4–6h, may give subsequent doses IM. ***Children, infants:*** Not less than 0.5 mg/kg/day.

Methylprednisolone Acetate:

Adrenogenital syndrome:
IM: Adults, elderly: 40 mg q2wks.

Rheumatoid arthritis:
IM: Adults: 40–120 mg/wk.

Dermatologic lesions:
IM: Adults, elderly: 40–120 mg/wk for 1–4 wks.

Asthma, allergic rhinitis:
IM: Adults, elderly: 80–120 mg/wk.

CONTRAINDICATIONS

Hypersensitivity to any corticosteroid, systemic fungal infection, peptic ulcers (except life-threatening situations). Avoid immunizations, smallpox vaccination.

CAUTIONS

History of tuberculosis (may reactivate disease), hypothyroidism, cirrhosis, nonspecific ulcerative colitis, CHF, hypertension, psychosis, renal insufficiency. Prolonged therapy should be discontinued slowly.

INTERACTIONS

DRUG: ***Amphotericin*** may increase hypokalemia. May decrease effect of ***oral hypoglycemics, insulin, diuretics, potassium supplements.*** May increase ***digoxin*** toxicity (due to hypokalemia). ***Hepatic enzyme inducers*** may decrease effect. ***Live virus vaccines*** may potentiate virus replication, increase vaccine side effects, decrease pt's antibody response to vaccine. **HERBAL:** None known. **FOOD:** None significant. **ALTERED LAB VALUES:** May decrease calcium, potassium, thyroxine. May increase cholesterol, lipids, glucose, sodium, amylase.

SIDE EFFECTS

FREQUENT: Insomnia, heartburn,

M

nervousness, abdominal distension, increased sweating, acne, mood swings, increased appetite, facial flushing, GI distress, delayed wound healing, increased susceptibility to infection, diarrhea/constipation. **OCCASIONAL:** Headache, edema, tachycardia, change in skin color, frequent urination, depression. **RARE:** Psychosis, increased blood coagulability, hallucinations.

ADVERSE REACTIONS/TOXIC EFFECTS

Long-term therapy: Muscle wasting (especially arms, legs), osteoporosis, spontaneous fractures, amenorrhea, cataracts, glaucoma, peptic ulcer, CHF. *Abrupt withdrawal following long-term therapy:* Anorexia, nausea, fever, headache, severe joint pain, rebound inflammation, fatigue, weakness, lethargy, dizziness, orthostatic hypotension.

PATIENT CONSIDERATIONS

Baseline Assessment

Question for hypersensitivity to any of the corticosteroids, components. Obtain baselines for height, weight, B/P, glucose, electrolytes. Check results of initial tests, (e.g., TB skin test, x-rays, EKG).

Intervention/Evaluation

Monitor I&O, weight; assess for edema. Evaluate food tolerance and bowel activity; report hyperacidity promptly. Check B/P, TPR at least 2 times/day. Be alert to infection: sore throat, fever, or vague symptoms. Monitor electrolytes. Watch for hypocalcemia (muscle twitching, cramps, positive Trousseau's or Chvostek's signs) or hypokalemia (weakness and muscle cramps, numbness/tingling [especially lower extremities], nausea and vomiting, irritability, EKG changes). Assess emotional status, ability to sleep. Check lab results for blood coagulability and clinical evidence of thromboembolism. Provide assistance w/ambulation.

Patient/Family Teaching

Take oral dose w/food or milk. For those on long-term therapy, carry identification of drug and dose, physician name and phone number. Do not change dose/schedule or stop taking drug; must taper off gradually under medical supervision. Notify physician of fever, sore throat, muscle aches, sudden weight gain/swelling. Obtain instructions for prescribed diet (usually sodium restricted w/high vitamin D, protein, and potassium). Maintain careful personal hygiene, avoid exposure to disease or trauma. Severe stress (serious infection, surgery or trauma) may require increased dosage. Do not take any other medication w/o consulting physician. Follow-up visits, lab tests are necessary; children must be assessed for growth retardation. Inform dentist or other physicians of methylprednisolone therapy now or within past 12 mos.

methysergide maleate

meth-i-**sir**-guide
(Sansert)

CANADIAN AVAILABILITY
Sansert

PREGNANCY CATEGORY X

CLASSIFICATION

Antimigraine

AVAILABILITY (Rx)

Tablets: 2 mg

PHARMACOKINETICS

Absorption: Rapidly absorbed from GI tract. Widely distributed. **Metabolism:** Metabolized in liver to active metabolite. **Excretion:** Primarily excreted in urine. **Half-life:** 10 hrs.

ACTION/ *THERAPEUTIC EFFECT*

Directly stimulates smooth muscle leading to vasoconstriction, *preventing or aborting vascular headaches.*

USES

Treatment of vascular headaches (e.g., migraine, cluster headaches).

ADMINISTRATION

ORAL:

- Give w/meals to avoid GI upset.

INDICATIONS/ROUTES/DOSAGE

Vascular headaches:

Oral: Adults: 4–8 mg/day in divided doses. Do not give continuously >6 mos w/o 3–4 wk drug-free interval between courses of therapy. Discontinue gradually over 2–3 wks (avoids rebound headaches).

CONTRAINDICATIONS

Hypersensitivity to ergot alkaloids, peripheral vascular disease (thromboangiitis obliterans, leutic arteritis, severe arteriosclerosis, Raynaud's disease), phlebitis or cellulitis of lower limbs, pulmonary disease, collagen diseases, fibrotic disease, impaired renal or hepatic function, severe pruritus, valvular heart disease, coronary artery disease, severe hypertension, debilitated, malnutrition, known or suspected pregnancy.

CAUTIONS

None significant.

INTERACTIONS

DRUG: ***Ergot alkaloids, systemic vasoconstrictors*** (e.g., ***norepinephrine***) may increase vasoconstrictor effect. **HERBAL:** None known. **FOOD:** None significant. **ALTERED LAB VALUES:** May increase BUN.

SIDE EFFECTS

FREQUENT: Dizziness, lightheadedness, diarrhea, drowsiness, nausea, vomiting, stomach pain, numbness in fingers, toes, face pain, cold hand or feet, weakness in legs. **OCCASIONAL:** Changes in vision, clumsiness, peripheral edema, fast or slow heartbeat, flushed face, rash, constipation, inability to sleep, heartburn. **RARE:** Pulmonary fibrosis.

ADVERSE REACTIONS/TOXIC EFFECTS

Prolonged administration or excessive dosage may produce ergotamine poisoning: nausea, vomiting, weakness of legs, pain in limb muscles, numbness and tingling of fingers/toes, precordial pain, tachycardia or bradycardia, hyper/hypotension. Localized edema, itching due to vasoconstriction of peripheral arteries and arterioles. Feet and hands will become cold, pale, numb. Muscle pain occurs when walking and, later, even at rest. Gangrene may occur. Occasionally, confusion, depression, drowsiness, convulsions may appear.

PATIENT CONSIDERATIONS

BASELINE ASSESSMENT

Question pt regarding history of peripheral vascular disease, renal or hepatic impairment, or possibility of pregnancy. Contact physician with findings before administering drug. Question pt regarding onset, location, and duration of migraine, and possible precipitating symptoms.

INTERVENTION/EVALUATION

Monitor closely for evidence of ergotamine overdosage as result of prolonged administration or excessive dosage (see Adverse Reactions/Toxic Effects). Contact physician if any signs and symptoms of ergotamine poisoning present.

PATIENT/FAMILY TEACHING

Initiate therapy at first sign of migraine attack. Inform physician if need to progressively increase dose in order to relieve vascular headaches or if irregular heartbeat, nausea, vomiting, numbness or tingling of fingers or toes or if pain or weakness of extremities is noted. Contraindicated in pregnancy; use nonhormonal contraception.

---

metipranolol

(OptiPranolol)

See Classification section under: Antiglaucoma agents

---

metoclopramide

meh-tah-**klo**-prah-myd

(Reglan)

CANADIAN AVAILABILITY

Apo-Metoclop, Maxeran, Reglan

PREGNANCY CATEGORY B

CLASSIFICATION

GI stimulant, antiemetic

AVAILABILITY (Rx)

Tablets: 5 mg, 10 mg. **Syrup:** 5 mg/5 ml. **Injection:** 5 mg/ml.

PHARMACOKINETICS

Absorption: Well absorbed from GI tract. **Metabolism:** Metabolized in liver. **Excretion:** Primarily excreted in urine. **Half-life:** 4–6 hrs.

ACTION/*THERAPEUTIC EFFECT*

Stimulates motility of upper GI tract, *accelerates intestinal transit and gastric emptying.* Decreases reflux into esophagus. Raises threshold activity of chemoreceptor trigger zone, *producing antiemetic activity.*

USES/*UNLABELED*

To facilitate small-bowel intubation, stimulate gastric emptying, intestinal transit. Relieves symptoms of acute, recurrent gastroparesis (nausea, vomiting, persistent fullness after meals). Prevents nausea, vomiting associated w/cancer chemotherapy. Treatment of heartburn, delayed gastric emptying secondary to reflux esophagitis. *Treatment of slow gastric emptying, vascular headaches, persistent hiccups, drug-related postop nausea/vomiting. Prophylaxis of aspiration pneumonia.*

STORAGE/HANDLING

Store tablets, syrup at room temperature. After reconstitution, IV infusion (piggyback) is stable for 48 hrs.

ADMINISTRATION

ORAL:

- Give 30 min before meals and at bedtime.
- Tablets may be crushed.

IV:

- For IV infusion (piggyback), may dilute w/5% dextrose or 0.9% NaCl.
- Infuse >15 min.
- May give slow IV push at rate of 10 mg over 1–2 min.
- A too rapid IV injection may produce intense feeling of anxiety or restlessness, followed by drowsiness.

INDICATIONS/ROUTES/DOSAGE

Note: May give orally, direct IV, IV infusion.

Diabetic gastroparesis:
Oral/IV: Adults: 10 mg 4 times/day for 2–8 wks.

Oral: Elderly: Initially, 5 mg 30 min before meals and at bedtime. May increase to 10 mg for 2–8 wks.

IV: Elderly: 5 mg over 1–2 min. May increase to 10 mg.

Symptomatic gastroesophageal reflux:
Oral: Adults: 10–15 mg up to 4 times/day; single doses up to 20 mg, as needed. ***Elderly:*** Initially, 5 mg 4 times/day. May increase to 10 mg.

Prevention of cancer chemotherapy-induced nausea and vomiting:
IV: Adults, elderly, children: 1–2 mg/kg 30 min prior to chemotherapy; repeat q2h for 2 doses, then q3h, as needed.

Facilitation of small-bowel intubation (single dose):
IV: Adults, elderly: 10 mg. ***Children 6–14 yrs:*** 2.5–5 mg. ***Children <6 yrs:*** 0.1 mg/kg.

CONTRAINDICATIONS

Pheochromocytoma, history of seizure disorders, concurrent use of medications likely to produce extrapyramidal reactions, GI obstruction or perforation, GI hemorrhage.

CAUTIONS

Impaired renal function, CHF, cirrhosis.

INTERACTIONS

DRUG: ***Alcohol*** may increase CNS depressant effect. ***CNS depressants*** may increase sedative effect. **HERBAL:** None known. **FOOD:** None significant. **ALTERED LAB VALUES:** May increase aldosterone, prolactin concentrations.

SIDE EFFECTS

Note: Doses of 2 mg/kg or higher or length of therapy may result in a greater incidence of side effects. **FREQUENT:** Diarrhea, drowsiness, restlessness, unusually tired. **OCCASIONAL:** Breast tenderness, swelling, altered menstruation, constipation, dizziness, headache, prolactin stimulation, nausea, rash, inability to sleep, dry mouth, galactorrhea, gynecomastia. **RARE:** Agranulocytosis (chills, fever, sore throat), hypotension, hypertension, tachycardia.

ADVERSE REACTIONS/TOXIC EFFECTS

Extrapyramidal reactions occur most frequently in children and young adults (age 18–30) receiving high doses (2 mg/kg) during cancer chemotherapy, and is usually limited to akathisia (motor restlessness), involuntary limb movement, and facial grimacing.

PATIENT CONSIDERATIONS

BASELINE ASSESSMENT

Antiemetic
Assess for dehydration (poor skin turgor, dry mucous membranes, longitudinal furrows in tongue).

INTERVENTION/EVALUATION

Monitor for anxiety, restlessness, extrapyramidal symptoms during IV administration. Monitor pattern of daily bowel activity and stool consistency. Assess for periorbital edema, skin for rash, hives. Evaluate for therapeutic response from gastroparesis (nausea, vomiting, persistent fullness after meals).

PATIENT/FAMILY TEACHING

Avoid tasks that require alertness, motor skills until drug response is established. Report involuntary eye, facial, or limb movement (extrapyramidal reaction). Avoid alcohol.

metolazone

me-**toh**-lah-zone
(Diulo, Mykrox, Zaroxolyn)

CANADIAN AVAILABILITY
Zaroxolyn

PREGNANCY CATEGORY D

CLASSIFICATION

Diuretic: Thiazide

AVAILABILITY (Rx)

Tablets: 2.5 mg, 5 mg, 10 mg. **Tablets (Mykrox):** 0.5 mg.

PHARMACODYNAMICS

	ONSET	PEAK	DURATION
Oral (diuretic)			
	1 hr	2 hrs	12–24 hrs

PHARMACOKINETICS

Absorption: Incompletely absorbed from GI tract. **Excretion:** Primarily excreted unchanged in urine. **Half-life:** 14 hrs.

ACTION/*THERAPEUTIC EFFECT*

Diuretic: Blocks reabsorption of sodium, potassium, chloride at distal convoluted tubule, promoting delivery of sodium to potassium side, increasing potassium excretion (Na–K) exchange, *producing renal excretion.* ***Antihypertensive:*** Reduces plasma, extracellular fluid volume. *Decreases peripheral vascular resistance, reduced B/P by direct effect on blood vessels.*

USES

Diulo, Zaroxolyn: Treatment of mild to moderate essential hypertension, edema of renal disease, edema due to CHF. ***Mykrox:*** Treatment of mild to moderate hypertension.

ADMINISTRATION

ORAL:

- May give w/food or milk if GI upset occurs, preferably w/breakfast (may prevent nocturia).

INDICATIONS/ROUTES/DOSAGE

DIULO, ZAROXOLYN:

Edema due to CHF:
Oral: Adults: 5–10 mg once daily in morning. Reduce dose to lowest maintenance level when dry weight is achieved (nonedematous state).

Edema due to renal disease:
Oral: Adults: 5–20 mg once daily in morning. Reduce dose to lowest maintenance level when dry

weight is achieved (nonedematous state).

Hypertension:
Oral: Adults: 2.5–5 mg once daily in morning.

Usual elderly dosage:
Oral: Initially, 2.5 mg/day or every other day.

MYKROX:

Hypertension:
Oral: Adults: 0.5 mg once daily in morning. Dose may be increased to 1 mg once daily if B/P response is insufficient.

CONTRAINDICATIONS

History of hypersensitivity to sulfonamides or thiazide diuretics, renal decompensation, anuria, hepatic coma or precoma.

CAUTIONS

Severe renal disease, impaired hepatic function, diabetes mellitus, elderly/debilitated, thyroid disorders.

INTERACTIONS

DRUG: ***Cholestyramine, colestipol*** may decrease absorption, effects. May increase ***digoxin*** toxicity (due to hypokalemia). May increase ***lithium*** toxicity. **HERBAL:** None known. **FOOD:** None significant. **ALTERED LAB VALUES:** May increase bilirubin, serum calcium, LDL, cholesterol, triglycerides, creatinine, glucose, uric acid. May decrease urinary calcium, magnesium, potassium, sodium.

SIDE EFFECTS

EXPECTED: Increase in urine frequency/volume. **FREQUENT:** Potassium depletion. **OCCASIONAL:** Postural hypotension, headache, abdominal bloating, palpitations, chills.

ADVERSE REACTIONS/TOXIC EFFECTS

Vigorous diuresis may lead to profound water loss and electrolyte depletion, resulting in hypokalemia, hyponatremia, dehydration. Acute hypotensive episodes may occur. Hyperglycemia may be noted during prolonged therapy. GI upset, pancreatitis, dizziness, paresthesias, headache, blood dyscrasias, pulmonary edema, allergic pneumonitis, dermatologic reactions occur rarely. Overdosage can lead to lethargy, coma w/o changes in electrolytes or hydration.

M

PATIENT CONSIDERATIONS

BASELINE ASSESSMENT

Check vital signs, especially B/P for hypotension prior to administration. Assess baseline electrolytes, particularly check for low potassium. Assess edema, skin turgor, mucous membranes for hydration status. Assess muscle strength, mental status. Note skin temperature, moisture. Obtain baseline weight. Initiate I&O.

INTERVENTION/EVALUATION

Continue to monitor B/P, vital signs, electrolytes, I&O, weight. Note extent of diuresis. Watch for electrolyte disturbances (hypokalemia may result in weakness, tremor, muscle cramps, nausea, vomiting, change in mental status, tachycardia; hyponatremia may result in confusion, thirst, cold/clammy skin).

PATIENT/FAMILY TEACHING

Expect increased frequency and volume of urination. To reduce hypotensive effect, rise slowly

from lying to sitting position and permit legs to dangle momentarily before standing. Eat foods high in potassium such as whole grains (cereals), legumes, meat, bananas, apricots, orange juice, potatoes (white, sweet), raisins.

metoprolol tartrate

meh-**toe**-pro-lol
(Lopressor, Toprol XL)

FIXED-COMBINATION(S)
W/hydrochlorothiazide, a diuretic **(Lopressor HCT)**

CANADIAN AVAILABILITY
Apo-Metoprolol, Betaloc, Lopressor, Novometoprol

PREGNANCY CATEGORY C
(D if used in second or third trimester)

CLASSIFICATION

Beta-adrenergic blocker

AVAILABILITY (Rx)

Tablets: 50 mg, 100 mg. **Tablets (extended-release):** 50 mg, 100 mg, 200 mg. **Injection:** 1 mg/ml.

PHARMACODYNAMICS

	ONSET	PEAK	DURATION
Oral	10–15 min	—	6 hrs
IV	—	20 min	5–8 hrs

PHARMACOKINETICS

Absorption: Well absorbed from GI tract. Widely distributed. **Metabolism:** Metabolized in liver (undergoes significant first-pass metabolism). **Excretion:** Primarily excreted in urine. **Half-life:** 3–7 hrs.

ACTION / *THERAPEUTIC EFFECT*

Selectively blocks $beta_1$-adrenergic receptors, *slowing sinus heart rate, decreasing cardiac output, decreasing B/P* (exact mechanism unknown but may block peripheral adrenergic receptors, decrease sympathetic outflow from CNS, or decrease renin release from kidney). Large dose may block $beta_2$-adrenergic receptors, *increasing airway resistance. Decreases myocardial ischemia* severity by decreasing oxygen requirements.

USES / *UNLABELED*

Management of mild to moderate hypertension. Used alone or in combination with diuretics, especially thiazide type. Management of chronic stable angina pectoris. Reduces cardiovascular mortality in those with definite or suspected acute MI. ***Extended-release:*** Management of hypertension, long-term treatment of angina pectoris. *Treatment/prophylaxis of cardiac arrhythmias, hypertrophic cardiomyopathy, pheochromocytoma, vascular headache, tremors, anxiety, thyrotoxicosis, mitral valve prolapse syndrome.* Increases survival rate in diabetics w/heart disease.

STORAGE/HANDLING

Store parenteral form at room temperature.

ADMINISTRATION

ORAL:

- Tablets may be crushed; do not crush or break extended-release tablets.
- Give at same time each day.
- May be given w/or immediately after meals (enhances absorption).

IV:

- Administer IV injection rapidly.
- Monitor EKG during administration.

INDICATIONS/ROUTES/DOSAGE

Hypertension, angina pectoris:
Oral: Adults: Initially, 100 mg/day as single or divided dose. Increase at weekly (or longer) intervals. *Maintenance:* 100–450 mg/day.

Usual elderly dosage:
Oral: Initially, 25 mg/day. *Range:* 25–300 mg/day.

Usual dosage for extended-release tablets:
Oral: Adults: Hypertension: 50–100 mg/day as single dose. May increase at least at weekly intervals until optimum B/P attained. *Angina:* Initially, 100 mg/day as single dose. May increase at least at weekly intervals until optimum clinical response achieved.

Myocardial infarction (early treatment):
IV: Adults: 5 mg q2min for 3 doses, followed by 50 mg orally q6h for 48 hrs. Begin oral dose 15 min after last IV dose. Alternatively, in those who do not tolerate full IV dose, give 25–50 mg orally q6h, 15 min after last IV dose.

Myocardial infarction (late treatment, maintenance):
Oral: Adults: 100 mg 2 times/day for at least 3 mos.

CONTRAINDICATIONS

Overt cardiac failure, cardiogenic shock, heart block greater than first degree, sinus bradycardia. *MI:* Heart rate <45 beats/min, systolic B/P <100 mm Hg.

CAUTIONS

Bronchospastic disease, impaired renal function, peripheral vascular disease, hyperthyroidism, diabetes, inadequate cardiac function.

INTERACTIONS

DRUG: ***Diuretics, other hypotensives*** may increase hypotensive effect; ***sympathomimetics, xanthines*** may mutually inhibit effects; may mask symptoms of hypoglycemia, prolong hypoglycemic effect of ***insulin, oral hypoglycemics; NSAIDs*** may decrease antihypertensive effect; ***cimetidine*** may increase concentration. **HERBAL:** None known. **FOOD:** None significant. **ALTERED LAB VALUES:** May increase ANA titer, SGOT (AST), SGPT (ALT), alkaline phosphatase, LDH, bilirubin, BUN, creatinine, potassium, uric acid, lipoproteins, triglycerides.

SIDE EFFECTS

Generally well tolerated, w/transient and mild side effects. **FREQUENT:** Decreased sexual ability, drowsiness, insomnia, unusually tired or weak. **OCCASIONAL:** Anxiety, nervousness, diarrhea, constipation, nausea, vomiting, nasal congestion, stomach discomfort, dizziness, difficulty breathing, cold hands or feet. **RARE:** Altered taste, dry eyes, itching, nightmares, numbness in fingers, feet, allergic reactions (rash, itching).

ADVERSE REACTIONS/TOXIC EFFECTS

Excessive dosage may produce profound bradycardia, hypotension, bronchospasm. Abrupt withdrawal may result in sweating, palpitations, headache, tremulousness, exacerbation of angina, MI, ventricular arrhythmias. May precipitate CHF, MI in those with cardiac disease, thyroid storm in those with thyrotoxicosis, peripheral ischemia in those

M

w/existing peripheral vascular disease. Hypoglycemia may occur in previously controlled diabetics.

PATIENT CONSIDERATIONS

Baseline Assessment

Assess baseline renal/liver function tests. Assess B/P, apical pulse immediately before drug is administered (if pulse is 60/min or below, or systolic B/P is below 90 mm Hg, withhold medication, contact physician).

Antianginal
Record onset, type (sharp, dull, squeezing), radiation, location, intensity, and duration of anginal pain, and precipitating factors (exertion, emotional stress).

Intervention/Evaluation

Measure B/P near end of dosing interval (determines if B/P is controlled throughout day). Monitor B/P for hypotension, respiration for shortness of breath. Assess pulse for strength/weakness, irregular rate, bradycardia. Assist w/ambulation if dizziness occurs. Check skin for evidence of rash. Assess for evidence of CHF: dyspnea (particularly on exertion or lying down), night cough, peripheral edema, distended neck veins. Monitor I&O (increase in weight, decrease in urine output may indicate CHF). Therapeutic response to hypertension noted in 1–2 wks.

Patient/Family Teaching

Do not abruptly discontinue medication. Compliance w/therapy regimen is essential to control hypertension, arrhythmias. If a dose is missed, take next scheduled dose (do not double dose). To avoid hypotensive effect, rise slowly from lying to sitting position, wait momentarily before standing. Avoid tasks that require alertness, motor skills until response to drug is established. Report excessive fatigue, dizziness. Do not use nasal decongestants, OTC cold preparations (stimulants) w/o physician approval. Outpatients should monitor B/P, pulse before taking medication. Restrict salt, alcohol intake.

metronidazole hydrochloride

meh-trow-**nye**-dah-zoll
(Flagyl, MetroCream, MetroGel, MetroLotion, Noritate, Protostat, Satric)

FIXED-COMBINATION(S)
W/bismuth subsalicylate and tetracycline, an anti-infective **(Helidac)**

CANADIAN AVAILABILITY
Apo-Metronidazole, Flagyl, MetroCream, MetroGel, NidaGel, Noritate, Novonidazol

PREGNANCY CATEGORY B

CLASSIFICATION

Antibacterial, antiprotozoal

AVAILABILITY (Rx)

Tablets: 250 mg, 500 mg. **Extended-Release Tablets:** 750 mg. **Capsules:** 375 mg. **Powder for Injection:** 500 mg. **Injection (infusion):** 500 mg/100 ml. **Lotion:** 0.75%. **Vaginal Gel:** 0.75%. **Topical Gel:** 0.75%. **Topical Cream:** 1%.

PHARMACOKINETICS

Absorption: Well absorbed from GI tract, minimal absorption after topical application. Widely distributed, crosses blood-brain barrier. **Metabolism:** Metabolized in liver to active metabolite. **Excretion:** Primarily excreted in urine; partially eliminated in feces. Removed by hemodialysis. **Half-life:** 8 hrs (increased in alcoholic liver disease, neonates).

ACTION/*THERAPEUTIC EFFECT*

Taken up by cells in susceptible microorganisms. Disrupts DNA, inhibits nucleic acid synthesis *producing bactericidal, amebicidal, trichomonacidal effects.* Produces anti-inflammatory, immunosuppressive effects when applied topically.

USES/*UNLABELED*

Treatment of anaerobic infections (skin/skin structure, CNS, lower respiratory tract, bone and joints, intra-abdominal, gynecologic, endocarditis, septicemia). Treatment of trichomoniasis, amebiasis, perioperatively for contaminated/potentially contaminated intra-abdominal surgery, antibiotic-associated pseudomembranous colitis. Treatment of *H. pylori*-associated gastritis/duodenal ulcer. Topical application in treatment of acne rosacea. Also used in treatment of grade III, IV decubitus ulcers w/anaerobic infection. Treatment of bacterial vaginosis. *Treatment of inflammatory bowel disease.*

ADMINISTRATION

ORAL:

- May give w/o regard to meals. Give w/food to decrease GI irritation.

IV:

- Infuse >30–60 min. Do not give bolus.
- Avoid prolonged use of indwelling catheters.

INDICATIONS/ROUTES/DOSAGE

Anaerobic bacterial infections:
IV: Adults, elderly: Initially, 1 g, then 500 mg q6–8h.
Oral: Adults, elderly: 500 mg q6–8h. ***Maximum:*** 4 g/24 hrs.

Antibiotic-associated pseudomembranous colitis:
Oral: Adults, elderly: 750 mg to 2 g/day in 3–4 divided doses for 7–14 days.

Trichomoniasis:
Oral: Adults: 2 g as single or in 2 divided doses for 1 day or 250 mg 3 times/day for 7 days or 375 mg 2 times/day for 7 days. ***Children:*** 15 mg/kg in 3 divided doses for 7–10 days. ***Infants:*** 10–30 mg/kg/day for 5–8 days.

Bacterial vaginosis:
Intravaginal: Adults: One applicatorful 2 times/day or once daily at bedtime for 5 days.
Oral: Adults: 750 mg once a day.

Amebiasis:
Oral: Adults, elderly: 500–750 mg 3 times/day for 5–10 days. ***Children:*** 35–50 mg/kg/day in 3 divided doses for 5 days.

Perioperative prophylaxis:
IV: Adults, elderly: 1 g 1 hr before surgery and 500 mg 6 and 12 hrs after initial dose.

Rosacea:
Topical: Adults: Thin application 2 times/day to affected area. ***Cream:*** Once daily. ***Lotion:*** Apply twice daily.

CONTRAINDICATIONS

Hypersensitivity to metronidazole or other nitroimidazole derivatives (also parabens w/topical application).

CAUTIONS

Blood dyscrasias, severe hepatic dysfunction, CNS disease, predisposition to edema, concurrent corticosteroid therapy. Safety and efficacy of topical administration in those <21 yrs of age not established.

INTERACTIONS

DRUG: ***Alcohol*** may cause disulfiram-type reaction. May increase effect of ***oral anticoagulants.*** May increase toxicity w/***disulfiram.*** **HERBAL:** None known. **FOOD:** None significant. **ALTERED LAB VALUES:** May increase SGOT (AST), SGPT (ALT), LDH.

SIDE EFFECTS

FREQUENT: Anorexia, nausea, dry mouth, metallic taste. ***Vaginal:*** Symptomatic cervicitis/vaginitis, abdominal cramps, uterine pain. **OCCASIONAL:** Diarrhea or constipation, vomiting, dizziness, erythematous rash, urticaria, reddish brown or dark urine. ***Topical:*** Transient redness, mild dryness, burning, irritation, stinging (also tearing when applied too close to eyes). ***Vaginal:*** Vaginal, perineal, vulvar itching, vulvar swelling. **RARE:** Mild, transient leukopenia, thrombophlebitis w/IV therapy.

ADVERSE REACTIONS/TOXIC EFFECTS

Oral therapy may result in furry tongue, glossitis, cystitis, dysuria, pancreatitis, flattening of T waves w/EKG readings. Peripheral neuropathy (numbness, tingling, paresthesia) is usually reversible if treatment is stopped immediately upon appearance of neurologic symptoms. Seizures occur occasionally.

PATIENT CONSIDERATIONS

Baseline Assessment

Question for history of hypersensitivity to metronidazole or other nitroimidazole derivatives (and parabens w/topical). Obtain specimens for diagnostic tests before giving first dose (therapy may begin before results are known).

Intervention/Evaluation

Evaluate food tolerance. Determine pattern of bowel activity. Check leukocyte counts frequently. Monitor I&O and assess for urinary problems. Be alert to neurologic symptoms: dizziness, numbness, tingling or paresthesia of extremities. Assess for rash, urticaria. Watch for onset of superinfection: ulceration or change of oral mucosa, furry tongue, vaginal discharge, genital/anal pruritus.

Patient/Family Teaching

Urine may be red-brown or dark because of metabolism of drug. Avoid alcohol and alcohol-containing preparations, (e.g., cough syrups, elixirs). Hard candy, gum, or tepid water may help w/dry mouth. If dizziness occurs, do not drive or use machines that require alertness. If taking metronidazole for trichomoniasis, refrain from sexual intercourse until physician advises. Report any new symptom to physician, especially dizziness, numbness, tingling. For amebiasis, frequent stool specimen checks will be necessary.

Topical
Avoid contact w/eyes. May apply cosmetics after application. Metronidazole acts on redness, papules, and pustules but has no effect on rhinophyma (hypertrophy of nose), telangiectasia, or ocular problems (conjunctivitis, keratitis, blepharitis). Other recommendations for rosacea

include avoidance of hot or spicy foods, alcohol, extremes of hot or cold temperatures, excessive sunlight.

mexiletine hydrochloride

mex-**ill**-eh-teen
(Mexitil)

CANADIAN AVAILABILITY
Mexitil

PREGNANCY CATEGORY C

CLASSIFICATION

Antiarrhythmic

AVAILABILITY (Rx)

Capsules: 150 mg, 200 mg, 250 mg

PHARMACODYNAMICS

	ONSET	PEAK	DURATION
Oral	0.5–2 hrs	2–3 hrs	8–12 hrs

PHARMACOKINETICS

Absorption: Well absorbed from upper intestinal section of GI tract. **Metabolism:** Metabolized in liver (undergoes first-pass effect). **Excretion:** Excreted via biliary system. Removed by hemodialysis. **Half-life:** 10–12 hrs (increase in liver disease, decreased renal function).

ACTION/*THERAPEUTIC EFFECT*

Shortens duration of action potential, decreases effective refractory period in His-Purkinje system of myocardium by blocking sodium transport across myocardial cell membranes, *suppressing ventricular arrhythmias.*

USES/*UNLABELED*

Suppress symptomatic ventricular arrhythmias (PVCs, unifocal or multifocal, couplets, and ventricular tachycardia). *Diabetic neuropathy.*

ADMINISTRATION

ORAL:

- Do not crush or break capsules.
- Give w/food or antacid to reduce GI distress.

INDICATIONS/ROUTES/DOSAGE

Usual dosage for arrhythmias:
Oral: Adults, elderly: Initially, 200 mg q8h. Adjust dose by 50–100 mg at 2–3 day intervals. ***Maintenance:*** 200–300 mg q8h. ***Maximum:*** 1,200 mg/day. **Note:** If 300 mg q8h or less controls arrhythmias, may give dose q12h. ***Maximum:*** 450 mg q12h.

Rapid control of arrhythmias:
Oral: Adults, elderly: Initially, 400 mg, then 200 mg q8h.

CONTRAINDICATIONS

Cardiogenic shock, preexisting second- or third-degree AV block (w/o presence of pacemaker).

CAUTIONS

Impaired myocardial function, second- or third-degree AV block (w/pacemaker), CHF, sick-sinus syndrome (bradycardia/tachycardia).

INTERACTIONS

DRUG: ***Urinary acidifiers*** may increase excretion, ***urinary alkalizers*** may decrease excretion. ***Hepatic enzyme inducers*** may decrease concentrations. ***Metoclopramide*** may increase absorption. **HERBAL:** None known. **FOOD:** None significant. **ALTERED LAB VALUES:** May cause positive ANA titers. May increase SGOT (AST).

SIDE EFFECTS

FREQUENT (>10%): GI distress (nausea, vomiting, heartburn), dizziness, lightheadedness, tremor. **OCCASIONAL (1–10%):** Nervousness, change in sleep habits, headache, visual disturbances, paresthesia, diarrhea/constipation, palpitations, chest pain, rash, respiratory difficulty, edema. **RARE (<1%):** Dry mouth, weakness, fatigue, tinnitus, depression, speech difficulties.

ADVERSE REACTIONS/TOXIC EFFECTS

Has ability to worsen existing arrhythmias or produce new ones. May produce or worsen CHF.

PATIENT CONSIDERATIONS

INTERVENTION/EVALUATION

Monitor EKG, vital signs closely during and after drug administration for cardiac performance. Assess pulse for irregular rate, strength/weakness. Observe for GI disturbances (high incidence). Monitor pattern of daily bowel activity and stool consistency. Assess for dizziness, syncope. Evaluate hand movement for tremor. Check for evidence of CHF (cough, dyspnea [particularly on exertion], rales at base of lungs, fatigue). Monitor fluid and electrolyte serum levels. Check for therapeutic serum level (0.5–2 mcg/ml).

PATIENT/FAMILY TEACHING

Compliance w/therapy regimen is essential to control cardiac arrhythmias. Report shortness of breath, cough, unexplained sore throat or fever, generalized fatigue. Do not use nasal decongestants, OTC cold preparations (stimulants) w/o physician approval. Restrict salt, alcohol intake.

mezlocillin sodium

mezz-low-**sill**-in
(Mezlin)

PREGNANCY CATEGORY B

CLASSIFICATION

Antibiotic: Penicillin

AVAILABILITY (Rx)

Powder for Injection: 1 g, 2 g, 3 g, 4 g, 10 g

PHARMACOKINETICS

Absorption: Well absorbed after IM administration. Widely distributed. **Excretion:** Primarily excreted unchanged in urine. Removed by hemodialysis. **Half-life:** 50–70 min.

ACTION/*THERAPEUTIC EFFECT*

Binds to bacterial membranes, *inhibiting cell wall synthesis. Bactericidal.*

USES

Treatment of gynecologic, skin/skin structure, respiratory, urinary tract, bone and joint, intra-abdominal infections, septicemia, gonorrhea (w/probenecid), perioperative prophylaxis, especially in abdominal surgery.

STORAGE/HANDLING

Solution appears clear, colorless to pale yellow; may darken slightly (does not indicate loss of potency). If precipitate forms, redissolve in warm water, agitate. IV infusion (piggyback) is stable for 24 hrs at room temperature.

ADMINISTRATION

- **Note:** Space doses evenly around the clock.

IM:
- For IM injection, inject slowly and deeply into gluteus maximus.
- Avoid IM injections >2 g.

IV:
- For IV injection, administer over 3–5 min.
- For intermittent IV infusion (piggyback), infuse over 30 min.
- Because of potential for hypersensitivity/anaphylaxis, start initial dose at few drops per minute, increase slowly to ordered rate; stay w/pt first 10–15 min, then check q10min.
- Alternating IV sites, use large veins to reduce risk of phlebitis.

INDICATIONS/ROUTES/DOSAGE

Uncomplicated UTI:
IM/IV: Adults, elderly: 1.5–2 g q6h.

Complicated UTI:
IM/IV: Adults, elderly: 3 g q6h.

Lower respiratory tract, intra-abdominal, gynecologic, skin/skin structure infections, septicemia:
IV: Adults, elderly: 4 g q6h or 3 g q4h.

Life-threatening infections:
IV: Adults, elderly: Up to 4 g q4h. *Maximum:* 24 g/day.

Acute, uncomplicated gonococcal urethritis:
IM/IV: Adults: 1–2 g one time w/1 g probenecid.

Perioperative prophylaxis:
IV: Adults, elderly: 4 g 30–90 min before surgery and 6 and 12 hrs after first dose.

Cesarean section:
IV: Adults: 4 g after umbilical cord clamped, then 4 and 8 hrs after first dose.

Usual dosage (children):
IM/IV: Children 1 mo–12 yrs: 50 mg/kg q4h.

Usual dosage (neonates):
IM/IV: Neonates 0–7 days: 75 mg/kg q8–12h. *Neonates 7–28 days:* 75 mg/kg q6–12h.

Dosage in renal impairment:
Dose and/or frequency modified on basis of creatinine clearance and/or severity of infection.

	CREATININE 10–30 ML/MIN	CLEARANCE <10 ML/MIN
Uncomplicated UTI	1.5 g q8h	1.5 g q8h
Complicated UTI	1.5 g q6h	1.5 g q8h
Serious infections	3 g q8h	2 g q8h
Life-threatening infections	3 g q6h	2 g q6h

CONTRAINDICATIONS

Hypersensitivity to any penicillin.

CAUTIONS

History of allergies, especially cephalosporins.

INTERACTIONS

DRUG: *Probenecid* may increase concentration, toxicity risk. **HERBAL:** None known. **FOOD:** None significant. **ALTERED LAB VALUES:** May increase SGOT (AST), SGPT (ALT), alkaline phosphatase, bilirubin, creatinine, sodium. May cause positive Coombs' test. May decrease potassium.

SIDE EFFECTS

FREQUENT: Rash, urticaria, pain, and induration at IM injection site; phlebitis, thrombophlebitis w/IV doses. OCCASIONAL: Nausea, vomiting, diarrhea, hypernatremia. RARE: Bleeding may occur w/high IV dosage; hypokalemia, headache, fatigue, dizziness.

ADVERSE REACTIONS/TOXIC EFFECTS

Superinfections, potentially fatal antibiotic-associated colitis may result from altered bacterial balance. Seizures, neurologic reactions may occur w/overdosage (most often w/renal impairment). Acute interstitial nephritis, severe hypersensitivity reactions occur rarely.

PATIENT CONSIDERATIONS

BASELINE ASSESSMENT

Question for history of allergies, especially penicillins, cephalosporins. Obtain specimen for culture and sensitivity before giving first dose (therapy may begin before results are known).

INTERVENTION/EVALUATION

Hold medication and promptly report rash (hypersensitivity) or diarrhea (w/fever, abdominal pain, mucus and blood in stool may indicate antibiotic-associated colitis). Assess food tolerance. Evaluate IV site for phlebitis (heat, pain, red streaking over vein). Check IM injection sites for pain, induration. Monitor I&O, urinalysis, renal function tests. Assess for bleeding: overt bleeding, bruising or tissue swelling; check hematology reports. Monitor electrolytes, particularly sodium, potassium. Be alert for superinfection: increased fever, onset sore throat, diarrhea, vomiting, ulceration or other oral changes, anal/genital pruritus.

PATIENT/FAMILY TEACHING

Continue antibiotic for full length of treatment. Space doses evenly. Discomfort may occur at IM injection site. Notify physician in event of rash, diarrhea, bleeding, bruising, other new symptom.

---

miconazole nitrate

mih-**kon**-nah-zoll

(Micatin, Monistat 3, 7, Monistat-Derm, M-Zole 3)

miconazole

(Monistat IV)

CANADIAN AVAILABILITY

Micatin, Micozole, Monistat

PREGNANCY CATEGORY C

CLASSIFICATION

Antifungal

AVAILABILITY (Rx)

Injection: 10 mg/ml. **Vaginal Suppository:** 100 mg, 200 mg. **Topical Cream:** 2%. **Vaginal Cream:** 2%. **Topical Powder:** 2%. **Topical Spray:** 2%.

PHARMACOKINETICS

Parenteral: Widely distributed in tissues. **Metabolism:** Metabolized in liver. **Excretion:** Primarily excreted in urine. **Half-life:** 24 hrs. *Topical:* **Absorption:** No systemic absorption following application to intact skin. *Intravaginal:* **Absorption:** Small amount absorbed systemically.

ACTION/THERAPEUTIC EFFECT

Inhibits synthesis of ergosterol (vital component of fungal cell formation), damaging fungal cell membrane. *Fungistatic; may be fungicidal, depending on concentration.*

USES

Treatment of coccidioidomycosis, paracoccidioidomycosis, cryptococcosis, petriellidiosis (allescheriosis), disseminated candidiasis, chronic mucocutaneous candidiasis. Fungal meningitis usually treated intrathecally as well as IV; urinary bladder infections w/installations as well as IV miconazole. ***Vaginally:*** Vulvovaginal candidiasis. ***Topical:*** Cutaneous candidiasis, tinea cruris, t. corporis, t. pedis, t. versicolor.

STORAGE/HANDLING

After reconstitution, IV solution is stable for 24 hrs at room temperature w/5% dextrose or 0.9% NaCl.

ADMINISTRATION

IV:

- Dilute each 200 mg ampoule w/at least 200 ml 5% dextrose or 0.9% NaCl to provide maximum concentration of 1 mg/ml.
- Give IV infusion (piggyback) over at least 30–60 min (rapid administration may cause arrhythmias).
- Because of incidence of phlebitis, central venous catheters are recommended.
- Initial treatment should be performed in hospital w/physician in attendance for first 200 mg dose.

INDICATIONS/ROUTES/DOSAGE

Note: IV doses may be divided over 3 IV infusions.

Coccidioidomycosis:
IV: Adults, elderly: 1.8–3.6 g/day for 3–20 wks or longer.

Cryptococcosis:
IV: Adults, elderly: 1.2–2.4 g/day for 3–12 wks or longer.

Petriellidiosis:
IV: Adults, elderly: 0.6–3.0 g/day for 5–20 wks or longer.

Candidiasis:
IV: Adults, elderly: 0.6–1.8 g/day for 1–20 wks or longer.

Paracoccidioidomycosis:
IV: Adults, elderly: 0.2–1.2 g/day for 2–16 wks or longer.

Usual dosage for children:
IV: 20–40 mg/kg/day in 3 divided doses. (Do not exceed 15 mg/kg for any 1 infusion.)

Vulvovaginal candidiasis:
Intravaginal: Adults, elderly: One 200 mg suppository at bedtime for 3 days; one 100 mg suppository or one applicatorful at bedtime for 7 days.

Topical fungal infections, cutaneous candidiasis:
Topical: Adults, elderly: Apply liberally 2 times/day, morning and evening.

CONTRAINDICATIONS

Hypersensitivity to miconazole. Children <1 yr; topically, children <2 yrs.

CAUTIONS

Hepatic insufficiency.

INTERACTIONS

DRUG: May increase effects of ***oral anticoagulants, oral hypoglycemics. Isoniazid, rifampin*** may decrease concentrations. May increase ***cisapride*** concentration, risk of cardiotoxicity. **HERBAL:** None known.

M

FOOD: None significant. ALTERED LAB VALUES: None significant.

SIDE EFFECTS

FREQUENT (>5%): Phlebitis, fever, chills, rash, itching, nausea, vomiting. OCCASIONAL (1–5%): Dizziness, drowsiness, headache, flushed face, abdominal pain, constipation, diarrhea, decreased appetite. ***Topical:*** Itching, burning, stinging, erythema, urticaria. ***Vaginal*** (2%): Vulvovaginal burning, itching, irritation, headache, skin rash. RARE: Anemia, liver toxicity, thrombocytopenia (bleeding, bruising).

ADVERSE REACTIONS/TOXIC EFFECTS

Anemia, thrombocytopenia occur rarely.

PATIENT CONSIDERATIONS

BASELINE ASSESSMENT

Question for history of allergies, especially to miconazole. Confirm that cultures or histologic tests were done. Check for/obtain orders for antiemetics, antihistamines (given before infusion to reduce nausea, vomiting).

INTERVENTION/EVALUATION

Check for nausea, vomiting (administer medication for symptomatic relief; avoid dosing at mealtimes, slow infusion rate). Assess skin for rash. Evaluate IV site for phlebitis. Determine pattern of bowel activity, stool consistency. Assess mental status (dizziness, drowsiness), provide assistance as needed. Monitor Hgb/Hct results, be alert for bleeding, bruising.

Topical/vaginal
Assess for burning, itching, irritation.

PATIENT/FAMILY TEACHING

Continue full length of treatment; prolonged therapy (weeks or months) may be necessary for some conditions. Discomfort may occur at IV site. Notify physician in event of bleeding, bruising, soft tissue swelling, or other new symptom. Do not ambulate w/o assistance or use any machinery if dizziness, drowsiness occur. Consult physician before taking any other medication.

Vaginal preparations
Base interacts w/certain latex products such as contraceptive diaphragm. Ask physician about douching, sexual intercourse.

Topical
Rub well into affected areas. Avoid getting in eyes. Do not apply any other preparations or occlusive covering w/o consulting physician. Use ointment (sparingly) or lotion in intertriginous areas. Keep areas clean, dry; wear light clothing for ventilation. Separate personal items in contact w/affected areas.

---

midazolam hydrochloride

my-**day**-zoe-lam
(Versed)

CANADIAN AVAILABILITY
Versed

PREGNANCY CATEGORY D

CLASSIFICATION

Sedative (Schedule IV)

AVAILABILITY (Rx)

Injection: 1 mg/ml, 5 mg/ml. **Syrup:** 2 mg/ml.

PHARMACODYNAMICS

	ONSET	PEAK	DURATION
IM			
	5–15 min	45 min	1–6 hrs
IV related			
	1–5 min	—	Dose related

PHARMACOKINETICS

Absorption: Well absorbed after IM administration. **Metabolism:** Metabolized in liver to active metabolite. **Excretion:** Primarily excreted in urine. **Half-life:** 1–5 hrs.

ACTION/*THERAPEUTIC EFFECT*

Enhances action of gamma-aminobutyric acid (GABA) neurotransmission at CNS, *producing sedative, anxiolytic effect due to CNS depressant action.* Inhibits spinal afferent pathways, *producing skeletal muscle relaxation.* Directly depresses motor nerve, muscle function effects.

USES/*UNLABELED*

IM: Preop for sedation, relief of anxiety; produces anterograde amnesia. *IV:* Sedation (w/o loss of consciousness) to relieve anxiety; produces anterograde amnesia for short diagnostic, endoscopic procedures, intubated/mechanical ventilator pts. *Adjunct to local anesthesia.*

STORAGE/HANDLING

Store at room temperature. Although undiluted solution should be protected from light, it is unnecessary to protect diluted solution from light.

ADMINISTRATION

- **Note:** Compatible w/5% dextrose, 0.9% NaCl, lactated Ringer's. Compatible for 30 min w/atropine, meperidine, morphine, scopolamine, low doses of opiate agonists.

IM:

- Give deep IM into large muscle mass.

IV:

- Oxygen, resuscitative equipment must be readily available before IV is administered.
- Administer by slow IV injection, in incremental dosages: Give each incremental dose over 2 or more minutes at intervals of at least 2 min.
- Reduce IV rate in those >60 yrs, and/or debilitated, those w/chronic disease states, and/or impaired pulmonary function.
- A too rapid IV rate, excessive doses, or a single large dose increases risk of respiratory depression/arrest.

INDICATIONS/ROUTES/DOSAGE

Preop:
IM: Adults >18 yrs: 70–80 mcg/kg (0.07–0.08 mg/kg) 30–60 min before surgery. ***Elderly/debilitated:*** Dosage should be lowered. ***Children:*** Individualized.

Conscious sedation:
*IV: **Adults:*** Initially, up to 2.5 mg. May further titrate in small increments to desired effect. Total dose rarely >5 mg. ***Elderly:*** Initially, up to 1.5 mg. May further titrate to desired effect. Total dose rarely >3.5 mg.

Adjunct to anesthesia:
*IV: **Adults:*** Initially, 150–350 mcg/kg. ***Elderly:*** Initially, 150–300 mcg/kg.

M

Additional doses, 25% of initial dose. ***Children:*** Individualized.

Usual oral dosage:
Children: 0.25–1 mg/kg. ***Maximum:*** 20 mg.

CONTRAINDICATIONS

Shock, comatose pts, acute alcohol intoxication, acute narrow-angle glaucoma.

CAUTIONS

Acute illness, severe fluid/electrolyte imbalance, impaired renal function, CHF, treated open-angle glaucoma.

INTERACTIONS

DRUG: *Alcohol, CNS depressants* may increase CNS, respiratory depression, hypotensive effects. *Hypotension-producing medications* may increase hypotensive effects. **HERBAL:** Kava kava, valerian may increase CNS depression. **FOOD:** Grapefruit juice increases absorption. **ALTERED LAB VALUES:** None significant.

SIDE EFFECTS

FREQUENT (3–10%): Hypotension (especially when pre-med w/narcotics), hiccups, pain at IM injection site or during IV injection, tenderness at IV site. **OCCASIONAL(1–3%):** Changes in vision, cough, dizziness, drowsiness, headache, hardness at injection site, nausea, numbness, muscle stiffness at injection site, vomiting. **RARE (<1%):** Delirium, hyperventilation, phlebitis, skin rash, hives, itching, wheezing.

ADVERSE REACTIONS/TOXIC EFFECTS

Too much or too little dosage, improper administration, or cerebral hypoxia may result in agitation, involuntary movements, hyperactivity, combativeness. Underventilation/apnea may produce hypoxia, cardiac arrest. A too rapid IV rate, excessive doses, or a single large dose increases risk of respiratory depression/arrest.

PATIENT CONSIDERATIONS

BASELINE ASSESSMENT

Resuscitative equipment, endotracheal tube, suction, oxygen must be available. Obtain vital signs before administration.

INTERVENTION/EVALUATION

Monitor respiratory rate continuously during parenteral administration for underventilation, apnea. Monitor vital signs q3–5min during recovery period.

PATIENT/FAMILY TEACHING

Discomfort may occur w/IM injection.

midodrine

my-dough-dreen
(Amatine)

CANADIAN AVAILABILITY
Amatine

PREGNANCY CATEGORY C

CLASSIFICATION

Vasopressor

AVAILABILITY (Rx)

Tablets: 2.5 mg, 5 mg

PHARMACODYNAMICS

	ONSET	PEAK	DURATION
Oral	15–30 min	1–2 hrs	2–3 hrs

PHARMACOKINETICS

Absorption: Well absorbed from GI tract. **Metabolism:** Metabolized in liver to active metabolite. **Excretion:** Eliminated by the kidneys. **Half-life:** 3–4 hrs.

ACTION/*THERAPEUTIC EFFECT*

Activates alpha-adrenergic receptors of arteriolar and venous vasculature, *producing elevation of standing, sitting, and supine systolic and diastolic blood pressure.*

USES/*UNLABELED*

Treatment of symptomatic orthostatic hypotension. *Management of urinary incontinence.*

ADMINISTRATION

ORAL:

- Give during daytime when the patient is upright, pursuing daily activities, (i.e., shortly before or upon arising in the morning, midday and late afternoon, no later than 6 PM).
- Do not give after the evening meal or <4 hrs before bedtime.
- May be given in 3 hr intervals, if necessary, to control symptoms.

INDICATIONS/ROUTES/DOSAGES

Orthostatic hypotension:
Oral: Adults, elderly: 10 mg, 3 times daily. *Renal impairment:* Starting dose of 2.5 mg.

CONTRAINDICATIONS

Severe organic heart disease, acute renal disease, urinary retention, pheochromocytoma, thyrotoxicosis, persistent and excessive supine hypertension.

CAUTIONS

Urinary retention problems, renal impairment, hepatic impairment, orthostatic hypotensive patients who are diabetic, history of visual problems, those taking fludrocortisone acetate.

INTERACTIONS

DRUG: Concurrent administration with ***cardiac glycosides, psychopharmacologic agents, beta blockers*** may precipitate bradycardia, A/V block or arrhythmia. ***Alpha-adrenergic agonists*** may potentiate pressor effect of midodrine. ***Fludrocortisone*** may produce increase in intraocular pressure, glaucoma. ***Alpha-adrenergic antagonists*** may antagonize effects of midodrine. **HERBAL:** None known. **FOOD:** None significant. **ALTERED LAB VALUES:** None significant.

SIDE EFFECTS

FREQUENT (12–18%): Paresthesia, piloerection (goose bumps), dysuria, pruritus. **OCCASIONAL (5–7%):** Supine hypertension, chills, pain. **RARE (<2%):** Rash, headache, feeling of pressure/fullness in the head, flushing of the face, confusion/abnormal thinking, dry mouth, anxiety/nervousness.

ADVERSE REACTIONS/TOXIC EFFECTS

Overdosage may produce hypertension, sensation of coldness, urinary retention. ***Antidote:*** Nemesis, phentolamine.

PATIENT CONSIDERATIONS

BASELINE ASSESSMENT

Obtain baseline B/P, pulse before therapy begins. Prevent patient from becoming fully supine (sleeping with head of bed elevated) in order to avoid risk of supine hypertension. Obtain renal and hepatic function studies before initial therapy begins and routinely thereafter during treatment.

M

Interventions/Evaluation

Monitor sitting and supine blood pressures in those beginning maintenance therapy and routinely thereafter, especially in those using concurrent agents that causes vasoconstriction. Assess for urinary retention; question for evidence of dysuria. A slight slowing of heart rate may occur after administration; if bradycardia occurs, therapy should be discontinued. Assess extremities for paresthesia, piloerection.

Patient/Family Teaching

Do not take other medications without physician's knowledge.

---

mifepristone

(Mifeprex)

See Supplement

---

miglitol

mig-lig-toll

(Glyset)

PREGNANCY CATEGORY B

CLASSIFICATION

Antidiabetic

AVAILABILITY (Rx)

Tablets: 25 mg, 50 mg, 100 mg

PHARMACOKINETICS

Absorption: Well absorbed from GI tract. Primarily distributed into extracellular fluid. **Metabolism:** Miglitol is not metabolized. **Excretion:** Excreted unchanged in the urine. **Half-life:** 2 hrs.

ACTION/*THERAPEUTIC EFFECT*

Delays ingestion of ingested carbohydrates *resulting in a smaller rise in blood glucose following meals.*

USES

Adjunct to diet to improve glycemic control in patients with Type II noninsulin-dependent diabetes mellitus (NIDDM). May also be used in combination with a sulfonylurea when diet plus miglitol does not result in adequate glycemic control.

ADMINISTRATION

ORAL:

- To be taken with the first bite of each main meal.

INDICATIONS/ROUTES/DOSAGES

Antidiabetic:

Oral: Adults, elderly: Initially, 25 mg 3 times/day with first bite of each main meal. ***Maintenance:*** 50 mg 3 times/day. ***Maximum:*** 100 mg 3 times/day.

CONTRAINDICATIONS

Diabetic ketoacidosis, inflammatory bowel disease, colonic ulceration, partial intestinal obstruction, predisposition to intestinal obstruction, chronic intestinal disease associated with marked disorders of digestion or absorption or with conditions that may deteriorate as a result of increased gas formation in the intestine.

CAUTIONS

Renal function impairment.

INTERACTIONS

DRUG: May reduce plasma concentrations of ***digoxin.*** May significantly reduce effect of ***propranolol, ranitidine. Digestive enzymes (amylase, pancreatin), intestinal***

adsorbents (charcoal) may reduce effect of miglitol. **HERBAL:** None known. **FOOD:** None significant. **ALTERED LAB VALUES:** May produce transient low serum iron (9%).

SIDE EFFECTS

Note: If side effects occur, they are generally transient, mild to moderate, and diminish in frequency and intensity with time. **FREQUENT (29–41%):** Flatulence, diarrhea. **OCCASIONAL (4–11%):** Abdominal pain, skin rash (usually transient).

ADVERSE REACTIONS/TOXIC EFFECTS

Overdosage does *not* cause hypoglycemia.

PATIENT CONSIDERATIONS

Baseline Assessment

Check blood glucose level. Discuss lifestyle to determine extent of learning, emotional needs. Assure follow-up instruction if pt/family do not thoroughly understand diabetes management or glucose-testing technique.

Interventions/Evaluation

Monitor blood glucose and food intake. Assess for hypoglycemia (cool wet skin, tremors, dizziness, anxiety, headache, tachycardia, numbness in mouth, hunger, diplopia) or hyperglycemia (polyuria, polyphagia, polydipsia, nausea, vomiting, dim vision, fatigue, deep rapid breathing). Be alert to conditions that alter glucose requirements: fever, increased activity or stress, surgical procedures.

Patient/Family Teaching

Diabetes mellitus requires lifelong control. Prescribed diet is principal part of treatment; do not skip or delay meals. Wear medical alert identification. Continue to adhere to dietary instructions, a regular exercise program and regular testing of urine or blood glucose. When taking combination drug therapy with a sulfonylurea or insulin, have a source of glucose available to treat symptoms of low blood sugar. Take with first bite of each meal.

M

milrinone lactate

mill-rih-known
(Primacor)

CANADIAN AVAILABILITY
Primacor

PREGNANCY CATEGORY C

CLASSIFICATION

Cardiotonic

AVAILABILITY (Rx)

Injection: 1 mg/ml. **Injection (premix):** 200 mcg/ml.

PHARMACODYNAMICS

	ONSET	PEAK	DURATION
IV	5–15 min	—	—

PHARMACOKINETICS

Metabolism: Metabolized in liver. **Excretion:** Excreted in urine. **Half-life:** 2.4 hrs.

ACTION/*THERAPEUTIC EFFECT*

Possesses positive inotropic effect (increases force of myocardial contraction), direct arterial vasodilation. Reduces preload and afterload by direct effect on vascular smooth muscle. *Increases cardiac output, decreases pulmonary capillary wedge pressure and vascular resistance.*

USES

Short-term management of congestive heart failure (CHF).

STORAGE/HANDLING

Store parenteral form at room temperature.

ADMINISTRATION

IV:

- Avoid furosemide injection into tubing of milrinone IV infusion (precipitate forms immediately).
- For IV injection (loading dose) administer slowly over 10 min.
- For IV infusion, dilute 20 mg (20 ml) vial with 80 or 180 ml diluent (0.9% NaCl, 5% dextrose) to provide concentration of 200 or 100 mcg/ml, respectively.
- Monitor for arrhythmias, hypotension during IV therapy. Reduce or temporarily discontinue infusion until condition stabilizes.

INDICATIONS/ROUTES/DOSAGE

Congestive heart failure:
*IV: **Adults:*** Initially, give 50 mcg/kg over 10 min. Continue w/maintenance infusion rate of 0.375–0.75 mcg/kg/min based on hemodynamic and clinical response (total daily dose: 0.59–1.13 mg/kg). Reduce dose to 0.2–0.43 mcg/kg/min in pts w/severe renal impairment.

CONTRAINDICATIONS

Severe obstructive aortic or pulmonic valvular disease.

CAUTIONS

Impaired renal, hepatic function.

INTERACTIONS

DRUG: Produces additive inotropic effects w/***cardiac glycosides.*** **HERBAL:** None known. **FOOD:** None significant. **ALTERED LAB VALUES:** None significant.

SIDE EFFECTS

OCCASIONAL (1–3%): Headache, hypotension. **RARE (<1%):** Angina, chest pain, thrombocytopenia.

ADVERSE REACTIONS/TOXIC EFFECTS

Supraventricular and ventricular arrhythmias occur in 12%; nonsustained ventricular tachycardia occurs in 2%, sustained ventricular tachycardia in 1% of those treated.

PATIENT CONSIDERATIONS

BASELINE ASSESSMENT

Offer emotional support (difficulty breathing may produce anxiety). Assess B/P, apical pulse rate before treatment begins and during IV therapy. Assess lung sounds, check edema.

INTERVENTION/EVALUATION

Monitor for hypotension during administration (discontinue or slow IV rate until condition stabilizes). Assess heart rate, serum electrolytes, I&O, renal function studies. Monitor CHF symptoms.

minocycline hydrochloride

min-know-**sigh**-clean
(Dynacin, Minocin)

CANADIAN AVAILABILITY
Minocin, Novo Minocycline

PREGNANCY CATEGORY D

CLASSIFICATION

Antibiotic: Tetracycline

AVAILABILITY (Rx)

Capsules: 50 mg, 75 mg, 100 mg. **Tablets:** 50 mg, 100 mg. **Oral Suspension:** 50 mg/5 ml. **Powder for Injection:** 100 mg.

PHARMACOKINETICS

Absorption: Well absorbed from GI tract. Widely distributed. **Metabolism:** Partially inactivated in liver. **Excretion:** Excreted in urine, eliminated in feces via biliary secretion. Minimally removed by hemodialysis. **Half-life:** 11–23 hrs.

ACTION/*THERAPEUTIC EFFECT*

Binds to ribosomes, *inhibiting protein synthesis. Bacteriostatic.*

USES/*UNLABELED*

Treatment of prostate, urinary tract, CNS infections (not meningitis), uncomplicated gonorrhea, inflammatory acne, brucellosis, skin granulomas, cholera, trachoma, nocardiasis, yaws, and syphilis when penicillins are contraindicated. *Treatment of atypical mycobacterial infections, scleroderma.*

STORAGE/HANDLING

Store capsules, oral suspension at room temperature. IV solution stable for 24 hrs at room temperature. Use IV infusion (piggyback) immediately after reconstitution. Discard if precipitate forms.

ADMINISTRATION

ORAL:

- Give oral capsules, tablets w/full glass of water.

IV:

- For intermittent IV infusion (piggyback), reconstitute each 100 mg vial w/5–10 ml sterile water for injection to provide concentration of 20 or 10 mg/ml, respectively.
- Further dilute w/500–1,000 ml 5% dextrose or 0.9% NaCl. Infuse over 6 hrs.
- Alternating IV sites, use large veins to reduce risk of phlebitis.

INDICATIONS/ROUTES/DOSAGE

Note: Space doses evenly around the clock.

Mild to moderate to severe infections:
Oral: Adults, elderly: Initially, 100–200 mg, then 100 mg q12h or 50 mg q6h.

IV: Adults, elderly: Initially, 200 mg, then 100 mg q12h up to 400 mg/day.

Oral/IV: Children >8 yrs: Initially, 4 mg/kg, then 2 mg/kg q12h.

CONTRAINDICATIONS

Hypersensitivity to tetracyclines, last half of pregnancy, children <8 yrs.

CAUTIONS

Renal impairment, sun or ultraviolet exposure (severe photosensitivity reaction).

INTERACTIONS

DRUG: ***Cholestyramine, colestipol*** may decrease absorption. May decrease effect of ***oral contraceptives. Carbamazepine, phenytoin*** may decrease concentrations. **HERBAL:** St. John's wort may increase risk of photosensitivity. **FOOD:** None significant. **ALTERED LAB VALUES:** May increase SGOT (AST), SGPT (ALT), alkaline phosphatase, amylase, bilirubin concentrations.

SIDE EFFECTS

FREQUENT: Dizziness, lightheadedness, diarrhea, nausea, vomiting, stomach cramps, increased sensitivity of skin to sunlight. **OCCASIONAL:** Pigmentation of skin, mucous membranes, itching in rectal/genital area, sore mouth/tongue.

ADVERSE REACTIONS/TOXIC EFFECTS

Superinfection (especially fungal), anaphylaxis, increased intracranial pressure, bulging fontanelles occur rarely in infants.

PATIENT CONSIDERATIONS

Baseline Assessment

Question for history of allergies, especially tetracyclines, sulfite. Obtain culture and sensitivity test before giving first dose (therapy may begin before results are known).

Intervention/Evaluation

Check IV site for phlebitis (heat, pain, red streaking over vein). Assess ability to ambulate: drowsiness, vertigo, dizziness. Determine pattern of bowel activity and stool consistency. Monitor food intake, tolerance. Assess skin for rash. Check B/P and level of consciousness for increased intracranial pressure. Be alert for superinfection: diarrhea, ulceration or changes of oral mucosa, anal/genital pruritus.

Patient/Family Teaching

Continue antibiotic for full length of treatment. Space doses evenly. Drink full glass of water w/capsules, tablets and avoid bedtime doses. Avoid tasks that require alertness, motor skills until response to drug is established. Notify physician if diarrhea, rash, other new symptom occurs. Protect skin from sun exposure. Consult physician before taking any other medication.

minoxidil

min-**ox**-ih-dill

(Loniten, Rogaine, Rogaine Extra Strength)

CANADIAN AVAILABILITY

Loniten, Rogaine

PREGNANCY CATEGORY C

CLASSIFICATION

Antihypertensive

AVAILABILITY (Rx)

Tablets: 2.5 mg, 10 mg. **Topical Solution (OTC):** 20 mg/ml, 50 mg/ml.

PHARMACODYNAMICS

	ONSET	PEAK	DURATION
Oral	0.5 hrs	2–8 hrs	2–5 days

PHARMACOKINETICS

Absorption: Well absorbed from GI tract, minimal absorption after topical application. Widely distributed. **Metabolism:** Metabolized in liver to active metabolite. **Excretion:** Primarily excreted in urine. Removed by hemodialysis. **Half-life:** 4.2 hrs.

ACTION/*THERAPEUTIC EFFECT*

Direct action of vascular smooth

muscle, producing vasodilation of arterioles, *decreasing peripheral vascular resistance, B/P.* ***Topical:*** Vasodilatory action *increases cutaneous blood flow, stimulates hair follicle epithelium, hair follicle growth.*

USES

Treatment of severe symptomatic hypertension, or hypertension associated w/organ damage. Used for those who fail to respond to maximal therapeutic dosages of diuretic and two other antihypertensive agents. Treatment of alopecia androgenetica (***males:*** baldness of vertex of scalp; ***females:*** diffuse hair loss or thinning of frontoparietal areas).

ADMINISTRATION

ORAL:

- Give w/o regard to food (w/food if GI upset occurs).
- Tablets may be crushed.

TOPICAL:

- Shampoo and dry hair before applying medication.
- Wash hands immediately after application.
- Do not use hair dryer after application (reduces effectiveness).

INDICATIONS/ROUTES/DOSAGE

Hypertension:

Oral: Adults: Initially, 5 mg/day. Increase w/at least 3 day intervals to 10 mg, 20 mg, up to 40 mg/day in 1–2 doses. ***Elderly:*** Initially, 2.5 mg/day. May increase gradually. ***Maintenance:*** 10–40 mg/day. ***Maximum:*** 100 mg/day. ***Children:*** Initially, 0.2 mg/kg (5 mg maximum) daily. Gradually increase at minimum 3 day intervals of 0.1–2 mg/kg. ***Maintenance:*** 0.25–1 mg/kg/day in 1–2 doses. ***Maximum:*** 50 mg/day.

Hair regrowth:

Topical: Adults: 1 ml to total affected areas of scalp 2 times/day. Total daily dose not to exceed 2 ml.

CONTRAINDICATIONS

Pheochromocytoma.

CAUTIONS

Severe renal impairment, chronic CHF, coronary artery disease, recent MI (1 mo).

INTERACTIONS

DRUG: ***Parenteral antihypertensives*** may increase hypotensive effect. ***NSAIDs*** may decrease effect. **HERBAL:** None known. **FOOD:** None significant. **ALTERED LAB VALUES:** May increase BUN, creatinine, plasma renin activity, alkaline phosphatase, sodium. May decrease Hgb, Hct, erythrocyte count.

SIDE EFFECTS

FREQUENT: ***Oral:*** Edema with concurrent weight gain, hypertrichosis (elongation, thickening, increased pigmentation of fine body hair) develops in 80% of pts within 3–6 wks after beginning therapy. **OCCASIONAL:** T wave changes but usually these revert to pretreatment state with continued therapy or drug withdrawal. ***Topical:*** Itching, skin rash, dry/flaking skin, erythema. **RARE:** Rash, pruritus, breast tenderness in male and female, headache. ***Topical:*** Allergic reaction, alopecia, burning scalp, soreness at hair root, headache, visual disturbances.

ADVERSE REACTIONS/TOXIC EFFECTS

Tachycardia and angina pectoris may occur because of increased oxygen demands associated w/increased heart rate, cardiac output. Fluid and electrolyte imbalance, CHF may be observed (especially if diuretic is not given concurrently). Too rapid reduction in B/P may result in syncope, cerebral vascular accident, MI, ischemia of special sense organs (vision, hearing). Pericardial effusion and tamponade may be seen in those w/impaired renal function not on dialysis.

PATIENT CONSIDERATIONS

BASELINE ASSESSMENT

Assess B/P on both arms and take pulse for 1 full min immediately before giving medication. If pulse increases 20 beats/min or more over baseline, or systolic or diastolic B/P decreases more than 20 mm Hg, withhold drug, contact physician.

INTERVENTION/EVALUATION

Assess for peripheral edema of hands, feet (usually, first area of low extremity swelling is behind medial malleolus in ambulatory, sacral area in bedridden). Assess for signs of CHF (cough, rales at base of lungs, cool extremities, dyspnea on exertion). Monitor fluid and electrolyte serum levels. Assess for distant or muffled heart sounds by auscultation (pericardial effusion, tamponade).

PATIENT/FAMILY TEACHING

Maximum B/P response occurs in 3–7 days. Reversible growth of fine body hair may begin 3–6 wks after treatment is initiated. When used topically for stimulation of hair growth, treatment must continue on a permanent basis—cessation of treatment will begin reversal of new hair growth.

mirtazapine

murr-**taz**-ah-peen
(Remeron)

PREGNANCY CATEGORY C

CLASSIFICATION

Antidepressant

AVAILABILITY (Rx)

Tablets: 15 mg, 30 mg

PHARMACOKINETICS

Absorption: Rapidly, completely absorbed following oral administration (not affected by food). **Metabolism:** Metabolized in liver. **Excretion:** Primarily excreted in urine. **Half-life:** 20–40 hrs (longer in males than females [37 hrs vs. 26 hrs]).

ACTION/*THERAPEUTIC EFFECT*

Acts as antagonist at presynaptic alpha$_2$-adrenergic receptors, increasing both norepinephrine and serotonin neurotransmission. *Produces antidepressant effect.* Prominent sedative effects, low anticholinergic activity.

USES

Treatment of depression.

ADMINISTRATION

ORAL:

- Give w/o regard to food.
- May crush or break scored tablets.

INDICATIONS/ROUTES/DOSAGE

Note: At least 14 days should elapse between discontinuing MAO inhibitors and instituting mirtazapine therapy. Also, allow at least 14 days after discontinuing mirtazapine and instituting MAO inhibitor therapy.

Depression:
Oral: Adults, elderly: 15 mg/day as single dose, preferably in evening prior to sleep (high sedative effect). ***Range:*** 15–45 mg/day. Dose adjustment should be no sooner than at 1–2 wk intervals.

CONTRAINDICATIONS

W/in 14 days of MAO inhibitor ingestion.

CAUTIONS

History of MI, angina, hypotensive episodes, history of mania/hypomania, hepatic/renal function impairment, elderly.

INTERACTIONS

DRUG: ***Alcohol, diazepam*** may increase impairment of cognition, motor skills. ***MAO inhibitors*** may increase risk of hypertensive crisis, severe convulsions. **HERBAL:** None known. **FOOD:** None significant. **ALTERED LAB VALUES:** May increase cholesterol, triglycerides, SGOT (ALT), SGPT (AST).

SIDE EFFECTS

FREQUENT: Somnolence (54%), dry mouth (25%), increase in appetite (17%), constipation (13%), weight gain (12%). **OCCASIONAL:** Asthenia (8%), dizziness (7%), flu syndrome (5%), abnormal dreams (4%). **RARE:** Abdominal discomfort, vasodilation, paresthesia, acne, dry skin, thirst, arthralgia.

ADVERSE REACTIONS/TOXIC EFFECTS

Higher incidence of seizures than w/tricyclic antidepressants (especially in those w/no previous history of seizures). High dosage may produce cardiovascular effects (severe postural hypotension, dizziness, tachycardia, palpitations, arrhythmias). Abrupt withdrawal from prolonged therapy may produce headache, malaise, nausea, vomiting, vivid dreams. Agranulocytosis occurs rarely.

PATIENT CONSIDERATIONS

Baseline Assessment

For those on long-term therapy, liver/renal function tests, blood counts should be performed periodically.

M

Intervention/Evaluation

Supervise suicidal risk pt closely during early therapy (as depression lessens, energy level improves, increasing suicide potential). Assess appearance, behavior, speech pattern, level of interest, mood. Monitor B/P, pulse for hypotension, arrhythmias.

Patient/Family Teaching

Avoid tasks that require alertness, motor skills until response to drug is established. Change positions slowly to avoid hypotensive effect. Tolerance to postural hypotension, sedative effects usually develops during early therapy. Do not abruptly discontinue medication. Report any sign of infection. Notify physician if pregnancy is planned or if pregnancy occurs.

---

misoprostol

mis-oh-**pros**-toll
(Cytotec)

FIXED-COMBINATION(S)
W/diclofenac, a NSAID **(Arthrotec)**

CANADIAN AVAILABILITY
Cytotec

PREGNANCY CATEGORY X

CLASSIFICATION

Antisecretory, gastric protectant

AVAILABILITY (Rx)

Tablets: 100 mcg, 200 mcg

PHARMACODYNAMICS

	ONSET	PEAK	DURATION
Oral	30 min	—	3–6 hrs

PHARMACOKINETICS

Absorption: Rapidly absorbed from GI tract. **Metabolism:** Rapidly converted to active metabolite. **Excretion:** Primarily excreted in urine. **Half-life:** 20–40 min.

ACTION/*THERAPEUTIC EFFECT*

Inhibits basal, nocturnal gastric acid secretion via direct action on parietal cells. *Increases production of protective gastric mucus.*

USES/*UNLABELED*

Prevention of NSAID-induced gastric ulcers and in those at high risk of developing gastric ulcer or gastric ulcer complication. *Treatment of duodenal ulcer.*

ADMINISTRATION

ORAL:

- Give w/or after meals (minimizes diarrhea).

INDICATIONS/ROUTES/DOSAGE

Prevention of NSAID-induced gastric ulcer:
Oral: Adults: 200 mcg 4 times/day w/food (last dose at bedtime). Continue for duration of NSAID therapy. May reduce dosage to 100 mcg if 200 mcg dose is not tolerable. ***Elderly:*** 100–200 mcg 4 times/day w/food.

CONTRAINDICATIONS

Pregnancy (produces uterine contractions), history of allergy to prostaglandins.

CAUTIONS

Impaired renal function.

INTERACTIONS

DRUG: None significant. **HERBAL:** None known. **FOOD:** None significant. **ALTERED LAB VALUES:** None significant.

SIDE EFFECTS

FREQUENT (>10%): Abdominal or stomach pain, diarrhea. **OCCASIONAL (1–3%):** Constipation, flatulence, headache, nausea, vomiting, vaginal bleeding, uterine stimulation, headache. **RARE (<1%):** Spotting, cramps.

ADVERSE REACTIONS/TOXIC EFFECTS

Overdosage may produce sedation, tremor, convulsions, dyspnea, palpitations, hypotension, bradycardia.

PATIENT CONSIDERATIONS

Baseline Assessment

Question for possibility of pregnancy before initiating therapy (Pregnancy Category X).

Patient/Family Teaching

Avoid magnesium-containing antacids (minimizes potential for diarrhea). Women of childbearing potential must not be pregnant before or during medication therapy (may result in hospitalization, surgery, infertility, fetal death).

mitomycin
(Mutamycin)
See Classification section under: Cancer chemotherapy

mitotane
(Lysodren)
See Classification section under: Cancer chemotherapy

mitoxantrone
(Novantrone)
See Classification section under: Cancer chemotherapy

mivacurium chloride
(Mivacron)
See Classification section under: Neuromuscular blocking agents

modafinil
mode-ah-**feen**-awl
(Provigil)

PREGNANCY CATEGORY C

CLASSIFICATION
$Alpha_1$ agonist: neurologic agent

AVAILABILITY (Rx)
Tablets: 100 mg, 200 mg

PHARMACOKINETICS
Absorption: Well absorbed following oral administration. Widely distributed. **Metabolism:** Metabolized in liver. **Excretion:** Kidney. **Half-life:** 8–10 hrs

ACTION / *THERAPEUTIC EFFECT*
Binds to dopamine reuptake carrier site, increasing alpha activity, decreasing delta, theta, and beta activity, *reducing the number of episodes of sleepiness and duration of daytime total sleep time.*

USES
Treatment of excessive daytime sleepiness associated with narcolepsy and other sleep disorders.

INDICATIONS/ROUTES/DOSAGES
Narcolepsy, sleep disorders:
Oral: Adults, elderly: 200–400 mg/day.

CONTRAINDICATIONS
Sensitivity to modanfinil.

CAUTIONS
None significant.

INTERACTIONS
DRUG: May increase effect of ***warfarin***. May reduce effectiveness of **oral contraceptives. HERBAL:** None known. **FOOD:** None significant. **ALTERED LAB VALUES:** None significant.

SIDE EFFECTS
Appear dose related: Dry mouth, dry eyes, nausea, poor sleep, sweating, headache, dizziness, hot flushes, hypersalivation, anorexia, anxiety, bad temper, choking, dysphoria/euphoria, increased B/P, fatigue, weight gain, sexual hyperactivity.

ADVERSE REACTIONS/TOXIC EFFECTS
Overdosage may produce tachycardia, excitation, insomnia.

PATIENT CONSIDERATIONS
BASELINE ASSESSMENT
Obtain baseline evidence of narcolepsy or other sleep disor-

ders, including pattern, environmental situations, lengths of time of sleep episodes. Question for sudden loss of muscle tone (cataplexy) precipitated by strong emotion such as laughter prior to sleep episode. Assess frequency and severity of sleep episodes prior to drug therapy.

INTERVENTIONS/EVALUATION

Monitor sleep pattern, evidence of restlessness during sleep, length of insomnia episodes during night. Assess for dizziness, anxiety; initiate fall precautions. Sugarless gum, sips of tepid water may relieve dry mouth.

PATIENT/FAMILY TEACHING

Avoid tasks that require alertness, motor skills until response to drug is established. Use alternative forms of contraception (to oral contraceptives).

moexipril hydrochloride

mow-**ex**-ih-prill
(Univasc)

FIXED-COMBINATION(S)
W/hydrochlorothiazide, a diuretic **(Uniretic)**

PREGNANCY CATEGORY C
First trimester

PREGNANCY CATEGORY D
Second and third trimesters

CLASSIFICATION

Angiotensin-converting enzyme (ACE) inhibitor

AVAILABILITY (Rx)

Tablets: 7.5 mg, 15 mg

PHARMACODYNAMICS

	ONSET	PEAK	DURATION
Oral	1 hr	3–6 hrs	24 hrs

PHARMACOKINETICS

Absorption: Incompletely absorbed from GI tract (food decreases absorption). **Metabolism:** Rapidly converted to active metabolite. **Excretion:** Primarily recovered in feces, partially excreted in urine. Unknown if removed by dialysis. **Half-life:** 1 hr (metabolite 2–9 hrs).

ACTION/*THERAPEUTIC EFFECT*

Suppresses renin-angiotensin-aldosterone system (prevents conversion of angiotensin I to angiotensin II, a potent vasoconstrictor; may also inhibit angiotensin II at local vascular and renal sites). *Reduces peripheral arterial resistance, B/P.*

USES

Treatment of hypertension. Used alone or in combination w/thiazide diuretics.

ADMINISTRATION

ORAL:

- Give 1 hr before meals.
- Tablets may be crushed.

INDICATIONS/ROUTES/DOSAGE

Hypertension (used alone):
Oral: Adults, elderly: Initially, 7.5 mg once daily 1 hr before meals. Adjust according to B/P effect. ***Maintenance:*** 7.5–30 mg/daily in 1–2 divided doses 1 hr before meals.

Hypertension (concurrent diuretic therapy):
Note: To reduce risk of hypotension, discontinue diuretic 2–3 days before initiating moexipril therapy. If B/P not controlled, resume diuretic. If diuretic cannot be dis-

continued, give initial dose of 3.75 mg moexipril.

Renal function impairment:
Oral: Adults, elderly: 3.75 mg once daily in pts w/creatinine clearance of ≤40 ml/min/1.73m^2. ***Maximum:*** May titrate up to 15 mg/day.

CONTRAINDICATIONS

History of angioedema w/previous treatment w/ACE inhibitors.

CAUTIONS

Renal impairment, those w/sodium depletion or on diuretic therapy, dialysis, hypovolemia, coronary or cerebrovascular insufficiency, hyperkalemia, aortic stenosis, ischemic heart disease, angina, severe CHF, cerebrovascular disease.

INTERACTIONS

DRUG: ***Alcohol, diuretics, hypotensive agents*** may increase effects. ***NSAIDs*** may decrease effect. ***Potassium-sparing diuretics, potassium supplements*** may cause hyperkalemia. May increase ***lithium*** concentration, toxicity. **HERBAL:** None known. **FOOD:** None significant. **ALTERED LAB VALUES:** May increase potassium, SGOT (AST), SGPT (ALT), alkaline phosphatase, bilirubin, BUN, creatinine. May decrease sodium. May cause positive ANA titer.

SIDE EFFECTS

OCCASIONAL: Cough, headache (6%), dizziness (4%), nausea, fatigue (3%). **RARE:** Flushing, rash, myalgia, nausea, vomiting.

ADVERSE REACTIONS/TOXIC EFFECTS

Excessive hypotension ("first-dose syncope") may occur in those w/CHF, severely salt/volume depleted. Angioedema (swelling of face/lips), hyperkalemia occur rarely. Agranulocytosis, neutropenia may be noted in those w/impaired renal function or collagen vascular disease (systemic lupus erythematosus, scleroderma). Nephrotic syndrome may be noted in those w/history of renal disease.

PATIENT CONSIDERATIONS

BASELINE ASSESSMENT

Obtain B/P and apical pulse immediately before each dose, in addition to regular monitoring (be alert to fluctuations). If excessive reduction in B/P occurs, place pt in supine position, feet slightly elevated. Renal function tests should be performed before therapy begins. In those w/renal impairment, autoimmune disease, or taking drugs that affect leukocytes or immune response, CBC and differential count should be performed before therapy begins and q2wks for 3 mos, then periodically thereafter.

INTERVENTION/EVALUATION

Monitor B/P, WBC count, serum potassium. Monitor for cough, question for headache. Assist w/ambulation if dizziness occurs.

PATIENT/FAMILY TEACHING

To reduce hypotensive effect, rise slowly from lying to sitting position and permit legs to dangle from bed momentarily before standing. Full therapeutic effect may take 2–4 wks. Report any sign of infection (sore throat, fever), swelling of hands or feet or face, chest pain, difficulty breathing or swallowing. Skipping doses or voluntarily discontinuing drug may produce severe, rebound hypertension.

Do not take cold preparations, nasal decongestants. Restrict sodium and alcohol as ordered.

molindone hydrochloride

mole-in-doan
(Moban)

PREGNANCY CATEGORY C

CLASSIFICATION

Antipsychotic

AVAILABILITY (Rx)

Tablets: 5 mg, 10 mg, 25 mg, 50 mg, 100 mg. **Oral Concentrate:** 20 mg/ml.

PHARMACODYNAMICS

	ONSET	PEAK	DURATION
Oral	—	—	36 hrs

PHARMACOKINETICS

Absorption: Rapidly absorbed from GI tract. Widely distributed. **Metabolism:** Metabolized in liver to active metabolite. **Excretion:** Primarily excreted in urine.

ACTION/*THERAPEUTIC EFFECT*

Acts on dopamine receptors in reticular activating, limbic systems in brain, decreases dopamine activity. *Suppresses locomotor activity, aggressiveness, suppresses conditioned responses. Produces tranquilization w/o compromising alertness.*

USES

Symptomatic management of schizophrenic disorders.

ADMINISTRATION

ORAL:
- Give w/o regard to meals.
- Give oral concentrate alone or mix w/water, milk, fruit juice, or carbonated beverages.

INDICATIONS/ROUTES/DOSAGE

Management of schizophrenia:
Oral: Adults: Initially, 50–75 mg/day in 3–4 divided doses. Increase to 100 mg/day in 3–4 days, if needed.

Maintenance (mild symptoms):
Oral: Adults: 5–15 mg 3–4 times/day.

Maintenance (moderate symptoms):
Oral: Adults: 10–25 mg 3–4 times/day.

Maintenance (severe symptoms):
Oral: Adults: Up to 225 mg may be needed.

Usual elderly dosage (nonpsychotic):
Oral: Initially, 5–10 mg 1–2 times/day. May increase by 5–10 mg every 4–7 days. ***Maximum:*** 112 mg/day.

CONTRAINDICATIONS

Severe CNS depression, comatose states.

CAUTIONS

Severe cardiovascular disorders, history of seizures.

INTERACTIONS

DRUG: ***Alcohol, CNS depression–producing medications*** may prolong CNS effects. ***Anticholinergics, antihistamines, MAO inhibitors, maprotiline, tricyclic antidepressants*** may increase anticholinergic, sedative effects. Extrapyramidal symptoms (EPS) may increase in severity, frequency w/***EPS-producing medications.*** May cause neurotoxic symptoms w/***lithium***. **HERBAL:** None known. **FOOD:** None significant. **ALTERED LAB VALUES:** May alter BUN, RBCs, glucose values. May increase prolactin concentration, WBCs.

SIDE EFFECTS

FREQUENT: Transient drowsiness, dry mouth, constipation, blurred vision, nasal congestion. **OCCASIONAL:** Diarrhea, peripheral edema, rash, urinary retention, nausea, mild/transient postural hypotension, tachycardia. **RARE:** Skin pigmentation, ocular changes.

ADVERSE REACTIONS/TOXIC EFFECTS

Frequently noted extrapyramidal symptom is akathisia (motor restlessness, anxiety). Occurring less frequently is akinesia (rigidity, tremor, salivation, mask-like facial expression, reduced voluntary movements). Infrequently noted are dystonias: torticollis (neck muscle spasm), opisthotonos (rigidity of back muscles), and oculogyric crisis (rolling back of eyes). Tardive dyskinesia (protrusion of tongue, puffing of cheeks, chewing/puckering of mouth) occurs rarely but may be irreversible. Risk is greater in female geriatric pts. Potentially fatal neuroleptic malignant syndrome (NMS) requires immediate discontinuation of the drug.

PATIENT CONSIDERATIONS

Baseline Assessment

Assess behavior, appearance, emotional status, response to environment, speech pattern, thought content.

Intervention/Evaluation

Supervise suicidal risk pt closely during early therapy (as depression lessens, energy level improves, increasing suicide potential). Monitor B/P for hypotension. Assess for peripheral edema behind medial malleolus (sacral area in bedridden pts). Monitor stools; avoid constipation. Assess for extrapyramidal symptoms (see Adverse Reactions/Toxic Effects), hyperthermia, altered mental status or level of consciousness, and autonomic instability (NMS); evaluate for evidence of tardive dyskinesia. Assess for therapeutic response (interest in surroundings, improvement in self-care, increased ability to concentrate, relaxed facial expression).

Patient/Family Teaching

Full therapeutic effects may take up to 6 wks. Report visual disturbances. Sugarless gum, sips of tepid water may relieve dry mouth. Drowsiness generally subsides during continued therapy. Avoid tasks that require alertness, motor skills until response to drug is established. Avoid alcohol and CNS depressants.

---

mometasone

(Elocon)

See Classification section under: Corticosteroids: topical

---

montelukast

mon-**tee**-leu-cast

(Singulair)

CANADIAN AVAILABILITY

Singulair

PREGNANCY CATEGORY B

CLASSIFICATION

Anti-asthmatic

AVAILABILITY (Rx)

Tablets: 10 mg. **Tablets, chewable:** 4 mg, 5 mg

PHARMACODYNAMICS

	ONSET	PEAK	DURATION
Oral	—	—	24 hrs
Oral, chewable	—	—	24 hrs

PHARMACOKINETICS

Absorption: Rapidly absorbed from GI tract. Bounds to plasma proteins. **Metabolism:** Extensively metabolized in the liver. **Excretion:** Excreted almost exclusively in the feces. **Half-life:** 2.7–5.5 hrs. Half-life slightly longer in the elderly.

ACTION/*THERAPEUTIC EFFECT*

A leukotriene receptor antagonist, inhibits airway edema, smooth muscle contraction, altered cellular activity associated with the inflammatory process, *relieving signs and symptoms of bronchial asthma.*

USES/*UNLABELED*

Prophylaxis and chronic treatment of asthma. Not for use in reversal of bronchospasm in acute asthma attacks, status asthmaticus, exercise-induced bronchospasm.

ADMINISTRATION

ORAL:

- Administer in the evening w/o regard to food ingestion.

INDICATIONS/ROUTES/DOSAGES

Bronchial asthma:

Oral: Adults, elderly, adolescents *≥15 yrs:* One 10 mg tablet daily, taken in the evening. ***Children 6–14 yrs:*** One 5 mg chewable tablet daily, taken in the evening.

CONTRAINDICATIONS

History of hypersensitivity to drug.

CAUTIONS

Systemic corticosteroid treatment reduction during montelukast therapy, impaired liver function.

INTERACTIONS

DRUG: *Phenobarbital, rifampin* may reduce duration of action of montelukast. **HERBAL:** None known. **FOOD:** None significant. **ALTERED LAB VALUES:** May increase SGOT (AST), SGPT (ALT).

SIDE EFFECTS

Adults, adolescents 15 yrs:
FREQUENT (18%): Headache. **OCCASIONAL (4%):** Influenza. **RARE (2–3%):** Abdominal pain, cough, dyspepsia, dizziness, fatigue, dental pain, systemic eosinophilia.

Children 6–14 yrs:
RARE (≤ 2%): Diarrhea, laryngitis, pharyngitis, nausea, otitis media, sinusitis, viral infection.

ADVERSE REACTIONS/TOXIC EFFECTS

None significant.

PATIENT CONSIDERATIONS

BASELINE ASSESSMENT

Chewable tablet contains phenylalanine (a component of aspartame); parents of phenylketonuric pts should be so informed. Montelukast should not be abruptly substituted for inhaled or oral corticosteroids.

INTERVENTIONS/EVALUATION

Monitor rate, depth, rhythm, type of respirations, quality and rate of pulse. Assess lung sounds

for rhonchi, wheezing, rales. Observe lips, fingernails for blue or dusky color in light-skinned patients, gray in dark-skinned patients.

PATIENT/FAMILY TEACHING

Increase fluid intake (decreases lung secretion viscosity). Take as prescribed, even during symptoms-free periods as well as during worsening asthma. Do not alter/stop other asthma medications. Drug is not for the treatment of acute asthma attacks. Patients sensitive to aspirin should avoid aspirin, NSAIDs while taking montelukast.

moricizine hydrochloride

mor-ih-**see**-zeen
(Ethmozine)

PREGNANCY CATEGORY B

CLASSIFICATION

Antiarrhythmic

AVAILABILITY (Rx)

Tablets: 200 mg, 250 mg, 300 mg

PHARMACODYNAMICS

	ONSET	PEAK	DURATION
Oral	—	2–4 hrs	—

PHARMACOKINETICS

Absorption: Well absorbed from GI tract. **Metabolism:** Undergoes significant first-pass metabolism. Metabolized in liver (induces own metabolism). **Excretion:** Primarily eliminated in feces via biliary system. Minimal removal by hemodialysis. **Half-life:** 1.5–3.5 hrs.

ACTION/*THERAPEUTIC EFFECT*

Prevents sodium current across myocardial cell membranes. Has potent local anesthetic activity and membrane stabilizing effects. Slows AV, Purkinje conduction, decreases action potential duration, effective refractory period, *suppressing ventricular arrhythmias.*

USES

Treatment of documented, life-threatening ventricular arrhythmias (e.g., sustained ventricular tachycardia).

ADMINISTRATION

ORAL:

- May be given w/o regard to food but give w/food if GI upset occurs.
- Monitor EKG for cardiac changes, particularly increase in PR and QRS intervals. Notify physician of any significant interval changes.

INDICATIONS/ROUTES/DOSAGE

Usual dosage for arrhythmias:
Oral: Adults, elderly: 200–300 mg q8h; may increase by 150 mg/day at 3 day intervals until desired effect achieved.

Dosage in hepatic/renal impairment:
Initially, 600 mg or less/day.

CONTRAINDICATIONS

Preexisting second- or third-degree AV block or right bundle-branch block associated w/left hemiblock (bifascicular block), w/o pacemaker; cardiogenic shock.

CAUTIONS

CHF, electrolyte imbalance, sick-sinus syndrome (bradycardia-tachycardia), impaired hepatic/renal function.

M

INTERACTIONS

DRUG: *Cimetidine* may increase concentrations; moricizine may decrease *theophylline* concentrations. **HERBAL:** None known. **FOOD:** None significant. **ALTERED LAB VALUES:** May cause EKG changes (prolong PR, QT intervals).

SIDE EFFECTS

FREQUENT (5–15%): Dizziness, nausea, headache, fatigue, dyspnea. **OCCASIONAL (2–5%):** Nervousness, paresthesia, sleep disturbances, dyspepsia, vomiting, diarrhea. **RARE (<2%):** Urinary retention/frequency, sweating, dry mouth, swelling of lips/tongue, periorbital edema, impotence, decreased libido, generalized body aches.

ADVERSE REACTIONS/TOXIC EFFECTS

Has ability to worsen existing arrhythmias or produce new ones. Jaundice w/hepatitis occurs rarely. Overdosage produces emesis, lethargy, syncope, hypotension, conduction disturbances, exacerbation of CHF, MI, sinus arrest.

PATIENT CONSIDERATIONS

Baseline Assessment

Correct electrolyte imbalance before administering medication.

Intervention/Evaluation

Monitor EKG for cardiac changes, particularly increase in PR and QRS intervals. Notify physician of any significant interval changes. Assess pulse for strength/weakness, irregular rate. Question for headache, GI upset, dizziness, nausea. Monitor fluid and electrolyte serum levels. Monitor pattern of daily bowel activity and stool consistency. Assess for dizziness, unsteadiness. Monitor liver enzyme results.

Patient/Family Teaching

Do not abruptly discontinue medication. Compliance w/therapy regimen is essential to control arrhythmias.

morphine sulfate

(Astramorph, Duramorph, Kadian, MS Contin, MSIR, RMS, Roxanol, Roxanol-T)

CANADIAN AVAILABILITY
Kadian, M.O.S., MSContin, MSIR, Oramorph

PREGNANCY CATEGORY B
(D if used for prolong periods or at high doses at term)

CLASSIFICATION

Opioid: Analgesic **(Schedule II)**

AVAILABILITY (Rx)

Injection: 0.5 mg/ml, 1 mg/ml, 2 mg/ml, 3 mg/ml, 4 mg/ml, 5 mg/ml, 8 mg/ml, 10 mg/ml, 15 mg/ml. **Tablets:** 15 mg, 30 mg. **Tablets (soluble):** 10 mg, 15 mg, 30 mg. **Tablets (controlled-release):** 30 mg, 60 mg. **Oral Solution:** 10 mg/5 ml, 20 mg/5 ml, 20 mg/ml, 100 mg/5 ml. **Suppositories:** 5 mg, 10 mg, 20 mg, 30 mg.

PHARMACODYNAMICS

	ONSET	PEAK	DURATION
Oral	Variable	60–120 min	4–5 hrs
Extended-release	—	60–120 min	8–12 hrs
SubQ	5–30 min	50–90 min	4–5 hrs

ONSET	PEAK	DURATION
IM		
5–30 min	30–60 min	3–7 hrs
IV Rapid	20 min	4–5 hrs
Rectal		
20–60 min	—	4–5 hrs
Epidural		
15–60 min	—	16–24 hrs
Intrathecal		
15–60 min	—	16–24 hrs

PHARMACOKINETICS

Absorption: Variably absorbed from GI tract. Readily absorbed after SubQ, IM administration. Widely distributed. **Metabolism:** Metabolized in liver. **Excretion:** Primarily excreted in urine. **Half-life:** 2–3 hrs.

ACTION/*THERAPEUTIC EFFECT*

Binds w/opioid receptors within CNS, *altering processes affecting pain perception, emotional response to pain. Decreases intestinal motility* by local, central actions.

USES

Relief of severe, acute, chronic pain, preop sedation, anesthesia supplement, analgesia during labor. Drug of choice for pain due to myocardial infarction, dyspnea from pulmonary edema not resulting from chemical respiratory irritant.

STORAGE/HANDLING

Store suppositories, parenteral, oral form at room temperature. Discard unused portion from pt-controlled IV infusion.

ADMINISTRATION

- **Note:** Give by IM injection if repeated doses necessary (repeated SubQ may produce local tissue irritation, induration). May also be given slow IV injection or IV infusion. Incompatible w/aminophylline, amobarbital, chlorothiazide, phenytoin, heparin, meperidine, methicillin, nitrofurantoin, pentobarbital, phenobarbital, sodium bicarbonate, sodium iodide, thiopental.

ORAL:

- Mix liquid form w/fruit juice to improve taste.
- Do not crush or break extended-release capsule.
- Kadian: May mix w/applesauce immediately prior to administration.

SUBQ/IM:

- Administer slowly, rotating injection sites.
- Pts with circulatory impairment experience higher risk of overdosage because of delayed absorption of repeated administration.

IV:

- For IV injection, dilute 2.5–15 mg morphine in 4–5 ml sterile water for injection.
- Always administer very slowly, over 4–5 min. Rapid IV increases risk of severe adverse reactions (apnea, chest wall rigidity, peripheral circulatory collapse, cardiac arrest, anaphylactoid effects).
- For multiple IV injections, may give pt-controlled analgesia, using pt-controlled infusion device.
- For continuous IV infusion, dilute to concentration of 0.1–1 mg/ml in 5% dextrose and give through controlled infusion device.

RECTAL:

- If suppository is too soft, chill for 30 min in refrigerator or run cold water over foil wrapper.
- Moisten suppository w/cold water before inserting well up into rectum.

INDICATIONS/ROUTES/DOSAGE

- **Note:** Reduce dosage in elderly/debilitated, those on concurrent CNS depressants.

Pain:
Oral: Adults, elderly: 10–30 mg q4h. ***Extended-release:*** 30 mg q8–12h.

Rectal: Adults, elderly: 10–30 mg q4h.

SubQ/IM: Adults, elderly: 10 mg q4h, as needed. ***Usual dosage range:*** 5–20 mg q4h. ***Children:*** 0.1–0.2 mg/kg per dose. Give q4h, as needed. Do not exceed single dose of 15 mg.

IV: Adults, elderly: 4–10 mg, given very slowly.

Severe, chronic pain associated w/cancer:
IV Infusion: Adults, elderly: 0.8–10 mg/hr. Increase to effective dosage level, as needed. ***Maintenance:*** 0.8–80 mg/hr. ***Children (Maintenance):*** 0.025–2.6 mg/kg/hr.

Epidural: Adults, elderly: Initially, 5 mg. If pain relief not obtained in 1 hr, may give additional doses in increments of 1–2 mg at sufficient intervals. ***Maximum total daily dose:*** 10 mg.

Continuous Epidural Infusion: Adults, elderly: Initially, 2–4 mg/day. May be increased by 1–2 mg/day if needed.

Intrathecal: Adults, elderly: 0.2–1 mg.

SubQ: Children: Usual maintenance level: 0.025–1.79 mg/kg/hr.

Myocardial infarction pain:
SubQ/IM/IV: Adults, elderly: 8–15 mg. Give additional smaller doses q3–4h.

Analgesia during labor:
SubQ/IM: Adults: 10 mg.

CONTRAINDICATIONS

Postop biliary tract surgery, surgical anastomosis.

EXTREME CAUTION

CNS depression, anoxia, hypercapnia, respiratory depression, seizures, acute alcoholism, shock, untreated myxedema, respiratory dysfunction.

CAUTIONS

Toxic psychoses, increased intracranial pressure, impaired hepatic function, acute abdominal conditions, hypothyroidism, prostatic hypertrophy, Addison's disease, urethral stricture, COPD.

INTERACTIONS

DRUG: ***Alcohol, CNS depressants*** may increase CNS or respiratory depression, hypotension. ***MAO inhibitors*** may produce severe, fatal reaction (reduce dose to $\frac{1}{4}$ usual dose). **HERBAL:** None known. **FOOD:** None significant. **ALTERED LAB VALUES:** May increase amylase, lipase.

SIDE EFFECTS

Note: Effects dependent on dosage amount, route of administration. Ambulatory pts, those not in severe pain may experience dizziness, nausea, vomiting, hypotension more frequently than those in supine position or who have severe pain. **FREQUENT:** Histamine reaction (decreased blood pressure, increased sweating, flushed face, wheezing), constipation, dizziness, drowsiness, hypotension, nausea, vomiting, unusually tired. **OCCASIONAL:** Allergic reaction (rash, itching), trouble breathing, confusion, pounding heartbeat, tremors, decreased urination, stomach cramps, vision changes, dry mouth, headache, decreased appetite, pain or burning at injection site. **RARE:** Paralytic ileus.

ADVERSE REACTIONS/TOXIC EFFECTS

Overdosage results in respiratory depression, skeletal muscle flaccidity, cold clammy skin, cyanosis, extreme somnolence progressing to convulsions, stupor, coma. Tolerance to analgesic effect, physical dependence may occur w/repeated use. Prolonged duration of action, cumulative effect may occur in those w/impaired hepatic, renal function.

PATIENT CONSIDERATIONS

BASELINE ASSESSMENT

Pt should be in a recumbent position before drug is given by parenteral route. Assess onset, type, location, and duration of pain. Obtain vital signs before giving medication. If respirations are 12/min or lower (20/min or lower in children), withhold medication, contact physician. Effect of medication is reduced if full pain recurs before next dose.

INTERVENTION/EVALUATION

Monitor vital signs 5–10 min after IV administration, 15–30 min after SubQ or IM. Be alert for decreased respirations or B/P. Check for adequate voiding; palpate bladder if output questionable. Monitor stools; avoid constipation. Initiate deep breathing and coughing exercises, particularly in those w/impaired pulmonary function. Assess for clinical improvement and record onset of pain relief. Consult physician if pain relief is not adequate.

PATIENT/FAMILY TEACHING

Discomfort may occur w/injection. Change positions slowly to avoid orthostatic hypotension. Avoid tasks that require alertness, motor skills until response to drug is established. Avoid alcohol and CNS depressants. Tolerance/dependence may occur with prolonged use of high doses.

---

moxifloxacin

(Avelox)

See Supplement and Classification section under: Antibiotics: quinolones

---

mupirocin

mew-**pie**-ro-sin

(Bactroban)

CANADIAN AVAILABILITY

Bactroban

PREGNANCY CATEGORY B

CLASSIFICATION

Topical antibacterial

AVAILABILITY (Rx)

Ointment: 2%. **Nasal Ointment:** 2%.

PHARMACOKINETICS

Metabolism: Metabolized in skin to inactive metabolite. **Excretion:** Transported to skin surface; removed by normal skin desquamation.

ACTION/*THERAPEUTIC EFFECT*

Inhibits bacterial protein, RNA synthesis. Less effective on DNA synthesis. ***Nasal:*** Eradicates nasal colonization of MRSA. *Prevents bacterial growth and replication. Bacteriostatic.*

USES / *UNLABELED*

Topical treatment of impetigo, infected traumatic skin lesions. ***Nasal:*** Reduces spread of MRSA (methicillin-resistant *S. aureus*). *Treatment of infected eczema, folliculitis, minor bacterial skin infections.*

ADMINISTRATION

TOPICAL:

- Gown and gloves are to be worn until 24 hrs after therapy is effective. Disease is spread by direct contact w/moist discharges.
- Apply small amount to affected areas.
- Cover affected areas w/gauze dressing if desired.

INDICATIONS / ROUTES / DOSAGE

Usual topical dosage:
Topical: Adults, elderly, children: Apply 3 times/day (may cover w/gauze).

Usual nasal dosage:
Intranasal: Adults, elderly, children: Apply 2 times/day for 5 days.

CONTRAINDICATIONS

Hypersensitivity to any of the components.

CAUTIONS

Impaired renal function. Safety of nasal preparation not established in children <12yrs.

INTERACTIONS

DRUG: None significant. **HERBAL:** None known. **FOOD:** None significant. **ALTERED LAB VALUES:** None significant.

SIDE EFFECTS

FREQUENT: ***Nasal (3–9%):*** Headache, rhinitis, upper respiratory congestion, pharyngitis, altered taste. **OCCASIONAL:** ***Nasal (2%):*** Burning, stinging, cough. ***Topical (1–2%):*** Pain, burning, stinging, itching. **RARE:** ***Nasal (<1%):*** Pruritis, diarrhea, dry mouth, epistaxis, nausea, rash. ***Topical (<1%):*** Rash, nausea, dry skin, contact dermatitis.

ADVERSE REACTIONS / TOXIC EFFECTS

Superinfection may result in bacterial or fungal infections, especially w/prolonged or repeated therapy.

PATIENT CONSIDERATIONS

BASELINE ASSESSMENT

Question for hypersensitivity to components. Assess skin for type and extent of lesions.

INTERVENTION / EVALUATION

Keep neonates or pts w/poor hygiene isolated. Wear gloves and gown if necessary when contact w/discharges is likely; continue until 24 hrs after therapy is effective. Cleanse/dispose of articles soiled with discharge according to institutional guidelines. In event of skin reaction, stop applications, cleanse area gently, and notify physician.

PATIENT / FAMILY TEACHING

For external use only. Avoid contact w/eyes. Explain precautions to avoid spread of infection; teach how to apply medication. If skin reaction, irritation develops, notify physician. If there is no improvement in 3–5 days, pt should be reevaluated.

muromonab-CD3

meur-**oh**-mon-ab
(Orthoclone, OKT3)

CANADIAN AVAILABILITY
Orthoclone

PREGNANCY CATEGORY C

CLASSIFICATION

Immunosuppressant

AVAILABILITY (Rx)

Injection: 1 mg/ml

ACTION/*THERAPEUTIC EFFECT*

Antibody (purified IgG_2 immune globulin) that reacts with T3 (CD3) antigen of human T cell membranes. Blocks function of T-cells (has major role in acute renal rejection). *Reverses graft rejection.*

USES

Treatment of acute allograft rejection in renal transplant pts, steroid-resistant acute allograft rejection in cardiac, hepatic transplant pts.

STORAGE/HANDLING

Refrigerate ampule. Do not shake ampule before using. Fine translucent particles may develop; does not affect potency.

ADMINISTRATION

IV:

- Administer direct IV over <1 min.
- Give methylprednisolone 1 mg/kg before and 100 mg hydrocortisone 30 min after dose (decreases adverse reaction to first dose).
- Draw solution into syringe through 0.22 micron filter. Discard filter; use needle for IV administration.

INDICATIONS/ROUTES/DOSAGE

Prevention of allograft rejection:
IV: Adults, elderly: 5 mg/day for 10–14 days. Begin when acute renal rejection is diagnosed.

CONTRAINDICATIONS

History of hypersensitivity to muromonab-CD3 or any murine origin product, those in fluid overload evidenced by chest x-ray or >3% weight gain within the week before initial treatment.

CAUTIONS

Impaired hepatic, renal, cardiac function.

INTERACTIONS

DRUG: Other ***immunosuppressants*** may increase risk of infection or development of lymphoproliferative disorders. ***Live virus vaccines*** may potentiate virus replication, increase vaccine side effects, decrease pt's antibody response to vaccine. **HERBAL:** Echinacea may decrease effect. **FOOD:** None significant. **ALTERED LAB VALUES:** None significant.

SIDE EFFECTS

FREQUENT: First-dose reaction: Fever, chills, dyspnea, malaise occurs 30 min to 6 hrs after first dose (reaction markedly reduced w/subsequent dosing after first 2 days of treatment). **OCCASIONAL:** Chest pain, nausea, vomiting, diarrhea, tremor.

ADVERSE REACTIONS/TOXIC EFFECTS

Cytokine release syndrome (CRS) may range from flulike illness to life-threatening shock-like reac-

M

tion. Occasionally fatal hypersensitivity reactions. Severe pulmonary edema occurs in <2% of those treated w/muromonab-CD3. Infection (due to immunosuppression) generally occurs within 45 days after initial treatment; cytomegalovirus occurs in 19%, herpes simplex in 27%. Severe and life-threatening infection occurs in <4.8%.

PATIENT CONSIDERATIONS

BASELINE ASSESSMENT

Chest x-ray must be taken within 24 hrs of initiation of therapy and be clear of fluid. Weight should be ≥3% above minimum weight the week before treatment begins (pulmonary edema occurs where fluid overload is present before treatment). Have resuscitative drugs and equipment immediately available.

INTERVENTION/EVALUATION

Monitor WBC, differential, platelet count, renal and hepatic function tests, and immunologic tests (plasma levels or quantitative T lymphocyte surface phenotyping) before and during therapy. If fever exceeds 100°F, antipyretics should be instituted. Monitor for fluid overload by chest x-ray and weight gain of >3% over weight before treatment began. Assess lung sounds for evidence of fluid overload. Monitor I&O. Assess stool frequency and consistency.

PATIENT/FAMILY TEACHING

Inform pt of first-dose reaction prior to treatment; headache, tremor may occur as a response to medication. Avoid crowds, those w/infections. Do not receive immunizations.

mycophenolate mofetil

my-koe-**phen**-oh-late
(CellCept)

CANADIAN AVAILABILITY
CellCept

PREGNANCY CATEGORY C

CLASSIFICATION

Immunosuppressant

AVAILABILITY (Rx)

Capsules: 250 mg. **Tablets:** 500 mg. **Oral Suspension, Injection.**

PHARMACOKINETICS

Absorption: Rapidly, extensively absorbed following oral administration (food does not alter the extent of absorption but plasma concentration decreased in presence of food). **Metabolism:** Completely hydrolyzed to active metabolite, mycophenolic acid (MPA). **Excretion:** Primarily excreted in urine. Usually not removed by hemodialysis. **Half-life:** 17.9 hrs.

ACTION

Inhibits inosine monophosphate dehydrogenase, an enzyme that deprives lymphocytes of nucleotides necessary for DNA and RNA synthesis. Inhibits proliferation of T- and B-lymphocytes. Suppresses immunologically mediated inflammatory response. *Prevents renal transplant rejection.*

USES/*UNLABELED*

Prophylaxis of organ rejection in pts receiving allogeneic renal transplants, liver transplants. Should be used concurrently w/cyclosporine and corticosteroids. *Prevention of organ rejection in pts undergoing heart transplants.*

ADMINISTRATION

ORAL:

- Give on an empty stomach.
- Do not open or crush capsules. Avoid inhalation of powder in capsules and avoid direct contact of powder on skin or mucous membranes. If contact occurs, wash thoroughly w/soap and water; rinse eyes profusely w/plain water.

INDICATIONS/ROUTES/DOSAGE

Kidney transplantation:
Oral: Adults, elderly: 1 g twice/day (2 g/day) w/initial dose given within 72 hrs after transplant. Give in combination w/corticosteroids and cyclosporine.

CONTRAINDICATIONS

Hypersensitivity to mycophenolate, mycophenolic acid, or any component of drug product.

CAUTIONS

Immunosuppressed pts, pts w/active, serious digestive system disease; renal function impairment.

INTERACTIONS

DRUG: *Acyclovir, ganciclovir* compete w/MPA (active metabolite) for renal excretion; may increase plasma concentration of each in presence of renal impairment. ***Antacids (magnesium, aluminum containing), cholestyramine*** may decrease absorption. Other ***immunosuppressants*** may increase risk of infection or development of lymphomas. ***Live virus vaccines*** may potentiate virus replication, increase vaccine side effects, decrease pt's antibody response to vaccine. ***Probenecid*** may increase concentration. **HERBAL:** Echinacea may interfere w/mycophenolate effect. **FOOD:** None significant. **ALTERED LAB VALUES:** May increase alkaline phosphatase, creatinine, SGOT (AST), SGPT (ALT). Alters calcium, glucose protein, uric acid, lipids levels.

M

SIDE EFFECTS

FREQUENT: Diarrhea/constipation, fever, headache, hypertension, UTI, peripheral edema, nausea, dyspepsia. **OCCASIONAL:** Asthenia, hematuria, vomiting, oral moniliasis, dyspnea, cough, acne, tremor, insomnia, pharyngitis. **RARE:** Dizziness, rash, back pain.

ADVERSE REACTIONS/TOXIC EFFECTS

Sepsis, infection occur occasionally, GI tract hemorrhage rarely. There is an increased risk of neoplasia (new, abnormal growth tumors). Significant anemia, leukopenia, thrombocytopenia, neutropenia, leukocytosis may occur, particularly in those undergoing kidney rejection.

PATIENT CONSIDERATIONS

Baseline Assessment

Women of childbearing potential should have a negative serum or urine pregnancy test within 1 wk prior to initiation of drug therapy. A negative pregnancy test report should be obtained before therapy is initiated. Assess medical history, especially renal function, existence of active digestive system

disease, drug history, especially other immunosuppressants.

INTERVENTION/EVALUATION

CBC should be performed weekly during first month of therapy, twice monthly during second and third months of treatment, then monthly throughout the first year. If rapid fall in WBC occurs, dosage should be reduced or discontinued. Assess particularly for delayed bone marrow suppression. Report any major change in assessment of pt. Routinely watch for any change from normal.

PATIENT/FAMILY TEACHING

Effective contraception should be used before, during, and for 6 wks after discontinuing therapy, even if there has been a history of infertility, other than hysterectomy. Two forms of contraception must be used concurrently unless abstinence is absolute. Contact physician if unusual bleeding or bruising, sore throat, mouth sores, abdominal pain, or fever occurs. Inform pts of need for laboratory tests while taking medication. Inform pts of risk of malignancies that may occur.

nabumetone

nah-**byew**-meh-tone
(Relafen)

CANADIAN AVAILABILITY
Relafen

PREGNANCY CATEGORY C
(D if used in third trimester or near delivery

CLASSIFICATION

Nonsteroidal anti-inflammatory

AVAILABILITY (Rx)

Tablets: 500 mg, 750 mg

PHARMACOKINETICS

Absorption: Readily absorbed from GI tract. Widely distributed. **Metabolism:** Metabolized in liver to active metabolite. **Excretion:** Primarily excreted in urine. **Half-life:** 22–30 hrs.

ACTION/*THERAPEUTIC EFFECT*

Produces analgesic and anti-inflammatory effect by inhibiting prostaglandin synthesis, *reducing inflammatory response and intensity of pain stimulus reaching sensory nerve endings.*

USES

Acute and chronic treatment of osteoarthritis, rheumatoid arthritis.

ADMINISTRATION

ORAL:

- Give w/food, milk, or antacids if GI distress occurs.
- Do not crush; swallow whole.

INDICATIONS/ROUTES/DOSAGE

Rheumatoid arthritis, osteoarthritis:
Oral: Adults, elderly: Initially, 1,000 mg as single dose or in 2 divided doses. May increase up to 2,000 mg/day as single or in 2 divided doses.

CONTRAINDICATIONS

Active peptic ulcer, GI ulceration, chronic inflammation of GI tract, GI bleeding disorders, history of hypersensitivity to aspirin or NSAIDs, history of significantly impaired renal function.

CAUTIONS

Impaired renal/hepatic function, history of GI tract disease, predisposition to fluid retention.

N

INTERACTIONS

DRUG: May increase effects of ***oral anticoagulants, heparin, thrombolytics.*** May decrease effect of ***antihypertensives, diuretics. Salicylates, aspirin*** may increase risk of GI side effects, bleeding. ***Bone marrow depressants*** may increase risk of hematologic reactions. May increase concentration, toxicity of ***lithium.*** May increase ***methotrexate*** toxicity. ***Probenecid*** may increase concentration. **HERBAL:** May decrease effect of feverfew. Ginkgo biloba may increase risk of bleeding. **FOOD:** None significant. **ALTERED LAB VALUES:** May increase alkaline phosphatase, LDH, serum transaminase, potassium, urine protein, BUN, serum creatinine. May decrease uric acid.

SIDE EFFECTS

FREQUENT (3–9%): Itching, rash, ringing in ears, edema, dizziness, headache, abdominal cramps, constipation, diarrhea, indigestion, nausea. **OCCASIONAL (1–3%):** Drowsiness, nervousness, vomiting, inability to sleep, dry mouth, increased sweating. **RARE (<1%):** Increased blood pressure, confusion, hives, blurred vision, shortness of breath, lightheadedness, unusually tired.

ADVERSE REACTIONS/TOXIC EFFECTS

Overdose may result in acute hypotension, tachycardia. Peptic ulcer, GI bleeding, nephrotoxicity (dysuria, cystitis, hematuria, proteinuria, nephrotic syndrome), gastritis, severe hepatic reaction (cholestasis, jaundice), severe hypersensitivity reaction (bronchospasm, angiofacial edema) occur rarely.

PATIENT CONSIDERATIONS

BASELINE ASSESSMENT

Assess onset, type, location, and duration of pain or inflammation. Inspect appearance of affected joints for immobility, deformities, and skin condition.

INTERVENTION/EVALUATION

Assist w/ambulation if somnolence/drowsiness/dizziness occurs. Monitor for evidence of dyspepsia. Monitor pattern of daily bowel activity and stool consistency. Check behind medial malleolus for fluid retention (usually first area noted). Evaluate for therapeutic response: relief of pain, stiffness, swelling, increase in joint mobility, reduced joint tenderness, improved grip strength.

PATIENT/FAMILY TEACHING

Swallow capsule whole; do not crush or chew. Avoid tasks that require alertness, motor skills until response to drug is established. If GI upset occurs, take w/food, milk. Avoid aspirin, alcohol during therapy (increases risk of GI bleeding). Report headache, GI distress, visual disturbances, edema, skin rash, itching, visual disturbances, increased wgt, black stools, or persistent headache.

nadolol

nay-**doe**-lol
(Corgard)

FIXED-COMBINATION(S)
W/bendroflumethiazide, a diuretic **(Corzide)**

CANADIAN AVAILABILITY
Apo-Nadol, Corgard, Novo-Nadolol

PREGNANCY CATEGORY C
(D if used in second or third trimester)

CLASSIFICATION

Beta-adrenergic blocker

AVAILABILITY (Rx)

Tablets: 20 mg, 40 mg, 80 mg, 120 mg, 160 mg

PHARMACODYNAMICS

	ONSET	PEAK	DURATION
Oral	—	—	24 hrs

PHARMACOKINETICS

Absorption: Partially absorbed from GI tract. **Excretion:** Primarily excreted unchanged in urine. Moderately removed by hemodialysis. **Half-life:** 20–24 hrs (increased in decreased renal function).

ACTION/*THERAPEUTIC EFFECT*

Nonselective beta blocker. Blocks $beta_1$-adrenergic receptors, *slowing sinus heart rate, decreasing cardiac output, decreasing B/P.* Blocks $beta_2$-adrenergic receptors, *increasing airway resistance. Decreases myocardial ischemia severity* by decreasing oxygen requirements.

USES/*UNLABELED*

Management of mild to moderate hypertension. Used alone or in combination w/diuretics, especially thiazide type. Management of chronic stable angina pectoris. *Treatment of cardiac arrhythmias, hypertrophic cardiomyopathy, myocardial infarction, pheochromocytoma, vascular headaches, migraines, tremors, thyrotoxicosis, mitral valve prolapse syndrome, neuroleptic-induced akathisia.*

ADMINISTRATION

ORAL:

- May be given w/o regard to meals.
- Tablets may be crushed.

INDICATIONS/ROUTES/DOSAGE

Hypertension:
Oral: Adults: Initially, 40 mg/day. Increase by 40–80 mg/day at 7 day intervals. ***Maintenance:*** 40–80 mg/day up to 240–320 mg/day.

Angina pectoris:
Oral: Adults: Initially, 40 mg/day. Increase by 40–80 mg/day at 3–7 day intervals. ***Maintenance:*** 40–80 mg/day up to 160–240 mg/day.

Usual elderly dosage:
Oral: Initially, 20 mg/day for angina/hypertension.

Dosage in renal impairment:
Dose is modified based on creatinine clearance.

CREATININE CLEARANCE	DOSAGE INTERVAL
>50 ml/min	q24h
31–50 ml/min	q24–36h
10–30 ml/min	q24–48h
<10 ml/min	q40–60h

CONTRAINDICATIONS

Bronchial asthma, COPD, uncontrolled cardiac failure, sinus bradycardia, heart block greater than first degree, cardiogenic shock, CHF unless secondary to tachyarrhythmias, those on MAO inhibitors.

CAUTIONS

Inadequate cardiac function, impaired renal/hepatic function, diabetes mellitus, hyperthyroidism.

INTERACTIONS

DRUG: ***Diuretics, other hypotensives*** may increase hypotensive effect; ***sympathomimetics, xanthines*** may mutually inhibit effects; may mask symptoms of hypoglycemia, prolong hypoglycemic effect of ***insulin, oral hypoglycemics; NSAIDs*** may decrease antihypertensive effect; ***cimetidine*** may increase concentration. **HERBAL:** None known. **FOOD:** None significant. **ALTERED LAB VALUES:** May increase ANA titer, SGOT (AST), SGPT (ALT), alkaline phosphatase, LDH, bilirubin, BUN, creatinine, potassium, uric acid, lipoproteins, triglycerides.

SIDE EFFECTS

Generally well tolerated, w/transient and mild side effects. **FREQUENT:** Decreased sexual ability, drowsiness, trouble sleeping, unusual tiredness or weakness. **OCCASIONAL:** Bradycardia, difficulty breathing, CHF (swelling of feet, shortness of breath), depression, cold hands/feet, diarrhea, constipation, anxiety, nasal congestion, nausea, vomiting. **RARE:** Altered taste, dry eyes, itching, numbness of fingers, toes, scalp.

ADVERSE REACTIONS/TOXIC EFFECTS

Excessive dosage may produce profound bradycardia, hypotension. Abrupt withdrawal may result in sweating, palpitations, headache, tremulousness, exacerbation of angina, MI, ventricular arrhythmias. May precipitate CHF, MI in those w/cardiac disease, thyroid storm in those w/thyrotoxicosis, peripheral ischemia in those w/existing peripheral vascular disease. Hypoglycemia may occur in previously controlled diabetics.

PATIENT CONSIDERATIONS

BASELINE ASSESSMENT

Assess baseline renal/liver function tests. Assess B/P, apical pulse immediately before drug is administered (if pulse is 60/min or below, or systolic B/P is below 90 mm Hg, withhold medication, contact physician).

Antianginal
Record onset, type (sharp, dull, squeezing), radiation, location, intensity, and duration of anginal pain, and precipitating factors (exertion, emotional stress).

INTERVENTION/EVALUATION

Monitor B/P for hypotension, respiration for shortness of breath. Assess pulse for strength/weakness, irregular rate, bradycardia. Assess fingers for color, numbness (Raynaud's). Assist w/ambulation if dizziness occurs. Assess for evidence of CHF: dyspnea (particularly on exertion or lying down), night cough, peripheral edema, distended neck veins. Monitor I&O (increase in weight, decrease in urine output may indicate CHF).

PATIENT/FAMILY TEACHING

Do not abruptly discontinue medication. Compliance w/therapy regimen is essential to control hypertension, arrhythmias. To avoid hypotensive effect, rise slowly from lying to sitting position; wait momentarily before standing. Avoid tasks that require alertness, motor skills until response to drug is established. Report excessive fatigue, dizziness. Do not use nasal decongestants, OTC cold preparations (stimulants) w/o physician approval. Outpatients should monitor B/P, pulse before taking medication. Restrict salt, alcohol intake.

nafarelin acetate

naf-ah-**rell**-in
(Synarel)

CANADIAN AVAILABILITY
Synarel

PREGNANCY CATEGORY X

CLASSIFICATION

Gonadotropin inhibitor

AVAILABILITY (Rx)

Nasal Solution: 2 mg/ml

PHARMACOKINETICS

Absorption: Well absorbed after intranasal administration. **Excretion:** Primarily eliminated in feces. **Half-life:** 3 hrs.

ACTION/*THERAPEUTIC EFFECT*

Initially stimulates the release of the pituitary gonadotropins, luteinizing hormone and follicle-stimulating hormone, *resulting in temporary increase of ovarian steroidogenesis.* Continued dosing *abolishes the stimulatory effect on the pituitary gland* and, after about 4 wks, leads to *decreased secretion of gonadal steroids.*

USES

Management of endometriosis, including dysmenorrhea, dyspareunia, and pelvic pain. Treatment of central precocious puberty.

ADMINISTRATION

INTRANASAL:

- Use metered spray pump to administer correct dose.
- When dose is given 2 times/day, alternate nostrils.
- When a topical nasal decongestant is necessary, do not use until at least 30 min after nafarelin dose.

INDICATIONS/ROUTES/DOSAGE

Endometriosis:
Note: Initiate treatment between days 2 and 4 of menstrual cycle. Duration of therapy is 6 mos.

Intranasal: Adults: 400 mcg/day: 200 mcg (1 spray) into 1 nostril in morning, 1 spray into other nostril in evening. For pts w/persistent regular menstruation after months of treatment, increase dose to 800 mcg/day (1 spray into each nostril in morning and evening).

Central precocious puberty:
Intranasal: Children: 1,600 mcg/day: 400 mcg (2 sprays into each nostril in morning and evening; total 8 sprays).

CONTRAINDICATIONS

Hypersensitivity to nafarelin, other agonist analogues and components of the preparation; undiagnosed abnormal vaginal bleeding, known or suspected pregnancy.

CAUTIONS

History of osteoporosis, chronic alcohol or tobacco use, intercurrent rhinitis.

INTERACTIONS

DRUG: None significant. **HERBAL:** None known. **FOOD:** None significant. **ALTERED LAB VALUES:** None significant.

SIDE EFFECTS

FREQUENT (>10%): Hot flashes (90%), nasal irritation, decreased libido, vaginal dryness, headache, acne, muscle pain, decreased breast size. **OCCASIONAL (1–10%):** Insomnia, edema, increased wgt, depression, hair growth. **RARE (<1%):** Palpitations, eye pain, hypersensitivity reaction (rash, itching).

ADVERSE REACTIONS/TOXIC EFFECTS

None significant.

PATIENT CONSIDERATIONS

Baseline Assessment

Quesiton for possibility of pregnancy before initiating therapy (Pregancy Category X). Question for hypersensitivity to any agonist analogue ingredients. Inquire about menstrual cycle; therapy should begin between days 2 and 4 of cycle.

Intervention/Evaluation

Check for pain relief as result of therapy. Inquire about menstrual cessation and other decreased estrogen effects.

Patient/Family Teaching

Pt should use nonhormonal contraceptive during therapy. Do not take drug, check w/physician if pregnancy is suspected (risk to fetus). Importance of full length of therapy, regular visits to physician's office. Notify physician if regular menstruation continues (menstruation should stop w/therapy).

---

nafcillin sodium

naph-**sill**-in
(Nafcil, Nallpen, Unipen)

N

PREGNANCY CATEGORY B

CLASSIFICATION

Antibiotic: Penicillin

AVAILABILITY (Rx)

Tablets: 500 mg. **Capsules:** 250 mg. **Powder for Injection:** 1 g, 2 g, 10 g.

PHARMACOKINETICS

Absorption: Poorly absorbed from GI tract (food decreases absorption). **Metabolism:** Metabolized in liver. **Excretion:** Primarily excreted in urine. Not removed by hemodialysis. **Half-life:** 0.5–1 hr (increased in decreased renal function, neonates).

ACTION/ *THERAPEUTIC EFFECT*

Binds to bacterial membranes, *inhibiting cell wall synthesis. Bactericidal.*

USES

Treatment of respiratory tract, skin/skin structure infections, osteomyelitis, endocarditis, meningitis; perioperatively, especially in cardiovascular, orthopedic procedures. Predominantly treatment of infections caused by penicillinase-producing staphylococci.

STORAGE/HANDLING

Store capsules, tablets at room temperature. ***Oral solution:*** After reconstitution, stable for 7 days if refrigerated. ***IV infusion (piggyback):*** Stable for 24 hrs at room temperature, 96 hrs if refrigerated. Discard if precipitate forms.

ADMINISTRATION

- **Note:** Space doses evenly around the clock.

ORAL:

- Give 1 hr before or 2 hrs after food/beverages.

IM:

- Reconstitute each 500 mg w/1.7 ml sterile water for injection or 0.9% NaCl injection to provide concentration of 250 mg/ml.
- Inject IM into large muscle mass.

IV:

- For IV injection, reconstitute as above, then further dilute each vial w/15–30 ml sterile water for injection or 0.9% NaCl injection. Administer over 5–10 min.
- For intermittent IV infusion (piggyback), further dilute with 50–100 ml 5% dextrose, 0.9% NaCl, or other compatible IV fluid. Infuse over 30–60 min.
- Because of potential for hypersensitivity/anaphylaxis, start initial dose at few drops per minute, increase slowly to ordered rate; stay w/pt first 10–15 min, then check q10min.
- Limit IV therapy to <48 hrs, if possible. Alternating IV sites, use large veins to reduce risk of phlebitis.
- Stop infusion if pt complains of pain.

INDICATIONS/ROUTES/DOSAGE

Usual dosage:
IV: Adults, elderly: 3–6 g/day in divided doses.

IM: Adults, elderly: 500 mg q4–6h.

Oral: Adults, elderly: 250 mg to 1 g q4–6h.

Usual pediatric dosage:
IM/IV: 25 mg/kg 2 times/day.

Oral: 25–50 mg/kg/day in 4 divided doses.

Usual neonate dosage:
IM/IV: Neonates <7 days: 50

mg/kg/day in 2–3 divided doses. *>7 days:* 75 mg/kg/day in 4 divided doses.

CONTRAINDICATIONS

Hypersensitivity to any penicillin.

CAUTIONS

History of allergies, particularly cephalosporins.

INTERACTIONS

DRUG: *Probenecid* may increase concentration, toxicity risk. **HERBAL:** None known. **FOOD:** None significant. **ALTERED LAB VALUES:** May cause positive Coombs' test.

SIDE EFFECTS

FREQUENT: Mild hypersensitivity reaction (fever, rash, pruritus), GI effects (nausea, vomiting, diarrhea) more frequent w/oral administration. **OCCASIONAL:** Hypokalemia w/high IV doses, phlebitis, thrombophlebitis (more common in elderly). **RARE:** Extravasation w/IV administration.

ADVERSE REACTIONS/TOXIC EFFECTS

Superinfections, potentially fatal antibiotic-associated colitis may result from altered bacterial balance. Hematologic effects (especially involving platelets, WBCs), severe hypersensitivity reactions, rarely anaphylaxis.

PATIENT CONSIDERATIONS

BASELINE ASSESSMENT

Question for history of allergies, especially penicillins, cephalosporins. Obtain specimen for culture and sensitivity before giving first dose (therapy may begin before results are known).

INTERVENTION/EVALUATION

Hold medication and promptly report rash (possible hypersensitivity) or diarrhea (w/fever, abdominal pain, mucus and blood in stool may indicate antibiotic-associated colitis). Assess food tolerance. Evaluate IV site frequently for phlebitis (heat, pain, red streaking over vein) and infiltration (potential extravasation). Check IM injection sites for pain, induration. Monitor potassium. Be alert for superinfection: increased fever, onset sore throat, vomiting, diarrhea, ulceration/changes of oral mucosa, anal/genital pruritus. Check hematology reports (especially WBCs), periodic renal or hepatic reports in prolonged therapy.

PATIENT/FAMILY TEACHING

Continue antibiotic for full length of treatment. Doses should be evenly spaced. Discomfort may occur w/IM injection. Report IV discomfort immediately. Notify physician in event of diarrhea, rash, other new symptom.

---

naftifine hydrochloride

(Naftin)

See Classification section under: Antifungals, topical

---

nalbuphine hydrochloride

nail-**byew**-phin

(Nubain)

CANADIAN AVAILABILITY

Nubain

PREGNANCY CATEGORY B
(D if used for prolonged periods or in high doses at term)

CLASSIFICATION

Opioid analgesic

AVAILABILITY (Rx)

Injection: 10 mg/ml, 20 mg/ml

PHARMACODYNAMICS

	ONSET	PEAK	DURATION
SubQ	<15 min	—	3–6 hrs
IM	<15 min	60 min	3–6 hrs
IV	2–3 min	30 min	3–6 hrs

PHARMACOKINETICS

Absorption: Well absorbed after SubQ, IM administration. **Metabolism:** Metabolized in liver. **Excretion:** Primarily eliminated in feces via biliary secretion. **Half-life:** 3.5–5 hrs.

ACTION/*THERAPEUTIC EFFECT*

Binds w/opioid receptors within CNS, *altering pain perception, emotional response to pain.* May displace opioid agonists and competitively inhibit their action (may precipitate withdrawal symptoms).

USES

Relief of moderate to severe pain, preop sedation, obstetrical analgesia, adjunct to anesthesia.

STORAGE/HANDLING

Store parenteral form at room temperature.

ADMINISTRATION

IM:

- Rotate IM injection sites.

IV:

- For IV injection, administer each 10 mg >3–5 min.

INDICATIONS/ROUTES/DOSAGE

Note: Dosage based on severity of pain, physical condition of pt, concurrent use of other medications.

Analgesia:
SubQ/IM/IV: Adults, elderly: 10 mg q3–6h, as necessary. Do not exceed maximum single dose of 20 mg, maximum daily dose of 160 mg. In pts chronically receiving narcotic analgesics of similar duration of action, give 25% of usual dosage.

Supplement to anesthesia:
IV: Adults, elderly: Induction: 0.3–3 mg/kg over 10–15 min. *Maintenance:* 0.25–0.5 mg/kg as necessary.

CONTRAINDICATIONS

Respirations <12/min.

CAUTIONS

Impaired hepatic/renal function, elderly, debilitated, head injury, increased intracranial pressure, MI w/nausea, vomiting, respiratory disease, hypertension, before biliary tract surgery (produces spasm of sphincter of Oddi).

INTERACTIONS

DRUG: *Alcohol, CNS depressants* may increase CNS or respiratory depression, hypotension. *MAO inhibitors* may produce severe, fatal reaction (reduce dose to ¼ usual dose). Effects may be decreased w/***buprenorphine.*** **HERBAL:** None known. **FOOD:** None significant. **ALTERED LAB VALUES:** May increase amylase, lipase, serum levels.

SIDE EFFECTS

FREQUENT (>10%): Histamine reaction (decreased blood pressure, increased sweating, flushing of skin, wheezing. **OCCASIONAL (1–10%):** Allergic reaction (rash, itching), dizziness, dry mouth, headache, decreased appetite, nausea, vomiting, redness, swelling at injection site, unusually tired. **RARE(<1%):** Trouble breathing, confusion, fast, pounding heartbeat, increased blood pressure, paralytic ileus, decreased urination, stomach cramps, blurred vision, insomnia.

ADVERSE REACTIONS/TOXIC EFFECTS

Abrupt withdrawal after prolonged use may produce symptoms of narcotic withdrawal (abdominal cramping, rhinorrhea, lacrimation, anxiety, increased temperature, piloerection [goose bumps]). Overdose results in severe respiratory depression, skeletal muscle flaccidity, cyanosis, extreme somnolence progressing to convulsions, stupor, coma. Tolerance to analgesic effect, physical dependence may occur w/chronic use.

PATIENT CONSIDERATIONS

Baseline Assessment

Raise bed rails. Obtain vital signs before giving medication. If respirations are 12/min or lower (20/min or lower in children), withhold medication, contact physician. Assess onset, type, location, and duration of pain. Effect of medication is reduced if full pain recurs before next dose. Low abuse potential.

Intervention/Evaluation

Increase fluid intake and environmental humidity to improve viscosity of lung secretions. Monitor for change in respirations, B/P, change in rate or quality of pulse. Monitor pattern of daily bowel activity and stool consistency. Initiate deep breathing and coughing exercises, particularly in those w/impaired pulmonary function. Change pt's position q2–4h. Assess for clinical improvement and record onset of relief of pain. Consult physician if pain relief is not adequate.

Patient/Family Teaching

Change positions slowly to avoid dizziness. Avoid tasks that require alertness, motor skills until response to drug is established. Note effects of abrupt withdrawal following long-term use. Avoid alcohol and CNS depressants.

nalmefene hydrochloride

nal-meh-feen
(Revex)

PREGNANCY CATEGORY B

CLASSIFICATION

Opioid antagonist

AVAILABILITY (Rx)

Injection: 100 mcg/ml (blue label in 1 ml amps); 1 mg/ml (green label in 2 ml amps)

PHARMACODYNAMICS

	ONSET	PEAK	DURATION
IV bolus	2–5 min	5–15 min	Variable
SubQ	5 min	5–15 min	Variable
IM	5 min	5–15 min	Variable

PHARMACOKINETICS

Absorption: Rapidly distributed

following parental administration by red blood cells and plasma. **Metabolism:** Metabolized by the liver. **Excretion:** Excreted in the urine. **Half-life:** 10.8 hrs. Half-life prolonged in renal/hepatic function impairment.

ACTION/ *THERAPEUTIC EFFECT*

Binds to opioid receptors, *preventing or reversing the effects of opioids, including respiratory depression, sedation, and hypotension.* No activity noted when administered in absence of opioid agonists.

USES

Complete or partial reversal of opioid drug effects induced by either natural or synthetic opioids; management of known or suspected opioid overdose.

ADMINISTRATION

- Should be given as an IV bolus but can be given either SubQ or IM if venous access is unavailable.
- The blue label ampoule contains 1 ml (100 mcg/ml) and is for postop use.
- The green label ample contains 2 ml (1 mg/ml) and is used for management of overdose.

INDICATIONS/ROUTES/DOSAGES

Postop patients:
SubQ/IM/IV: Adults: Initially, 0.25 mcg/kg followed by additional 0.25 mcg doses at 2–5 min intervals until desired response is attained. Cumulative doses > 1 mcg/kg do not provide additional therapeutic effect.

Known/suspected overdose:
SubQ/IM/IV: Adults: Initially, 0.5 mg/70 kg. May be followed by a second dose of 1 mg/70 kg 2–5 min later. If physical opioid dependence is suspected, give challenge dose of 0.1 mg/70 kg. If no evidence of withdrawal is noted, follow recommended dose.

Cardiovascular risk patients:
SubQ/IM/IV: Adults: May dilute nalmefene 1:1 with saline or sterile water; use smaller initial and incremental doses of 0.1 mcg/kg.

Patients with renal failure:
SubQ/IM/IV: Adults: Give incremental doses over 60 sec (minimizes risk of hypertension, dizziness).

CONTRAINDICATIONS

History of hypersensitivity to drug.

CAUTIONS

High cardiovascular risk, those who have received potentially cardiotoxic drugs, known physical opioid dependence , following surgery involving high uses of opioids, renal/hepatic function impairment.

INTERACTIONS

DRUG: Potential risk of seizures with ***flumazenil.*** May produce incomplete reversal of ***buprenorphine***-induced respiratory depression. **HERBAL:** None known. **FOOD:** None significant. **ALTERED LAB VALUES:** May increase SGOT (AST).

SIDE EFFECTS

None significant (little or no pharmacologic effect in absence of narcotics). **FREQUENT (>5%):** Vomiting, nausea. **OCCASIONAL (1–5%):** Tachycardia, hypertension, postop pain, fever, dizziness, headache, chills, hypotension, vasodilation.

ADVERSE REACTIONS/TOXIC EFFECTS

Can produce acute withdrawal

symptoms in those who are opioid dependent (nausea, vomiting, elevated B/P, anxiety, chills, abdominal cramps, myalgia, tachycardia). Those at high cardiovascular risk may experience hypotension, hypertension, pulmonary edema, cardiovascular instability as a result of abrupt reversal of opioid effects.

PATIENT CONSIDERATIONS

Baseline Assessment

Establish patent airway, ventilator assistance, oxygen administration. Establish circulatory access, if possible.

Interventions/Evaluation

Monitor vital signs especially rate, depth, and rhythm of respiration during and frequently after administration. Carefully observe patient after satisfactory response for recurrence of respiratory depression.

naloxone hydrochloride

nay-**lox**-own
(Narcan)

CANADIAN AVAILABILITY
Narcan

PREGNANCY CATEGORY B

CLASSIFICATION

Opioid antagonist

AVAILABILITY (Rx)

Injection: 0.02 mg/ml, 0.4 mg/ml, 1 mg/ml

PHARMACODYNAMICS

	ONSET	PEAK	DURATION
SubQ			
	2–5 min	—	1–4 hrs
IM	2–5 min	—	1–4 hrs
IV	1–2 min	—	1–4 hrs

PHARMACOKINETICS

Absorption: Well absorbed after SubQ, IM administration. **Metabolism:** Metabolized in liver. **Excretion:** Primarily excreted in urine. **Half-life:** 60–100 min.

ACTION/*THERAPEUTIC EFFECT*

Displaces opiates at opiate-occupied receptor sites in CNS, *blocking narcotic effects. Reverses opiate-induced sleep or sedation. Increases respiratory rate, returns depressed B/P to normal rate.*

USES

Diagnosis and treatment of opioid toxicity, treatment of opioid induced respiratory depression, and other effects (e.g., sedation, coma, convulsions). Used in neonates to reverse respiratory depression caused by opioids given to mother during labor and delivery. Adjunctive therapy to treat hypotension in management of septic shock.

STORAGE/HANDLING

Store parenteral form at room temperature. Use mixture within 24 hrs; discard unused solution.

ADMINISTRATION

IM:

- Give in upper, outer quadrant of buttock.

IV:

- May dilute 1 mg/ml with 50 ml sterile water for injection to provide a concentration of 0.02 mg/ml.
- Use the 0.4 mg/ml and 1 mg/ml

for injection for adults, the 0.02 mg/ml concentration for neonates.
- For continuous IV infusion, dilute each 2 mg of naloxone with 500 ml of 5% dextrose in water or 0.9% NaCl, producing solution containing 0.004 mg/ml.

INDICATIONS/ROUTES/DOSAGE

Opioid toxicity (IV route preferred):
IM/IV/SubQ: Adults: 0.4–2 mg as single dose. May repeat at 2–3 min intervals. ***Children:*** 0.01 mg/kg. May repeat w/0.1 mg/kg.
Note: AAP recommends initial dose of 0.1 mg/kg for infants and children up to 5 yrs and weighing <20 kg. Children >5 yrs or >20 kg recommended initial dose 2 mg.

Opioid respiratory depression:
IV: Adults: 0.1–0.2 mg q2–3min until adequate. ventilation and alertness w/o pain are obtained. May repeat dose at 1–2 hr intervals. ***Children:*** 5–10 mcg (0.005–0.01 mg) q2–3min. ***Neonates:*** 10 mcg (0.01 mg)/kg. May repeat q2–3min.

Septic shock:
IV: Adults: 0.03–0.2 mg/kg initially, then IV infusion of 0.03–0.3 mg/kg/hr for 1–20 hrs.

CONTRAINDICATIONS

Respiratory depression due to nonopiate drugs.

CAUTIONS

Opiate-dependent pt, cardiovascular disorders.

INTERACTIONS

DRUG: Reverses analgesic/side effects, may precipitate withdrawal symptoms of ***butorphanol, nalbuphine, pentazocine, opioid agonist analgesics.*** **HERBAL:** None known. **FOOD:** None significant. **ALTERED LAB VALUES:** None significant.

SIDE EFFECTS

None significant (little or no pharmacologic effect in absence of narcotics).

ADVERSE REACTIONS/TOXIC EFFECTS

Too rapid reversal of narcotic depression may result in nausea, vomiting, tremulousness, sweating, increased B/P, tachycardia. Excessive dosage in postop pts may produce significant reversal of analgesia, excitement, tremulousness. Hypotension or hypertension, ventricular tachycardia and fibrillation, pulmonary edema may occur in those w/cardiovascular disease.

PATIENT CONSIDERATIONS

Baseline Assessment

Maintain clear airway. Obtain weight of children to calculate drug dosage.

Intervention/Evaluation

Monitor vital signs especially rate, depth, and rhythm of respiration during and frequently after administration. Carefully observe pt after satisfactory response (duration of opiate may exceed duration of naloxone, resulting in recurrence of respiratory depression). Assess for increased pain w/reversal of opiate.

---

naltrexone hydrochloride

nal-**trex**-own
(ReVia)

CANADIAN AVAILABILITY
ReVia

PREGNANCY CATEGORY C

CLASSIFICATION

Opioid antagonist

AVAILABILITY (Rx)

Tablets: 50 mg

PHARMACODYNAMICS

	ONSET	PEAK	DURATION
Oral	—	—	24–72 hrs

PHARMACOKINETICS

Absorption: Rapid, complete absorption following oral administration. **Metabolism:** Undergoes extensive first-pass hepatic metabolism. Metabolized in liver to active metabolite. **Excretion:** Excreted in urine. **Half-life:** 4–13 hrs.

ACTION / *THERAPEUTIC EFFECT*

Opioid antagonist: Binds to opioid receptors, *blocking physical effects of morphine, heroin, other opioids.* ***Alcohol deterrent:*** Exact mechanism unknown. *Decreases craving, drinking days, relapse rate.*

USES / *UNLABELED*

Blockade of effects of exogenously administered opioids. Treatment of alcohol dependence. *Treatment of postconcussional syndrome unresponsive to other treatments; eating disorders.*

ADMINISTRATION

SubQ/IM/IV:

- In those w/narcotic dependence, do not attempt treatment until pt has remained opioid free for 7–10 days. Test urine for opioids for verification. Pt should not be experiencing withdrawal symptoms.
- Administer a naloxone challenge test (see Indications/Dosage/Routes). If pt experiences any signs/symptoms of withdrawal, withhold treatment (challenge test can be repeated in 24 hrs). Naloxone challenge test must be negative before naltrexone therapy is initiated.

INDICATIONS/ROUTES/DOSAGE

Naloxone challenge test:
IV: Adults, elderly: Draw 2 ampules naloxone, 2 ml (0.8 mg) into syringe. Inject 0.5 ml (0.2 mg); while needle is still in vein, observe for 30 sec for withdrawal signs/symptoms (see Adverse Reactions/Toxic Effects). If no evidence of withdrawal, inject remaining 1.5 ml (0.6 mg); observe for additional 20 min for withdrawal signs/symptoms.
SubQ: Adults, elderly: Give 2 ml (0.8 mg); observe for 45 min for withdrawal signs/symptoms.

Opioid-free state:
Oral: Adults, elderly: Initially, 25 mg. Observe pt for 1 hr. If no withdrawal signs appear, give another 25 mg. May be given as 100 mg every other day or 150 mg q3days.

Adjunct in treatment of alcohol dependence:
Oral: Adults, elderly: 50 mg once daily.

CONTRAINDICATIONS

Pts experiencing opiate withdrawal, opioid dependent, acute opioid withdrawal, failed naloxone challenge, positive urine screen for opioids, history of sensitivity to naltrexone, acute hepatitis, liver failure.

CAUTIONS

Active liver disease.

INTERACTIONS

DRUG: Concurrent use w/***thioridazine*** may produce lethargy, somnolence. Benefits of ***opioid-containing products*** (cough and cold preparations, antidiarrheal preparations, opioid analgesics) are negated. **HERBAL:** None

N

known. **FOOD:** None significant. **ALTERED LAB VALUES:** May increase serum transaminase, SGOT (AST), SGPT (ALT).

SIDE EFFECTS

FREQUENT: *Alcoholism:* Nausea (10%), headache (7%), depression (5–7%). *Narcotic addiction:* Insomnia, anxiety, nervousness, headache, low energy, abdominal cramps, nausea, vomiting, joint/muscle pain (>10%). **OCCASIONAL:** *Alcoholism:* Dizziness, nervousness, fatigue (4%), insomnia, vomiting (3%), anxiety, suicidal ideation (2%). *Narcotic addiction:* Irritability, increased energy, dizziness, anorexia, diarrhea or constipation, rash, chills, increased thirst.

ADVERSE REACTIONS/TOXIC EFFECTS

Signs and symptoms of opioid withdrawal include stuffy or runny nose, tearing, yawning, sweating, tremor, vomiting, piloerection (goose bumps), feeling of temperature change, joint/bone/muscle pain, abdominal cramps, feeling of skin crawling. May cause hepatocellular injury if given in large doses. Accidental naltrexone overdosage produces withdrawal symptoms within 5 min of ingestion, lasts up to 48 hrs. Symptoms present as confusion, visual hallucinations, somnolence, significant vomiting and diarrhea.

PATIENT CONSIDERATIONS

BASELINE ASSESSMENT

If there is any question of opioid dependence, a naloxone challenge test (see Indications/Dosage/Routes) should be performed. Treatment w/naltrexone should not be instituted unless pt is opioid free for 7–10 days before therapy begins. Pt should wear identification indicating naltrexone therapy. Obtain medication history (especially opioids), other medical conditions (especially hepatitis, other liver disease).

INTERVENTION/EVALUATION

Monitor closely for evidence of hepatotoxicity (abdominal pain that lasts longer than a few days, white bowel movements, dark urine, jaundice), SGOT, SGPT, bilirubin, creatinine clearance lab values.

PATIENT/FAMILY TEACHING

If heroin or other opiates are self-administered, there will be no effect. However, any attempt to overcome naltrexone's prolonged 24–72 hr blockade of opioid effect by taking large amounts of opioids is very dangerous and may result in coma, serious injury, or fatal overdose. Naltrexone also blocks effects of opioid-containing medicine (cough and cold preparations, antidiarrheal preparations, opioid analgesics). Contact physician if abdominal pain that lasts longer than 3 days, white bowel movements, dark-colored urine, yellow eyes occurs. Periodic blood testing should be performed to detect liver toxicity. Stress importance of compliance/support groups/counseling. Carry identification card indicating use of naltrexone.

naphazoline

na-**faz**-oh-leen

(Albalon, Estivin, Naphcon, Vasocon)

FIXED-COMBINATION(S)
W/pheniramine maleate, an antihistamine **(Naphcon-A)**

CANADIAN AVAILABILITY
Albalon, Naphcon, Vasocon

PREGNANCY CATEGORY C

CLASSIFICATION

Sympathomimetic, decongestant

AVAILABILITY (OTC)

Nasal Solution: 0.05%. **Ophthalmic Solution:** 0.012%, 0.02%, 0.03%, 0.1% (Rx).

ACTION/*THERAPEUTIC EFFECT*

Directly acts on alpha-adrenergic receptors in arterioles of conjunctiva, *causing vasoconstriction, w/subsequent decreased congestion to area.*

USES

Ophthalmic: Relief of itching, congestion, and minor irritation; to control hyperemia in pts with superficial corneal vascularity. Occasionally may be used during some ocular diagnostic procedures. ***Intranasal:*** Relief of nasal congestion due to common cold, acute or chronic rhinitis, hay fever or other allergies.

STORAGE/HANDLING

Do not store in aluminum containers (degraded by aluminum). Do not use if cloudy or discolored solution.

ADMINISTRATION

OPHTHALMIC:

- Follow manufacturer's directions regarding contact lenses.
- Tilt pt's head back; place solution in conjunctival sac.
- Have pt close eyes; press gently on lacrimal sac for 1 min.
- Take care not to touch any area w/the applicator.
- Remove excess solution by gently blotting w/tissue.

INTRANASAL:

- **Note:** Applicator should not touch any surface; rinse tip of dispenser or dropper w/hot water following use. Use for only 1 person.

DROPS:

- Position pt in lateral, head-low position or reclining w/head tilted as far back as possible.
- Apply drops to one nostril and maintain position for 5 min. Then apply drops to second nostril and maintain position for 5 min.

SPRAY:

- Administer spray into each nostril w/pt's head erect so that excess solution is not released.
- After 2–3 min, have pt blow nose thoroughly.

INDICATIONS/ROUTES/DOSAGE

Usual nasal dosage:
Intranasal: Adults, elderly, children >12 yrs: 2 drops/sprays (0.05%) in each nostril q3–6h.

Usual ophthalmic dosage:
Ophthalmic: Adults, elderly: 1–2 drops q3–4h for 3–4 days.

CONTRAINDICATIONS

Hypersensitivity to naphazoline or any component of the preparation; narrow-angle glaucoma or those w/a narrow angle who do not have glaucoma; before peripheral iridectomy; eyes capable of angle closure.

CAUTIONS

Hypertension, diabetes, hyperthyroidism, heart disease, hypertensive cardiovascular disease, coronary artery disease, cerebral arteriosclerosis, long-standing bronchial asthma. Consider precautions for individual components.

INTERACTIONS

DRUG: ***Tricyclic antidepressants, maprotiline*** may increase effect. **HERBAL:** Ma Huang (Ephedra) may increase CNS stimulation. **FOOD:** None significant. **ALTERED LAB VALUES:** None significant.

SIDE EFFECTS

OCCASIONAL: *Nasal:* Burning, stinging, drying nasal mucosa, sneezing, rebound congestion. *Ophthalmic:* Blurred vision, large pupils, increased eye irritation. **Note:** ***Systemic absorption:*** Fast/irregular/pounding heartbeat, headache, lightheadedness, nervousness, trembling, insomnia, nausea.

ADVERSE REACTIONS/TOXIC EFFECTS

Large doses may produce tachycardia, palpitations, lightheadedness, nausea, vomiting. Overdosage in pts >60 yrs: hallucinations, CNS depression, seizures.

PATIENT CONSIDERATIONS

Baseline Assessment

Question for hypersensitivity to naphazoline or any component of preparation.

Patient/Family Teaching

Teach correct application (see Ophthalmic/Intranasal Administration). Do not use beyond 72 hrs w/o consulting a physician. Use caution w/activities that require visual acuity. Discontinue and consult physician if the following occur: vision changes, headache, eye pain, floating spots, pain w/light exposure, acute eye redness, insomnia, dizziness, weakness, tremor, irregular heartbeat. Too frequent use may result in rebound effect.

naproxen

nah-**prox**-en

(EC-Naprosyn, Naprelan, Naprosyn)

naproxen sodium

(Aleve, Anaprox)

CANADIAN AVAILABILITY

Anaprox, Apo-Napro, Naprosyn, Naxen, Novonaprox, Synflex

PREGNANCY CATEGORY B

(D if used in third trimester or near delivery)

CLASSIFICATION

Nonsteroidal anti-inflammatory

AVAILABILITY (Rx)

Gelcap: 200 mg **(OTC). Tablets:** 200 mg **(OTC):** 250 mg, 375 mg, 500 mg. **Tablets (delayed-release):** 375 mg, 500 mg. **Oral Suspension:** 125 mg/5 ml.

PHARMACODYNAMICS

	ONSET	PEAK	DURATION
Oral (analgesic)			
	<1 hr	—	Up to 7 hrs
Oral (antirheumatic)			
	Up to 2–4 wks	14 days	—

PHARMACOKINETICS

Absorption: Completely absorbed from GI tract. **Metabolism:** Metabolized in liver. **Excretion:** Primarily excreted in urine. **Half-life:** 13 hrs.

ACTION/*THERAPEUTIC EFFECT*

Produces analgesic and anti-inflammatory effect by inhibiting prostaglandin synthesis, *reducing inflammatory response and intensity of pain stimulus reaching sensory nerve endings.*

USES/*UNLABELED*

Treatment of acute or long-term mild to moderate pain, primary dysmenorrhea, mild to moderately severe pain, rheumatoid arthritis, juvenile rheumatoid arthritis, osteoarthritis, ankylosing spondylitis, acute gouty arthritis, bursitis, tendinitis. *Treatment of vascular headaches.*

ADMINISTRATION

ORAL:

- Do not crush or break enteric-coated form.
- May give with food, milk, or antacids if GI distress occurs.

INDICATIONS/ROUTES/DOSAGE

Note: Each 275 or 550 mg tablet of naproxen sodium equals 250 or 500 mg naproxen, respectively.

Rheumatoid arthritis, osteoarthritis, ankylosing spondylitis:
Oral: Adults, elderly: 250–500 mg (275–550 mg) 2 times/day or 250 mg (275 mg) in morning and 500 mg (550 mg) in evening. ***Naprelan:*** 750–1,000 mg daily as single dose.

Juvenile rheumatoid arthritis (naproxen only):
Oral: Children: 10 mg/kg/day in 2 divided doses.

Acute gouty arthritis:
Oral: Adults, elderly: Initially, 750 (825) mg, then 250 (275) mg q8h until attack subsides. ***Naprelan:*** Initially, 1,000–1,500 mg, then 1,000 mg/day as single dose until attack subsides.

Mild to moderate pain, dysmenorrhea, bursitis, tendinitis:
Oral: Adults, elderly: Initially, 500 (550) mg, then 250 (275) mg q6–8h as needed. Total daily dose not to exceed 1.25 (1.375) g. ***Naprelan:*** 1,000 mg/day as single dose.

CONTRAINDICATIONS

GI ulceration, chronic inflammation of GI tract, bleeding disorders, history of hypersensitivity to aspirin or NSAIDs.

CAUTIONS

Impaired renal/hepatic function, history of GI tract disease, predisposition to fluid retention.

INTERACTIONS

DRUG: May increase effects of ***oral anticoagulants, heparin, thrombolytics.*** May decrease effect of ***antihypertensives, diuretics. Salicylates, aspirin*** may increase risk of GI side effects, bleeding. ***Bone marrow depressants*** may increase risk of hematologic reactions. May increase concentration, toxicity of ***lithium.*** May increase ***methotrexate*** toxicity. ***Probenecid*** may increase concentration. **HERBAL:** May decrease effects of feverfew. Ginkgo biloba may increase risk of bleeding. **FOOD:** None significant. **ALTERED LAB VALUES:** May prolong bleeding time, alter blood glucose levels. May increase liver function tests. May decrease sodium, uric acid.

SIDE EFFECTS

FREQUENT (3–9%): Rash, ringing in ears, edema, shortness of breath, dizziness, headache, abdominal cramps, constipation, heartburn, nausea. **OCCASIONAL (1–3%):**

Blurred/double vision, stomatitis, lightheadedness, diarrhea, indigestion. **RARE (<1%):** Confusion, itching, muscle cramps/pain, insomnia, vomiting.

ADVERSE REACTIONS/TOXIC EFFECTS

Peptic ulcer, GI bleeding, gastritis, severe hepatic reaction (cholestasis, jaundice) occur rarely. Nephrotoxicity (dysuria, hematuria, proteinuria, nephrotic syndrome) and severe hypersensitivity reaction (fever, chills, bronchospasm) occur rarely.

PATIENT CONSIDERATIONS

BASELINE ASSESSMENT

Assess onset, type, location, and duration of pain or inflammation. Inspect appearance of affected joints for immobility, deformities, and skin condition.

INTERVENTION/EVALUATION

Assist w/ambulation if dizziness occurs. Monitor pattern of daily bowel activity and stool consistency. Check behind medial malleolus for fluid retention (usually first area noted). Evaluate for therapeutic response: relief of pain, stiffness, swelling, increase in joint mobility, reduced joint tenderness, improved grip strength.

PATIENT/FAMILY TEACHING

Avoid tasks that require alertness, motor skills until response to drug is established. If GI upset occurs, take w/food, milk. Avoid aspirin, alcohol during therapy (increases risk of GI bleeding). Report headache, rash, visual disturbances, increased wgt, black stools, persistent headache. Scored tablets may be broken or crushed; swallow enteric-coated form whole.

naratriptan

nar-ah-**trip**-tan
(Amerge)

CANADIAN AVAILABILITY
Amerge

PREGNANCY CATEGORY C

CLASSIFICATION

Antimigraine

AVAILABILITY (Rx)

Tablets: 1 mg, 2.5 mg

PHARMACOKINETICS

Absorption: Well absorbed following oral administration. **Metabolism:** Metabolized by the liver to inactive metabolite. **Excretion:** Eliminated primarily in the urine with lesser amount excreted in the feces. **Half-life:** 6 hrs. Half-life increased in renal/hepatic impairment.

ACTION/*THERAPEUTIC EFFECT*

Binds selectively to vascular receptors producing a vasoconstrictive effect on cranial blood vessels, *producing relief of migraine headache.*

USES

Treatment of acute migraine attack with or without aura in adults.

INDICATIONS/ROUTES/DOSAGES

Migraine:
Oral: Adults: Give 1 or 2.5 mg. If headache returns or patient received only a partial response to initial dose, may repeat dose once after 4 hrs. *Maximum:* 5 mg per 24 hr period.

Mild-to-moderate renal/hepatic impairment:
Oral: Adults: Consider with low starting dose. Do not exceed 2.5 mg over a 24 hr period.

CONTRAINDICATIONS

Coronary artery disease, uncontrolled hypertension, severe renal impairment (Ccr <15 ml/min), severe hepatic impairment (Child-Pugh grade C), cerebrovascular or peripheral vascular syndromes, ischemic heart disease (angina pectoris, history of MI, silent ischemia), Prinzmetal's angina, concurrent use (or within 24 hrs) of ergotamine-containing preparations, concurrent (or within 2 wks) of MAO therapy, hemiplegic or basilar migraine, within 24 hrs of another serotonin receptor agonist.

CAUTIONS

Mild-to-moderate renal/hepatic impairment, pt profile suggesting cardiovascular risks.

INTERACTIONS

DRUG: *Ergotamine*-containing drugs may produce vasospastic reaction. ***Oral contraceptives*** reduces naratriptan's clearance, volume of distribution. Combined use of ***fluoxetine, fluvoxamine, paroxetine, sertraline*** may produce weakness, hyperreflexia, incoordination. **HERBAL:** None known. **FOOD:** None significant. **ALTERED LAB VALUES:** None significant.

SIDE EFFECTS

OCCASIONAL (5%): Nausea. RARE (2%): Paresthesia, dizziness, fatigue, drowsiness, fatigue, neck/throat/jaw pressure.

ADVERSE REACTIONS/TOXIC EFFECTS

May produce corneal opacities and defects. Cardiac events (ischemia, coronary artery vasospasm, MI), noncardiac vasospasm-related reactions (hemorrhage, stroke) occur rarely but particularly in those with hypertension, obesity, smokers, diabetes, strong family history of coronary artery disease, male > 40 yrs, postmenopausal women.

PATIENT CONSIDERATIONS

BASELINE ASSESSMENT

Question regarding history of peripheral vascular disease, renal/hepatic impairment, possibility of pregnancy. Question pt regarding onset, location, and duration of migraine and possible precipitating symptoms.

INTERVENTIONS/EVALUATION

Assess for relief of migraine headache and potential for photophobia, phonophobia (sound sensitivity, nausea, vomiting).

PATIENT/FAMILY TEACHING

Take a single dose as soon as symptoms of an actual migraine attack appears. Medication is intended to relieve migraine headaches, not to prevent or reduce number of attacks. If heart throbbing, pain/tightness in chest or throat, sudden or severe abdominal pain, or pain or weakness of extremities occurs, contact physician immediately.

---

natamycin

(Natacyn)
See Classification section under: Antifungals: topical

---

nateglinide

(Starlix)
See Supplement

N

nedocromil sodium

ned-oh-**crow**-mul
(Tilade)

CANADIAN AVAILABILITY
Mireze, Tilade

PREGNANCY CATEGORY B

CLASSIFICATION

Anti-inflammatory

AVAILABILITY (Rx)

Inhalation Aerosol: 1.75 mg/activation

PHARMACODYNAMICS

	ONSET	PEAK	DURATION
Inhalation			
	30 min	—	—

PHARMACOKINETICS

Absorption: Minimal absorption from GI tract after inhalation. Distributed to plasma. **Excretion:** Primarily excreted unchanged in urine or via biliary system. **Half-life:** 1.5–3.3 hrs.

ACTION/*THERAPEUTIC EFFECT*

Prevents activation, release of mediators of inflammation (e.g., histamine, leukotrienes, mast cells, eosinophils, monocytes). *Prevents both early and late asthmatic responses.*

USES/*UNLABELED*

Maintenance therapy for preventing airway inflammation, bronchoconstriction in pts w/mild to moderate bronchial asthma. *Prevents bronchospasm in pts w/reversible obstructive airway disease.*

ADMINISTRATION

INHALATION:

- Shake container well, then remove cap from mouthpiece.
- Position mouthpiece to bottom, tilt head back.
- Breathe out through mouth to functional volume.
- Place mouthpiece in mouth or hold 1–2 inches away from open mouth.
- Activate inhaler while breathing in slowly and deeply.
- Hold breath 5–10 sec (or as long as possible).
- Remove inhaler from mouth and breathe out slowly.
- Wait 1–10 min before second inhalation.

INDICATIONS/ROUTES/DOSAGE

Asthma:
Oral Inhalation: Adults, elderly, children >6 yrs: Two inhalations (4 mg) 4 times/day. May decrease to 3 times/day then 2 times/day as control of asthma occurs. ***Maximum:*** 16 mg/24 hrs.

CONTRAINDICATIONS

Hypersensitivity to nedocromil.

CAUTIONS

Not for reversing acute bronchospasm.

INTERACTIONS

DRUG: None significant. **HERBAL:** None known. **FOOD:** None significant. **ALTERED LAB VALUES:** None significant.

SIDE EFFECTS

FREQUENT (5–10%): Cough, pharyngitis, bronchospasm, headache, unpleasant taste. **OCCASIONAL (1–5%):** Rhinitis, upper respiratory tract infection, dyspnea, nausea, vomiting, abdominal pain, fatigue. **RARE (<1%):** Diarrhea, dizziness.

ADVERSE REACTIONS/TOXIC EFFECTS

None significant.

PATIENT CONSIDERATIONS

BASELINE ASSESSMENT

Assess sensitivity to nedocromil.

INTERVENTION/EVALUATION

Evaluate therapeutic response: reduced dependence on antihistamine, less frequent/less severe asthmatic attacks.

PATIENT/FAMILY TEACHING

Increase fluid intake (decreases lung secretion viscosity). Must be administered at regular intervals (even when symptom free) to achieve optimal results of therapy. Proper inhalation technique is essential (illustrated pt information leaflet accompanies medication). Do not increase or decrease dosage w/o consulting physician. Unpleasant taste after inhalation may be relieved by rinsing mouth w/water immediately, using sugarless hard candy or gum.

nefazodone hydrochloride

nef-**aye**-zoh-doan
(Serzone)

CANADIAN AVAILABILITY
Serzone

PREGNANCY CATEGORY C

CLASSIFICATION

Antidepressant

AVAILABILITY (Rx)

Tablets: 100 mg, 150 mg, 200 mg, 250 mg

PHARMACOKINETICS

Absorption: Rapidly, completely absorbed from GI tract. Food delays absorption. Widely distributed in body tissues, including CNS. **Metabolism:** Extensively metabolized to active metabolites. **Excretion:** Excreted in urine and eliminated in feces. **Half-life:** 2–4 hrs.

ACTION/*THERAPEUTIC EFFECT*

Exact mechanism unknown. Appears to inhibit neuronal uptake of serotonin and norepinephrine, antagonize alpha$_1$-adrenergic receptors, *producing antidepressant effect.*

USES

Treatment of depression exhibited as persistent, prominent dysphoria (occurring nearly every day for at least 2 wks) manifested by 4 of 8 symptoms: change in appetite, change in sleep pattern, increased fatigue, impaired concentration, feelings of guilt or worthlessness, loss of interest in usual activities, psychomotor agitation or retardation, or suicidal tendencies. Maintenance treatment to prevent relapse of acute depressive episode.

ADMINISTRATION

ORAL:

- Give w/o regard to meals.

INDICATIONS/ROUTES/DOSAGE

Note: At least 14 days should elapse between discontinuing

MAO inhibitors and initiation of nefazodone therapy. At least 7 days should elapse after discontinuing nefazodone and initiation of MAO inhibitor therapy.

Depression, prevention of relapse acute episodes:
Oral: Adults: Initially, 200 mg/day, given in two divided doses. Gradually increase dose in increments of 100–200 mg/day on a twice daily schedule, at intervals of at least 1 wk. ***Elderly:*** Initially, 100 mg/day on a twice daily schedule. Adjust the rate of subsequent dose titration based on clinical response. ***Range:*** 300–600 mg/day.

CONTRAINDICATIONS

Within 14 days of MAO inhibitor ingestion, coadministration w/astemizole, cisapride or terfenadine therapy, hypersensitivity to nefazodone.

CAUTIONS

Recent MI, unstable heart disease, hepatic cirrhosis, dehydration, hypovolemia, cerebrovascular disease, history of mania/hypomania, history of seizures.

INTERACTIONS

DRUG: May increase concentration, toxicity of ***alprazolam triazolam*** (dosage reduction advised). ***MAOIs*** may produce severe reactions (see Adverse Reactions/Toxic Effects). At least 14 days should elapse between discontinuing MAO inhibitors and initiation of nefazodone therapy. At least 7 days should elapse after discontinuing nefazodone and initiation of MAO inhibitor therapy. **HERBAL:** St. John's wort may increase side effects (nausea, vomiting, restlessness). **FOOD:** None significant. **ALTERED LAB VALUES:** None significant.

SIDE EFFECTS

Elderly/debilitated experience increased susceptibility to side effects. **FREQUENT:** Headache (36%), dry mouth, somnolence (25%), nausea (22%), dizziness (17%), constipation (14%), insomnia, asthenia (loss of strength, energy), lightheadedness (10%). **OCCASIONAL:** Dyspepsia, blurred vision (9%), diarrhea, infection (8%), confusion, abnormal vision (7%), pharyngitis (6%), increased appetite (5%), postural hypotension, vasodilation (flushing, feeling of warmth) (4%), peripheral edema, cough, flu syndrome (3%).

ADVERSE REACTIONS/TOXIC EFFECTS

Concurrent MAO inhibitor administration or if time frame between discontinuation and initiation of drug therapy (see Indications/Dosage/Routes) is not followed, serious reactions (hyperthermia, rigidity, myoclonus, extreme agitation, delirium, coma) occur. Coadministration w/astemizole or terfenadine therapy may produce serious cardiovascular abnormalities.

PATIENT CONSIDERATIONS

Baseline Assessment

Question for history of sensitivity to nefazodone or trazodone, other medication (especially alprazolam, astemizole, MAOIs, terfenadine, triazolam). Obtain history of cardiovascular or cerebrovascular disease, mania/hypomania, seizures.

Intervention/Evaluation

Supervise suicidal risk pt closely during early therapy (as energy level improves, suicide

potential increases). Assess appearance, behavior, speech pattern, level of interest, mood. Assist w/ambulation if dizziness, lightheadedness occurs. Monitor stool frequency and consistency.

PATIENT/FAMILY TEACHING

Maximum therapeutic response may require several weeks of therapy. If orthostatic hypotension occurs, rise very slowly from lying to sitting, sitting to standing position. Dry mouth may be relieved by sugarless gum, sips of tepid water. Report headache, nausea, visual disturbances. Avoid tasks that require alertness, motor skills until response to drug is established. Avoid alcohol.

nelfinavir mesylate

nell-**fine**-ah-veer
(Viracept)

PREGNANCY CATEGORY B

CLASSIFICATION

Antiviral

AVAILABILITY (Rx)

Tablets: 250 mg. **Powder:** 50 mg/g.

PHARMACOKINETICS

Absorption: Well absorbed following oral administration. Absorption increased w/food. **Metabolism:** Metabolized by the liver. Highly bound to plasma proteins. **Excretion:** Eliminated primarily in feces. **Half-life:** 3.5–5 hrs.

ACTION/*THERAPEUTIC EFFECT*

Inhibits activity of HIV-1 protease, the enzyme necessary for the formation of infectious HIV, *resulting in formation of immature noninfectious viral particles rather than HIV replication.*

USES/*UNLABELED*

Treatment of HIV infection when antiretoviral therapy is warranted.

ADMINISTRATION

ORAL POWDER:

- Take with food (light meal or snack).
- Mix oral powder with small amount of water, milk, formula, soy formula, soy milk or dietary supplement.
- Entire contents must be consumed in order to ingest full dose.
- Do not mix with acidic food, orange juice, apple juice or applesauce (bitter taste) or with water in its original container.

INDICATIONS/DOSAGE/ROUTES

HIV infection:

Oral: Adults: 750 mg (three 250 mg tablets) 3 times/day or 1,250 mg 2 times/day in combination with nucleoside analogues (enhances antiviral activity). ***Children 2–13 yrs:*** 20–30 mg/kg/dose, 3 times daily.

CONTRAINDICATIONS

History of hypersensitivity to medication, concurrent administration with astemizole, cisapride, midazolam, triazolam, rifampin, terfenadine.

CAUTIONS

Hepatic function impairment

INTERACTIONS

DRUG: ***Astemizole, terfenadine*** may create serious or life-threatening events (cardiac arrhythmias). ***Alcohol, psychoactive drugs*** may produce additive CNS effects. ***Anticonvulsants, rifampin, rifabutin*** lowers nelfinavir plasma concentration. Increases ***indinavir, saquinavir*** plasma concentration. ***Ritonavir*** increases nelfinavir plasma concentration. Decreases effects of ***oral contraceptives.*** **HERBAL:** None known. **FOOD:** Food increases plasma concentration. **ALTERED LAB VALUES:** May decrease Hgb, WBCs, neutrophils; increase SGOT (AST), SGPT (ALT), creatine kinase.

SIDE EFFECTS

FREQUENT (20%): Diarrhea. **OCCASIONAL (3–7%):** Nausea, rash. **RARE (1–2%):** Flatulence, asthenia.

ADVERSE REACTIONS/TOXIC EFFECTS

None significant.

PATIENT CONSIDERATIONS

Baseline Assessment

Offer emotional support. Check hematology, liver function tests for accurate baseline.

Intervention/Evaluation

Determine pattern of bowel activity and stool consistency. Monitor liver enzyme studies for abnormalities. Be alert to development of opportunistic infections, (e.g., fever, chills, cough, myalgia).

Patient/Family Teaching

Take with food (optimizes absorption). Take medication every day as prescribed. Doses should be evenly spaced around the clock. Do not alter dose or discontinue medication w/o informing physician. Medication is not a cure for HIV infection, and patient may continue to experience illnesses, including opportunistic infections, nor does it reduce risk of transmission to others. Diarrhea can be controlled with OTC medication. Use alternative/additional contraceptive measures if taking oral contraceptives.

---

neomycin sulfate

ne-oh-**my**-sin
(Mycifradin, Myciguent)

FIXED-COMBINATION(S)

W/polymyxin B, an anti-infective **(Neosporin, Neosporin G.U. Irrigant)**; w/polymyxin B and bacitracin, an antibiotic **(Mycitracin, Neosporin, Neo-Polycin)**; w/polymyxin B and hydrocortisone, a steroid **(Cortisporin)**; w/gramicidin, an anti-infective **(Spectrocin)**.

CANADIAN AVAILABILITY

Mycifradin, Myciguent

PREGNANCY CATEGORY C

CLASSIFICATION

Antibiotic: Aminoglycoside

AVAILABILITY (Rx)

Tablets: 500 mg. **Oral Solution:** 125 mg/5 ml. **Ointment. Cream. Ophthalmic (combination).**

PHARMACOKINETICS

Absorption: Minimal absorption from GI tract, after ophthalmic, topical administration. **Excretion:** Primarily eliminated unchanged in feces. **Half-life:** 2–3 hrs.

ACTION/*THERAPEUTIC EFFECT*

Irreversibly binds to protein on bacterial ribosome, *interfering in protein synthesis of susceptible microorganisms.* Decreases ammonia production in intestine (inhibits bacteria from ammonia synthesis), *suppressing bacterial growth in bowel.*

USES/*UNLABELED*

Irrigation of wounds, surgical sites, bladder; preop use for intestinal antisepsis; diarrhea due to enteropathogenic *Escherichia coli,* adjunctive therapy for hepatic encephalopathy. ***Ophthalmic:*** Ointment/solution for superficial eye infections. ***Topical:*** Prevention or treatment of superficial skin infections. Not for long-term therapy due to associated toxicities. ***Topical:*** *Treatment of minor bacterial skin infections, dermal ulcer.*

ADMINISTRATION

- **Note:** Given orally, as retention enema, bladder irrigation, ophthalmic, otic, or topical. Neomycin frequently combined w/corticosteroids, anesthetics, other antiinfectives when applied in topical/ophthalmic form.

ORAL:

- Give w/o regard to meals.
- If GI upset occurs, give w/food or milk.
- Tablets may be crushed.

OPHTHALMIC:

- Place finger on lower eyelid and pull out until a pocket is formed between eye and lower lid.
- Hold dropper above pocket and place correct number of drops ($^1/_4$–$^1/_2$ inch ointment) into pocket.
- Close eye gently.
- *Solution:* Apply digital pressure to lacrimal sac for 1–2 min (minimizes drainage into nose and throat, reducing risk of systemic effects). Ointment: Close eye for 1–2 min, rolling eyeball (increases contact area of drug to eye).
- Remove excess solution or ointment around eye w/tissue.

N

INDICATIONS/ROUTES/DOSAGE

Hepatic encephalopathy, adjunctive therapy:
Oral: Adults, elderly: 4–12 g/day in 4 divided doses.

Preop intestinal antisepsis:
Oral: Adults, elderly: 1 g every hour for 4 doses; then 1 g q4h for balance of 24 hrs, or 1 g at 1, 2, and 11 PM on day before surgery (w/erythromycin).

Continuous bladder irrigation:
Adults, elderly: 1 ml of urogenital concentrate (contains 200,000 units polymyxin B and 57 mg neomycin) added to 1,000 ml 0.9% NaCl given over 24 hrs for up to 10 days (may increase to 2,000 ml/day).

Usual ophthalmic dosage:
Ointment: Adults, elderly, children: Thin strip to conjunctiva q3–4h.

Liquid: Adults, elderly, children: 1 drop to conjunctiva q3–4h.

Usual topical dosage:
Topical: Adults, elderly, children: Apply gently 1–3 times/day up to 5 times/day. Apply no more than once daily in pts w/>20% burns.

CONTRAINDICATIONS

Hypersensitivity to neomycin, other aminoglycosides (cross-sensitivity). Oral administration contraindicated in intestinal obstruction.

CAUTIONS

Elderly, infants w/renal insufficiency/immaturity; neuromuscular disorders (potential for respiratory depression), prior hearing loss, vertigo, renal impairment.

INTERACTIONS

DRUG: If significant systemic absorption occurs, may increase nephrotoxicity, ototoxicity w/***aminoglycosides,*** other ***nephrotoxic, ototoxic medications.*** HERBAL: None known. FOOD: None significant. ALTERED LAB VALUES: None significant.

SIDE EFFECTS

FREQUENT: *Systemic:* Nausea, vomiting, diarrhea, irritation of mouth/rectal area. *Ophthalmic:* Hypersensitivity (itching, rash, redness, swelling). *Ophthalmic/Topical:* Itching, redness, swelling, rash. OCCASIONAL: *Ophthalmic:* Itching, burning, redness. RARE: *Systemic:* Malabsorption syndrome, neuromuscular blockade (drowsiness, weakness, difficulty breathing).

ADVERSE REACTIONS/TOXIC EFFECTS

Nephrotoxicity (evidenced by increased BUN and serum creatinine, decreased creatinine clearance) may be reversible if drug stopped at first sign of symptoms; irreversible ototoxicity (tinnitus, dizziness, ringing/roaring in ears, reduced hearing) and neurotoxicity (headache, dizziness, lethargy, tremors, visual disturbances) occur occasionally. Risk is greater with higher dosages, prolonged therapy, or if preparation applied directly to mucosa (particularly extensive areas). Severe respiratory depression, anaphylaxis occur rarely. Superinfections, particularly w/fungi, may result from bacterial imbalance following administration via any route.

PATIENT CONSIDERATIONS

BASELINE ASSESSMENT

Dehydration must be treated before aminoglycoside therapy. Establish pt's baseline hearing acuity before beginning therapy. Cumulative effects may occur when given via more than one route. Question for history of allergies, especially aminoglycosides. Obtain specimens for culture, sensitivity before giving first dose (therapy may begin before results are known).

INTERVENTION/EVALUATION

Monitor I&O (maintain hydration), urinalysis (casts, RBCs, WBCs, decrease in specific gravity). Monitor results of peak/trough blood tests. Be alert to ototoxic and neurotoxic symptoms (see Adverse Reactions/Toxic Effects). Assess for rash (*ophthalmic*—assess for redness, burning, itching, tearing; *topical*—assess for redness, itching). Be alert for superinfection, particularly genital/anal pruritus, changes of oral mucosa, diarrhea. When treating pts w/neuromuscular disorders, assess respiratory response carefully.

PATIENT/FAMILY TEACHING

Continue antibiotic for full length of treatment. Space doses evenly. Notify physician in event

of hearing, visual, balance, urinary problems, even after therapy is completed. Do not take other medication w/o consulting physician.

Ophthalmic
Blurred vision or tearing may occur briefly after application. Contact physician if tearing, redness, irritation continue.

Topical
Cleanse area gently before application; report redness, itching.

neostigmine bromide

nee-oh-**stig**-meen
(Prostigmin [oral])

neostigmine methylsulfate

(Prostigmin [parenteral])

CANADIAN AVAILABILITY
Prostigmin

PREGNANCY CATEGORY C

CLASSIFICATION

Anticholinesterase agent

AVAILABILITY (Rx)

Tablets: 15 mg. **Injection:** 1:1,000, 1:2,000, 1:4,000.

PHARMACODYNAMICS

	ONSET	PEAK	DURATION
Oral	2–4 hrs	—	—
IM	10–30 min	20–30 min	2.5–4 hrs

PHARMACOKINETICS

Absorption: Poorly absorbed from GI tract. Rapid absorption following IM administration. **Metabolism:** Metabolized in liver, plasma. **Excretion:** Primarily excreted in urine. **Half-life:** 24–79 min.

ACTION/*THERAPEUTIC EFFECT*

Prevents destruction of acetylcholine by attaching to enzyme, anticholinesterase. *Improves intestinal/skeletal muscle tone, increases secretions, salivation.*

USES

Improvement of muscle strength in control of myasthenia gravis, to diagnose myasthenia gravis, prevention/treatment of postop distension and urinary retention, as antidote for reversal of effects of nondepolarizing neuromuscular blocking agents after surgery.

STORAGE/HANDLING

Store parenteral, oral form at room temperature.

ADMINISTRATION

ORAL:

- For those w/difficulty chewing, give dose 30–45 min before meals, preferably w/milk (drug produces fewer cholinergic effects if taken w/milk or food).

SubQ/IM/IV:

- **Note:** May be given undiluted. Do not add to IV solutions.
- When given as curariform block antidote following surgery (unless tachycardia is present), give 0.6–1.2 mg atropine concurrently w/neostigmine to prevent bradycardia.
- If bradycardia is present, increase pulse rate to 80/min w/atropine before administering neostigmine.
- Administer IV very slowly (0.5 mg or less over 1 min).

INDICATIONS/ROUTES/DOSAGE

Note: Dosage, frequency of administration dependent on daily clinical pt response (remissions, exacerbations, physical and emotional stress).

Myasthenia gravis:
Oral: Adults, elderly: Initially, 15–30 mg 3–4 times/day. Increase dose gradually until therapeutic response achieved. ***Usual maintenance dose:*** 150 mg/day w/range of 15–375 mg. ***Children:*** Initially, 2 mg/kg/day divided q3–4h. ***Neonatal:*** 1–4 mg q2–3h.

SubQ/IM/IV: Adults: 0.5–2.5 mg as needed. ***Neonatal:*** 0.1–0.2 mg SubQ or 0.03 mg/kg IM q2–4h.

Diagnosis of myasthenia gravis:
Note: Discontinue all anticholinesterase therapy at least 8 hrs before testing. Give 0.011 mg/kg atropine sulfate IV simultaneously w/neostigmine or IM 30 min before administering neostigmine (prevents adverse effects).

IM: Adults, elderly: 0.022 mg/kg. If cholinergic reaction occurs, discontinue tests and administer 0.4–0.6 mg or more atropine sulfate IV. ***Children:*** 0.025–0.04 mg/kg IM preceded by atropine sulfate 0.011 mg/kg SubQ.

Prevention of postop urinary retention:
SubQ/IM: Adults, elderly: 0.25 mg q4–6h for 2–3 days.

Postop distension, urinary retention:
SubQ/IM: Adults, elderly: 0.5–1 mg. Catheterize if voiding does not occur within 1 hr. After voiding, continue 0.5 mg q3h for 5 injections.

Reversal of neuromuscular blockade:
IV: Adults, elderly: 0.5–2.5 mg given slowly.

CONTRAINDICATIONS

Concurrent use of high doses of halothane, cyclopropane, mechanical GI or GU obstruction, peritonitis, doubtful bowel viability.

CAUTIONS

Bronchial asthma, bradycardia, epilepsy, coronary occlusion, vagotonia, hyperthyroidism, cardiac arrhythmias, peptic ulcer.

INTERACTIONS

DRUG: ***Anticholinergics*** reverse/prevent effects. ***Cholinesterase inhibitors*** may increase toxicity. Antagonizes **neuromuscular blocking agents.** ***Quinidine, procainamide*** may antagonize action. **HERBAL:** None known. **FOOD:** None significant. **ALTERED LAB VALUES:** None significant.

SIDE EFFECTS

FREQUENT: Muscarinic effects (diarrhea, increased sweating/watering of mouth, nausea, vomiting, stomach cramps/pain). **OCCASIONAL:** Muscarinic effects (increased frequency/urge to urinate, increased bronchial secretions, unusually small pupils/watering of eyes).

ADVERSE REACTIONS/TOXIC EFFECTS

Overdose produces a cholinergic reaction manifested as abdominal discomfort/cramping, nausea, vomiting, diarrhea, flushing, feeling of warmth/heat about face, excessive salivation and sweating, lacrimation, pallor, bradycardia/tachycardia, hypotension, urinary urgency, blurred vision, bronchospasm, pupillary contraction, involuntary muscular contraction visible under the skin (fasciculation).

Overdose may also produce ***cholinergic crisis,*** manifested by increasingly severe muscle weakness (appears first in muscles involving chewing, swallowing, followed by muscular weakness of shoulder girdle and upper extremities), respiratory muscle paralysis followed by pelvic girdle and leg muscle paralysis. Requires a withdrawal of all cholinergic drugs and immediate use of 0.6–1.2 mg atropine sulfate IV for adults, 0.01 mg/kg in infants, children under 12 yrs.

Myasthenic crisis (due to underdose) also produces extreme muscle weakness but requires a *more* intensive drug therapy program (differentiation between the two crises is imperative for accurate treatment). Weakness beginning 1 hr after drug administration suggests overdosage; weakness occurring 3 hrs or more after administration suggests underdosage or resistance to anticholinesterase drugs. Extremely high doses may produce CNS stimulation followed by CNS depression.

PATIENT CONSIDERATIONS

BASELINE ASSESSMENT

Larger doses should be given at time of greatest fatigue. Assess muscle strength before testing for diagnosis of myasthenia gravis, as well as after drug administration. Avoid large doses in those w/megacolon or reduced GI motility. Have tissues readily available at pt's bedside.

INTERVENTION/EVALUATION

Monitor vital capacity during myasthenia gravis testing or if dosage is increased. Distinguish carefully between cholinergic crisis and myasthenic crisis (see Adverse Reactions/Toxic Effects). Monitor for therapeutic response to medication (increased muscle strength, decreased fatigue, improved chewing, swallowing functions).

PATIENT/FAMILY TEACHING

Report nausea, vomiting, diarrhea, sweating, increased salivary secretions, irregular heartbeat, muscle weakness, severe abdominal pain, or difficulty in breathing.

N

netilmicin sulfate

neh-till-**my**-sin
(Netromycin)

CANADIAN AVAILABILITY
Netromycin

PREGNANCY CATEGORY D

CLASSIFICATION

Antibiotic: Aminoglycoside

AVAILABILITY (Rx)

Injection: 100 mg/ml

PHARMACOKINETICS

Absorption: Rapid, complete absorption after IM administration. Widely distributed (does not cross blood-brain barrier, low concentrations in CSF). **Excretion:** Excreted unchanged in urine. Removed by hemodialysis. **Half-life:** 2–4 hrs (increased in decreased renal function, neonates; decreased in cystic fibrosis, burn or febrile pts).

ACTION/*THERAPEUTIC EFFECT*

Irreversibly binds to protein on bacterial ribosome, *interfering in protein synthesis of susceptible microorganisms.*

USES

Treatment of skin/skin structure, bone, joint, lower respiratory tract, intra-abdominal, complicated urinary tract infections; burns, septicemia.

STORAGE/HANDLING

Store parenteral form at room temperature. Solutions appear clear, colorless to pale yellow. May be discolored by light, air (does not affect potency). Intermittent IV infusion (piggyback) stable for 72 hrs at room temperature, or refrigerated. Discard if precipitate forms.

ADMINISTRATION

- **Note:** Coordinate peak and trough lab draws w/administration times.

IM:

- To minimize discomfort, give deep IM slowly. Less painful if injected into gluteus maximus rather than lateral aspect of thigh.

IV:

- Dilute with 50–200 ml 5% dextrose, 0.9% NaCl, or other compatible IV fluid.
- Infuse over 30–60 min for adults, older children, and over 60–120 min for infants, young children.
- Alternating IV sites, use large veins to reduce risk of phlebitis.

INDICATIONS/ROUTES/DOSAGE

Note: Space doses evenly around the clock. Dosage based on ideal body weight. Peak, trough serum concentrations determined periodically to maintain desired serum concentrations (minimizes risk of toxicity). ***Recommended peak level:*** 6–12 mcg/ml; ***trough level:*** 0.5–2 mcg/ml.

Complicated urinary tract infections:

IM/IV: Adults, elderly: 3–4 mg/kg/day in divided doses q12h.

Septicemia, skin/skin structure, intra-abdominal, lower respiratory infections:

IM/IV: Adults, elderly: 4–6.5 mg/kg/day in divided doses q8–12h. ***Children >6 wks:*** 5.5–8 mg/kg/day in divided doses q8–12h. ***Neonates:*** 4–6.5 mg/kg/day in divided doses q12h.

Dosage in renal impairment:

Dose and/or frequency is modified based on degree of renal impairment, serum concentration of drug. After loading dose of 1.3–2.2 mg/kg, maintenance doses, intervals are based on serum creatinine or creatinine clearance.

CONTRAINDICATIONS

Hypersensitivity to netilmicin, other aminoglycosides (cross-sensitivity). Sulfite sensitivity may result in anaphylaxis, especially in asthmatics.

CAUTIONS

Elderly, neonates w/renal insufficiency/immaturity; neuromuscular disorders (potential for respiratory depression), prior hearing loss, vertigo, renal impairment.

INTERACTIONS

DRUG: Other ***aminoglycosides, nephrotoxic, ototoxic-producing medications*** may increase toxicity. May increase effects of ***neuromuscular blocking agents.*** **HERBAL:** None known. **FOOD:** None significant. **ALTERED LAB VALUES:** May increase BUN, SGPT (ALT), SGOT (AST), bilirubin, creatinine, LDH concentrations; may decrease serum calcium, magnesium, potassium, sodium concentrations.

SIDE EFFECTS

OCCASIONAL: Pain, induration at IM injection site; phlebitis, thrombophlebitis w/IV administration; hypersensitivity reactions: rash, fever, urticaria, pruritus. **RARE:** Headache.

ADVERSE REACTIONS/TOXIC EFFECTS

Nephrotoxicity (evidenced by increased BUN and serum creatinine, decreased creatinine clearance) may be reversible if drug stopped at first sign of symptoms; irreversible ototoxicity (tinnitus, dizziness, ringing/roaring in ears, reduced hearing) and neurotoxicity (headache, dizziness, lethargy, tremors, visual disturbances) occur occasionally. Risk is greater w/higher dosages, prolonged therapy. Superinfections, particularly w/fungi, may result from bacterial imbalance.

PATIENT CONSIDERATIONS

BASELINE ASSESSMENT

Dehydration must be treated before aminoglycoside therapy. Establish pt's baseline hearing acuity before beginning therapy. Question for history of allergies, especially aminoglycosides, sulfite. Obtain specimens for culture, sensitivity before giving first dose (therapy may begin before results are known).

INTERVENTION/EVALUATION

Monitor I&O (maintain hydration), urinalysis (casts, RBCs, WBCs, decrease in specific gravity). Monitor results of peak/trough blood tests. Be alert to ototoxic and neurotoxic symptoms (see Adverse Reactions/Toxic Effects). Check IM injection site for pain, induration. Evaluate IV site for phlebitis (heat, pain, red streaking over vein). Assess for rash. Assess for superinfection, particularly genital/anal pruritus, changes of oral mucosa, diarrhea.

PATIENT/FAMILY TEACHING

Continue antibiotic for full length of treatment. Space doses evenly. Discomfort may occur with IM injection. Notify physician in event of headache, shortness of breath, dizziness, hearing, urinary problem even after therapy is completed. Do not take other medication w/o consulting physician. Lab tests are an essential part of therapy.

nevirapine

neh-**vear**-ah-peen
(Viramune)

PREGNANCY CATEGORY C

CLASSIFICATION

Antiviral

AVAILABILITY (Rx)

Tablets: 200 mg. **Oral Suspension:** 50 mg/5 ml.

PHARMACOKINETICS

Absorption: Readily absorbed following oral administration (unaffected by food). Widely distributed. **Metabolism:** Extensively metabolized in liver. **Excretion:** Primarily excreted in urine.

ACTION/*THERAPEUTIC EFFECT*

Binds directly to virus type 1 (HIV-1) reverse transcriptase (RT), blocking RNA and DNA-dependent DNA polymerase activity (changes the shape of RT enzyme), *slowing HIV replication, reducing progression of HIV infection.*

USES/ *UNLABELED*

Used in combination w/nucleoside analogues or protease inhibitors for treatment of HIV-1 infected adults who have experienced clinical and immunologic deterioration. *Reduces risk of transmitting HIV from infected mother to newborn.*

ADMINISTRATION

ORAL:

- May give w/o regard to meals.

INDICATIONS/ROUTES/DOSAGE

Note: Always administer nevirapine in combination with at least one additional antiretroviral agent (resistant HIV virus appears rapidly when nevirapine is given as monotherapy).

HIV-1 infection:
Oral: Adults: 200 mg daily for 14 days (reduces risk of rash). ***Maintenance:*** 200 mg twice daily in combination w/nucleoside analogue antiretroviral agents. ***Children, 2 mos–8 yrs:*** 4 mg/kg once daily for 14 days, then 7 mg/kg 2 times/day. ***Children >8 yrs:*** 4 mg/kg once daily for 14 days then 4 mg/kg 2 times/day. ***Maximum:*** 400 mg/day.

CONTRAINDICATIONS

None significant.

CAUTIONS

Renal or hepatic function impairment.

INTERACTIONS

DRUG: May decrease ***protease inhibitors, oral contraceptives,*** plasma concentration. **HERBAL:** St. John's wort may decrease concentration, effect. **FOOD:** None significant. **ALTERED LAB VALUES:** May significantly increase SGPT (ALT), SGOT (AST), bilirubin, GGT. May significantly decrease Hgb, platelets, neutrophil count.

SIDE EFFECTS

FREQUENT (3–8%): Rash (may become severe), fever, headache, nausea. **OCCASIONAL (1–3%):** Stomatitis (erythema/irritation of oral mucous membranes, gingivitis, glossitis). **RARE (<1%):** Paresthesia, myalgia, abdominal pain.

ADVERSE REACTIONS/TOXIC EFFECTS

Rash may become severe and life threatening. Hepatitis occurs rarely.

PATIENT CONSIDERATIONS

BASELINE ASSESSMENT

Offer emotional support. Establish baseline lab values, especially liver function tests, prior to initiating therapy and at intervals during therapy. Obtain medication history (especially use of oral contraceptives).

INTERVENTION/EVALUATION

Closely monitor for evidence of rash (usually appears on trunk, face, and extremities; occurs within first 6 wks of drug initiation). Observe for rash accompanied by fever, blistering, oral lesions, conjunctivitis, swelling, muscle or joint aches, general malaise. Monitor clinical chemistry tests for marked laboratory abnormalities. Assess for fever, headache, nausea.

PATIENT/FAMILY TEACHING

If nevirapine therapy is missed for more than 7 days, restart by using one 200 mg tablet daily for

first 14 days, followed by one 200 mg tablet twice daily. Continue therapy for full length of treatment. Doses should be evenly spaced. Do not take any medications w/o consulting physician. Nevirapine is not a cure for HIV infection, nor does it reduce risk of transmission to others. If rash appears, contact physician before continuing therapy.

niacin, nicotinic acid

(Niacor, Niaspan, Nicobid, Nico-400, Nicotinex)

PREGNANCY CATEGORY A
(C if used in doses above RDA)

CLASSIFICATION

Antihyperlipoproteinemic

AVAILABILITY (OTC)

Tablets: 25 mg, 50 mg, 100 mg, 250 mg, 500 mg. **Tablets (timed-release):** 250 mg, 500 mg, 750 mg. **Capsules (timed-release):** 125 mg, 250 mg, 300 mg, 400 mg, 500 mg. **Elixir:** 50 mg/5 ml. **Injection: (Rx)** 100 mg/ml.

PHARMACOKINETICS

Absorption: Readily absorbed from GI tract. Widely distributed. **Metabolism:** Metabolized in liver. **Excretion:** Primarily excreted in urine. **Half-life:** 45 min.

ACTION/*THERAPEUTIC EFFECT*

Inhibits free fatty acid release in fat tissue, decreases rate of VLDL, LDL synthesis in liver, increases lipoprotein lipase activity. Component of coenzymes that are necessary for *lipid metabolism, tissue respiration, and glycogenolysis. Lowers serum cholesterol and triglycerides (decreases LDL, VLDL, increases HDL).*

USES

Adjunct to diet therapy to decrease elevated serum cholesterol and triglyceride concentrations (elevated LDL, VLDL in treatment of Type II, III, IV, or V hyperlipoproteinemia). Extended-release tablets increase HDL cholesterol. Prevention and treatment of vitamin B_3 deficiency states (i.e., pellagra).

N

ADMINISTRATION

ORAL:

- Preferably given w/or after meals (decreases GI upset).

INDICATIONS/ROUTES/DOSAGE

Hyperlipoproteinemia:
Oral: Adults, elderly: Initially, 100 mg 3 times/day. Increase by 300 mg/day at 4–7 day intervals. ***Maintenance:*** 1–2 g 3 times/day. ***Maximum:*** 8 g/day. ***Extended-Release:*** Initially, 375 mg/day. Maintenance: 1,000–2,000 mg/day at bedtime.

Nutritional supplement:
Oral: Adults, elderly: 10–20 mg/day.

CONTRAINDICATIONS

Hypersensitivity to niacin or tartrazine (frequently seen in pts sensitive to aspirin), active peptic ulcer, severe hypotension, hepatic dysfunction, arterial hemorrhaging.

CAUTIONS

Diabetes mellitus, gallbladder disease, gout, history of jaundice or liver disease.

INTERACTIONS

DRUG: ***Lovastatin, pravastatin, simvastatin*** may increase risk of rhabdomyolysis and acute renal failure. **HERBAL:** None known. **FOOD:** None significant. **ALTERED LAB VALUES:** May increase uric acid.

SIDE EFFECTS

FREQUENT: Flushing (especially of face, neck) occurring within 20 min of administration and lasting for 30–60 min, GI upset, pruritus. **OCCASIONAL:** Dizziness, hypotension, headache, blurred vision, burning or tingling of skin, flatulence, nausea, vomiting, diarrhea. **RARE:** Hyperglycemia, glycosuria, rash, hyperpigmentation, dry skin.

ADVERSE REACTIONS/TOXIC EFFECTS

Cardiac arrhythmias, particularly in those w/CHD, occur rarely.

PATIENT CONSIDERATIONS

Baseline Assessment

Question for history of hypersensitivity to niacin, tartrazine, or aspirin. Assess baselines: cholesterol, triglyceride, blood glucose, liver function tests.

Intervention/Evaluation

Evaluate flushing and degree of discomfort. Check for headache, dizziness, blurred vision. Monitor B/P at least 2 times/day. Assess food tolerance. Determine pattern of bowel activity. Monitor liver function test results, cholesterol and triglyceride. Check blood glucose levels carefully in those on insulin or oral antihyperglycemics. Assess skin for rash, dryness.

Patient/Family Teaching

Take w/meals to decrease GI upset. Follow special diet (important part of treatment). Do not alter dosage. Consult physician before taking other medication. In event of new symptoms, notify physician. If dizziness occurs, avoid sudden posture changes and activities that require steady/alert response. Flushing may decrease w/continued therapy; however, discuss considerable discomfort w/physician.

nicardipine hydrochloride

nigh-**car**-dih-peen
(Cardene, Cardene SR)

CANADIAN AVAILABILITY
Cardene

PREGNANCY CATEGORY C

CLASSIFICATION

Calcium channel blocker

AVAILABILITY (Rx)

Capsules: 20 mg, 30 mg. **Capsules (sustained-release):** 30 mg, 45 mg, 60 mg. **Injection:** 2.5 mg/ml.

PHARMACODYNAMICS

	ONSET	PEAK	DURATION
Oral	—	1–2 hrs	8 hrs

PHARMACOKINETICS

Absorption: Rapidly, completely absorbed from GI tract. **Metabolism:** Undergoes first-pass metabolism in liver. Metabolized in liver. **Excretion:** Primarily excreted in urine. **Half-life:** 8.6 hrs.

ACTION/*THERAPEUTIC EFFECT*

Inhibits calcium ion movement across cell membrane, depressing contraction of cardiac and vascular smooth muscle. *Increases heart rate, cardiac output. Decreases systemic vascular resistance, B/P.*

USES / *UNLABELED*

Oral: Treatment of chronic stable (effort-associated) angina or essential hypertension. ***Sustained-release:*** Treatment of essential hypertension. ***Parenteral:*** Short-term treatment of hypertension when oral therapy not feasible or desirable. *Treatment of vasospastic angina, Raynaud's phenomena, subarachnoid hemorrhage, associated neurologic deficits.*

STORAGE/HANDLING

Store oral, parenteral forms at room temperature. Diluted IV solution is stable for 24 hrs at room temperature.

ADMINISTRATION

ORAL:

- Do not crush or break oral, sustained-release capsules.
- May take w/o regard to food.

IV:

- Dilute each 25 mg ampule w/240 ml 5% dextrose, 0.9% NaCl, or other compatible IV to provide a concentration of 1 mg/10 ml.
- Change IV site q12h if administered peripherally.

INDICATIONS/ROUTES/DOSAGE

Chronic stable angina:
Oral: Adults, elderly: Initially, 20 mg 3 times/day. ***Range:*** 20–40 mg 3 times/day.

Essential hypertension:
Oral: Adults, elderly: Initially, 20 mg 3 times/day. ***Range:*** 20–40 mg 3 times/day.

Sustained-release: Adults, elderly: Initially, 30 mg 2 times/day. ***Range:*** 30–60 mg 2 times/day.

Dosage in liver impairment:
Initially, 20 mg 2 times/day, then titrate.

Dosage in renal impairment:
Initially, 20 mg q8h (30 mg 2 times/day sustained-release), then titrate.

Usual parenteral dosage: Substitute for oral nicardipine:
IV: Adults, elderly: 0.5 mg/hr (20 mg q8h); 1.2 mg/hr (30 mg q8h); 2.2 mg/hr (40 mg q8h).

Drug-free pt:
IV: Adults, elderly: (Gradual B/P decrease): Initially, 5 mg/hr. May increase by 2.5 mg/hr q15 min. ***(Rapid B/P decrease):*** Initially, 5 mg/hr. May increase by 2.5 mg/hr q5min. ***Maximum:*** 15 mg/hr until desired B/P attained.

Note: After B/P goal achieved, decrease rate to 3 mg/hr.

Changing to oral antihypertensive therapy:
Begin 1 hr after IV discontinued; for nicardipine, give first dose 1 hr before discontinuing IV.

CONTRAINDICATIONS

Severe hypotension, advanced aortic stenosis.

CAUTIONS

Impaired renal, hepatic function.

INTERACTIONS

DRUG: Beta blockers may have additive effect. May increase ***digoxin*** concentration. ***Procainamide, quinidine*** may increase risk of QT interval prolongation. ***Hypokalemia-producing agents*** may increase risk of arrhythmias. **HERBAL:** None known. **FOOD:** Grapefruit/grapefruit juice may affect absorption. **ALTERED LAB VALUES:** None significant.

SIDE EFFECTS

FREQUENT (5–10%): Flushing of

skin, feeling of warmth. **OCCASIONAL (1–5%):** Angina (chest pain), peripheral edema, tachycardia, dizziness, headache, nausea, palpitations. **RARE (<1%):** Allergic reaction, pulmonary edema, diarrhea, constipation, drowsiness, dry mouth.

ADVERSE REACTIONS/TOXIC EFFECTS

Marked hypotension, CHF.

PATIENT CONSIDERATIONS

Baseline Assessment

Concurrent therapy of sublingual nitroglycerin may be used for relief of anginal pain. Record onset, type (sharp, dull, squeezing), radiation, location, intensity, and duration of anginal pain, and precipitating factors (exertion, emotional stress).

Intervention/Evaluation

Monitor B/P during and after IV infusion. Assist w/ambulation if dizziness occurs. Assess for peripheral edema behind medial malleolus (sacral area in bedridden pts). Assess skin for facial flushing, dermatitis, rash. Question for asthenia, headache. Monitor liver enzyme results. Assess EKG, pulse for tachycardia, palpitations.

Patient/Family Teaching

Do not abruptly discontinue medication. Compliance w/therapy regimen is essential to control anginal pain. To avoid hypotensive effect, rise slowly from lying to sitting position; wait momentarily before standing. Avoid tasks that require alertness, motor skills until response to drug is established. Contact physician/nurse if irregular heartbeat, shortness of breath, pronounced dizziness, or nausea occurs.

nicotine polacrilex

nick-oh-teen
(Nicorette)

nicotine transdermal system

(Habitrol, Nicoderm, Nicotrol)

CANADIAN AVAILABILITY
Habitrol, Nicoderm, Nicorette, Nicotrol

PREGNANCY CATEGORY X
Nicotine polacrilex

PREGNANCY CATEGORY D
Transdermal nicotine

CLASSIFICATION

Smoking deterrent

AVAILABILITY (OTC)

Transdermal: Habitrol (Rx): 7 mg/day, 14 mg/day, 21 mg/day. **Nicoderm (OTC):** 7 mg/day, 14 mg/day, 21 mg/day. **Nicotrol (Rx):** 5 mg/day, 10 mg/day; **(OTC):** 15 mg/day. **Chewing Gum (OTC):** 2 mg, 4 mg squares. **Nasal Spray (Rx). Inhaler (Rx).**

PHARMACOKINETICS

Absorption: Not absorbed from GI tract. Absorption increased from buccal mucosa, well absorbed after topical administration. **Metabolism:** Metabolized in liver. **Excretion:** Primarily excreted in urine. **Half-life:** 1–2 hrs.

ACTION/*THERAPEUTIC EFFECT*

Nicotine, a cholinergic-receptor agonist, produces autonomic effects by binding to acetylcholine receptors. Produces both stimulating and depressant effects on peripheral and central nervous systems; respiratory stimulant; low amounts increase heart rate, B/P; high doses may decrease B/P; may increase motor activity of GI smooth muscle. Nicotine produces psychological and physical dependence.

USES

An alternative, less potent form of nicotine (w/o tar, carbon monoxide, carcinogenic substances of tobacco) used as part of a smoking cessation program.

ADMINISTRATION

TRANSDERMAL:

- Apply promptly upon removal from protective pouch (prevents evaporation, loss of nicotine). Use only intact pouch.
- Apply only once/day to hairless, clean, dry skin on upper body or outer arm.
- Replace daily at different sites; do not use same site within 7 days; do not use same patch >24 hrs.
- Wash hands after applying patch. Wash w/water alone (soap may increase nicotine absorption).
- Discard used patch by folding patch in half (sticky side together), placing in pouch of new patch, and throwing away in such a way as to prevent child/pet accessibility.

GUM:

- Do not swallow.
- Chew 1 piece whenever urge to smoke present.
- Chew slowly/intermittently for 30 min.
- Chew until distinctive nicotine taste (peppery) or slight tingling in mouth perceived, then stop; when tingling almost gone (about 1 min) repeat chewing procedure (this allows constant slow buccal absorption).
- Too rapid chewing may cause excessive release of nicotine, resulting in adverse effects similar to oversmoking (e.g., nausea, throat irritation).

INHALER:

- Insert cartridge into mouthpiece.
- Vigorously puff for 20 min.

INDICATIONS/ROUTES/DOSAGE

Smoking deterrent:
Note: Individualize dose; stop smoking immediately.

Transdermal: Adults, elderly: (Habitrol/Nicoderm): 21 mg/day for 6 wks; then 14 mg/day for 2 wks; then 7 mg/day for 2 wks.

Gum: Adults, elderly: Usually, 10–12 pieces/day. ***Maximum:*** 30 pieces/day.

Nasal Spray: Adults, elderly: (1 dose = 2 sprays = 1 mg) 1–2 doses/hr up to 40 doses/day.

Inhaler: Adults, elderly: Puff on nicotine cartridge mouthpiece for about 20 min as needed.

CONTRAINDICATIONS

During immediate post-MI period, life-threatening arrhythmias, severe or worsening angina, active temporomandibular joint disease.

CAUTIONS

Hyperthyroidism, pheochromocytoma, insulin-dependent diabetes mellitus, severe renal impairment, eczematous dermatitis, oral or pharyngeal inflammation, esophagitis, peptic ulcer (delays healing in peptic ulcer disease).

INTERACTIONS

DRUG: Smoking cessation may increase effects of ***beta-adrenergic blockers, bronchodilators (e.g., theophylline), insulin, propoxy-***

N

phene. HERBAL: None known. **FOOD:** None significant. **ALTERED LAB VALUES:** None significant.

SIDE EFFECTS

FREQUENT: Fast heartbeat, headache, increased appetite. *Gum:* Mouth or throat soreness, nausea, hiccups, injury to mouth, teeth, dental work. *Transdermal:* Erythema, pruritus, burning at application site. OCCASIONAL: Constipation, coughing, diarrhea, dizziness, drowsiness, dry mouth, menstrual pain, insomnia, decreased appetite, muscle/joint pain, stomach indigestion, sweating, irritability. *Gum:* Hiccups, hoarseness. *Inhaler:* Mouth or throat irritation or cough. RARE: Irregular heartbeat, hypersensitivity reaction (redness, swelling, hives, itching).

ADVERSE REACTIONS/TOXIC EFFECTS

Overdose produces palpitations, tachyarrhythmias, convulsions, depression, confusion, profuse diaphoresis, hypotension, rapid/weak pulse, difficulty breathing. Lethal dose, adults: 40–60 mg. Death results from respiratory paralysis.

PATIENT CONSIDERATIONS

BASELINE ASSESSMENT

Screen, evaluate those w/coronary heart disease (history of MI, angina pectoris), serious ardiac arrhythmias, Buerger's disease, Prinzmetal's variant angina.

INTERVENTION/EVALUATION

If increase in cardiovascular symptoms occurs, discontinue use. Assess all symptoms carefully w/regard to method of medication (see Side Effects).

PATIENT/FAMILY TEACHING

Give instruction sheet to pt; review proper application and disposal of transdermal system. Gradually withdraw or stop nicotine gum usage <3 mos, transdermal nicotine after 4–8 wks of use, progressively decreasing dose q2–4wks. Do not eat or drink anything during or immediately before nicotine gum use (reduces salivary pH). Use contraceptive measures during therapy.

nifedipine

nye-**fed**-ih-peen
(Adalat, Procardia)

CANADIAN AVAILABILITY
Adalat, Apo-Nifed, Novonifedin

PREGNANCY CATEGORY C

CLASSIFICATION

Calcium channel blocker

AVAILABILITY (Rx)

Capsules: 10 mg, 20 mg. **Tablets (extended-release):** 30 mg, 60 mg, 90 mg.

PHARMACODYNAMICS

	ONSET	PEAK	DURATION
Oral	20 min	30–60 min	—

PHARMACOKINETICS

Absorption: Rapidly, completely absorbed from GI tract. **Metabolism:** Undergoes first-pass metabolism in liver. Metabolized in liver. **Excretion:** Primarily excreted in urine. **Half-life:** 2–5 hrs.

ACTION/*THERAPEUTIC EFFECT*

Inhibits calcium ion movement across cell membrane, depressing contraction of cardiac and vascular smooth muscle. *Increases heart rate, cardiac output. Decreases systemic vascular resistance, B/P.*

USES / *UNLABELED*

Treatment of angina due to coronary artery spasm (Prinzmetal's variant angina), chronic stable angina (effort-associated angina). ***Extended-release:*** Treatment of essential hypertension. *Treatment of Raynaud's phenomena.*

ADMINISTRATION

ORAL:

- Do not crush or break film-coated tablet or sustained-release capsule.
- May give w/o regard to meals.
- Do not give w/grapefruit or grapefruit juice (alters absorption).

SUBLINGUAL:

- Capsule must be punctured, chewed, and/or squeezed to express liquid into mouth.

INDICATIONS / ROUTES / DOSAGE

Note: May give 10–20 mg sublingual as needed for acute attacks of angina.

Prinzmetal's variant angina, chronic stable angina:
Oral: Adults, elderly: Initially, 10 mg 3 times/day. Increase at 7–14 day intervals. ***Maintenance:*** 10 mg 3 times/day up to 30 mg 4 times/day.

Extended-release: Adults, elderly: Initially, 30–60 mg/day. ***Maintenance:*** Up to 120 mg/day.

Hypertension:
Oral: Extended-release: Adults, elderly: Initially, 30–60 mg/day. ***Maintenance:*** Up to 120 mg/day.

CONTRAINDICATIONS

Severe hypotension, advanced aortic stenosis.

CAUTIONS

Impaired renal/hepatic function.

INTERACTIONS

DRUG: ***Beta blockers*** may have additive effect. May increase ***digoxin*** concentration. ***Hypokalemia-producing agents*** may increase risk of arrhythmias. **HERBAL:** None known. **FOOD:** Grapefruit/grapefruit juice may increase absorption. **ALTERED LAB VALUES:** May cause positive ANA, direct Coombs' test.

SIDE EFFECTS

FREQUENT (>10%): Peripheral edema (swelling of ankles, feet), headache, flushed skin, nausea, dizziness. **OCCASIONAL (3–10%):** Constipation, unusually tired, muscle cramps or pain, shortness of breath, wheezing, cough, palpitations, nasal congestion. **RARE (<3%):** Allergic reaction (rash, hives), angina (chest pain), arthritis, gingival hyperplasia.

ADVERSE REACTIONS / TOXIC EFFECTS

May precipitate CHF, MI in those w/cardiac disease, peripheral ischemia. Overdose produces nausea, drowsiness, confusion, slurred speech.

PATIENT CONSIDERATIONS

BASELINE ASSESSMENT

Concurrent therapy of sublingual nitroglycerin may be used for relief of anginal pain. Record onset, type (sharp, dull, squeezing), radiation, location, intensity, and duration of anginal pain, and precipitating factors (exertion, emotional stress). Check B/P for hypotension immediately before giving medication.

INTERVENTION / EVALUATION

Observe for giddiness (common

effect). Assist w/ambulation if lightheadedness, dizziness occurs. Assess for peripheral edema behind medial malleolus (sacral area in bedridden pts). Assess skin for flushing. Monitor liver enzyme tests.

PATIENT/FAMILY TEACHING

Rise slowly from lying to sitting position and permit legs to dangle from bed momentarily before standing to reduce hypotensive effect. Contact physician/nurse if irregular heartbeat, shortness of breath, pronounced dizziness, or nausea occurs. Avoid concomitant grapefruit/grapefruit juice use.

nilutamide

nih-**lute**-ah-myd
(Nilandron)

CANADIAN AVAILABILITY
Anandron

PREGNANCY CATEGORY C

CLASSIFICATION

Antineoplastic: hormone

AVAILABILITY (Rx)

Tablets: 50 mg, 100 mg

PHARMACOKINETICS

Absorption: Rapidly, completely absorbed following oral administration. **Metabolism:** Extensively metabolized in liver to inactive metabolites. **Excretion:** Primarily excreted in urine. **Half-life:** 23–72 hrs.

ACTION/*THERAPEUTIC EFFECT*

Competitively inhibits androgen action by binding to androgen receptors in target tissue. *Decreases growth of prostatic carcinoma.*

USES

Treatment of metastatic prostatic carcinoma (stage D_2) in combination w/surgical castration. For maximum benefit, begin on same day or day after surgical castration.

ADMINISTRATION

ORAL:

- May be given w/ or w/o food.
- Take at same time each day.

INDICATIONS/ROUTES/DOSAGE

Prostatic carcinoma:
Oral: Adults, elderly: 300 mg once a day for 30 days, then 150 mg once a day. Begin on same day or day after surgical castration.

CONTRAINDICATIONS

Hypersensitivity to nilutamide, severe liver impairment, severe respiratory insufficiency.

CAUTIONS

Hepatitis, marked increase in liver enzymes.

INTERACTIONS

DRUG: None significant. **HERBAL:** None known. **FOOD:** None significant. **ALTERED LAB VALUES:** May increase SGOT (AST), SGPT (ALT), bilirubin, creatinine.

SIDE EFFECTS

FREQUENT (>10%): Hot flashes, delay in recovering vision after bright illumination (sun, television, bright lights), loss of libido, sexual potency, mild nausea, gynecomastia, alcohol intolerance. **OCCASIONAL (<10%):** Constipation, hypertension, dizziness, dyspnea, urinary tract infections.

ADVERSE REACTIONS/TOXIC EFFECTS

Interstitial pneumonitis may occur.

PATIENT CONSIDERATIONS

BASELINE ASSESSMENT

Baseline chest x-ray, hepatic enzyme levels should be obtained before therapy begins. Question for hypersensitivity to nilutamide. Assess medical condition (especially liver function).

INTERVENTION/EVALUATION

Monitor B/P periodically and hepatic function tests in long-term therapy.

PATIENT/FAMILY TEACHING

Do not stop taking medication. Contact physician if any side effects occur at home, especially signs of liver toxicity (jaundice, dark urine, fatigue, abdominal pain). Explain side effects and action on carcinoma. Report any dyspnea or aggravation of preexisting dyspnea. Caution about driving at night (tinted glasses may help). Avoid alcohol.

nimodipine

nih-**moad**-ih-peen
(Nimotop)

CANADIAN AVAILABILITY
Nimotop

PREGNANCY CATEGORY C

CLASSIFICATION

Calcium channel blocker

AVAILABILITY (Rx)

Capsules: 30 mg

PHARMACOKINETICS

Absorption: Rapidly absorbed from GI tract. **Metabolism:** Metabolized in liver. **Excretion:** Excreted in urine, eliminated in feces. **Half-life:** 8–9 hrs.

ACTION/*THERAPEUTIC EFFECT*

Inhibits movement of calcium ions across cellular membranes in vascular smooth muscle. *Produces favorable effect on severity of neurologic deficits due to cerebral vasospasm. Greatest effect on cerebral arteries; may prevent cerebral spasm.*

N

USES/*UNLABELED*

Improvement of neurologic deficits due to spasm following subarachnoid hemorrhage from ruptured congenital intracranial aneurysms in pts in good neurologic condition. *Treatment of chronic and classic migraine, chronic cluster headaches.*

ADMINISTRATION

ORAL:

- If pt unable to swallow, place hole in both ends of capsule with 18 gauge needle to extract contents into syringe.
- Empty into nasogastric tube; wash tube w/30 ml normal saline.

INDICATIONS/ROUTES/DOSAGE

Subarachnoid hemorrhage:
Oral: Adults, elderly: 60 mg q4h for 21 days. Begin within 96 hrs of subarachnoid hemorrhage.

CONTRAINDICATIONS

Severe hypotension.

CAUTIONS

Impaired renal/hepatic function.

INTERACTIONS

DRUG: None significant. **HERBAL:** None known. **FOOD:** None significant. **ALTERED LAB VALUES:** None significant.

SIDE EFFECTS

OCCASIONAL (2–6%): Hypotension, peripheral edema (swelling of ankles, feet), diarrhea, dizziness, headache, nausea. **RARE (<2%):** Allergic reaction (rash, hives), tachycardia, flushing of skin, thrombocytopenia, pulmonary edema.

ADVERSE REACTIONS/TOXIC EFFECTS

Overdosage produces nausea, weakness, dizziness, drowsiness, confusion, slurred speech.

PATIENT CONSIDERATIONS

Baseline Assessment

Assess level of consciousness, neurologic response, initially and throughout therapy. Monitor baseline liver function tests. Assess B/P, apical pulse immediately before drug is administered (if pulse is 60/min or below, or systolic B/P is below 90 mm Hg, withhold medication, contact physician).

Intervention/Evaluation

Monitor pulse rate for bradycardia. Assess skin for dermatitis, rash, flushing. Monitor daily bowel activity and stool consistency. Assess for headache.

Patient/Family Teaching

To avoid hypotensive effect, rise slowly from lying to sitting position; wait momentarily before standing. Avoid tasks that require alertness, motor skills until response to drug is established. Contact physician/nurse if irregular heartbeat, shortness of breath, pronounced dizziness, or nausea occurs.

---

nisoldipine

nye-**soul**-dih-peen
(Sular)

PREGNANCY CATEGORY C

CLASSIFICATION

Calcium channel blocker

AVAILABILITY (Rx)

Tablets (extended-release): 10 mg, 20 mg, 30 mg, 40 mg

PHARMACODYNAMICS

	ONSET	PEAK	DURATION
Oral	—	1–2 hrs	8 hrs

PHARMACOKINETICS

Absorption: Rapidly, completely absorbed from GI tract. **Metabolism:** Undergoes first-pass metabolism in liver. Metabolized in liver. **Excretion:** Primarily excreted in urine. **Half-life:** 7–12 hrs.

ACTION/*THERAPEUTIC EFFECT*

Inhibits calcium ion movement across cell membrane, depressing contraction of cardiac and vascular smooth muscle. *Increases heart rate, cardiac output. Decreases systemic vascular resistance, B/P.*

USES/*UNLABELED*

Treatment of hypertension, alone or in combination w/other antihypertensive agents, *stable angina pectoris, CHF.*

ADMINISTRATION

ORAL:

- Do not crush or break sustained-release capsule.

- May give w/o regard to meals.
- Avoid grapefruit products before or after giving medication.

INDICATIONS/ROUTES/DOSAGE

Hypertension:
Extended-Release: ***Adults:*** Initially, 20 mg once daily, then increase by 10 mg per week, or longer intervals until therapeutic B/P response is attained. ***Elderly:*** Initially, 10 mg once daily. Increase by 10 mg per week to therapeutic response. ***Maintenance:*** 20–40 mg once daily. ***Maximum:*** 60 mg once daily.

CONTRAINDICATIONS

Sick-sinus syndrome/second- or third-degree AV block (except in presence of pacemaker).

CAUTIONS

Impaired renal/hepatic function, aortic stenosis, elderly, cirrhosis.

INTERACTIONS

DRUG: None significant. **HERBAL:** None known. **FOOD:** Grapefruit/grapefruit juice may alter absorption. **ALTERED LAB VALUES:** None significant.

SIDE EFFECTS

FREQUENT: Giddiness, dizziness, lightheadedness, peripheral edema, headache, flushing, weakness, nausea. **OCCASIONAL:** Transient hypotension, heartburn, muscle cramps, nasal congestion, cough, wheezing, sore throat, palpitations, nervousness, mood changes. **RARE:** Increase in frequency, intensity, duration of anginal attack during initial therapy.

ADVERSE REACTIONS/TOXIC EFFECTS

May precipitate CHF, MI in those w/cardiac disease, peripheral ischemia. Overdose produces nausea, drowsiness, confusion, slurred speech.

PATIENT CONSIDERATIONS

BASELINE ASSESSMENT

Concurrent therapy of sublingual nitroglycerin may be used for relief of anginal pain. Record onset, type (sharp, dull, squeezing), radiation, location, intensity, and duration of anginal pain, and precipitating factors (exertion, emotional stress). Check B/P for hypotension immediately before giving medication.

INTERVENTION/EVALUATION

Monitor B/P closely during dosage adjustment. Observe for giddiness (common effect). Assist w/ambulation if lightheadedness, dizziness occurs. Assess for peripheral edema behind medial malleolus (sacral area in bedridden pts). Assess skin for flushing. Monitor liver enzyme tests.

PATIENT/FAMILY TEACHING

Avoid eating grapefruit, high-fat meal before and after taking medication. Swallow capsule whole; do not chew, divide, or crush. Rise slowly from lying to sitting position and permit legs to dangle from bed momentarily before standing to reduce hypotensive effect. Contact physician/nurse if irregular heartbeat, shortness of breath, pronounced dizziness, or nausea occurs.

nitrofurantoin sodium

ny-tro-feur-**an**-twon
(Furadantin, Furalan, Macrodantin)

CANADIAN AVAILABILITY
Apo-Nitrofurantoin, Macrodantin

N

PREGNANCY CATEGORY B

CLASSIFICATION

Antibacterial

AVAILABILITY (Rx)

Capsules: 25 mg, 50 mg, 100 mg. **Capsules:** 100 mg (25 mg as macrocrystals/75 mg as microcrystals). **Oral Suspension:** 25 mg/5 ml.

PHARMACOKINETICS

Absorption: Microcrystalline: rapidly, completely absorbed; macrocrystalline: more slowly absorbed. Food increases absorption. Primarily concentrated in urine, kidneys. **Metabolism:** Metabolized in most body tissues. **Excretion:** Primarily excreted in urine. **Half-life:** 20–60 min.

ACTION/*THERAPEUTIC EFFECT*

Bactericidal. Inactivates or alters bacterial ribosomal proteins, *producing bacteriostatic activity; bactericidal at high concentrations.*

USES/*UNLABELED*

Treatment of urinary tract infections, initial and chronic. *Prophylaxis of bacterial UTIs.*

ADMINISTRATION

ORAL:

- Give w/food, milk to enhance absorption, reduce GI upset.

INDICATIONS/ROUTES/DOSAGE

Initial or recurrent urinary tract infection (UTI):

Oral: Adults, elderly: 50–100 mg 4 times/day. *Maximum:* 400 mg/day. *Children >1 mo:* 5–7 mg/kg in 4 divided doses.

Long-term prophylactic therapy of UTI:

Oral: Adults, elderly: 50–100 mg as single evening dose. *Children:* 1–2 mg/kg in 1–2 divided doses.

CONTRAINDICATIONS

Hypersensitivity to nitrofurantoin, infants <1 mo of age because of hemolytic anemia, anuria, oliguria, substantial renal impairment (creatinine clearance <40 ml/min).

CAUTIONS

Renal impairment, diabetes mellitus, electrolyte imbalance, anemia, vitamin B deficiency, debilitated (greater risk of peripheral neuropathy), glucose 6-phosphate dehydrogenase (G-6-PD) deficiency (greater risk of hemolytic anemia).

INTERACTIONS

DRUG: *Hemolytics* may increase risk of toxicity. ***Neurotoxic medications*** may increase risk of neurotoxicity. *Probenecid* may increase concentration, toxicity. HERBAL: None known. FOOD: None significant. ALTERED LAB VALUES: None significant.

SIDE EFFECTS

FREQUENT: Abdominal or stomach pain, diarrhea, nausea, vomiting, decreased appetite, pneumonitis (chest pain, chills, fever, trouble breathing). OCCASIONAL: Hematologic reactions: granulocytopenia, leukopenia (sore throat, fever), megaloblastic anemia (unusually tired); neurotoxicity (dizziness, drowsiness, headache), polyneuropathy (numbness of face, mouth, muscle weakness). RARE: Hypersensitivity reaction (rash, itching, arthalgia, fever, chills).

ADVERSE REACTIONS/TOXIC EFFECTS

Superinfection, hepatotoxicity, peripheral neuropathy (may be irreversible), Stevens-Johnson syndrome, permanent pulmonary function impairment (rarely respiratory failure, death), anaphylaxis occur rarely.

PATIENT CONSIDERATIONS

Baseline Assessment

Question for history of asthma, hypersensitivity to nitrofurantoin. Obtain urine specimens for culture and sensitivity before giving first dose (therapy may begin before results are known). Evaluate lab test results for renal and hepatic baselines.

Intervention/Evaluation

Monitor I&O, renal function results. Evaluate food tolerance. Determine pattern of bowel activity. Assess skin for rash, urticaria. Be alert for numbness or tingling, especially of lower extremities (may signal onset of peripheral neuropathy). Watch for signs of hepatotoxicity: fever, rash, arthralgia, hepatomegaly. Check B/P at least 2 times/day. Perform respiratory assessment: Auscultate lungs, check for cough, chest pain, difficulty breathing.

Patient/Family Teaching

Urine may become dark yellow or brown. Take with food or milk for best results and to reduce GI upset. Complete full course of therapy. Avoid sun and ultraviolet light; use sunscreens, wear protective clothing. Notify physician if cough, fever, chest pain, difficult breathing, numbness/tingling of fingers or toes occurs. Rare occurrence of alopecia is transient.

---

nitroglycerin intravenous

nigh-trow-**glih**-sir-in
(Nitro-Bid, Nitrostat, Tridil)

nitroglycerin sublingual

(Nitrostat)

nitroglycerin sustained-release

(Nitro-Bid, Nitroglyn)

nitroglycerin topical

(Nitro-Bid, Nitrol)

nitroglycerin transdermal

(Minitran, Nitrek, Nitro-Dur, Transderm Nitro, Nitrodisc)

nitroglycerin translingual

(Nitrolingual)

nitroglycerin transmucosal

(Nitrogard)

CANADIAN AVAILABILITY

Minitran, Nitro-Dur, Nitrol, Nitrolingual, Nitrong, Nitrostat, Transderm Nitro, Trinipatch

PREGNANCY CATEGORY B

CLASSIFICATION

Nitrate

AVAILABILITY (Rx)

Tablets (sublingual): 0.4 mg. **Spray:** 0.4 mg/dose. **Tablets (buccal, controlled-release):** 1 mg, 2 mg, 3 mg. **Tablets (sustained-release):** 2.6 mg, 6.5 mg, 9 mg. **Capsules (sustained-release):** 2.5 mg, 6.5 mg, 9 mg, 13 mg. **Transdermal:** 0.1 mg/hr, 0.2 mg/hr, 0.3 mg/hr, 0.4 mg/hr, 0.6 mg/hr, 0.8 mg/hr. **Topical Ointment:** 2%.

Injection: 0.5 mg/ml, 5 mg/ml. **Injection Solution:** 100 mcg/ml, 200 mcg/ml.

PHARMACODYNAMICS

	ONSET	PEAK	DURATION
Sublingual	2–5 min	4–8 min	30–60 min
Transmucosal	2–5 min	4–10 min	3–5 hrs
Extended-release	20–45 min	—	3–8 hrs
Topical	15–60 min	0.5–2 hrs	3–8 hrs
Patch	30–60 min	1–3 hrs	8–12 hrs
IV	1–2 min	—	3–5 min

PHARMACOKINETICS

Absorption: Well absorbed after oral, sublingual, topical administration. **Metabolism:** Undergoes extensive first-pass metabolism. Metabolized in liver, enzymes in bloodstream. **Excretion:** Primarily excreted in urine. **Half-life:** 1–4 min.

ACTION/*THERAPEUTIC EFFECT*

Decreases myocardial oxygen demand. Reduces left ventricular preload and afterload. *Dilates coronary arteries, improves collateral blood flow to ischemic areas within myocardium.* ***Intravenous:*** *Produces peripheral vasodilation.*

USES

Lingual/sublingual/buccal dose used for acute relief of angina pectoris. Extended-release, topical forms used for prophylaxis, long-term angina management. IV form used in treatment of CHF associated w/acute MI.

STORAGE/HANDLING

Store tablets/capsules at room temperature. Keep sublingual tablets in original container.

ADMINISTRATION

ORAL:
- Do not chew extended-release form.
- Do not shake oral aerosol canister before lingual spraying.

SUBLINGUAL:
- Do not swallow; dissolve under the tongue.
- Administer while seated.
- Slight burning sensation under tongue may be lessened by placing tablet in buccal pouch.

TOPICAL:
- Spread thin layer on clean/dry/hairless skin of upper arm or body (not below knee or elbow), using applicator or dose-measuring papers. Do not use fingers; do not rub or massage into skin.

TRANSDERMAL:
- Apply patch on clean/dry/hairless skin of upper arm or body (not below knee or elbow).

IV:
- Dilute in given amount of 5% dextrose in water or 0.9% NaCl.
- Use microdrop or infusion pump.

INDICATIONS/ROUTES/DOSAGE

Acute angina, acute prophylaxis: ***Lingual Spray: Adults, elderly:*** 1 spray onto or under tongue q3–5min until relief is noted (no more than 3 sprays in 15 min period).

Sublingual: Adults, elderly: 0.4 mg q5min until relief is noted (no more than 3 doses in 15 min period). Use prophylactically 5–10 min before activities that may cause an acute attack.

Long-term prophylaxis of angina: ***Oral (Extended-Release): Adults, elderly:*** Initially, 2.5 mg 3–4 times/day. Increase by 2.5 mg 2–4 times/day at intervals of several days or weeks.

Topical: Adults, elderly: Initially, 1/2 inch q8h. Increase by 1/2 inch w/each application. ***Range:*** 1–2 inches q8h up to 4–5 inches q4h.

Transdermal Patch: Adults, elderly: Initially, 0.2–0.4 mg/hr. ***Maintenance:*** 0.4–0.8 mg/hr. Consider patch on 12–14 hrs, patch off 10–12 hrs (prevents tolerance).

Usual parenteral dosage:
IV: Adults, elderly: Initially, 5 mcg/min via infusion pump. Increase in 5 mcg/min increments at 3–5 min intervals until B/P response is noted or until dosage reaches maximum of 20 mcg/min. Dosage may be further titrated according to pt, therapeutic response.

CONTRAINDICATIONS

Hypersensitivity to nitrates, severe anemia, closed-angle glaucoma, postural hypotension, head trauma, increased intracranial pressure. ***Sublingual:*** Early MI. ***Transdermal:*** Allergy to adhesives. ***Extended-release:*** GI hypermotility/malabsorption, severe anemia. ***IV:*** Uncorrected hypovolemia, hypotension, inadequate cerebral circulation, constrictive pericarditis, pericardial tamponade.

CAUTIONS

Acute MI, hepatic/renal disease, glaucoma (contraindicated in closed-angle glaucoma), blood volume depletion from diuretic therapy, systolic B/P below 90 mm Hg.

INTERACTIONS

DRUG: ***Alcohol, antihypertensives, vasodilators*** may increase risk of orthostatic hypotension. **HERBAL:** None known. **FOOD:** None significant. **ALTERED LAB VALUES:** May increase methemoglobin, urine catecholamines, urine VMA.

SIDE EFFECTS

FREQUENT: Headache (may be severe) occurs mostly in early therapy, diminishes rapidly in intensity, usually disappears during continued treatment; transient flushing of face and neck, dizziness (especially if pt is standing immobile or is in a warm environment), weakness, postural hypotension. ***Sublingual:*** Burning, tingling sensation at oral point of dissolution. ***Ointment:*** Erythema, pruritus. **OCCASIONAL:** GI upset. ***Transdermal:*** Contact dermatitis.

ADVERSE REACTIONS/TOXIC EFFECTS

Drug should be discontinued if blurred vision, dry mouth occurs. Severe postural hypotension manifested by fainting, pulselessness, cold/clammy skin, profuse sweating. Tolerance may occur w/repeated, prolonged therapy (minor tolerance w/intermittent use of sublingual tablets). High dose tends to produce severe headache.

PATIENT CONSIDERATIONS

BASELINE ASSESSMENT

Record onset, type (sharp, dull, squeezing), radiation, location, intensity, and duration of anginal pain, and precipitating factors (exertion, emotional stress). Assess B/P and apical pulse before administration and periodically after dose. Pt must have continuous EKG monitoring for IV administration.

INTERVENTION/EVALUATION

Assist w/ambulation if lightheadedness, dizziness occurs. Assess

for facial/neck flushing. Cardioverter/defibrillator must not be discharged through paddle electrode overlying nitroglycerin system (may cause burns to pt or damage to paddle via arcing).

PATIENT/FAMILY TEACHING

Rise slowly from lying to sitting position and dangle legs momentarily before standing. Take oral form on empty stomach (however, if headache occurs during therapy, take medication w/meals). Use inhalants only when lying down. Dissolve sublingual tablet under tongue; do not swallow. Take at first sign of angina. If not relieved within 5 min, dissolve second tablet under tongue. Repeat if no relief in another 5 min. If pain continues, contact physician or go immediately to emergency room. Do not change brands. Keep container away from heat, moisture. Do not inhale lingual aerosol but spray onto or under tongue (avoid swallowing after spray is administered). Expel from mouth any remaining lingual/sublingual/intrabuccal tablet after pain is completely relieved. Place transmucosal tablets under upper lip or buccal pouch (between cheek and gum); do not chew or swallow tablet. Avoid alcohol (intensifies hypotensive effect). If alcohol is ingested soon after taking nitroglycerin, possible acute hypotensive episode (marked drop in B/P, vertigo, pallor) may occur.

nitroprusside sodium

nigh-troe-**pruss**-eyd
(Nipride, Nitropress)

CANADIAN AVAILABILITY
Nipride

PREGNANCY CATEGORY C

CLASSIFICATION

Antihypertensive

AVAILABILITY (Rx)

Powder for Injection: 50 mg

PHARMACODYNAMICS

ONSET	PEAK	DURATION
IV		
1–2 min	Dependent on infusion rate	Dissipates rapidly after stopping IV

PHARMACOKINETICS

Reacts w/hemoglobin in erythrocytes, producing cyanmethemoglobin, cyanide ions. **Excretion:** Primarily excreted in urine. **Half-life:** 2 min.

ACTION/*THERAPEUTIC EFFECT*

Direct vasodilating action on arterial, venous smooth muscle. Decreases peripheral vascular resistance, preload, afterload, improves cardiac output. *Dilates coronary arteries, decreases oxygen consumption, relieves persistent chest pain.*

USES/*UNLABELED*

Immediate reduction of B/P in hypertensive crisis. Produces controlled hypotension in surgical procedures to reduce bleeding. Treatment of acute CHF. *Controls paroxysmal hypertension prior to/during surgery for pheochromocytoma; treatment adjunct for myocardial infarction, valvular regurgitation, peripheral vasospasm caused by ergot alkaloid overdose.*

STORAGE/HANDLING

Protect solution from light. Solution should appear very faint brown in color. Use only freshly prepared solution. Once prepared, do not keep or use longer than 24 hrs. Deterioration evidenced by color change from brown to blue, green, or dark red. Discard unused portion.

ADMINISTRATION

IV:

- Give by IV infusion only.
- Reconstitute 50 mg vial with 2–3 ml 5% dextrose or sterile water for injection w/o preservative.
- Further dilute w/250–1,000 ml of 5% dextrose to provide concentration of 200 mcg, 50 mcg/ml, respectively.
- Wrap infusion bottle in aluminum foil immediately after mixing.
- Administer using IV infusion pump or microdrip (60 gtt/ml).
- Be alert for extravasation (produces severe pain, sloughing).

INDICATIONS/ROUTES/DOSAGE

Usual parenteral dosage:
IV: Adults, elderly, children: Initially, 0.3 mcg/kg/min. ***Range:*** 0.5–10 mcg/kg/min. Do not exceed 10 mcg/kg/min (risk of precipitous drop in B/P).

CONTRAINDICATIONS

Compensatory hypertension (arteriovenous shunt or coarctation of aorta), inadequate cerebral circulation, moribund pts.

CAUTIONS

Severe hepatic, renal impairment, hypothyroidism, hyponatremia, elderly. Except at low concentrations or brief use, may cause increased quantities of cyanide ion (may be toxic, lethal).

INTERACTIONS

DRUG: *Dobutamine* may increase cardiac output, decrease pulmonary wedge pressure. ***Hypotensive-producing medications*** may increase hypotensive effect. **HERBAL:** None known. **FOOD:** None significant. **ALTERED LAB VALUES:** None significant.

SIDE EFFECTS

OCCASIONAL: Flushing of skin, increased intracranial pressure, rash, pain, redness at injection site. *Too rapid IV administration:* Excessive fall in blood pressure, stomach pain, dizziness, headache, muscle twitching, restlessness, reflex tachycardia.

N

ADVERSE REACTIONS/TOXIC EFFECTS

A too rapid IV rate reduces B/P too quickly. Nausea, retching, diaphoresis (sweating), apprehension, headache, restlessness, muscle twitching, dizziness, palpitation, retrosternal pain, and abdominal pain may occur. Symptoms disappear rapidly if rate of administration is slowed or temporarily discontinued. Overdosage produces metabolic acidosis, tolerance to therapeutic effect.

PATIENT CONSIDERATIONS

Baseline Assessment

Pt must have continuous EKG monitoring and B/P monitoring (using either continually reinflated sphygmomanometer or an intra-arterial pressure sensor). Check w/physician for desired B/P level (B/P is normally maintained about 30–40% below pretreatment levels). Medication should be discontinued if thera-

peutic response is not achieved within 10 min following IV infusion at 10 mcg/kg/min.

Intervention/Evaluation

Assess IV site for extravasation. Monitor rate of infusion frequently. Monitor blood acid-base balance, electrolytes, laboratory results, I&O. Assess for metabolic acidosis (weakness, disorientation, headache, nausea, hyperventilation, vomiting). Assess for therapeutic response to medication. B/P for potential rebound hypertension after infusion is discontinued.

nizatidine

nye-**zaye**-tih-deen
(Axid, Axid AR))

CANADIAN AVAILABILITY
Axid

PREGNANCY CATEGORY B

CLASSIFICATION

H_2 receptor antagonist

AVAILABILITY (Rx)

Capsules: 75 mg **(OTC)**, 150 mg, 300 mg

PHARMACOKINETICS

Absorption: Rapidly, well absorbed from GI tract. **Metabolism:** Metabolized in liver. **Excretion:** Primarily excreted in urine. **Half-life:** 1–2 hrs (increased in decreased renal function).

ACTION/*THERAPEUTIC EFFECT*

Inhibits histamine action at H-2 receptors of parietal cells, *inhibiting basal and nocturnal gastric acid secretion.*

USES/*UNLABELED*

Short-term treatment of active duodenal ulcer, active benign gastric ulcer. Prevention of duodenal ulcer recurrence. Treatment of gastroesophageal reflux disease (GERD) including erosive esophagitis. *Treatment of gastric hypersecretory conditions, Zollinger-Ellison syndrome, multiple endocrine adenoma.*

ADMINISTRATION

ORAL:

- Give w/o regard to meals. Best given after meals or at bedtime.
- Do not administer within 1 hr of magnesium or aluminum-containing antacids (decreases absorption).
- May take right before eating for heartburn prevention.

INDICATIONS/ROUTES/DOSAGE

Active duodenal ulcer:
Oral: Adults, elderly: 300 mg at bedtime or 150 mg 2 times/day.

Maintenance of healed ulcer:
Oral: Adults, elderly: 150 mg at bedtime.

GERD:
Oral: Adults, elderly: 150 mg 2 times/day.

Active benign gastric ulcer:
Oral: Adults, elderly: 150 mg 2 times/day or 300 mg at bedtime.

Dosage in renal impairment:

CREATININE CLEARANCE	ACTIVE ULCER	MAINTENANCE THERAPY
20–50 ml/min	150 mg at bedtime	150 mg every other day
<20 ml/min	150 mg every other day	150 mg every 3 days

CONTRAINDICATIONS

None significant.

CAUTIONS

Impaired renal/hepatic function.

INTERACTIONS

DRUG: ***Antacids*** may decrease absorption (do not give within 1 hr). May decrease absorption of ***ketoconazole*** (give at least 2 hrs after). **HERBAL:** None known. **FOOD:** None significant. **ALTERED LAB VALUES:** Interferes w/skin tests using allergen extracts. May increase SGOT (AST), SGPT (ALT), alkaline phosphatase.

SIDE EFFECTS

OCCASIONAL: Somnolence, fatigue. **RARE:** Sweating, rash.

ADVERSE REACTIONS/TOXIC EFFECTS

Asymptomatic ventricular tachycardia, hyperuricemia (not associated w/gout), nephrolithiasis occur rarely.

PATIENT CONSIDERATIONS

INTERVENTION/EVALUATION

Assess for abdominal pain, GI bleeding (overt blood in emesis or stool, tarry stools). Monitor blood tests for elevated SGOT (AST), SGPT (ALT), alkaline phosphatase (hepatocellular injury).

PATIENT/FAMILY TEACHING

Avoid tasks that require alertness, motor skills until drug response is established. Avoid alcohol, aspirin, and smoking.

---

norepinephrine bitartrate

nor-eh-pih-**nef**-rin
(Levophed)

CANADIAN AVAILABILITY
Levophed

PREGNANCY CATEGORY C

CLASSIFICATION

Sympathomimetic

AVAILABILITY (Rx)

Injection: 1 mg/ml

PHARMACODYNAMICS

	ONSET	PEAK	DURATION
IV	Rapid	1–2 min	—

PHARMACOKINETICS

Localized in sympathetic tissue. **Metabolism:** Metabolized in liver. **Excretion:** Primarily excreted in urine.

ACTION/*THERAPEUTIC EFFECT*

Stimulates beta$_1$-adrenergic receptors, *enhancing contractile myocardial force, increasing cardiac output.* Stimulates alpha-adrenergic receptors, *constricting resistance and capacitance vessels, resulting in increased systemic B/P, coronary artery blood flow.* Pressor effect primarily due to increased peripheral resistance.

USES

Corrects hypotension unresponsive to adequate fluid volume replacement, as part of shock syndrome, caused by myocardial infarction, bacteremia, open heart surgery, renal failure.

STORAGE/HANDLING

Do not use if brown in color or contains precipitate.

ADMINISTRATION

IV:

- **Note:** Blood, fluid volume depletion should be corrected before drug is administered.

N

- Add 4 ml to 250 ml (16 mcg base/ml)–1,000 ml (4 mcg base/ml) of D_5W.
- Infuse through plastic catheter, using antecubital vein of arm.
- Avoid catheter tie-in technique (encourages stasis, increases local drug concentration).
- Closely monitor IV infusion flow rate (use microdrip or infusion pump).
- Monitor B/P q2min during IV infusion until desired therapeutic response is achieved, then q5min during remaining IV infusion. Never leave pt unattended.
- Maintain B/P at 80–100 mm Hg in previously normotensive pts, and 30–40 mm Hg below preexisting B/P in previously hypertensive pts.
- Reduce IV infusion gradually. Avoid abrupt withdrawal.
- It is imperative to check the IV site frequently for free flow and infused vein for blanching, hardness to vein, coldness, pallor to extremity.
- If extravasation occurs, area should be infiltrated w/10–15 ml sterile saline containing 5–10 mg phentolamine (does not alter pressor effects of norepinephrine).

INDICATIONS/ROUTES/DOSAGE

Acute hypotension:
IV: Adults, elderly: Initially, administer at 0.5–1 mcg/min. Adjust rate of flow to establish, maintain desired B/P (40 mm Hg below preexisting systolic pressure). ***Average maintenance dose:*** 2–12 mcg/min. ***Children:*** Administer at rate of 0.1 mcg/kg/min. Adjust rate of flow to establish, maintain desired B/P, up to 1 mcg/kg/min.

CONTRAINDICATIONS

Hypovolemic states (unless an emergency measure), mesenteric/peripheral vascular thrombosis, profound hypoxia.

CAUTIONS

Severe cardiac disease, hypertensive and hypothyroid pts, those on MAO inhibitors.

INTERACTIONS

DRUG: ***Tricyclic antidepressants, maprotiline*** may increase cardiovascular effects. May decrease effect of ***methyldopa.*** May have mutually inhibitory effects w/***beta blockers.*** May increase risk of arrhythmias w/***digoxin. Ergonovine, oxytocin*** may increase vasoconstriction. **HERBAL:** Ma Huang (Ephedra) may increase CNS stimulation. **FOOD:** None significant. **ALTERED LAB VALUES:** None significant.

SIDE EFFECTS

Norepinephrine produces less pronounced and less frequent side effects than epinephrine. **FREQUENT (5%):** Increased heart rate, blood pressure, hypotension, PVCs. **OCCASIONAL (3–5%):** Pain at injection site. **RARE (1–3%):** Nausea, headache, anginal pain, shortness of breath, fever.

ADVERSE REACTIONS/TOXIC EFFECTS

Extravasation may produce tissue necrosis, sloughing. Overdosage manifested as severe hypertension w/violent headache (may be first clinical sign of overdosage), arrhythmias, photophobia, retrosternal/pharyngeal pain, pallor, excessive sweating, vomiting. Prolonged therapy may result in plasma volume depletion. Hypotension may recur if plasma volume is not maintained.

PATIENT CONSIDERATIONS

BASELINE ASSESSMENT

Assess EKG and B/P continuously (be alert to precipitous B/P drop). Never leave pt alone during IV infusion. Be alert to pt complaint of headache.

INTERVENTION/EVALUATION

Monitor IV flow rate diligently. Assess for extravasation characterized by blanching of skin over vein, coolness (results from local vasoconstriction); color and temperature of IV site extremity (pallor, cyanosis, mottling). Assess nailbed capillary refill. Monitor I&O; measure output hourly and report <30 cc. IV should not be reinstated unless systolic B/P falls below 70–80 mm Hg.

norfloxacin

nor-**flocks**-ah-sin
(Chibroxin, Noroxin)

CANADIAN AVAILABILITY
Noroxin

PREGNANCY CATEGORY C

CLASSIFICATION

Anti-infective: Quinolone

AVAILABILITY (Rx)

Tablets: 400 mg. **Ophthalmic Solution:** 3 mg/ml.

PHARMACOKINETICS

Absorption: Rapidly, incompletely absorbed from GI tract. Widely distributed. **Metabolism:** Possibly metabolized in liver. **Excretion:** Primarily excreted in urine. **Half-life:** 3–4 hrs (increased in decreased renal function).

ACTION/*THERAPEUTIC EFFECT*

Inhibits DNA replication and repair by interfering w/DNA-gyrase in susceptible microorganisms, *producing bactericidal activity.*

USES

Treatment of complicated and uncomplicated urinary tract infections, uncomplicated gonococcal infections, acute/chronic prostatitis. *Ophthalmic:* Conjunctival keratitis, keratoconjunctivitis, corneal ulcers, blepharitis, blepharoconjunctivitis, acute meibomianitis, dacryocystitis.

ADMINISTRATION

ORAL:

- Give 1 hr before or 2 hrs after meals, w/8 oz water.
- Encourage additional glasses of water between meals.
- Do not administer antacids w/or within 2 hrs of norfloxacin dose.
- Encourage cranberry juice, citrus fruits (to acidify urine).

OPHTHALMIC:

- Tilt pt's head back; place solution in conjunctival sac.
- Have pt close eyes; press gently on lacrimal sac for 1 min.
- Do not use ophthalmic solutions for injection.

INDICATIONS/ROUTES/DOSAGE

Complicated or uncomplicated urinary tract infections:
Oral: Adults, elderly: 400 mg 2 times/day for 7–21 days.

Prostatitis:
Oral: Adults: 400 mg 2 times/day for 28 days.

Uncomplicated gonococcal infections:
Oral: Adults: 800 mg as single dose.

Dosage in renal impairment: The dose and/or frequency is modified based on degree of renal impairment.

CREATININE CLEARANCE	DOSAGE
>30 ml/min	400 mg 2 times/day
<30 ml/min	400 mg once daily

Usual ophthalmic dosage: *Ophthalmic: Adults, elderly:* 1–2 drops 4 times/day up to 7 days. For severe infections, may give 1–2 drops q2h while awake the first day.

CONTRAINDICATIONS

Hypersensitivity to norfloxacin, quinolones, or any component of preparation. Do not use in children <18 yrs of age—produces arthropathy. *Ophthalmic:* Epithelial herpes simplex, keratitis, vaccinia, varicella, mycobacterial infection, fungal disease of ocular structure. Do not use after uncomplicated removal of foreign body.

CAUTIONS

Impaired renal function; any predisposition to seizures.

INTERACTIONS

DRUG: ***Antacids, sucralfate*** may decrease absorption. Decrease clearance, may increase concentration, toxicity of ***theophylline.*** May increase effects of ***oral anticoagulants.*** **HERBAL:** None known. **FOOD:** None significant. **ALTERED LAB VALUES:** May increase SGOT (AST), SGPT (ALT), alkaline phosphatase, LDH, bilirubin, BUN, creatinine.

SIDE EFFECTS

FREQUENT: Nausea, headache, dizziness, eosinophilia. *Ophthalmic:* Bad taste in mouth. **OCCASIONAL:** *Ophthalmic:* Temporary blurring of vision, irritation, burning, stinging, itching. **RARE:** Vomiting, diarrhea, dry mouth, bitter taste, nervousness, drowsiness, insomnia, photosensitivity, tinnitus, crystalluria, rash, fever, seizures. *Ophthalmic:* Conjunctival hyperemia, photophobia, decreased vision, pain.

ADVERSE REACTIONS/TOXIC EFFECTS

Superinfection, anaphylaxis, Stevens-Johnson syndrome, arthropathy (joint disease) occurs rarely.

PATIENT CONSIDERATIONS

Baseline Assessment

Question for history of hypersensitivity to norfloxacin, quinolones, any component of preparation. Obtain specimens for diagnostic tests before giving first dose (therapy may begin before results are known).

Intervention/Evaluation

Evaluate food tolerance, taste sensation, and dryness of mouth. Determine pattern of bowel activity. Assess skin for rash. Check for headache, dizziness. Monitor level of consciousness, pattern of sleep. Assess temperature at least 2 times/day.

Ophthalmic
Check for therapeutic response, side effects (see Side Effects).

Patient Familty Teaching

Take 1 hr before or 2 hrs after meals. Complete full course of therapy. Take w/8 oz of water, drink several glasses of water between meals. Eat/drink high sources of ascorbic acid, (e.g., cranberry juice, citrus fruits). Do not take antacids w/or within 2

hrs of norfloxacin dose. Avoid sunlight/ultraviolet exposure; wear sunscreen and protective clothing if photosensitivity develops. Avoid tasks that require alert response if dizziness/drowsiness occur. Sugarless gum or hard candy, ice chips may help dry mouth and bitter taste. Notify nurse/physician if headache, dizziness, or other symptoms occur. Report inflammation or tendon pain.

Ophthalmic
Report any increased burning, itching, or other discomfort promptly.

nortriptyline hydrochloride

nor-**trip**-teh-leen
(Aventyl, Pamelor)

CANADIAN AVAILABILITY
Aventyl

PREGNANCY CATEGORY D

CLASSIFICATION

Antidepressant: Tricyclic

AVAILABILITY (Rx)

Capsules: 10 mg, 25 mg, 50 mg, 75 mg. **Oral Solution:** 10 mg/5 ml.

PHARMACOKINETICS

Absorption: Rapidly, well absorbed from GI tract. **Metabolism:** Metabolized in liver, undergoes first-pass metabolism. **Excretion:** Primarily excreted in urine. Minimal removal by hemodialysis. **Half-life:** 18–44 hrs.

ACTION / *THERAPEUTIC EFFECT*

Blocks reuptake of neurotransmitters (norepinephrine, serotonic) at neuronal presynaptic membranes, increasing availability at postsynaptic receptor sites. *Resulting enhancements of synaptic activity produces antidepressant effect.*

USES / *UNLABELED*

Treatment of various forms of depression, often in conjunction w/psychotherapy. *Treatment of panic disorder, neurogenic pain, prophylaxis of headache, migraines.*

ADMINISTRATION

ORAL:

- Give w/food or milk if GI distress occurs.

INDICATIONS / ROUTES / DOSAGE

Oral: Adults: 75–100 mg/day in 1–4 divided doses until therapeutic response achieved. Reduce dosage gradually to effective maintenance level. ***Elderly:*** Initially, 10–25 mg at bedtime. May increase by 25 mg q3–7days. ***Maximum:*** 150 mg/day.

CONTRAINDICATIONS

Acute recovery period following MI, within 14 days of MAO inhibitor ingestion.

CAUTIONS

Prostatic hypertrophy, history of urinary retention or obstruction, glaucoma, diabetes mellitus, history of seizures, hyperthyroidism, cardiac/hepatic/renal disease, schizophrenia, increased intraocular pressure, hiatal hernia.

INTERACTIONS

DRUG: *Alcohol, CNS depressants*

may increase CNS, respiratory depression, hypotensive effects. ***Antithyroid agents*** may increase risk of agranulocytosis. ***Phenothiazines*** may increase sedative, anticholinergic effects. ***Cimetidine*** may increase concentration, toxicity. May decrease effects of ***clonidine, guanadrel.*** May increase cardiac effects w/***sympathomimetics.*** May increase risk of hypertensive crisis, hyperpyretic convulsions w/***MAOIs.*** **HERBAL:** St. John's wort may decrease concentration. **FOOD:** None significant. **ALTERED LAB VALUES:** May alter EKG readings, glucose.

SIDE EFFECTS

FREQUENT: Drowsiness, fatigue, dry mouth, blurred vision, constipation, delayed micturition, postural hypotension, excessive sweating, disturbed concentration, increased appetite, urinary retention. **OCCASIONAL:** GI disturbances (nausea, GI distress, metallic taste sensation). **RARE:** Paradoxical reaction (agitation, restlessness, nightmares, insomnia), extrapyramidal symptoms (particularly fine hand tremor).

ADVERSE REACTIONS/TOXIC EFFECTS

High dosage may produce cardiovascular effects (severe postural hypotension, dizziness, tachycardia, palpitations, arrhythmias) and seizures. May also result in altered temperature regulation (hyperpyrexia or hypothermia). Abrupt withdrawal from prolonged therapy may produce headache, malaise, nausea, vomiting, vivid dreams.

PATIENT CONSIDERATIONS

BASELINE ASSESSMENT

For those on long-term therapy, liver/renal function tests, blood counts should be performed periodically.

INTERVENTION/EVALUATION

Supervise suicidal risk pt closely during early therapy (as depression lessens, energy level improves, increasing suicide potential). Assess appearance, behavior, speech pattern, level of interest, mood. Monitor stools; avoid constipation w/increased fluids, bulky foods. Monitor B/P pulse for hypotension, arrhythmias. Assess for urinary retention including output estimate and bladder palpation if indicated.

PATIENT/FAMILY TEACHING

Change positions slowly to avoid hypotensive effect. Tolerance to postural hypotension, sedative, and anticholinergic effects usually develops during early therapy. Therapeutic effect may be noted in 2 or more weeks. Photosensitivity to sun may occur. Use sunscreens, protective clothing. Dry mouth may be relieved by sugarless gum, sips of tepid water. Report visual disturbances. Do not abruptly discontinue medication. Avoid tasks that require alertness, motor skills until response to drug is established.

---

nystatin

nigh-**stat**-in

(Mycostatin, Nilstat, Nystop)

FIXED-COMBINATION(S)

W/triamcinolone, a steroid **(Mycolog II, Myco-Triacet II, Mykacet, Mytrex F)**

CANADIAN AVAILABILITY
Mycostatin, Nadostine, Nilstat

PREGNANCY CATEGORY B

CLASSIFICATION

Antifungal

AVAILABILITY (Rx)

Tablets: 500,000 units. **Oral Suspension:** 100,000 units/ml. **Troches:** 200,000 units. **Vaginal Tablets:** 100,000 units. **Cream. Ointment. Powder.**

PHARMACOKINETICS

Oral: **Absorption:** Poorly absorbed from GI tract. **Excretion:** Eliminated unchanged in feces. *Topical:* **Absorption:** Not absorbed systemically from intact skin.

ACTION/*THERAPEUTIC EFFECT*

Binds to sterols in cell membrane increasing permeability, permitting loss of potassium, other cell components. *Fungistatic.*

USES/*UNLABELED*

Treatment of intestinal and oral candidiasis, cutaneous/mucocutaneous mycotic infections caused by *Candida albicans* (oral thrush, paronychia, vulvovaginal candidiasis, diaper rash, perleche). *Prophylaxis/treatment of oropharyngeal candidiasis, tinea barbae, capitis.*

ADMINISTRATION

ORAL:

- Dissolve lozenges (troches) slowly/completely in mouth (optimal therapeutic effect). Do not chew or swallow lozenges whole.
- Shake suspension well before administration.
- Place and hold suspension in mouth or swish throughout mouth as long as possible before swallowing.

INDICATIONS/ROUTES/DOSAGE

Intestinal candidiasis:
Oral: Adults, elderly: 500,000–1,000,000 units 3 times/day. *Children:* 500,000 units 4 times/day.

Oral candidiasis:
Oral: Adults, elderly, children: Oral suspension: 400,000–600,000 units 4 times/day. *Infants:* 100,000–200,000 units 4 times/day.
Oral: Adults, elderly, children: Troches: 200,000–400,000 units 4–5 times/day up to 14 days.

Vulvovaginal candidiasis:
Intravaginal: Adults, elderly: 1 tablet high in vagina 1–2 times/day for 14 days.

Topical fungal infections:
Topical: Adults, elderly: Apply 2–3 times/day.

CONTRAINDICATIONS

Hypersensitivity to nystatin or components of preparation.

INTERACTIONS

DRUG: None significant. **HERBAL:** None known. **FOOD:** None significant. **ALTERED LAB VALUES:** None significant.

SIDE EFFECTS

OCCASIONAL: *Oral:* Nausea, vomiting, diarrhea, and GI distress with high dosage. *Topical:* Skin irritation. *Vaginal:* Vaginal irritation.

ADVERSE REACTIONS/TOXIC EFFECTS

None significant.

PATIENT CONSIDERATIONS

BASELINE ASSESSMENT

Question for history of allergies,

N

especially to nystatin. Confirm that cultures or histologic tests were done for accurate diagnosis.

INTERVENTION/EVALUATION

Evaluate food intake, tolerance. Determine pattern of bowel activity and stool consistency. Assess for increased irritation w/topical, increased vaginal discharge with vaginal application.

PATIENT/FAMILY TEACHING

Do not miss dose; complete full length of treatment (continue vaginal use during menses). Notify physician if nausea, vomiting, diarrhea, stomach pain develop.

Vaginal
Insert high in vagina. Check w/physician regarding douching, sexual intercourse.

Topical
Rub well &into affected areas. Must not contact eyes. Do not apply any other preparations or occlusive covering w/o consulting physician. Use cream (sparingly)/powder on erythematous areas. Keep areas clean, dry; wear light clothing for ventilation. Separate personal items in contact w/affected areas.

octreotide acetate

ock-**tree**-oh-tide
(Sandostatin, Sandostatin LAR Depot)

CANADIAN AVAILABILITY
Sandostatin

PREGNANCY CATEGORY B

CLASSIFICATION

Secretory inhibitor

AVAILABILITY (Rx)

Injection: 0.05 mg/ml, 0.1 mg/ml, 0.2 mg/ml, 0.5 mg/ml, 1 mg/ml. **Suspension for Injection.**

PHARMACODYNAMICS

	ONSET	PEAK	DURATION
SubQ	—	—	Up to 12 hrs

PHARMACOKINETICS

Absorption: Rapidly, completely absorbed from injection site. **Excretion:** Excreted in urine. **Half-life:** 1.5 hrs.

ACTION/*THERAPEUTIC EFFECT*

Suppresses secretion of serotonin, gastroenteropancreatic peptides. Enhances fluid/electrolyte absorption from GI tract; *prolongs intestinal transit time.*

USES/*UNLABELED*

Symptomatic treatment of pts w/metastatic carcinoid tumors or vasoactive intestinal peptide tumors. Treatment of acromegaly. *Treatment of hypotension due to carcinoid crises during anesthesia induction, adjunct in treatment of symptoms of hyperinsulinemia from severe refractory metastatic insulinoma, AIDS-associated diarrhea.*

STORAGE/HANDLING

Refrigerate ampules. Ampules may be kept at room temperature on day to be used. Do not use if discolored, contains particulates.

ADMINISTRATION

SubQ:

- Recommended route of administration is SubQ (IV bolus has been given in emergency conditions).
- Do not use if particulates and/or discoloration are noted.
- Avoid multiple injections at the same site within short periods.

INDICATIONS/ROUTES/DOSAGE

Note: Initial dose is 50 mcg 1–2 times/day; then dose is increased based on response/tolerability of pt to medication.

Carcinoid tumors:
SubQ: Adults, elderly: 100–600 mcg/day in 2–4 divided doses during first 2 wks of therapy. ***Maintenance:*** 450 mcg/day (range: 50–750 mcg).

Vasoactive intestinal peptide tumors:
SubQ: Adults, elderly: 200–300 mcg/day in 2–4 divided doses during first 2 wks of therapy (range: 150–750 mcg/day). Dosage adjusted to achieve therapeutic response, usually not above 450 mcg/day.

Acromegaly:
SubQ: Adults, elderly: Initially, 50 mcg 3 times/day. Up to 100 mcg 3 times/day.

Usual maintenance dosage:
IM: Adults, elderly: 20 mg q4wks for 2 mos. May increase to 30 mg q4wks.

CONTRAINDICATIONS

Hypersensitivity to drug or any of its components.

CAUTIONS

Insulin-dependent diabetes, renal failure.

INTERACTIONS

DRUG: May alter glucose concentrations w/*insulin*, ***oral hypoglycemics, glucagon, growth hormone.*** **HERBAL:** None known. **FOOD:** None significant. **ALTERED LAB VALUES:** May decrease T_4 concentration.

SIDE EFFECTS

FREQUENT (>10%): Diarrhea, nausea, abdominal discomfort, increased glucose. **OCCASIONAL (1–10%):** Vomiting, flatulence, constipation, headache, alopecia, flushing, itching, dizziness, fatigue, arrhythmias, pain at injection site, bruising, blurred vision. **RARE (<1%):** Hepatitis, jaundice, GI bleeding, depression, decreased libido, seizures, vertigo, palpitations, shortness of breath.

ADVERSE REACTIONS/TOXIC EFFECTS

Increased risk of cholelithiasis. Potential for hypothyroidism w/prolonged high therapy.

PATIENT CONSIDERATIONS

BASELINE ASSESSMENT

Question for hypersensitivity to drug, components. Establish baseline B/P, weight, blood glucose, electrolytes.

INTERVENTION/EVALUATION

Evaluate blood glucose levels (especially w/diabetics), electrolytes (therapy generally reduces abnormalities). Weigh every 2–3 days, report >5 lbs gain/week. Monitor B/P, pulse, respirations periodically during treatment. Be alert for decreased urinary output, swelling of ankles, fingers. Check food tolerance. Monitor stools for frequency, consistency.

PATIENT/FAMILY TEACHING

Careful instruction on SubQ injection. Follow-up by physician and tests are essential. Report jaundice (yellow eyes or skin, dark urine, clay-colored stools), abdominal pain, edema. Therapy should provide significant improvement of symptoms.

ocular lubricant

ock-you-lar **lube**-rih-cant
(Hypotears, Lacrilube)

CANADIAN AVAILABILITY
Tears Naturale

CLASSIFICATION

Ophthalmic lubricant

AVAILABILITY (OTC)

Ophthalmic Ointment. Solution.

ACTION/*THERAPEUTIC EFFECT*

Maintains ocular tonicity (0.9% NaCl equivalent); buffers to adjust pH, viscosity agents to prolong eye contact time. *Protects and lubricates eye.*

USES

Protection and lubrication of the eye in exposure keratitis, decreased corneal sensitivity, recurrent corneal erosions, keratitis sicca (particularly for nighttime use), after removal of a foreign body, during and following surgery.

ADMINISTRATION

OPHTHALMIC:

- Do not use w/contact lenses.
- *Ointment:* Hold tube in hand for a few minutes to warm ointment.
- Avoid touching tip of tube or dropper to any surface.

- Gently pull lower lid down to form pouch.
- Have pt tilt head backward and look up.
- *Ointment:* Place ordered amount of ointment in pouch w/a sweeping motion. Instruct pt to close the eye for 1–2 min and roll the eyeball around in all directions.
- *Drops:* Instill drop(s); have pt close eye gently for 1–2 min. Apply gentle pressure w/fingers to bridge of nose (inside corner of eye).
- Wipe away excess around eye w/a tissue.

INDICATIONS/ROUTES/DOSAGE

Usual ophthalmic dosage:
Adults, elderly: Small amount in conjunctival cul-de-sac.

CONTRAINDICATIONS

Hypersensitivity to any component of preparation.

CAUTIONS

None significant.

INTERACTIONS

DRUG: None significant. **HERBAL:** None known. **FOOD:** None significant. **ALTERED LAB VALUES:** None significant.

SIDE EFFECTS

FREQUENT: Temporary blurring after administration, especially w/ointment.

ADVERSE REACTIONS/TOXIC EFFECTS

None significant.

PATIENT CONSIDERATIONS

PATIENT/FAMILY TEACHING

Teach proper application. Do not use contact lenses. Temporary blurring will occur especially w/administration of ointment. Avoid activities requiring visual acuity until blurring clears. If eye pain, change of vision, or worsening of condition occurs, or if condition is unchanged after 72 hrs, notify physician. Do not touch to any surface (may contaminate).

ofloxacin

oh-**flocks**-ah-sin
(Floxin, Floxin Otic, Ocuflox)

O

CANADIAN AVAILABILITY
Apo-Oflox, Floxin, Ocuflox

PREGNANCY CATEGORY C

CLASSIFICATION

Anti-infective: Quinolone

AVAILABILITY (Rx)

Tablets: 200 mg, 300 mg, 400 mg. **Injection:** 200 mg, 400 mg. **Ophthalmic Solution:** 3 mg/ml. **Otic Solution:** 0.3%.

PHARMACOKINETICS

Absorption: Rapidly, well absorbed from GI tract. Widely distributed (penetrates CSF). **Metabolism:** Metabolized in liver. **Excretion:** Primarily excreted in urine. Minimally removed by hemodialysis. **Half-life:** 4.7–7 hrs (increased in decreased renal function, elderly, cirrhosis).

ACTION/*THERAPEUTIC EFFECT*

Inhibits DNA-gyrase in susceptible microorganisms, *interfering w/bacterial DNA replication and repair. Bactericidal.*

USES

Treatment of infections of urinary tract, skin/skin structure, sexually transmitted diseases, lower respiratory tract, prostatitis due to

Escherichia coli, PID. ***Ophthalmic:*** Bacterial conjunctivitis, corneal ulcers. ***Otic:*** Otitis externa, acute/chronic otitis media.

STORAGE/HANDLING

Store oral, parenteral forms at room temperature. After dilution, IV stable for 72 hrs at room temperature; 14 days refrigerated. Discard unused portions.

ADMINISTRATION

ORAL:

- Do not give w/food; preferred dosing time: 1 hr before or 2 hrs after meals.
- Do not administer antacids (aluminum, magnesium) or iron-/zinc-containing products within 2 hrs of ofloxacin.
- Encourage cranberry juice, citrus fruits (to acidify urine).
- Give w/8 oz water and encourage fluid intake.

IV:

- Give only by IV infusion; avoid rapid or bolus IV administration. Must dilute the 20 mg/ml or 40 mg/ml vial.
- Infuse over at least 60 min.
- Must dilute each 200 mg w/50 ml 5% dextrose or 0.9% NaCl (400 mg w/100 ml) to provide concentration of 4 mg/ml.
- Do not add or infuse other medication through same IV line at same time.

OPHTHALMIC:

- Tilt pt's head back; place solution in conjunctival sac.
- Have pt close eyes; press gently on lacrimal sac for 1 min.
- Do not use ophthalmic solutions for injection.
- Unless infection very superficial, systemic administration generally accompanies ophthalmic.

INDICATIONS/ROUTES/DOSAGE

Urinary tract infection:
Oral/IV Infusion: Adults: 200 mg q12h.

Lower respiratory tract, skin/skin structure infections:
Oral/IV Infusion: Adults: 400 mg q12h for 10 days.

Prostatitis, sexually transmitted diseases (cervicitis, urethritis):
Oral: Adults: 300 mg q12h.

PID:
Oral: Adults: 400 mg q12h for 10–14 days.

Prostatitis:
IV Infusion: Adults: 300 mg q12h.

Sexually transmitted diseases:
IV Infusion: Adults: 400 mg as single dose.

Acute, uncomplicated gonorrhea:
Oral: Adults: 400 mg 1 time.

Usual elderly dosage:
Oral: 200–400 mg q12–24h for 7 days up to 6 wks.

Dosage in renal impairment:
After a normal initial dose, dosage/interval based on creatinine clearance.

CREATININE CLEARANCE	ADJUSTED DOSE	DOSAGE INTERVAL
>50 ml/min	none	12 hrs
10–50 ml/min	none	24 hrs
<10 ml/min	1/2	24 hrs

Bacterial conjunctivitis:
Ophthalmic: Adults, elderly: 1–2 drops q2–4h for 2 days, then 4 times/day for 5 days.

Corneal ulcers:
Ophthalmic: Adults: 1–2 drops q30min while awake for 2 days, then q60min while awake for 5–7 days, then 4 times/day.

Usual otic dosage:
Adults, elderly, children: Twice daily. Warm drops before administering.

CONTRAINDICATIONS

Syphilis, hypersensitivity to ofloxacin or any quinolones. Children <18 yrs.

CAUTIONS

Renal impairment, CNS disorders, seizures, those taking theophylline or caffeine. May mask or delay symptoms of syphilis; serologic test for syphilis should be done at diagnosis and 3 mos after treatment.

INTERACTIONS

DRUG: ***Antacids, sucralfate*** may decrease absorption, effect of ofloxacin. May increase ***theophylline*** concentrations, toxicity. **HERBAL:** None known. **FOOD:** None significant. **ALTERED LAB VALUES:** None significant.

SIDE EFFECTS

FREQUENT (5–10%): Nausea, headache, seizures. **OCCASIONAL (1–5%):** Abdominal pain, diarrhea, vomiting, dry mouth, flatulence, dizziness, fatigue, drowsiness, rash, itching, fever. **RARE (<1%):** Constipation, numbness of hands, feet.

ADVERSE REACTIONS/TOXIC EFFECTS

Superinfection, severe hypersensitivity reaction occur rarely. Arthropathy (joint disease w/swelling, pain, clubbing of fingers and toes, degeneration of stress-bearing portion of a joint) may occur if given to children.

PATIENT CONSIDERATIONS

Baseline Assessment

Question for history of hypersensitivity to ofloxacin or any quinolones. Obtain specimen for diagnostic tests before giving first dose (therapy may begin before results are known).

Intervention/Evaluation

Assess skin and discontinue medication at first sign of rash or other allergic reaction. Evaluate food tolerance. Determine pattern of bowel activity, stool consistency. Assess during the night for sleeplessness, restlessness, complaint of dreaming. Check for dizziness, headache, visual difficulties, tremors; provide ambulation assistance as needed. Monitor TPR, B/P at least 2 times/day. Be alert for superinfection, (e.g., genital pruritus, vaginitis, fever, sores, and discomfort in mouth).

Patient/Family Teaching

Do not skip dose; take full course of therapy. Take w/8 oz water; drink several glasses of water between meals. Eat/drink high sources of ascorbic acid (cranberry juice, citrus fruits). Do not take antacids (reduces/destroys effectiveness). Avoid tasks that require alertness, motor skills until response to drug is established. Avoid sunlight/ultraviolet exposure; wear sunscreen, protective clothing if photosensitivity develops. Notify physician if new symptoms occur. Report inflammation or tendon pain. *Otic:* Warm drops in hands 1–2 min before administering (prevents dizziness).

---

olanzapine

oh-**lan**-sah-peen
(Zyprexa)

CANADIAN AVAILABILITY
Zyprexa

PREGNANCY CATEGORY C

CLASSIFICATION

Antipsychotic

AVAILABILITY (Rx)

Tablets: 5 mg, 7.5 mg, 10 mg. **Disintegrating Tablets:** 5 mg, 10 mg.

PHARMACOKINETICS

Absorption: Well absorbed following oral administration. Extensively distributed throughout body. **Metabolism:** Extensively metabolized by first-pass liver metabolism. **Excretion:** Excreted in urine, w/lesser amount eliminated in feces. Not removed by dialysis. **Half-life:** 21–54 hrs.

ACTION/*THERAPEUTIC EFFECT*

Antagonizes dopamine, serotonin, muscarinic, histamine, and alpha$_1$-adrenergic receptors, *diminishing psychotic disorders.* Produces anticholinergic, histaminic, CNS depressant effects.

USES

Management of manifestations of psychotic disorders. Treatment of acute mania associated w/bipolar disorder; maintenance treatment in schizophrenia.

ADMINISTRATION

ORAL:

- May give w/o regard to meals.

INDICATIONS/ROUTES/DOSAGE

Psychotic disorders:
Oral: Adults, elderly: Initially, 5–10 mg once daily w/target dose of 10 mg/day within several days after initiation. If needed, dose increments/decrements of 5 mg once daily but not less than 1 wk intervals.

Debilitated, predisposition to hypotensive reactions, elderly >65 yrs:
Oral: Adults, elderly: Initially, 5 mg/day.

CONTRAINDICATIONS

Hypersensitivity to olanzapine.

CAUTIONS

Hypersensitivity to clozapine, pts who should avoid anticholinergics (e.g., pts w/benign prostatic hypertrophy), hepatic function impairment, elderly, concurrent potentially hepatotoxic drugs, dose escalation, known cardiovascular disease (history of MI or ischemia, heart failure, conduction abnormalities), cerebrovascular disease, conditions predisposing pts to hypotension (dehydration, hypovolemia, hypertensive medications), history of seizures, conditions lowering seizure threshold (e.g., Alzheimer's dementia), those at risk of aspiration pneumonia.

INTERACTIONS

DRUG: ***Alcohol, CNS depressants*** may increase CNS depressant effects. ***Antihypertensive agents*** increase risk of hypotensive effect. May inhibit metabolism of ***theophylline, imipramine. Fluvoxamine; ciprofloxacin (quinolone)*** may increase olanzapine blood levels. Antagonizes effects of ***levodopa, dopamine agonists. Carbamazepine*** increases olanzapine clearance. **HERBAL:** None known. **FOOD:** None significant. **ALTERED LAB VALUES:** May significantly increase SGPT (ALT), SGOT (AST), GGT levels, prolactin levels.

SIDE EFFECTS

FREQUENT: Somnolence (26%), agitation (23%), insomnia (20%), headache (17%), nervousness (16%), hostility (15%), dizziness (11%), rhinitis (10%). **OCCASIONAL:** Anxiety, constipation (9%), nonaggressive objectionable behavior (8%), dry mouth (7%), weight gain (6%), postural hypotension, fever, joint pain, restlessness, cough, pharyngitis, dimness of vision (5%). **RARE:** Tachycardia, back/chest/abdominal pain, tremor, extremity pain.

ADVERSE REACTIONS/TOXIC EFFECTS

Seizures occur rarely. Neuroleptic malignant syndrome (NMS), a potentially fatal syndrome, occurs rarely and may present as hyperpyrexia, muscle rigidity, irregular pulse or B/P, tachycardia, diaphoresis, cardiac dysrhythmias. Extrapyramidal symptoms may occur. Dysphagia (esophageal dysmotility, aspiration) may be noted. Overdosage (300 mg) produces drowsiness, slurred speech.

PATIENT CONSIDERATIONS

Baseline Assessment

Obtain baseline hepatic function lab values before initiating treatment. Assess behavior, appearance, emotional status, response to environment, speech pattern, thought content.

Intervention/Evaluation

Supervise suicidal risk pt closely during early therapy (as depression lessens, energy level improves, increasing suicide potential). Periodically reassess need for maintenance treatment. Assess for therapeutic response (interest in surroundings, improvement in self-care, increased ability to concentrate, relaxed facial expression). Question bowel activity for evidence of constipation. Assist w/ambulation if dizziness occurs. Notify physician if extrapyramidal symptoms occur. Monitor liver function tests.

Patient/Family Teaching

Avoid dehydration, particularly during exercise, exposure to extreme heat, concurrent medication causing dry mouth, other drying effects. Notify physician if pregnancy occurs or if there is intention to become pregnant during olanzapine therapy. Take medication as ordered; do not stop taking or increase dosage. Report visual disturbances. Sugarless gum, sips of tepid water may relieve dry mouth. Drowsiness generally subsides during continued therapy. Avoid driving or performing tasks that require alertness, motor skills until response to drug is established. Avoid alcohol. Change positions slowly to reduce hypotensive effect.

olopatadine hydrochloride

owe-low-**pay**-tah-deen
(Patanol)

CANADIAN AVAILABILITY
Patanol

PREGNANCY CATEGORY C

CLASSIFICATION

Ophthalmic antihistamine

AVAILABILITY (Rx)

Ophthalmic Solution: 0.1%

PHARMACODYNAMICS

Absorption: Absorbed into the conjunctiva. Usually does not produce measurable plasma concentration. **Metabolism:** Converts to metabolites. **Excretion:** Excreted predominately in the urine. **Half-life:** 3 hrs.

ACTION/*THERAPEUTIC EFFECT*

A selective histamine H_1 antagonist, inhibits immediate hypersensitivity reaction, blocks histamine release from the mast cell, *preventing hypersensitivity reaction.*

USES

Temporary relief of signs and symptoms of allergic conjunctivitis.

ADMINISTRATION

OPHTHALMIC:

- Place finger on lower eyelid and pull out until pocket is formed between eye and lower lid.
- Hold dropper above pocket and place drop into center of pocket.
- Instruct patient to close eye gently so medication will not be squeezed out of sac.
- Apply digital pressure to lacrimal sac at inner canthus for 1–2 min (promotes absorption, minimizes drainage into nose and throat).
- Remove excess solution around eye with tissue.
- Do not apply medication while pt is wearing soft contact lenses (absorbs drug preservative). Lenses may be reinserted 10 min after drug is administered.

INDICATIONS/DOSAGE/ROUTES

Allergic conjunctivitis:
Ophthalmic: Adults, elderly: Apply 1–2 drops into affected eye(s) 2 times/day at 6–8 hr intervals.

CONTRAINDICATIONS

History of hypersensitivity to medication.

CAUTIONS

None significant.

INTERACTIONS

DRUG: None significant. **HERBAL:** None known. **FOOD:** None significant.**ALTERED LAB VALUES:** None significant.

SIDE EFFECTS

FREQUENT (7%): Headache. **OCCASIONAL (1–5%):** Burning or stinging, dry eye, foreign body sensation, lid edema, pruritus, asthenia, cold syndrome, abnormal taste.

ADVERSE REACTIONS/TOXIC EFFECTS

None significant.

PATIENT CONSIDERATIONS

INTERVENTION/EVALUATION

Monitor for headache, burning or stinging, dry eye, foreign body sensation, lid edema, pruritus, asthenia, cold syndrome, abnormal taste.

PATIENT/FAMILY TEACHING

Do not touch eyelids or surrounding area with dropper tip of the bottle. Keep bottle tightly closed when not is use. Do not apply medication while wearing soft contact lenses (absorbs drug preservative). Reinsert lenses ≥10 min after drug is administered. Check with physician if condition does not improve or worsens.

---

olsalazine sodium

ol-**sal**-ah-zeen
(Dipentum)

CANADIAN AVAILABILITY
Dipentum

PREGNANCY CATEGORY C

CLASSIFICATION

Anti-inflammatory agent

AVAILABILITY (Rx)

Capsules: 250 mg

PHARMACOKINETICS

Absorption: Minimally absorbed from GI tract (99% reaches colon). **Metabolism:** Converted to mesalamine in colon. **Excretion:** Primarily eliminated in feces. **Half-life:** 0.9 hrs.

ACTION/*THERAPEUTIC EFFECT*

Converted in colon by bacterial action to mesalamine, *reducing colonic inflammation* by blocking prostaglandin production in bowel mucosa.

USES/*UNLABELED*

Maintenance of remission of ulcerative colitis in those intolerant of sulfasalazine medication. *Treatment of inflammatory bowel disease.*

ADMINISTRATION

ORAL:

- Give w/food in evenly divided doses.

INDICATIONS/ROUTES/DOSAGE

Maintenance of controlled ulcerative colitis:
Oral: Adults, elderly: 1 g/day in 2 divided doses (preferably q12h).

CONTRAINDICATIONS

History of hypersensitivity to salicylates.

CAUTIONS

Preexisting renal disease.

INTERACTIONS

DRUG: None significant. **HERBAL:** None known. **FOOD:** None significant. **ALTERED LAB VALUES:** May increase SGOT (AST), SGPT (ALT).

SIDE EFFECTS

FREQUENT (5–10%): Headache, diarrhea, abdominal pain or cramps, nausea. **OCCASIONAL (1–5%):** Depression, fatigue, dyspepsia, upper respiratory infection, decreased appetite, rash, itching, arthralgia. **RARE (<1%):** Dizziness, vomiting, stomatitis.

ADVERSE REACTIONS/TOXIC EFFECTS

Sulfite sensitivity in susceptible pts noted as cramping, headache, diarrhea, fever, rash, hives, itching, wheezing. Discontinue drug immediately. Excessive diarrhea associated w/extreme fatigue noted rarely.

PATIENT CONSIDERATIONS

Baseline Assessment

Discontinue medication if rash, fever, cramping, or diarrhea occurs.

Intervention/Evaluation

Encourage adequate fluid intake. Assess bowel sounds for peristalsis. Monitor daily bowel activity and stool consistency (watery, loose, soft, semisolid, solid) and record time of evacuation. Assess for abdominal disturbances. Assess skin for rash, hives.

Patient/Family Teaching

Notify physician if diarrhea continues or increases, rash or pruritus occurs.

omeprazole

oh-**mep**-rah-zole
(Prilosec)

CANADIAN AVAILABILITY
Losec

PREGNANCY CATEGORY C

CLASSIFICATION

Gastric acid pump inhibitor

AVAILABILITY (Rx)

Capsules (delayed-release): 10 mg, 20 mg, 40 mg

PHARMACOKINETICS

Absorption: Rapidly absorbed from GI tract. Primarily distributed into gastric parietal cells. **Metabolism:** Metabolized extensively in liver. **Excretion:** Primarily excreted in urine. **Half-life:** 0.5–1 hr (increased in decreased liver function).

ACTION/*THERAPEUTIC EFFECT*

Converted to active metabolites that irreversibly bind to and inhibit H+/K+ ATPase (an enzyme on surface of gastric parietal cells). Inhibits hydrogen ion transport into gastric lumen, *increasing gastric pH, reducing gastric acid production.*

USES

Short-term treatment (4–8 wks) of erosive esophagitis (diagnosed by endoscopy); symptomatic gastroesophageal reflux disease (GERD) poorly responsive to other treatment. Long-term treatment of pathologic hypersecretory conditions; treatment of active duodenal ulcer. Maintenance healing of erosive esophagitis. Treatment of *H. pylori*–associated duodenal ulcer (combination therapy), active benign gastric ulcers. Prevention/treatment NSAID-induced ulcers.

ADMINISTRATION

ORAL:

- Give before meals.
- Do not crush or chew capsule; swallow whole.

INDICATIONS/ROUTES/DOSAGE

Erosive esophagitis, poorly responsive GERD, active duodenal ulcer, prevent/treat MSAID induced ulcers:
Oral: Adults, elderly: 20 mg/day.

Maintenance healing of erosive esophagitis:
Oral: Adults, elderly: 20 mg/day.

Pathologic hypersecretory conditions:
Oral: Adults, elderly: Initially, 60 mg/day up to 120 mg, 3 times/day.

***H. pylori* duodenal ulcer:**
Oral: Adults, elderly: 20 mg 2 times/day for 10 days.

Active benign gastric ulcer:
Oral: Adults, elderly: 40 mg/day for 4–8 wks.

CONTRAINDICATIONS

None significant.

CAUTIONS

None significant.

INTERACTIONS

DRUG: May increase concentration of ***oral anticoagulants, diazepam, phenytoin.*** **HERBAL:** None known. **FOOD:** None significant. **ALTERED LAB VALUES:** May increase SGOT (AST), SGPT (ALT), alkaline phosphatase.

SIDE EFFECTS

FREQUENT (>5%): Headache.

OCCASIONAL (1–5%): Dizziness, asthenia (loss of strength), diarrhea, abdominal pain, nausea, vomiting, back pain, constipation, rash, cough, upper respiratory infection.

ADVERSE REACTIONS/TOXIC EFFECTS

None significant.

PATIENT CONSIDERATIONS

INTERVENTION/EVALUATION

Evaluate for therapeutic response, (i.e., relief of GI symptoms). Question if GI discomfort, nausea, diarrhea occurs.

PATIENT/FAMILY TEACHING

Report headache. Swallow capsules whole, do not chew or crush. Take prior to eating.

ondansetron hydrochloride

on-**dan**-sah-tron
(Zofran)

CANADIAN AVAILABILITY
Zofran

PREGNANCY CATEGORY B

CLASSIFICATION

Antiemetic

AVAILABILITY (Rx)

Tablets: 4 mg, 8 mg, 24 mg. **Oral Disintegrating Tablets:** 4 mg, 8 mg. **Oral Solution:** 4 mg/5ml. **Injection:** 2 mg/ml. **Injection (Premix):** 32 mg/50 ml.

PHARMACOKINETICS

Absorption: Readily absorbed from GI tract. **Metabolism:** Metabolized in liver. **Excretion:** Primarily excreted in urine. **Half-life:** 4 hrs.

ACTION/*THERAPEUTIC EFFECT*

Exhibits selective 5-HT_3 receptor antagonism for *preventing nausea/vomiting associated w/cancer chemotherapy.* Action may be central (CTZ) or peripheral (vagus nerve terminal).

USES/*UNLABELED*

Prevention, treatment of nausea and vomiting due to cancer chemotherapy, including high-dose cisplatin. Prevention of postop nausea, vomiting. Prevention of radiation-induced nausea, vomiting. *Treatment of postop nausea/vomiting.*

ADMINISTRATION

ORAL:

- May give w/o regard to food.

IM:

- Inject into large muscle mass.

IV:

- For IV infusion, dilute w/50 ml 5% dextrose or 0.9% NaCl before administration.
- Infuse over 15 min.

STORAGE/HANDLING

Store parenteral form at room temperature. After dilution, stable at room temperature for 48 hrs.

INDICATIONS/ROUTES/DOSAGE

Nausea, vomiting: Chemotherapy
IV: Adults, elderly, children (4–18 yrs): 3 doses 0.15 mg/kg. First dose given 30 min before chemotherapy; then 4 and 8 hrs after first dose of ondansetron.

Oral: Adults, elderly: 24 mg once a

day; 8 mg 30 min before start of chemotherapy, then 4 and 8 hrs after first dose; then, 8 mg q8h for 1–2 days after completion of chemotherapy. *Children:* 4 mg using same regimen as for adults.

Nausea, vomiting: Postop
IM/IV: Adults, elderly: 4 mg undiluted over 2–5 min. *Children <40 kg:* 0.1 mg/kg. *>40 kg:* 4 mg.

Nausea, vomiting: Radiation
Oral: Adults, elderly: 8 mg 3 times/day.

CONTRAINDICATIONS

None significant.

CAUTIONS

None significant.

INTERACTIONS

DRUG: None significant. **HERBAL:** None known. **FOOD:** None significant. **ALTERED LAB VALUES:** May transiently increase SGOT (AST), SGPT (ALT), bilirubin.

SIDE EFFECTS

FREQUENT (5–10%): Anxiety, dizziness, drowsiness, headache, fatigue, constipation, diarrhea, arrhythmias, chills. **OCCASIONAL (1–5%):** Abdominal pain, xerotomia (diminished saliva secretion), hypotension, feeling of cold, redness, pain at injection site, numbness of hands, feet, weakness. **RARE (<1%):** Hypersensitivity reaction (rash, itching), blurred vision.

ADVERSE REACTIONS/TOXIC EFFECTS

Overdose may produce combination of CNS stimulation and depressant effects.

PATIENT CONSIDERATIONS

Baseline Assessment

Assess for dehydration if excessive vomiting occurs (poor skin turgor, dry mucous membranes, longitudinal furrows in tongue). Provide emotional support.

Intervention/Evaluation

Monitor pt in environment. Assess bowel sounds for peristalsis. Provide supportive measures. Assess mental status. Monitor daily bowel activity and stool consistency (watery, loose, soft, semisolid, solid) and record time of evacuation.

Patient/Family Teaching

Relief from nausea/vomiting generally occurs shortly after drug administration (check w/physician if vomiting persists). Avoid alcohol, barbiturates.

---

oprelvekin

oh-**prell**-veh-kin
(Neumega, Interleukin 11, IL-11)

PREGNANCY CATEGORY C

CLASSIFICATION

Platelet growth factor

AVAILABILITY (Rx)

Powder for Injection: 5 mg

PHARMACODYNAMICS

	ONSET	PEAK	DURATION
SubQ	—	5–9 days after initiation	Up to 7 days after discontinuing

PHARMACOKINETICS

Rapidly cleared from serum and distributed to highly perfused organs. **Metabolism:** Metabolized by the liver to inactive metabolite. **Excretion:** Eliminated primarily in the urine. **Half-life:** 6.9 hrs.

ACTION/*THERAPEUTIC EFFECT*

Stimulates production of hematopoietic stem cells and megakaryocyte cells, *resulting in increased platelet production. Improves platelet nadirs, accelerates platelet recovery.*

USES

Prevention of severe thrombocytopenia and reduction of need for platelet transfusions following myelosuppressive chemotherapy in patients with nonmyeloid malignancies.

ADMINISTRATION

SUBQ:

- May give in abdomen, thigh, or hip (upper arm if not self-injecting).
- Reconstitute with 1 ml sterile water for injection; direct stream from needle to the side of the vial.
- Swirl contents gently (avoid agitation). The reconstituted solution contains 5 mg/ml.
- Reconstituted solution must be used within 3 hrs.

INDICATIONS/ROUTES/DOSAGES

Prevention of thrombocytopenia: **Note:** Begin dosing 6–24 hrs after chemotherapy is completed; discontinue at least 2 days before starting next cycle of chemotherapy.

SubQ: Adults: 50 mcg/kg once daily. ***Pediatric:*** 75–100 mcg/kg.

CONTRAINDICATIONS

History of hypersensitivity to oprelvekin.

CAUTIONS

Clinically evident CHF, those susceptible to developing CHF, history of heart failure who are well compensated and receiving appropriate medical treatment, history of atrial arrhythmia, preexisting papilledema (blurring of vision) or tumors involving CNS.

INTERACTIONS

DRUG: None significant. **HERBAL:** None known. **FOOD:** None significant. **ALTERED LAB VALUES:** May moderately decrease Hgb, Hct, and RBC (due to increase in plasma volume related to sodium and water retention). Hgb decrease begins 3–5 days after initiation of treatment and is reversible about 1 wk after cessation of treatment.

SIDE EFFECTS

FREQUENT (77%): Nausea, vomiting. **(59–33%):** Fluid retention (peripheral edema, dyspnea upon exertion), neutropenic fever, diarrhea, mucositis, rhinitis, headache, dizziness, fever, insomnia. **OCCASIONAL (29–10%):** Cough, rash, pharyngitis, tachycardia, vasodilation, oral moniliasis, palpitations, syncope. **RARE (<10%):** Asthenia, pain, chills, abdominal pain, anorexia, constipation, dyspepsia, ecchymosis, myalgia, bone pain, nervousness, alopecia.

ADVERSE REACTIONS/TOXIC EFFECTS

Transient atrial arrhythmias (atrial fibrillation or flutter) occur occasionally. They are usually brief in duration; some are asymptomatic.

PATIENT CONSIDERATIONS

BASELINE ASSESSMENT

Platelet counts begin to increase between 5 and 9 days after initiat-

ing of treatment. After cessation of treatment, platelet counts continue to increase for 7 days, then return to baseline count within 14 days. Obtain CBC prior to chemotherapy and at regular intervals thereafter. In those also receiving diuretic therapy, include the monitoring of electrolyte status. Monitor platelet counts during time of expected nadir and until postnadir counts ≥50,000.

INTERVENTION/EVALUATION

Closely monitor fluid balance. Include preexisting fluid collections, including pleural effusions or ascites. Assess for peripheral edema, dyspnea on exertion. Monitor platelet counts periodically. Treatment to continue until postnadir platelet count is ≥50,000 cells/mcL.

orlistat

ore-leh-stat
(Xenical)

PREGNANCY CATEGORY B

CLASSIFICATION

Weight reduction

AVAILABILITY (Rx)

Tablets: 120 mg

PHARMACOKINETICS

Absorption: Minimal absorption following administration. **Excretion:** Primarily eliminated unchanged in feces.

ACTION/*THERAPEUTIC EFFECT*

A gastric/pancreatic lipase inhibitor *reducing absorption of fat.*

USES

Weight reduction.

ADMINISTRATION

ORAL:

- May take w/ or w/o food.

INDICATIONS/ROUTES/DOSAGE

Weight reduction:
Oral: Adults, elderly: 120 mg three times/day.

CONTRAINDICATIONS

History of hypersensitivity to medication, chronic malabsorption syndrome, cholestasis.

CAUTIONS

None significant.

INTERACTIONS

DRUG: May increase concentration, risk of rhabdomyolysis with ***pravastatin.*** **HERBAL:** None known. **FOOD:** None significant. **ALTERED LAB VALUES:** Decreases total cholesterol, LDL, glucose.

SIDE EFFECTS

FREQUENT: Gastrointestinal (mild, moderate, transient) including abdominal pain, flatulence, fecal urgency, fatty evacuation, nausea. Decreases absorption/levels of vitamins A and E.

ADVERSE REACTIONS/TOXIC EFFECTS

None significant.

PATIENT CONSIDERATIONS

INTERVENTION/EVALUATION

Monitor cholesterol, LDL, glucose.

PATIENT/FAMILY TEACHING

High-fiber, low-fat diet decreases fat evacuation.

orphenadrine citrate

(Norflex)

FIXED-COMBINATION(S)

W/aspirin, nonnarcotic analgesic and caffeine, a stimulant **(Norgesic)**

See Classification section under: Skeletal muscle relaxants

oseltamivir

(Tamiflu)

See Supplement

oxacillin sodium

ox-ah-**sill**-in

(Bactocill, Prostaphlin)

PREGNANCY CATEGORY B

CLASSIFICATION

Antibiotic: Penicillin

AVAILABILITY (Rx)

Capsules: 250 mg, 500 mg. **Oral Suspension:** 250 mg/5 ml. **Powder for Injection:** 250 mg, 500 mg, 1 g, 2 g, 4 g, 10 g.

PHARMACOKINETICS

Absorption: Moderately absorbed from GI tract (food decreases absorption). Widely distributed. **Metabolism:** Metabolized in liver. **Excretion:** Primarily excreted in urine. **Half-life:** 0.5–0.7 hrs (increased in decreased renal function, neonates).

ACTION/*THERAPEUTIC EFFECT*

Binds to bacterial membranes, *inhibiting cell wall synthesis. Bactericidal.*

USES

Treatment of respiratory tract, skin/skin structure infections, osteomyelitis, endocarditis, meningitis, perioperatively, especially in cardiovascular, orthopedic procedures. Predominantly used in treatment of infections caused by penicillinase-producing staphylococci.

STORAGE/HANDLING

Store capsules at room temperature. After reconstitution, oral solution is stable for 3 days at room temperature, 14 days if refrigerated; IV infusion (piggyback) is stable for at least 6 hrs at room temperature, 8 days if refrigerated. Discard if precipitate forms.

ADMINISTRATION

- **Note:** Space doses evenly around the clock.

ORAL:

- Give 1 hr before or 2 hrs after food.

IM:

- Dilute 250 mg vial w/1.4 ml (500 mg with 2.7 ml, 1 g w/5.7 ml, 2 g w/11.4 ml, or 4 g w/21.8 ml) sterile water for injection or 0.9% NaCl injection to provide concentration of 250 mg/1.5 ml.
- Inject IM into large muscle mass.

IV:

- For IV injection, dilute each 250 or 500 mg vial w/5 ml (1 g w/10 ml, 2 g w/20 ml) sterile water for injection or 0.9% NaCl injection. Administer over 10 min.
- For intermittent IV infusion (piggyback), further dilute w/50–100 ml 5% dextrose, 0.9% NaCl, or other compatible IV fluid. Infuse over 30–60 min.
- Because of potential for hypersensitivity/anaphylaxis, start initial dose at few drops per minute, increase slowly to ordered rate; stay w/pt first 10–15 min, then check q10min.

- Alternating IV sites, use large veins to reduce risk of phlebitis.

INDICATIONS/ROUTES/DOSAGE

Mild to moderate infections of upper respiratory tract, skin/skin structure infections:
Oral: Adults, elderly, children >20 kg: 500 mg q4–6h. *Children <20 kg:* 50 mg/kg/day in divided doses q6h.

IM/IV: Adults, elderly, children >40 kg: 250–500 mg q4–6h. *Children <40 kg:* 50 mg/kg/day in divided doses q6h.

Lower respiratory tract, disseminated infections, serious infections:
Oral: Adults, elderly: 1 g q4–6h. *Children:* 100 mg/kg/day in divided doses q4–6h.

IM/IV: Adults, elderly, children >40 kg: 1 g q4–6h. *Maximum:* 12 g/day. *Children <40 kg:* 100 mg/kg/day in divided doses q4–6h. *Maximum:* 300 mg/kg/day.

Usual dosage (neonates):
IM/IV: Neonates 0–7 days: 50–75 mg/kg/day in 2–3 divided doses. *Neonates 7–28 days:* 100–150 mg/kg/day in 3–4 divided doses.

CONTRAINDICATIONS

Hypersensitivity to any penicillin.

CAUTIONS

History of allergies, especially cephalosporins.

INTERACTIONS

DRUG: *Probenecid* may increase concentration, toxicity risk. **HERBAL:** None known. **FOOD:** None significant. **ALTERED LAB VALUES:** May increase SGOT (AST). May cause positive Coombs' test.

SIDE EFFECTS

FREQUENT: Mild hypersensitivity reaction (fever, rash, pruritus), GI effects (nausea, vomiting, diarrhea) more frequent w/oral administration. **OCCASIONAL:** Phlebitis, thrombophlebitis (more common in elderly), hepatotoxicity w/high IV dosage.

ADVERSE REACTIONS/TOXIC EFFECTS

Superinfections, antibiotic-associated colitis may result from altered bacteria balance; hypersensitivity reaction ranging from mild to severe may occur in those allergic to penicillin.

PATIENT CONSIDERATIONS

Baseline Assessment

Question for history of allergies, especially penicillins, cephalosporins. Obtain specimen for culture and sensitivity before giving first dose (therapy may begin before results are known).

Intervention/Evaluation

Hold medication and promptly report rash (possible hypersensitivity) or diarrhea (w/fever, abdominal pain, blood and mucus in stool may indicate antibiotic-associated colitis). Assess food tolerance. Evaluate IV site frequently for phlebitis (heat, pain, red streaking over vein). Monitor I&O, urinalysis, renal function tests. Be alert for superinfection: vomiting, diarrhea, black/hairy tongue, ulceration/changes of oral mucosa, anal/genital pruritus. Check hematology reports (especially WBCs), periodic renal or hepatic reports in prolonged therapy.

Patient/Family Teaching

Continue antibiotic for full length of treatment. Space doses evenly. Discomfort may occur

w/IM injection. Notify physician in event of diarrhea, rash, or other new symptom.

oxaprozin

ox-ah-**pro**-zin
(Daypro)

CANADIAN AVAILABILITY
Daypro

PREGNANCY CATEGORY C
(D if used in third trimester or near delivery)

CLASSIFICATION

Nonsteroidal anti-inflammatory

AVAILABILITY (Rx)

Tablets: 600 mg

PHARMACOKINETICS

Absorption: Well absorbed from GI tract. Widely distributed. **Metabolism:** Metabolized in liver. **Excretion:** Primarily excreted in urine; partially eliminated in feces. **Half-life:** 42–50 hrs.

ACTION/*THERAPEUTIC EFFECT*

Produces analgesic and anti-inflammatory effect by inhibiting prostaglandin synthesis, *reducing inflammatory response and intensity of pain stimulus reaching sensory nerve endings.*

USES

Acute and chronic treatment of osteoarthritis, rheumatoid arthritis.

ADMINISTRATION

ORAL:

- May give w/food, milk, or antacids if GI distress occurs.

INDICATIONS/ROUTES/DOSAGE

Osteoarthritis:
Oral: Adults, elderly: 1,200 mg once daily; 600 mg in pts w/low body weight, mild disease. *Maximum:* 1,800 mg/day.

Rheumatoid arthritis:
Oral: Adults, elderly: 1,200 mg once daily. *Range:* 600–1,800 mg/day.

CONTRAINDICATIONS

Active peptic ulcer, GI ulceration, chronic inflammation of GI tract, GI bleeding disorders, history of hypersensitivity to aspirin or NSAIDs.

CAUTIONS

Impaired renal/hepatic function, history of GI tract disease, predisposition to fluid retention.

INTERACTIONS

DRUG: May increase effects of ***oral anticoagulants, heparin, thrombolytics.*** May decrease effect of ***antihypertensives, diuretics. Salicylates, aspirin*** may increase risk of GI side effects, bleeding. ***Bone marrow depressants*** may increase risk of hematologic reactions. May increase concentration, toxicity of ***lithium.*** May increase ***methotrexate*** toxicity. ***Probenecid*** may increase concentration. **HERBAL:** May decrease effects of feverfew. Ginkgo biloba may increase risk of bleeding. **FOOD:** None significant. **ALTERED LAB VALUES:** May increase SGOT (AST), SGPT (ALT), serum creatinine, BUN.

SIDE EFFECTS

FREQUENT (3–9%): Rash, constipation, diarrhea, nausea, indigestion. **OCCASIONAL (1–3%):** Confusion, ringing in ears, insomnia, abdominal cramps, decreased appetite. **RARE (<1%):** Increased blood pressure, hives, itching, bruising, blurred vision, stomatitis, decreased hearing.

ADVERSE REACTIONS/TOXIC EFFECTS

GI bleeding, coma may occur. Hypertension, acute renal failure, respiratory depression occur rarely.

PATIENT CONSIDERATIONS

Baseline Assessment

Assess onset, type, location, and duration of pain or inflammation.

Intervention/Evaluation

Assist w/ambulation if dizziness occurs. Monitor stools; avoid constipation through high-fiber diet, appropriate exercise, and increased fluids. Check for rash. Evaluate for therapeutic response: relief of pain, stiffness, swelling, increase in joint mobility, reduced joint tenderness, improved grip strength.

Patient/Family Teaching

Avoid aspirin, alcohol during therapy (increases risk of GI bleeding). Report tarry stools. If GI upset occurs, take w/food, milk. Avoid tasks that require alertness, motor skills until response to drug is established.

---

oxazepam

ox-**az**-eh-pam
(Serax)

CANADIAN AVAILABILITY
Apo-Oxazepam, Serax

PREGNANCY CATEGORY D

CLASSIFICATION

Antianxiety: Benzodiazepine

AVAILABILITY (Rx)

Capsules: 10 mg, 15 mg, 30 mg. **Tablets:** 15 mg.

PHARMACOKINETICS

Absorption: Well absorbed from GI tract. **Metabolism:** Metabolized in liver. **Excretion:** Primarily excreted in urine. **Half-life:** 5–15 hrs.

ACTION/*THERAPEUTIC EFFECT*

Enhances inhibitory gamma-aminobutyric acid (GABA) neurotransmission at CNS, *producing anxiolytic effect.* Inhibits spinal afferent pathways, *producing skeletal muscle relaxation.* Depressant effects occur at all levels of CNS. Directly depresses motor nerve, muscle function.

USES

Management of acute alcohol withdrawal symptoms (tremulousness, anxiety on withdrawal). Treatment of anxiety associated w/depressive symptoms.

ADMINISTRATION

ORAL:

- Give w/o regard to meals.
- Capsules may be emptied and mixed w/food.

INDICATIONS/ROUTES/DOSAGE

Note: Use smallest effective dose in elderly, debilitated, those w/liver disease, low serum albumin.

Mild to moderate anxiety:
Oral: Adults: 10–15 mg 3–4 times/day.

Severe anxiety:
Oral: Adults: 15–30 mg 3–4 times/day.

Alcohol withdrawal:
Oral: Adults: 15–30 mg 3–4 times/day.

Usual elderly dosage:
Oral: Initially, 10 mg 2–3 times/day. May gradually increase up to 30–45 mg/day.

CONTRAINDICATIONS

Acute narrow-angle glaucoma.

CAUTIONS

Impaired renal/hepatic function.

INTERACTIONS

DRUG: Potentiated effects when used w/other *CNS depressants,* including *alcohol.* HERBAL: Kava kava, valerian may increase effects of CNS depression. FOOD: None significant. ALTERED LAB VALUES: May produce abnormal renal function tests, elevate SGOT (AST), SGPT (ALT), LDH, alkaline phosphatase, serum bilirubin.

SIDE EFFECTS

FREQUENT: Mild, transient drowsiness at beginning of therapy. OCCASIONAL: Dizziness, headache. RARE: Paradoxical CNS hyperactivity/nervousness in children, excitement/restlessness in elderly/debilitated (generally noted during first 2 wks of therapy, particularly noted in presence of uncontrolled pain).

ADVERSE REACTIONS/TOXIC EFFECTS

Abrupt or too rapid withdrawal may result in pronounced restlessness, irritability, insomnia, hand tremors, abdominal/muscle cramps, sweating, vomiting, seizures. Overdose results in somnolence, confusion, diminished reflexes, coma.

PATIENT CONSIDERATIONS

Baseline Assessment

Offer emotional support to anxious pt. Assess motor responses (agitation, trembling, tension) and autonomic responses (cold, clammy hands, sweating).

Intervention/Evaluation

For those on long-term therapy, liver/renal function tests, blood counts should be performed periodically. Assess for paradoxical reaction, particularly during early therapy. Assist w/ambulation if drowsiness, lightheadedness occur. Evaluate for therapeutic response: a calm facial expression, decreased restlessness, and/or insomnia.

Patient/Family Teaching

Drowsiness usually disappears during continued therapy. If dizziness occurs, change positions slowly from recumbent to sitting position before standing. Avoid tasks that require alertness, motor skills until response to drug is established. Smoking reduces drug effectiveness. Do not abruptly withdraw medication after long-term therapy.

---

oxcarbazepine

(Trileptal)

See Supplement

---

oxiconazole

(Oxistat)

See Classification section under: Antifungals: topical

---

oxybutynin chloride

ox-ee-**byoo**-tih-nin

(Ditropan)

CANADIAN AVAILABILITY

Ditropan

PREGNANCY CATEGORY B

CLASSIFICATION

Antispasmodic

AVAILABILITY (Rx)

Tablets: 5 mg. **Syrup:** 5 mg/5 ml. **Extended-Release Tablets:** 5 mg, 10 mg, 15 mg.

PHARMACODYNAMICS

	ONSET	PEAK	DURATION
Oral	0.5–1 hr	3–6 hrs	6–10 hrs

PHARMACOKINETICS

Absorption: Rapid absorption from GI tract. **Metabolism:** Metabolized in liver. **Excretion:** Primarily excreted in urine. **Half-life:** 1–2.3 hrs.

ACTION/*THERAPEUTIC EFFECT*

Exerts antispasmodic (papaverinelike) and antimuscarinic (atropinelike) action on detrusor smooth muscle of bladder. *Increases bladder capacity, diminishes frequency of uninhibited detrusor muscle contraction, delays desire to void.*

USES

Relief of symptoms (urgency, incontinence, frequency, nocturia, urge incontinence) associated w/uninhibited neurogenic bladder or reflex neurogenic bladder.

ADMINISTRATION

ORAL:

- Give w/o regard to meals.

INDICATIONS/ROUTES/DOSAGE

Neurogenic bladder:
Oral: Adults: 5 mg 2–3 times/day. *Maximum:* 5 mg 4 times/day. *Children >5 yrs:* 5 mg 2 times/day. *Maximum:* 5 mg 3 times/day.

Usual elderly dosage:
Oral: Initially, 2.5–5 mg/day. May increase by 2.5 mg q1–2days.

Usual extended-release dosage:
Oral: Adults, elderly: 5–30 mg/day as single daily dose.

CONTRAINDICATIONS

Angle-closure glaucoma, GI obstruction, myasthenia gravis, paralytic ileus, megacolon, ulcerative colitis, intestinal atony, unstable cardiovascular disease.

CAUTIONS

Impaired renal or hepatic function, elderly, autonomic neuropathy.

INTERACTIONS

DRUG: Medication w/***anticholinergic*** effects (e.g., ***antihistamines***) may increase effects. **HERBAL:** None known. **FOOD:** None significant. **ALTERED LAB VALUES:** None significant.

SIDE EFFECTS

FREQUENT: Constipation, dry mouth, drowsiness, decreased sweating. **OCCASIONAL:** Decreased lacrimation, salivary/sweat gland secretion, sexual ability. Urinary hesitancy/retention, suppressed lactation, blurred vision, mydriasis, nausea or vomiting, insomnia.

ADVERSE REACTIONS/TOXIC EFFECTS

Overdosage produces CNS excitation (nervousness, restlessness, hallucinations, irritability), hypo/hypertension, confusion, fast heartbeat or tachycardia, flushed or red face, respiratory depression (shortness of breath or troubled breathing).

PATIENT CONSIDERATIONS

INTERVENTION/EVALUATION

Assess pulse periodically. Monitor I&O; palpate bladder for retention. Monitor stools; avoid consti-

pation w/fluids, bulk, and exercise. Hold medication and notify physician of diarrhea at once.

PATIENT/FAMILY TEACHING

May cause dry mouth. Avoid alcohol and sedatives. Report diarrhea promptly (may be early symptom of incomplete intestinal obstruction, especially those w/ileostomy or colostomy). Do not take medication in high environmental temperature (heat prostration may occur due to decreased sweating). Avoid tasks that require alertness, motor skills until response to drug is established.

oxycodone

ox-ih-**koe**-doan
(Oxycontin, Perolone, Roxicodone)

FIXED-COMBINATION(S)
W/acetaminophen **(Percocet, Roxicet, Tylox)**; w/aspirin **(Percodan, Roxiprin)**

CANADIAN AVAILABILITY
Oxy Contin, Supeudol

PREGNANCY CATEGORY B
(D if used for prolonged periods or in high doses at term)

CLASSIFICATION

Opioid analgesic **(Schedule II)**

AVAILABILITY (Rx)

Tablets: 5 mg. **Tablets (controlled-release):** 10 mg, 20 mg, 40 mg, 80 mg, 160 mg. **Oral Solution:** 5 mg/5 ml. **Oral Concentrate:** 20 mg/ml.

PHARMACODYNAMICS

	ONSET	PEAK	DURATION
Oral	10–15 min	30–60 min	3–6 hrs

PHARMACOKINETICS

Absorption: Moderately absorbed from GI tract. Widely distributed. **Metabolism:** Metabolized in liver. **Excretion:** Excreted in urine. **Half-life:** 2–3 hrs.

ACTION/*THERAPEUTIC EFFECT*

Binds w/opioid receptors within CNS, *altering processes affecting pain perception, emotional response to pain.*

USES

Relief of mild to moderately severe pain.

ADMINISTRATION

ORAL:
- Give w/o regard to meals.
- Tablets may be crushed.
- *Controlled-Release:* Swallow whole; do not crush, break, chew.

INDICATIONS/ROUTES/DOSAGE

Note: Reduce initial dosage in those w/hypothyroidism, concurrent CNS depressants, Addison's disease, renal insufficiency, elderly/debilitated.

Analgesia:
Oral: Adults: 5 mg q6h as needed. *Elderly:* 2.5–5 mg q6h as needed. *Controlled-Release:* 10–30 mg q12h.

CONTRAINDICATIONS

None significant.

EXTREME CAUTION

CNS depression, anoxia, hypercapnia, respiratory depression, seizures, acute alcoholism, shock, untreated myxedema, respiratory dysfunction.

CAUTIONS

Increased intracranial pressure, impaired hepatic function, acute abdominal conditions, hypothyroidism, prostatic hypertrophy, Addison's disease, urethral stricture, COPD.

INTERACTIONS

DRUG: *Alcohol, CNS depressants* may increase CNS or respiratory depression, hypotension. ***MAO inhibitors*** may produce severe, fatal reaction (reduce dose to $^1/_4$ usual dose). **HERBAL:** None known. **FOOD:** None significant. **ALTERED LAB VALUES:** May increase amylase, lipase.

SIDE EFFECTS

Note: Effects are dependent on dosage amount. Ambulatory pts and those not in severe pain may experience dizziness, nausea, vomiting, hypotension more frequently than those in supine position or having severe pain. **FREQUENT:** Dizziness, drowsiness, hypotension, nausea, vomiting, unusually tired. **OCCASIONAL:** Histamine reaction (decreased blood pressure, increased sweating, flushing, wheezing), decreased urination, constipation, dry mouth, headache, nervousness. **RARE:** Allergic reactions (rash, hives), trouble breathing, shortness of breath, confusion, paralytic ileus, ringing in ears, inability to sleep.

ADVERSE REACTIONS/TOXIC EFFECTS

Overdose results in respiratory depression, skeletal muscle flaccidity, cold, clammy skin, cyanosis, extreme somnolence progressing to convulsions, stupor, coma. Hepatotoxicity may occur w/overdosage of acetaminophen component. Tolerance to analgesic effect, physical dependence may occur w/repeated use.

PATIENT CONSIDERATIONS

BASELINE ASSESSMENT

Assess onset, type, location, and duration of pain. Effect of medication is reduced if full pain recurs before next dose. Obtain vital signs before giving medication. If respirations are 12/min or lower (20/min or lower in children), withhold medication, contact physician.

INTERVENTION/EVALUATION

Palpate bladder for urinary retention. Monitor pattern of daily bowel activity and stool consistency. Initiate deep breathing and coughing exercises, particularly in those w/impaired pulmonary function. Assess for clinical improvement and record onset of relief of pain.

PATIENT/FAMILY TEACHING

Change positions slowly to avoid orthostatic hypotension. Avoid tasks that require alertness, motor skills until response to drug is established. Tolerance/dependence may occur w/prolonged use of high doses. Avoid alcohol and CNS depressants.

---

oxytocin

ox-ih-**toe**-sin
(Pitocin)

CLASSIFICATION

Oxytocic

AVAILABILITY (Rx)

Injection: 10 units/ml. **Nasal Spray:** 40 units/ml.

PHARMACODYNAMICS

	ONSET	PEAK	DURATION
IM	3–5 min	—	2–3 hrs
IV	Immediate	—	1 hr
Intranasal			
	Few minutes	—	20 min

PHARMACOKINETICS

Absorption: Rapidly absorbed through nasal mucous membranes. Distributed in extracellular fluid. **Metabolism:** Metabolized in liver, kidney. **Excretion:** Primarily excreted in urine.

ACTION / *THERAPEUTIC EFFECT*

Acts on uterine myofibril activity, *stimulates contraction of uterine smooth muscle* (augments number of contracting myofibrils). Stimulates mammary smooth muscle to *enhance milk ejection from breasts.*

USES

Parenteral (Antepartum): To initiate or improve uterine contraction to achieve early vaginal delivery; stimulate or reinforce labor; management of incomplete or inevitable abortion. ***(Postpartum):*** To produce uterine contractions during third stage of labor; control uterine bleeding. ***Nasal:*** To promote breast milk ejection.

ADMINISTRATION

IV:

- Requires qualified personnel, hospitalization w/availability of surgical facilities and intensive care.
- Continuous monitoring of uterine contractions, fetal and maternal heart rates, maternal B/P, and, if possible, intrauterine pressure.
- Dilute 10 units (1 ml) in 1,000 ml of 0.9% NaCl, lactated Ringer's, or 5% dextrose injection to provide a concentration of 10 milliunits/ml solution.
- Give by IV infusion (use infusion device to carefully control rate of flow).

NASAL SPRAY:

- W/pt in sitting position, spray in one or both nostrils.
- Give 2–3 min before nursing or pumping breasts.

INDICATIONS / ROUTES / DOSAGE

Induction/stimulation of labor:
IV Infusion: Adults: Initially, 1–2 milliunits/min; gradually increase in increments of 1–2 milliunits/min q15–30min (until contraction pattern similar to spontaneous labor reached). ***Maximum:*** Rarely >20 milliunits/min.

Incomplete/inevitable abortion:
IV Infusion: Adults: 10 units in 500 ml (20 milliunits/ml) 5% dextrose in water or 0.9% NaCl infused at 10–20 milliunits/min.

Control of postpartum bleeding:
IV Infusion: Adults: 10–40 units (maximum: 40 units/1,000 ml) infused at rate of 20–40 milliunits/min after delivery of infant.

IM: Adults: 10 units after delivery of placenta.

Promotion of milk ejection:
Nasal: Adults: 1 spray to one or both nostrils 2–3 min before nursing or pumping breasts.

CONTRAINDICATIONS

Hypersensitivity to oxytocin, cephalopelvic disproportion, unfavorable fetal position or presentation, unengaged fetal head, fetal distress w/o imminent delivery, prematurity, when vaginal delivery is contraindicated (e.g., active genital herpes infection, placenta previa, cord presentation), obstetric emergencies that favor surgical intervention, grand multiparity, hypertonic or hyperactive uterus, adequate uterine activity that fails to progress. Nasal spray during pregnancy.

CAUTIONS

Induction should be for medical, not elective reasons.

INTERACTIONS

DRUG: *Caudal block anesthetics, vasopressors* may increase pressor effects. *Other oxytocics* may cause uterine hypertonus, uterine rupture, or cervical lacerations. **HERBAL:** Ma Huang (Ephedra) may cause hypertension. **FOOD:** None significant. **ALTERED LAB VALUES:** None significant.

SIDE EFFECTS

OCCASIONAL: Tachycardia, PVCs, hypotension, nausea, vomiting. **RARE:** Hypertonicity with tearing of uterus, increased bleeding, abruptio placenta, cervical and vaginal lacerations. ***Fetus:*** Bradycardia, CNS or brain damage, trauma due to rapid propulsion, low Apgar at 5 min, retinal hemorrhage. ***Nasal:*** Lacrimation (tearing), nasal irritation, rhinorrhea, unexpected uterine bleeding or contractions.

ADVERSE REACTIONS/TOXIC EFFECTS

Prolonged IV infusion of oxytocin w/excessive fluid volume has caused severe water intoxication w/seizures, coma, and death. Anaphylaxis that may rarely be fatal.

PATIENT CONSIDERATIONS

Baseline Assessment

Question for hypersensitivity to oxytocin. Assess baselines for TPR, B/P, and fetal heart rate. Determine frequency, duration, and strength of contractions.

Intervention/Evaluation

Monitor B/P, pulse, respirations, fetal heart rate, intrauterine pressure, contractions (duration, strength, frequency) q15min. Notify physician of contractions that last >1 min, occur more frequently than every 2 min, or stop. Maintain careful I/O; be alert to potential water intoxication. Check for blood loss.

Patient/Family Teaching

Keep pt, family informed of labor progress.

Nasal spray
Teach proper use.

paclitaxel

(Paxene, Taxol)

See Classification section under: Cancer chemotherapy

palivizumab

pal-ih-**vih**-zoo-mab

(Synagis)

PREGNANCY CATEGORY C

CLASSIFICATION

Monoclonal antibody: immunization agent

AVAILABILITY (Rx)

Injection: 100 mg vials

PHARMACOKINETICS

Half-life: 20 days (children <24 mos).

ACTION/*THERAPEUTIC EFFECT*

Exhibits neutralizing activity against respiratory syncytial virus (RSV) in infants, *inhibiting RSV replication in the lower respiratory tract.*

USES

Prevention of serious lower respiratory tract disease caused by respiratory syncytial virus in infants and children w/bronchopulmonary dysplasia (BPD) and infants w/history of premature birth.

ADMINISTRATION

IM:

- Add 1 ml sterile water for injection to 100 mg vial.
- Swirl vial for 30 sec (avoids foaming). *Do not shake vial.*
- Let vial stand at room temperature for minimum of 20 min before administration (allows solution to clarify).
- Administer in lateral aspect of thigh (do not use gluteal muscle).

INDICATIONS/ROUTES/DOSAGES

Prevention of respiratory syncytial virus (RSV):

IM: Pediatric: 15 mg/kg. Give monthly doses throughout RSV season using following calculation: Dose per month = (pt weight (kg) × 15 mg/kg ÷ 100 mg/ml palivizumab.

CONTRAINDICATIONS

History of hypersensitivity to drug.

CAUTIONS

Thrombocytopenia, coagulation disorders (because of IM injection).

INTERACTIONS

DRUG: None significant. **HERBAL:** None known. **FOOD:** None significant. **ALTERED LAB VALUES:** May increase AST (SGPT).

SIDE EFFECTS

FREQUENT (20–50%): Upper respiratory tract infection, otitis media, rhinitis, rash. **OCCASIONAL (2–10%):** Pain, hernia, pharyngitis. **RARE (<2%):** Cough, diarrhea, vomiting, injection site reaction, flu syndrome.

ADVERSE REACTIONS/TOXIC EFFECTS

None significant.

PATIENT CONSIDERATIONS

None significant.

P

pamidronate disodium

pam-ih-**drow**-nate
(Aredia)

CANADIAN AVAILABILITY
Aredia

PREGNANCY CATEGORY C

CLASSIFICATION

Hypocalcemic

AVAILABILITY (Rx)

Powder for Injection: 30 mg, 60 mg, 90 mg

PHARMACOKINETICS

Absorption: After IV administration, rapidly absorbed by bone. **Excretion:** Slowly excreted unchanged in urine.

ACTION/*THERAPEUTIC EFFECT*

Decreases release of phosphates, calcium from bone and increases renal excretion as parathyroid levels (usually suppressed in hypercalcemia in malignancy) return to normal levels. *Inhibits accelerated bone resorption* (bone formation and mineralization not inhibited).

USES

Treatment of moderate to severe hypercalcemia associated w/malignancy (w/o or w/bone metastases). Treatment of moderate to severe Paget's disease, osteolytic bone lesions of multiple myeloma, breast cancer.

STORAGE/HANDLING

Store parenteral form at room temperature. Reconstituted vials stable for 24 hrs refrigerated; IV solution stable for 24 hrs after dilution.

ADMINISTRATION

IV:

- Adequate hydration is essential in conjunction w/pamidronate therapy (avoid overhydration in pts w/potential for cardiac failure).
- Reconstitute each 30 mg vial w/10 ml sterile water for injection to provide concentration of 3 mg/ml.
- Allow drug to dissolve before withdrawing.
- Further dilute w/1,000 ml sterile 0.45% or 0.9% NaCl or 5% dextrose.
- Do not mix w/Ringer's solution or other calcium-containing solutions.

INDICATIONS/ROUTES/DOSAGE

Hypercalcemia:
IV Infusion: Adults, elderly: **Moderate (corrected serum calcium 12–13.5 mg/dl):** 60 mg over 4–24 hrs. **Severe (corrected serum calcium >13.5 mg/dl):** 90 mg over 24 hrs.

Paget's disease
IV Infusion: Adults, elderly: 30 mg/day for 3 days. Infuse over 4 hrs.

Osteolytic bone lesion:
IV Infusion: Adults, elderly: 90 mg over 4 hrs every mo.

Osteolytic bone metastasis breast cancer:
IV Infusion: Adults, elderly: 90 mg over 2 hrs every 3–4 wks.

CONTRAINDICATIONS

Hypersensitivity to biphosphonates.

CAUTIONS

Safety and efficacy in children not established. Cardiac failure, renal function impairment.

INTERACTIONS

DRUG: *Calcium-containing medications, vitamin D* may antagonize effects in treatment of hypercalcemia. **HERBAL:** None known. **FOOD:** None significant. **ALTERED LAB VALUES:** May decrease phosphate, potassium, magnesium, calcium levels.

SIDE EFFECTS

FREQUENT (>10%): 27% of pts have temperature elevation (at least 1° C) 24–48 hrs after administration. Drug-related redness, swelling, induration, pain at catheter site (18% of pts receiving 90 mg). Anorexia, nausea, fatigue, hypophosphatemia, hypokalemia, hypomagnesemia, hypocalcemia occur more frequently w/higher dosage. **OCCASIONAL (1–10%):** Constipation, GI hemorrhage, rales, rhinitis, anemia, hypertension, tachycardia, atrial fibrillation, somnolence occur more often w/90 mg dosages.

ADVERSE REACTIONS/TOXIC EFFECTS

None significant.

PATIENT CONSIDERATIONS

Baseline Assessment

Obtain electrolyte and CBC levels; check B/P, pulse, temperature. Assess lungs for rales, dependent parts of the body for edema.

Intervention/Evaluation

Provide adequate hydration; avoid overhydration. Monitor I&O carefully; check lungs for rales, dependent body parts for edema. Monitor B/P, temperature, pulse. Assess catheter site for redness, swelling, pain. Check electrolytes (especially calcium and potassium) and CBC results. Monitor food intake and stool frequency. Be alert for potential GI hemorrhage w/90 mg dosage.

Patient/Family Teaching

Explain the rationale for the therapy and how to assist in maintaining an accurate I&O.

pancreatin

pan-kree-**ah**-tin
(Pancreatin)

pancrelipase

pan-kree-**lie**-pace
(Cotazym, Creon, Ilozyme, Pancrease MT, Ultrase, Viokase)

CANADIAN AVAILABILITY
Cotazym, Creon, Pancrease, Ultrase, Viokase

PREGNANCY CATEGORY C

CLASSIFICATION

Digestive enzyme

AVAILABILITY (Rx)

Tablets. Capsules.

ACTION/*THERAPEUTIC EFFECT*

Aids in digestion of protein, carbohydrate, fat in GI tract (primarily in duodenum, upper jejunum).

USES

Pancreatic enzyme replacement/supplement when enzymes are absent or deficient (i.e., chronic pancreatitis, cystic fibrosis, ductal obstruction from pancreatic cancer, common bile duct). Treatment of steatorrhea associated w/postgastrectomy syndrome, bowel resection; reduces malabsorption.

ADMINISTRATION

ORAL:

- Give before or w/meals. Tablets may be crushed. Do not crush enteric-coated tablets. Instruct pt not to chew (minimizes irritation to mouth, lips, tongue).

INDICATIONS/ROUTES/DOSAGE

Usual oral dosage:
Oral: Adults, elderly: 1–3 capsules or tablets before or w/meals, snacks. May increase up to 8 tablets/dose.

CONTRAINDICATIONS

Hypersensitivity to pork protein.

CAUTIONS

None significant.

INTERACTIONS

DRUG: *Antacids* may decrease effect. May decrease absorption of *iron supplements.* HERBAL: None known. FOOD: None significant. ALTERED LAB VALUES: May increase uric acid.

SIDE EFFECTS

RARE: Allergic reaction, mouth irritation, shortness of breath, wheezing.

ADVERSE REACTIONS/TOXIC EFFECTS

Excessive dosage may produce nausea, cramping, and/or diarrhea. Hyperuricosuria, hyperuricemia reported w/extremely high doses.

PATIENT CONSIDERATIONS

Baseline Assessment

Spilling powder on hands (Viokase) may irritate skin. Inhaling powder may irritate mucous membranes, produce bronchospasm.

Intervention/Evaluation

Question for therapeutic relief from GI symptoms.

Patient/Family Teaching

Take before or w/meals. Do not change brands w/o consulting physician.

---

pancuronium bromide
(Pavulon)
See Classification section under: Neuromuscular blockers

---

pantoprazole
(Protonix)
See Supplement

---

paricalcitol

pear-ee-**kal**-cih-toll
(Zempler)

PREGNANCY CATEGORY C

CLASSIFICATION

Vitamin D analogue

AVAILABILITY (Rx)

Injection: 0.005 mg/ml (5 mcg/ml)

PHARMACOKINETICS

Highly protein bound (>99%). **Metabolism:** Extensively metabolized in the liver. **Excretion:** Eliminated primarily in the feces. **Half-life:** 14 hrs (chronic renal failure pts).

ACTION/*THERAPEUTIC EFFECT*

A vitamin D analogue, reduces parathyroid hormone levels w/only small changes in serum calcium or phosphorous. Exact mechanism unknown.

USES

Treatment and prevention of secondary hyperparathyroidism associated w/chronic renal failure.

ADMINISTRATION

IV:

- Give as IV bolus injection.

INDICATIONS/ROUTES/DOSAGES

Hyperparathyroidism:
IV bolus: Adults, elderly: 0.04 mcg/kg to 0.1 mcg/kg (2.8–7 mcg) no more than every other day at any time during dialysis. May increase by 2–4 mcg increments at 2–4 wk intervals.

CONTRAINDICATIONS

History of hypersensitivity to paricalcitol. Hypercalcemia.

CAUTIONS

Children, pregnancy, breast-feeding, hypervitaminosis D.

INTERACTIONS

DRUG: *Vitamin D, phosphate salts* may increase effect, toxicity. *Calcium-containing antacids, thiazide diuretics* may cause hypercalcemia. Use of *magnesium-containing antacids* w/paricalcitol may increase serum magnesium levels. **HERBAL:** None known. **FOOD:** None significant. **ALTERED LAB VALUES:** May increase serum calcium, phosphorous levels.

SIDE EFFECTS

FREQUENT (10–19%): Headache, somnolence/drowsiness, dizziness. **OCCASIONAL (3–9%):** Constipation, postural hypotension, tachycardia, dry mouth, dyspepsia, rash, weakness, abdominal pain, rhinitis. **RARE (2%):** Back pain, fever, weight gain.

ADVERSE REACTIONS/TOXIC EFFECTS

Overdosage produces fatigue, weakness, drowsiness, confusion, dehydration, nausea, vomiting, headache, constipation, metallic taste, bone pain, dry mouth. Later effects include anorexia, weight loss, somnolence, cardiac arrhythmias.

PATIENT CONSIDERATIONS

BASELINE ASSESSMENT

Assess baseline calcium, phosphorous, parathyroid (PTH) levels.

INTERVENTION/EVALUATION

Monitor PTH, calcium phosphorous levels.

PATIENT/FAMILY TEACHING

Avoid vitamin D–related compounds while taking paricalcitol. Do not take antacids or calcium supplements w/o consulting physician. Report fever, increased weakness, headache, nausea, vomiting, constipation, muscle pain, confusion, metallic taste, increased thirst, increased need to urinate.

paroxetine hydrochloride

pear-**ox**-eh-teen
(Paxil, Paxil CR)

CANADIAN AVAILABILITY
Paxil

PREGNANCY CATEGORY B

CLASSIFICATION

Antidepressant

AVAILABILITY (RX)

Tablets: 10 mg, 20 mg, 30 mg, 40 mg. **Controlled-Release Tablets:** 12.5 mg, 25 mg

PHARMACOKINETICS

Absorption: Well absorbed from GI tract. Widely distributed. **Metabolism:** Metabolized in liver. **Excretion:** Excreted in urine. **Half-life:** 24 hrs.

ACTION/*THERAPEUTIC EFFECT*

Selectively blocks uptake of neurotransmitter serotonin at CNS neuronal presynaptic membranes, thereby increasing availability at postsynaptic neuronal receptor sites. Resulting enhancement of synaptic activity *produces antidepressant effect, reduces obsessive-compulsive behavior, decreases anxiety.*

USES

Treatment of major depression exhibited as persistent, prominent dysphoria (occurring nearly every day for at least 2 wks) manifested by 4 of 8 symptoms: change in appetite, change in sleep pattern, increased fatigue, impaired concentration, feelings of guilt or worthlessness, loss of interest in usual activities, psychomotor agitation or retardation, or suicidal tendencies. Treatment of panic disorder, obsessive-compulsive disorder manifested as repetitive tasks producing marked distress, time consuming, or significantly interfering w/social or occupational behavior. Treatment of social anxiety disorder.

ADMINISTRATION

ORAL:

- Give w/food or milk if GI distress occurs.
- Scored tablet may be crushed.
- Best if given as single morning dose.

INDICATIONS/ROUTES/DOSAGE

Note: Reduce dosage in elderly, pts w/severe renal, hepatic impairment. Dose changes should occur at 1 wk intervals.

Depression:
Oral: Adults: Initially, 20 mg/day, usually in morning. Dosage may be gradually increased in 10 mg/day increments to 50 mg/day. **Extended-Release:** Initially, 12.5 mg. ***Maximum:*** 60 mg/day. ***Elderly, debilitated, those w/severe hepatic, renal impairment:*** Initially, 10 mg/day. Do not exceed maximum 40 mg/day. **Extended-Release:** Initially, 12.5 mg. ***Maximum:*** 50 mg/day.

Panic disorder:
Oral: Adults: Initially, 10 mg/day; increase 10 mg/day at intervals of at least 1 wk up to 40 mg/day. ***Maximum:*** 60 mg/day. ***Elderly:*** Initially 10 mg/day. ***Maximum:*** 40 mg/day.

Obsessive-compulsive disorder:
Oral: Adults: Initially, 20 mg/day; increase 10 mg/day at intervals of at least 1 wk. ***Elderly:*** Initially, 10 mg/day. ***Maximum:*** 40 mg/day.

Social anxiety disorder:
Oral: Adults: 20 mg/day.

CONTRAINDICATIONS

Within 14 days of MAO inhibitor therapy.

CAUTIONS

Severe renal, hepatic impairment. History of mania, seizures, those w/metabolic or hemodynamic disease, history of drug abuse.

INTERACTIONS

DRUG: ***MAO inhibitors*** may cause serotonergic syndrome (excitement, diaphoresis, rigidity, hyperthermia, autonomic hyperactivity, coma). ***Cimetidine*** may increase concentrations; ***phenytoin*** may decrease concentrations. **HERBAL:** St. John's wort may increase adverse effects (e.g., nausea, weakness). **FOOD:** None significant. **ALTERED LAB VALUES:** May increase liver enzymes. May decrease Hb, Hct, WBC.

SIDE EFFECTS

FREQUENT: Nausea (26%), somnolence (23%), headache, dry mouth (18%), weakness (15%), constipation (15%), dizziness, insomnia (13%), diarrhea (12%), excessive sweating (11%), tremor (8%). **OCCASIONAL:** Decreased appetite, respiratory disturbance (6%), anxiety, nervousness (5%), flatulence, paresthesia, yawning (4%), decreased libido/sexual dysfunction, abdominal discomfort (3%). **RARE:** Palpitations, vomiting, blurred vision, taste change, confusion.

ADVERSE REACTIONS/TOXIC EFFECTS

None significant.

PATIENT CONSIDERATIONS

Baseline Assessment

Assess appearance, behavior, speech pattern, level of interest, mood. Assess for history of drug abuse.

Intervention/Evaluation

For those on long-term therapy, liver/renal function tests, blood counts should be performed periodically. Supervise suicidal risk pt closely during early therapy (as depression lessens, energy level improves, increasing suicide potential). Assess appearance, behavior, speech pattern, level of interest, mood.

Patient/Family Teaching

Therapeutic effect may be noted within 1–4 wks. Dry mouth may be relieved by sugarless gum, sips of tepid water. Do not abruptly discontinue medication. Avoid tasks that require alertness, motor skills until response to drug is established. Inform physician of intention of pregnancy or if pregnancy occurs. Avoid alcohol.

---

pegasparagase

(Oncaspar)

See Classification section under: Cancer chemotherapy

---

pemirolast

(Alamast)

See Supplement

---

pemoline

pem-oh-leen
(Cylert)

CANADIAN AVAILABILITY
Cylert

PREGNANCY CATEGORY B

CLASSIFICATION

CNS stimulant

AVAILABILITY (Rx)

Tablets: 18.75 mg, 37.5 mg, 75 mg. **Tablets (chewable):** 37.5 mg.

PHARMACODYNAMICS

	ONSET	PEAK	DURATION
Oral (adults)			
	Gradual	4 hrs	8 hrs
Oral (children)			
	Gradual	—	—

PHARMACOKINETICS

Absorption: Readily absorbed from GI tract. **Metabolism:** Metabolized in liver. **Excretion:** Primarily excreted in urine. **Half-life:** 12 hrs.

ACTION/*THERAPEUTIC EFFECT*

Appears to act through dopaminergic receptor sites. In children, *appears to reduce motor restlessness, increases mental alertness, provides mood elevation, reduces sense of fatigue.*

USES

Treatment of attention deficit disorder in children w/moderate to severe distraction, short attention span, hyperactivity, emotional impulsiveness.

ADMINISTRATION

ORAL:

- Do not administer in afternoon or evening (to avoid insomnia).
- Tablets may be crushed.

INDICATIONS/ROUTES/DOSAGE

Attention deficit disorder:
Oral: Children >6 yrs: Initially, 37.5 mg/day given as single dose in morning. May increase by 18.75 mg at weekly intervals until therapeutic response is achieved. ***Range:*** 56.25–75 mg/day. ***Maximum:*** 112.5 mg/day.

CONTRAINDICATIONS

Impaired hepatic function, pts w/motor tics, family history of Tourette's disorder.

CAUTIONS

Impaired renal function.

INTERACTIONS

DRUG: *CNS-stimulating medications* may increase CNS stimulation. **HERBAL:** Ma Huang (Ephedra) may increase CNS stimulation. **FOOD:** None significant. **ALTERED LAB VALUES:** May increase SGOT (AST), SGPT (ALT), LDH.

SIDE EFFECTS

FREQUENT: Anorexia, insomnia. **OCCASIONAL:** Nausea, abdominal discomfort, diarrhea, headache, dizziness, drowsiness.

ADVERSE REACTIONS/TOXIC EFFECTS

Dyskinetic movements of tongue, lips, face, and extremities, and visual disturbances, rash have occurred. Large doses may produce extreme nervousness, tachycardia. Hepatic effects (hepatitis, jaundice) appear to be reversible when drug is discontinued. Prolonged administration to children w/attention deficit disorder may produce a temporary suppression of weight and/or height patterns.

PATIENT CONSIDERATIONS

BASELINE ASSESSMENT

Liver function tests should be performed before therapy begins and periodically during therapy.

PATIENT/FAMILY TEACHING

Therapeutic response to medication may take 3–4 wks. Insomnia, anorexia usually disappear during continued therapy. Anorexia usually accompanied by weight loss. Return to normal weight usually occurs within 3–6 mos.

---

penbutolol

pen-**beaut**-oh-lol
(Levatol)

PREGNANCY CATEGORY C
(D if used in second or third trimester)

CLASSIFICATION

Beta-adrenergic blocker

AVAILABILITY (Rx)

Tablets: 20 mg

PHARMACODYNAMICS

	ONSET	PEAK	DURATION
Oral	—	1 hr	24 hrs

PHARMACOKINETICS

Absorption: Completely absorbed from GI tract. **Metabolism:** Metabolized in liver. **Excretion:** Primarily excreted in urine. **Half-life:** 5 hrs (increased in decreased renal function).

ACTION / *THERAPEUTIC EFFECT*

Nonselective beta blocker. Blocks beta$_1$-adrenergic receptors, *slowing sinus heart rate, decreasing cardiac output, decreasing B/P.* Blocks beta$_2$-adrenergic receptors, *increasing airway resistance. Decreases myocardial ischemia severity* by decreasing oxygen requirements. Has moderate intrinsic sympathomimetic activity.

USES / *UNLABELED*

Treatment of mild to moderate hypertension. *Treatment of chronic angina pectoris.*

ADMINISTRATION

ORAL:

- May give w/o regard to food.
- Tablets may be crushed.

INDICATIONS/ROUTES/DOSAGE

Hypertension:

Oral: Adults: Initially, 20 mg/day as single dose. May increase to 40–80 mg/day. ***Elderly:*** Initially, 10 mg/day.

CONTRAINDICATIONS

Bronchial asthma, COPD, sinus bradycardia, heart block greater than first degree, cardiogenic shock, CHF (unless secondary to tachyarrhythmias), overt cardiac failure.

CAUTIONS

Inadequate cardiac function, impaired renal/hepatic function, diabetes mellitus, hyperthyroidism.

INTERACTIONS

DRUG: *Diuretics, other hypotensives* may increase hypotensive effect; ***sympathomimetics, xanthines*** may mutually inhibit effects; may mask symptoms of hypoglycemia, prolong hypoglycemic effect of ***insulin, oral hypoglycemics; NSAIDs*** may decrease antihypertensive effect; ***cimetidine*** may increase concentration. **HERBAL:** None known. **FOOD:** None significant. **ALTERED LAB VALUES:** May increase ANA titer, SGOT (AST), SGPT (ALT), alkaline phosphatase, LDH, bilirubin, BUN, creatinine, potassium, uric acid, lipoproteins, triglycerides.

SIDE EFFECTS

FREQUENT: Decreased sexual ability, drowsiness, trouble sleeping, unusually tired/weak. **OCCASIONAL:** Bradycardia, difficulty breathing, CHF(swelling of feet, shortness of breath), depression, cold hands/feet, diarrhea, constipation, anxiety, nasal congestion, nausea, vomiting. **RARE:** Altered taste, dry eyes, itching, numbness of fingers, toes, scalp.

ADVERSE REACTIONS/TOXIC EFFECTS

Abrupt withdrawal (particularly in those w/coronary artery disease) may produce angina or precipitate MI. May precipitate thyroid crisis in those w/thyrotoxicosis.

PATIENT CONSIDERATIONS

BASELINE ASSESSMENT

Assess baseline renal/liver function tests. Assess B/P, apical pulse immediately before drug is administered (if pulse is 60/min or below or systolic B/P is below 90 mm Hg, withhold medication, contact physician).

INTERVENTION/EVALUATION

Assess pulse for strength/weak-

ness, irregular rate, bradycardia. Monitor EKG for cardiac changes. Assist w/ambulation if dizziness occurs. Assess for peripheral edema of hands, feet (usually, first area of low extremity swelling is behind medial malleolus in ambulatory, sacral area in bedridden). Monitor pattern of daily bowel activity, stool consistency. Assess skin for development of rash. Monitor any unusual changes in pt.

PATIENT/FAMILY TEACHING

Do not abruptly discontinue medication. Compliance w/therapy regimen is essential to control hypertension. If dizziness occurs, sit or lie down immediately. Full therapeutic response may not occur for up to 2 wks. Avoid tasks that require alertness, motor skills until response to drug is established. Report excessively slow pulse rate (<60 beats/min), peripheral numbness, dizziness. Do not use nasal decongestants, OTC cold preparations (stimulants) w/o physician approval. Outpatients should monitor B/P, pulse before taking medication. Restrict salt, alcohol intake.

penciclovir

pen-**sigh**-klo-vear
(Denavir)

PREGNANCY CATEGORY B

CLASSIFICATION
Antiviral

AVAILABILITY (Rx)

Cream: 1%

PHARMACOKINETICS

Not detected in plasma or urine.

ACTION / *THERAPEUTIC EFFECT*

Inhibits antiviral activity against herpes simples virus (HSV). *DNA synthesis, and therefore HSV replication, is prevented.*

USES

Treatment of recurrent herpes labialis (cold sores).

STORAGE/HANDLING

Store at room temperature. Do not freeze.

INDICATIONS/ROUTES/DOSAGE

Note: Begin treatment as soon as possible (as soon as symptom indicating immediate onset of virus is evident or when lesions appear).

Herpes labialis (cold sores):
Topical: Adults, elderly: Apply q2h during waking hours for 4 days.

CONTRAINDICATIONS

Known hypersensitivity to product.

CAUTIONS

None significant.

INTERACTIONS

DRUG: None significant. **HERBAL:** None known. **FOOD:** None significant. **ALTERED LAB VALUES:** None significant.

SIDE EFFECTS

FREQUENT (>5%): Headache, mild erythema. **OCCASIONAL (1–5%):** Application site reaction. **RARE (<1%):** Altered taste, rash.

ADVERSE REACTIONS/TOXIC EFFECTS

None significant.

PATIENT CONSIDERATIONS

BASELINE ASSESSMENT

Use only on lips or face. Do not apply to oral mucous membranes. Avoid application in or near eyes (produces irritation).

PATIENT/FAMILY TEACHING

Observe precautions to avoid exposure of cold sores to direct sunlight.

penicillamine

pen-ih-**sill**-ah-mine
(Cuprimine, Depen)

CANADIAN AVAILABILITY
Cuprimine, Depen

PREGNANCY CATEGORY D

CLASSIFICATION

Chelating agent, anti-inflammatory

AVAILABILITY (Rx)

Capsules: 125 mg, 250 mg. **Tablets:** 250 mg.

PHARMACOKINETICS

Absorption: Well absorbed from GI tract. **Metabolism:** Metabolized in liver. **Excretion:** Primarily excreted in urine. **Half-life:** 1.7–3.2 hrs.

ACTION/*THERAPEUTIC EFFECT*

Chelates copper, iron, mercury, lead to form complexes, *promoting excretion of copper.* Combines with cystine-forming complex, thus reducing concentration of cystine to below levels for formation of cystine stones. *Prevents renal calculi. May dissolve existing stones.* ***Rheumatoid arthritis:*** Exact mechanism unknown. May decrease cell-mediated immune response; *acts as anti-inflammatory drug;* may inhibit collagen formation.

USES/*UNLABELED*

Promotes excretion of copper in treatment of Wilson's disease; decreases excretion of cystine, prevents renal calculi in cystinuria associated w/nephrolithiasis; treatment of active rheumatoid arthritis not controlled w/conventional therapy. *Treatment of rheumatoid vasculitis, heavy metal toxicity.*

ADMINISTRATION

ORAL:

- Preferably give on empty stomach (1 hr before or 2 hrs after meals) or at least 1 hr from any drug, food, or milk.
- Take w/large amounts of water when treating cystinuria.
- Largest single dose is 500 mg; give larger amounts in divided doses.
- Tablets may be crushed; do not crush or break capsules.

INDICATIONS/ROUTES/DOSAGE

Wilson's disease:

Note: Base dosage on urinary copper excretion, serum-free copper concentration that produces/maintains negative copper balance. Give w/10–40 mg sulfurated potash at each meal for 6–12 mos.

Oral: Adults, elderly, children: Initially, 250 mg 4 times/day (some pts may begin at 250 mg/day; gradually increase). Dosages of 750–1,500 mg/day that produce initial 24 hr cupruresis >2 mg should be continued for 3 mos. **Maintenance:** Based on serum-free copper concentration (<10 mcg/dl indicative of

P

adequate maintenance). ***Maximum:*** 2 g/day.

Cystinuria:
Note: Give in 4 equal doses; if not feasible, give larger dose at bedtime. Dose based on urinary cystine excretion. Maintain high fluid intake.

Oral: Adults, elderly: Initially, 250 mg/day. Gradually increase dose. ***Maintenance:*** 2 g/day. ***Range:*** 1–4 g/day. ***Children:*** 30 mg/kg/day.

Rheumatoid arthritis:
Oral: Adults, elderly: Initially, 125–250 mg/day. May increase by 125–250 mg/day at 1–3 mo intervals. ***Maintenance:*** 500–750 mg/day. After 2–3 mos w/no improvement or toxicity, may increase by 250 mg/day at 2–3 mo intervals until remission or toxicity. ***Maximum:*** 1 g up to 1.5 g/day.

CONTRAINDICATIONS

History of penicillamine-related aplastic anemia or agranulocytosis, rheumatoid arthritis pts w/history or evidence of renal insufficiency, pregnancy, breast feeding.

CAUTIONS

Elderly, debilitated, impaired renal/hepatic function, penicillin allergy.

INTERACTIONS

DRUG: ***Iron supplements, antacids*** may decrease absorption. ***Bone marrow depressants, gold compounds, immunosuppressants*** may increase risk of hematologic, renal adverse effects. **HERBAL:** None known. **FOOD:** May decrease absorption. **ALTERED LAB VALUES:** None significant.

SIDE EFFECTS

FREQUENT: Rash (pruritic, erythematous, maculopapular, morbilliform), reduced/altered sense of taste (hypogeusia), GI disturbances (anorexia, epigastric pain, nausea, vomiting, diarrhea), oral ulcers, glossitis. **OCCASIONAL:** Proteinuria, hematuria, hot flashes, drug fever. **RARE:** Alopecia, tinnitus, pemphigoid rash (water blisters).

ADVERSE REACTIONS/TOXIC EFFECTS

Aplastic anemia, agranulocytosis, thrombocytopenia, leukopenia, myasthenia gravis, bronchiolitis, erythematouslike syndrome, evening hypoglycemia, skin friability at sites of pressure/trauma producing extravasation or white papules at venipuncture, surgical sites reported. Iron deficiency (particularly children, menstruating women) may develop.

PATIENT CONSIDERATIONS

BASELINE ASSESSMENT

Baseline WBC, differential, hemoglobin, platelet count should be performed before therapy begins, every 2 wks thereafter for first 6 mos, then monthly during therapy. Liver function tests (GGT, SGOT, SGPT, LDH) and x-ray for renal stones should also be ordered. A 2 hr interval is necessary between iron and penicillamine therapy. In event of upcoming surgery, dosage should be reduced to 250 mg/day until wound healing is complete.

INTERVENTION/EVALUATION

Encourage copious amounts of water in those w/cystinuria. Monitor WBC, differential, platelet count. If WBC <3,500, neutrophils <2,000/mm^3, monocytes

>500/mm^3, or platelet counts <100,000, or if a progressive fall in either platelet count or WBC in three successive determinations noted, inform physician (drug withdrawal necessary). Assess for evidence of hematuria. Monitor urinalysis for hematuria, proteinuria (if proteinuria exceeds 1 g/24 hrs, inform physician).

PATIENT/FAMILY TEACHING

Promptly report any missed menstrual periods/other indications of pregnancy, fever, sore throat, chills, bruising, bleeding, difficulty breathing on exertion, unexplained cough or wheezing. Take medication 1 hr before or 2 hrs after meals or at least 1 hr from any other drug, food, or milk.

---

penicillin G benzathine

pen-ih-**sil**-lin G **benz**-ah-thene
(Bicillin)

FIXED-COMBINATION(S)
W/penicillin G procaine, an antibiotic (**Bicillin CR**)

CANADIAN AVAILABILITY
Bicillin

penicillin G potassium, sodium

(Pentids, Pfizerpen)

CANADIAN AVAILABILITY
Crystapen

penicillin G procaine

(Crystacillin, Duracillin, Pfizerpen, Wycillin)

FIXED-COMBINATION(S)
W/probenecid, a renal tubular blocking agent (**Wycillin & Probenecid**); w/penicillin G benzathine, an antibiotic (**Bicillin-CR**)

PREGNANCY CATEGORY B

CLASSIFICATION

Antibiotic: Penicillin

AVAILABILITY (Rx)

Benzathine: 300,000 units/ml, 600,000 units/ml

PCN-G Potassium: Powder for Injection: 1 million units, 5 million units, 10 million units, 20 million units

PCN-G Sodium: Powder for Injection: 5 million units

Procaine: 300,000 units/ml, 500,000 units/ml, 600,000 units/ml

PHARMACOKINETICS

Absorption: Slowly absorbed after IM administration. Widely distributed. **Metabolism:** Metabolized in liver. **Excretion:** Primarily excreted in urine. Moderately removed by hemodialysis. **Half-life:** 0.5–0.7 hrs (increased in decreased renal function).

ACTION/*THERAPEUTIC EFFECT*

Binds to bacterial membranes, *inhibiting cell wall synthesis. Bactericidal.*

USES

Benzathine, procaine: Mild to moderate infections of respiratory tract, skin and skin structure, rheumatic fever prophylaxis, early syphilis, yaws, bejel, pinta. Follow-up to IM/IV therapy w/penicillin G potassium, sodium. ***PCN-G:*** Treatment of infections of respiratory tract, skin and skin structure, bone and joints;

P

septicemia, meningitis, endocarditis, pericarditis, diphtheria, Listeria, clostridium, disseminated gonococcal infections, actinomycosis, rheumatic fever prophylaxis, syphilis, necrotizing ulcerative gingivitis, anthrax, Lyme disease.

STORAGE/HANDLING

Benzathine, procaine: Refrigerate. *PCN-G:* IV infusion (piggyback) is stable for 24 hrs at room temperature, 7 days if refrigerated. Discard if precipitate forms.

ADMINISTRATION

- **Note:** *Benzathine, procaine:* Do not give IV, intra-arterially, intravascularly, or SubQ. Space doses evenly around the clock.

IM:

- Give IM injection deeply into gluteus maximus or midlateral thigh.
- Do not administer if blood is aspirated; draw up new dose; select another site.
- Avoid areas of nerves, repeated IM injections into anterolateral thigh.
- Administer IM injection slowly; stop if pt complains of severe pain.

IV:

- After reconstitution, dilute w/50–100 ml 5% dextrose, 0.9% NaCl, or other compatible IV fluid. Infuse over 1–2 hrs in adults, 15–30 min in neonates, children.
- Because of potential for hypersensitivity/anaphylaxis, start initial dose at few drops/min, increase slowly to ordered rate; stay w/pt first 10–15 min, then check q10min.
- Alternating IV sites, use large veins to reduce risk of phlebitis.

INDICATIONS/ROUTES/DOSAGE

Usual parenteral dosage (benzathine):
IM: Adults, elderly: 1.2 million units one time. *Children >27 kg:* 900,000–1.2 million units one time. *Children <27 kg, infants:* 300,000–600,000 units/kg one time. *Neonates:* 50,000 units/kg one time.

Usual parenteral dosage (PCN-G):
IV: Adults, elderly: 5 million units/day minimum. *Children:* 100,000–250,000 units/kg/day in divided doses q4h. *Infants:* 50,000–100,000 units/kg/day in divided doses q6–12h.

PENICILLIN G PROCAINE:

Moderate to severe upper respiratory tract, otitis media, tonsillitis, pharyngitis, skin/skin structure infections, uncomplicated pneumonia:
IM: Adults, elderly, children: 600,000–1.2 million units/day. *Children <60 lbs:* 300,000 units/day.

Acute uncomplicated gonorrhea:
IM: Adults, elderly: 4.8 million units one time in divided doses (w/1 g probenecid 30 min before penicillin).

Syphilis:
IM: Adults, elderly: 600,000 units/day for 8 days.

Neurosyphilis:
IM: Adults, elderly: 2.4 million units/day and probenecid 500 mg 4 times/day for 10 days; follow w/penicillin G benzathine 2.4 million units weekly for 3 wks.

Congenital syphilis:
IM: Children <70 lbs, neonates: 50,000 units/kg/day for 10–14 days.

CONTRAINDICATIONS

Hypersensitivity to any penicillin.

CAUTIONS

Renal impairment, history of allergies, particularly cephalosporins, aspirin (tartrazine reaction may occur in those sensitive to aspirin).

INTERACTIONS

DRUG: *Probenecid* may increase concentration, toxicity risk. *Angiotensin-converting enzyme inhibitors, potassium-sparing diuretics, potassium supplements* may increase risk of hyperkalemia. HERBAL: None known. FOOD: None significant. ALTERED LAB VALUES: May cause positive Coombs' test.

SIDE EFFECTS

FREQUENT: GI reactions (nausea, vomiting, diarrhea). OCCASIONAL: Pain, induration at IM injection site. *PCN-G potassium, sodium:* High IV dosage may cause electrolyte imbalance, phlebitis, thrombophlebitis. RARE: Bleeding.

ADVERSE REACTIONS/TOXIC EFFECTS

Hypersensitivity reactions occur frequently, ranging from rash, fever/chills to anaphylaxis. Nephrotoxicity may occur w/high parenteral dosages, preexisting renal disease. Superinfections, potentially fatal antibiotic-associated colitis may result from altered bacterial balance. Toxic reaction to procaine (confusion, combativeness, seizures) w/large doses.

PATIENT CONSIDERATIONS

Baseline Assessment

Question for history of allergies, particularly penicillins, cephalosporins, aspirin, procaine. Obtain specimen for culture and sensitivity before giving first dose (therapy may begin before results are known).

Intervention/Evaluation

Hold medication and promptly report rash (hypersensitivity) or diarrhea (w/fever, abdominal pain, mucus and blood in stool may indicate antibiotic-associated colitis). Assess for food tolerance. Check IM injection sites for induration, tenderness. Check for wheezing, respiratory difficulty due to tartrazine sensitivity. Monitor I&O, urinalysis, renal function tests for nephrotoxicity. Be alert for superinfection: increased fever, sore throat, nausea, vomiting, diarrhea, ulceration or changes of oral mucosa, vaginal discharge, anal/genital pruritus. Evaluate hemoglobin levels and assess for signs of bleeding: overt bleeding, bruising/swelling of tissue.

Patient/Family Teaching

Continue antibiotic for full length of treatment. Space doses evenly. Discomfort may occur w/IM injection. Notify physician in event of rash, diarrhea, bleeding, bruising, other new symptom. Sodium content of penicillin G sodium must be considered for those on sodium-restricted diets.

penicillin V potassium

(Pen Vee K, V-Cillin-K, Veetids)

CANADIAN AVAILABILITY

Apo-Pen VK, Nadopen-V, Novopen VK

PREGNANCY CATEGORY B

CLASSIFICATION

Antibiotic: Penicillin

AVAILABILITY (RX)

Tablets: 125 mg, 250 mg, 500 mg. **Powder for Oral Solution:** 125 mg/5 ml, 250 mg/5 ml.

PHARMACOKINETICS

Absorption: Moderately absorbed from GI tract. Widely distributed. **Metabolism:** Metabolized in liver. **Excretion:** Primarily excreted in urine. **Half-life:** 1 hr (increased in decreased renal function).

ACTION/*THERAPEUTIC EFFECT*

Binds to bacterial membranes, *inhibiting cell wall synthesis. Bactericidal.*

USES

Treatment of mild to moderate infections of respiratory tract and skin/skin structure, otitis media, necrotizing ulcerative gingivitis, prophylaxis for rheumatic fever, dental procedures.

STORAGE/HANDLING

Store tablets at room temperature. Oral solution, after reconstitution, is stable for 14 days if refrigerated.

ADMINISTRATION

ORAL:

- Space doses evenly around the clock.
- Give w/o regard to meals.

INDICATIONS/ROUTES/DOSAGE

Usual adult, elderly dosage
Oral: 125–500 mg 4 times/day.

Usual children's dosage
Oral: 15–50 mg/kg/day in divided doses q6–8h.

CONTRAINDICATIONS

Hypersensitivity to any penicillin.

CAUTIONS

Renal impairment, history of allergies, particularly cephalosporins, aspirin.

INTERACTIONS

DRUG: *Probenecid* may increase concentration, toxicity risk. **HERBAL:** None known. **FOOD:** None significant. **ALTERED LAB VALUES:** May cause positive Coombs' test.

SIDE EFFECTS

FREQUENT: Mild hypersensitivity reaction (rash, fever/chills), nausea, vomiting, diarrhea. RARE: Bleeding, allergic reactions.

ADVERSE REACTIONS/TOXIC EFFECTS

Severe hypersensitivity reaction, including anaphylaxis, may occur. Nephrotoxicity, superinfections (including potentially fatal antibiotic-associated colitis) may result from high dosages, prolonged therapy.

PATIENT CONSIDERATIONS

BASELINE ASSESSMENT

Question for history of allergies, particularly penicillins, cephalosporins. Obtain specimen for culture and sensitivity before giving first dose (therapy may begin before results are known).

INTERVENTION/EVALUATION

Hold medication and promptly report rash (hypersensitivity) or diarrhea (w/fever, abdominal pain, mucus and blood in stool may indicate antibiotic-associated colitis). Assess food tolerance. Monitor I&O, urinalysis, renal function tests for nephrotoxicity. Be alert for superinfection: increased fever, sore throat, nausea, vomiting, diarrhea, ulceration or changes of oral mucosa, vaginal discharge, anal/genital pruritus. Review hemoglobin levels; check for bleeding: overt bleeding, bruising or swelling of tissue.

PATIENT/FAMILY TEACHING

Continue antibiotic for full length of treatment. Space doses evenly. Notify physician immediately in event of rash, diarrhea, bleeding, bruising, or other new symptom.

pentaerythritol tetranitrate (P.E.T.N.)

(Duotrate, Peritrate)

See Classification section under: Nitrates

pentamidine isethionate

pen-**tam**-ih-deen

(NebuPent, Pentam-300)

CANADIAN AVAILABILITY

Pentacarinat

PREGNANCY CATEGORY C

CLASSIFICATION

Anti-infective

AVAILABILITY (Rx)

Injection: 300 mg. **Aerosol:** 300 mg.

PHARMACOKINETICS

Absorption: Minimal absorption following inhalation, well absorbed after IM administration. Widely distributed. **Excretion:** Primarily excreted in urine. Minimally removed by hemodialysis. **Half-life:** 6.5 hrs (increased in decreased renal function).

ACTION/*THERAPEUTIC EFFECT*

Exact mechanism unknown. May interfere w/incorporation of nucleotides; *inhibits DNA, RNA, phospholipid, protein synthesis.*

USES/*UNLABELED*

Treatment of pneumonia caused by *Pneumocystis carinii* (PCP). Prevention of PCP in high-risk HIV-infected pts. *Treatment of visceral/cutaneous Leishmaniasis, African Trypanosomiasis.*

STORAGE/HANDLING

Store vials at room temperature. After reconstitution, IV solution and aerosol are stable for 48 hrs at room temperature. Use freshly prepared aerosol solution. Discard unused portion.

ADMINISTRATION

- **Note:** Pt must be in supine position during administration w/frequent B/P checks until stable (potential for life-threatening hypotensive reaction). Have resuscitative equipment nearby.

IM:

- Reconstitute 300 mg vial w/3 ml sterile water for injection to provide concentration of 100 mg/ml.

IV:

- For intermittent IV infusion (piggyback), reconstitute each vial w/3–5 ml 5% dextrose or sterile water for injection.
- Withdraw desired dose and

P

further dilute w/50–250 ml 5% dextrose; infuse over 60 min.

- Do not give by IV injection or rapid IV infusion (increases potential for severe hypotension).

AEROSOL (NEBULIZER):

- Reconstitute 300 mg vial w/6 ml sterile water for injection. Avoid saline (may cause precipitate).
- Do not mix w/other medication in nebulizer reservoir.

INDICATIONS/ROUTES/DOSAGE

Pneumocystis carinii pneumonia: *IM/IV: Adults, elderly, children:* 4 mg/kg/day once daily for 14 days.

Prevention of ***P. carinii*** **pneumonia:** *Aerosol (Nebulizer): Adults, elderly:* 300 mg once q4wks via nebulizer.

CONTRAINDICATIONS

When PCP has been firmly established, there are no absolute contraindications. Inhalation of drug is contraindicated in those w/history of severe asthma or anaphylactic reaction to drug by any route.

CAUTIONS

Hyper/hypotension, hepatic/renal dysfunction, hyper/hypoglycemia, hypocalcemia, thrombocytopenia, leukopenia, anemia.

INTERACTIONS

DRUG: *Blood dyscrasias–producing medication, bone marrow depressants* may increase abnormal hematologic effects. *Didanosine* may increase risk of pancreatitis. *Foscarnet* may increase hypocalcemia, hypomagnesemia, nephrotoxicity. *Nephrotoxic medications* may increase risk of nephrotoxicity. HERBAL: None known. FOOD: None significant. ALTERED LAB VALUES: May increase SGOT (AST), SGPT (ALT), alkaline phosphatase, bilirubin, BUN, creatinine. May decrease calcium, magnesium. May alter glucose levels.

SIDE EFFECTS

FREQUENT (Injection >10%): Abscess, pain at injection site, increased creatinine. **(Inhalation >5%):** Fatigue, metallic taste, shortness of breath, decreased appetite, dizziness, rash, cough, nausea, vomiting, chills. **OCCASIONAL (Injection 1–10%):** Increased liver function tests, leukopenia, nausea, decreased appetite, hypotension, fever, rash, bad taste, anemia, confusion. **(Inhalation 1–5%):** Diarrhea, headache, anemia, muscle pain. **RARE (Injection <1%):** Neuralgia, thrombocytopenia, phlebitis, dizziness.

ADVERSE REACTIONS/TOXIC EFFECTS

Life-threatening/fatal hypotension, arrhythmias, hypoglycemia, or leukopenia; nephrotoxicity and renal failure; anaphylactic shock; Stevens-Johnson syndrome; toxic epidural necrolysis. Hyperglycemia and insulin-dependent diabetes mellitus (often permanent) may occur even months after therapy.

PATIENT CONSIDERATIONS

BASELINE ASSESSMENT

Question history of anaphylactic reaction to pentamidine isethionate. Avoid concurrent use of nephrotoxic drugs. Establish baseline for B/P, blood glucose. Obtain specimens for diagnostic tests before giving first dose.

INTERVENTION/EVALUATION

Monitor B/P during administration until stable for both IM and IV administration (pt should remain supine). Check glucose levels and clinical signs for hypoglycemia (sweating, nervousness, tremor, tachycardia, palpitation, light-

headedness, headache, numbness of lips, double vision, incoordination), hyperglycemia (polyuria, polyphagia, polydipsia, malaise, visual changes, abdominal pain, headache, nausea/vomiting). Evaluate IM sites for pain, redness, and induration; IV sites for phlebitis (heat, pain, red streaking over vein). Monitor renal, hepatic, and hematology test results. Assess skin for rash. Determine food tolerance. Evaluate equilibrium during ambulation. Be alert for respiratory difficulty when administering by inhalation route.

PATIENT/FAMILY TEACHING

Remain flat in bed during administration of medication and get up slowly w/assistance when B/P stable. Notify nurse immediately of sweating, shakiness, lightheadedness, palpitations. Even several months after therapy stops, drowsiness, increased urination, thirst, anorexia may develop—notify nurse/physician immediately. Mouthwash, hard candy, or gum may help w/unpleasant taste that can occur.

pentazocine

pen-**tah**-zoe-seen
(Talwin [parenteral])

FIXED-COMBINATION(S)
W/naloxone, a narcotic antagonist (oral) **(Talwin NX)**; w/aspirin (oral) **(Talwin Compound)**; w/acetaminophen (oral) **(Talacen)**

CANADIAN AVAILABILITY
Talwin

PREGNANCY CATEGORY C
(D if used for prolonged periods or in high doses at term)

CLASSIFICATION

Opioid analgesic **(Schedule IV)**

AVAILABILITY (Rx)

Injection: 30 mg

PHARMACODYNAMICS

	ONSET	PEAK	DURATION
Oral	15–30 min	1–3 hrs	>3 hrs
SubQ	15–20 min	—	—
IM	15–20 min	1 hr	2 hrs
IV	2–3 min	15 min	1 hr

PHARMACOKINETICS

Absorption: Well absorbed from GI tract after IM, SubQ administration. Widely distributed. **Metabolism:** Metabolized in liver. **Excretion:** Primarily excreted in urine. **Half-life:** 2–3 hrs.

ACTION/*THERAPEUTIC EFFECT*

Binds w/opioid receptors within CNS, *altering processes affecting pain perception, emotional response to pain.* May displace opioid agonists and competitively inhibit their action (may precipitate withdrawal symptoms).

USES

Relief of moderate to severe pain. Parenteral form used preop or preanesthetic or as supplement to surgical anesthesia.

STORAGE/HANDLING

Store oral, parenteral form at room temperature.

ADMINISTRATION

ORAL:

- Scored tablets may be crushed; do not crush or break Talwin Compound caplets.
- May give w/o regard to meals

but give w/food or milk if GI distress is evident.

SubQ:
- Give SubQ only if absolutely necessary (severe tissue damage possible at injection sites).

IM:
- Give deep into upper outer quadrant of buttock, always rotating sites (severe sclerosing of skin, tissue and muscle damage may occur at repeated injection site).

IV:
- Do not mix in same syringe w/soluble barbiturates (precipitation will occur).
- May be given undiluted or diluted (each 5 mg w/1 ml sterile water for direct injection).
- Administer each 5 mg or fraction thereof >1 min.

INDICATIONS/ROUTES/DOSAGE

Analgesia:
Oral: Adults: 50 mg q3–4h. May increase to 100 mg q3–4h, if needed. ***Maximum:*** 600 mg/day.

SubQ/IM/IV: Adults: 30 mg q3–4h. Do not exceed 30 mg IV or 60 mg SubQ/IM per dose. ***Maximum:*** 360 mg/day.

Usual elderly dosage:
Oral: 50 mg q4h as needed.

IM: 25 mg q4h as needed.

Obstetric labor:
IM: Adults: 30 mg.

IV: Adults: 20 mg when contractions are regular. May repeat 2–3 times q2–3h.

CONTRAINDICATIONS

Hypersensitivity to pentazocine.

CAUTIONS

Impaired hepatic/renal function, elderly, debilitated, head injury, respiratory disease, prior to biliary tract surgery (produces spasm of sphincter of Oddi), MI w/nausea, vomiting.

INTERACTIONS

DRUG: ***Alcohol, CNS depressants*** may increase CNS or respiratory depression, hypotension. ***MAO inhibitors*** may produce severe, fatal reaction (reduce dose to 1/4 usual dose). Effects may be decreased w/***buprenorphine.*** **HERBAL:** None known. **FOOD:** None significant. **ALTERED LAB VALUES:** May increase amylase, lipase.

SIDE EFFECTS

FREQUENT: Drowsiness, euphoria, nausea, vomiting. **OCCASIONAL:** Allergic reaction, shortness of breath, pounding heartbeat, histamine reaction (decreased blood pressure, increased sweating, flushing, wheezing), decreased urination, altered vision, constipation, dizziness, dry mouth, headache, hypotension, pain/burning at injection site. **RARE:** Confusion, seizures, paralytic ileus, ringing in ears, trembling, stomach cramps, decreased appetite, insomnia.

ADVERSE REACTIONS/TOXIC EFFECTS

Overdosage results in severe respiratory depression, skeletal muscle flaccidity, cyanosis, extreme somnolence progressing to convulsions, stupor, coma. Abrupt withdrawal after prolonged use may produce symptoms of narcotic withdrawal (abdominal cramps, rhinorrhea, lacrimation, nausea, vomiting, restlessness, anxiety, increased temperature, piloerection [goose bumps]). Tolerance to analgesic effect and physical dependence may occur w/chronic use.

PATIENT CONSIDERATIONS

BASELINE ASSESSMENT

Raise bed rails. Obtain vital signs before giving medication. If respirations are 12/min or lower, withhold medication, contact physician. Assess onset, type, location, and duration of pain. Effect of medication is reduced if full pain recurs before next dose.

INTERVENTION/EVALUATION

Encourage deep breathing and coughing exercises. Check vital signs periodically (5–10 min after IV dose). Monitor for change in respirations, B/P, change in rate/quality of pulse. Initiate deep breathing and coughing exercises, particularly in those w/impaired pulmonary function. Change pt's position q2–4h. Assess for clinical improvement and record onset of relief of pain. Contact physician if pain is not adequately relieved.

PATIENT/FAMILY TEACHING

Change positions slowly to avoid dizziness. Head-low position may help relieve lightheadedness, nausea. Explain need for assistance if ambulating. Avoid alcohol. Request pain medication before pain fully recurs.

---

pentobarbital

(Nembutal)

See Classification section under: Sedative-hypnotics

---

pentosan

(Elmiron)

See Supplement

---

pentostatin

(Nipent)

See Classification section under: Cancer chemotherapy

---

pentoxifylline

pen-**tox**-ih-fill-in

(Pentoxil, Trental)

CANADIAN AVAILABILITY

Trental

PREGNANCY CATEGORY C

CLASSIFICATION

Hemorheologic

AVAILABILITY (Rx)

Tablets (controlled-release): 400 mg

PHARMACOKINETICS

Absorption: Completely absorbed from GI tract. Bound to erythrocyte membrane. **Metabolism:** Metabolized in erythrocytes, liver to active metabolite. **Excretion:** Primarily excreted in urine. **Half-life:** 0.4–0.8 hrs; metabolite: 1–1.6 hrs.

ACTION/*THERAPEUTIC EFFECT*

Improves erythrocyte flexibility, microcirculatory flow, tissue oxygen concentration; *reduces blood viscosity.*

USES

Symptomatic treatment of intermittent claudication associated w/occlusive peripheral vascular disease, diabetic angiopathies.

P

ADMINISTRATION

ORAL:

- Do not crush or break film-coated tablets.
- Give w/meals to avoid GI upset.

INDICATIONS/ROUTES/DOSAGE

Intermittent claudication:
Oral: Adults, elderly: 400 mg 3 times/day. Decrease to 400 mg 2 times/day if GI or CNS side effects occur. Continue for at least 8 wks.

CONTRAINDICATIONS

History of intolerance to xanthine derivatives (caffeine, theophylline, theobromine).

CAUTIONS

Coronary artery disease, cerebrovascular disease, impaired renal function.

INTERACTIONS

DRUG: May increase effect of ***antihypertensives.*** **HERBAL:** None known. **FOOD:** None significant. **ALTERED LAB VALUES:** None significant.

SIDE EFFECTS

FREQUENT (2–5%): Nausea, dyspepsia. **OCCASIONAL (1–2%):** Vomiting, dizziness, headache. **RARE (<1%):** Bad taste, itching, rash, decreased appetite, constipation, dry mouth, blurred vision, angina, edema, nasal congestion, dyspnea, tremors, anxiety.

ADVERSE REACTIONS/TOXIC EFFECTS

Angina, chest pain occur rarely. May be accompanied by palpitations, tachycardia, arrhythmias. Overdosage (flushing, hypotension, nervousness, agitation, hand tremor, fever, somnolence) noted 4–5 hrs after ingestion, lasts 12 hrs.

PATIENT CONSIDERATIONS

INTERVENTION/EVALUATION

Assist w/ambulation if dizziness occurs. Assess for hand tremor. Monitor for relief of symptoms of intermittent claudication (pain, aching, cramping in calf muscles, buttocks, thigh, feet). Symptoms generally occur while walking/exercising and not at rest or w/weight bearing in absence of walking/exercising. Monitor B/P, EKG.

PATIENT/FAMILY TEACHING

Therapeutic effect generally noted in 2–4 wks. Avoid driving, tasks requiring alert response until response to drug known. Do not smoke (causes constriction and occlusion of peripheral blood vessels).

pergolide mesylate

purr-go-lied
(Permax)

CANADIAN AVAILABILITY
Permax

PREGNANCY CATEGORY B

CLASSIFICATION

Antiparkinson

AVAILABILITY (Rx)

Tablets: 0.05 mg, 0.25 mg, 1 mg

PHARMACOKINETICS

Absorption: Well absorbed from GI tract. **Metabolism:** Metabolized in liver (undergoes extensive first-pass effect). **Excretion:** Primarily excreted in urine.

ACTION/*THERAPEUTIC EFFECT*

Inhibits prolactin secretion; directly stimulates postsynaptic dopamine receptors, *assisting in reduction in tremor, improvement in akinesia (absence of movement), posture and equilibrium disorders, rigidity of parkinsonism.*

USES

Adjunctive treatment w/levodopa/carbidopa in those w/Parkinson's disease.

ADMINISTRATION

ORAL:

- Scored tablets may be crushed.
- May be given w/o regard to meals.

INDICATIONS/ROUTES/DOSAGE

Note: Daily doses usually given in 3 divided doses.

Parkinsonism:

Oral: Adults, elderly: Initially, 0.05 mg/day for 2 days. Increase by 0.1–0.15 mg/day q3days over the following 12 days; then may increase by 0.25 mg/day q3days. ***Maximum:*** 5 mg/day. ***Range:*** 3–4.6 mg/day.

CONTRAINDICATIONS

None significant.

CAUTIONS

Cardiac dysrhythmias.

INTERACTIONS

DRUG: *Haloperidol, loxapine, methyldopa, metoclopramide, phenothiazines* may decrease effect. *Hypotension-producing medications* may increase hypotensive effect. **HERBAL:** None known. **FOOD:** None significant. **ALTERED LAB VALUES:** May increase plasma growth hormone.

SIDE EFFECTS

FREQUENT (>10%): Confusion, dyskinesia, uncontrolled body movements, UTI, abdominal or stomach pain, constipation, dizziness, drowsiness, flulike symptoms, hypotension, nausea, low back pain, rhinitis, weakness. **OCCASIONAL (2–10%):** Chills, diarrhea, dry mouth, edema of face, vomiting, decreased appetite. **RARE (<2%):** Headache, seizures, change in vision, myocardial infarction.

ADVERSE REACTIONS/TOXIC EFFECTS

Overdosage may require supportive measures to maintain arterial B/P (monitor cardiac function, vital signs, blood gases, serum electrolytes). Activated charcoal may be more effective than emesis or lavage.

PATIENT CONSIDERATIONS

INTERVENTION/EVALUATION

Be alert to neurologic effects: headache, lethargy, mental confusion, agitation. Monitor for evidence of dyskinesia (difficulty w/movement). Assess for clinical reversal of Parkinson symptoms (improvement of tremor of head/hands at rest, mask-like facial expression, shuffling gait, muscular rigidity).

PATIENT/FAMILY TEACHING

Tolerance to feeling of lightheadedness develops during therapy. To reduce hypotensive effect, rise slowly from lying to sitting position and permit legs to dangle momentarily before standing. Avoid tasks that require alertness, motor skills until response to drug is established. Dry mouth, drowsiness, dizziness may be expected responses of drug. Avoid alcoholic beverages

P

during therapy. Coffee or tea may help reduce drowsiness.

perindopril

(Aceon)

See Supplement

perphenazine

per-**fen**-ah-zeen

(Trilafon)

FIXED-COMBINATION(S)

W/amitriptyline, a tricyclic antidepressant **(Etrafon, Triavil)**

CANADIAN AVAILABILITY

Apo-Perphenazine, Trilafon

PREGNANCY CATEGORY C

CLASSIFICATION

Antipsychotic

AVAILABILITY (Rx)

Tablets: 2 mg, 4 mg, 8 mg, 16 mg. **Oral Concentrate:** 16 mg/5 ml. **Injection:** 5 mg/ml.

PHARMACOKINETICS

Absorption: Well absorbed from GI tract. Widely distributed. **Metabolism:** Metabolized in liver to active metabolite. **Excretion:** Primarily excreted in urine.

ACTION/*THERAPEUTIC EFFECT*

Blocks postsynaptic dopamine receptor sites in brain. *Suppresses behavioral response in psychosis, produces antiemetic effect, terminates intractable hiccups.*

USES

Management of psychotic disorders; control of nausea, vomiting, intractable hiccups.

STORAGE/HANDLING

Store oral, parenteral form at room temperature. Yellow discoloration of solution does not affect potency, but discard if markedly discolored or if precipitate forms.

ADMINISTRATION

ORAL:

- Do not mix oral concentrate w/caffeine (coffee, cola, tea), apple juice because of physical incompatibility.
- Mix each 5 ml oral concentrate w/60 ml water, carbonated lemon-lime or orange drink, milk, vegetable, pineapple, apricot, prune, orange, tomato, grapefruit juice.
- **Parenteral Administration:** Pt must remain recumbent for 30–60 min in head-low position w/legs raised, to minimize hypotensive effect.

IM:

- Inject slow, deep IM into upper outer quadrant of gluteus maximus. If irritation occurs, dilute further injections w/0.9% NaCl or 2% procaine hydrochloride.
- Massage IM injection site to reduce discomfort.

IV:

- **Note:** Give by fractional IV injection or IV infusion.
- For fractional IV, dilute each 5 mg (1 ml) w/9 ml 0.9% NaCl, producing final concentration of 0.5 mg/ml.
- Do not give more than 1 mg per injection at slow rate at not less than 1–2 min intervals.
- For IV infusion, dilute further and give at rate of 0.5 mg or less/min.

INDICATIONS/ROUTES/DOSAGE

Note: Decrease dose gradually to optimum response. Decrease to lowest effective level for maintenance. Replace parenteral therapy w/oral therapy as soon as possible.

Hospitalized psychotic:
Oral: Adults, children >12 yrs: 8–16 mg 2–4 times/day.

IM: Adults, children >12 yrs: 5 mg q6h, as needed.

Nonhospitalized:
Oral: Adults, children >12 yrs: 4–8 mg 3 times/day.

Severe nausea, vomiting, intractable hiccups:
Oral: Adults: 8–16 mg/day.

IM: Adults: 5 mg.

IV: Adults: Up to 5 mg.

Usual elderly dosage (nonpsychotic):
Oral: Initially, 2–4 mg/day. May increase by 2–4 mg/day q4–7days. *Maximum:* 32 mg/day.

CONTRAINDICATIONS

Severe CNS depression, comatose states, severe cardiovascular disease, bone marrow depression, subcortical brain damage.

CAUTIONS

Impaired respiratory/hepatic/renal/cardiac function, alcohol withdrawal, history of seizures, urinary retention, glaucoma, prostatic hypertrophy, hypocalcemia (increases susceptibility to dystonias).

INTERACTIONS

DRUG: *Alcohol, CNS depressants* may increase CNS, respiratory depression, hypotensive effects. *Tricyclic antidepressants, MAO inhibitors* may increase sedative, anticholinergic effects. *Antithyroid agents* may increase risk of agranulocytosis. Extrapyramidal symptoms (EPS) may increase *w/ EPS-producing medications. Hypotensives* may increase hypotension. May decrease *levodopa* effects. *Lithium* may decrease absorption, produce adverse neurologic effects. **HERBAL:** None known. **FOOD:** None significant. **ALTERED LAB VALUES:** May produce false-positive pregnancy test, phenylketonuria (PKU). EKG changes may occur, including Q and T wave disturbances.

SIDE EFFECTS

FREQUENT: Hypotension, dizziness, fainting occur frequently after parenteral form is given and occasionally thereafter but rarely w/oral dosage. **OCCASIONAL:** Marked photosensitivity. Drowsiness during early therapy, dry mouth, blurred vision, lethargy, constipation/diarrhea, nasal congestion, peripheral edema, urinary retention. **RARE:** Ocular changes, skin pigmentation (those on high doses for prolonged periods).

P

ADVERSE REACTIONS/TOXIC EFFECTS

Extrapyramidal symptoms appear dose related (particularly high dosage) and are divided into 3 categories: akathisia (inability to sit still, tapping of feet, urge to move around), parkinsonian symptoms (mask-like face, tremors, shuffling gait, hypersalivation), and acute dystonias: torticollis (neck muscle spasm), opisthotonos (rigidity of back muscles), and oculogyric crisis (rolling back of eyes). Dystonic reaction may also produce profuse sweating, pallor. Tardive dyskinesia (protrusion of tongue, puffing of cheeks, chewing/puckering of the mouth) occurs rarely (may be irreversible). Abrupt withdrawal following long-term therapy may precipitate nausea, vomiting, gastritis, dizziness, tremors. Blood dyscrasias, particularly agranulocytosis, mild leukopenia may occur. May lower seizure threshold.

PATIENT CONSIDERATIONS

BASELINE ASSESSMENT

Avoid skin contact w/solutions (contact dermatitis).

Antiemetic
Assess for dehydration (poor skin turgor, dry mucous membranes, longitudinal furrows in tongue).

Antipsychotic
Assess behavior, appearance, emotional status, response to environment, speech pattern, thought content.

INTERVENTION/EVALUATION

Monitor B/P for hypotension. Assess for extrapyramidal symptoms. Monitor WBC, differential count for blood dyscrasias. Monitor for fine tongue movement (may be early sign of tardive dyskinesia). Supervise suicidal risk pt closely during early therapy (as depression lessens, energy level improves increasing suicide potential). Assess for therapeutic response (interest in surroundings, improvement in self-care, increased ability to concentrate, relaxed facial expression).

Antiemetic
Monitor I&O and food tolerance.

PATIENT/FAMILY TEACHING

Full therapeutic effect may take up to 6 wks. Urine may turn pink or reddish brown. Do not abruptly withdraw from long-term drug therapy. Report visual disturbances. Sugarless gum, sips of tepid water may relieve dry mouth. Drowsiness generally subsides during continued therapy. Avoid tasks that require alertness, motor skills until response to drug is established. Avoid alcohol and CNS depressants. Wear protective clothing, sunscreens in sunlight.

phenazopyridine hydrochloride

feen-ah-zoe-**peer**-ih-deen
(Pyridium, Urodine)

CANADIAN AVAILABILITY
Phenazo, Pyridium

PREGNANCY CATEGORY B

CLASSIFICATION

Urinary analgesic

AVAILABILITY (Rx)

Tablets: 100 mg, 200 mg

PHARMACOKINETICS

Absorption: Well absorbed from GI tract. **Metabolism:** Partially metabolized in liver. **Excretion:** Primarily excreted in urine.

ACTION/*THERAPEUTIC EFFECT*

Exact mechanism unknown. *Excreted in urine where it produces topical analgesic effect on urinary tract mucosa.*

USES

Symptomatic relief of pain, burning, urgency, frequency resulting from lower urinary tract mucosa irritation (may be caused by infection, trauma, surgery).

ADMINISTRATION

ORAL:
- Give after meals.

INDICATIONS/ROUTES/DOSAGE

Analgesic:
Oral: Adults: 200 mg 3 times/day. *Children >6 yrs:* 12 mg/kg/day in 3 divided doses for 3–15 days.

CONTRAINDICATIONS

Renal insufficiency.

CAUTIONS

None significant.

INTERACTIONS

DRUG: None significant. **HERBAL:** None known. **FOOD:** None significant. **ALTERED LAB VALUES:** May interfere w/urinalysis color reactions, (e.g., urinary glucose, ketone tests, urinary protein, or determination of urinary steroids).

SIDE EFFECTS

OCCASIONAL: Headache, GI disturbance, rash, pruritus.

ADVERSE REACTIONS/TOXIC EFFECTS

Overdosage levels or those w/impaired renal function or severe hypersensitivity may develop renal toxicity, hemolytic anemia, hepatic toxicity. Methemoglobinemia generally occurs as result of massive, acute overdosage.

PATIENT CONSIDERATIONS

INTERVENTION/EVALUATION

Assess for therapeutic response: relief of pain, burning, urgency, frequency of urination.

PATIENT/FAMILY TEACHING

A reddish orange discoloration of urine should be expected. May stain fabric. Take after meals (reduces possibility of GI upset).

phenobarbital

feen-oh-**bar**-bih-tall
(Barbita, Sulfoton)

phenobarbital sodium

(Luminal)

FIXED-COMBINATION(S)
W/phenytoin sodium, an anticonvulsant **(Dilantin w/Phenobarbital Kapseals)**; w/belladonna, an anticholinergic and ergotamine **(Bellergal-S)**.

P

PREGNANCY CATEGORY D

CLASSIFICATION

Anticonvulsant, hypnotic

AVAILABILITY (Rx)

Tablets: 15 mg, 30 mg, 60 mg, 100 mg. **Elixir:** 15 mg/5 ml, 20 mg/5 ml. **Injection:** 30 mg/ml, 60 mg/ml, 130 mg/ml.

PHARMACOKINETICS

Absorption: Well absorbed after oral, parenteral administration. Rapidly, widely distributed. **Metabolism:** Metabolized in liver. **Excretion:** Primarily excreted in urine. **Half-life:** 53–118 hrs.

ACTION/*THERAPEUTIC EFFECT*

Decreases motor activity to electrical/chemical stimulation, *producing anticonvulsant effect.* CNS depressant effect produces all levels from mild sedation, hypnosis to deep coma.

USES/*UNLABELED*

Management of generalized tonic-clonic (grand mal) seizures, partial seizures, control of acute convulsive episodes (status epilepticus, eclampsia, febrile seizures). Relieves anxiety, provides preop sedation. *Prophylaxis/treatment of hyperbilirubinemia.*

ADMINISTRATION

ORAL:

- Give w/o regard to meals. Tablets may be crushed.
- Elixir may be mixed w/water, milk, fruit juice.

IM:

- Do not inject more than 5 ml in any one IM injection site (produces tissue irritation).
- Inject IM deep into gluteus maximus or lateral aspect of thigh.

IV:

- Administer at rate not greater than 60 mg/min (too rapid IV may produce severe hypotension, marked respiratory depression).
- Monitor vital signs q3–5min during and q15min for 1–2 hrs after administration.
- Inadvertent intra-arterial injection may result in arterial spasm w/severe pain, tissue necrosis. Extravasation in subcutaneous tissue may produce redness, tenderness, tissue necrosis. If either occurs, treat w/injection of 0.5% procaine solution into affected area, apply moist heat.

INDICATIONS/ROUTES/DOSAGE

Note: When replacement by another anticonvulsant is necessary, decrease phenobarbital over 1 wk as therapy begins w/low replacement dose.

Anticonvulsant:
Oral: Adults, elderly: 60–250 mg/day as single or divided doses. *Children:* 1–6 mg/kg/day as single or divided doses.

IV: Adults, elderly: 100–320 mg. May repeat up to total daily dose of 600 mg/24 hrs. *Children:* Initially, 20 mg/kg as single dose, then 1–6 mg/kg/day.

Hypnotic:
Oral/IM/IV: Adults, elderly: 100–320 mg at bedtime.

Sedative:
Oral/IM/IV: Adults, elderly: 30–120 mg in 2–3 divided doses per day. *Children:* 2 mg/kg 3 times/day.

Status epilepticus:
IV: Adults, elderly: 10–20 mg/kg; may repeat. *Children:* 15–20 mg/kg, given over 10–15 min.

CONTRAINDICATIONS

History of porphyria, bronchopneumonia.

CAUTIONS

Uncontrolled pain (may produce paradoxical reaction), impaired liver function.

INTERACTIONS

DRUG: May decrease effects of ***glucocorticoids, digoxin, metronidazole, oral anticoagulants, quinidine, tricyclic antidepressants. Alcohol, CNS depressants*** may increase effect. May increase metabolism of ***carbamazepine. Valproic acid*** decreases metabolism, increases concentration, toxicity. **HERBAL:** None known. **FOOD:** None known. **ALTERED LAB VALUES:** May decrease bilirubin.

SIDE EFFECTS

FREQUENT: Drowsiness, sedation, irritability, headache, restlessness, ataxia (muscular incoordination), joint aches, vertigo, anorexia, nausea, gastric distress. **OCCASIONAL:** Paradoxical CNS hyperactivity/nervousness in children, excitement/restlessness in elderly (generally noted during first 2 wks of therapy, particularly noted in presence of uncontrolled pain).

ADVERSE REACTIONS/TOXIC EFFECTS

Abrupt withdrawal after prolonged therapy may produce effects ranging from markedly increased dreaming, nightmares and/or insomnia, tremor, sweating, vomiting, to hallucinations, delirium, seizures, status epilepticus. Skin eruptions appear as hypersensitivity reaction. Blood dyscrasias, liver disease, hypocalcemia occur rarely. Overdosage produces cold, clammy skin, hypothermia, severe CNS depression, cyanosis, rapid pulse, Cheyne-Stokes respirations. Toxicity may result in severe renal impairment.

PATIENT CONSIDERATIONS

BASELINE ASSESSMENT

Assess B/P, pulse, respirations immediately before administration. Liver function tests, blood counts should be performed before therapy begins and periodically during therapy.

Hypnotic
Raise bed rails, provide environment conducive to sleep (back rub, quiet environment, low lighting).

Seizures
Review history of seizure disorder (length, presence of auras, level of consciousness). Observe frequently for recurrence of seizure activity. Initiate seizure precautions.

INTERVENTION/EVALUATION

Assess elderly, debilitated, children for evidence of paradoxical reaction, particularly during early therapy. Evaluate for therapeutic response: decrease in length, number of seizures. Monitor for therapeutic serum level (10–30 mcg/ml).

PATIENT/FAMILY TEACHING

Drowsiness may gradually decrease/disappear w/continued use. Do not abruptly withdraw medication following long-term use (may precipitate seizures). Avoid tasks that require alertness, motor skills until response to drug is established. Tolerance/dependence may occur w/prolonged use of high doses. Strict maintenance of drug therapy is essential for seizure control. Avoid alcohol and other CNS depressants. Notify physician promptly of pregnancy.

phenytoin

phen-**ih**-toyn
(Dilantin)

CANADIAN AVAILABILITY
Dilantin

PREGNANCY CATEGORY D

CLASSIFICATION

Anticonvulsant, antiarrhythmic

AVAILABILITY (Rx)

Capsules: 30 mg, 100 mg. **Tablets (chewable):** 50 mg. **Oral Suspension:** 30 mg/5 ml, 125 mg/5 ml. **Injection:** 50 mg/ml.

PHARMACOKINETICS

Absorption: Slow, variably absorbed after oral administration; slow but complete absorption following IM administration. Widely distributed. **Metabolism:** Metabolized in liver. **Excretion:** Primarily excreted in urine. **Half-life:** 22 hrs.

ACTION/*THERAPEUTIC EFFECT*

Anticonvulsant: Stabilizes neuronal membranes in motor cortex, *limits spread of seizure activity. Stabilizes threshhold against hyperexcitability. Decreases post-tetanic potentiation and repetitive discharge.* **Antiarrhythmic:** Decreases abnormal ventricular automaticity *(shortens refractory period, QT interval, action potential duration).*

USES / *UNLABELED*

Management of generalized tonic-clonic sezures (grand mal), complex partial seizures (psychomotor), cortical focal seizures, status epilepticus. Combination therapy in absence seizures, myoclonic seizures, atonic epilepsy. Treatment of cardiac arrhythmias due to digitalis intoxication. *Treatment of digoxin-induced arrhythmias, trigeminal neuralgia; muscle relaxant in treatment of muscle hyperirritability; adjunct in treatment of tricyclic antidepressant toxicity.*

ADMINISTRATION

ORAL:

- Give w/ food if GI distress occurs.
- Do not chew/break capsules. Tablets may be chewed.
- Shake oral suspension well before using.

IV:

- Severe hypotension, cardiovascular collapse occurs if rate of IV injection exceeds 50 mg/min for adults. Administer 50 mg > 2–3 min for elderly. In neonates, administer at rate not exceeding 1–3 mg/kg/min.
- IV injection very painful (chemical irritation of vein due to alkalinity of solution). To minimize effect, flush vein w/ sterile saline solution through same IV needle/catheter following each IV injection.
- IV toxicity characterized by CNS depression, cardiovascular collapse.

INDICATIONS / ROUTES / DOSAGE

Seizure control:
Oral: Adults, elderly: Initially, 100 mg 3 times/day. May increase in 100 mg increments q2–4 wks. ***Range:*** 300–400 mg/day. ***Maximum:*** 600 mg/day (300 mg for extended-release). ***Children:*** Initially, 5 mg/kg/day in 2–3 equally divided doses. ***Maintenance:*** 4–8 mg/kg. ***Maximum:*** 300 mg/day.

Status epilepticus:
IV: Adults, elderly: 15–20 mg/kg. ***Children:*** 15–20 mg/kg in divided doses of 5–10 mg/kg.

Arrhythmias:
IV: Adults, elderly: 100 mg at 5 min intervals until arrhythmias disappear or undesirable effects occur. ***Maximum:*** 15 mg/kg total dose.

Management of arrhythmias:
Oral: Adults, elderly: 100 mg 2–4 times/day.

CONTRAINDICATIONS

Seizures due to hypoglycemia, hydantoin hypersensitivity. ***IV route only:*** Sinus bradycardia, sinoatrial block, second- and third-degree heart block, Adam-Stokes syndrome.

CAUTIONS

Impaired hepatic/renal function, severe myocardial insufficiency, hypotension, hyperglycemia. ***IV only:*** Respiratory depression, myocardial infarction, CHF, damaged myocardium.

INTERACTIONS

DRUG: Increase phenytoin effects: ***Allopurinol, amiodarone, benzodiazepines, cimetidine, fluconazole, metronidazole, omeprazole, co-trimethoxazole.*** Decrease phenytoin effects: ***Carbamazepine, chronic alcohol use, antacids, sucralfate.*** May decrease effects of ***amiodarone, carbamazepine, corticosteroids, oral***

contraceptives, theophylline, valproic acid. **HERBAL:** None known. **FOOD:** None significant. **ALTERED LAB VALUES:** May increase alkaline phosphatase, GGT, glucose

SIDE EFFECTS

FREQUENT: Nystagmus, ataxia, confusion, slurred speech, tremors, gingival hyperplasia, hypersensitivity reaction, constipation, dizziness, drowsiness, nausea, vomiting. **OCCASIONAL:** Enlarged facial features (e.g., thickening lips), gynecomastia, headache, hair growth, insomnia, muscle twitching, pain at injection site. **RARE:** Jaundice, hepatitis, impaired cognition.

ADVERSE REACTIONS/TOXIC EFFECTS

Abrupt withdrawal may precipitate status epilepticus. Blood dyscrasias, lymphadenopathy, osteomalacia (due to interference of vitamin D metabolism) may occur. Phenytoin blood concentration of 25 mcg/ml (toxic) may produce ataxia (muscular incoordination), nystagmus (rhythmic oscillation of eyes), double vision. As level increases, extreme lethargy to comatose states occur.

PATIENT CONSIDERATIONS

Baseline Assessment

Anticonvulsant: Review history of seizure disorder (intensity, frequency, duration, level of consciousness). Initiate seizure precautions. Liver function tests, CBC, platelet count should be performed before therapy begins and periodically during therapy. Repeat CBC, platelet count 2 wks after therapy begins and 2 wks after maintenance dose is given.

Intervention/Evaluation

Observe frequently for recurrence of sezure activity. Assess for clinical improvement (decrease in intensity/frequency of seizures). Monitor EKG for cardiac arrhythmias. Assess B/P, EKG diligently w/IV administration. Assist w/ambulation if drowsiness, lethargy, vertigo occur. Monitor for therapeutic serum level (10–20 mcg/ml).

Patient/Family Teaching

Pain may occur w/IV injection. To prevent gingival hyperplasia (bleeding, tenderness, swelling of gums), encourage good oral hygiene care, gum massage, regular dental visits. CBC should be performed every month for 1 yr after maintenance dose is established and q3mos thereafter. Urine may appear pink, red, or red brown. Report sore throat, fever, glandular swelling, skin reaction (hematologic toxicity). Drowsiness usually diminishes w/continued therapy. Do not abruptly withdraw medication following long-term use (may precipitate seizures). Strict maintenance of drug therapy is essential for seizure control, arrhythmias. Avoid tasks that require alertness, motor skills until response to drug is established. Avoid alcohol.

---

pioglitazone
(Actos)
See Supplement

---

piperacillin sodium/ tazobactam sodium

pip-ur-ah-**sill**-in/tay-zoe-**back**-tam
(Zosyn)

P

CANADIAN AVAILABILITY
Tazocin

PREGNANCY CATEGORY B

CLASSIFICATION

Antibiotic: Penicillin

AVAILABILITY (Rx)

Powder for Injection: 2.25 g, 3.375 g, 4.5 g

PHARMACOKINETICS

Widely distributed. **Excretion:** Primarily excreted unchanged in urine. Removed by hemodialysis. **Half-life:** 0.7–1.2 hrs (increased in decreased renal function, hepatic cirrhosis).

ACTION/*THERAPEUTIC EFFECT*

Piperacillin: Binds to bacterial membranes, *inhibiting cell wall synthesis. Bactericidal.* ***Tazobactam:*** Inactivates bacterial beta-lactamase enzymes. *Protects piperacillin from inactivation by beta-lactamase-producing organisms, extends spectrum of activity, prevents bacterial overgrowth.*

USES

Treatment of appendicitis (complicated by rupture or abscess), peritonitis, uncomplicated and complicated skin and skin structure infections including cellulitis, cutaneous abscesses, ischemic/diabetic foot infections, postpartum endometritis, pelvic inflammatory disease, community-acquired pneumonia (moderate severity only), moderate to severe nosocomial pneumonia.

STORAGE/HANDLING

Reconstituted vials stable for 24 hrs at room temperature or 48 hrs if refrigerated. After further dilution, stable for 24 hrs at room temperature or 7 days if refrigerated.

ADMINISTRATION

IV:

- Reconstitute each 1 g w/5 ml diluent.
- Further dilute w/at least 50 ml 5% dextrose, 0.9% NaCl, or other compatible diluent.
- Infuse over 30 min.
- Alternating IV sites, use large veins to prevent phlebitis.

INDICATIONS/ROUTES/DOSAGE

Usual parenteral dosage:
IV: Adults, elderly: 12 g/1.5 g/day as 3.375 g q6hrs.

Dosage in renal impairment:
Dose and/or frequency based on creatinine clearance.

CREATININE CLEARANCE	DOSAGE
20–40 ml/min	8 g/1 g/day (2.25 g q6h)
<20 ml/min	6 g/0.75 g/day (2.25 g q8h)

CONTRAINDICATIONS

Hypersensitivity to any penicillin.

CAUTIONS

History of allergies, especially cephalosporins, other drugs.

INTERACTIONS

DRUG: ***Probenecid*** may increase concentration, risk of toxicity. ***Hepatotoxic medications*** may increase hepatotoxicity. **HERBAL:** None known. **FOOD:** None significant. **ALTERED LAB VALUES:** May increase SGOT (AST), SGPT (ALT), alkaline phosphatase, bilirubin, LDH, sodium. May cause positive Coombs' test. May decrease potassium.

SIDE EFFECTS

FREQUENT: Diarrhea, headache, constipation, nausea, insomnia, rash. **OCCASIONAL:** Vomiting, dyspepsia, pruritus, fever, agitation, pain, moniliasis, dizziness, abdominal pain, edema, anxiety, dyspnea, rhinitis.

ADVERSE REACTIONS/TOXIC EFFECTS

Superinfections, potentially fatal antibiotic-associated colitis may result from bacterial imbalance. Seizures, neurologic reactions w/overdosage (more often w/renal impairment). Severe hypersensitivity reactions, including anaphylaxis, occur rarely.

PATIENT CONSIDERATIONS

Baseline Assessment

Question for history of allergies, especially penicillins, cephalosporins, other drugs. Obtain specimen for culture and sensitivity before giving first dose (may begin therapy before results are known).

Intervention/Evaluation

Hold medication and promptly report rash (hypersensitivity) or diarrhea (w/fever, abdominal pain, mucus and blood in stool may indicate antibiotic-associated colitis). Evaluate IV site for phlebitis (heat, pain, red streaking over vein). Monitor I&O, urinalysis, renal function tests. Monitor electrolytes, especially potassium. Be alert for superinfection: increased fever, onset of sore throat, diarrhea, vomiting, ulceration, or other oral changes, anal/genital pruritus.

Patient/Family Teaching

Continue antibiotic for full length of treatment. Space doses evenly. Notify physician in event of rash, diarrhea, bleeding, bruising, other new symptom.

piroxicam

purr-**ox**-i-kam
(Feldene)

CANADIAN AVAILABILITY
Apo-Piroxicam, Feldene, Fexicam, Novopirocam

PREGNANCY CATEGORY C
(D if used in third trimester or near delivery)

CLASSIFICATION

Nonsteroidal anti-inflammatory

AVAILABILITY (Rx)

Capsules: 10 mg, 20 mg

PHARMACODYNAMICS

	ONSET	PEAK	DURATION
Oral (analgesic)			
	1 hr	—	48–72 hrs
Oral (antirheumatic)			
	7–12 days	2–3 wks	—

PHARMACOKINETICS

Absorption: Well absorbed from GI tract. **Metabolism:** Metabolized in liver. **Excretion:** Primarily excreted in urine. **Half-life:** 30–86 hrs (increased in decreased renal function).

ACTION/*THERAPEUTIC EFFECT*

Produces analgesic and anti-inflammatory effect by inhibiting prostaglandin synthesis, *reducing inflammatory response and intensity of pain stimulus reaching sensory nerve endings.*

USES/*UNLABELED*

Symptomatic treatment of acute/chronic rheumatoid arthritis, osteoarthritis. *Treatment of ankylosing spondylitis, acute gouty arthritis, dysmenorrhea.*

ADMINISTRATION

ORAL:

- Do not crush or break capsule form.
- May give w/food, milk, or antacids if GI distress occurs.

INDICATIONS/ROUTES/DOSAGE

Acute/chronic rheumatoid arthritis, osteoarthritis:
Oral: Adults, elderly: Initially, 20 mg/day as single/divided doses. Some pts may require up to 30–40 mg/day.

CONTRAINDICATIONS

Active peptic ulcer, GI ulceration, chronic inflammation of GI tract, GI bleeding disorders, history of hypersensitivity to aspirin/NSAIDs.

CAUTIONS

Impaired renal/hepatic function, history of GI tract disease, predisposition to fluid retention.

INTERACTIONS

DRUG: May increase effects of ***oral anticoagulants, heparin, thrombolytics.*** May decrease effect of ***antihypertensives, diuretics. Salicylates, aspirin*** may increase risk of GI side effects, bleeding. ***Bone marrow depressants*** may increase risk of hematologic reactions. May increase concentration, toxicity of ***lithium.*** May increase ***methotrexate*** toxicity. ***Probenecid*** may increase concentration. **HERBAL:** May decrease effects of feverfew. Ginkgo biloba may increase risk of bleeding. **FOOD:** None significant.

ALTERED LAB VALUES: May increase serum transaminase activity. May decrease uric acid.

SIDE EFFECTS

FREQUENT (3–9%): Abdominal cramps or pain, epigastric pain, nausea. **OCCASIONAL (1–3%):** Itching, rash, stomatitis, ringing in ears, edema, dizziness, drowsiness, headache, lightheadedness, constipation, diarrhea, decreased appetite, indigestion, flulike symptoms. **RARE (<1%):** Chest pain, increased blood pressure, hives, painful or difficult urination, bruising, ecchymosis, trouble breathing, blurred vision, inability to sleep.

ADVERSE REACTIONS/TOXIC EFFECTS

Peptic ulcer, GI bleeding, gastritis, severe hepatic reaction (cholestasis, jaundice) occur rarely. Nephrotoxicity (dysuria, hematuria, proteinuria, nephrotic syndrome), severe hypersensitivity reaction (fever, chills, bronchospasm), hematologic toxicity (anemia, leukopenia, eosinophilia, thrombocytopenia) may occur rarely w/long-term treatment.

PATIENT CONSIDERATIONS

BASELINE ASSESSMENT

Assess onset, type, location, duration of pain/inflammation. Inspect appearance of affected joints for immobility, deformities, and skin condition.

INTERVENTION/EVALUATION

Assist w/ambulation if dizziness occurs. Monitor pattern of daily bowel activity, stool consistency. Check behind medial malleolus for fluid retention (usually first area noted). Monitor for evidence of nausea, GI distress. Assess skin for evidence of rash. Evaluate for

therapeutic response (relief of pain, stiffness, swelling, increase in joint mobility, reduced joint tenderness, improved grip strength).

Patient/Family Teaching

Avoid aspirin, alcohol during therapy (increases risk of GI bleeding). If GI upset occurs, take w/food, milk, or antacids. Avoid tasks that require alertness until response to drug is established. Do not crush or chew capsule form.

plasma protein fraction

(Plasmanate, Plasma-Plex, Plasmatein)

PREGNANCY CATEGORY C

CLASSIFICATION

Plasma volume expander

AVAILABILITY (Rx)

Injection: 5%

ACTION/*THERAPEUTIC EFFECT*

Regulates both the volume of circulating blood and tissue fluid balance. *Binds and functions as a carrier of intermediate metabolites (hormones, enzymes, drugs) in the transport and exchange of tissue products.*

USES

Plasma volume expansion in treatment of shock complicated by circulatory volume deficit. Management of protein deficiencies in pts with hypoproteinemia.

STORAGE/HANDLING

Store at room temperature. Liquid is typically transparent, slightly brown, and odorless. Do not use if solution has been frozen, if solution appears turbid or contains sediment, or if not used within 4 hrs of opening vial.

ADMINISTRATION

IV:

- Give by IV infusion.
- May be administered w/o regard to pt's blood group/Rh factor.
- Do not administer near site of any trauma/infection.
- Monitor blood pressure during infusion.

P

INDICATIONS/ROUTES/DOSAGE

Hypovolemic shock:
IV: Adults, elderly: Initially, 250–500 ml at a rate not exceeding 10 ml/min (minimizes hypotension). ***Infants, children:*** 20–30 ml/kg at a rate not to exceed 10 ml/min.

Hypoproteinemia:
IV: Adults, elderly: 1,000–1,500 ml/day at a rate not to exceed 5–8 ml/min (prevents hypervolemia).

CONTRAINDICATIONS

Severe anemia, cardiac failure, history of allergic reactions to albumin, renal insufficiency, no albumin deficiency.

CAUTIONS

Low cardiac reserve, pulmonary disease, hepatic/renal failure.

INTERACTIONS

DRUG: None significant. **HERBAL:** None known. **FOOD:** None significant. **ALTERED LAB VALUES:** None significant.

SIDE EFFECTS

OCCASIONAL: Hypotension. ***High dosage, repeated therapy:*** Allergy or protein overload (chills, fever, flushing, low back pain, nausea, urticaria, vital sign changes).

ADVERSE REACTIONS/TOXIC EFFECTS

Fluid overload (headache, weakness, blurred vision, behavioral changes, incoordination, isolated muscle twitching) and pulmonary edema (rapid breathing, rales, wheezing, coughing, increased B/P, distended neck veins) may occur.

PATIENT CONSIDERATIONS

BASELINE ASSESSMENT

Obtain B/P, pulse, respirations immediately before administration. There should be adequate hydration before administration.

INTERVENTION/EVALUATION

Monitor B/P for hypotension. Assess frequently for evidence of fluid overload, pulmonary edema (see Adverse Reactions/Toxic Effects). Check skin for flushing, urticaria. Monitor hemoglobin, hematocrit. Monitor I&O ratio (watch for decreased output). Assess for therapeutic response (increased B/P, decreased edema).

---

plicamycin

(Mithracin)

See Classification section under: Cancer chemotherapy

---

podofilox

(Condylox)

See Supplement

---

polycarbophil

polly-**car**-bow-fill

(Fibercon, Mitrolan)

CANADIAN AVAILABILITY

Replens

PREGNANCY CATEGORY C

CLASSIFICATION

Laxative: Bulk-forming

AVAILABILITY (OTC)

Tablets: 500 mg, 1,000 mg. **Tablets (chewable):** 500 mg.

PHARMACODYNAMICS

	ONSET	PEAK	DURATION
Oral	12–72 hrs	—	—

PHARMACOKINETICS

Acts in small/large intestine.

ACTION/*THERAPEUTIC EFFECT*

Laxative: Retains water in intestine, opposes dehydrating forces of the bowel (promotes well-formed stools). **Antidiarrheal:** Absorbs free fecal water (forms gel, producing formed stool). *Restores normal moisture level, provides bulk.*

USES

Treatment of diarrhea associated w/irritable bowel syndrome, diverticulosis, acute nonspecific diarrhea. Relieves constipation associated w/irritable or spastic bowel.

INDICATIONS/ROUTES/DOSAGE

Note: For severe diarrhea, give every $\frac{1}{2}$ hr up to maximum daily dosage; for laxative, give w/8 oz liquid.

Laxative, antidiarrheal:

Oral: Adults, elderly: 1 g 4 times/day, or as needed. ***Maximum:***

6 g/24 hrs. ***Children 6–12 yrs:*** 500 mg 1–3 times/day, or as needed. ***Maximum:*** 3 g/24 hrs. ***Children 2–6 yrs:*** 500 mg 1–2 times/day, or as needed. ***Maximum:*** 1.5 g/24 hrs.

CONTRAINDICATIONS

Abdominal pain, nausea, vomiting, symptoms of appendicitis, partial bowel obstruction, dysphagia.

CAUTIONS

None significant.

INTERACTIONS

DRUG: May interfere w/effects of ***potassium-sparing diuretics, potassium supplements.*** May decrease effects of ***oral anticoagulants, digoxin, salicylates, tetracyclines*** by decreasing absorption. **HERBAL:** None known. **FOOD:** None significant. **ALTERED LAB VALUES:** May increase glucose. May decrease potassium.

SIDE EFFECTS

RARE: Some degree of abdominal discomfort, nausea, mild cramps, griping, faintness.

ADVERSE REACTIONS/TOXIC EFFECTS

Esophageal/bowel obstruction may occur if administered with insufficient liquid (less than 250 ml or 1 full glass).

PATIENT CONSIDERATIONS

INTERVENTION/EVALUATION

Encourage adequate fluid intake. Assess bowel sounds for peristalsis. Monitor daily bowel activity, stool consistency (watery, loose, soft, semisolid, solid) and record time of evacuation. Monitor serum electrolytes in those exposed to prolonged, frequent, or excessive use of medication.

PATIENT/FAMILY TEACHING

Institute measures to promote defecation (increase fluid intake, exercise, high-fiber diet). Drink 6–8 glasses of water/day when used as laxative (aids stool softening).

polyethylene glycol-electrolyte solution (PEG-ES)

poly-**eth**-ah-leen
(Colovage, CoLyte, GoLYTELY, MiraLax, NuLytely, OCL)

CANADIAN AVAILABILITY
CoLyte, Golytely, Klean-Prep, Peglyte, Pro-Lax

PREGNANCY CATEGORY C

CLASSIFICATION

Bowel evacuant

AVAILABILITY (Rx)

Powder for Oral Solution. Oral Solution.

PHARMACODYNAMICS

	ONSET	PEAK	DURATION
Oral	30–60 min	—	Completed: 4 hrs

ACTION/*THERAPEUTIC EFFECT*

Osmotic effect. *Induces diarrhea, cleanses bowel* (electrolytes in solution prevent water/electrolyte imbalance).

USES

Bowel cleansing before GI examination and colon surgery. **Miralax:** Treatment of occasional constipation.

P

STORAGE/HANDLING

Refrigerate reconstituted solutions; use within 48 hrs.

ADMINISTRATION

ORAL:

- May use tap water to prepare solution. Shake vigorously several minutes to ensure complete dissolution of powder.
- Fasting should occur at least 3 hrs before ingestion of solution (solid food should always be avoided <2 hrs before administration).
- Only clear liquids permitted after administration.
- May give via N-G tube.
- Rapid drinking preferred.

INDICATIONS/ROUTES/DOSAGE

Bowel evacuant:
Oral: Adults: 4 L prior to GI examination: 240 ml (8 oz) q10 min until 4 L consumed or rectal effluent clear. *N-G tube:* 20–30 ml/min.

Constipation:
Oral: Adults: 17 g/day.

CONTRAINDICATIONS

GI obstruction, gastric retention, bowel perforation, toxic colitis, toxic megacolon, ileus.

CAUTIONS

Ulcerative colitis.

INTERACTIONS

DRUG: May decrease absorption of ***oral medications*** if given within 1 hr (may be flushed from GI tract). **HERBAL:** None known. **FOOD:** None significant. **ALTERED LAB VALUES:** None significant.

SIDE EFFECTS

FREQUENT (>10%): Some degree of abdominal fullness, nausea, bloating. **OCCASIONAL (1–10%):** Abdominal cramping, vomiting, anal irritation. **RARE (<1%):** Urticaria, rhinorrhea, dermatitis.

ADVERSE REACTIONS/TOXIC EFFECTS

None significant.

PATIENT CONSIDERATIONS

BASELINE ASSESSMENT

Do not give oral medication within 1 hr of start of therapy (may not adequately be absorbed before GI cleansing).

INTERVENTION/EVALUATION

Assess bowel sounds for peristalsis. Monitor bowel activity, stool consistency (watery, loose, soft, semisolid, solid) and record time of evacuation. Assess for abdominal disturbances.

polymyxin B sulfate

polly-**mix**-in
(Aerosporin)

FIXED-COMBINATION(S)

Ophthalmic: W/bacitracin, an anti-infective **(Ocumycin, Polysporin Ophthalmic, AK-Poly-Bac)**; w/neomycin, an aminoglycoside **(Statrol)**; w/neomycin and bacitracin, anti-infectives **(Neosporin, AK-Spore, Ocutricin)**; w/neomycin and bacitracin, anti-infectives, and hydrocortisone, a corticosteroid **(Coracin)**; w/dexamethasone, a corticosteroid, and neomycin, an aminoglycoside **(AK-Trol, Dexacidin, Dex-Ide, Maxitrol)**; w/chloramphenicol, an antibiotic **(Ophthocort)**. *Misc:* W/neomycin, an aminoglycoside **(Neosporin GU irrigant)**.

PREGNANCY CATEGORY B

CLASSIFICATION

Antibiotic

AVAILABILITY (Rx)

Injection: 500,000 units. **Ophthalmic Powder for Solution.**

PHARMACOKINETICS

Widely distributed in tissues. **Excretion:** Excreted unchanged in urine. Serum concentration increased, half-life prolonged in those w/renal impairment. **Half-life:** 4–6 hrs (increased in decreased renal function).

ACTION/*THERAPEUTIC EFFECT*

Alters cell membrane permeability in susceptible microorganisms, *producing bactericidal activity.*

USES

Septicemia, infections of skin, urinary tract, meninges; treatment of superficial ocular infections, minor skin abrasions, external ear canal infections, mastoidectomy cavity infections. Prevents bacteriuria/bacteremia associated w/indwelling catheters (combination w/neomycin) as irrigating solution.

STORAGE/HANDLING

After reconstitution, solution stable for 72 hrs if refrigerated. Discard if precipitate forms.

ADMINISTRATION

- **Note:** Pts must be hospitalized, closely supervised by physician for parenteral administration.

IM:

- Reconstitute each 500,000 unit vial w/2 ml sterile water for injection, 0.9% NaCl injection, or 1% procaine to provide concentration of 250,000 units/ml.
- Administer deeply into upper outer quadrant of gluteus maximus.
- Repeat IM injections at same site not recommended (produces tissue irritation, pain).

IV:

- For IV infusion (piggyback), further dilute w/300–500 ml 5% dextrose. Infuse over 60–90 min.
- Alternating IV sites, use large veins to reduce risk of phlebitis.

OPHTHALMIC:

- Place finger on lower eyelid and pull out until a pocket is formed between eye and lower lid. Hold dropper above pocket and place correct number of drops (1/4–1/2 inch ointment) into pocket.
- Have pt close eye gently; *w/solution,* apply digital pressure to lacrimal sac for 1–2 min (minimizes draining into nose and throat, reducing risk of systemic effects).
- *W/ointment,* have pt close and roll eyes in all directions (increases contact area of drug to eye).
- Remove excess solution or ointment around eye w/tissue.

INDICATIONS/ROUTES/DOSAGE

Mild to moderate infections:
IV: Adults, elderly, children >2 yrs: 15,000–25,000 units/kg/day in divided doses q12h. ***Infants:*** Up to 40,000 units/kg/day.

IM: Adults, elderly, children >2 yrs: 25,000–30,000 units/kg/day in divided doses q4–6h. ***Infants:*** Up to 40,000 units/kg/day.

Usual irrigation dosage:
Continuous bladder irrigation: Adults, elderly: 1 ml urogenital concentrate (contains 200,000 units

polymyxin B, 57 mg neomycin) added to 1,000 ml 0.9% NaCl. Give each 1,000 ml >24 hrs for up to 10 days (may increase to 2,000 ml/day when urine output >2 L/day).

Usual ophthalmic dosage:
Adults, elderly, children: 1 drop q3–4h.

CONTRAINDICATIONS

Hypersensitivity to polymyxins or other components in fixed-combinations.

CAUTIONS

Renal impairment, neuromuscular disorders.

INTERACTIONS

DRUG: May produce muscle paralysis, prolonged or increased skeletal muscle relaxation w/***neuromuscular blocking agents or anesthetics. Aminoglycosides, other nephrotoxic drugs*** may increase nephrotoxicity. **HERBAL:** None known. **FOOD:** None significant. **ALTERED LAB VALUES:** None significant.

SIDE EFFECTS

FREQUENT: Severe pain, irritation at IM injection sites, phlebitis, thrombophlebitis w/IV administration. **OCCASIONAL:** Fever, urticaria.

ADVERSE REACTIONS/TOXIC EFFECTS

Nephrotoxicity, especially w/concurrent/sequential use of other nephrotoxic drugs, renal impairment, concurrent/sequential use of muscle relaxants. Neurotoxicity may occur, especially w/other neurotoxic medications, following anesthesia. Superinfection, especially w/fungi, may occur.

PATIENT CONSIDERATIONS

BASELINE ASSESSMENT

Question pt for history of allergies to polymyxins, other ingredients when used in fixed-combinations. Avoid concurrent administration of other nephrotoxic, neurotoxic drugs if possible. Obtain specimens for culture, sensitivity before giving first dose (therapy may begin before results are known).

INTERVENTION/EVALUATION

Evaluate IV sites for phlebitis (heat, pain, red streaking over vein). Assess pain, irritation from IM injections. Check I&O, renal function tests. Monitor level of consciousness. Assess for muscle weakness, steadiness on ambulation (support as needed). Obtain vital signs, be especially alert to respiratory depression.

PATIENT/FAMILY TEACHING

Therapy must be continued for full length of treatment. Discomfort may occur at IM injection sites. Notify physician in event of dizziness, drowsiness, difficulty breathing, or other new symptoms: w/ophthalmic therapy, report any increased irritation, inflammation, itching, burning.

---

poractant

(Curosurf)

See Supplement

---

porfimer sodium

(Photofrin)

See Classification section under: Cancer chemotherapy

---

potassium acetate

(Potassium acetate)

potassium bicarbonate/citrate

(K-Lyte)

potassium chloride

(K-Lor, K-Lyte-Cl, Klotrix, K-Dur, Kaochlor, Micro-K, Slow-K)

potassium gluconate

(Kaon)

potassium phosphate

(Potassium phosphate)

CANADIAN AVAILABILITY
Apo-K, Kaochlor, K-Dur, K-Lor, Micro-K, Slow-K

PREGNANCY CATEGORY A

CLASSIFICATION

Electrolyte

AVAILABILITY (Rx)

Acetate: Injection: 2 mEq/ml

Bicarbonate/Citrate: Effervescent Tablets: 25 mEq, 50 mEq

Chloride: Tablets: 6.7 mEq, 8 mEq, 10 mEq, 20 mEq. **Liquid:** 20 mEq/15 ml, 30 mEq/15 ml, 40 mEq/15 ml, 45 mEq/15 ml. **Oral Powder:** 15 mEq, 20 mEq, 25 mEq. **Injection:** 2 mEq/ml, 4 mEq/ml.

Gluconate: Liquid: 20 mEq/15 ml

Phosphate: Injection: 3 mM/ml (mM = millimoles)

PHARMACOKINETICS

Absorption: Well absorbed from GI tract. Enters cells via active transport from extracellular fluid. **Excretion:** Primarily excreted in urine.

ACTION/*THERAPEUTIC EFFECT*

Necessary for multiple cellular metabolic processes. Primary action intracellular. Necessary *for nerve impulse conduction, contraction of cardiac, skeletal, smooth muscle; maintains normal renal function, acid-base balance.*

USES

Treatment of potassium deficiency found in severe vomiting, diarrhea, loss of GI fluid, malnutrition, prolonged diuresis, debilitated, poor GI absorption, metabolic alkalosis, prolonged parenteral alimentation; prevents hypokalemia in risk pts.

STORAGE/HANDLING

Store oral, parenteral forms at room temperature.

ADMINISTRATION

ORAL:

- Take w/or after meals and w/full glass of water (decreases GI upset).
- Liquids, powder, or effervescent tablets: Mix, dissolve w/juice, water before administering.
- Do not chew, crush tablets; swallow whole.

IV:

- For IV infusion only, must dilute before administration/mixed well/infused slowly.
- Generally, no more than 40 mEq/L; no faster than 20 mEq/hr. (Higher concentrations/faster rates may sometimes be necessary.)
- Use largest peripheral vein/ small-bore needle.
- Avoid adding potassium to hanging IV.
- Check IV site closely during infusion for evidence of phlebitis (heat, pain, red streaking of skin over vein, hardness to

vein), extravasation (swelling, pain, cool skin, little or no blood return).

INDICATIONS/ROUTES/DOSAGE

Treatment/prevention of hypokalemia:
Note: Dosage is individualized.

Oral: Adults, elderly: Prevention: 20 mEq/day. ***Treatment:*** 40–100 mEq/day. ***Children:*** No more than 3 mEq/kg/day. ***Infants:*** 2–3 mEq/kg/day. Give in 2–4 divided doses.

IV: Adults, elderly, children: Individualize based on EKG, serum potassium concentrations.

CONTRAINDICATIONS

Severe renal impairment, untreated Addison's disease, postop oliguria, shock w/hemolytic reaction and/or dehydration, hyperkalemia, those receiving potassium-sparing diuretics, digitalis toxicity, heat cramps, severe burns.

CAUTIONS

Cardiac disease, tartrazine sensitivity (mostly noted in those w/aspirin hypersensitivity).

INTERACTIONS

DRUG: ***Angiotensin-converting enzyme (ACE) inhibitors, NSAIDs, beta-adrenergic blockers, potassium-sparing diuretics, heparin, potassium-containing medications, salt substitutes*** may increase potassium concentration. ***Anticholinergics*** may increase risk of GI lesions. **HERBAL:** None known. **FOOD:** None significant. **ALTERED LAB VALUES:** None significant.

SIDE EFFECTS

OCCASIONAL: Nausea, vomiting, diarrhea, flatulence, abdominal discomfort w/distension, phlebitis w/IV administration (particularly when potassium concentration of more than 40 mEq/L is infused). **RARE:** Rash, irritation GI tract.

ADVERSE REACTIONS/TOXIC EFFECTS

Hyperkalemia (observed particularly in elderly or in those w/impaired renal function) manifested as paresthesia of extremities, heaviness of legs, cold skin, grayish pallor, hypotension, mental confusion, irritability, flaccid paralysis, cardiac arrhythmias.

PATIENT CONSIDERATIONS

BASELINE ASSESSMENT

Oral dose should be given w/food or after meals w/full glass of water or fruit juice (minimizes GI irritation).

INTERVENTION/EVALUATION

Monitor serum potassium level (particularly in renal function impairment). If GI disturbance is noted, dilute preparation further or give w/meals. Be alert to decrease in urinary output (may be indication of renal insufficiency). Monitor daily bowel activity, stool consistency. Assess I&O diligently during diuresis, IV site for extravasation, phlebitis. Be alert to evidence of hyperkalemia (skin pallor/coldness, complaints of paresthesia of extremities, feeling of heaviness of legs).

PATIENT/FAMILY TEACHING

Foods rich in potassium include beef, veal, ham, chicken, turkey, fish, milk, bananas, dates, prunes, raisins, avocado, watermelon, cantaloupe, apricots, molasses, beans, yams, broccoli, brussel sprouts, lentils, potatoes,

spinach. Report paresthesia of extremities, feeling of heaviness of legs.

pramipexole

pram-ih-**pecks**-all
(Mirapex)

CANADIAN AVAILABILITY
Mirapex

PREGNANCY CATEGORY C

CLASSIFICATION

Antiparkinson agent

AVAILABILITY (Rx)

Tablets: 0.125 mg, 0.25 mg, 1 mg, 1.5 mg

PHARMACOKINETICS

Absorption: Rapid, extensive absorption following oral administration. Widely distributed. **Metabolism:** Distributed into red blood cells. Steady-state concentrations achieved within 2 days. No metabolites identified. **Excretion:** Primarily eliminated in the urine. **Half-life:** 8 hrs (12 hrs in elderly >65 yrs).

ACTION/*THERAPEUTIC EFFECT*

Stimulates dopamine receptors in the striatum, *relieving signs/symptoms of Parkinson's disease.*

USES/*UNLABELED*

Treatment of signs and symptoms of idiopathic Parkinson's disease.

ADMINISTRATION

ORAL:

- May take w/o regard to food.

INDICATIONS/ROUTES/DOSAGES

Parkinson's disease:
Oral: Adults, elderly: Initially, 0.375 mg/day in 3 divided doses. Do not increase dose more frequently than every 5–7 days. *Maintenance:* 1.5–4.5 mg/day in equally divided doses 3 times/day.

Renal function impairment:
Oral: Adults, elderly, creatinine clearance >60 ml/min: Initially, 0.125 mg 3 times/day. ***Maximum:*** 1.5 mg 3 times/day. ***Creatinine clearance 35–59 ml/min:*** Initially, 0.125 mg 2 times/day. ***Maximum:*** 1.5 mg twice daily. ***Creatinine clearance 15–34 ml/min:*** Initially, 0.125 mg 1 time/day. ***Maximum:*** 1.5 mg once daily.

CONTRAINDICATIONS

History of hypersensitivity to medication.

CAUTIONS

History of orthostatic hypotension, syncope, hallucinations, renal function impairment, use of concomitant CNS depressants.

INTERACTIONS

DRUG: *Cimetidine* increases pramipexole's plasma concentration and increases its half-life. Combined use of ***cimetidine, ranitidine, diltiatem, triamterene, verapamil, quinidine, quinine*** may decrease pramipexole clearance. May increase plasma levels of ***carbidopa or levodopa combinations.*** **HERBAL:** None known. **FOOD:** Time to maximum plasma levels is increased by 1 hr when taken with food (extent of absorption not affected). **ALTERED LAB VALUES:** None significant.

SIDE EFFECTS

Early Parkinson's disease:
FREQUENT (10–30%): Asthenia

P

(weakness), dizziness, somnolence, insomnia, nausea, constipation. **OCCASIONAL (1–10%):** Edema, malaise, fever, confusion, amnesia, akathisia (restlessness), anorexia, dysphagia, peripheral edema, decreased weight, altered vision, impotence.

Advanced Parkinson's disease: FREQUENT (>25%): Postural hypotension, dyskinesia, extrapyramidal signs, insomnia, dizziness, hallucinations. **OCCASIONAL (10–25%):** Accidental injury, asthenia, somnolence, confusion, constipation. **RARE (1–10%):** Edema, malaise, chest pain, gait abnormality, amnesia, tremors, restlessness, urinary frequency/incontinence, urinary tract infection, arthritis, dyspnea, rhinitis, vision changes, dry mouth.

ADVERSE REACTIONS/TOXIC EFFECTS

None significant.

PATIENT CONSIDERATIONS

INTERVENTION/EVALUATION

Instruct patient to rise from lying to sitting or sitting to standing position slowly to prevent risk of postural hypotension. Assess for clinical improvement. Assist with ambulation if dizziness occurs. Assess for constipation; encourage fiber, fluids, and exercise.

PATIENT/FAMILY TEACHING

Inform patient that hallucination may occur, more so in the elderly than in younger patients with Parkinson's disease. Postural hypotension may occur more frequently during initial therapy. Avoid tasks that require alertness, motor skills until response to drug is established. If nausea occurs, take medication with food. Do not abruptly discontinue medication.

pravastatin

pra-vah-**stah**-tin
(Pravachol)

CANADIAN AVAILABILITY
Pravachol

PREGNANCY CATEGORY X

CLASSIFICATION

Antihyperlipoproteinemic

AVAILABILITY (Rx)

Tablets: 10 mg, 20 mg, 40 mg

PHARMACOKINETICS

Absorption: Poorly absorbed from GI tract. **Metabolism:** Metabolized in liver (minimal active metabolites). **Excretion:** Primarily excreted in feces via biliary system. **Half-life:** 2.7 hrs.

ACTION/*THERAPEUTIC EFFECT*

Interferes w/cholesterol biosynthesis by preventing the conversion of HMG-CoA reductase to mevalonate, a precursor to cholesterol. *Lowers LDL cholesterol, VLDL, plasma triglycerides; increases HDL concentration.*

USES

Preventive therapy to reduce risks of the following in pts w/previous myocardial infarction (MI) and normal cholesterol levels: recurrent MI, undergoing myocardial revascularization procedures, stroke or transient ischemic attack. Prevents CV events in pts w/elevated cholesterol levels.

ADMINISTRATION

ORAL:
- Give w/o regard to meals.
- Administer in evening.

INDICATIONS/ROUTES/DOSAGE

Note: Before initiating therapy, pt should be on standard cholesterol-lowering diet for minimum of 3–6 mos. Continue diet throughout pravastatin therapy.

Usual dosage:
Oral: Adults: Initially, 10–20 mg/day at bedtime. ***Elderly:*** Initially, 10 mg/day at bedtime. ***Range:*** 10–40 mg/day at bedtime.

CONTRAINDICATIONS

Hypersensitivity to pravastatin or any component of the preparation, active liver disease or unexplained, persistent elevations of liver function tests. Safety and efficacy in individuals less than 18 yrs of age has not been established.

CAUTIONS

History of liver disease, substantial alcohol consumption. Withholding/discontinuing pravastatin may be necessary when pt at risk for renal failure secondary to rhabdomyolysis. Severe metabolic, endocrine, or electrolyte disorders.

INTERACTIONS

DRUG: Increased risk of rhabdomyolysis, acute renal failure ***w/cyclosporine, erythromycin, gemfibrozil, niacin, other immunosuppressants.*** **HERBAL:** None known. **FOOD:** None significant. **ALTERED LAB VALUES:** May increase creatinine kinase, serum transaminase concentrations.

SIDE EFFECTS

Generally well tolerated. Side effects usually mild and transient. **FREQUENT (5–10%):** Nausea, vomitng, diarrhea, abdominal pain, headache, rhinitis. **OCCASIONAL (1–5%):** Constipation, heartburn, dyspepsia, muscle pain, dizziness, cough, rash, itching, fatigue, flulike symptoms.

ADVERSE REACTIONS/TOXIC EFFECTS

Potential for malignancy, cataracts. Hypersensitivity syndrome has been reported rarely.

PATIENT CONSIDERATIONS

BASELINE ASSESSMENT

Question for possibility of pregnancy before initiating therapy (Pregnancy Category X). Question history of hypersensitivity to pravastatin. Assess baseline lab results: cholesterol, triglycerides, liver function tests.

INTERVENTION/EVALUATION

Monitor cholesterol and triglyceride lab results for therapeutic response. Monitor liver function tests. Evaluate food tolerance. Determine pattern of bowel activity. Check for headache, dizziness (provide assistance as needed). Assess for rash, pruritus. Be alert for malaise, muscle cramping/weakness; if accompanied by fever, may require discontinuation of medication.

PATIENT/FAMILY TEACHING

Take w/o regard to meals. Follow special diet (important part of treatment). Periodic lab tests are essential part of therapy. Do not take other medications w/o physician's knowledge. Do not stop medication w/o consulting physician. Report promptly any muscle pain/weakness, especially if accompanied by fever or malaise. Do not drive/perform activities that require alert response if dizziness occurs. Use nonhormonal contraception.

praziquantel

pray-zih-**kwon**-tel
(Biltricide)

CANADIAN AVAILABILITY
Biltricide

PREGNANCY CATEGORY B

CLASSIFICATION

Anthelmintic

AVAILABILITY (Rx)

Tablets: 600 mg

PHARMACOKINETICS

Absorption: Rapidly absorbed from GI tract (undergoes extensive first-pass metabolism). Distributed in serum, CSF. **Metabolism:** Metabolized in liver. **Excretion:** Primarily excreted in urine. **Half-life:** 0.8–1.5 hrs (metabolite: 4–6 hrs).

ACTION/*THERAPEUTIC EFFECT*

Vermicidal. Increases cell permeability in susceptible helminths resulting in loss of intracellular calcium, massive contractions and paralysis of their musculature, followed by attachment of phagocytes to the parasites, *dislodging the dead and dying worms.*

USES

Treatment of all stages of schistosomiasis (bilharziasis or fluke infections), infections due to liver flukes, clonorchiasis and opisthorchiasis.

ADMINISTRATION

ORAL:

- Tablets must not be chewed, but can be halved or quartered.
- Give w/meals, w/sufficient fluid to swallow w/o gagging.

INDICATIONS/ROUTES/DOSAGE

Schistosomiasis:
Oral: Adults, elderly: 3 doses of 20 mg/kg as 1 day treatment. Do not give doses <4 hrs or >6 hrs apart.

Clonorchiasis/opisthorchiasis:
Oral: Adults, elderly: 3 doses of 25 mg/kg as 1 day treatment.

CONTRAINDICATIONS

Ocular cysticercosis, hypersensitivity to praziquantel.

CAUTIONS

None significant.

INTERACTIONS

DRUG: None significant. **HERBAL:** None known. **FOOD:** None significant. **ALTERED LAB VALUES:** None significant.

SIDE EFFECTS

FREQUENT: Headache, dizziness, malaise, abdominal pain occur in 90% of pts. **OCCASIONAL:** Anorexia, vomiting, diarrhea. Severe cramping abdominal pain may occur within 1 hr of administration w/fever, sweating, bloody stools. **RARE:** Giddiness, urticaria.

ADVERSE REACTIONS/TOXIC EFFECTS

Overdose should be treated w/fast-acting laxative.

PATIENT CONSIDERATIONS

BASELINE ASSESSMENT

Question for history of hypersensitivity to praziquantel. Obtain

stool, urine specimens to confirm diagnosis.

INTERVENTION/EVALUATION

Collect stool, urine specimens as required to monitor effectiveness of therapy. Assess food tolerance, encourage adequate nutrition. Monitor CNS reactions, provide safety measures for ambulation. Check hematology results for anemia. Assess for urticaria.

PATIENT/FAMILY TEACHING

Complete full course of therapy. If iron supplements are ordered, continue as directed (may be up to 6 mos post therapy). Notify physician if symptoms do not improve in a few days, or if they become worse. Follow-up office visits (several months after therapy is complete) are essential to assure cure. Don't drive, use machinery if dizzy or drowsy.

prazosin hydrochloride

pray-zoe-sin
(Minipress)

FIXED-COMBINATION(S)
W/polythiazide, a diuretic **(Minizide)**

CANADIAN AVAILABILITY
Minipress

PREGNANCY CATEGORY C

CLASSIFICATION

Antihypertensive

AVAILABILITY (Rx)

Capsules: 1 mg, 2 mg, 5 mg

PHARMACODYNAMICS

	ONSET	PEAK	DURATION
Oral	2 hrs	2–4 hrs	24 hrs

PHARMACOKINETICS

Absorption: Well absorbed from GI tract. Widely distributed. **Metabolism:** Metabolized in liver. **Excretion:** Primarily eliminated in feces and bile. Not removed by hemodialysis. **Half-life:** 2–3 hrs.

ACTION/*THERAPEUTIC EFFECT*

Blocks alpha-adrenergic receptors. *Produces vasodilation, decreases peripheral resistance.*

P

USES/*UNLABELED*

Treatment of mild to moderate hypertension. Used alone or in combination w/other antihypertensives. *Treatment of CHF, ergot alkaloid toxicity, pheochromocytoma, Raynaud's phenomena, benign prostate hypertrophy.*

ADMINISTRATION

ORAL:

- May give w/o regard to food.
- Administer first dose at bedtime (minimizes risk of fainting due to "first-dose syncope").

INDICATIONS/ROUTES/DOSAGE

Hypertension (alone):
Oral: Adults: Initially, 0.5–1 mg 2–3 times/day. Increase gradually up to 20–40 mg/day in divided doses. ***Maintenance:*** 6–15 mg/day in divided doses.

Hypertension (in combinations w/antihypertensives):
Oral: Adults: 1–2 mg 3 times/day and retitrate.

Usual elderly dosage:
Oral: Initially, 1 mg 1–2 times/day.

CONTRAINDICATIONS

None significant.

CAUTIONS

Chronic renal failure, impaired hepatic function.

INTERACTIONS

DRUG: *Estrogen, NSAIDs, sympathomimetics* may decrease effect. *Hypotension-producing medications* may increase antihypertensive effect. **HERBAL:** None known. **FOOD:** None significant. **ALTERED LAB VALUES:** None significant.

SIDE EFFECTS

FREQUENT (3–9%): Dizziness, orthostatic hypotension, drowsiness, headache, malaise, asthma. OCCASIONAL (1–3%): Dry mouth, fatigue, nervousness, palpitations. **RARE (<1%):** Angina, dyspnea, nausea, frequent urge to urinate.

ADVERSE REACTIONS/TOXIC EFFECTS

"First-dose syncope" (hypotension w/sudden loss of consciousness) generally occurs 30–90 min after giving initial dose of 2 mg or greater, a too rapid increase in dose, or addition of another hypotensive agent to therapy. May be preceded by tachycardia (120–160 beats/min).

PATIENT CONSIDERATIONS

Baseline Assessment

Give first dose at bedtime. If initial dose is given during daytime, pt must remain recumbent for 3–4 hrs. Assess B/P, pulse immediately before each dose and q15–30min until stabilized (be alert to B/P fluctuations).

Intervention/Evaluation

Monitor pulse diligently (first-dose syncope may be preceded by tachycardia). Monitor pattern of daily bowel activity and stool consistency. Assist w/ambulation if dizziness, lightheadedness occurs.

Patient/Family Teaching

Dry mouth may be relieved by sugarless gum/sips of tepid water. Carbonated beverage, unsalted crackers, dry toast may relieve nausea. Nasal congestion may occur. Full therapeutic effect may not occur for 3–4 wks. May cause syncope (fainting). Avoid driving for 12–24 hrs after first dose or increase in dosage. Use caution driving or operating machinery. Use caution when rising from sitting or lying position. Report dizziness or palpitations if bothersome.

---

prednicarbate

(Dermatop)

See Supplement
See Classification section under: Corticosteroids: topical

---

prednisolone

pred-**niss**-oh-lone
(Prelone, Delta-Cortef)

prednisolone acetate

(Econopred, Inflamase, Pred Mild, Pred Forte, Predolone)

prednisolone sodium phosphate

(Hydeltrasol, Pediapred)

prednisolone tebutate

(Hydeltra TBA, Predalone TBA)

FIXED-COMBINATION(S)

Prednisolone acetate w/sulfacetamide sodium, a sulfonamide **(Blephamide Liquifilm, Isopto Cetopred)**; w/atropine sulfate, a mydriatic **(Mydrapred)**; w/neomycin and polymyxin B, anti-infectives **(Poly-Pred Liquifilm).**

Prednisolone sodium phosphate w/sulfacetamide, a sulfonamide **(Vasocidin, Optimyd).**

CANADIAN AVAILABILITY

Inflamase, Pediapred

PREGNANCY CATEGORY B

CLASSIFICATION

Corticosteroid

AVAILABILITY (Rx)

Tablets: 5 mg. **Syrup:** 15 mg/5 ml. **Ophthalmic Suspension:** 0.125%, 1%. **Ophthalmic Solution:** 1%.

Acetate: Injection: 25 mg/ml, 50 mg/ml

Phosphate: Injection: 20 mg/ml. **Oral Liquid:** 5 mg/5 ml.

Tebutate: Injection: 20 mg/ml

PHARMACOKINETICS

Absorption: Well absorbed from GI tract, after IM administration. Widely distributed. **Metabolism:** Metabolized in liver, tissues. **Excretion:** Primarily excreted in urine. **Half-life:** 3–6 hrs.

ACTION / *THERAPEUTIC EFFECT*

Inhibits accumulation of inflammatory cells at inflammation sites, phagocytosis, lysosomal enzyme release and synthesis, and/or release of mediators of inflammation. *Prevents/suppresses cell-mediated immune reactions. Decreases/prevents tissue response to inflammatory process.*

USES

Substitution therapy in deficiency states: Acute/chronic adrenal insufficiency, congenital adrenal hyperplasia, adrenal insufficiency secondary to pituitary insufficiency. ***Nonendocrine disorders:*** Arthritis, rheumatic carditis; allergic, collagen, intestinal tract, liver, ocular, renal, skin diseases; bronchial asthma, cerebral edema, malignancies.

ADMINISTRATION

ORAL:

- Give w/food or milk.
- Single doses given before 9 AM; multiple doses at evenly spaced intervals.

IM:

- Give deep IM in gluteus maximus.

IV:

- May add to 5% dextrose in water or 0.9% NaCl; use within 24 hrs.
- Prednisolone tebutate not for IV use.

OPHTHALMIC:

- Place finger on lower eyelid and pull out until a pocket is formed between eye and lower lid. Hold dropper above pocket and place correct number of drops (1/4–1/2 inch ointment) into pocket. Close eye gently. *Solution: Apply digital pressure to lacrimal sac for 1–2 min (minimizes drainage into nose and throat, reducing risk of systemic*

effects). Remove excess solution around eye w/tissue.
- *As w/other corticosteroids, taper dosage slowly when discontinuing.*

INDICATIONS/ROUTES/DOSAGE

Note: Individualize dose based on disease, pt, and response.

Usual Oral Dosage:

Oral: Adults, elderly: 5–60 mg/day.

Multiple sclerosis:
Oral: Adults, elderly: 200 mg/day for 1 wk; then 80 mg every other day for 1 mo.

Prednisolone Acetate:

IM: Adults, elderly: 4–60 mg/day.

Intralesional, Intra-articular, Soft Tissue: Adults, elderly: 5 mg up to 100 mg/day.

Multiple sclerosis:
IM: Adults, elderly: 200 mg/day for 7 days; then 80 mg every other day for 30 days.

Prednisolone Tebutate:

Intralesional, Intra-articular, Soft Tissue: Adults, elderly: 4–30 mg.

Prednisolone Sodium Phosphate:

IM/IV Adults, elderly: 4–60 mg/day.

Intralesional, Intra-articular, Soft Tissue: Adults, elderly: 2–30 mg.

Multiple sclerosis:
IM: Adults, elderly: 200 mg/day for 7 days; then 80 mg every other day for 30 days.

Usual Ophthalmic Dosage:

Adults, elderly: Solution: 1–2 drops q1h during day; q2h during night; after response, decrease dose to 1 drop q4h, then 1 drop 3–4 times/day. ***Ointment:*** thin coat 3–4 times/day; after response, decrease to 2 times/day; then once daily.

CONTRAINDICATIONS

Hypersensitivity to any corticosteroid or tartrazine, systemic fungal infection, peptic ulcers (except life-threatening situations). Avoid live virus vaccine such as smallpox.

CAUTIONS

Thromboembolic disorders, history of tuberculosis (may reactivate disease), hypothyroidism, cirrhosis, nonspecific ulcerative colitis, CHF, hypertension, psychosis, renal insufficiency, seizure disorders. Prolonged therapy should be discontinued slowly.

INTERACTIONS

DRUG: ***Amphotericin*** may increase hypokalemia. May decrease effect of ***oral hypoglycemics, insulin, diuretics, potassium supplements***. May increase ***digoxin*** toxicity (due to hypokalemia). ***Hepatic enzyme inducers*** may decrease effect. ***Live virus vaccines*** may potentiate virus replication, increase vaccine side effects, decrease pt's antibody response to vaccine. **HERBAL:** None known. **FOOD:** None significant. **ALTERED LAB VALUES:** May decrease calcium, potassium, thyroxine. May increase cholesterol, lipids, glucose, sodium, amylase.

SIDE EFFECTS

FREQUENT: Insomnia, heartburn, nervousness, abdominal distension, increased sweating, acne, mood swings, increased appetite, facial flushing, delayed wound healing, increased susceptibility to infection, diarrhea/constipation. **OCCASIONAL:** Headache, edema, change in skin color, frequent urination. **RARE:** Tachycardia, allergic reaction (rash, hives), psychic changes, hallucinations, depression. *Ophthalmic:* Stinging or burning, posterior subcapsular cataracts.

ADVERSE REACTIONS/TOXIC EFFECTS

Long-term therapy: Hypocalcemia, hypokalemia, muscle wasting (especially arms, legs), osteoporosis, spontaneous fractures, amenorrhea, cataracts, glaucoma, peptic ulcer, CHF. *Abrupt withdrawal following long-term therapy:* Anorexia, nausea, fever, headache, sudden, severe joint pain, rebound inflammation, fatigue, weakness, lethargy, dizziness, orthostatic hypotension. Sudden discontinuance may be fatal.

PATIENT CONSIDERATIONS

Baseline Assessment

Question for hypersensitivity to any corticosteroids. Obtain baselines for height, weight, B/P, glucose, electrolytes. Check results of initial tests, (e.g., TB skin test, x-rays, EKG). Never give live virus vaccine (i.e., smallpox).

Intervention/Evaluation

Evaluate food tolerance and bowel activity; report hyperacidity promptly. Check B/P, temperature, pulse, respiration at least 2 times/day. Be alert to infection (sore throat, fever, or vague symptoms); assess mouth daily for signs of candida infection (white patches, painful tongue and mucous membranes). Monitor electrolytes. Monitor I&O, daily weight; assess for edema. Watch for hypokalemia (weakness and muscle cramps, numbness/tingling especially lower extremities, nausea and vomiting, irritability, EKG changes) or hypocalcemia (muscle twitching, cramps, positive Trousseau's or Chvostek's signs). Assess emotional status, ability to sleep.

Patient/Family Teaching

Carry identification of drug and dose, physician's name and phone number. Do not change dose/schedule or stop taking drug; must taper off gradually under medical supervision. Notify physician of fever, sore throat, muscle aches, sudden weight gain/swelling. W/dietician give instructions for prescribed diet (may be sodium restricted, high protein and potassium). Maintain careful personal hygiene, avoid exposure to disease or trauma. Severe stress (serious infection, surgery, or trauma) may require increased dosage. Do not take any other medication w/o consulting physician. Follow-up visits, lab tests are necessary; children must be assessed for growth retardation. Inform dentist or other physicians of prednisolone therapy now or within past 12 mos. Caution against overuse of joints injected for symptomatic relief.

Ophthalmic

Teach proper administration.

prednisone

pred-nih-sewn

(Orasone, Deltasone, Meticorten)

CANADIAN AVAILABILITY

Apo-Prednisone, Deltasone, Winpred

PREGNANCY CATEGORY B

CLASSIFICATION

Corticosteroid

AVAILABILITY (Rx)

Tablets: 1 mg, 2.5 mg, 5 mg, 10 mg, 20 mg, 50 mg. **Oral Solution:** 5 mg/5 ml, 5 mg/ml. **Syrup:** 5 mg/5 ml.

PHARMACOKINETICS

Absorption: Well absorbed from GI tract. Widely distributed. **Metabolism:** Metabolized in liver (converted to prednisolone). **Excretion:** Primarily excreted in urine. **Half-life:** 3.4–3.8 hrs.

ACTION/*THERAPEUTIC EFFECT*

Inhibits accumulation of inflammatory cells at inflammation sites, phagocytosis, lysosomal enzyme release and synthesis, and/or release of mediators of inflammation. *Prevents/suppresses cell-mediated immune reactions. Decreases/prevents tissue response to inflammatory process.*

USES

Substitution therapy in deficiency states: Acute/chronic adrenal insufficiency, congenital adrenal hyperplasia, adrenal insufficiency secondary to pituitary insufficiency. *Nonendocrine disorders:* Arthritis, rheumatic carditis; allergic, collagen, intestinal tract, liver, ocular, renal, skin diseases; bronchial asthma, cerebral edema, malignancies.

ADMINISTRATION

ORAL:

- Give w/o regard to meals (give w/food if GI upset occurs).
- Give single doses before 9 AM, multiple doses at evenly spaced intervals.

INDICATIONS/ROUTES/DOSAGE

Usual oral dosage:
Oral: Adults, elderly: 5–60 mg/day.
Children: 0.14–2 mg/kg/day.

CONTRAINDICATIONS

Hypersensitivity to any corticosteroid, systemic fungal infection, peptic ulcer (except life-threatening situations), breast feeding.

CAUTIONS

Thromboembolic disorders, history of tuberculosis (may reactivate disease), hypothyroidism, cirrhosis, nonspecific ulcerative colitis, CHF, hypertension, psychosis, renal insufficiency, seizure disorders.

INTERACTIONS

DRUG: *Amphotericin* may increase hypokalemia. May decrease effect of ***oral hypoglycemics, insulin, diuretics, potassium supplements.*** May increase ***digoxin*** toxicity (due to hypokalemia). ***Hepatic enzyme inducers*** may decrease effect. ***Live virus vaccines*** may potentiate virus replication, increase vaccine side effects, decrease pt's antibody response to vaccine. **HERBAL:** None known. **FOOD:** None significant. **ALTERED LAB VALUES:** May decrease calcium, potassium, thyroxine. May increase cholesterol, lipids, glucose, sodium, amylase.

SIDE EFFECTS

FREQUENT: Insomnia, heartburn, nervousness, abdominal distension, increased sweating, acne, mood swings, increased appetite, facial flushing, delayed wound healing, increased susceptibility to infection, diarrhea/constipation. **OCCASIONAL:** Headache, edema, change in skin color, frequent urination. **RARE:** Tachycardia, allergic reaction (rash, hives), psychic changes, hallucinations, depression.

ADVERSE REACTIONS/TOXIC EFFECTS

Long-term therapy: Muscle wasting (especially arms, legs), osteoporosis, spontaneous fractures, amenorrhea, cataracts, glaucoma, peptic ulcer, CHF. ***Abrupt withdrawal following long-term therapy:*** Anorexia, nausea, fever, headache, sudden or severe joint pain, rebound inflammation, fatigue, weakness, lethargy, dizziness, orthostatic hypotension. Sudden discontinuance may be fatal.

PATIENT CONSIDERATIONS

Baseline Assessment

Question for hypersensitivity to any corticosteroids. Obtain baselines for height, weight, B/P, glucose, electrolytes. Check results of initial tests, (e.g., TB skin test, x-rays, EKG). Never give live virus vaccine.

Intervention/Evaluation

Monitor I&O, daily weight; assess for edema. Check lab results for blood coagulability, clinical evidence of thromboembolism. Evaluate food tolerance, bowel activity; report hyperacidity promptly. Check B/P, temperature, pulse, respiration, at least 2 times/day. Be alert to infection: sore throat, fever/vague symptoms. Assess mouth daily for signs of candida infection (white patches, painful tongue and mucous membranes). Monitor electrolytes. Watch for hypocalcemia (muscle twitching, cramps, positive Trousseau's or Chvostek's signs) or hypokalemia (weakness and muscle cramps, numbness/tingling, especially lower extremities, nausea and vomiting, irritability, EKG changes). Assess emotional status, ability to sleep.

Patient/Family Teaching

Carry identification of drug and dose, physician's name and phone number. Do not change dose/schedule or stop taking drug (must taper off gradually under medical supervision). Notify physician of fever, sore throat, muscle aches, sudden weight gain/swelling. Give instructions for prescribed diet (may be sodium restricted, high protein and potassium). Maintain careful personal hygiene, avoid exposure to disease/trauma. Severe stress (serious infection, surgery, or trauma) may require increased dosage. Do not take any other medication w/o consulting physician. Follow-up visits, lab tests are necessary; children must be assessed for growth retardation. Inform dentist or other physicians of prednisone therapy now or within past 12 mos. Caution against overuse of joints injected for symptomatic relief.

P

primidone

prih-mih-doan
(Mysoline)

CANADIAN AVAILABILITY
Apo-Primidone, Mysoline

PREGNANCY CATEGORY D

CLASSIFICATION

Anticonvulsant

AVAILABILITY (Rx)

Tablets: 50 mg, 250 mg. **Oral Suspension:** 250 mg/5 ml.

PHARMACOKINETICS

Absorption: Rapidly, completely absorbed from GI tract. Widely distributed. **Metabolism:** Metabolized in liver to active metabolite (phenobarbital). **Excretion:** Primarily excreted in urine. **Half-life:** 3–23 hrs; metabolite: 75–126 hrs.

ACTION/*THERAPEUTIC EFFECT*

Decreases motor activity to electrical/chemical stimulation, stabilizes threshhold against hyperexcitability, *producing anticonvulsant effect.*

USES/*UNLABELED*

Management of partial seizures w/complex symptomatology (psychomotor seizures), generalized tonic-clonic (grand mal) seizures. *Treatment of essential tremor.*

ADMINISTRATION

ORAL:

- Give w/o regard to meals.
- Shake oral suspension well before administering (may be mixed w/food).
- Tablets may be crushed.

INDICATIONS/ROUTES/DOSAGE

Note: When replacement by another anticonvulsant is necessary, decrease primidone gradually as therapy begins w/low replacement dose.

Anticonvulsant:

Oral: Adults, elderly, children >8 yrs: 100–125 mg daily for 3 days at bedtime, then 100–125 mg 2 times/day for days 4–6, then 100–125 mg 3 times/day for days 7–9, then maintenance of 250 mg 3 times/day. ***Children <8 yrs:*** 50 mg at bedtime for 3 days, then 50 mg 2 times/day for days 4–6, then 100 mg 2 times/day for days 7–9, then maintenance of 125–250 mg 3 times/day.

CONTRAINDICATIONS

History of porphyria, bronchopneumonia.

EXTREME CAUTION

Nephritis, renal insufficiency.

CAUTIONS

Uncontrolled pain (may produce paradoxical reaction), impaired liver function.

INTERACTIONS

DRUG: May decrease effects of ***glucocorticoids, digoxin, metronidazole, oral anticoagulants, quinidine, tricyclic antidepressants. Alcohol, CNS depressants*** may increase effect. May increase metabolism of ***carbamazepine. Valproic acid*** decreases metabolism, increases concentration, toxicity. **HERBAL:** None known. **FOOD:** None significant. **ALTERED LAB VALUES:** May decrease bilirubin.

SIDE EFFECTS

FREQUENT: Ataxia, dizziness. **OCCASIONAL:** Loss of appetite, drowsiness, mental changes, nausea, vomiting, paradoxical excitement. **RARE:** Skin rash.

ADVERSE REACTIONS/TOXIC EFFECTS

Abrupt withdrawal after prolonged therapy may produce effects ranging from markedly increased dreaming, nightmares and/or insomnia, tremor, sweating, vomiting, to hallucinations, delirium, seizures, status epilepticus. Skin eruptions may appear as hypersensitivity reaction. Blood dyscrasias, liver disease, hypocalcemia occur rarely. Overdosage produces cold clammy skin, hypothermia, severe CNS depression followed by high fever, coma.

PATIENT CONSIDERATIONS

BASELINE ASSESSMENT

Review history of seizure disorder (intensity, frequency, duration, level of consciousness). Observe frequently for recurrence of seizure activity. Initiate seizure precautions.

INTERVENTION/EVALUATION

For those on long-term therapy, liver/renal function tests, blood counts should be performed periodically. Assist w/ambulation if dizziness, ataxia occurs. Assess children, elderly for paradoxical reaction (particularly during early therapy). Assess for clinical improvement (decrease in intensity/frequency of seizures). Monitor for therapeutic serum level (5–12 mcg/ml).

PATIENT/FAMILY TEACHING

Do not abruptly withdraw medication following long-term use (may precipitate seizures). Strict maintenance of drug therapy is essential for seizure control. Drowsiness usually disappears during continued therapy. If dizziness occurs, change positions slowly from recumbent to sitting position before standing. Avoid tasks that require alertness, motor skills until response to drug is established. Avoid alcohol.

probenecid

pro-**ben**-ah-sid
(Benemid, Probalan)

FIXED-COMBINATION(S)
W/colchicine, antigout agent (**Col-Benemid, Proben-C**)

CANADIAN AVAILABILITY
Benemid, Benuryl

PREGNANCY CATEGORY B

CLASSIFICATION

Uricosuric

AVAILABILITY (Rx)

Tablets: 500 mg

PHARMACOKINETICS

Absorption: Rapidly, completely absorbed from GI tract. Widely distributed. **Metabolism:** Metabolized in liver to active metabolite. **Excretion:** Primarily excreted in urine. **Half-life:** 3–12 hrs.

ACTION/*THERAPEUTIC EFFECT*

Inhibits tubular reabsorption of urate at proximal renal tubule, *increasing urinary excretion of uric acid.*

USES

Treatment of hyperuricemia associated w/gout or gouty arthritis. Adjunctive therapy w/penicillins or cephalosporins to elevate and prolong antibiotic plasma levels.

ADMINISTRATION

ORAL:

- May give w/or immediately after meals or milk.
- Instruct pt to drink at least 6–8 glasses (8 oz) of water/day (prevents kidney stone development).

INDICATIONS/ROUTES/DOSAGE

Gout:
Note: Do not start until acute gout attack subsides; continue if acute attack occurs during therapy.

P

Oral: Adults, elderly: Initially, 250 mg 2 times/day for 1 wk; then 500 mg 2 times/day. May increase by 500 mg q4wks. ***Maximum:*** 2–3 g/day. ***Maintenance:*** Dosage that maintains normal uric acid levels.

Penicillin/cephalosporin therapy: Note: Do not use in presence of renal impairment.

Oral: Adults, elderly: 2 g/day in divided doses. ***Children (2–14 yrs):*** Initially, 25 mg/kg. ***Maintenance:*** 40 mg/kg/day in 4 divided doses. ***Children >50 kg:*** Receive adult dosage.

CONTRAINDICATIONS

Blood dyscrasias, uric acid kidney stones, concurrent use w/penicillin in presence of renal impairment.

CAUTIONS

Impaired renal function, history of peptic ulcer.

INTERACTIONS

DRUG: May increase concentrations of ***cephalosporins, methotrexate, NSAIDs, nitrofurantoin, penicillins, zidovudine. Antineoplastics*** may increase risk of uric acid nephropathy. ***Salicylates*** may decrease uricosuric effect. May increase, prolong effects of ***heparin***. **HERBAL:** None known. **FOOD:** None significant. **ALTERED LAB VALUES:** May inhibit renal excretion of PSP (phenolsulfonphthalein), 17-ketosteroids, BSP (sulfobromophthalein) tests.

SIDE EFFECTS

FREQUENT (5–10%): Acute attack gouty arthritis (joint pain, swelling, redness), headache, decreased appetite, nausea, vomiting. **OCCASIONAL (1–5%):** Lower back or side pain, rash, hives, itching, dizziness, flushed face, frequent urge to urinate, sore gums. **RARE (<1%):** Fever, anemia, leukopenia, nephrotic syndrome, aplastic anemia.

ADVERSE REACTIONS/TOXIC EFFECTS

Severe hypersensitivity reactions (including anaphylaxis) occur rarely (usually within a few hours after readministration following previous use). Discontinue immediately, contact physician. Pruritic maculopapular rash should be considered a toxic reaction. May be accompanied by malaise, fever, chills, joint pain, nausea, vomiting, leukopenia.

PATIENT CONSIDERATIONS

BASELINE ASSESSMENT

Do not initiate therapy until acute gouty attack has subsided. Question pt for hypersensitivity to probenecid or if taking penicillin or cephalosporin antibiotics. Instruct pt to drink 6–8 glasses (8 oz) of fluid daily while on medication.

INTERVENTION/EVALUATION

If exacerbation of gout recurs following therapy, use other agents for gout. Discontinue medication immediately if rash or other evidence of allergic reaction appears. Encourage high fluid intake (3,000 ml/day). Monitor I&O (output should be at least 2,000 ml/day). Assess CBC, serum uric acid levels. Assess urine for cloudiness, unusual color, odor. Assess for therapeutic response (reduced joint tenderness, swelling, redness, limitation of motion).

PATIENT/FAMILY TEACHING

Encourage low-purine food

intake (reduce/omit meat, fowl, fish; use eggs, cheese, vegetables). Foods high in purine: kidneys, liver, sweetbreads, sardines, anchovies, meat extracts. May take 1 or more wks for full therapeutic effect. Drink 6–8 glasses (8 oz) of fluid daily while on medication. Avoid tasks that require alertness, motor skills until response to drug is established. Contact physician, nurse if rash, irritation of eyes, swelling of lips/mouth occurs.

procainamide hydrochloride

pro-**cane**-ah-myd
(ProcanBid, Procan-SR, Pronestyl, Rhythmin)

CANADIAN AVAILABILITY
Pronestyl, Procan SR

PREGNANCY CATEGORY C

CLASSIFICATION

Antiarrhythmic

AVAILABILITY (Rx)

Capsules: 250 mg, 375 mg, 500 mg. **Tablets:** 250 mg, 375 mg, 500 mg. **Tablets (sustained-release):** 250 mg, 500 mg, 750 mg, 1,000 mg. **Injection:** 100 mg/ml, 500 mg/ml.

PHARMACOKINETICS

Absorption: Rapidly, completely absorbed from GI tract. Widely distributed. **Metabolism:** Metabolized in liver to active metabolite. **Excretion:** Primarily excreted in urine. Removed by hemodialysis. **Half-life:** 2.5–4.5 hrs; metabolite: 6 hrs.

ACTION/*THERAPEUTIC EFFECT*

Prolongs refractory period by direct effect, decreasing myocardial excitability and conduction velocity. *Depresses myocardial contractility.*

USES/*UNLABELED*

Prophylactic therapy to maintain normal sinus rhythm after conversion of atrial fibrillation and/or flutter. Treatment of premature ventricular contractions, paroxysmal atrial tachycardia, atrial fibrillation, ventricular tachycardia. *Conversion/management of atrial fibrillation and PAT.*

STORAGE/HANDLING

Solution appears clear, colorless to light yellow. Discard if solution darkens/appears discolored or if precipitate forms. When diluted w/5% dextrose, solution is stable for 24 hrs at room temperature or for 7 days if refrigerated.

ADMINISTRATION

ORAL:

- Do not crush or break sustained-release tablets.

IM/IV:

- **Note:** May give by IM, IV injection, or IV infusion.
- B/P, EKG should be monitored continuously during IV administration and rate of infusion adjusted to eliminate arrhythmias.
- For direct IV injection, dilute w/5% dextrose and, w/pt in supine position, administer at rate not exceeding 25–50 mg/min.
- For initial loading infusion, add 1 g to 50 ml 5% dextrose to

provide a concentration of 20 mg/ml. Infuse 1 ml/min for up to 25–30 min.

- For IV infusion, add 1 g to 250–500 ml 5% dextrose to provide concentration of 2–4 mg/ml. Infuse at 1–3 ml/min.
- Check B/P q5–10min during infusion. If fall in B/P exceeds 15 mm Hg, discontinue drug, contact physician.
- Monitor EKG for cardiac changes, particularly widening of QRS, prolongation of PR and QT interval. Notify physician of any significant interval changes.

INDICATIONS/ROUTES/DOSAGE

Note: Dose, interval of administration individualized based on underlying myocardial disease, pt's age, renal function, clinical response. Extended-release capsules used for maintenance therapy.

Usual oral dosage (to provide 50 mg/kg/day):
Oral: Adults, elderly (40–50 kg): 250 mg q3h up to 500 mg q6h. ***(60–70 kg):*** 375 mg q3h up to 750 mg q6h. ***(80–90 kg):*** 500 mg q3h up to 1 g q6h. ***(>100 kg):*** 625 mg q3h up to 1.25 g q6h.

Oral (extended-release): Adults, elderly (40–50 kg): 500 mg q6h. ***(60–70 kg):*** 750 mg q6h. ***(80–90 kg):*** 1 g q6h. ***(>100 kg):*** 1.25 g q6h. ***ProCanbid:*** 500–1,000 mg q12h.

Usual parenteral dosage:
IM: Adults, elderly: 50 mg/kg/day in divided doses q3–6h.

IV: Adults, elderly: 100 mg q5min until arrhythmias suppressed or 500 mg administered.

IV Infusion: Adults, elderly: Initially, loading infusion of 20 mg/ml at 1 ml/min for 25–30 min to deliver 500–600 mg procainamide. ***Maintenance:*** Infusion of 2 mg/ml at 1–3 ml/min to deliver 2–6 mg/min.

CONTRAINDICATIONS

Complete AV block, second- and third-degree AV block w/o pacemaker, abnormal impulses/rhythms because of escape mechanism.

CAUTIONS

Ventricular tachycardia during coronary occlusion, renal/hepatic disease, incomplete AV nodal block, digitalis intoxication, CHF, preexisting hypotension.

INTERACTIONS

DRUG: ***Pimozide, other antiarrhythmics*** may increase cardiac effects. May increase effects of ***antihypertensives (IV procainamide), neuromuscular blockers.*** May decrease antimyasthenic effect on skeletal muscle. **HERBAL:** None known. **FOOD:** None significant. **ALTERED LAB VALUES:** May cause positive ANA, Coombs' test, EKG changes. May increase SGOT (AST), SGPT (ALT), alkaline phosphatase, bilirubin, LDH.

SIDE EFFECTS

FREQUENT: *Oral:* Abdominal pain/cramping, nausea, diarrhea, vomiting. **OCCASIONAL:** Dizziness, giddiness, weakness, hypersensitivity reaction (rash, urticaria, pruritus, flushing). *IV:* Transient, but at times, marked hypotension. **RARE:** Confusion, mental depression, psychosis.

ADVERSE REACTIONS/TOXIC EFFECTS

Paradoxical, extremely rapid ventricular rate may occur during treatment of atrial fibrillation/flutter. Systemic lupus erythematosus–like syndrome (fever, joint pain, pleuritic chest pain) w/prolonged therapy. Cardiotoxic effects occur most commonly w/IV administration, observed as conduction changes (50% widening of QRS complex, frequent ventricular premature contractions, ventricular tachycardia, complete AV block). Prolonged PR and QT intervals, flattened T waves occur less frequently (discontinue drug immediately).

PATIENT CONSIDERATIONS

BASELINE ASSESSMENT

Check B/P and pulse for 1 full min (unless pt is on continuous monitor) before giving medication.

INTERVENTION/EVALUATION

Monitor EKG for cardiac changes, particularly widening of QRS, prolongation of PR and QT interval. Assess pulse for strength/weakness, irregular rate. Monitor I&O, electrolyte serum level (potassium, chloride, sodium). Assess for complaints of GI upset, headache, dizziness, joint pain. Monitor pattern of daily bowel activity, stool consistency. Assess for dizziness. Monitor B/P for hypotension. Assess skin for evidence of hypersensitivity reaction (especially in those on high-dose therapy). Monitor for therapeutic serum level (3–10 mcg/ml).

PATIENT/FAMILY TEACHING

Take medication at evenly spaced doses around the clock. Contact physician if fever, joint pain/stiffness, signs of upper respiratory infection occur. Do not abruptly discontinue medication. Compliance w/therapy regimen is essential to control arrhythmias. Do not use nasal decongestants, OTC cold preparations (stimulants) w/o physician approval. Restrict salt, alcohol intake. Report any arthralgia, myalgia, fever, chills, rash, easy bruising, sore throat, dark urine, nausea, vomiting, diarrhea, palpitations, dizziness.

---

procaine hydrochloride

(Novocain)

See Classification section under: Anesthetics: local

---

procarbazine hydrochloride

(Matulane)

See Classification section under: Cancer chemotherapy

---

prochlorperazine

pro-klor-**pear**-ah-zeen

(Compazine suppositories)

prochlorperazine edisylate

(Compazine syrup, injection)

prochlorperazine maleate

(Compazine spansule, tablets)

CANADIAN AVAILABILITY

Stemetil

PREGNANCY CATEGORY C

CLASSIFICATION

Antiemetic, antipsychotic

AVAILABILITY (Rx)

Tablets: 5 mg, 10 mg, 25 mg. **Capsules (sustained-release):** 10 mg, 15 mg, 30 mg. **Syrup:** 5 mg/5 ml. **Suppository:** 2.5 mg, 5 mg, 25 mg. **Injection:** 5 mg/ml.

PHARMACODYNAMICS

	ONSET	PEAK	DURATION
Tablets, syrup (antiemetic)			
	30–40 min	—	3–4 hrs
Extended-Release (antiemetic)			
	30–40 min	—	10–12 hrs
IM (antiemetic)			
	10–20 min	—	3–4 hrs
Rectal (antiemetic)			
	60 min	—	3–4 hrs

PHARMACOKINETICS

Absorption: Variably absorbed after oral administration, well absorbed after IM administration. Widely distributed. **Metabolism:** Metabolized in liver, GI mucosa. **Excretion:** Primarily excreted in urine. **Half-life:** 23 hrs.

ACTION/*THERAPEUTIC EFFECT*

Antiemetic: Acts centrally to inhibit/block dopamine receptors in chemoreceptor trigger zone and peripherally to block vagus nerve in GI tract. *Relieves nausea and vomiting.* ***Antipsychotic:*** Antagonizes dopamine neurotransmission at synapses by blocking postsynaptic dopaminergic receptors in brain. *Suppresses behavioral response in psychosis.*

USES

Control of severe nausea and vomiting, management of psychotic disorders, moderate to severe anxiety and tension in psychoneurotic pts.

STORAGE/HANDLING

Store at room temperature (including suppositories), protect from light (darkens on exposure). Slight yellow discoloration of solution does not affect potency, but discard if markedly discolored or precipitate forms.

ADMINISTRATION

ORAL:

- Give w/o regard to meals.
- **Parenteral Administration:** Pt must remain recumbent for 30–60 min in head-low position w/legs raised to minimize hypotensive effect.

IM:

- Inject slow, deep IM into upper outer quadrant of gluteus maximus. If irritation occurs, further injections may be diluted w/0.9% NaCl or 2% procaine hydrochloride.
- Massage IM injection site to reduce discomfort.

IV:

- **Note:** Give by direct IV injection or IV infusion.
- For direct IV, administer each 5 mg >1 min.
- For IV infusion, dilute 20 mg (4 ml) prochlorperazine w/0.9% NaCl and administer 5 mg/min rate of infusion.
- Monitor B/P diligently for hypotension during IV administration.

RECTAL:

- Moisten suppository w/cold water before inserting well up into rectum.

INDICATIONS/ROUTES/DOSAGE

Severe nausea, vomiting:
Oral: Adults, elderly: 5–10 mg 3–4 times/day. ***Oral/Rectal: Children >2***

yrs, 20–29 lbs: 2.5 mg q12–24h. Do not exceed 7.5 mg/day. ***Children 30–39 lbs:*** 2.5 mg 2–3 times/day. Do not exceed 10 mg/day. ***Children 40–85 lbs:*** 2.5 mg 3 times/day or 5 mg 2 times/day. Do not exceed 15 mg/day.

IM: ***Adults, elderly:*** 5–10 mg q3–4h. Do not exceed 40 mg/day. ***Children >20 lbs, >2 yrs:*** 0.13 mg/kg.

Rectal: ***Adults, elderly:*** 25 mg 2 times/day.

Severe nausea, vomiting after surgery:
IM: ***Adults, elderly:*** 5–10 mg. Repeat once in 30 min, if needed.

IV: ***Adults, elderly:*** 5–10 mg. Repeat once, if needed.

Psychotic disorders, outpatient:
Oral: ***Adults, elderly:*** 5–10 mg 3–4 times/day. Increase dosage gradually every 2–3 days until therapeutic response noted.

Oral/Rectal: ***Children 2–12 yrs:*** 2.5 mg 2–3 times/day. Increase gradually to therapeutic response. ***Maximum: Children 2–5 yrs:*** 20 mg/day. ***6–12 yrs:*** 25 mg/day.

Psychotic disorders, inpatient:
Oral: ***Adults, elderly:*** 10 mg 3–4 times/day.

IM: ***Adults, elderly:*** 10–20 mg q1–4h to control symptoms.

CONTRAINDICATIONS

Suspected Reye's syndrome, severe CNS depression, comatose states, severe cardiovascular disease, bone marrow depression, subcortical brain damage.

CAUTIONS

Impaired respiratory/hepatic/renal/cardiac function, alcohol withdrawal, history of seizures, urinary retention, glaucoma, prostatic hypertrophy, hypocalcemia (increases susceptibility to dystonias).

INTERACTIONS

DRUG: ***Alcohol, CNS depressants*** may increase CNS, respiratory depression, hypotensive effects. ***Tricyclic antidepressants, MAO inhibitors*** may increase sedative, anticholinergic effects. ***Antithyroid agents*** may increase risk of agranulocytosis. Extrapyramidal symptoms (EPS) may increase w/***EPS-producing medications. Hypotensives*** may increase hypotension. May decrease ***levodopa*** effects. ***Lithium*** may decrease absorption, produce adverse neurologic effects. **HERBAL:** None known. **FOOD:** None significant. **ALTERED LAB VALUES:** None significant.

SIDE EFFECTS

FREQUENT: Hypotension, dizziness, fainting occur frequently after first injection, occasionally after subsequent injections, and rarely w/oral dosage. **OCCASIONAL:** Drowsiness during early therapy, dry mouth, blurred vision, lethargy, constipation/diarrhea, muscular aches, nasal congestion, peripheral edema, urinary retention.

ADVERSE REACTIONS/TOXIC EFFECTS

Extrapyramidal symptoms appear dose related (particularly w/high dosage) and are divided into 3 categories: akathisia (inability to sit still, tapping of feet, urge to move around), parkinsonian symptoms (mask-like face, tremors, shuffling gait, hypersalivation), and acute dystonias: torticollis (neck muscle spasm), opisthotonos (rigidity of back muscles), and oculogyric crisis (rolling

P

back of eyes). Dystonic reaction may also produce profuse sweating, pallor. Tardive dyskinesia (protrusion of tongue, puffing of cheeks, chewing/puckering of the mouth) occurs rarely (may be irreversible). Abrupt withdrawal following long-term therapy may precipitate nausea, vomiting, gastritis, dizziness, tremors. Blood dyscrasias, particularly agranulocytosis, mild leukopenia (sore mouth/gums/throat) may occur. May lower seizure threshold.

PATIENT CONSIDERATIONS

BASELINE ASSESSMENT

Avoid skin contact w/solution (contact dermatitis).

Antiemetic
Assess for dehydration (poor skin turgor, dry mucous membranes, longitudinal furrows in tongue).

Antipsychotic
Assess behavior, appearance, emotional status, response to environment, speech pattern, thought content.

INTERVENTION/EVALUATION

Monitor B/P for hypotension. Assess for extrapyramidal symptoms. Monitor WBC, differential count for blood dyscrasias. Monitor for fine tongue movement (may be early sign of tardive dyskinesia). Supervise suicidal risk pt closely during early therapy (as depression lessens, energy level improves, increasing suicide potential). Assess for therapeutic response (interest in surroundings, improvement in self-care, increased ability to concentrate, relaxed facial expression).

PATIENT/FAMILY TEACHING

Urine may turn pink or reddish brown. Do not abruptly withdraw from long-term drug therapy. Report visual disturbances. Sugarless gum, sips of tepid water may relieve dry mouth. Drowsiness generally subsides during continued therapy. Avoid tasks that require alertness, motor skills until response to drug is established. Avoid alcohol, CNS depressants. Use sunscreen, protective clothing in sun or ultraviolet light. Use caution in hot weather (possibility of heat stroke).

progesterone

proe-**jess**-ter-one
(Crinone, Gesterol, Prometrium)

CANADIAN AVAILABILITY
Prometrium

PREGNANCY CATEGORY D

CLASSIFICATION

Progestin

AVAILABILITY (Rx)

Injection: 50 mg/ml. **Intrauterine System. Soft Gel Capsule:** 400 mg. **Vaginal Gel:** 4%, 8%.

PHARMACOKINETICS

Absorption: Slow absorption after IM administration. **Metabolism:** Metabolized in liver. **Excretion:** Primarily excreted in urine.

ACTION/*THERAPEUTIC EFFECT*

Transforms endometrium from proliferative to secretory (in an estrogen-primed endometrium); inhibits secretion of pituitary gonadotropins, preventing follicular maturation and ovulation. Stimulates the growth of mammary alveolar tissue; relaxes uterine smooth muscle. *Restores hormonal balance.*

USES/*UNLABELED*

Treatment of primary or secondary amenorrhea. Prevention of endometrial hyperplasia in estrogen recipients, abnormal uterine bleeding due to hormonal imbalance, endometriosis. ***Vaginal Gel (8%):*** Treatment of infertility. *Treatment of corpus luteum dysfunction.*

ADMINISTRATION

IM:

- Administer deep IM in large muscle.

INDICATIONS/ROUTES/DOSAGE

Amenorrhea:
IM: Adults: 5–10 mg for 6–8 days. Withdrawal bleeding expected in 48–72 hrs if ovarian activity produced proliferative endometrium.

Vaginal: Adults: Apply every other day for up to 6 doses.

Oral: Adults: 400 mg daily in evening for 10 days.

Abnormal uterine bleeding:
IM: Adults: 5–10 mg for 6 days. (When estrogen given concomitantly, begin progesterone after 2 wks of estrogen therapy; discontinue when menstrual flow begins.)

Prevention of endometrial hyperplasia:
Oral: Adults: 200 mg/day for 12 days per 28-day cycle taken as single dose in evening in combination w/daily conjugated estrogen.

CONTRAINDICATIONS

Hypersensitivity to progestins; thrombophlebitis, thromboembolic disorders, cerebral apoplexy or history of these conditions; severe liver dysfunction; breast cancer; undiagnosed vaginal bleeding; missed abortion; use as a diagnostic test for pregnancy.

CAUTIONS

Diabetes, conditions aggravated by fluid retention (e.g., asthma, epilepsy, migraine, cardiac/renal dysfunction), history of mental depression.

INTERACTIONS

DRUG: May interfere w/effects of ***bromocriptine.*** **HERBAL:** None known. **FOOD:** None significant. **ALTERED LAB VALUES:** May increase alkaline phosphatase, LDL. May decrease HDL. May cause abnormal thyroid, metapyrone, liver, endocrine function tests, decrease glucose tolerance.

P

SIDE EFFECTS

FREQUENT: Breakthrough bleeding or spotting at beginning of therapy. Amenorrhea, change in menstrual flow, breast tenderness. **OCCASIONAL:** Edema, weight gain or loss, rash, pruritus, photosensitivity, skin pigmentation. **RARE:** Pain/swelling at injection site, acne, mental depression, alopecia, hirsutism.

ADVERSE REACTIONS/TOXIC EFFECTS

Thrombophlebitis, cerebrovascular disorders, retinal thrombosis, pulmonary embolism occurs rarely.

PATIENT CONSIDERATIONS

BASELINE ASSESSMENT

Question for possibility of pregnancy or hypersensitivity to progestins before initiating therapy. Obtain baseline weight, blood glucose level, B/P.

INTERVENTION/EVALUATION

Check weight daily; report weekly gain of 5 lbs or more. Assess skin for rash, hives.

Immediately report the development of chest pain, sudden shortness of breath, sudden decrease in vision, migraine headache, pain (especially w/swelling, warmth, and redness) in calves, numbness of an arm/leg (thrombotic disorders). Check B/P periodically. Note progesterone therapy on pathology specimens.

PATIENT/FAMILY TEACHING

Importance of medical supervision. Do not take other medications w/o physician's approval. Use sunscreens, protective clothing to protect from sunlight/ultraviolet light until tolerance determined. Notify physician of abnormal vaginal bleeding or other symptoms. Teach how to perform Homans' test, signs and symptoms of blood clots (report these to physician immediately). Teach breast self-exam. Stop taking medication and contact physician at once if pregnancy suspected. Give labeling from drug package.

promethazine hydrochloride

pro-**meth**-ah-zeen
(Phenergan)

FIXED-COMBINATION(S)

W/codeine, a narcotic analgesic **(Phenergan w/Codeine)**; w/dextromethorphan, an antitussive **(Phenergan w/Dextromethorphan)**; w/meperidine, a narcotic analgesic **(Mepergan)**; w/phenylephrine, a nasal vasoconstrictor **(Phenergan VC)**; w/phenylephrine and codeine **(Phenergan VC w/Codeine)**

CANADIAN AVAILABILITY

Phenergan

PREGNANCY CATEGORY C

CLASSIFICATION

Antihistamine

AVAILABILITY (Rx)

Tablets: 12.5 mg, 25 mg, 50 mg. **Syrup:** 6.25 mg/5 ml, 25 mg/5 ml. **Suppository:** 12.5 mg, 25 mg, 50 mg. **Injection:** 25 mg/ml, 50 mg/ml.

PHARMACODYNAMICS

	ONSET	PEAK	DURATION
Oral	20 min	—	2–8 hrs
IM	20 min	—	2–8 hrs
Rectal	20 min	—	2–8 hrs
IV	3–5 min	—	2–8 hrs

PHARMACOKINETICS

Absorption: Well absorbed from GI tract, after IM administration. Widely distributed. **Metabolism:** Metabolized in liver. **Excretion:** Primarily excreted in urine.

ACTION / *THERAPEUTIC EFFECT*

Antihistamine: Inhibits histamine at histamine receptor sites, *preventing, antagonizing most allergic effects (e.g., urticaria, pruritus).* ***Antiemetic:*** Diminishes vestibular stimulation, depresses labyrinthine function, acts on chemoreceptor trigger zone, *producing antiemetic effect.* ***Sedative-hypnotic:*** Decreases stimulation to brain stem reticular formation, *producing CNS depression.*

USES

Provides symptomatic relief of

allergic symptoms; sedative/antiemetic in surgery/labor; decreases postop nausea/vomiting; adjunct to analgesics in control of pain; management of motion sickness.

STORAGE/HANDLING

Store oral, parenteral forms at room temperature. Refrigerate suppositories.

ADMINISTRATION

ORAL:

- Give w/o regard to meals. Scored tablets may be crushed.

IM:

- **Note:** Significant tissue necrosis may occur if given SubQ. Inadvertent intra-arterial injection may produce severe arteriospasm, resulting in severe circulation impairment.
- May be given undiluted.
- Inject deep IM.

IV:

- Final dilution should not exceed 25 mg/ml.
- Administer at 25 mg/min rate thru IV infusion tube.
- A too rapid rate of infusion may result in transient fall in blood pressure, producing orthostatic hypotension, reflex tachycardia.
- If pt complains of pain at IV site, stop injection immediately (possibility of intra-arterial needle placement/perivascular extravasation).

RECTAL:

- Moisten suppository w/cold water before inserting well up into rectum.

INDICATIONS/ROUTES/DOSAGE

Allergic symptoms:
Oral: Adults, elderly: 25 mg at bedtime or 12.5 mg 4 times/day. *Children:* Up to 25 mg at bedtime or up to 12.5 mg 3 times/day.
Rectal/IM/IV: Adults, elderly: 25 mg, may repeat in 2 hrs.

Motion sickness:
Oral: Adults, elderly: 25 mg 30–60 min before departure; may repeat in 8–12 hrs, then every morning on arising and before evening meal. *Children:* 12.5–25 mg (same regimen).

Prevention of nausea, vomiting:
Oral/IM/IV/Rectal: Adults, elderly: 12.5–25 mg q4–6h as needed. *Children:* 0.25–0.5 mg/kg q4–6h as needed.

Pre- and postop sedation; adjunct to analgesics:
IM/IV: Adults, elderly: 25–50 mg. *Children:* 12.5–25 mg.

CONTRAINDICATIONS

Comatose, those receiving large doses of other CNS depressants, acutely ill/dehydrated children, acute asthmatic attack, vomiting of unknown etiology in children, Reye's syndrome, those receiving MAO inhibitors.

EXTREME CAUTION

History of sleep apnea, young children, family history of sudden infant death syndrome (SIDS), those difficult to arouse from sleep.

CAUTIONS

Narrow-angle glaucoma, peptic ulcer, prostatic hypertrophy, pyloroduodenal/bladder neck obstruction, asthma, COPD, increased intraocular pressure, cardiovascular disease, hyperthyroidism, hypertension, seizure disorders.

INTERACTIONS

DRUG: *Alcohol, CNS depressants*

may increase CNS depressant effects. ***Anticholinergics*** may increase anticholinergic effects. ***MAO inhibitors*** may prolong, intensify anticholinergic, CNS depressant effects. **HERBAL:** None known. **FOOD:** None significant. **ALTERED LAB VALUES:** May suppress wheal and flare reactions to antigen skin testing, unless discontinued 4 days before testing.

SIDE EFFECTS

FREQUENT: Hypotension, confusion, syncope more likely noted in elderly. Drowsiness, disorientation, dry mouth, urinary retention, thickening of bronchial secretions. **OCCASIONAL:** Epigastric distress, flushing, visual disturbances, hearing disturbances, wheezing, paresthesia, sweating, chills. **RARE:** Dizziness, urticaria, photosensitivity, nightmares. Fixed-combination form with pseudoephedrine may produce mild CNS stimulation.

ADVERSE REACTIONS/TOXIC EFFECTS

Paradoxical reaction (particularly in children) manifested as excitation, nervousness, tremor, hyperactive reflexes, convulsions. CNS depression has occurred in infants and young children (respiratory depression, sleep apnea, SIDS). Long-term therapy may produce extrapyramidal symptoms noted as dystonia (abnormal movements), pronounced motor restlessness (most frequently occurs in children), and parkinsonian symptoms (especially noted in elderly). Blood dyscrasias, particularly agranulocytosis, have occurred.

PATIENT CONSIDERATIONS

BASELINE ASSESSMENT

Assess B/P and pulse for bradycardia/tachycardia if pt is given parenteral form. If used as an antiemetic, assess for dehydration (poor skin turgor, dry mucous membranes, longitudinal furrows in tongue).

INTERVENTION/EVALUATION

Monitor serum electrolytes in pts w/severe vomiting. Assist w/ambulation if drowsiness, lightheadedness occurs.

PATIENT/FAMILY TEACHING

Drowsiness, dry mouth may be an expected response to drug. Sugarless gum, sips of tepid water may relieve dry mouth. Coffee/tea may help reduce drowsiness. Report visual disturbances. Avoid tasks that require alertness, motor skills until response to drug is established. Avoid alcohol and other CNS depressants. Use caution in sun; wear protective clothing and use sunscreens.

propafenone hydrochloride

pro-**pah**-phen-own
(Rythmol)

CANADIAN AVAILABILITY
Rythmol

PREGNANCY CATEGORY C

CLASSIFICATION

Antiarrhythmic

AVAILABILITY (Rx)

Tablets: 150 mg, 300 mg

PHARMACOKINETICS

Absorption: Well absorbed from GI tract (undergoes first-pass effect). Distributed primarily to heart, liver, lung. **Metabolism:** Metabolized in liver to active metabolite. **Excretion:** Primarily eliminated in feces. **Half-life:** 2–10 hrs.

ACTION / *THERAPEUTIC EFFECT*

Decreases the fast sodium current in Purkinje/myocardial cells. *Decreases excitability, automaticity; prolongs conduction velocity, refractory period.* Greatest effects on Purkinje system.

USES / *UNLABELED*

Treatment of documented, life-threatening ventricular arrhythmias (e.g., sustained ventricular tachycardias). Prolong time to recurrence of paroxysmal supraventricular tachycardia (PSVT) and paroxysmal atrial fibrillation/fluttrer (PAF) associated w/disabling symptoms. *Treatment of supraventricular arrhythmias.*

ADMINISTRATION

ORAL:

- Scored tablets may be crushed.
- Give w/o regard to meals (food may increase serum concentrations).

INDICATIONS / ROUTES / DOSAGE

Usual dosage:
Oral: Adults, elderly: Initially, 150 mg q8h, may increase at 3–4 day intervals to 225 mg q8h, then to 300 mg q8h. ***Maximum:*** 900 mg/day.

CONTRAINDICATIONS

Uncontrolled CHF, cardiogenic shock, sinoatrial, AV and intraventricular disorders of impulse/conduction (sick-sinus syndrome [bradycardia-tachycardia], AV block) w/o presence of pacemaker, bradycardia, marked hypotension, bronchospastic disorders, manifest electrolyte imbalance.

CAUTIONS

Impaired renal/hepatic function, recent myocardial infarction, CHF, conduction disturbances.

INTERACTIONS

DRUG: May increase concentrations of ***digoxin, propranolol.*** May increase effects of ***warfarin.*** **HERBAL:** None known. **FOOD:** None significant. **ALTERED LAB VALUES:** May cause EKG changes (e.g., QRS widening, PR prolongation), positive ANA titers.

P

SIDE EFFECTS

FREQUENT (>5%): Dizziness, unusual taste, nausea, vomiting, constipation, blurred vision. **OCCASIONAL (1–5%):** Headache, dyspepsia, weakness. **RARE (<1%):** Dry mouth, diarrhea, rash, edema, hot flashes.

ADVERSE REACTIONS / TOXIC EFFECTS

May produce/worsen existing arrhythmias. Overdosage may produce hypotension, somnolence, bradycardia, intra-atrial and intraventricular conduction disturbances.

PATIENT CONSIDERATIONS

BASELINE ASSESSMENT

Correct electrolyte imbalance before administering medication.

INTERVENTION/EVALUATION

Assess pulse for strength/weakness, irregular rate. Monitor EKG for cardiac performance/changes, particularly widening of QRS, prolongation of PR interval. Question for visual distur-

bances, headache, GI upset. Monitor fluid, electrolyte serum levels. Monitor pattern of daily bowel activity, stool consistency. Assess for dizziness, unsteadiness. Monitor liver enzymes results. Monitor for therapeutic serum level (0.06–1 μ/ml).

PATIENT/FAMILY TEACHING

Compliance w/therapy regimen is essential to control arrhythmias. Unusual taste sensation may occur. Report headache, blurred vision. Report fever, sore throat, chills, unusual bleeding/bruising. If bothersome, report palpitations, change in vision, difficulty breathing.

proparacaine

(Ophthaine, AK-Taine, Alcaine, I-Paracaine, Kainair, Ophthetic)

FIXED-COMBINATION(S)

W/fluorescein, a water-soluble dye (Fluoracaine, Parascein, Ocu-Flurcaine)

See Classification section under: Anesthetics: local

propofol

pro-**poe**-foal

(Diprivan)

CANADIAN AVAILABILITY

Diprivan

PREGNANCY CATEGORY B

CLASSIFICATION

Anesthetic: General

AVAILABILITY (Rx)

Injection: 10 mg/ml

PHARMACODYNAMICS

	ONSET	PEAK	DURATION
IV	40 sec	—	—

PHARMACOKINETICS

Rapidly, extensively distributed. **Metabolism:** Metabolized in liver. **Excretion:** Primarily excreted in urine. **Half-life:** 3–12 hrs.

ACTION/*THERAPEUTIC EFFECT*

Unknown. *Produces hypnosis rapidly.*

USES

Induction and maintenance of anesthesia. Continuous sedation in intubated/respiratory controlled adult pts in ICU.

STORAGE/HANDLING

Store at room temperature. Discard unused portions. Do not use if emulsion separates. Shake well before using.

ADMINISTRATION

IV:

- **Note:** Do not give through same IV line w/blood or plasma.
- Dilute only w/5% dextrose.
- Do not dilute to concentration <2 mg/ml.
- Use larger veins of forearm or antecubital fossa to minimize IV pain.
- Transient, local pain at IV site may be reduced w/1 ml of 1% IV lidocaine solution.
- A too rapid IV may produce marked severe hypotension, respiratory depression, irregular muscular movements.
- Observe for signs of intra-arterial injection (pain, discolored skin patches, white/blue color to hand, delayed onset of drug action).

- Inadvertent intra-arterial injection may result in arterial spasm w/severe pain, thrombosis, gangrene.

INDICATIONS/ROUTES/DOSAGE

ICU sedation:
IV: Adults, elderly: Initially, 5 mcg/kg/min for at least 5 min until onset of peak effect. May increase by increments of 5–10 mcg/kg/min over 5–10 min intervals. ***Maintenance:*** 5–50 mcg/kg/min (some pts may require higher dosage).

Anesthesia:
IV: Adults ASA I & II: 2–2.5 mg/kg (about 40 mg q10sec until onset of anesthesia). ***IV: Elderly, debilitated, hypovolemic, or ASA III or IV:*** 1–1.5 mg/kg q10sec until onset of anesthesia.

Maintenance:
IV: Adults ASA I & II: 0.1–0.2 mg/kg/min. ***IV: Elderly, debilitated, hypovolemic, or ASA III or IV:*** 0.05–0.1 mg/kg/min.

CONTRAINDICATIONS

Increased intracranial pressure, impaired cerebral circulation.

CAUTIONS

Debilitated, impaired respiratory, circulatory, renal, hepatic, lipid metabolism disorders.

INTERACTIONS

DRUG: *Alcohol, CNS depressants* may increase CNS, respiratory, depression, hypotensive effect. **HERBAL:** None known. **FOOD:** None significant. **ALTERED LAB VALUES:** None significant.

SIDE EFFECTS

FREQUENT: Involuntary muscular movement, apnea (common during induction; lasts >60 sec), hypotension, nausea, vomiting, burning/stinging at IV site. **OCCASIONAL:** Twitching, bucking, jerking, thrashing, headache, dizziness, bradycardia, hypertension, fever, abdominal cramping, tingling, numbness, coldness, cough, hiccups, facial flushing. **RARE:** Rash, dry mouth, agitation, confusion, myalgia, thrombophlebitis.

ADVERSE REACTIONS/TOXIC EFFECTS

Continuous/repeated intermittent infusion may result in extreme somnolence, respiratory/circulatory depression. A too rapid IV may produce marked severe hypotension, respiratory depression, irregular muscular movements. Acute allergic reaction (erythema, pruritus, urticaria, rhinitis, dyspnea, hypotension, restlessness, anxiety, abdominal pain) may occur.

PATIENT CONSIDERATIONS

Baseline Assessment

Resuscitative equipment, endotracheal tube, suction, oxygen must be available. Obtain vital signs before administration.

Intervention/Evaluation

Monitor for hypotension, bradycardia q3–5min during and after administration until recovery is achieved. Assess diligently for apnea during administration. Monitor for involuntary skeletal muscle movement.

Patient/Family Teaching

Discomfort along IV route may occur. Activities requiring mental alertness may be impaired after sedation.

propoxyphene hydrochloride

pro-**pox**-ih-feen
(Darvon)

FIXED-COMBINATION(S)
W/aspirin, caffeine **(Darvon Compound-65)**; w/acetaminophen **(Wygesic)**

propoxyphene napsylate

(Darvon-N)

FIXED-COMBINATION(S)
W/acetaminophen **(Darvocet-N)**

CANADIAN AVAILABILITY
Darvon-N

PREGNANCY CATEGORY C
(D if used for prolonged periods)

CLASSIFICATION

Opioid analgesic

AVAILABILITY (Rx)

Hydrochloride: Capsules: 32 mg, 65 mg

Napsylate: Tablets: 100 mg. **Suspension:** 10 mg/ml.

PHARMACODYNAMICS

	ONSET	PEAK	DURATION
Oral	15–60 min	—	4–6 hrs

PHARMACOKINETICS

Absorption: Well absorbed from GI tract. Widely distributed. **Metabolism:** Metabolized in liver. **Excretion:** Primarily excreted in urine. **Half-life:** 6–12 hrs; metabolite: 30–36 hrs.

ACTION / *THERAPEUTIC EFFECT*

Binds w/opioid receptors within CNS, *altering processes affecting pain perception, emotional response to pain.*

USES

Relief of mild to moderate pain.

ADMINISTRATION

ORAL:

- Give w/o regard to meals.
- Capsules may be emptied and mixed w/food.
- Shake oral suspension well.
- Do not crush or break film-coated tablets.

INDICATIONS / ROUTES / DOSAGE

Note: Reduce initial dosage in those w/hypothyroidism, concurrent CNS depressants, Addison's disease, renal insufficiency, elderly/debilitated.

Propoxyphene hydrochloride:
Oral: Adults, elderly: 65 mg q4h, as needed. ***Maximum:*** 390 mg/day.

Propoxyphene napsylate:
Oral: Adults, elderly: 100 mg q4h, as needed. ***Maximum:*** 600 mg/day.

CONTRAINDICATIONS

None significant.

EXTREME CAUTION

Severe CNS depression, anoxia, hypercapnia, respiratory depression, seizures, acute alcoholism, shock, untreated myxedema, respiratory dysfunction.

CAUTIONS

Increased intracranial pressure, impaired hepatic function, acute abdominal conditions, hypothyroidism, prostatic hypertrophy,

Addison's disease, urethral stricture, COPD.

INTERACTIONS

DRUG: ***Alcohol, CNS depressants*** may increase CNS or respiratory depression, risk of hypotension. May increase concentration, toxicity of ***carbamazepine.*** Effects may be decreased w/***buprenorphine. MAO inhibitors*** may produce severe, fatal reaction (reduce dose to 1/4 usual dose). **HERBAL:** None known. **FOOD:** None significant. **ALTERED LAB VALUES:** May increase amylase, lipase, SGOT (AST), SGPT (ALT), LDH, alkaline phosphatase, bilirubin.

SIDE EFFECTS

Note: Effects dependent on dosage amount. Ambulatory pts and those not in moderate pain may experience dizziness, nausea, vomiting, hypotension more frequently than those in supine position or having moderate pain. **FREQUENT:** Dizziness, drowsiness, dry mouth, euphoria, hypotension, nausea, vomiting, unusually tired. **OCCASIONAL:** Histamine reaction (decreased blood pressure, increased sweating, flushing, wheezing), ringing in ears, trembling, decreased urination, altered vision, constipation, headache. **RARE:** Confusion, liver toxicity, increased blood pressure, depression, paralytic ileus, stomach cramps, decreased appetite.

ADVERSE REACTIONS/TOXIC EFFECTS

Overdosage results in respiratory depression, skeletal muscle flaccidity, cold clammy skin, cyanosis, extreme somnolence progressing to convulsions, stupor, coma. Hepatotoxicity may occur w/overdosage of acetaminophen component. Tolerance to analgesic effect, physical dependence may occur w/repeated use.

PATIENT CONSIDERATIONS

Baseline Assessment

Obtain vital signs before giving medication. If respirations are 12/min or lower (20/min or lower in children), withhold medication, contact physician. Assess onset, type, location, and duration of pain. Effect of medication is reduced if full pain recurs before next dose.

Intervention/Evaluation

Palpate bladder for urinary retention. Monitor pattern of daily bowel activity, stool consistency. Initiate deep breathing and coughing exercises, particularly in those w/impaired pulmonary function. Assess for clinical improvement, record onset of relief of pain. Contact physician if pain is not adequately relieved.

Patient/Family Teaching

Change positions slowly to avoid orthostatic hypotension. Avoid tasks that require alertness, motor skills until response to drug is established. Tolerance/dependence may occur w/prolonged use of high doses.

propranolol hydrochloride

pro-**pran**-oh-lol
(Inderal)

FIXED-COMBINATION(S)
W/hydrochlorothiazide, a diuretic **(Inderide)**

CANADIAN AVAILABILITY
Apo-Propranolol, Inderal

PREGNANCY CATEGORY C
(D if used in second or third trimester)

CLASSIFICATION

Beta-adrenergic blocker

AVAILABILITY (Rx)

Tablets: 10 mg, 20 mg, 40 mg, 60 mg, 80 mg, 90 mg. **Capsules (sustained-release):** 60 mg, 80 mg, 120 mg, 160 mg. **Oral Solution:** 4 mg/ml, 8 mg/ml. **Solution (concentrate):** 80 mg/ml. **Injection:** 1 mg/ml.

PHARMACODYNAMICS

	ONSET	PEAK	DURATION
Oral	—	60–90 min	—
Oral (long-acting)	—	6 hrs	—
IV	Immediate	1 min	—

PHARMACOKINETICS

Absorption: Almost completely absorbed from GI tract. Widely distributed. **Metabolism:** Metabolized in liver. **Excretion:** Primarily excreted in urine. Not removed by hemodialysis. **Half-life:** 3–5 hrs.

ACTION / *THERAPEUTIC EFFECT*

Nonselective beta blocker. Blocks beta$_1$-adrenergic receptors, *slowing sinus heart rate, decreasing cardiac output, decreasing B/P.* Blocks beta$_2$-adrenergic receptors, *increasing airway resistance. Decreases myocardial ischemia severity* by decreasing oxygen requirements. Slows AV conduction, increases refractory period in AV node; *exhibits antiarrhythmic activity.*

USES / *UNLABELED*

Treatment of hypertension, angina, various cardiac arrhythmias, hypertrophic subaortic stenosis, migraine headache, essential tremor, and as an adjunct to alpha-blocking agents in the treatment of pheochromocytoma. Used to reduce risk of cardiovascular mortality and reinfarction in pts who have previously suffered a myocardial infarction (MI). *Treatment of adjunct anxiety, thyrotoxicosis, mitral valve prolapse syndrome, migraines.*

ADMINISTRATION

ORAL:

- May crush scored tablets.
- Give at same time each day.

IV:

- Give undiluted for direct injection.
- Do not exceed 1 mg/min injection rate.
- For IV infusion, may dilute each 1 mg in 10 ml 5% dextrose in water.
- Give 1 mg over 10–15 min.

INDICATIONS / ROUTES / DOSAGE

Hypertension:
Oral: Adults, elderly: Initially, 40 mg 2 times/day or 80 mg daily as extended-release capsule. Increase at 3–7 day intervals. ***Maintenance:*** 120–240 mg/day as tablets or oral solution, 120–160 mg/day as extended-release capsules. ***Maximum:*** 640 mg/day. ***Children:*** Initially, 1 mg/kg/day in 2 equally divided doses. Increase at 3–5 day intervals up to 2 mg/kg/day.

Angina pectoris:
Oral: Adults, elderly: Initially, 80–320 mg/day in 2–4 divided doses or 80 mg/day (sustained-release). ***Maximum:*** 320 mg/day. ***Maintenance:*** 160 mg/day.

Cardiac arrhythmias:
Oral: Adults, elderly: 10–30 mg 3–4 times/day.

Life-threatening arrhythmias:
IV: Adults, elderly: 0.5–3 mg. Repeat once in 2 min. Give additional doses at intervals of at least 4 hrs.

Hypertrophic subaortic stenosis:
Oral: Adults, elderly: 20–40 mg in 3–4 divided doses or 80–160 mg/day as extended-release capsule.

Pheochromocytoma:
Oral: Adults, elderly: 60 mg/day in divided doses w/alpha blocker for 3 days before surgery. ***Maintenance (inoperable tumor):*** 30 mg/day w/alpha blocker.

Migraine headache:
Oral: Adults, elderly: 80 mg/day in divided doses or 80 mg once daily as extended-release capsule. Increase up to 160–240 mg/day in divided doses.

Myocardial infarction:
Oral: Adults, elderly: 180–240 mg/day in divided doses beginning 5–21 days after MI.

Essential tremor:
Oral: Adults, elderly: Initially, 40 mg 2 times/day increased up to 120–320 mg/day in 3 divided doses.

Usual pediatric dosage:
Oral: 2–4 mg/kg/day in 2 equally divided doses up to 16 mg/kg/day in divided doses.

CONTRAINDICATIONS

Bronchial asthma, COPD, uncontrolled cardiac failure, sinus bradycardia, heart block greater than first degree, cardiogenic shock, CHF, unless secondary to tachyarrhythmias, those on MAO inhibitors.

CAUTIONS

Inadequate cardiac function, impaired renal/hepatic function, those w/Wolff-Parkinson-White syndrome, diabetes mellitus, hyperthyroidism.

INTERACTIONS

DRUG: ***Diuretics, other hypotensives*** may increase hypotensive effect. ***Sympathomimetics, xanthines*** may mutually inhibit effects. May mask symptoms of hypoglycemia, prolong hypoglycemic effect of ***insulin, oral hypoglycemics. NSAIDs*** may decrease antihypertensive effect. May increase cardiac depressant effect w/***IV phenytoin.*** **HERBAL:** None known. **FOOD:** None significant. **ALTERED LAB VALUES:** May increase ANA titer, SGOT (AST), SGPT (ALT), alkaline phosphatase, LDH, bilirubin, BUN, creatinine, potassium, uric acid, lipoproteins, triglycerides.

SIDE EFFECTS

FREQUENT: Decreased sexual ability, drowsiness, touble sleeping, unusually tired/weak. **OCCASIONAL:** Bradycardia, difficulty breathing, CHF (swelling of feet, shortness of breath), depression, cold hands/feet, diarrhea, constipation, anxiety, nasal congestion, nausea, vomiting. **RARE:** Altered taste, dry eyes, itching, numbness of fingers, toes, scalp.

ADVERSE REACTIONS/TOXIC EFFECTS

May produce profound bradycardia, hypotension. Abrupt withdrawal may result in sweating, palpitations, headache, tremulousness. May precipitate CHF, MI in those w/cardiac disease, thyroid storm in those w/thyrotoxicosis, peripheral ischemia in those w/existing peripheral vascular disease. Hypoglycemia may occur in previously controlled diabetics.

PATIENT CONSIDERATIONS

BASELINE ASSESSMENT

Assess baseline renal/liver function tests. Assess B/P, apical pulse immediately before drug is administered (if pulse is 60/min or below or systolic B/P is below 90 mm Hg, withhold medication, contact physician). *Anginal:* Record onset, type (sharp, dull, squeezing), radiation, location, intensity, and duration of anginal pain and precipitating factors (exertion, emotional stress).

INTERVENTION/EVALUATION

Assess pulse for strength/weakness, irregular rate, bradycardia. Monitor EKG for cardiac arrhythmias. Assess fingers for color, numbness (Raynaud's). Assist w/ambulation if dizziness occurs. Assess for evidence of CHF (dyspnea [particularly on exertion or lying down], night cough, peripheral edema, distended neck veins). Monitor I&O (increase in weight, decrease in urine output may indicate CHF). Assess for rash, fatigue, behavioral changes. Therapeutic response ranges from a few days to several weeks. Measure B/P near end of dosing interval (determines if B/P is controlled throughout day).

PATIENT/FAMILY TEACHING

Do not abruptly discontinue medication. Compliance w/therapy regimen is essential to control hypertension, arrhythmia, anginal pain. To avoid hypotensive effect, rise slowly from lying to sitting position, wait momentarily before standing. Avoid tasks that require alertness, motor skills until response to drug is established. Report excessively slow pulse rate (<60 beats/min), peripheral numbness, dizziness. Do not use nasal decongestants, OTC cold preparations (stimulants) w/o physician approval. Outpatients should monitor B/P, pulse before taking medication. Restrict salt, alcohol intake.

---

propylthiouracil

pro-pill-thye-oh-**your**-ah-sill
(Propylthiouracil)

CANADIAN AVAILABILITY
Propyl-Thyracil

PREGNANCY CATEGORY D

CLASSIFICATION

Antithyroid

AVAILABILITY (Rx)

Tablets: 50 mg

PHARMACOKINETICS

Absorption: Readily absorbed from GI tract. Concentrated in thyroid. **Metabolism:** Metabolized in liver. **Excretion:** Primarily excreted in urine. Minimally removed by hemodialysis. **Half-life:** 1–2 hrs.

ACTION / *THERAPEUTIC EFFECT*

In hyperthyroidism, *inhibits synthesis of thyroid hormone.* Diverts iodine from thyroid hormone synthesis.

USES

Palliative treatment of hyperthyroidism; adjunct to ameliorate hyperthyroidism in preparation for surgical treatment or radioactive iodine therapy.

ADMINISTRATION

ORAL:
- Space doses evenly.

INDICATIONS/ROUTES/DOSAGE

Hyperthyroidism:
Oral: Adults, elderly: Initially: 300–400 mg/day. *Maintenance:* 100–150 mg/day. *Children (6–10 yrs):* Initially: 50–150 mg/day; *(>10 yrs):* 150–300 mg/day. *Maintenance:* Determined by pt response.

CONTRAINDICATIONS

Hypersensitivity to the drug.

CAUTIONS

Pts over 40 years of age or in combination w/other agranulocytosis-inducing drugs.

INTERACTIONS

DRUG: *Amiodarone, iodinated glycerol, iodine, potassium iodide* may decrease response. May decrease effect of ***oral anticoagulants.*** May increase concentration of ***digoxin*** (as pt becomes euthyroid). May decrease ***thyroid uptake of*** I^{131}. HERBAL: None known. FOOD: None significant. ALTERED LAB VALUES: May increase SGOT (AST), SGPT (ALT), alkaline phosphatase, LDH, bilirubin, prothrombin time.

SIDE EFFECTS

FREQUENT: Urticaria, rash, pruritus, nausea, skin pigmentation, hair loss, headache, paresthesia. OCCASIONAL: Drowsiness, lymphadenopathy, vertigo. RARE: Drug fever, lupus-like syndrome.

ADVERSE REACTIONS/TOXIC EFFECTS

Agranulocytosis (which may occur as long as 4 mos after therapy), pancytopenia, fatal hepatitis have occurred.

PATIENT CONSIDERATIONS

Baseline Assessment

Question for hypersensitivity. Obtain baseline weight, pulse.

Intervention/Evaluation

Monitor pulse, weight daily. Assess food tolerance. Check for skin eruptions, itching, swollen lymph glands. Be alert to hepatitis (nausea, vomiting, drowsiness, jaundice). Monitor hematology results for bone marrow suppression; check for signs of infection/bleeding.

Patient/Family Teaching

Do not exceed ordered dose; follow-up w/physician is essential. Space evenly around the clock. Take resting pulse daily (teach pt/family), report as directed. Do not take other medications w/o approval of physician. Seafood, iodine products may be restricted. Report illness, unusual bleeding/bruising immediately. Inform physician of sudden/continuous weight gain, cold intolerance, or depression.

protamine sulfate

pro-tah-meen
(Protamine sulfate)

CANADIAN AVAILABILITY
Protamine

PREGNANCY CATEGORY C

CLASSIFICATION

Heparin antagonist

AVAILABILITY (Rx)

Injection: 10 mg/ml

PHARMACODYNAMICS

	ONSET	PEAK	DURATION
IV	5 min	—	2 hrs

PHARMACOKINETICS

After IV administration, protamine neutralizes heparin within 5 min (forms complex).

ACTION/*THERAPEUTIC EFFECT*

Complexes w/heparin to form a stable salt, *resulting in reduction of anticoagulant activity of heparin.*

USES/*UNLABELED*

Treatment of severe heparin overdose (causing hemorrhage). Neutralizes effects of heparin administered during extracorporeal circulation. *Treatment of enoxaparin toxicity.*

STORAGE/HANDLING

Keep at room temperature. Use only colorless solutions. Discard unused portions.

ADMINISTRATION

IV:

- Administer *slowly,* over 1–3 min (less than 50 mg over any 10 min period).
- Give by IV injection only.
- May be administered undiluted or diluted w/5% dextrose/0.9% NaCl fluid for injection.

INDICATIONS/ROUTES/DOSAGE

Antidote:

IV: Adults, elderly: 1 mg protamine sulfate neutralizes 90–115 units of heparin. Heparin disappears rapidly from circulation, reducing the dosage demand for protamine as time elapses.

CONTRAINDICATIONS

None significant.

CAUTIONS

History of allergy to fish, vasectomized/infertile men, those on isophane (NPH) insulin or previous protamine therapy (propensity to hypersensitivity reaction).

INTERACTIONS

DRUG: None significant. **HERBAL:** None known. **FOOD:** None significant. **ALTERED LAB VALUES:** None significant.

SIDE EFFECTS

FREQUENT: Decreased B/P, dyspnea. **OCCASIONAL:** Hypersensitivity reaction: urticaria, angioedema; nausea, vomiting (generally occurs in those sensitive to fish, vasectomized or infertile men, those on isophane [NPH], insulin, or previous protamine therapy). **RARE:** Back pain.

ADVERSE REACTIONS/TOXIC EFFECTS

A too rapid IV administration may produce acute hypotension, bradycardia, pulmonary hypertension, dyspnea, transient flushing, feeling of warmth. Heparin rebound may occur several hours after heparin has been neutralized by protamine (usually evident 8–9 hrs after protamine administration). Occurs most often following arterial/cardiac surgery.

PATIENT CONSIDERATIONS

Baseline Assessment

Check prothrombin time, activated partial thromboplastin time (APTT), hematocrit; assess for bleeding.

Intervention/Evaluation

Monitor pts closely after cardiac surgery for evidence of hyperheparinemia/bleeding. Monitor APTT or activated coagulation time (ACT) 5–15 min after protamine administration. Because of possibility of heparin rebound, repeat tests in 2–8 hrs. Assess hematocrit, platelet count, urine/stool culture for occult blood. Assess for decrease in B/P, increase in pulse rate, complaint of abdominal/back pain, severe headache (may be evidence of hemorrhage). Question for increase in amount of discharge during menses. Assess peripheral pulses; skin for bruises, petechiae. Check for excessive bleeding from minor cuts, scratches. Assess gums for erythema, gingival bleeding. Assess urine output for hematuria.

protriptyline hydrochloride

pro-**trip**-teh-leen
(Vivactil)

CANADIAN AVAILABILITY
Triptil

PREGNANCY CATEGORY C

CLASSIFICATION

Antidepressant: Tricyclic

AVAILABILITY (Rx)

Tablets: 5 mg, 10 mg

PHARMACOKINETICS

Absorption: Well absorbed from GI tract. Widely distributed. **Metabolism:** Metabolized in liver (undergoes first-pass effect). **Excretion:** Primarily excreted in urine. **Half-life:** 67–89 hrs.

ACTION/*THERAPEUTIC EFFECT*

Blocks reuptake of neurotransmitters (norepinephrine, serotonin) at neuronal presynaptic membranes, increasing availability at postsynaptic receptor sites. *Resulting enhancements of synaptic activity produce antidepressant effect.*

USES

Treatment of various forms of depression, often in conjunction w/psychotherapy.

ADMINISTRATION

ORAL:

- Give w/food or milk if GI distress occurs.
- Do not break or chew tablets.

INDICATIONS/ROUTES/DOSAGE

Depression:
Oral: Adults: Initially, 15–40 mg daily, given in 1–4 divided doses. Increase dosage gradually to 60 mg daily, then reduce dosage to lowest effective maintenance level. ***Adolescents:*** Initially, 5 mg 3 times daily.

Usual elderly dosage:
Oral: Initially, 5–10 mg/day. May increase by 5–10 mg/day q3–7days. ***Maintenance:*** 10–20 mg/day.

CONTRAINDICATIONS

Acute recovery period following

P

MI, within 14 days of MAO inhibitor therapy.

CAUTIONS

Prostatic hypertrophy, history of urinary retention/obstruction, glaucoma, diabetes mellitus, history of seizures, hyperthyroidism, cardiac/hepatic/renal disease, schizophrenia, increased intraocular pressure, hiatal hernia.

INTERACTIONS

DRUG: ***Alcohol, CNS depressants*** may increase CNS, respiratory depression, hypotensive effects. ***Antithyroid agents*** may increase risk of agranulocytosis. ***Phenothiazines*** may increase sedative, anticholinergic effects. ***Cimetidine*** may increase concentration, toxicity. May decrease effects of ***clonidine, guanadrel.*** May increase cardiac effects w/***sympathomimetics.*** May increase risk of hypertensive crisis, hyperpyretic convulsions w/***MAO inhibitors.*** **HERBAL:** St. John's wort may increase risk of adverse effect. **FOOD:** None significant. **ALTERED LAB VALUES:** May alter EKG readings, glucose.

SIDE EFFECTS

FREQUENT: Drowsiness, fatigue, dry mouth, blurred vision, constipation, delayed micturition, postural hypotension, excessive sweating, disturbed concentration, increased appetite, urinary retention. **OCCASIONAL:** GI disturbances (nausea, GI distress, metallic taste sensation). **RARE:** Paradoxical reaction (agitation, restlessness, nightmares, insomnia), extrapyramidal symptoms (particularly fine hand tremor).

ADVERSE REACTIONS/TOXIC EFFECTS

High dosage may produce cardiovascular effects (severe postural hypotension, dizziness, tachycardia, palpitations, arrhythmias) and seizures. May also result in altered temperature regulation (hyperpyrexia/hypothermia). Abrupt withdrawal from prolonged therapy may produce headache, malaise, nausea, vomiting, vivid dreams.

PATIENT CONSIDERATIONS

BASELINE ASSESSMENT

For those on long-term therapy, liver/renal function tests, blood counts should be performed periodically.

INTERVENTION/EVALUATION

Supervise suicidal risk patient closely during early therapy (as depression lessens, energy level improves, increasing suicide potential). Assess appearance, behavior, speech pattern, level of interest, mood. Monitor stools; avoid constipation. Monitor B/P, pulse for hypotension, arrhythmias. Closely monitor for cardiac disturbances in elderly pts receiving more than 20 mg daily. Assess for urinary retention by bladder palpation.

PATIENT/FAMILY TEACHING

Change positions slowly to avoid hypotensive effect. Tolerance to postural hypotension, sedative and anticholinergic effects usually develops during early therapy. Therapeutic effect may be noted within 2–5 days, maximum effect within 2–3 wks. Photosensitivity to sun may occur; use sunscreens, wear protective clothing. Dry mouth may be relieved by sugarless gum, sips of tepid water. Report visual disturbances. Do not abruptly discontinue medication. Avoid tasks that require alertness, motor skills until response to drug is established. Avoid alcohol and other CNS depressants.

pseudoephedrine hydrochloride

su-do-eh-**fed**-rin
(Novafed, Sudafed)

pseudoephedrine sulfate

(Afrinol Repetabs)

FIXED-COMBINATION(S)
W/acrivastine, an antihistamine **(Semprex-D)**; w/fexofenidine, an antihistamine **(Allegra-D)**; w/loratidine, an antihistamine **(Claritin-D)**

CANADIAN AVAILABILITY

Eltor, Sudafed

PREGNANCY CATEGORY C

CLASSIFICATION

Sympathomimetic

AVAILABILITY (OTC)

Tablets: 30 mg, 60 mg. **Tablets (extended-release):** 120 mg. **Capsules:** 60 mg. **Capsules (extended-release):** 120 mg. **Liquid:** 15 mg/5 ml, 30 mg/5 ml. **Drops:** 7.5 mg/0.8 ml.

PHARMACODYNAMICS

	ONSET	PEAK	DURATION
Tablets, syrup			
	15–30 min	—	4–6 hrs
Extended-release			
	—	—	8–12 hrs

PHARMACOKINETICS

Absorption: Well absorbed from GI tract. **Metabolism:** Partially metabolized in liver. **Excretion:** Primarily excreted in urine. **Half-life:** 9–16 hrs.

ACTION/*THERAPEUTIC EFFECT*

Acts directly on alpha-adrenergic receptors and, to lesser extent, on beta-adrenergic receptors, *producing vasoconstriction of respiratory tract mucosa, resulting in shrinkage of nasal mucous membranes, edema, nasal congestion.* Produces little, if any, rebound nasal congestion.

USES

For nasal congestion, treatment of obstructed eustachian ostia in those w/otic inflammation, infection.

P

ADMINISTRATION

ORAL:

- Do not crush, chew extended-release tablets; swallow whole.

INDICATIONS/ROUTES/DOSAGE

Decongestant:
Oral: Adults, children >12 yrs: 60 mg q4–6h. *Maximum:* 240 mg/day. *Children 6–12 yrs:* 30 mg q6h. *Maximum:* 120 mg/day. *Children 2–5 yrs:* 15 mg q6h. *Maximum:* 60 mg/day.

Usual elderly dose:
Oral: 30–60 mg q6h as needed.

Extended-release:
Oral: Adults, children >12 yrs: 120 mg q12h.

CONTRAINDICATIONS

Severe hypertension, coronary artery disease, lactating women, MAO inhibitor therapy.

CAUTIONS

Elderly, hyperthyroidism, diabetes, ischemic heart disease, prostatic hypertrophy.

INTERACTIONS

DRUG: May decrease effects of *antihypertensive, diuretics, beta-adrenergic blockers. MAO inhibitors* may increase cardiac stimulant, vasopressor effects. HERBAL: Ma Huang (Ephedra) may increase CNS stimulation. FOOD: None significant. ALTERED LAB VALUES: None significant.

SIDE EFFECTS

FREQUENT (5–10%): Nervousness, restlessness, insomnia. OCCASIONAL (1–5%): Trembling, fast, pounding heartbeat, headache, increased sweating, nausea, vomiting, trouble breathing, weakness. RARE (<1%): Seizures, irregular hearbeat, shortness of breath.

ADVERSE REACTIONS/TOXIC EFFECTS

Large doses may produce tachycardia, palpitations (particularly in those with cardiac disease), lightheadedness, nausea, vomiting. Overdosage in those >60 yrs may result in hallucinations, CNS depression, seizures.

PATIENT CONSIDERATIONS

PATIENT/FAMILY TEACHING

Discontinue drug if adverse reactions occur. Report insomnia, dizziness, tremor, irregular heartbeat.

psyllium

sill-ee-um

(Fiberall, Hydrocil, Konsyl, Metamucil, Perdiem)

CANADIAN AVAILABILITY

Metamucil, Prodiem Plain

PREGNANCY CATEGORY C

CLASSIFICATION

Laxative: Bulk forming

AVAILABILITY (OTC)

Powder. Wafer.

PHARMACODYNAMICS

	ONSET	PEAK	DURATION
Oral	12–72 hrs	—	—

PHARMACOKINETICS

Acts in small/large intestine.

ACTION/*THERAPEUTIC EFFECT*

Powder, wafer dissolves and swells in water (provides increased bulk, moisture content in stool). *Increased bulk promotes peristalsis, bowel motility.*

USES

Prophylaxis in those who should not strain during defecation. Facilitates defecation in those w/diminished colonic motor response.

ADMINISTRATION

ORAL:

- Drink 6–8 glasses of water/day (aids stool softening).
- Do not swallow in dry form; mix w/at least 1 full glass (8 oz) liquid.

INDICATIONS/DOSAGE/ROUTES

Laxative:

Oral: Adults, elderly: 1 rounded tsp, packet, or wafer in water 1–3 times/day.

CONTRAINDICATIONS

Abdominal pain, nausea, vomiting, symptoms of appendicitis, partial bowel obstruction, dysphagia.

CAUTIONS

None significant.

INTERACTIONS

DRUG: May interfere w/effects of ***potassium-sparing diuretics, potassium supplements.*** May decrease effect of ***oral anticoagulants, digoxin, salicylates*** by decreasing absorption. **HERBAL:** None known. **FOOD:** None significant. **ALTERED LAB VALUES:** May increase glucose. May decrease potassium.

SIDE EFFECTS

RARE: Some degree of abdominal discomfort, nausea, mild cramps, griping, faintness.

ADVERSE REACTIONS/TOXIC EFFECTS

Esophageal/bowel obstruction may occur if administered with insufficient liquid (less than 250 ml or 1 full glass).

PATIENT CONSIDERATIONS

INTERVENTION/EVALUATION

Encourage adequate fluid intake. Assess bowel sounds for peristalsis. Monitor daily bowel activity, stool consistency (watery, loose, soft, semisolid, solid). Monitor serum electrolytes in those exposed to prolonged, frequent, or excessive use of medication.

PATIENT/FAMILY TEACHING

Institute measures to promote defecation (increase fluid intake, exercise, high-fiber diet).

---

pyrazinamide

peer-a-**zin**-a-mide
(Pyrazinamide)

FIXED-COMBINATION(S)
W/ioniazid and rifampin, antituberculars **(Rifater)**

CANADIAN AVAILABILITY
Tebrazid

PREGNANCY CATEGORY C

CLASSIFICATION

Antitubercular

AVAILABILITY (Rx)

Tablets: 500 mg

PHARMACOKINETICS

Absorption: Rapidly, completely absorbed from GI tract. Widely distributed. **Metabolism:** Metabolized in liver to active metabolite. Removed by hemodialysis. **Half-life:** 9.5 hrs (increased in decreased renal function).

ACTION/*THERAPEUTIC EFFECT*

Exact mechanism unknown. *Either bacteriostatic or bactericidal, depending on its concentration at infection site and susceptibility of infecting bacteria.*

USES

In conjunction w/at least one other antitubercular agent in treatment of clinical tuberculosis after failure of primary agents (isoniazid, rifampin).

INDICATIONS/ROUTES/DOSAGE

Tuberculosis:
Oral: Adults: 20–35 mg/kg/day as single dose. ***Maximum:*** 3 g/day. ***Children:*** 15–30 mg/kg/day in 1 or 2 doses. ***Maximum:*** 1.5 g/day.

CONTRAINDICATIONS

Hypersensitivity to pyrazinamide, severe hepatic dysfunction.

P

CAUTIONS

Diabetes mellitus, renal impairment, history of gout, children (safety not established). Possible cross-sensitivity w/isoniazid, ethionamide, niacin.

INTERACTIONS

DRUG: May decrease effects of ***allopurinol, colchicine, probenecid, sulfinpyrazone.*** **HERBAL:** None known. **FOOD:** None significant. **ALTERED LAB VALUES:** May increase SGOT (AST), SGPT (ALT), uric acid concentrations.

SIDE EFFECTS

FREQUENT: Arthralgia, myalgia (usually mild and self-limiting). **RARE:** Hypersensitivity (rash, urticaria, pruritus), photosensitivity.

ADVERSE REACTIONS/TOXIC EFFECTS

Hepatoxicity, thrombocytopenia, anemia occurs rarely.

PATIENT CONSIDERATIONS

Baseline Assessment

Question for hypersensitivity to pyrazinamide, isoniazid, ethionamide, niacin. Assure collection of specimens for culture, sensitivity. Evaluate results of initial CBC, hepatic function tests, uric acid levels.

Intervention/Evaluation

Monitor hepatic function results and be alert for hepatic reactions: jaundice, malaise, fever, liver tenderness, anorexia/nausea/vomiting (stop drug, notify physician promptly). Check serum uric acid levels and assess for hot, painful, swollen joints, especially big toe, ankle, or knee (gout). Evaluate blood sugars, diabetic status carefully (pyrazinamide makes management difficult). Assess for rash, skin eruptions. Monitor CBC results for thrombocytopenia, anemia.

Patient/Family Teaching

Do not skip doses; complete full length of therapy (may be months, years). Office visits, lab tests are essential part of treatment. Take w/food to reduce GI upset. Do not take any other medications w/o consulting physician. Avoid too much sun or ultraviolet light until photosensitivity is determined. Notify physician of any new symptom, immediately for yellow eyes or skin; unusual tiredness; fever; loss of appetite; hot, painful, or swollen joints.

pyridostigmine bromide

pier-id-oh-**stig**-meen
(Mestinon, Regonol)

CANADIAN AVAILABILITY
Mestinon

PREGNANCY CATEGORY C

CLASSIFICATION

Anticholinesterase agent

AVAILABILITY (Rx)

Tablets: 60 mg. **Tablets (sustained-release):** 180 mg. **Syrup:** 60 mg/5 ml. **Injection:** 5 mg/ml.

PHARMACODYNAMICS

	ONSET	PEAK	DURATION
Oral	30–45 min	—	3–6 hrs
IM	<15 min	—	2–4 hrs
IV	2–5 min	—	2–3 hrs

PHARMACOKINETICS

Absorption: Minimally absorbed from GI tract. **Metabolism:** Metabolized in liver, by plasma cholinesterases. **Excretion:** Primarily excreted in urine. **Half-life:** 63–112 min.

ACTION/*THERAPEUTIC EFFECT*

Prevents destruction of acetylcholine by enzyme, anticholinesterase. *Produces miosis, increases tone of intestinal and skeletal muscles, stimulates salivary, sweat gland secretions.*

USES

Improvement of muscle strength in control of myasthenia gravis, reversal of effects of nondepolarizing neuromuscular blocking agents after surgery.

STORAGE/HANDLING

Store oral, parenteral forms at room temperature.

ADMINISTRATION

ORAL:

- Give w/food or milk.
- Tablets may be crushed; do not chew, crush extended-release tablets (may be broken).
- Give larger dose at times of increased fatigue (e.g., for those w/difficulty in chewing, 30–45 min before meals).

IM/IV:

- Give large parenteral doses concurrently w/0.6–1.2 mg atropine sulfate IV to minimize side effects.

INDICATIONS/ROUTES/DOSAGE

Note: Dosage, frequency of administration dependent on daily clinical pt response (remissions, exacerbations, physical and emotional stress).

Myasthenia gravis:
Oral: Adults, elderly: Initially, 60 mg 3 times/day. Increase dose at intervals of 48 hrs or more until therapeutic response is achieved. When increased dosage does not produce further increase in muscle strength, reduce dose to previous dosage level. ***Maintenance:*** 60–1,500 mg/day. ***Children:*** Initially, 7 mg/kg/day in 5–6 divided doses.

Extended-Release: Adults, elderly: 180–540 mg 1–2 times/day (must maintain at least 6 hrs between doses).

IM/IV: Adults, elderly: 2 mg q2–3h.

Oral: Neonates: 5 mg q4–6h.

IM: Neonates: 0.05–0.15 mg/kg q4–6h.

Reversal of nondepolarizing muscle relaxants:
IV: Adults, elderly: 10–20 mg with, or shortly after, 0.6–1.2 mg atropine sulfate or 0.2–0.6 mg glycopyrrolate.

CONTRAINDICATIONS

Mechanical GI, urinary obstruction.

CAUTIONS

Bronchial asthma, bradycardia, epilepsy, recent coronary occlusion, vagotonia, hyperthyroidism, cardiac arrhythmias, peptic ulcer.

INTERACTIONS

DRUG: ***Anticholinergics*** reverse/prevent effects. ***Cholinesterase inhibitors*** may increase toxicity. Antagonizes ***neuromuscular blocking agents. Quinidine, procainamide*** may antagonize action. **HERBAL:** None known. **FOOD:** None significant. **ALTERED LAB VALUES:** None significant.

P

SIDE EFFECTS

FREQUENT: Miosis, increased GI and skeletal muscle tone, reduced pulse rate, constriction of bronchi and ureters, salivary and sweat gland secretion. **OCCASIONAL:** Headache, slight temporary decrease in diastolic B/P w/mild reflex tachycardia, short periods of atrial fibrillation in hyperthyroid pts. Hypertensive pts may react w/marked fall in B/P. **RARE:** Rash.

ADVERSE REACTIONS/TOXIC EFFECTS

Overdosage produces cholinergic reaction manifested as abdominal discomfort/cramping, nausea, vomiting, diarrhea, flushing, feeling of warmth/heat about face, excessive salivation and sweating, lacrimation, pallor, bradycardia/tachycardia, hypotension, urinary urgency, blurred vision, bronchospasm, pupillary contraction, involuntary muscular contraction visible under the skin (fasciculation).

Overdosage may also produce a ***cholinergic crisis,*** manifested by increasingly severe muscle weakness (appears first in muscles involving chewing, swallowing, followed by muscular weakness of shoulder girdle and upper extremities), respiratory muscle paralysis followed by pelvis girdle and leg muscle paralysis. Requires withdrawal of all cholinergic drugs and immediate use of 1–4 mg atropine sulfate IV for adults, 0.01 mg/kg in infants and children under 12 yrs.

Myasthenic crisis (due to underdosage) also produces extreme muscle weakness but requires a *more* intensive drug therapy program (differentiation between the two crises is imperative for accurate treatment). Weakness beginning 1 hr after drug administration suggests overdosage; weakness occurring 3 hrs or more after administration suggests underdosage/resistance to anticholinesterase drugs. Extremely high doses may produce CNS stimulation followed by CNS depression. Resistance to pyridostigmine therapy may occur following prolonged treatment in myasthenic pts. Responsiveness may be restored by decreasing dose/temporarily discontinuing therapy for several days.

PATIENT CONSIDERATIONS

BASELINE ASSESSMENT

Larger doses should be given at time of greatest fatigue. Assess muscle strength before testing for diagnosis of myasthenia gravis and after drug administration. Avoid large doses in those w/megacolon or reduced GI motility. Have tissues readily available at pt's bedside.

INTERVENTION/EVALUATION

Monitor respirations closely during myasthenia gravis testing or if dosage is increased. Assess diligently for cholinergic reaction, as well as bradycardia in the myasthenic pt in crisis. Coordinate dosage time vs. periods of fatigue and increased/decreased muscle strength. Monitor for therapeutic response to medication (increased muscle strength, decreased fatigue, improved chewing, swallowing functions).

PATIENT/FAMILY TEACHING

Report nausea, vomiting, diarrhea, sweating, increased salivary secretions, irregular heartbeat, muscle weakness, severe abdominal pain, or difficulty in breathing.

pyridoxine hydrochloride (vitamin B_6)

pie-rih-**docks**-in
(Pyridoxine)

CANADIAN AVAILABILITY
Hexa-Betalin

PREGNANCY CATEGORY A
(C if doses above RDA)

CLASSIFICATION

Vitamin (B_6), coenzyme

AVAILABILITY (OTC)

Tablets: 25 mg, 50 mg, 100 mg. **Tablets (time-release):** 100 mg. **Injection (Rx):** 100 mg/ml.

PHARMACOKINETICS

Absorption: Readily absorbed primarily in jejunum. Stored in liver, muscle, brain. **Metabolism:** Metabolized in liver. **Excretion:** Primarily excreted in urine. Removed by hemodialysis. **Half-life:** 15–20 days.

ACTION/*THERAPEUTIC EFFECT*

Coenzyme for various metabolic functions *affecting protein, carbohydrate, lipid utilization.*

USES

Prevention, treatment of pyridoxine deficiency caused by inadequate diet, drug-induced (e.g., INH, penicillamine, cyclosporine) or inborn error of metabolism. Treatment of INH poisoning. Treatment of seizures in neonate unresponsive to conventional therapy. Treatment of sideroblastic anemia associated w/increased serum iron concentrations.

ADMINISTRATION

- **Note:** Give orally unless nausea, vomiting, or malabsorption occurs. Avoid IV use in cardiac pts.

IV:

- Give undiluted or add to IV solutions and give as infusion.

INDICATIONS/ROUTES/DOSAGE

Pyridoxine deficiency:
Oral: Adults, elderly: (Diet): 2.5–10 mg/day; after signs of deficiency decrease, 2.5–5 mg/day for several wks. *(Drug-induced):* 10–50 mg/day (INH, penicillamine); 100–300 mg/day (cyclosporine). *(Error metabolism):* 100–500 mg/day.

INH toxicity (>10 g); with other anticonvulsants:
IV: Adults, elderly: 4 g, then 1 g q30min until entire dose given. *Total dose:* Equal to amount INH ingested.

Seizures in neonates:
IM/IV: Neonates: 10–100 mg/day; then oral therapy of 2–100 mg/day for life.

Sideroblastic anemia:
Oral: Adults, elderly: 200–600 mg/day. After adequate response, 30–50 mg/day for life.

CONTRAINDICATIONS

IV therapy in cardiac pts.

CAUTIONS

Megadosage in pregnancy.

INTERACTIONS

DRUG: *Immunosuppressants, isoniazid, penicillamine* may antagonize pyridoxine (may cause ane-

P

mia/peripheral neuritis). Reverses effects of ***levodopa.*** **HERBAL:** None known. **FOOD:** None significant. **ALTERED LAB VALUES:** None significant.

SIDE EFFECTS

OCCASIONAL: Stinging at IM injection site. **RARE:** Headache, nausea, somnolence; high doses cause sensory neuropathy (paresthesia, unstable gait, clumsiness of hands).

ADVERSE REACTIONS/TOXIC EFFECTS

Long-term megadoses (2–6 g more than 2 mos) may produce sensory neuropathy (reduced deep tendon reflex, profound impairment of sense of position in distal limbs, gradual sensory ataxia). Toxic symptoms reverse w/drug discontinuance. Seizures have occurred following IV megadoses.

PATIENT CONSIDERATIONS

INTERVENTION/EVALUATION

Observe for improvement of deficiency symptoms, including nervous system abnormalities (anxiety, depression, insomnia, motor difficulty, peripheral numbness and tremors), skin lesions (glossitis, seborrhealike lesions around mouth, nose, eyes). Evaluate for nutritional adequacy.

PATIENT/FAMILY TEACHING

Discomfort may occur w/IM injection. Foods rich in pyridoxine include legumes, soybeans, eggs, sunflower seeds, hazelnuts, organ meats, tuna, shrimp, carrots, avocado, banana, wheat germ, bran.

quazepam

(Doral)

See Classification section under: Sedative-hypnotics

quetiapine

kwe-**tie**-ah-peen

(Seroquel)

CANADIAN AVAILABILITY

Seroquel

PREGNANCY CATEGORY C

CLASSIFICATION

Antipsychotic

AVAILABILITY (Rx)

Tablets: 25 mg, 100 mg, 200 mg

PHARMACOKINETICS

Absorption: Well absorbed following oral administration. Highly bound to plasma proteins. Widely distributed in tissues; CNS concentrations exceed those in plasma. **Metabolism:** Extensively metabolized by first-pass liver metabolism. **Excretion:** Primarily excreted in the urine. **Half-life:** 6 hrs.

ACTION/*THERAPEUTIC EFFECT*

Interacts with neurotransmitter receptors, including dopamine, serotonin, histamine and alpha$_1$-adrenergic receptors, *diminishing psychotic disorders.* Produces moderate sedation, few extrapyramidal effects, no anticholinergic effects.

USES

Management of manifestations of psychotic disorders.

ADMINISTRATION

ORAL:

- Dosage adjustments should occur at 2 day intervals.
- Initial dose and dose titration should occur at a lower dose in elderly, those with hepatic impairment, debilitated or those predisposed to hypotensive reactions.
- When restarting patients who have been off quetiapine for less than 1 wk, titration is not required and maintenance dose can be reinstituted.
- When restarting patients who have been off quetiapine for more than 1 wk, follow initial titration schedule.
- May take w/o regard to food.

INDICATIONS/ROUTES/DOSAGES

Psychotic disorder:

Oral: Adults: Initially 25 mg 2 times/day, then 25–50 mg 2–3 times daily on second and third days, up to 300–400 mg/day by the fourth day, given 2–3 times daily. Further adjustments of 25–50 mg 2 times/day made at 2 day intervals.

CONTRAINDICATIONS

History of hypersensitivity to quetiapine.

CAUTIONS

Alzheimer's dementia, history of breast cancer, cardiovascular disease (e.g., CHF, history myocardial infarction), cerebrovascular disease, impaired liver function, dehydration, hypovolemia, history of drug abuse or drug dependence, seizures, hypothyroidism.

INTERACTIONS

DRUG: ***Alcohol, CNS depressants*** may increase CNS depression. May increase effects of ***antihypertensives. Hepatic enzyme induces (e.g., phenytoin),*** may increase drug clearance. **HERBAL:** None known. **FOOD:** None significant. **ALTERED LAB VALUES:** May produce false-positive pregnancy test. May decrease total and free thyroxine (T_4) levels. May increase cholesterol, triglycerides, transaminase levels (e.g., ALT, AST).

SIDE EFFECTS

FREQUENT (10–19%): Headache, somnolence/drowsiness, dizziness. **OCCASIONAL (3–9%):** Constipation, postural hypotension, tachycardia, dry mouth, dyspepsia, rash, weakness, abdominal pain, rhinitis. **RARE (2%):** Back pain, fever, weight gain.

ADVERSE REACTIONS/TOXIC EFFECTS

Overdosage produces drowsiness, heart block (slow/irregular), decreased B/P, hypokalemia (weakness), tachycardia.

PATIENT CONSIDERATIONS

Baseline Assessment

Assess behavior, appearance, emotional status, response to environment, speech pattern, thought content. Obtain baseline CBC, hepatic function serum levels prior to initiation of treatment and periodically thereafter.

Intervention/Evaluation

Assist with ambulation if dizziness occurs. Supervise suicidal risk patient closely during early therapy (as psychosis, depression lessens, energy level improves, increasing suicide potential). Monitor B/P for hypo/hypertension. Assess pulse for tachycardia (especially with rapid increase in dosage). Monitor blood serum levels for evidence of blood dyscrasias. Question bowel activity for evidence of constipation. Assess for therapeutic response (improved thought content, increased ability to concentrate, improvement in self-care).

Patient/Family Teaching

Avoid exposure to extreme heat. Drink fluids often, especially during physical activity. Take medication as ordered; do not stop taking or increase dosage. Drowsiness generally subsides during continued therapy. Avoid driving or performing tasks that require alertness, motor skills until response to drug is established. Avoid alcohol. Change positions slowly to reduce hypotensive effect.

quinapril hydrochloride

quin-ah-prill
(Accupril)

CANADIAN AVAILABILITY
Accupril

PREGNANCY CATEGORY D

CLASSIFICATION

Angiotensin-converting enzyme (ACE) inhibitor

AVAILABILITY (Rx)

Tablets: 5 mg, 10 mg, 20 mg, 40 mg

PHARMACODYNAMICS

	ONSET	PEAK	DURATION
Oral	1 hr	2–4 hrs	—

PHARMACOKINETICS

Absorption: Readily absorbed from GI tract. **Metabolism:** Metabolized in liver, GI tract, extravascular tissue to active metabolite. **Excretion:** Primarily excreted in urine. Minimal removal by hemodialysis. **Half-life:** 1–2 hrs; metabolite: 3 hrs (increased in decreased renal function).

ACTION/*THERAPEUTIC EFFECT*

Suppresses renin-angiotensin-aldosterone system (prevents conversion of angiotensin I to angiotensin II, a potent vasoconstrictor; may also inhibit angiotensin II at local vascular and renal sites). *Reduces peripheral arterial resistance, B/P, pulmonary capillary wedge pressure; improves cardiac output.*

USES/*UNLABELED*

Treatment of hypertension. Used alone or in combination w/other antihypertensives. Adjunctive therapy in management of heart failure. *Treatment of hypertension/renal crisis in scleroderma.*

ADMINISTRATION

ORAL:

- May give w/o regard to food.
- Tablets may be crushed.

INDICATIONS/ROUTES/DOSAGE

Hypertension (used alone):
Oral: Adults: Initially, 10–20 mg/day. May adjust dose after at least 2 wk intervals. ***Maintenance:*** 20–80 mg/day as single or 2 divided doses. ***Maximum:*** 80 mg/day.

Hypertension (combination therapy):
Note: Discontinue diuretic 2–3 days before initiating quinapril therapy.

Oral: Adults: Initially, 5 mg/day titrated to pt's needs.

Usual elderly dose:
Oral: Initially, 2.5–5 mg/day. May increase by 2.5–5 mg q1–2wks.

Heart failure:
Oral: Adults, elderly: Initially, 5 mg 2 times/day. ***Range:*** 20–40 mg/day.

Dosage in renal impairment:
Titrate to pt need after following initial doses:

CREATININE CLEARANCE	INITIAL DOSE
>60 ml/min	10 mg
30–60 ml/min	5 mg
10–30 ml/min	2.5 mg

CONTRAINDICATIONS

MI, coronary insufficiency, angina, evidence of coronary artery disease, hypersensitivity to phentolamine, history of angioedema w/previous treatment w/ACE inhibitors.

CAUTIONS

Renal impairment, those w/sodium depletion or on diuretic therapy, dialysis, hypovolemia, coronary/cerebrovascular insufficiency.

INTERACTIONS

DRUG: ***Alcohol, diuretics, hypotensive agents*** may increase effects. ***NSAIDs*** may decrease effect. ***Potassium-sparing diuretics, potassium supplements*** may cause hyperkalemia. May increase ***lithium*** concentration, toxicity. **HERBAL:** None known. **FOOD:** None significant. **ALTERED LAB VALUES:** May increase potassium, SGOT (AST), SGPT (ALT), alkaline phosphatase, bilirubin, BUN, creatinine. May decrease sodium. May cause positive ANA titer.

SIDE EFFECTS

FREQUENT (>5%): Headache, dizziness. **OCCASIONAL (1–5%):** Chest pain, hypotension, fatigue, vomiting, nausea, diarrhea, cough, dyspnea, rash, syncope, muscle pain. **RARE (<1%):** Palpitations, angina, tachycardia, inability to sleep, drowsiness, malaise, flushed skin.

ADVERSE REACTIONS/TOXIC EFFECTS

Excessive hypotension ("first-dose syncope") may occur in those w/CHF, severely salt/volume depleted. Angioedema (swelling of face/lips), hyperkalemia occur rarely. Agranulocytosis, neutropenia may be noted in those w/impaired renal function or collagen vascular disease (systemic lupus erythematosus, scleroderma). Nephrotic syndrome may be noted in those w/history of renal disease.

PATIENT CONSIDERATIONS

BASELINE ASSESSMENT

Obtain B/P immediately before each dose in addition to regular monitoring (be alert to fluctuations). If excessive reduction in B/P occurs, place pt in supine position w/legs slightly elevated. Renal function tests should be performed before therapy begins. In those w/prior renal disease, urine test for protein by dipstick method should be made w/first urine of day before therapy begins and periodically thereafter. In those w/renal impairment, autoimmune disease or those taking drugs that affect leukocytes/immune response, CBC and differential count should be performed before therapy begins and q2wks for 3 mos, then periodically thereafter.

INTERVENTION/EVALUATION

Assist w/ambulation if dizziness occurs. Question for evidence of headache.

PATIENT/FAMILY TEACHING

To reduce hypotensive effect, rise slowly from lying to sitting position and permit legs to dangle from bed momentarily before standing. Noncola carbonated beverage, unsalted crackers, dry toast may relieve nausea. Full therapeutic effect may take 1–2 wks. Report any sign of infection (sore throat, fever). Skipping doses or voluntarily discontinuing drug may produce severe rebound hypertension. Avoid driving and other tasks that require alert responses until reaction to drug is known. Do not use salt substitutes w/o consulting physician.

quinidine gluconate

kwin-ih-deen
(Duraquin, Quinaglute)

quinidine polygalacturonate

(Cardioquin)

quinidine sulfate

(Cin-quin, Quinidex)

CANADIAN AVAILABILITY
Apo-Quinidine, Cardioquin, Quinate, Quinidex

PREGNANCY CATEGORY C

CLASSIFICATION

Antiarrhythmic

AVAILABILITY (Rx)

Gluconate: Tablets (sustained-release): 324 mg. **Injection:** 80 mg/ml (50 mg/ml quinidine).

Polygalacturonate: Tablets: 275 mg (200 mg quinidine)

Sulfate: Tablets: 200 mg, 300 mg. **Tablets (sustained-release):** 300 mg.

PHARMACODYNAMICS

	ONSET	PEAK	DURATION
Oral	1–3 hrs	—	6–8 hrs

PHARMACOKINETICS

Absorption: Completely absorbed from GI tract. Widely distributed. **Metabolism:** Metabolized in liver. **Excretion:** Primarily excreted in urine. Small amounts removed by hemodialysis. **Half-life:** 6 hrs (increased in CHF, cirrhosis, elderly).

ACTION/*THERAPEUTIC EFFECT*

Direct cardiac effects *(decreases excitability, conduction velocity, automaticity, membrane responsiveness; prolongs refractory period).*

USES/*UNLABELED*

Prophylactic therapy to maintain normal sinus rhythm after conversion of atrial fibrillation and/or flutter. Prevention of premature atrial, AV and ventricular contractions, paroxysmal atrial tachycardia, paroxysmal AV junctional rhythm, atrial fibrillation, atrial flutter, paroxysmal ventricular tachycardia not associated w/complete heart block. *Treatment of malaria (IV only).*

STORAGE/HANDLING

For parenteral form, use only clear, colorless solution. Solution is stable for 24 hrs at room temperature when diluted w/5% dextrose.

ADMINISTRATION

ORAL:

- Do not crush or chew sustained-release tablets.
- GI upset can be reduced if given w/food.

IV:

- **Note:** B/P, EKG should be monitored continuously during IV administration and rate of infusion adjusted to eliminate arrhythmias.
- For IV infusion, dilute 800 mg w/40 ml 5% dextrose to provide concentration of 16 mg/ml.
- Administer w/pt in supine position.
- For IV injection, give at rate of 1 ml (16 mg)/min (too rapid IV rate may markedly decrease arterial pressure).
- Monitor EKG for cardiac changes, particularly prolongation of PR, QT interval, widening of QRS complex. Notify physician of any significant interval changes.

Q

INDICATIONS/ROUTES/DOSAGE

Note: Extended-release tablets used only for maintenance therapy; 267 mg quinidine gluconate = 275 mg quinidine polygalacturonate or 200 mg quinidine sulfate.

Conversion of atrial fibrillation:
Oral: Adults, elderly: 200 mg q2–3h for 5–8 doses. Increase dose until sinus rhythm achieved/toxicity occurs. ***Maximum:*** 4 g/day. Control ventricular rate w/digoxin before quinidine administration.

Atrial flutter:
Oral: Adults, elderly: Individualize, give after digitalization.

Paroxysmal supraventricular tachycardia:
Oral: Adults, elderly: 400–600 mg q2–3h.

Premature atrial/ventricular contractions:
Oral: Adults, elderly: 200–300 mg 3–4 times/day.

Maintenance therapy:
Oral: Adults, elderly: 200–400 mg 3–4 times/day or 300–600 mg (as extended-release tablets) q8–12h.

Usual parenteral dosage:
IM: Adults, elderly: Initially, 600 mg, then 400 mg q2h adjusting each subsequent dose according to effect achieved by previous dose.

IV: Adults, elderly: 300 mg (may give 500–750 mg) infused at initial rate of 16 mg/min (1 ml/min).

CONTRAINDICATIONS

Complete AV block, intraventricular conduction defects, abnormal impulses and rhythms due to escape mechanism, myasthenia gravis.

EXTREME CAUTION

Incomplete AV block, digitalis intoxication, CHF, preexisting hypotension.

CAUTIONS

Preexisting asthma, muscle weakness, infection w/fever, hepatic/renal insufficiency.

INTERACTIONS

DRUG: May increase concentration of ***digoxin. Pimozide, other antiarrhythmics*** may increase cardiac effects. ***Urinary alkalizers (e.g., antacids)*** may decrease excretion. May increase effects of ***oral anticoagulants, neuromuscular blockers.*** May decrease effects of ***antimyasthenics*** on skeletal muscle. **HERBAL:** None known. **FOOD:** None significant. **ALTERED LAB VALUES:** None significant.

SIDE EFFECTS

FREQUENT: Abdominal pain/cramps, nausea, diarrhea, vomiting (can be immediate, intense). **OCCASIONAL:** Mild cinchonism (ringing in ears, blurred vision, hearing loss) or severe cinchonism (headache, vertigo, sweating, lightheadedness, photophobia, confusion, delirium). **RARE:** Hypotension (particularly w/IV administration), hypersensitivity reaction (fever, anaphylaxis, thrombocytopenia).

ADVERSE REACTIONS/TOXIC EFFECTS

Cardiotoxic effects occur most commonly w/IV administration, particularly at high concentration, observed as conduction changes (50% widening of QRS complex, prolonged QT interval, flattened T waves, disappearance of P wave), ventricular tachycardia/flutter, frequent PVCs, complete AV block. Quinidine-induced syncope may occur w/usual dosage (discontinue drug). Severe hypotension may result from high doses. Atrial flutter/fibrillation pts may experience a paradoxical, extremely rapid ventricular rate (may be prevented by prior digitalization). Hepatotoxicity w/jaundice due to drug hypersensitivity.

PATIENT CONSIDERATIONS

Baseline Assessment

Check B/P and pulse for 1 full min (unless pt is on continuous monitor) before giving medication. For those on long-term therapy, CBC and liver/renal function tests should be performed periodically.

Intervention/Evaluation

Monitor EKG for cardiac changes, particularly prolongation of PR, QT interval, widening of QRS complex. Monitor I&O, CBC, serum potassium, hepatic/renal function tests. Monitor pattern of daily bowel activity, stool consis-

tency. Assess for dizziness, syncope. Monitor B/P for hypotension (especially in those on high-dose therapy). If cardiotoxic effect occurs (see Adverse Reactions/Toxic Effects), notify physician immediately. Monitor for therapeutic serum level (2–6 mcg/ml).

PATIENT/FAMILY TEACHING

Report rash, fever, unusual bleeding or bruising, visual disturbances, ringing in ears. Teach pt/family to take pulse properly. Photophobia may occur—sunglasses will provide some relief.

quinine sulfate

kwye-nine
(Quinine)

FIXED-COMBINATION(S)
W/vitamin E for nocturnal leg cramps **(M-KYA, Q-vel)**

CANADIAN AVAILABILITY
Quinine

PREGNANCY CATEGORY D

CLASSIFICATION

Antimalarial, antimyotonic

AVAILABILITY (Rx)

Capsules: 65 mg, 200 mg, 300 mg, 325 mg. **Tablets:** 162.5 mg, 260 mg.

PHARMACOKINETICS

Absorption: Rapidly, completely absorbed from GI tract. Widely distributed. **Metabolism:** Metabolized in liver. **Excretion:** Primarily excreted in urine. Minimal removal by hemodialysis. **Half-life:** 11 hrs.

ACTION/*THERAPEUTIC EFFECT*

Myotonia: *Relaxes skeletal muscle* by increasing the refractory period, decreasing excitability of motor end plates (curarelike), and affecting distribution of calcium w/muscle fiber. ***Antimalaria:*** Elevates pH in intracellular organelles of parasites, *producing parasitic death.*

USES

Prevention, treatment of nocturnal recumbency leg cramps. Generally replaced by more effective, less toxic antimalarials. Used alone, w/pyrimethamine and sulfonamide (or w/oral tetracycline) for treatment of chloraquine-resistant falciparum malaria.

Q

ADMINISTRATION

ORAL:

- Do *not* crush tablets (irritating to gastric mucosa, bitter).
- Give w/or after meals to reduce GI distress.
- Bedtime dose should be given w/milk or snack.

INDICATIONS/ROUTES/DOSAGE

Nocturnal leg cramps:
Oral: Adults, elderly: 260–300 mg at bedtime as needed.

Treatment of malaria:
Oral: Adults, elderly: 260–650 mg 3 times a day for 6–12 days. ***Children:*** 10 mg/kg q8h for 5–7 days.

CONTRAINDICATIONS

Hypersensitivity to quinine (possible cross-sensitivity to quinidine), G-6-PD deficiency, tinnitus, optic neuritis, history of thrombocytopenia during previous quinine therapy, blackwater fever.

CAUTIONS

Cardiovascular disease (as w/quinidine), myasthenia gravis, asthma.

INTERACTIONS

DRUG: May increase concentration of ***digoxin. Mefloquine*** may increase seizures, EKG abnormalities. **HERBAL:** None known. **FOOD:** None significant. **ALTERED LAB VALUES:** May interfere w/17-OH steroid determinations.

SIDE EFFECTS

FREQUENT: Nausea, headache, tinnitus, slight visual disturbances (mild cinchonism). **OCCASIONAL:** Extreme flushing of skin w/intense generalized pruritus is most typical hypersensitivity reaction; also rash, wheezing, dyspnea, angioedema. Prolonged therapy: cardiac conduction disturbances, decreased hearing.

ADVERSE REACTIONS/TOXIC EFFECTS

Overdosage (severe cinchonism): cardiovascular effects, severe headache, intestinal cramps w/vomiting and diarrhea, apprehension, confusion, seizures, blindness, respiratory depression. Hypoprothrombinemia, thrombocytopenic purpura, hemoglobinuria, asthma, agranulocytosis, hypoglycemia, deafness, optic atrophy occur rarely.

PATIENT CONSIDERATIONS

Baseline Assessment

Question for possibility of pregnancy before initiating therapy (Pregnancy Category X). Question for hypersensitivity to quinine, quinidine. Evaluate initial EKG, CBC results.

Intervention/Evaluation

Check for hypersensitivity: flushing, rash/urticaria, itching, dyspnea, wheezing (hold drug, inform physician at once). Assess level of hearing, visual acuity, presence of headache/tinnitus, nausea, and report adverse effects promptly (possible cinchonism). Monitor CBC results for blood dyscrasias; be alert to infection (fever, sore throat) and bleeding/bruising or unusual tiredness/weakness. Assess pulse, EKG for arrhythmias. Check FBS levels and watch for hypoglycemia (cold sweating, tremors, tachycardia, hunger, anxiety).

Patient/Family Teaching

Use appropriate contraceptive measures (Pregnancy Category X). Use nonhormonal contraception. Take w/food; do not crush tablets. Do not take any other medication w/o consulting physician. Report *any* new symptom immediately, especially visual/hearing difficulties, shortness of breath, rash/itching, nausea. Periodic lab tests are part of therapy.

---

quinupristin-dalfopristin

quin-you-**pris**-tin/dal-foh-**pris**-tin (Synercid)

PREGNANCY CATEGORY B

CLASSIFICATION

Antimicrobial

AVAILABILITY (Rx)

Injection: 500 mg vial (350 mg dalfopristin/150 mg quinupristin)

PHARMACOKINETICS

Metabolism: After IV administration, both are extensively metabolized in the liver, with dalfopristin to active metabolite. **Excretion:** Primarily eliminated in feces. **Half-life:** 1–2 hrs.

ACTION/*THERAPEUTIC EFFECT*

Bactericidal (in combination). Two chemically distinct compounds that, when given together, bind to different sites on bacterial ribosomes forming a drug-ribosome complex. Protein synthesis is interrupted, *resulting in bacterial cell death.*

USES

Treatment of intra-abdominal, skin/skin structure, urinary tract, central catheter, bone and joint, respiratory infections, endocarditis, bacteremia.

STORAGE/HANDLING

Refrigerate vials. Reconstitute w/5% dextrose (compatibility w/0.9% NaCl unknown). After reconstitution, stable for 6 hrs at room temperature, 72 hrs refrigerated.

ADMINISTRATION

- **Note:** Space doses evenly around the clock for full effectiveness.

IV:

- For intermittent IV infusion (piggyback), infuse over 1 hr.
- Alternating IV sites, use large veins to reduce risk of phlebitis.

INDICATIONS/ROUTES/DOSAGE

Usual adult dosage:
IV Infusion: Adults, elderly: 7.5 mg/kg q8–12h.

CONTRAINDICATIONS

Hypersensitivity to quinupristin-dalfopristin.

CAUTIONS

Liver/renal dysfunction.

INTERACTIONS

DRUG: None significant. **HERBAL:** None known. **FOOD:** None significant. **ALTERED LAB VALUES:** May increase SGOT (AST), SGPT (ALT), LDH, serum creatinine, bilirubin.

SIDE EFFECTS

FREQUENT: Mild erythema, itching, pain, or burning at infusion site for doses of 7 mg/kg or higher. **OCCASIONAL:** Headache, diarrhea. **RARE:** Vomiting, arthralgia, myalgia.

ADVERSE REACTIONS/TOXIC EFFECTS

Superinfection, including antibiotic-associated colitis, may result from bacterial imbalance. Liver function abnormalities, peripheral venous intolerability may occur.

PATIENT CONSIDERATIONS

BASELINE ASSESSMENT

Question history of allergies, especially penicillins, cephalosporins. Obtain specimen for culture and sensitivity before giving first dose (therapy may begin before results are known). Assess temperature, B/P, respiratory rate, pulse. Obtain baseline liver function tests, BUN, CBC w/differential, urinalysis.

INTERVENTION/EVALUATION

Hold medication and promptly inform physician of diarrhea (w/fever, abdominal pain, mucus and blood in stool may indicate antibiotic-associated colitis). Evaluate IV site for mild erythema, itching, pain, or burning. Be alert for superinfection: increased fever, onset sore throat, nausea, vomiting, diarrhea, ulceration or changes of oral mucosa, anal/genital pruritus. Check liver function studies. Assess cultures of infection site. Monitor temperature for sign of infection.

rabeprazole

(Aciphex)

See Supplement

raloxifene

rah-**lock**-sih-feen

(Evista)

CANADIAN AVAILABILITY

Evista

PREGNANCY CATEGORY X

CLASSIFICATION

Selective estrogen receptor modulator

AVAILABILITY (Rx)

Tablets: 60 mg

PHARMACOKINETICS

Absorption: Rapidly absorbed following oral administration. Highly bound to plasma proteins (>95%) and albumin. **Metabolism:** Undergoes extensive first-pass metabolism in the liver. **Excretion:** Excreted mainly in the feces with a lesser amount in the urine. **Half-life:** 27.7 hrs.

ACTION/*THERAPEUTIC EFFECT*

Increases bone density, lowers LDL and total cholesterol, *preventing bone loss and lowering cholesterol w/o stimulating the endometrium.*

USES/*UNLABELED*

Treatment and prevention of osteoporosis in postmenopausal women. *Prevention of fractures, breast cancer in postmenopausal women*

ADMINISTRATION

ORAL:

- Give at any time of day w/o regard to meals.

INDICATIONS/ROUTES/DOSAGES

Prevention/treatment of osteoporosis:

Oral: Adults: 60 mg daily.

CONTRAINDICATIONS

Pregnancy, those who may become pregnant, active or those who have history of venous thromboembolic events (deep vein thrombosis, pulmonary embolism, retinal vein thrombosis), history of hypersensitivity to drug.

CAUTIONS

Hepatic function impairment.

INTERACTIONS

DRUG: ***Cholestyramine, ampicillin*** reduces raloxifene peak levels, extent of absorption. May decrease effect of ***warfarin*** (decreases prothrombin time). Do not use concurrently with systemic ***estrogen*** or ***hormone*** replacement therapy. **HERBAL:** None known. **FOOD:** None significant. **ALTERED LAB VALUES:** Lowers serum total and LDL cholesterol (does not affect HDL cholesterol or triglycerides). Slight decrease in serum total calcium, inorganic phosphate, total protein, albumin, platelet count.

SIDE EFFECTS

FREQUENT (10–25%): Hot flashes, flu syndrome, arthralgia, sinusitis. **OCCASIONAL (5–9%):** Weight gain, nausea, myalgia, pharyngitis, cough, dyspepsia, leg cramps, rash, depression. **RARE (3–4%):** Vaginitis, urinary tract infection, peripheral edema, flatulence, vomiting, fever, migraine, sweating.

ADVERSE REACTIONS/TOXIC EFFECTS

Pneumonia, gastroenteritis, chest pain, vaginal bleeding, breast pain occur rarely.

PATIENT CONSIDERATIONS

BASELINE ASSESSMENT

Question for possibility of pregnancy (Pregnancy Category X). Drug should be discontinued 72 hours before and during prolonged immobilization (postop recovery, prolonged bed rest). Therapy may be resumed only after pt is fully ambulatory. Determine total and LDL cholesterol serum blood levels prior to therapy and routinely thereafter.

INTERVENTION/EVALUATION

Monitor total and LDL cholesterol, total calcium, inorganic phosphate, total protein, albumin, and platelet count.

PATIENT/FAMILY TEACHING

Avoid prolonged restriction of movement during travel (increased risk of venous thromboembolic events). Take supplemental calcium, vitamin D if daily dietary intake is inadequate. Weight-bearing exercise, decrease or modification of cigarette smoking, alcohol consumption is advised.

ramipril

ram-ih-prill
(Altace)

CANADIAN AVAILABILITY
Altace

PREGNANCY CATEGORY D

CLASSIFICATION

Angiotensin-converting enzyme (ACE) inhibitor

AVAILABILITY (Rx)

Capsules: 1.25 mg, 2.5 mg, 5 mg, 10 mg

PHARMACODYNAMICS

	ONSET	PEAK	DURATION
Oral	1–2 hrs	3–6 hrs	24 hrs

PHARMACOKINETICS

Absorption: Well absorbed from GI tract. **Metabolism:** Metabolized in liver to active metabolite. **Excretion:** Primarily excreted in urine. **Half-life:** 5.1 hrs.

ACTION/*THERAPEUTIC EFFECT*

Suppresses renin-angiotensin-aldosterone system. Decreases plasma angiotensin II, increases plasma renin activity, decreases aldosterone secretion. *Reduces peripheral arterial resistance.*

USES/*UNLABELED*

Treatment of hypertension. Used alone or in combination w/other antihypertensives. Treatment of CHF. *Treatment of hypertension/renal crisis in scleroderma. Preventional of heart attacks, stroke.*

ADMINISTRATION

ORAL:

- May give w/o regard to food.
- Do not chew or break capsules.
- May mix w/water, apple juice/sauce.

INDICATIONS/ROUTES/DOSAGE

Hypertension (used alone):
Oral: Adults, elderly: Initially, 2.5 mg/day. ***Maintenance:*** 2.5–20 mg/day as single or in 2 divided doses.

Hypertension (combination therapy):
Note: Discontinue diuretic 2–3 days before initiating ramipril therapy.

Oral: Adults, elderly: Initially, 1.25 mg/day titrated to pt's needs.

CHF:
Oral: Adults, elderly: Initially, 1.25–2.5 mg 2 times/day. ***Maximum:*** 5 mg 2 times/day.

Dosage in renal impairment (Ccr <40 ml/min; serum creatinine >2.5 mg/dl):
Initially, 1.25 mg/day titrated up to maximum of 5 mg/day.

CONTRAINDICATIONS

History of angioedema w/previous treatment w/ACE inhibitors.

CAUTIONS

Renal impairment, those w/sodium depletion or on diuretic therapy, dialysis, hypovolemia, coronary/cerebrovascular insufficiency.

INTERACTIONS

DRUG: ***Alcohol, diuretics, hypotensive agents*** may increase effects. ***NSAIDs*** may decrease effect. ***Potassium-sparing diuretics, potassium supplements*** may cause hyperkalemia. May increase ***lithium*** concentration, toxicity. **HERBAL:** None known. **FOOD:** None significant. **ALTERED LAB VALUES:** May increase potassium, SGOT (AST), SGPT (ALT), alkaline phosphatase, bilirubin, BUN, creatinine. May decrease sodium. May cause positive ANA titer.

SIDE EFFECTS

FREQUENT (5–10%): Hypotension, cough. **OCCASIONAL (1–5%):** Angina, dizziness, fatigue, nausea, vomiting, asthenia (loss of strength). **RARE (<1%):** Palpitations, insomnia, nervousness, malaise, abdominal pain, muscle pain.

ADVERSE REACTIONS/TOXIC EFFECTS

Excessive hypotension ("first-dose syncope") may occur in those w/CHF, severely salt/volume depleted. Angioedema (swelling of face/lips), hyperkalemia occur rarely. Agranulocytosis, neutropenia may be noted in those w/impaired renal function or collagen vascular disease (systemic lupus erythematosus, scleroderma). Nephrotic syndrome may be noted in those w/history of renal disease.

PATIENT CONSIDERATIONS

BASELINE ASSESSMENT

Obtain B/P immediately before each dose, in addition to regular monitoring (be alert to fluctuations). If excessive reduction in B/P occurs, place pt in supine position w/legs elevated. Renal function tests should be performed before therapy begins. In those w/prior renal disease, urine test for protein by dipstick method should be made w/first urine of day before therapy begins and periodically thereafter. In those w/renal impairment, autoimmune disease, or taking drugs that affect leukocytes/immune response, CBC and differential count should be performed before therapy begins and q2wks for 3 mos, then periodically thereafter.

INTERVENTION/EVALUATION

Assess for cough (common effect). Assist w/ambulation if dizziness occurs. Assess lung sounds for rales, wheezing in those w/CHF. Monitor urinalysis for proteinuria. Monitor serum potassium levels in those on concurrent diuretic therapy. Monitor pattern of daily bowel activity, stool consistency.

PATIENT/FAMILY TEACHING

Report any sign of infection (sore throat, fever). Several weeks may be needed for full therapeutic effect of B/P reduction. Skipping doses or voluntarily discontinuing drug may produce severe, rebound hypertension. To reduce

hypotensive effect, rise slowly from lying to sitting position and permit legs to dangle from bed momentarily before standing.

ranitidine

rah-**nih**-tih-deen
(Zantac)

ranitidine bismuth citrate

(Tritec)

CANADIAN AVAILABILITY
Apo-Ranitidine, Novo-Ranidine, Zantac

PREGNANCY CATEGORY B

CLASSIFICATION

Histamine H-2 receptor antagonist

AVAILABILITY (Rx)

Tablets: 75 mg **(OTC),** 150 mg, 300 mg. **Tablets (effervescent):** 150 mg. **Capsules:** 150 mg, 300 mg. **Syrup:** 15 mg/ml. **Granules (effervescent):** 150 mg. **Injection:** 25 mg/ml, 0.5 mg/ml, 100 ml infusion.

Bismuth citrate: Tablets: 400 mg.

PHARMACOKINETICS

Absorption: Rapidly absorbed from GI tract. Widely distributed. **Metabolism:** Metabolized in liver. **Excretion:** Primarily excreted in urine. **Half-life:** *Oral:* 2.5 hrs; *IV:* 2–2.5 hrs (increased in decreased renal function).

ACTION/*THERAPEUTIC EFFECT*

Inhibits histamine action at H-2 receptors of parietal cells, *inhibiting basal and nocturnal gastric acid secretion.*

USES/*UNLABELED*

Short-term treatment of active duodenal ulcer. Prevention of duodenal ulcer recurrence. Treatment of active benign gastric ulcer, pathologic GI hypersecretory conditions, acute gastroesophageal reflux disease (GERD) including erosive esophagitis. Maintenance of healed erosive esophagitis. ***Bismuth citrate:*** Treatment of duodenal ulcers associated w/*H. pylori. Prophylaxis of aspiration pneumonia.*

STORAGE/HANDLING

Store tablets, syrup at room temperature. IV solutions appear clear, colorless to yellow (slight darkening does not affect potency). IV infusion (piggyback) is stable for 48 hrs at room temperature (discard if discolored or precipitate forms).

ADMINISTRATION

ORAL:

- Give w/o regard to meals. Best given after meals or at bedtime.
- Do not administer within 1 hr of magnesium- or aluminum-containing antacids (decreases absorption by 33%).

IM:

- May be given undiluted.
- Give deep IM into large muscle mass.

IV:

- For direct IV, dilute w/20 ml NaCl or other compatible IV fluid. Administer over minimum of 5 min (prevents arrhythmias, hypotension).
- For intermittent IV infusion (piggyback), dilute w/50 ml 0.9% NaCl, 5% dextrose, or other compatible IV fluid. Infuse over 15–20 min.

- For IV infusion, dilute w/100–1,000 ml 0.9% NaCl, 5% dextrose solution. Infuse over 24 hrs.

INDICATIONS/ROUTES/DOSAGE

Active duodenal ulcer:
Oral: Adults, elderly: 150 mg 2 times/day or 300 mg at bedtime. ***Maintenance:*** 150 mg at bedtime.

Pathologic hypersecretory conditions:
Oral: Adults, elderly: 150 mg 2 times/day up to 6 g/day.

Benign gastric ulcer, GERD:
Oral: Adults, elderly: 150 mg 2 times/day.

Erosive esophagitis:
Oral: Adults, elderly: 150 mg 4 times/day. ***Maintenance:*** 150 mg 2 times/day.

H. pylori **duodenal ulcer:**
Oral: Adults, elderly: 400 mg 2 times/day for 28 days (days 1–14 w/clarithromycin).

Usual parenteral dosage:
IM/IV: Adults, elderly: 50 mg q6–8h. ***Maximum:*** 400 mg/day.

IV Infusion: Adults, elderly: 150 mg/day up to 2.5 mg/kg/hr (Zollinger-Ellison).

Dosage in renal impairment (creatinine clearance <50 ml/min):
Oral: 150 mg q24h.

IM/IV: 50 mg q18–24h.

CONTRAINDICATIONS

None significant.

CAUTIONS

Impaired renal/hepatic function, elderly.

INTERACTIONS

DRUG: ***Antacids*** may decrease absorption (do not give within 1 hr). May decrease absorption of ***ketoconazole*** (give at least 2 hrs after). **HERBAL:** None known. **FOOD:** None significant. **ALTERED LAB VALUES:** Interferes w/skin tests using allergen extracts. May increase liver function tests, creatinine, gamma-glutamyl transpeptidase.

SIDE EFFECTS

FREQUENT: Headache. **OCCASIONAL:** Constipation, diarrhea, dizziness, drowsiness, nausea, vomiting, skin rash. **RARE:** Confusion, fever, blurred vision, joint or muscle pain, loss of hair, tachycardia, bronchospasm.

ADVERSE REACTIONS/TOXIC EFFECTS

Reversible hepatitis, blood dyscrasias occur rarely.

PATIENT CONSIDERATIONS

BASELINE ASSESSMENT

Do not confuse medication w/Xanax (alprazolam).

INTERVENTION/EVALUATION

Monitor serum SGOT (AST), SGPT (ALT) levels. Assess mental status in elderly.

PATIENT/FAMILY TEACHING

Smoking decreases effectiveness of medication. Do not take medicine within 1 hr of magnesium- or aluminum-containing antacids. Transient burning/itching may occur w/IV administration. Report headache. Avoid alcohol, aspirin.

remifentanil hydrochloride

(Ultiva)
See Classification section under: Opioid analgesics

repaglinide

reh-**pah**-glih-nide
(Prandin)

PREGNANCY CATEGORY C

CLASSIFICATION

Antidiabetic

AVAILABILITY (Rx)

Tablets: 0.5 mg, 1 mg, 2 mg

PHARMACOKINETICS

Absorption: Rapidly and completely absorbed from GI tract. Highly protein bound. **Metabolism:** Metabolized in liver to inactive metabolites. **Excretion:** Excreted primarily in the feces with a lesser amount in the urine. **Half-life:** 1 hr.

ACTION/*THERAPEUTIC EFFECT*

Stimulates release of insulin from beta cells of the pancreas by depolarizing beta cells, leading to an opening of calcium channels. Resulting calcium influx induces insulin secretion, *lowering glucose concentration.*

USES

Adjunct to diet and exercise to lower blood glucose in pts with type 2 diabetes mellitus (formerly known as NIDDM). Used as monotherapy or in combination with metformin (Glucophage).

ADMINISTRATION

ORAL:

- Ideally, give within 15 min of a meal but may be given immediately before a meal to as long as 30 min before a meal.

INDICATIONS/ROUTES/DOSAGES

Diabetes mellitus:
Oral: Adults, elderly: 0.5–4 mg 2–4 times/day. ***Maximum:*** 16 mg/day.

CONTRAINDICATIONS

Diabetic ketoacidosis, type 1 diabetes mellitus, history of hypersensitivity to drug.

CAUTIONS

Hepatic/renal function impairment.

INTERACTIONS

DRUG: Antifungal agents ***ketoconazole, miconazole),*** antibacterial agents ***(erythromycin)*** may reduce repaglinide metabolism. ***Troglitazone, rifampin, barbiturates, carbamazepine*** increase repaglinide metabolism. ***NSAIDs, salicylates, sulfonamides, chloramphenicol, warfarin, probenecid, MAOIs, beta blockers*** may increase effect. ***Diuretics, corticosteroids, phenothiazines, thyroid medication, estrogens, oral contraceptives, phenytoin, nicotinic acid, sympathomimetics, calcium channel blockers, isoniazid*** may produce hyperglycemia. **HERBAL:** None known. **FOOD:** Food decreases repaglinide plasma concentration. **ALTERED LAB VALUES:** None significant.

SIDE EFFECTS

FREQUENT (6–10%): Upper respiratory infection, headache, rhinitis, bronchitis, back pain. **OCCASIONAL (3–5%):** Diarrhea,

R

dyspepsia, sinusitis, nausea, arthralgia, urinary tract infection, weight gain. **RARE (2%):** Constipation, vomiting, paresthesia, allergy.

ADVERSE REACTIONS/TOXIC EFFECTS

Hypoglycemia occurs in 16% of pts. Chest pain occurs rarely.

PATIENT CONSIDERATIONS

BASELINE ASSESSMENT

Check fasting blood glucose and glycosylated Hgb (HbA_1C) periodically to determine minimum effective dose. Discuss lifestyle to determine extent of learning, emotional needs. Assure follow-up instruction if pt/family do not thoroughly understand diabetes management or glucose-testing technique. At least 1 wk should elapse to assess response to drug before new dose adjustment is made.

INTERVENTION/EVALUATION

Monitor blood glucose and food intake. Assess for hypoglycemia (cool wet skin, tremors, dizziness, anxiety, headache, tachycardia, numbness in mouth, hunger, diplopia) or hyperglycemia (polyuria, polyphagia, polydipsia, nausea, vomiting, dim vision, fatigue, deep rapid breathing). Be alert to conditions that alter glucose requirements: fever, increased activity or stress, surgical procedures.

PATIENT/FAMILY TEACHING

Diabetes mellitus requires lifelong control. Prescribed diet and exercise is principal part of treatment; do not skip or delay meals. Wear medical alert identification. Continue to adhere to dietary instructions, a regular exercise program, and regular testing of urine or blood glucose. When taking combination drug therapy with a sulfonylurea or insulin, have a source of glucose available to treat symptoms of low blood sugar.

---

respiratory syncytial virus immune globulin

(Respigam)

See Supplement

---

reteplase, recombinant

rhet-eh-place

(Retavase)

PREGNANCY CATEGORY C

CLASSIFICATION

Thrombolytic

AVAILABILITY (Rx)

Powder for Injection: 10.8 units (18.8 mg)

PHARMACOKINETICS

Metabolism: Rapidly cleared from plasma. **Excretion:** Eliminated primarily by the liver and kidney. **Half-life:** 13–16 min.

ACTION/*THERAPEUTIC EFFECT*

Activates fibrinolytic system by directly cleaving plasminogen to generate plasmin, an enzyme that *degrades the fibrin of the thrombus, exerting thrombolytic action.*

USES

Management of acute myocardial infarction (AMI) for improvement of ventricular function following AMI, reduction of incidence of CHF and reduction of mortality associated with AMI.

STORAGE/HANDLING

Use within 4 hrs of reconstitution. Discard any unused portion.

ADMINISTRATION

IV:

- Reconstitute only with sterile water for injection immediately before use. Reconstituted solution contains 1U/ml. Slight foaming may occur; let stand for a few minutes to allow bubbles to dissipate.
- Give through an IV line in which no other medications are being administered simultaneously.
- Give as a 10 unit plus 10 unit double bolus, with each IV bolus administered over 2 min period.
- Give the second bolus 30 min after the first bolus injection.
- Do not add other medications to the bolus injection solution.
- Do not give second bolus if serious bleeding occurs after first IV bolus is given

INDICATIONS/ROUTES/DOSAGES

Acute MI:

IV bolus: Adults, elderly: 10 units over 2 min, then repeat 10 units 30 min after initiation of first bolus injection.

CONTRAINDICATIONS

Active internal bleeding, history of CVA, recent intracranial or intraspinal surgery or trauma, intracranial neoplasm, arteriovenous malformation or aneurysm, bleeding diathesis or severe uncontrolled hypertension (increases risk of bleeding).

CAUTIONS

Recent major surgery (coronary artery bypass graft, OB delivery, organ biopsy), cerebrovascular disease, recent GI or GU bleeding, hypertension, mitral stenosis with atrial fibrillation, acute pericarditis, bacterial endocarditis, hepatic/renal impairment, diabetic retinopathy, ophthalmic hemorrhaging, septic thrombophlebitis, occluded AV cannula at an infected site, advanced age, those receiving oral anticoagulants.

R

INTERACTIONS

DRUG: ***Heparin, warfarin platelet aggregation antagonists (e.g., aspirin, dipyridamole, abciximab)*** increases risk of bleeding. **HERBAL:** None known. **FOOD:** None significant. **ALTERED LAB VALUES:** Plasminogen and fibrinogen levels may decrease.

SIDE EFFECTS

FREQUENT: Bleeding at superficial sites (venous injection sites, catheter insertion sites, venous cutdowns, arterial punctures, sites of recent surgical procedures).

ADVERSE REACTIONS/TOXIC EFFECTS

Bleeding at internal sites (intracranial, retroperitoneal, GI, GU or respiratory) occurs occasionally. Lysis or coronary thrombi may produce atrial or ventricular dysrhythmias, stroke.

PATIENT CONSIDERATIONS

BASELINE ASSESSMENT

Obtain baseline B/P, apical pulse.

Evaluate 12 lead EKG, CPK, CPK-MB, electrolytes. Assess hematocrit, platelet count, thrombin (TT), activated thromboplastin (APTT), prothrombin time (PT), plasminogen and fibrinogen level before therapy is instituted. Type and hold blood.

INTERVENTION/EVALUATION

Carefully monitor all needle puncture sites, catheter insertion sites for bleeding. Continuous cardiac monitoring for arrhythmias, B/P, pulse, respiration is essential until pt is stable. Check peripheral pulses, lung sounds. Monitor for chest pain relief; notify physician of continuation or recurrence of chest pain (note location, type, intensity). Avoid any trauma that may increase risk of bleeding (injections, shaving).

Rho (D) immune globulin IV

(WinRho SD)
See Supplement

ribavirin

rye-bah-**vi**-rin
(Virazole)

FIXED-COMBINATION(S)
W/interferon alpha 2b (**Rebetron**)

CANADIAN AVAILABILITY
Virazole

PREGNANCY CATEGORY X

CLASSIFICATION

Antiviral

AVAILABILITY (Rx)

Powder for Reconstitution (Aerosol): 6 g/100 ml

PHARMACOKINETICS

Absorption: Small amount systemically absorbed after inhalation. Rapidly absorbed from GI tract. Primarily distributed to plasma, respiratory tract secretions, RBCs. **Metabolism:** Metabolized in liver to active metabolite. **Excretion:** Primarily excreted in urine. **Half-life:** 9.5 hrs.

ACTION/*THERAPEUTIC EFFECT*

Appears to be virustatic through disruption of RNA and DNA synthesis, *interfering with viral replication, protein synthesis.*

USES/*UNLABELED*

Severe lower respiratory tract infections due to respiratory syncytial viruses in select infants, children. *Treatment of influenza A or B.*

STORAGE/HANDLING

Solutions appear clear and colorless, are stable for 24 hrs at room temperature. Discard solutions for nebulization after 24 hrs. Discard if discolored or cloudy.

ADMINISTRATION

INHALATION:

- **Note:** May be given via nasal or oral inhalation.
- Add 50–100 ml sterile water for injection or inhalation to 6 g vial.
- Transfer to a flask, serving as reservoir for aerosol generator.
- Further dilute to final volume of 300 ml, giving a solution concentration of 20 mg/ml.
- Use only aerosol generator available from manufacturer of drug.
- Do not give concomitantly

w/other drug solutions for nebulization.

- Discard reservoir solution when fluid levels are low and at least q24h.
- Controversy over safety in ventilator-dependent pts; only experienced personnel should administer.

INDICATIONS/ROUTES/DOSAGE

Severe lower respiratory tract infection caused by RSV:

Inhalation: Children, infants: Deliver mist containing 190 mcg/L at rate of 12.5 L of mist/min continuously for 12–18 hrs/day for 3–7 days.

CONTRAINDICATIONS

Hypersensitivity to drug, potential for pregnancy.

CAUTIONS

Use care in assisted ventilation because of mechanical problems associated w/precipitate and "rainout" when fluid accumulates in tubing.

INTERACTIONS

DRUG: May have antagonistic effect w/***zidovudine.*** **HERBAL:** None known. **FOOD:** None significant. **ALTERED LAB VALUES:** None significant.

SIDE EFFECTS

OCCASIONAL: Rash, conjunctivitis, reticulocytosis. **RARE:** Hypotension, digitalis toxicity.

ADVERSE REACTIONS/TOXIC EFFECTS

Cardiac arrest, apnea and ventilator dependence, bacterial pneumonia, pneumonia, pneumothorax occur rarely. If therapy exceeds 7 days, anemia may occur.

PATIENT CONSIDERATIONS

BASELINE ASSESSMENT

Obtain respiratory tract secretions before giving first dose or at least during first 24 hrs of therapy. Assess respiratory status for baseline.

INTERVENTION/EVALUATION

Monitor I&O, fluid balance carefully. Check hematology reports for anemia due to reticulocytosis when therapy exceeds 7 days. For ventilator-assisted pts watch for "rainout" in tubing and empty frequently; be alert to impaired ventilation and gas exchange due to drug precipitate. Assess skin for rash. Monitor B/P, respirations; assess lung sounds.

PATIENT/FAMILY TEACHING

Therapy must be continued for full length of treatment. Report immediately any difficulty breathing, chest discomfort or itching/swelling/redness of eyes.

rifabutin

rye-fah-**byew**-tin
(Mycobutin)

CANADIAN AVAILABILITY
Mycobutin

PREGNANCY CATEGORY B

CLASSIFICATION

Antibacterial (antimycobacterial)

AVAILABILITY (Rx)

Capsules: 150 mg

PHARMACOKINETICS

Absorption: Readily absorbed

from GI tract (high-fat meals slow absorption). Widely distributed. Crosses blood-brain barrier. Extensive intracellular tissue uptake. **Metabolism:** Metabolized in liver to active metabolite. **Excretion:** Excreted in urine; eliminated in feces. **Half-life:** 16–69 hrs.

ACTION/*THERAPEUTIC EFFECT*

Inhibits DNA-dependent RNA polymerase, an enzyme in susceptible strains of *E. coli* and *Bacillus subtilis, preventing M avium complex (MAC) disease.*

USES

Prevention of disseminated *Mycobacterium avium* complex (MAC) disease in those w/advanced HIV infection.

ADMINISTRATION

ORAL:

- May take w/o regard to food. Give w/food to decrease GI irritation.
- May mix w/applesauce if pt is unable to swallow capsules whole.

INDICATIONS/ROUTES/DOSAGE

MAC:

Oral: Adults, elderly, adolescents: 300 mg/day as single dose or in two divided doses.

CONTRAINDICATIONS

Hypersensitivity to rifabutin, other rifamycins (e.g., rifampin). Active tuberculosis.

CAUTIONS

Safety in children not established.

INTERACTIONS

DRUG: May decrease effects of ***oral contraceptives.*** May decrease concentration of ***zidovudine*** (does not affect inhibition of HIV by zidovudine). **HERBAL:** None known. **FOOD:** None significant. **ALTERED LAB VALUES:** May increase SGOT (AST), SGPT (ALT), alkaline phosphatase. May cause anemia, neutropenia, leukopenia, thrombocytopenia.

SIDE EFFECTS

FREQUENT (>10%): Skin rash, red-orange-red-brown discoloration of urine, feces, saliva, skin, sputum, sweat or tears. **OCCASIONAL (2–10%):** Arthralgia, altered taste, muscle pain, uveitis (eye pain, loss of vision), nausea, diarrhea, decreased appetite. **RARE (<1%):** Vomiting, insomnia.

ADVERSE REACTIONS/TOXIC EFFECTS

Hepatitis, thrombocytopenia occur rarely.

PATIENT CONSIDERATIONS

BASELINE ASSESSMENT

Chest x-ray, sputum or blood cultures, biopsy of suspicious node must be done to rule out active tuberculosis (given in active tuberculosis may cause resistance to both rifabutin and rifampin). Obtain baseline CBC, platelets, differential count, hepatic function tests.

INTERVENTION/EVALUATION

Monitor CBC, platelets, differential count. Avoid IM injections, rectal temperatures, other trauma that may induce bleeding. Check temperature and notify physician of flulike syndrome, rash, or GI intolerance. If jaundice occurs w/nausea, vomiting, and fatigue, may indicate hepatitis.

PATIENT/FAMILY TEACHING

Urine, feces, saliva, sputum, perspiration, tears, skin may be discolored brown orange. Soft contact lenses may be permanently discolored. Rifabutin may decrease efficacy of oral contraceptives; nonhormonal methods should be considered. Avoid crowds, those w/infections. Notify physician immediately of signs and symptoms of MAC and tuberculosis: night sweats, fatigue, fever, weight loss, abdominal pain. Report any yellowing of skin or eyes.

rifampin

rif-**am**-pin
(Rifadin, Rimactane)

FIXED-COMBINATION(S)
W/isoniazid, an antitubercular **(Rifamate)**; w/isoniazid and pyrazinamide, antituberculars **(Rifater)**

CANADIAN AVAILABILITY
Rifadin, Rimactane, Rofact

PREGNANCY CATEGORY C

CLASSIFICATION

Antitubercular

AVAILABILITY (Rx)

Capsules: 150 mg, 300 mg. **Powder for Injection:** 600 mg.

PHARMACOKINETICS

Absorption: Well absorbed from GI tract (food delays absorption). Widely distributed. **Metabolism:** Metabolized in liver to active metabolite. **Excretion:** Primarily eliminated via biliary system. Not removed by hemodialysis. **Half-life:** 3–5 hrs.

ACTION/*THERAPEUTIC EFFECT*

Interferes bacterial RNA synthesis by binding to DNA-dependent RNA polymerase, preventing attachment of the enzyme to DNA, thereby blocking RNA transcription. *Bactericidal activity occurs in susceptible microorganisms.*

USES/*UNLABELED*

In conjunction w/at least one other antitubercular agent for initial treatment and retreatment of clinical tuberculosis. Eliminates *Neisseria* meningococci from the nasopharynx of asymptomatic carriers in situations w/high risk of meningococcal meningitis (prophylaxis, not cure). Recommended by WHO as adjunctive therapy w/dapsone for leprosy. *Prophylaxis of H. influenza type b infection, treatment of atypical mycobacterial infection, serious infections caused by Staphylococcus species.*

STORAGE/HANDLING

Store capsules at room temperature. Reconstituted vial stable for 24 hrs. Use diluted solution within 4 hrs.

ADMINISTRATION

ORAL:
- Preferably give 1 hr before or 2 hrs after meals w/8 oz water (may give w/food to decrease GI upset; will delay absorption).
- For those unable to swallow capsules, contents may be mixed w/applesauce, jelly.
- Administer at least 1 hr before antacids, especially those containing aluminum.

IV:
- For IV infusion only. Avoid IM, SubQ administration.
- Avoid extravasation (local irritation, inflammation).

- Reconstitute 600 mg vial w/10 ml sterile water to provide concentration of 60 mg/ml.
- Withdraw desired dose and further dilute w/500 ml 5% dextrose; infuse over 3 hrs (may dilute w/100 ml D_5W and infuse over 30 min).

INDICATIONS/ROUTES/DOSAGE

Tuberculosis:
Oral/IV: Adults, elderly: 600 mg/day. ***Children:*** 10–20 mg/kg/day. ***Maximum:*** 600 mg/day.

Meningococcal carrier:
Oral: Adults, elderly: 600 mg/day. ***Children:*** 10–20 mg/kg/day. ***Maximum:*** 600 mg for 4 consecutive days.

CONTRAINDICATIONS

Hypersensitivity to rifampin or any rifamycin, intermittent therapy.

CAUTIONS

Hepatic dysfunction, active/treated alcoholism. Dosage not established in children under 5 yrs of age.

INTERACTIONS

DRUG: ***Alcohol, hepatotoxic medications*** may increase risk of hepatotoxicity. May increase clearance of ***aminophylline, theophylline.*** May decrease effects of ***oral anticoagulants, oral hypoglycemics, chloramphenicol, digoxin, disopyramide, mexiletine, quinidine, tocainide, fluconazole, methadone, phenytoin, verapamil.*** **HERBAL:** None known. **FOOD:** None significant. **ALTERED LAB VALUES:** May increase SGOT (AST), SGPT (ALT), alkaline phosphatase, bilirubin, BUN, uric acid.

SIDE EFFECTS

FREQUENT: Red-orange-brown discoloration of urine, feces, saliva, skin, sputum, sweat or tears, diarrhea, stomach cramps. **OCCASIONAL:** Flulike symptoms, hypersensitivity reaction (itching, redness, rash), fungal overgrowth (sore mouth, tongue). **RARE:** Interstitial nephritis, sore throat, bleeding, bruising.

ADVERSE REACTIONS/TOXIC EFFECTS

Hepatotoxicity (risk increased w/isoniazid combination), hepatitis, blood dyscrasias, Stevens-Johnson syndrome, antibiotic-associated colitis occur rarely.

PATIENT CONSIDERATIONS

Baseline Assessment

Question for hypersensitivity to rifampin, rifamycins. Assure collection of diagnostic specimens. Evaluate initial hepatic function and CBC results.

Intervention/Evaluation

Assess IV site at least hourly during infusion; restart at another site at the first sign of irritation/inflammation. Monitor hepatic function tests and assess for hepatitis: jaundice, anorexia/nausea/vomiting, fatigue, weakness (hold rifampin and inform physician at once). Report hypersensitivity reactions promptly: any type skin eruption, pruritus, flulike syndrome w/high dosage. Monitor frequency, consistency of stools especially w/potential for antibiotic-associated colitis. Evaluate mental status. Check for visual difficulties. Assess for dizziness, assist w/ambulation as needed. Monitor CBC results for blood dyscrasias and be alert for infection (fever, sore throat),

bleeding/bruising, or unusual tiredness/weakness.

PATIENT/FAMILY TEACHING

Do not skip doses, take full length of treatment (may take for months, years). Office visits, vision and lab tests are important part of treatment. Preferably take on empty stomach w/8 oz water 1 hr before or 2 hrs after meal (w/food if GI upset). Avoid alcohol during treatment. Do not take *any* other medications w/o consulting physician, including antacids; must take rifampin at least 1 hr before antacid. Urine, feces, sputum, sweat, tears may become red orange; soft contact lenses may be permanently stained. Notify physician of *any* new symptom, immediately for yellow eyes/skin, fatigue, weakness, nausea/vomiting, sore throat, fever, "flu," unusual bruising/bleeding. Be certain no vision difficulty, dizziness, or other impairment exists before driving, using machinery. If taking oral contraceptives check w/physician (reliability may be affected).

rifapentine

(Priftin)

See Supplement

rimantadine

rye-**man**-tah-deen

(Flumadine)

PREGNANCY CATEGORY C

CLASSIFICATION

Antiviral

AVAILABILITY (Rx)

Tablets: 100 mg. **Syrup:** 50 mg/5 ml.

PHARMACOKINETICS

Absorption: Readily absorbed from GI tract. **Metabolism:** Metabolized in liver. **Excretion:** Primarily excreted in urine. **Half-life:** 20–65 hrs (increased in severe liver and/or renal impairment).

ACTION / *THERAPEUTIC EFFECT*

Exact mechanism unknown. Appears to exert inhibitory effect early in viral replication cycle. May inhibit uncoating of virus, *preventing replication of influenza A virus.*

USES

Adults: Prophylaxis and treatment of illness due to influenza A virus. *Children:* Prophylaxis against influenza A virus.

ADMINISTRATION

ORAL:

- May give w/o regard to food.

INDICATIONS/ROUTES/DOSAGE

Prophylaxis against influenza A virus:

Oral: Adults, elderly, children >10 yrs: 100 mg 2 times/day. *Severe hepatic/renal impairment, elderly nursing home pts:* 100 mg/day. *Children <10 yrs:* 5 mg/kg once daily. *Maximum:* 150 mg.

Treatment of influenza virus A:

Oral: Adults, elderly: 100 mg 2 times/day for 7 days. *Severe hepatic/renal impairment, elderly nursing home pts:* 100 mg/day for 7 days.

CONTRAINDICATIONS

Hypersensitivity to amantadine, rimantadine.

CAUTIONS

Pts w/renal, liver impairment; history of seizures (increased incidence of seizures).

INTERACTIONS

DRUG: *Acetaminophen, aspirin* may decrease concentrations. *Cimetidine* may increase concentrations. **HERBAL:** None known. **FOOD:** None significant. **ALTERED LAB VALUES:** None significant.

SIDE EFFECTS

OCCASIONAL (1–3%): Insomnia, dizziness, headache, nervousness, fatigue, asthenia. Nausea, vomiting, anorexia, dry mouth, abdominal pain. **RARE (<1%):** Diarrhea, dyspepsia, agitation, impaired concentration, ringing in ears, dyspnea.

ADVERSE REACTIONS/TOXIC EFFECTS

None significant.

PATIENT CONSIDERATIONS

Intervention/Evaluation

Assess for nervousness and evaluate sleep pattern for insomnia. Provide assistance if dizziness occurs. Check food tolerance. When administering for illness, monitor temperature.

Patient/Family Teaching

Avoid contact w/those who are at high risk for influenza A (rimantadine-resistant virus may be shed during therapy). Do not drive or perform tasks that require alert response if dizziness or decreased concentration occurs. *Do not* take aspirin, acetaminophen, or compounds containing these drugs.

rifapentine

rye-fah-**pen**-teen
(Priftin)

PREGNANCY CATEGORY C

CLASSIFICATION

Antituberculous antibiotic

AVAILABILITY (Rx)

Tablets: 150 mg

PHARMACOKINETICS

Absorption: Well absorbed following oral administration. Highly bound to plasma proteins. **Metabolism:** Hydrolyzed by an esterase enzyme. **Excretion:** Excreted primarily in the feces with lesser amount eliminated in the urine. **Half-life:** 13 hrs.

ACTION/*THERAPEUTIC EFFECT*

Inhibits DNA dependent RNA polymerase *exhibiting bactericidal activity against intracellular and extracellular M. tuberculosis organisms.*

USES/*UNLABELED*

Used in conjunction with at least one other antituberculosis agent for the treatment of pulmonary tuberculosis (TB). *Treatment/prophylaxis of MAC in pts with AIDS.*

ADMINISTRATION

- Advise pt that a red-orange discoloration to urine, sweat, sputum and tears may occur. Contact lenses may become permanently stained.
- Always use in combination with

other antitubercular drugs to ensure early sputum conversion and protection against relapse.

- In those predisposed to neuropathy (alcoholism, diabetes mellitus), adolescents and malnourished, use concurrently with pyridoxine (vitamin B_6).
- Give with food if stomach upset, nausea, vomiting occurs.
- More frequent dosing is recommended in HIV-infected pts.

INDICATIONS/ROUTES/DOSAGES

Tuberculosis, intensive phase: *Oral: Adults, elderly:* 600 mg (four 150 mg tablets twice weekly) with an interval of ≥3 days (72 hrs) between doses. Continue for 2 mos.

Tuberculosis, continuation phase: *Oral: Adults, elderly:* 600 mg/week for 4 mos in combination with other appropriate antitubercular drug.

CONTRAINDICATIONS

History of hypersensitivity to medication, rifampin or rifabutin.

CAUTIONS

Hepatic function impairment, those taking protease inhibitors, alcoholism (active or in remission).

INTERACTIONS

DRUG: Effectiveness is significantly decreased with ***indinavir.*** Accelerates metabolism and reduces activity of ***amitriptyline, barbiturates, cardiac glycosides, chloramphenicol, clarithromycin, clofibrate, corticosteroids, cyclosporine, dapsone, delavirdine, diazepam, diltiazem, disopyramide, doxycycline, fluconazole, fluoroquinolones, haloperidol, indinavir, itraconazole, ketoconazole, levothyroxine, methadone, mexiletine, nelfinavir, nifedipine, nortriptyline, oral contraceptives, phenytoin, progestins, quinidine, quinine, ritonavir, saquinavir, sildenafil, sulfonylureas, tacrolimus, theophylline, tocainide, verapamil, warfarin, zidovudine.*** **HERBAL:** None known. **FOOD:** None significant. **ALTERED LAB VALUES:** Alters test results for serum folate, vitamin B_{12} determinations. May increase bilirubin, SGOT (AST), SGPT (ALT), BUN, uric acid.

SIDE EFFECTS

FREQUENT (10–15%): Proteinuria, hematuria, pyuria. **OCCASIONAL (4–9%):** Arthralgia, rash, pruritus, nausea, anorexia, acne, dizziness, vomiting, diarrhea. **RARE (2–3%):** Headache, dyspepsia, hypertension.

ADVERSE REACTIONS/TOXIC EFFECTS

May produce blood dyscrasias (neutropenia, lymphopenia, anemia, leukopenia, thrombocytosis), hepatotoxicity. Pseudomembranous colitis may occur. If persistent or severe diarrhea occur, rifapentine should be stopped immediately and oral vancomycin initiated. Medication inhibiting peristalsis is contraindicated in this condition.

PATIENT CONSIDERATIONS

BASELINE ASSESSMENT

Emphasize diligent compliance with dosage regimen (poor compliance associated with late sputum conversion and high relapse rate). Obtain baseline hepatic function tests (especially hepatic enzymes, bilirubin), CBC, platelet count and periodically thereafter.

Intervention/Evaluation

Monitor liver function tests (especially serum transaminase) before initial therapy and q2–4wks during treatment. Assess for hepatitis (jaundice, anorexia, nausea, vomiting, fatigue, weakness). Monitor frequency, consistency of stools especially with potential for pseudomembranous colitis. Monitor CBC, platelet count for blood dyscrasias and be alert for infection.

Patient/Family Teaching

May produce a red-orange discoloration to skin, teeth, tongue, urine, feces, saliva, sputum, tears, sweat). Contact lenses may be permanently stained. Use alternative birth control measures because reliability of oral or systemic hormonal contraceptives may be affected by medication. It is imperative not to miss any doses; absolute compliance is an essential part of treatment. Take with food if GI upset occurs. Report fever, decreased appetite, nausea, vomiting, malaise, darkened urine, pain or swelling at joints, yellowing of skin/eyes. Avoid alcohol.

---

risedronate sodium

rise-droh-nate
(Actonal)

PREGNANCY CATEGORY C

CLASSIFICATION

Bone resorption inhibitor

AVAILABILITY (Rx)

Tablets: 5 mg, 30 mg

PHARMACOKINETICS

Absorption: Rapidly absorbed following oral administration and distributed to bone with uptake greatest at sites of active bone turnover. **Excretion:** Absorbed dose excreted in urine with unabsorbed drug eliminated unchanged in feces. **Half-life:** 1.5 hrs (initial), 220 hrs (terminal).

ACTION/*THERAPEUTIC EFFECT*

Inhibits abnormal bone resorption, evidenced by significant decrease in serum alkaline phosphatase (marker of bone formation) and urinary creatinine (marker of bone resorption), *decreasing osteolysis of both axial and appedicular skeleton.*

USES/*UNLABELED*

Treatment of those with Paget's disease of bone having alkaline phosphatase at least two times the upper limit of normal, or those symptomatic or at risk for future complications from Paget's disease. *Prevention of bone loss in menopausal women. Prevention and treatment of postmenopausal osteoporosis and corticosteroid-induced osteoporosis.*

ADMINISTRATION

ORAL:

- Give ≥30 min before first food, medication, or drink of day other than water.
- Patient to take medication while in an upright position with a full glass (6–8 oz) of plain water (mineral water, coffee, tea, juice will decrease absorption).
- Avoid lying down for 30 min (allows medication to reach stomach quickly, minimizes esophageal irritation).

INDICATIONS/ROUTES/DOSAGES

Note: Take with full glass of plain water only, 30 minutes before first food, beverage, or medication.

Paget's disease:
Oral: Adults: 30 mg once daily first thing in the morning for 2 mos.

CONTRAINDICATIONS

Severe renal impairment (creatinine clearance <30 ml/min), history of hypersensitivity to biphosphates.

CAUTIONS

Gastrointestinal diseases (duodenitis, dysphagia, esophagitis, gastritis, ulcers) may be exacerbated by risedronate.

INTERACTIONS

DRUG: ***Antacids, calcium supplements*** interferes with absorption. **HERBAL:** None known. **FOOD:** Effectiveness is decreased when taken with food; must be taken ≥30 min before first food, medication, or drink of day other than water. **ALTERED LAB VALUES:** May decrease serum alkaline phosphatase, urinary creatinine, serum calcium, phosphates.

SIDE EFFECTS

FREQUENT (11–33%): Arthralgia, diarrhea, headache, abdominal cramping, rash. **OCCASIONAL (5–9%):** Flulike symptoms, nausea, constipation, peripheral edema, dizziness. **RARE (3–4%):** Weakness, sinusitis, belching, leg cramps, dry eye, tinnitus.

ADVERSE REACTIONS/TOXIC EFFECTS

Bone pain, chest pain, colitis, bronchitis occur rarely.

PATIENT CONSIDERATIONS

Baseline Assessment

Hypocalcemia, vitamin D deficiency must be corrected before therapy begins. Obtain baseline alkaline phosphatase, urinary creatinine, serum calcium, phosphates.

Intervention/Evaluation

Monitor electrolytes, especially calcium and alkaline phosphatase serum levels. Monitor stool frequency and consistency (watery, loose, soft, semisolid, solid). Evaluate pain in those with Paget's disease. Monitor serum alkaline phosphatase, urinary creatinine, serum calcium, phosphates.

Patient/Family Teaching

Expected benefits occur only when medication is taken with a full glass (6–8 oz) of plain water only, 30 min before first food, beverage, or medication. Take medication while in an upright position (decreases risk of GI upset) with a full glass of plain water (mineral water, coffee, tea, juice will decrease absorption). Take supplemental calcium, vitamin D if daily dietary intake is inadequate. Weight-bearing exercise, decrease or modification of cigarette smoking, alcohol consumption is advised. Take antacids at a different time of day than risedronate ingestion (antacids prevents risedronate absorption).

risperidone

ris-**pear**-ih-doan
(Risperdal)

CANADIAN AVAILABILITY
Risperdal

PREGNANCY CATEGORY C

CLASSIFICATION

Antipsychotic

AVAILABILITY (Rx)

Tablets: 0.25 mg, 0.5 mg, 1 mg, 2 mg, 3 mg, 4 mg. **Oral Solution:** 1 mg/ml.

PHARMACOKINETICS

Absorption: Well absorbed from GI tract (unaffected by food). **Metabolism:** Extensively metabolized in liver to active metabolite. **Excretion:** Primarily excreted in urine. **Half-life:** 3–20 hrs; metabolite: 21–30 hrs (increased in elderly).

ACTION / *THERAPEUTIC EFFECT*

Exact mechanism unknown. Action may be due to dopamine and serotonin receptor antagonism. *Suppresses behavioral response in psychosis.*

USES

Management of manifestations of psychotic disorders.

ADMINISTRATION

ORAL:

- May take w/o regard to food.

INDICATIONS / ROUTES / DOSAGE

Antipsychotic:

Oral: Adults: Initially, 1 mg 2 times/day for 1 day; then, 2 mg 2 times/day for 1 day; then, 3 mg 2 times/day for 1 day. Further adjustments of 1 mg 2 times/day made at at least 1 wk intervals. Maximum effect in range of 4–6 mg/day. ***Elderly, debilitated, pts w/severe liver/renal impairment, risk of hypotension:*** Initially, 0.5 mg 2 times/day for 1 day; then, 1 mg 2 times/day for 1 day; then, 1.5 mg 2 times/day for 1 day. Further adjustments: at least 1 wk intervals.

CONTRAINDICATIONS

Hypersensitivity to risperidone.

CAUTIONS

Cardiac pts (e.g., history of MI, ischemia, CHF, conduction abnormality); pts w/cerebrovascular disease, dehydration, hypovolemia, use of antihypertensives. History of seizures. Safety in children unknown. May mask signs of drug overdose, intestinal obstruction.

INTERACTIONS

DRUG: May decrease effects of ***levodopa, dopamine agonists. Carbamazepine*** may decrease concentration. ***Clozapine*** may increase concentration. ***Alcohol, CNS depressants*** may increase CNS depression. **HERBAL:** None known. **FOOD:** None significant. **ALTERED LAB VALUES:** May increase creatine phosphokinase, uric acid, triglycerides, SGOT (AST), SGPT (ALT), prolactin. May decrease potassium, sodium, protein, glucose. May cause EKG changes.

SIDE EFFECTS

FREQUENT (>10%): Extrapyramidal symptoms (akathisia, dystonia, parkinsonism), anxiety, change in vision, dizziness, insomnia, mental changes, skin rash, unusually tired, constipation, cough, diarrhea, drowsiness, headache, nausea, rhinitis. **OCCASIONAL (2–10%):** Amenorrhea, back pain, dyspnea, galactorrhea, abdominal pain, arthralgia, dry skin, darkening of skin, vomiting. **RARE (<2%):** Loss of appetite, mania, increased thirst, seizures.

ADVERSE REACTIONS/TOXIC EFFECTS

Neuroleptic malignant syndrome (NMS): hyperpyrexia, muscle rigidity, change in mental status, irregular pulse or B/P, tachycardia, diaphoresis, cardiac dysrhythmias, elevated creatine phosphokinase, rhabdomyolysis, acute renal failure. Tardive dyskinesia: irreversible, involuntary, dyskinetic movements. Extension of action: drowsiness, sedation, tachycardia, hypotension, EPS.

PATIENT CONSIDERATIONS

BASELINE ASSESSMENT

Renal and liver function tests should be done before therapy. Assess behavior, appearance, emotional status, response to environment, speech pattern, thought content.

INTERVENTION/EVALUATION

Monitor for fine tongue movement (may be first sign of tardive dyskinesia, which may be irreversible: protrusion of tongue, puffing of cheeks, chewing/puckering of the mouth). Supervise suicidal risk pt closely during early therapy (as depression lessens, energy level improves, increasing suicide potential). Smallest prescription possible reduces risk of overdose. Assess for therapeutic response (greater interest in surroundings, improved self-care, increased ability to concentrate, relaxed facial expression). Monitor for potential NMS: fever, muscle rigidity, irregular B/P or pulse, altered mental status. Possible antiemetic effect may mask signs and symptoms of other conditions.

PATIENT/FAMILY TEACHING

Change positions slowly to prevent hypotensive effect. Wear protective clothing, use sunscreens to protect from sunlight, ultraviolet light. Do not drive or perform tasks requiring alert response until assured that drug does not cause impairment. Consult physician before taking any other medications. Inform physician if become or plan to become pregnant; do not breast-feed.

ritodrine

rih-toe-dreen
(Yutopar)

R

CANADIAN AVAILABILITY
Yutopar

PREGNANCY CATEGORY B

CLASSIFICATION

Uterine relaxant

AVAILABILITY (Rx)

Injection: 10 mg/ml, 15 mg/ml

PHARMACOKINETICS

Metabolism: Undergoes first-pass metabolism. Metabolized in liver. **Excretion:** Primarily excreted in urine. Removed by hemodialysis. **Half-life:** 15–17 hrs.

ACTION/*THERAPEUTIC EFFECT*

Beta$_2$-adrenergic stimulant that relaxes uterine muscle, *suppresses uterine contractions.*

USES

To prolong gestation by inhibiting uterine contractions in preterm labor.

STORAGE/HANDLING

Stable for 48 hrs at room temperature after dilutions of 150 mg in 500 ml 0.9% NaCl or 5% dextrose in water. Do not use if discolored or if precipitate forms.

ADMINISTRATION

IV:

- Hospitalization advised.
- Place pt in left lateral position to prevent hypotension.
- Dilute 15 ml of concentrate for injection (150 mg) in 500 ml of 5% dextrose injection (provides solution of 0.3 mg/ml). Because of potential for pulmonary edema, NaCl-containing solutions are used only when dextrose medically undesirable (e.g., diabetes mellitus).
- Use infusion device to carefully control rate of flow.

INDICATIONS/ROUTES/DOSAGE

Usual parenteral dosage:

IV Infusion: Adults: Initially, 0.05 mg/min (10 ml/hr); gradually increase by 0.05 mg/min (10 ml/hr) q10min until desired result reached. ***Range:*** 0.15–0.35 mg/min (30–70 ml/hr). Continue for 12 hrs after uterine contractions cease.

CONTRAINDICATIONS

Before 20th week of pregnancy. Preexisting medical conditions for mother that would be adversely affected by the effects of ritodrine: cardiac arrhythmias, uncontrolled hypertension, bronchial asthma treated w/betamimetics or steroids, hypovolemia. When continuation of pregnancy is hazardous to mother or fetus: eclampsia, severe pre-eclampsia, antepartum hemorrhage, intrauterine fetal death, pulmonary hypertension, pheochromocytoma, hyperthyroidism, cardiac disease, chorioamnionitis, uncontrolled diabetes mellitus. W/injection, sulfite sensitivity (often w/aspirin sensitivity).

CAUTIONS

Migraine headache, diabetes mellitus, concomitant use of potassium-depleting diuretics.

INTERACTIONS

DRUG: ***Beta-adrenergic blockers*** antagonize effects. ***Glucocorticoids*** enhance fetal lung maturity; may increase risk of pulmonary edema in mother. **HERBAL:** None known. **FOOD:** None significant. **ALTERED LAB VALUES:** May increase SGOT (AST), SGPT (ALT), FFA, blood glucose, serum insulin. May decrease potassium.

SIDE EFFECTS

FREQUENT: Increased maternal and fetal heart rates widening maternal pulse pressure (80–100%); palpitations (33%); nausea, vomiting, headache, erythema (10–15%). **OCCASIONAL (3–10%):** Tremors, jitteriness, chest pain/tightness, constipation, diarrhea, bloating, sweating, chills, weakness. ***Neonate:*** Hypo/hyperglycemia, ileus, hypocalcemia, hypotension. **RARE (<1%):** Impaired liver function.

ADVERSE REACTIONS/TOXIC EFFECTS

Ketoacidosis occurs infrequently. Pulmonary edema (may be fatal, especially w/preexisting cardiopulmonary disease or concomitant use of corticosteroids), anaphylactic shock, hepatitis occur rarely.

PATIENT CONSIDERATIONS

BASELINE ASSESSMENT

Question for hypersensitivity to ritodrine, sulfite, or aspirin.

Assess baselines for temperature, pulse, respiration, B/P, glucose and potassium levels, EKG, fetal heart rate. Check lungs, determine hydration status. Determine frequency, duration, and strength of contractions.

INTERVENTION/EVALUATION

Take temperature at start and conclusion of IV infusion. B/P, pulse, respirations, and fetal heart rate are monitored q15min until stable, then hourly until infusion complete. Check uterine contractions frequently throughout the infusion. Assess lungs for rales; pay particular attention to evidence of impending pulmonary edema (persistent tachycardia, fluid retention [I&O], increased respiratory rate/shortness of breath). Monitor potassium and glucose levels. Evaluate for palpitations, chest pain/tightness, nausea/vomiting, headache, jitteriness.

PATIENT/FAMILY TEACHING

Keep pt, family informed of therapeutic response during infusion. Explain importance of left lateral position during IV infusion.

ritonavir

rih-**tone**-ah-vir
(Norvir)

CANADIAN AVAILABILITY
Norvir

FIXED-COMBINATION(S)
W/lopinavir, an antiviral **(Kaletra)**

PREGNANCY CATEGORY B

CLASSIFICATION

Antiviral

AVAILABILITY (Rx)

Soft Gelatin Capsules: 100 mg. **Oral Solution:** 80 mg/ml.

PHARMACOKINETICS

Absorption: Slowly absorbed following oral administration (extent of absorption increased with food). **Metabolism:** Extensively metabolized by liver to active metabolite. **Excretion:** Primarily eliminated in feces. **Half-life:** 2.7–5 hrs.

ACTION/*THERAPEUTIC EFFECT*

Inhibits HIV-1 and HIV-2 proteases, rendering the enzymes incapable of processing the polypeptide precursor that leads to production of immature HIV particles, *slowing HIV replication, reducing progression of HIV infection.*

R

USES

Used in combination w/nucleoside analogues or as monotherapy for treatment of HIV infection.

STORAGE/HANDLING

Store capsules, solution in refrigerator. Protect from light. Refrigeration of oral solution by pt is recommended but not necessary if used within 30 days and stored below 77°F.

ADMINISTRATION

ORAL:

- May give w/o regard to meals (preferably give w/food).
- May improve taste of oral solution by mixing w/chocolate milk, Ensure, or Advera within 1 hr of dosing.

INDICATIONS/ROUTES/DOSAGE

HIV infection:
Oral: Adults: 600 mg 2 times/day. If nausea becomes apparent upon initiation of 600 mg twice daily, give 300 mg twice daily for 1 day, 400 mg twice daily for 2 days, 500 mg twice daily for 1 day, then 600 mg twice daily thereafter. ***Children:*** 400 mg/m^2 twice daily. ***Maximum:*** 600 mg twice daily.

CONTRAINDICATIONS

Hypersensitivity to drug; amiodarone, astemizole, bepridil, bupropion, cisapride, clozapine, encainide, flecainide, meperidine, piroxicam, propafenone, propoxyphene, quinidine, rifabutin, and terfenadine increase risk of arrhythmias, hematologic abnormalities, seizures. Alprazolam, clorazepate, diazepam, estrazolam, flurazepam, midazolam, triazolam and zolpidem may produce extreme sedation and respiratory depression.

CAUTIONS

Impaired hepatic function.

INTERACTIONS

DRUG: May produce disulfiramlike reaction if taken w/***disulfiram or drugs causing disulfiramlike reaction (e.g., metronidazole). Enzyme inducers (e.g., nevirapine, phenobarbital, carbamazepine, dexamethasone, phenytoin, rifampin, rifabutin)*** may increase metabolism, decrease efficacy. May decrease effectiveness of ***theophylline, oral contraceptives.*** May increase concentration of ***desipramine, other antidepressants.*** **HERBAL:** St. John's wort may decrease concentration, effect. **FOOD:** None significant. **ALTERED LAB VALUES:** May alter SGPT (ALT), SGOT (AST), creatinine clearance, GGT, CPK, uric acid, triglycerides.

SIDE EFFECTS

FREQUENT: GI disturbances (nausea, diarrhea, vomiting, anorexia, abdominal pain), neurologic disturbances (taste perversion, circumoral and peripheral paresthesias), headache, dizziness, paresthesia (especially around lips, hands, or feet), fatigue, weakness. **OCCASIONAL:** Allergic reaction, flu syndrome, hypotension.

ADVERSE REACTIONS/TOXIC EFFECTS

Numerous body system effects may occur (<2%).

PATIENT CONSIDERATIONS

Baseline Assessment

Pts beginning combination therapy w/ritonavir and nucleosides may promote GI tolerance by beginning ritonavir alone and subsequently adding nucleosides before completing 2 wks of ritonavir monotherapy. Obtain baseline laboratory testing, especially liver function tests, triglycerides before beginning ritonavir therapy and at periodic intervals during therapy. Offer emotional support. Obtain medication history.

Intervention/Evaluation

Closely monitor for evidence of GI disturbances or neurologic abnormalities (particularly paresthesias). Monitor clinical chemistry tests for marked laboratory abnormalities.

Patient/Family Teaching

Continue therapy for full length of treatment. Doses should be evenly spaced. Do not take any medications, including OTC drugs, w/o consulting physician (many interacting medications). Ritonavir is not a cure for HIV infection, nor does it reduce risk of transmission to others. Pts may continue to acquire illnesses associated w/advanced HIV infection. If possible, take ritonavir w/food. Taste of solution may be mixed w/chocolate, Ensure, or Advera.

rituximab

(Rituxan)

See Supplement

rivastigmine

(Exelon)

See Supplement

rizatriptan

rise-ah-**trip**-tan

(Maxalt, Maxalt-MLT)

PREGNANCY CATEGORY C

CLASSIFICATION

Antimigraine

AVAILABILITY (Rx)

Tablets: 5 mg, 10 mg. **Orally Disintegrating Tablets:** 5 mg, 10 mg.

PHARMACOKINETICS

Absorption: Well absorbed following oral administration. Crosses blood-brain barrier. **Metabolism:** Metabolized by the liver to inactive metabolite. **Excretion:** Eliminated primarily in the urine with lesser amount excreted in the feces. **Half-life:** 2–3 hrs.

ACTION/*THERAPEUTIC EFFECT*

Binds selectively to vascular receptors producing a vasoconstrictive effect on cranial blood vessels, *producing relief of migraine headache.*

USES

Treatment of acute migraine attack w/ or w/o aura.

ADMINISTRATION

- The oral disintegrating tablet is packaged in an individual aluminum pouch.
- Open packet with dry hands and place tablet onto tongue to be dissolved and swallowed with saliva. Administration w/water is not necessary.

INDICATIONS/ROUTES/DOSAGES

Migraine:

Oral: Adults, adolescents: 5–10 mg. Separate doses by at least 2 hrs. ***Maximum:*** 30 mg/24 hrs.

CONTRAINDICATIONS

Coronary artery disease, uncontrolled hypertension, ischemic heart disease (angina pectoris, history of MI, silent ischemia), Prinzmetal's angina, concurrent use (or within 24 hrs) of ergotamine-containing preparations, concurrent (or within 2 wks) of MAO therapy, hemiplegic or basilar migraine, within 24 hrs of another serotonin receptor agonist.

CAUTIONS

Mild-to-moderate renal/hepatic impairment, pt profile suggesting cardiovascular risks.

INTERACTIONS

DRUG: *Ergotamine*-containing drugs may produce vasospastic reaction. ***MAO inhibitors, propranolol*** may dramatically increase plasma concentration of rizatriptan. Combined use of ***fluoxetine, fluvoxamine, paroxetine, sertraline*** may produce weakness, hyperreflexia, incoordination. **HERBAL:** None known. **FOOD:** Food delays peak drug concentrations by 1 hr. **ALTERED LAB VALUES:** None significant.

SIDE EFFECTS

FREQUENT (7–9%): Dizziness, somnolence, tingling, fatigue. **OCCASIONAL (3–6%):** Nausea, paresthesia, sensation of chest pressure, dry mouth. **RARE (2%):** Headache, neck/throat/jaw pressure, photosensitivity.

ADVERSE REACTIONS/TOXIC EFFECTS

Cardiac events (ischemia, coronary artery vasospasm, MI), noncardiac vasospasm-related reactions (hemorrhage, stroke) occur rarely but particularly in those with hypertension, obesity, smokers, diabetes, strong family history of coronary artery disease, male > 40 yrs, postmenopausal women.

PATIENT CONSIDERATIONS

BASELINE ASSESSMENT

Question regarding history of peripheral vascular disease, renal/hepatic impairment, possibility of pregnancy. Question pt regarding onset, location, and duration of migraine and possible precipitating symptoms.

INTERVENTION/EVALUATION

Monitor for evidence of dizziness. Assess for relief of migraine headache and potential for photophobia, phonophobia (sound sensitivity, nausea, vomiting).

PATIENT/FAMILY TEACHING

Take a single dose as soon as symptoms of an actual migraine attack appear. Medication is intended to relieve migraine, not to prevent or reduce number of attacks. Avoid tasks that require alertness, motor skills until response to drug is established. If heart throbbing, pain/tightness in chest or throat, or pain or weakness of extremities occurs, contact physician immediately. Do not use if pregnant, planning to become pregnant, or not using adequate contraception. Do not remove the blister from the orally disintegrating tablet until just prior to dosing. Orally disintegrating tablet contains phenylalanine. Take protective measures (e.g., sunscreen, protective clothing) against exposure to UV/sunlight.

---

rocuronium bromide

(Zemuron)

See Classification section under: Neuromuscular blockers

---

rofecoxib

(Vioxx)

See Supplement

---

ropinirole hydrochloride

roh-**pin**-ih-role

(Requip)

CANADIAN AVAILABILITY

Requip

PREGNANCY CATEGORY C

CLASSIFICATION

Antiparkinson agent (dopamine agonist)

AVAILABILITY (Rx)

Tablets: 0.25 mg, 0.5 mg, 1 mg, 2 mg, 4 mg, 5 mg

PHARMACOKINETICS

Absorption: Rapidly absorbed after oral administration. Extensively distributed throughout the body. **Metabolism:** Extensively metabolized. Steady-state concentrations achieved within 2 days. **Excretion:** Eliminated in the urine. **Half-life:** 6 hrs.

ACTION/*THERAPEUTIC EFFECT*

Stimulates dopamine receptors in the striatum, *relieving signs/symptoms of Parkinson's disease.*

USES

Treatment of signs and symptoms of idiopathic Parkinson's disease.

ADMINISTRATION

ORAL:

- Ascending-dose schedule should increase very gradually at weekly intervals: ***Week 1:*** 0.25 mg 3 times/day to total daily dose 0.75 mg. ***Week 2:*** 0.5 mg 3 times/day to total daily dose 1.5 mg. ***Week 3:*** 0.75 mg 3 times/day to total daily dose 2.25 mg. ***Week 4:*** 1 mg 3 times/day to total daily dose 3 mg.
- Discontinue medication gradually at 7 day intervals. Decrease frequency from 3 times/day to 2 times/day for 4 days. For the remaining 3 days, decrease frequency to once daily prior to complete withdrawal.

INDICATIONS/ROUTES/DOSAGES

Parkinson's disease:
Oral: Initially, 0.25 mg 3 times/day. Do not increase dose more frequently than q7days. After week 4, daily dosage may be increased, if needed, by 1.5–3 mg/day per week to total daily dose of 24 mg/day.

CONTRAINDICATIONS

History of hypersensitivity to ropinirole.

CAUTIONS

History of orthostatic hypotension, syncope, hallucinations, especially in elderly, CNS depressants.

INTERACTIONS

DRUG: Additive side effects with ***CNS depressants.*** Increases ***levodopa*** concentration. ***Estrogens*** reduce ropinirole clearance. ***Ciprofloxacin*** increases ropinirole concentration. ***Cimetidine, diltiazem, enoxacin, erythromycin, fluvoxamine, mexiletine, norfloxacin, tacrine*** alters ropinirole's concentration. ***Phenothiazines, butyrophenones, thioxanthenes, metaclopramide*** diminishes effectiveness of ropinirole. **HERBAL:** None known. **FOOD:** Time to maximum plasma levels is increased by 2.5 hours when taken with food (extent of absorption not affected). Food may decrease the occurrence of nausea. **ALTERED LAB VALUES:** May increase alkaline phosphatase.

SIDE EFFECTS

FREQUENT (40–60%): Nausea, dizziness, excessive drowsiness. **OCCASIONAL (5–12%):** Syncope, vomiting, fatigue, viral infection, dyspepsia, increased sweating, weakness, orthostatic hypotension, abdominal discomfort, pharyngitis, abnormal vision, dry mouth, hypertension, hallucinations, confusion.

RARE (≤4%): Anorexia, peripheral edema, memory loss, rhinitis, sinusitis, palpitations, impotence.

ADVERSE REACTIONS/TOXIC EFFECTS

None significant.

PATIENT CONSIDERATIONS

INTERVENTION/EVALUATION

Instruct pt to rise from lying to sitting or sitting to standing position slowly to prevent risk of postural hypotension. Assess for clinical improvement. Assist with ambulation if dizziness occurs. Assess for clinical reversal of symptoms (improvement of tremor of head/hands at rest, mask-like facial expression, shuffling gait, muscular rigidity).

PATIENT/FAMILY TEACHING

Drowsiness, dizziness may be an initial response of drug. Postural hypotension may occur more frequently during initial therapy. Avoid tasks that require alertness, motor skills until response to drug is established. If nausea occurs, take medication with food. Inform pt that hallucinations may occur, more so in the elderly than in younger pts with Parkinson's disease. Postural hypotension may occur more frequently during initial therapy. Avoid tasks that require alertness, motor skills until response to drug is established. If nausea occurs, take medication with food.

---

rosiglitazone

(Avandia)

See Supplement

salicylate salts

sal-**ih**-sah-late

choline salicylate

(Arthropan)

magnesium salicylate

(Magan, Mobidin)

sodium salicylate

(Trilisate combination)

PREGNANCY CATEGORY C

CLASSIFICATION

Nonsteroidal anti-inflammatory

AVAILABILITY (OTC)

Choline: Liquid: 870 mg/5 ml **Magnesium: Caplets:** 325 mg, 500 mg. **Tablets (Rx):** 545 mg, 600 mg. **Sodium: Tablets:** 325 mg, 650 mg

PHARMACOKINETICS

Absorption: Rapidly, completely absorbed from GI tract. **Metabolism:** Hydrolyzed in GI tract, liver, blood; further metabolized in liver. **Excretion:** Primarily excreted in urine. Removed by hemodialysis. **Half-life:** dose dependent (*low dose: 2–3 hrs;* high dose: 20 hrs).

ACTION/*THERAPEUTIC EFFECT*

Produces analgesic and anti-inflammatory effect by inhibiting prostaglandin synthesis, *reducing inflammatory response and intensity of pain stimulus reaching sensory nerve endings.* Antipyresis produced by drug's effect on hypothalamus, producing vasodilation, *decreasing elevated body temperature.*

USES

Relieves mild to moderate musculoskeletal, arthritic pain of low to moderate intensity; reduces fever.

ADMINISTRATION

ORAL:

- May give w/food, milk, or antacids if GI distress occurs.
- Choline salicylate may be mixed w/water, fruit juice, carbonated beverage to mask taste (do not mix w/antacid).

INDICATIONS/ROUTES/DOSAGE

Analgesic, Antipyretic:

Choline salicylate:
Oral: Adults, elderly, children >11 yrs: 2.5–5 ml q4h as needed. *Children 2–11 yrs:* 11.5 ml/m^2/day in 4–6 divided doses.

Magnesium salicylate:
Oral: Adults, elderly, children >11 yrs: 300–600 mg q4h as needed. *Children 2–11 yrs:* 150–450 mg q4h as needed.

S

Sodium salicylate:
Oral: Adults, elderly, children >11 yrs: 325–650 mg q4h as needed. *Children 2–11 yrs:* 25–50 mg/kg/day in 4–6 divided doses.

Rheumatoid Arthritis, Osteoarthritis, Inflammatory Conditions:

Choline salicylate:
Oral: Adults, elderly: 5–10 ml up to 20–40 ml/day in divided doses. *Children:* 0.6–0.8 ml/kg/day in divided doses.

Magnesium salicylate:
Oral: Adults, elderly: 545–1,200 mg 3–4 times/day.

Sodium salicylate:
Oral: Adults, elderly: 3.6–5.4 g/day in divided doses. *Children:* 80–100 mg/kg/day up to 130 mg/kg/day in divided doses.

CONTRAINDICATIONS

Chicken pox or flu in children/teenagers, GI bleeding/ulceration, bleeding disorders, history of hypersensitivity to aspirin/NSAIDs, impaired hepatic function.

CAUTIONS

Vitamin K deficiency, chronic renal insufficiency, those w/"aspirin triad" (rhinitis, nasal polyps, asthma).

INTERACTIONS

DRUG: ***Alcohol, NSAIDs*** may increase risk of GI effects (e.g., ulceration). ***Urinary alkalinizer, antacids*** increase excretion. ***Anticoagulants, heparin, thrombolytics*** increase risk of bleeding. Large dose may increase effect of ***insulin, oral hypoglycemics. Valproic acid, platelet aggregation inhibitors*** may increase risk of bleeding. May increase toxicity of ***methotrexate, zidovudine. Ototoxic medications, vancomycin*** may increase ototoxicity. May decrease effect of ***probenecid, sulfinpyrazone.*** **HERBAL:** Ginkgo biloba may increase risk of bleeding. **FOOD:** None significant. **ALTERED LAB VALUES:** May alter SGOT (AST), SGPT (ALT), alkaline phosphatase, uric acid; prolong prothrombin time, bleeding time. May decrease cholesterol, potassium, T_3, T_4.

SIDE EFFECTS

FREQUENT (5–25%): Nausea, dyspepsia. **OCCASIONAL (1–5%):** Heartburn, loss of appetite, epigastric distress, GI bleeding, hives, rash, fever, thirst.

ADVERSE REACTIONS/TOXIC EFFECTS

High doses may produce GI bleeding and/or gastric mucosal lesions. Low-grade toxicity characterized by ringing in ears, generalized pruritus (may be severe), decreased hearing ability, headache, dizziness, flushing, tachycardia, hyperventilation, sweating, thirst. Febrile, dehydrated children can reach toxic levels quickly. Marked intoxication may be manifested by hyperthermia, restlessness, abnormal breathing pattern, convulsions, respiratory failure, coma.

PATIENT CONSIDERATIONS

BASELINE ASSESSMENT

Do not give to children/teenagers who have flu/chicken pox (increases risk of Reye's syndrome). Assess onset, type, location, and duration of pain, fever, or inflammation. Inspect appearance of affected joints for immobility, deformities, and skin condition.

INTERVENTION/EVALUATION

In long-term therapy, monitor plasma salicylic acid concentration. Monitor urinary pH (sudden acidification [pH from 6.5 to 5.5] may result in toxicity). Assess skin for evidence of bruising. If given as an antipyretic, assess temperature directly before and 1 hr after giving medication. Evaluate for therapeutic response: relief of pain/stiffness/swelling, increase in joint mobility, reduced joint tenderness, improved grip strength.

PATIENT/FAMILY TEACHING

Take w/food if GI distress is noted. Minimize or avoid other NSAIDs, alcohol during therapy (increases possibility of GI irritation). Report ringing in ears, persistent GI pain.

---

salmeterol

sal-**met**-er-all
(Serevent, Serevent Diskus)

CANADIAN AVAILABILITY
Serevent

FIXED-COMBINATION(S)
W.fluticasone, a corticosteroid **(Advair)**

PREGNANCY CATEGORY C

CLASSIFICATION

Bronchodilator

AVAILABILITY (Rx)

Aerosol. Aerosol Powder: 50 mcg.

PHARMACODYNAMICS

	ONSET	PEAK	DURATION
Inhalation			
	10–20 min	3 hrs	12 hrs

PHARMACOKINETICS

Absorption: Primarily acts in lung; low systemic absorption. **Metabolism:** Metabolized by hydroxylation. **Excretion:** Primarily eliminated in feces. **Half-life:** 5.5 hrs.

ACTION / *THERAPEUTIC EFFECT*

Stimulates beta$_2$-adrenergic receptors resulting in relaxation of bronchial smooth muscle, *relieving bronchospasm; reduces airway resistance.*

USES

Maintenance treatment of asthma, bronchospasm associated w/COPD. Prevention of exercise-induced bronchospasm, bronchospasm in pts w/reversible obstructive airway disease.

ADMINISTRATION

INHALATION:

- Shake container well, then remove cap from mouthpiece.
- Position mouthpiece to bottom, tilt head back.
- Breathe out through mouth to functional volume.
- Place mouthpiece in mouth or hold 1–2 inches away from open mouth.
- Activate inhaler while breathing in slowly and deeply.
- Hold breath 5–10 sec (or as long as possible).
- Remove inhaler from mouth and breathe out slowly.
- Wait 1–10 min before second inhalation.

INDICATIONS/ROUTES/DOSAGE

Maintenance of bronchodilation, prevention of asthma symptoms:
Inhalation: Adults, elderly, children >4 yrs: 1 50 mcg inhalation 2 times/day, morning and evening about 12 hrs apart.

Prevention of exercise-induced bronchospasm:
Inhalation: Adults, elderly, children >4 yrs: 1 50 mcg inhalation at least 30–60 min before exercise.

Long-term maintenance for treatment of COPD-induced bronchospasm:
Inhalation: Adults: 2 inhalations q12h.

CONTRAINDICATIONS

History of hypersensitivity to salmeterol.

CAUTIONS

Not for acute symptoms. May cause paradoxical bronchospasm. Pts w/cardiovascular disorders (e.g., coronary insufficiency, arrhythmias, hypertension), seizure disorder, thyrotoxicosis. Safety in children <12 yrs not known.

INTERACTIONS

DRUG: May decrease effects of ***beta-adrenergic blockers.*** **HERBAL:** None known. **FOOD:** None significant. **ALTERED LAB VALUES:** May decrease serum potassium levels.

SIDE EFFECTS

FREQUENT (>3%): Headache (28%), cough. **OCCASIONAL (1–3%):** Abdominal pain, heartburn, dizziness, diarrhea, dry throat or irritation, shakiness, vomiting, muscle cramps, nausea, nervousness, palpitations, tachycardia, trembling. **RARE (<1%):** Paradoxical bronchospasm, dermatitis (skin rash, urticaria, hives, angioedema), arrhythmias.

ADVERSE REACTIONS/TOXIC EFFECTS

Tachycardia, arrhythmias, tremor, headache, muscle cramps. May prolong QT interval (may lead to ventricular arrhythmias). May cause hypokalemia, hyperglycemia.

PATIENT CONSIDERATIONS

INTERVENTION/EVALUATION

Monitor rate, depth, rhythm, tape of respiration; quality and rate of pulse, B/P. Assess lungs for wheezing, rales, rhonchi. Periodically evaluate potassium levels.

PATIENT/FAMILY TEACHING

Not for relief of acute episodes. Keep canister at room temperature (cold decreases effects). Teach pt correct use of aerosol. Do not stop medication or exceed recommended dosage. Notify physician promptly of chest pain, dizziness, or failure to respond to medication. Wait at least one full minute before second inhalation. Administer dose 30 to 60 min before exercise when used to prevent exercise-induced bronchospasm. Avoid excessive use of caffeine derivatives: coffee, tea, colas, chocolate.

---

salsalate

sal-sah-late
(Disalcid, Mono-Gesic)

CANADIAN AVAILABILITY
Disalcid

PREGNANCY CATEGORY C

CLASSIFICATION

Nonsteroidal anti-inflammatory

AVAILABILITY (Rx)

Capsules: 500 mg. **Tablets:** 500 mg, 750 mg.

PHARMACOKINETICS

Absorption: Rapidly, completely absorbed from GI tract. **Metabolism:** Hydrolyzed in GI tract, liver, blood; further metabolized in liver. **Excretion:** Primarily excreted in urine. Removed by hemodialysis. **Half-life:** Dose dependent (*low dose: 7–8 hrs;* high dose: 15–30 hrs).

ACTION/*THERAPEUTIC EFFECT*

Produces analgesic, anti-inflammatory effect by inhibiting prostaglandin synthesis, reducing inflammatory response and intensity of pain stimulus reaching sensory nerve endings.

USES

Symptomatic treatment of acute and/or chronic rheumatoid arthritis and osteoarthritis, related inflammatory conditions.

ADMINISTRATION

ORAL:

- Give w/food/large amount of water.

INDICATIONS/ROUTES/DOSAGE

Rheumatoid arthritis, osteoarthritis:
Oral: Adults, elderly: Initially, 3 g/day in 2–3 divided doses. ***Maintenance:*** 2–4 g/day.

CONTRAINDICATIONS

History of hypersensitivity to salicylates; chicken pox/flu in children/teenagers.

CAUTIONS

None significant.

INTERACTIONS

DRUG: *Alcohol, NSAIDs* may increase risk of GI effects (e.g., ulceration). ***Urinary alkalinizers, antacids*** increase excretion. ***Anticoagulants, heparin, thrombolytics*** increase risk of bleeding. Large dose may increase effect of ***insulin, oral hypoglycemics. Valproic acid, platelet aggregation inhibitors*** may increase risk of bleeding. May increase toxicity of ***methotrexate, zidovudine. Ototoxic medications, vancomycin*** may increase ototoxicity. May decrease effect of ***probenecid, sulfinpyrazone.*** HERBAL: Ginkgo biloba may increase risk of bleeding. FOOD: None significant. ALTERED LAB VALUES: May alter SGOT (AST), SGPT (ALT), alkaline phosphatase, uric acid; prolong prothrombin time, bleeding time. May decrease cholesterol, potassium, T_3, T_4.

SIDE EFFECTS

OCCASIONAL: Nausea, dyspepsia (heartburn, indigestion, epigastric pain).

ADVERSE REACTIONS/TOXIC EFFECTS

Tinnitus may be first sign that blood salicylic acid concentration is reaching/exceeding upper therapeutic range. May also produce vertigo, headache, confusion, drowsiness, sweating, hyperventilation, vomiting, diarrhea. Severe overdosage may result in electrolyte imbalance, hyperthermia, dehydration, blood pH imbalance. Low incidence of GI bleeding, peptic ulcer.

PATIENT CONSIDERATIONS

BASELINE ASSESSMENT

Do not give to children/teenagers who have flu/chicken pox (increases risk of Reye's syndrome). Assess type, location, duration of pain, inflammation. Inspect appearance of affected joints for immobility, deformities, and skin condition.

INTERVENTION/EVALUATION

Monitor pattern of daily bowel activity, stool consistency. Assess skin for evidence of bruising. Check behind medial malleolus for evidence of fluid retention. Assess for evidence of nausea, dyspepsia. Evaluate for therapeutic response: relief of pain/stiffness/swelling, increase in joint mobility, reduced joint tenderness, improved grip strength.

PATIENT/FAMILY TEACHING

Do not crush/chew capsules or film-coated tablets. Avoid antacids (decreases drug effectiveness). Report ringing in ears, persistent GI pain. Avoid alcohol.

S

saquinavir mesylate

sah-**quin**-ah-vir
(Fortovase, Invirase)

CANADIAN AVAILABILITY
Invirase

PREGNANCY CATEGORY B

CLASSIFICATION

Antiviral

AVAILABILITY (Rx)

Capsules, Soft Gelatin Capsules: 200 mg

PHARMACOKINETICS

Absorption: Poorly absorbed following oral administration (high-caloric/high-fat meal increases absorption). **Metabolism:** Metabolized in liver to inactive metabolite. **Excretion:** Primarily eliminated in feces.

ACTION/*THERAPEUTIC EFFECT*

Inhibits HIV protease, rendering the enzyme incapable of processing the polyprotein precursor to generate functional proteins in HIV-infected cells, *slowing HIV replication, reducing progression of HIV infection.*

USES

Used in combination w/nucleoside analogues for treatment of advanced HIV infection in selected pts.

ADMINISTRATION

ORAL:

- Give within 2 hrs after a full meal (if taken w/o food in stomach, may result in no antiviral activity).

INDICATIONS/ROUTES/DOSAGE

Note: Complete prescribing information for saquinavir should be consulted before concurrent therapy w/zidovudine (AZT), zalcitabine (ddC).

HIV infection (combination therapy):

Oral: Adults, elderly: Fortovase: 1,200 mg 3 times/day. ***Saquinavir:*** Three 200 mg capsules given 3 times daily within 2 hrs after a full meal. Do not give <600 mg/day (does not produce antiviral activity). Recommended daily doses of ddC or AZT: ddC 0.75 mg 3 times daily; AZT 200 mg 3 times daily.

CONTRAINDICATIONS

Clinically significant hypersensitivity to drug.

CAUTIONS

Impaired hepatic function.

INTERACTIONS

DRUG: ***Ketoconazole*** increases saquinavir concentration. ***Rifampin, phenobarbital, phenytoin, dexamethasone, carbamazepine*** may reduce saquinavir plasma concentration. May increase ***terfenadine, astemizole, calcium channel blockers, clindamycin, dapsone, quinidine, triazolam*** plasma concentrations. **HERBAL:** St. John's wort may decrease concentration, effect. **FOOD:** Grapefruit juice may increase saquinavir concentrations. **ALTERED LAB VALUES:** May elevate serum transaminase, lower glucose level, alter CPK.

SIDE EFFECTS

OCCASIONAL: Diarrhea, abdominal discomfort or pain, nausea, photosensitivity, buccal mucosa ulceration. **RARE:** Confusion, ataxia, weakness, headache, rash.

ADVERSE REACTIONS/TOXIC EFFECTS

None significant.

PATIENT CONSIDERATIONS

BASELINE ASSESSMENT

Obtain baseline laboratory testing, especially liver function tests, before beginning saquinavir therapy and at periodic intervals during therapy. Offer emotional support. Obtain medication history.

INTERVENTION/EVALUATION

Closely monitor for evidence of GI discomfort. Monitor stool frequency and consistency (watery, loose, soft). Inspect mouth for signs of mucosal ulceration. Monitor clinical chemistry tests for marked laboratory abnormalities. If serious or severe toxicities occur, interrupt therapy, contact physician.

PATIENT/FAMILY TEACHING

Continue therapy for full length of treatment. Doses should be evenly spaced. Do not take any medications, including OTC drugs, w/o consulting physician. Saquinavir is not a cure for HIV infection, nor does it reduce risk of transmission to others. Pts may continue to acquire illnesses associated w/advanced HIV infection. Take within 2 hrs after a full meal. Take protective measures against exposure to ultraviolet or sunlight (i.e., sunscreens, protective clothing) until tolerance is established. Avoid coadministration w/grapefruit products.

sargramostim

sar-**gra**-moh-stim
(Leukine, Prokine)

PREGNANCY CATEGORY C

CLASSIFICATION

Colony-stimulating factor

AVAILABILITY (Rx)

Powder for Injection: 250 mcg, 500 mcg. **Liquid for Injection:** 500 mcg/ml.

PHARMACOKINETICS

Half-life: *IV:* 2 hrs; *SubQ:* 3 hrs.

ACTION/*THERAPEUTIC EFFECT*

Stimulates proliferation/differentiation of hematopoietic cells to activate mature granulocytes and macrophages, *assisting bone marrow in making new WBCs.* Chemotactic, antifungal, and antiparasite activities increase. Increases cytotoxicity of monocytes to certain neoplastic cells; *activates neutrophils to inhibit tumor cell growth.*

USES/*UNLABELED*

Accelerates myeloid recovery in pt w/non-Hodgkin's lymphoma, acute lymphoblastic leukemia, and Hodgkin's disease undergoing autologous bone marrow transplantation. Used in pts w/allogenic or autologous bone marrow transplantation where engraftment is delayed or has failed. Shortens time of neutrophil recovery following induction chemotherapy in pts w/AML. Mobilizes autologous peripheral blood progenitor cells (PBPC) following induction of chemotherapy in pt >55 yrs w/acute myelogenous leukemia; used in myeloid reconstitution after allogenic bone marrow transplantation. *Treatment of AIDS-related neutropenia; chronic, severe neutropenia, drug-induced neutropenia; myelodysplastic syndrome.*

STORAGE/HANDLING

Refrigerate powder, reconstituted solution, diluted solution for injection. Do not shake. Do not use past expiration date. Reconstituted solutions are clear, colorless. Use within 6 hrs; discard unused portions. Use 1 dose/vial; do not reenter vial.

ADMINISTRATION

IV:

- To 250 mcg/500 mcg vial, add 1 ml sterile water for injection (preservative free).
- Direct sterile water to side of vial, gently swirl contents to avoid foaming; do not shake/vigorously agitate.
- After reconstitution, further dilute w/0.9% NaCl. If final concentration <10 mcg/ml, add 1 mg albumin/ml 0.9% NaCl to provide a final albumin concentration of 0.1%. **Note:** Albumin is added before addition of sar-

gramostim (prevents drug adsorption to components of drug delivery system).

- Administer within 6 hrs of preparation/dilution.
- Monitor for supraventricular arrhythmias during administration (particularly in those w/history of cardiac arrhythmias).
- Assess closely for dyspnea during and immediately following infusion (particularly in those w/history of lung disease). If dyspnea occurs during infusion, cut infusion rate by half. If dyspnea continues, stop infusion immediately.
- If neutrophil count exceeds 20,000 cells/mm^3 or platelet count exceeds 500,000/mm^3, stop infusion or reduce dose by half, based on clinical condition of pt.

INDICATIONS/ROUTES/DOSAGE

Usual parenteral dosage:
IV Infusion: Adults, elderly: 250 mcg/m^2/day for 21 days (as a 2 hr infusion). Begin 2–4 hrs after autologous bone marrow infusion and not less than 24 hrs after last dose of chemotherapy or not less than 12 hrs after last radiation treatment. Discontinue if blast cells appear or underlying disease progresses.

Bone marrow transplantation failure/engraftment delay:
IV Infusion: Adults, elderly: 250 mcg/m^2/day for 14 days. Infuse over 2 hrs. May repeat after 7 days of therapy if engraftment not occurred w/500 mcg/m^2/day for 14 days.

Mobilization or post PBPC transplant:
IV/SubQ: Adults: 250 mcg/m^2/day.

Allogeneic transplantation:
IV Infusion: Adults: 250 mcg/m^2/day × 21 days starting 2–4 hrs after bone marrow infusion and not less than 24 hrs after last chemotherapy dose or 12 hrs after last radiation dose.

CONTRAINDICATIONS

Excessive leukemic myeloid blasts in bone marrow/peripheral blood (greater than/equal to 10%), known hypersensitivity to GM-CSF, yeast-derived products, any component of drug, 24 hrs before/after chemotherapy, 12 hrs before/after radiation therapy.

CAUTIONS

Preexisting cardiac disease, hypoxia, preexisting fluid retention, pulmonary infiltrates, CHF, impaired renal/hepatic function.

INTERACTIONS

DRUG: ***Lithium, steroids*** may increase effect. **HERBAL:** None known. **FOOD:** None significant. **ALTERED LAB VALUES:** May decrease albumin. May increase bilirubin, creatinine, liver enzymes.

SIDE EFFECTS

FREQUENT: GI disturbances, arthralgia/myalgia, headache, rash, pruritus. **OCCASIONAL:** Peripheral edema, weight gain, SOB, fever, leukocytosis, capillary leak syndrome (e.g., fluid retention, irritation at local injection site, peripheral edema, rash). **RARE:** Wheezing, rapid/irregular heartbeat, thrombophlebitis.

ADVERSE REACTIONS/TOXIC EFFECTS

Pleural/pericardial effusion occurs rarely following infusion.

PATIENT CONSIDERATIONS

BASELINE ASSESSMENT

Assess renal, hepatic function tests before initial therapy and biweekly. Note that excessive blood counts return to normal or

baseline 3–7 days after discontinuation of therapy. Obtain baseline weight.

INTERVENTION/EVALUATION

Monitor urinalysis reports, alkaline phosphatase, serum creatinine, bilirubin, SGOT (AST), SGPT (ALT) levels, CBC w/differential diligently. Monitor body weight. Assess for peripheral edema, particularly behind medial malleolus (usually first area showing peripheral edema), skin turgor, mucous membranes for hydration status. Note skin temperature, moisture. Assess muscle strength. Monitor daily bowel activity, stool consistency (watery, loose, soft, semisolid, solid). Assess injection site for redness, irritation.

scopolamine

(Scopolamine, Transderm Scop)
See Supplement

scopolamine bromide

(Isopto Hyoscine)
See Classification section under: Anticholinergics

secobarbital sodium

(Seconal)
See Classification section under: Sedative-hypnotics

selegiline hydrochloride

sell-**eh**-geh-leen
(Eldepryl)

CANADIAN AVAILABILITY
Eldepryl, Novo-Selegiline

PREGNANCY CATEGORY C

CLASSIFICATION

Antiparkinson

AVAILABILITY (Rx)

Capsules: 5 mg. **Tablets:** 5 mg.

PHARMACOKINETICS

Absorption: Rapidly absorbed from GI tract. Crosses blood-brain barrier. **Metabolism:** Metabolized in liver to active metabolites. **Excretion:** Primarily excreted in urine. **Half-life:** 16–69 hrs.

ACTION/*THERAPEUTIC EFFECT*

Irreversibly inhibits monoamine oxidase type B activity. Increases dopaminergic action, *assisting in reduction in tremor, akinesia (absence of sense of movement), posture and equilibrium disorders, rigidity of parkinsonism.*

USES

Adjunctive to levodopa/carbidopa in treatment of Parkinson's disease.

ADMINISTRATION

ORAL:
- May be given w/meals.

INDICATIONS/ROUTES/DOSAGE

Note: Therapy should begin w/lowest dosage, then be increased in gradual increments over 3–4 wks.

Parkinsonism:
Oral: Adults: 10 mg/day in divided doses (5 mg at breakfast and lunch). ***Elderly:*** Initially, 5 mg in morning. May increase up to 10 mg/day.

CONTRAINDICATIONS

None significant.

CAUTIONS

Cardiac dysrhythmias, history peptic ulcer disease, dementia, psychosis, tardive dyskinesia, profound tremor.

INTERACTIONS

DRUG: *Fluoxetine* may cause mania, serotonin syndrome (mental changes, restlessness, diaphoresis, diarrhea, fever). ***Meperidine*** may cause a potentially fatal reaction (e.g., excitation, sweating, rigidity, hypertension or hypotension, coma, and death). **HERBAL:** None known. **FOOD:** Tyramine-rich foods may produce hypertensive reactions. **ALTERED LAB VALUES:** None significant.

SIDE EFFECTS

FREQUENT (>3%): Nausea, dizziness, lightheadedness, faintness, abdominal discomfort. **OCCASIONAL (2–3%):** Confusion, hallucinations, dry mouth, vivid dreams, dyskinesia (impairment of voluntary movement). **RARE (1%):** Headache, generalized aches.

ADVERSE REACTIONS/TOXIC EFFECTS

Overdosage may vary from CNS depression (sedation, apnea, cardiovascular collapse, death) to severe paradoxical reaction (hallucinations, tremor, seizures). Impaired motor coordination (loss of balance, blepharospasm [blinking], facial grimace, feeling of heavy leg/stiff neck, involuntary movements), hallucinations, confusion, depression, nightmares, delusions, overstimulation, sleep disturbance, anger occurs in some pts.

PATIENT CONSIDERATIONS

Intervention/Evaluation

Be alert to neurologic effects (headache, lethargy, mental confusion, agitation). Monitor for evidence of dyskinesia (difficulty w/movement). Assess for clinical reversal of symptoms (improvement of tremor of head/hands at rest, mask-like facial expression, shuffling gait, muscular rigidity).

Patient/Family Teaching

Tolerance to feeling of lightheadedness develops during therapy. To reduce hypotensive effect, rise slowly from lying to sitting position and permit legs to dangle momentarily before standing. Avoid tasks that require alertness, motor skills until response to drug is established. Dry mouth, drowsiness, dizziness may be an expected response of drug. Avoid alcoholic beverages during therapy. Coffee/tea may help reduce drowsiness. Inform other physicians, dentist of Eldepryl therapy.

---

senna

sen-ah
(Senokot, Senolax)

FIXED-COMBINATION(S)
W/docusate, a stool softener **(Gentlax-S, Senokap DSS, Senokot-S)**

CANADIAN AVAILABILITY
Senokot

PREGNANCY CATEGORY C

CLASSIFICATION

Laxative: Stimulant

AVAILABILITY (OTC)

Tablets: 187 mg, 217 mg, 374 mg, 600 mg. **Granules:** 326 mg/tsp. **Suppository:** 652 mg. **Syrup:** 218 mg/5 ml. **Liquid:** 33.3 mg/ml.

PHARMACODYNAMICS

	ONSET	PEAK	DURATION
Oral	6–12 hrs	—	—
Rectal	0.5–2 hrs	—	—

PHARMACOKINETICS

Absorption: Minimal absorption after oral administration. **Metabolism:** Hydrolyzed to active form by enzymes of colonic flora. Absorbed drug metabolized in liver. **Excretion:** Eliminated in feces via biliary system.

ACTION/*THERAPEUTIC EFFECT*

Increases peristalsis by direct effect on intestinal smooth musculature (stimulates intramural nerve plexi). Builds fluid and ion accumulation in colon, *promoting laxative effect.*

USES

Facilitates defecation in those w/diminished colonic motor response, for evacuation of colon for rectal, bowel examination, elective colon surgery.

ADMINISTRATION

ORAL:

- Give on an empty stomach (faster results).
- Offer at least 6–8 glasses of water/day (aids stool softening).
- Avoid giving within 1 hr of other oral medication (decreases drug absorption).

RECTAL:

- If suppository is too soft, chill for 30 min in refrigerator or run cold water over foil wrapper.
- Moisten suppository w/cold water before inserting well up into rectum.

INDICATIONS/ROUTES/DOSAGE

Laxative:

Oral: Adults, elderly: 2 tablets (or 1 tsp granules) at bedtime. ***Maximum:*** 4 tablets (2 tsp) 2 times/day. ***Children:*** 1 tablet (1/2 tsp granules) at bedtime.

Oral: Adults, elderly: (Syrup): 10–15 ml at bedtime. ***Children 5–15 yrs:*** 5–10 ml at bedtime. ***Children 1–5 yrs:*** 2.5–5 ml at bedtime. ***Children 1 mo–1 yr:*** 1.25–2.5 ml at bedtime.

Rectal: Adults, elderly: 1 suppository at bedtime, may repeat in 2 hrs. ***Children:*** 1/2 suppository at bedtime.

CONTRAINDICATIONS

Abdominal pain, nausea, vomiting, appendicitis, intestinal obstruction.

CAUTIONS

None significant.

INTERACTIONS

DRUG: May decrease transit time of concurrently administered ***oral medication,*** decreasing absorption. **HERBAL:** None known. **FOOD:** None significant. **ALTERED LAB VALUES:** May increase glucose, may decrease potassium.

SIDE EFFECTS

FREQUENT: Pink red, red violet, red brown, or yellow brown discoloration of urine. **OCCASIONAL:** Some degree of abdominal discomfort, nausea, mild cramps, griping, faintness.

ADVERSE REACTIONS/TOXIC EFFECTS

Long-term use may result in laxative dependence, chronic constipation, loss of normal bowel function. Chronic use/overdosage may result in electrolyte disturbances (hypokalemia, hypocalcemia, metabolic acidosis/alkalosis), persistent diarrhea, malabsorption, weight loss. Electrolyte disturbance may produce vomiting, muscle weakness.

PATIENT CONSIDERATIONS

INTERVENTION/EVALUATION

Encourage adequate fluid intake. Assess bowel sounds for peristalsis. Monitor stool frequency, consistency (watery, loose, soft, semisolid, solid). Assess for abdominal disturbances. Monitor serum electrolytes in those exposed to prolonged, frequent, or excessive use of medication.

PATIENT/FAMILY TEACHING

Urine may turn pink red, red violet, red brown, or yellow brown (only temporary and not harmful). Institute measures to promote defecation (increase fluid intake, exercise, high-fiber diet). Laxative effect generally occurs in 6–12 hrs, but may take 24 hrs. Suppository produces evacuation in 30 min to 2 hrs. Do not take other oral medication within 1 hr of taking this medicine (decreased effectiveness).

---

sermorelin
(Geref)
See Supplement

---

sertraline hydrochloride

sir-trah-leen
(Zoloft)

CANADIAN AVAILABILITY
Zoloft

PREGNANCY CATEGORY B

CLASSIFICATION

Antidepressant

AVAILABILITY (Rx)

Tablets: 50 mg, 100 mg. **Oral Concentrate.**

PHARMACOKINETICS

Absorption: Incompletely, slowly absorbed from GI tract (food increases absorption). Widely distributed. **Metabolism:** Undergoes extensive first-pass metabolism in liver to active compound. **Excretion:** Excreted in urine, eliminated in feces. **Half-life:** 26 hrs.

ACTION/*THERAPEUTIC EFFECT*

Blocks reuptake of the neurotransmitter serotonin at CNS neuronal presynaptic membranes, increasing availability at postsynaptic receptor sites, *producing antidepressant, anxiolytic effect.*

USES

Treatment of major depressive disorders, panic disorder, obsessive compulsive disorder (OCD), post-traumatic stress disorder.

ADMINISTRATION

ORAL:
- Give w/food or milk if GI distress occurs.

INDICATIONS/ROUTES/DOSAGE

Antidepressant:
Oral: Adults: Initially, 50 mg/day w/morning or evening meal. May increase at intervals no sooner than 1 wk. ***Elderly:*** Initially, 25 mg/day. May increase by 25 mg q2–3days. ***Maximum:*** 200 mg/day.

Panic disorder:
Oral: Adults: Initially, 25 mg/day titrated individually.

OCD:
Oral: Adults: Initially, 50 mg/day titrated individually. ***Children 13–17 yrs:*** Initially, 50 mg/day. ***Children 6–12 yrs:*** Initially, 25 mg/day.

CONTRAINDICATIONS

During or within 14 days of MAO inhibitor antidepressant therapy.

CAUTIONS

Severe hepatic/renal impairment.

INTERACTIONS

DRUG: May increase concentration, toxicity of ***highly protein-bound medications (e.g., digoxin, warfarin). MAO inhibitors, erythromycin*** may cause serotonin syndrome (mental changes, restlessness, diaphoresis, shivering, diarrhea, fever), confusion, agitation, hyperpyretic convulsions. **HERBAL:** St. John's wort may increase adverse effects (e.g., dizziness, nausea, vomiting, anxiety). **FOOD:** None significant. **ALTERED LAB VALUES:** May increase SGOT (AST), SGPT (ALT), total cholesterol, triglycerides. May decrease uric acid.

SIDE EFFECTS

FREQUENT: Decreased appetite, decreased sexual drive, diarrhea, dizziness, drowsiness, dry mouth, headache, increased sweating, inability to sleep, nausea, stomach pain, unusually tired, tremors. **OCCASIONAL:** Anxiety, nervousness, change in vision, constipation, flushed skin w/feeling of warmth, vomiting, palpitations, increased appetite. **RARE:** Fever, mania, skin rash, hives, itching.

ADVERSE REACTIONS/TOXIC EFFECTS

None significant.

PATIENT CONSIDERATIONS

BASELINE ASSESSMENT

For those on long-term therapy, liver/renal function tests, blood counts should be performed periodically.

INTERVENTION/EVALUATION

Supervise suicidal risk pt closely during early therapy (as depression lessens, energy level improves, increasing suicide potential). Assess appearance, behavior, speech pattern, level of interest, mood. Monitor pattern of daily bowel activity, stool consistency. Assist w/ambulation if dizziness occurs.

PATIENT/FAMILY TEACHING

Dry mouth may be relieved by sugarless gum, sips of tepid water. Report headache, fatigue, tremor, sexual dysfunction. Avoid tasks that require alertness, motor skills until response to drug is established. Take w/food if nausea occurs. Inform physician if become pregnant. Avoid alcohol. Do not take OTC medications w/o consulting physician.

---

sevelamer
(Renagel)
See Supplement

---

sibutramine

sigh-**bew**-trah-meen
(Meridia)

PREGNANCY CATEGORY C

CLASSIFICATION

Anorexiant

AVAILABILITY (Rx)

Capsules: 5 mg, 10 mg, 15 mg

PHARMACOKINETICS

Absorption: Rapidly absorbed

from GI tract following oral administration. Extensively distributed throughout the body. **Metabolism:** Undergoes extensive first-pass metabolism in liver to active metabolite. Highly bound to plasma proteins. **Excretion:** Primarily excreted in urine. **Half-life:** 1.1 hrs (metabolite: 14–16 hrs).

ACTION/*THERAPEUTIC EFFECT*

Inhibits reuptake of serotonin and norepinephrine, *enhancing satiety and raising the metabolic rate. Induces and maintains weight loss.*

USES

Management of obesity, including weight loss and maintenance of weight loss, when used in conjunction with a reduced-calorie diet.

INDICATIONS/DOSAGE/ROUTES

Weight loss:
Oral: Adults: Initially, 10 mg/day. May be titrated after 4 wks to total 15 mg once daily.

CONTRAINDICATIONS

Concurrent use of MAO inhibitors, history of hypersensitivity to sibutramine, those with anorexia nervosa, those taking other appetite suppressant drugs. Should not be used in those with history of coronary artery disease, congestive heart failure, arrhythmias, stroke, renal or hepatic function impairment, uncontrolled hypertension.

CAUTIONS

Those concurrently taking decongestants, and cough, cold and allergy medication that contain phenylpropanolamine, ephedrine, pseudoephedrine (may significantly raise B/P, heart rate), narrow-angle glaucoma, elderly, history of seizures.

INTERACTIONS

DRUG: ***MAO inhibitors*** may cause serious reactions and at least 2 wks should elapse before starting treatment with sibutramine and at least a 2 wk interval after stopping sibutramine before beginning treatment with MAO inhibitors. ***Fluoxetine, paroxetine*** may increase risk of serotonin syndrome (see Adverse Reactions/Toxic Effects). **HERBAL:** None known. **FOOD:** None significant. **ALTERED LAB VALUES:** May increase SGOT (AST), SGPT (ALT), alkaline phosphatase, bilirubin, HDL. May decrease LDL, triglycerides, cholesterol, uric acid.

SIDE EFFECTS

FREQUENT (11–30%): Headache, dry mouth, constipation, insomnia, rhinitis, dizziness, pharyngitis. **OCCASIONAL (4–9%):** Back pain, weakness, nausea, arthralgia, dyspepsia, sinusitis, nervousness, abdominal discomfort, anxiety. **RARE (2–3%):** Depression, rash, cough, dysmenorrhea, alteration in taste, migraine, paresthesia, sweating.

ADVERSE REACTIONS/TOXIC EFFECTS

Increased blood pressure, tachycardia, vasodilation, palpitations occur rarely. "Serotonin syndrome" is a very rare but serious toxic effect manifested as excitement, hypomania, restlessness, confusion, agitation, tremor, hyperthermia, vomiting, motor weakness, myoclonus, loss of consciousness.

PATIENT CONSIDERATIONS

BASELINE ASSESSMENT

Regular monitoring of B/P, pulse is required part of treatment. In pts taking MAO inhibitors, there should be 2 wk interval after stopping MAO inhibitors before

starting treatment with sibutramine and at least a 2 wk interval after stopping sibutramine before beginning treatment with MAO inhibitors. Question pt if concurrently taking other weight-reducing agents, decongestants, antidepressants, cough suppressants, lithium, dihydroergotamine, sumatriptan or tryptophan (potential for interactions).

PATIENT/FAMILY TEACHING

Contact physician if rash or other allergic condition occurs. Inform physician if taking other weight-reducing agents, decongestants, antidepressants, cough suppressants, lithium, Migranol nasal spray, Imitrex or tryptophan (potential for interactions). Regular monitoring of blood pressure and pulse is an essential part of therapy.

sildenafil

sill-**den**-ah-fill
(Viagra)

CLASSIFICATION

Cardiovascular agent

AVAILABILITY (Rx)

Tablets: 25 mg, 50 mg, 100 mg

PHARMACOKINETICS

Absorption: Rapidly absorbed from GI tract following oral administration. Highly bound to plasma proteins. Distributed into tissue. **Metabolism:** Metabolized in liver to active metabolite. **Excretion:** Primarily eliminated in feces. **Half-life:** 4 hrs.

ACTION/*THERAPEUTIC EFFECT*

Inhibits type V cyclic GMP, a specific phosphodiesterase and the predominant isoenzyme in human corpus cavernosum in the penis. *Relaxes smooth muscle, increasing blood flow, facilitating an erection.*

USES/*UNLABELED*

Treatment of male erectile dysfunction. *Treatment of sexual dysfunction from SSRI (antidepressants), diabetic gastroparesis.*

ADMINISTRATION

ORAL:

- May be taken approximately 1 hr before sexual activity but may take as long as 4 hrs to 30 min before sexual activity.

INDICATIONS/ROUTES/DOSAGES

Erectile dysfunction:
PO: Adults: 50 mg 1 hr before sexual activity. Dosage may be increased to maximum of 100 mg or decreased to 25 mg. Maximum frequency is once/day.

CONTRAINDICATIONS

Those concurrently using sodium nitroprusside or organic nitrates in any form, history of hypersensitivity to sildenafil.

CAUTIONS

Renal or hepatic function impairment, anatomic deformation of the penis, those that may be predisposed to priapism (sickle-cell anemia, multiple myeloma, leukemia). Pts w/angina, CHF w/low B/P, on multiple drugs for hypertension.

INTERACTIONS

DRUG: ***Cimetidine, erythromycin, itraconazole, ketoconazole*** may increase sildenafil plasma concentration. Potentiates hypotensive effects of *nitrates.* HERBAL: None known. **FOOD:** Rate of absorption is reduced and time to maximum effectiveness is delayed by 1 hr when taken with a high-fat meal. **ALTERED LAB VALUES:** None significant.

SIDE EFFECTS

FREQUENT: Headache (16%), flushing (10%). OCCASIONAL (3–7%): Dyspepsia, nasal congestion, urinary tract infection, abnormal vision, diarrhea. RARE (2%): Dizziness, rash.

ADVERSE REACTIONS/TOXIC EFFECTS

None significant.

PATIENT CONSIDERATIONS

Baseline Assessment

Assess cardiovascular status before initiating treatment for erectile dysfunction.

Patient/Family Teaching

Sildenafil has no effect in the absence of sexual stimulation.

silver sulfadiazine

sul-fah-**dye**-ah-zeen

(Silvadene, Flint SSD)

CANADIAN AVAILABILITY
Flamazine

PREGNANCY CATEGORY B

CLASSIFICATION

Burn preparation

AVAILABILITY (Rx)

Cream

PHARMACOKINETICS

Absorption: Variably absorbed. Significant systemic absorption may occur if applied to extensive burns. **Excretion:** Absorbed medication excreted unchanged in urine. **Half-life:** 10 hrs (increased in decreased renal function).

ACTION/*THERAPEUTIC EFFECT*

Acts on cell wall and cell membrane to *produce bactericidal effect.* Silver is released slowly in concentrations selectively toxic to bacteria.

USES/*UNLABELED*

Prevention, treatment of infection in second- and third-degree burns, protection against conversion from partial- to full-thickness wounds (infection causes extended tissue destruction). *Treatment of minor bacterial skin infection, dermal ulcer.*

ADMINISTRATION

TOPICAL:

- Apply to cleansed, debrided burns using sterile glove.
- Keep burn areas covered w/silver sulfadiazine cream at all times; reapply to areas where removed by pt activity.
- Dressings may be ordered on individual basis.

INDICATIONS/ROUTES/DOSAGE

Usual topical dosage:
Topical: Adults, elderly: Apply 1–2 times/day.

CONTRAINDICATIONS

Hypersensitivity to silver sulfadiazine, components of preparation.

CAUTIONS

Impaired renal/hepatic function, G-6-PD deficiency, premature neonates, infants <2 mos. Cross-sensitivity w/other sulfonamides unknown.

INTERACTIONS

DRUG: *Collagenase, papain, sutilains* may be inactivated. **HERBAL:** None known. **FOOD:** None significant. ALTERED LAB VALUES: None significant.

SIDE EFFECTS

Side effects characteristic of all sulfonamides may occur when systemically absorbed, e.g., extensive burn areas (over 20% of body surface): anorexia, nausea, vomiting, headache, diarrhea, dizziness, photosensitivity, joint pain. **FREQUENT:** Burning feeling at treatment site. **OCCASIONAL:** Brown-gray skin discoloration, rash, itching. **RARE:** Increased skin sensitivity to sunlight.

ADVERSE REACTIONS/TOXIC EFFECTS

If significant systemic absorption occurs, less often but serious are hemolytic anemia, hypoglycemia, diuresis, peripheral neuropathy, Stevens-Johnson syndrome, agranulocytosis, disseminated lupus erythematosus, anaphylaxis, hepatitis, toxic nephrosis. Fungal superinfections may occur. Interstitial nephritis occurs rarely.

PATIENT CONSIDERATIONS

Baseline Assessment

Question for hypersensitivity to silver sulfadiazine/components, other sulfonamides. Determine initial CBC, renal/hepatic function test results.

Intervention/Evaluation

Evaluate fluid balance, renal function: Check I&O, renal function tests and report changes promptly. Monitor vital signs. Check serum sulfonamide concentrations carefully. Assess burns, surrounding areas for pain, burning, itching, rash (antihistamines may provide relief, silver sulfadiazine therapy continued unless reactions severe). Check CBC results.

Patient/Family Teaching

Therapy must be continued until healing is satisfactory or the site is ready for grafting.

simethicone

sye-**meth**-ih-cone
(Mylicon, Phazyme, Silain)

FIXED-COMBINATION(S)
W/aluminum and magnesium hydroxide, antacids **(Digel, Gelusil, Maalox Plus, Mylanta)**; w/loperamide, an antidiarrheal **(Imodium Advanced)**; w/magaldrate, an antacid **(Riopan)**

CANADIAN AVAILABILITY
Ovol, Phazyme

PREGNANCY CATEGORY C

CLASSIFICATION

Antiflatulent

AVAILABILITY (OTC)

Tablets: 60 mg, 95 mg. **Tablets (chewable):** 40 mg, 80 mg, 125 mg. **Capsules:** 125 mg. **Drops:** 40 mg/0.6 ml.

PHARMACOKINETICS

Absorption: Does not appear to be absorbed from GI tract. **Excretion:** Excreted unchanged in feces.

ACTION/*THERAPEUTIC EFFECT*

Changes surface tension of gas bubbles allowing for easier elimination of gas. *Disperses, prevents formation of gas pockets in GI tract.*

USES/*UNLABELED*

Treatment of flatulence, gastric bloating, postop gas pain or when gas retention may be problem (i.e., peptic ulcer, spastic colon, air swallowing). *Adjunct to gastroscopy, bowel radiography.*

ADMINISTRATION

ORAL:

- Give after meals and at bedtime as needed. Chewable tablets are to be chewed thoroughly before swallowing. Enteric-coated tablets are swallowed whole; do not crush.
- Shake suspension well before using.

INDICATIONS/ROUTES/DOSAGE

Antiflatulent:
Oral: Adults, elderly: (capsules): 125 mg 4 times/day; ***(tablets):*** 50–125 mg 4 times/day; ***(suspension):*** 40 mg (0.6 ml) 4 times/day; ***(chewable tablets):*** 40–80 mg 4 times/day.

CONTRAINDICATIONS

None significant.

CAUTIONS

None significant.

INTERACTIONS

DRUG: None significant. **HERBAL:** None known. **FOOD:** None significant. **ALTERED LAB VALUES:** None significant.

SIDE EFFECTS

None significant.

ADVERSE REACTIONS/TOXIC EFFECTS

None significant.

PATIENT CONSIDERATIONS

INTERVENTION/EVALUATION

Evaluate for therapeutic response: relief of flatulence, abdominal bloating.

simvastatin

sim-vah-**stay**-tin
(Zocor)

CANADIAN AVAILABILITY
Zocor

PREGNANCY CATEGORY X

CLASSIFICATION

Antihyperlipoproteinemic

AVAILABILITY (RX)

Tablets: 5 mg, 10 mg, 20 mg, 40 mg, 80 mg

PHARMACOKINETICS

Absorption: Well absorbed from GI tract. **Metabolism:** Undergoes extensive first-pass metabolism. Hydrolyzed to active metabolite. **Excretion:** Primarily eliminated in feces.

ACTION/*THERAPEUTIC EFFECT*

Interferes w/cholesterol biosynthesis by inhibiting the conversion of the enzyme HMG-CoA to mevalonate. *Decreases LDL, cholesterol, VLDL, plasma triglycerides, slight increase in HDL concentration.*

USES

Adjunct to diet therapy to decrease elevated total and LDL cholesterol concentrations in those w/primary hypercholesterolemia (types IIa and IIb), lowers triglyceride levels, increases HDL. Reduces deaths, prevents heart attacks in pts w/heart disease, high cholesterol. Decreases risk of mortality by decreasing coronary death, risk of nonfatal myocardial infarction, need for myocardial revascularization procedures. Decreases risk for stroke/TIA.

ADMINISTRATION

ORAL:

- Give w/o regard to meals.
- Administer in evening.

INDICATIONS/ROUTES/DOSAGE

Note: Before initiating therapy, pt should be on standard cholesterol-lowering diet for minimum of 3–6 mos. Continue diet throughout simvastatin therapy.

Hyperlipidemia/decreased mortality:
Oral: Adults: Initially, 10–20 mg/day in evening. Dosage adjustment at 4 wk intervals. ***Elderly:*** Initially, 10 mg/day. May increase by 5–10 mg/day q4wks. ***Range:*** 5–80 mg/day. ***Maximum:*** 80 mg/day.

CONTRAINDICATIONS

Pregnancy, hypersensitivity to simvastatin/any component of the preparation, active liver disease or unexplained, persistent elevations of liver function tests, <18 yrs.

CAUTIONS

History of liver disease, substantial alcohol consumption. Withholding/discontinuing simvastatin may be necessary when pt at risk for renal failure secondary to rhabdomyolysis. Severe metabolic, endocrine, or electrolyte disorders.

INTERACTIONS

DRUG: Increased risk of rhabdomyolysis, acute renal failure w/***cyclosporine, erythromycin, gemfibrozil, niacin, other immunosuppressants. Erythromycin, itraconazole, ketoconazole*** may increase concentration, cause muscle pain, inflammation or weakness. **HERBAL:** None known. **FOOD:** None significant. **ALTERED LAB VALUES:** May increase creatinine kinase, serum transaminase concentrations.

SIDE EFFECTS

Generally well tolerated. Side effects usually mild and transient. **OCCASIONAL:** Abdominal pain, headache, constipation, upper respiratory infection. **RARE:** Diarrhea, flatulence, asthenia (loss of strength and energy), nausea/vomiting.

ADVERSE REACTIONS/TOXIC EFFECTS

Potential for lens opacities. Hypersensitivity reaction, hepatitis occurs rarely.

PATIENT CONSIDERATIONS

S

BASELINE ASSESSMENT

Question for possibility of pregnancy before initiating therapy (Pregnancy Category X). Question history of hypersensitivity to simvastatin. Assess baseline lab results: cholesterol, triglycerides, liver function tests.

INTERVENTION/EVALUATION

Monitor cholesterol and triglyceride lab results for therapeutic response. Monitor liver function tests. Evaluate food tolerance. Determine pattern of bowel activity. Check for headache, dizziness (provide assistance as needed). Assess for rash, pruritus. Be alert for malaise, muscle cramping/weakness; if accompanied by fever, may require discontinuation of medication.

PATIENT/FAMILY TEACHING

Take w/o regard to meals. Use appropriate contraceptive measures (Pregnancy Category X). Follow special diet (important

part of treatment). Periodic lab tests are essential part of therapy. Do not take other medications w/o physician knowledge. Do not stop medication w/o consulting physician. Report promptly any muscle pain/weakness, especially if accompanied by fever/malaise. Do not drive or perform activities that require alert response if dizziness occurs.

---

sirolimus

(Rapamune)

See Supplement

---

sodium bicarbonate

(Sodium bicarbonate)

CANADIAN AVAILABILITY

Sodium bicarbonate

PREGNANCY CATEGORY C

CLASSIFICATION

Antacid, alkalinizing agent

AVAILABILITY (OTC)

Tablets: 325 mg, 520 mg, 650 mg. **Injection (Rx):** 0.5 mEq/ml (4.2%), 0.6 mEq/ml (5%), 0.9 mEq/ml (7.5%), 1 mEq/ml (8.4%).

PHARMACOKINETICS

After administration, sodium bicarbonate dissociates to sodium and bicarbonate ions. Forms/excretes CO_2 (w/increased hydrogen ions combines to form carbonic acid, then dissociates to carbon dioxide, which is excreted by lungs). Plasma concentration regulated by kidney (ability to excrete/make bicarbonate).

ACTION/*THERAPEUTIC EFFECT*

Systemic alkalizer. Increases plasma bicarbonate, buffers excess hydrogen ion concentration, *increases pH, reverses acidosis.* ***Urinary alkalizer:*** Increases excretion of free bicarbonate in urine, *increases urinary pH.* ***Antacid:*** Neutralizes existing quantities of stomach acid, *increases pH of stomach contents.*

USES

Corrects metabolic acidosis occurring in severe renal disease and for advanced cardiac life support during cardiopulmonary resuscitation. Used in treatment of drug intoxicants and hyperacidity, associated stomach upset. Treatment of symptoms of peptic ulcer disease; reduces uric acid crystallization (prophylactic).

ADMINISTRATION

ORAL:

- Individualize dose (based on neutralizing capacity of antacids).
- *Chewable tablets:* Thoroughly chew tablets before swallowing (follow w/glass of water or milk).

IV:

- The 4.2%, 7.5%, and 8.4% solutions can be used for direct IV administration.
- For IV injection, give up to 1 mEq/kg over 1–3 min for cardiac arrest.
- The 5% solution is administered by IV piggyback.
- For IV infusion, do not exceed rate of infusion of 50 mEq/hr. For children <2 yrs, premature infants, neonates, administer by slow infusion, up to 8 mEq/daily.

INDICATIONS/ROUTES/DOSAGE

Note: May give by direct IV, IV infusion, or orally. Dose individualized (based on severity of acidosis, laboratory values, pt age, weight, clinical conditions). Do not fully correct bicarbonate deficit during first 24 hrs (may cause metabolic alkalosis).

Cardiac arrest:
IV: Adults, elderly: Initially, 1 mEq/kg (as 7.5–8.4% solution). May repeat w/0.5 mEq/kg q10min during continued arrest. Postresuscitation phase based on arterial blood pH, $PaCO_2$ base deficit. ***Children, infants:*** Initially, 1 mEq/kg.

Metabolic acidosis (less severe):
IV Infusion: Adults, elderly, older children: 2–5 mEq/kg over 4–8 hrs. May repeat based on laboratory values.

Acidosis (associated w/chronic renal failure):
Note: Give when plasma bicarbonate <15 mEq/L.

Oral: Adults, elderly: Initially, 20–36 mEq/day in divided doses.

Renal tubular acidosis (prevents renal failure, osteomalacia):
Oral: Adults, elderly: 4–6 g/day in divided doses or 0.5–10 mEq/kg/day in divided doses (higher doses for proximal renal tubular acidosis).

Alkalinization of urine:
Oral: Adults, elderly: Initially, 4 g, then 1–2 g q4h. ***Maximum:*** 16 g/day. ***Children:*** 84–840 mg/kg/day in divided doses.

Antacid:
Oral: Adults, elderly: 300 mg to 2 g 1–4 times/day.

CONTRAINDICATIONS

Metabolic/respiratory alkalosis, hypocalcemia, excessive chloride loss due to vomiting/diarrhea/GI suction.

CAUTIONS

CHF, edematous states, renal insufficiency, those on corticosteroid therapy.

INTERACTIONS

DRUG: May decrease excretion of ***quinidine, ketoconazole, tetracyclines. Calcium-containing products, milk, milk products*** may result in milk-alkali syndrome. May increase excretion of ***salicylates, lithium.*** May decrease effect of ***methenamine.*** **HERBAL:** None known. **FOOD:** Milk, milk products may result in milk-alkali syndrome. **ALTERED LAB VALUES:** May increase serum, urinary pH.

S

SIDE EFFECTS

FREQUENT: Abdominal distension, flatulence, belching. Extravasation may occur at IV site, resulting in necrosis, ulceration.

ADVERSE REACTIONS/TOXIC EFFECTS

Excessive/chronic use may produce metabolic alkalosis (irritability, twitching, numbness/tingling of extremities, cyanosis, slow/shallow respiration, headache, thirst, nausea). Fluid overload results in headache, weakness, blurred vision, behavioral changes, incoordination, muscle twitching, rise in B/P, decrease in pulse rate, rapid respirations, wheezing, coughing, distended neck veins.

PATIENT CONSIDERATIONS

BASELINE ASSESSMENT

Do not give other oral medication within 1–2 hrs of antacid administration.

Intervention/Evaluation

Monitor blood and urine pH, CO_2 level, serum electrolytes, plasma bicarbonate, and $PaCO_2$ levels. Watch for signs of metabolic alkalosis, fluid overload. Assess for clinical improvement of metabolic acidosis (relief from hyperventilation, weakness, disorientation). Assess pattern of daily bowel activity, stool consistency. Monitor serum phosphate, calcium, uric acid levels. Assess for relief of gastric distress.

Patient/Family Teaching

Chewable tablets: Chew tablets thoroughly before swallowing (may be followed by water or milk). Tablets may discolor stool. Maintain adequate fluid intake.

sodium chloride

(Salinex, Ocean Mist)

CANADIAN AVAILABILITY
Salinex, Sodium chloride

PREGNANCY CATEGORY C

CLASSIFICATION

Electrolyte

AVAILABILITY (OTC)

Tablets: 650 mg, 1 g, 2.25 g. **Tablets (slow-release):** 600 mg. **Nasal Solution:** 0.4%, 0.6%, 0.75%. **Ophthalmic Solution:** 2%, 5%. **Ophthalmic Ointment:** 5%. **Injection (concentrate) (Rx):** 14.6%, 23.4%. **Injection (Infusion) (Rx):** 0.45%, 0.9%, 3%, 5%. **Irrigation (Rx):** 0.45%, 0.9%.

PHARMACOKINETICS

Absorption: Well absorbed from GI tract. Widely distributed. **Excretion:** Primarily excreted in urine.

ACTION/*THERAPEUTIC EFFECT*

Sodium (a major cation of extracellular fluid) primarily *controls water distribution, fluid/electrolyte balance, osmotic pressure of body fluids.* Associated w/chloride and bicarbonate, *maintains acid-base balance.*

USES

Parenteral: Source of hydration; prevent/treats sodium and chloride deficiencies (hypertonic for severe deficiencies). Prevents muscle cramps/heat prostration occurring w/excessive perspiration. ***Hypotonic:*** Hydrating solution, used to assess renal function status and manage hyperosmolar diabetes. Diluent for reconstitution. ***Nasal:*** Restores moisture, relieves dry and inflamed nasal membranes. ***Ophthalmic:*** Therapy in reduction of corneal edema, diagnostic aid in ophthalmoscopic exam.

STORAGE/HANDLING

Store nasal, ophthalmic, parenteral forms at room temperature.

ADMINISTRATION

ORAL:

- Do not crush or break enteric-coated or extended-release tablets.

NASAL:

- Instruct pt to begin inhaling slowly just before releasing medication into nose.
- Inhale slowly, then release air gently through mouth.
- Continue technique for 20–30 sec.

OPHTHALMIC:

- Position pt w/head tilted back, looking up.
- Gently pull lower lid down to form pouch and instill drops (or apply thin strip of ointment).
- Do not touch tip of applicator to lids or any surface.
- When lower lid is released, have pt keep eye open w/o blinking for at least 30 sec for solution; for ointment have pt close eye and roll eyeball around to distribute medication.
- Apply gentle finger pressure to lacrimal sac (bridge of the nose, inside corner of the eye) for 1–2 min after administration of solution.
- Remove excess solution around eye w/tissue.

IV:

- Hypertonic solutions (3 or 5%) administered via large vein; avoid infiltration; do not exceed 100 ml/hr.
- Vials containing 2.5–4 mEq/ml (concentrated NaCl) must be diluted before administration.

INDICATIONS/ROUTES/DOSAGE

Usual parenteral dosage:
Note: Dosage based on age, weight, clinical condition, fluid, electrolyte, acid-base status.

IV Infusion: Adults, elderly: (0.9 or 0.45%): 1–2 L/day. *(3 or 5%):* 100 ml over 1 hr; assess serum electrolyte concentration before additional fluid given.

Usual oral dosage:
Oral: Adults, elderly: 1–2 g 3 times/day.

Usual nasal dosage:
Intranasal: Adults, elderly: Take as needed.

Usual ophthalmic dosage:
Ophthalmic: Adults, elderly: (Solution): 1–2 drops q3–4h. ***(Ointment):*** Once/day or as directed.

CONTRAINDICATIONS

Hypernatremia, fluid retention.

CAUTIONS

CHF, circulatory insufficiency, kidney dysfunction, hypoproteinemia. Do not use NaCl preserved w/benzyl alcohol in neonates.

INTERACTIONS

DRUG: ***Hypertonic saline and oxytocics*** may cause uterine hypertonus, possible uterine ruptures or lacerations. **HERBAL:** None known. **FOOD:** None significant. **ALTERED LAB VALUES:** None significant.

SIDE EFFECTS

FREQUENT: Flushed face. **OCCASIONAL:** Fever, irritation/phlebitis/extravasation at injection site. *Ophthalmic:* Temporary burning/irritation.

ADVERSE REACTIONS/TOXIC EFFECTS

Too rapid administration may produce peripheral edema, CHF, pulmonary edema. Excessive dosage produces hypokalemia, hypervolemia, hypernatremia.

PATIENT CONSIDERATIONS

Baseline Assessment

Assess fluid balance (I&O, edema).

Intervention/Evaluation

Monitor fluid balance (e.g., I&O, daily weight, edema, lung sounds), IV site for extravasation. Monitor serum electrolytes, acid-base balance, B/P. Hypernatremia associated w/edema,

S

weight gain, elevated B/P; hyponatremia associated w/muscle cramps, nausea, vomiting, dry mucous membranes.

PATIENT/FAMILY TEACHING

Temporary burning, irritation may occur upon instillation of eye medication. Discontinue eye medication if severe pain, headache, rapid change in vision (side and straight ahead), sudden appearance of floating spots, acute redness of eyes, pain on exposure to light, or double vision occurs and contact physician.

sodium polystyrene sulfonate

sew-dee-um poly-**sty**-reen **sul**-foe-nate
(SPS, Kayexalate)

CANADIAN AVAILABILITY
Kayexalate

PREGNANCY CATEGORY N/A

CLASSIFICATION

Cation exchange resin

AVAILABILITY (Rx)

Suspension: 15 g/60 ml. **Powder.**

ACTION/*THERAPEUTIC EFFECT*

Resin either passes through intestine or is retained in colon; *releases sodium ions in exchange for primarily potassium ions.* Occurs from 2–12 hrs after oral administration, longer after rectal administration.

USES

Treatment of hyperkalemia.

STORAGE/HANDLING

After preparation, suspension stable for 24 hrs.

ADMINISTRATION

ORAL:

- Give w/20–100 ml sorbitol (facilitates passage of resin through intestinal tract, prevents constipation, aids in potassium removal, increases palatability).
- Do not mix w/foods, liquids containing potassium.

RECTAL:

- Initial cleansing enema, then insert large rubber tube into rectum well into sigmoid colon, tape in place.
- Introduce suspension (w/100 ml sorbitol) via gravity.
- Flush w/50–100 ml fluid and clamp.
- Retain for several hours if possible.
- Irrigate colon w/nonsodium-containing solution to remove resin.

INDICATIONS/ROUTES/DOSAGE

Hyperkalemia:
Oral: Adults, elderly: 60 ml (15 g) 1–4 times/day.

Rectal: Adults, elderly: 30–50 g as needed q6h.

Usual pediatric dosage:
Oral/Rectal: Based on 1 g resin binding approx. 1 mEq potassium: 1 g/kg q6h.

CONTRAINDICATIONS

None significant.

CAUTIONS

Those who cannot tolerate increase in sodium (CHF, severe hypertension, marked edema).

INTERACTIONS

DRUG: ***Cation-donating antacids, laxatives (e.g., magnesium hydroxide)*** may decrease effect, cause systemic alkalosis (pts w/renal impairment). **HERBAL:** None known. **FOOD:** None significant. **ALTERED LAB VALUES:** May decrease magnesium, calcium.

SIDE EFFECTS

High dosage: Anorexia, nausea, vomiting, constipation. High dosage in elderly: Fecal impaction (severe stomach pain w/nausea/vomiting). **OCCASIONAL:** Diarrhea, sodium retention (decreased urination, swelling hands/feet, increased weight), hypocalcemia (abdominal/muscle cramps).

ADVERSE REACTIONS/TOXIC EFFECTS

Serious potassium deficiency may occur. Early signs of hypokalemia: irritable confusion, delayed thought processes, often associated w/lengthened QT interval and widening, flattening, or conversion of T wave and prominent U waves. Arrhythmias, severe muscle weakness may be noted.

PATIENT CONSIDERATIONS

BASELINE ASSESSMENT

Does not rapidly correct severe hyperkalemia (may take hours to days). Consider other measures in medical emergency (IV calcium, IV sodium bicarbonate, glucose, insulin, dialysis).

INTERVENTION/EVALUATION

Frequent potassium levels within each 24 hrs should be maintained, monitored. Assess pt's clinical condition, EKG (valuable in determining when treatment should be discontinued). In addition to checking serum potassium, monitor magnesium, calcium levels. Monitor daily bowel activity, stool consistency (fecal impaction may occur in those on high doses, particularly in elderly).

---

somatrem

soe-ma-trem
(Protropin)

CANADIAN AVAILABILITY
Protropin

CLASSIFICATION

Growth stimulator

AVAILABILITY (Rx)

Powder for Injection: 5 mg, 10 mg

PHARMACOKINETICS

Absorption: Well absorbed following SubQ, IM administration. **Metabolism:** Metabolized in liver. **Excretion:** Eliminated in feces via biliary system, excreted in urine. **Half-life:** 3–5 hrs.

ACTION/*THERAPEUTIC EFFECT*

Stimulates linear growth. Increases number, size of muscle cells, increases red cell mass. Affects carbohydrate metabolism (antagonizes action of insulin), fats (increases mobilization of fats), and proteins (increases cellular protein synthesis).

USES

Long-term treatment of children who have growth failure due to endogenous growth hormone deficiency.

STORAGE/HANDLING

Refrigerate vials. After reconstitution, use within 7 days. Avoid freezing.

ADMINISTRATION

IM:

- Reconstitute each 5 mg vial w/1–5 ml of bacteriostatic water for injection (benzyl alcohol preserved only). For newborns (because of toxicity w/benzyl alcohol), reconstitute w/water for injection.
- To prepare solution, inject diluent into vial aiming the stream of liquid against the glass wall. Swirl gently until dissolved. *Do Not Shake.*
- Use one dose per vial; discard unused portion.
- Do not administer if solution is cloudy/contains particulate matter.
- To prevent contamination, use disposable needle/syringe for each entry into vial.

INDICATIONS/ROUTES/DOSAGE

Usual parenteral dosage:
IM/SubQ: Up to 0.1 mg/kg (0.26 IU/kg) 3 times/wk.

CONTRAINDICATIONS

Pts w/closed epiphyses, known sensitivity to benzyl alcohol, active neoplasia (intracranial tumors must be inactive and antitumor therapy complete before somatrem therapy; discontinue if tumor growth recurs).

CAUTIONS

Diabetes mellitus, hypothyroidism, pts whose growth hormone deficiency is secondary to an intracranial lesion.

INTERACTIONS

DRUG: *Glucocorticoids* (chronic use) may decrease effects. **HERBAL:** None known. **FOOD:** None significant. **ALTERED LAB VALUES:** May increase fatty acid, phosphate concentration. May decrease glucose tolerance, thyroid function tests.

SIDE EFFECTS

FREQUENT: 30% of pts develop persistent antibodies to growth hormone (generally does not cause failure to respond to somatrem). **OCCASIONAL:** Headache, muscle pain, weakness, mild hyperglycemia, allergic reaction (rash, itching), pain, swelling at injection site, pain in hip or knee.

ADVERSE REACTIONS/TOXIC EFFECTS

Hypothyroidism (must be treated or will interfere w/response to somatrem).

PATIENT CONSIDERATIONS

Baseline Assessment

Question sensitivity to benzyl alcohol. Baseline blood glucose, thyroid function, and bone age determinations should be established.

Intervention/Evaluation

Monitor blood glucose levels and check for hyperglycemia (polyuria, polydipsia, polyphagia). Assess for developing hypothyroidism: forgetfulness, dry skin and hair, feeling cold, apathy, lethargy, weight gain, bradycardia.

Patient/Family Teaching

Somatrem therapy may continue for years, as long as pt is responsive, until mature adult height is reached or epiphyses close. Importance of regular visits to the physician, tests during thera-

py. Record height, weight as directed by physician. Signs and symptoms of hypothyroidism, hyperglycemia: Report promptly.

somatropin

soe-mah-**troe**-pin
(Humatrope, Norditropin, Nutropin, Nutropin AQ, Saizen)

CANADIAN AVAILABILITY

Humatrope, Nutropin, Saizen

CLASSIFICATION

Growth stimulator

AVAILABILITY (Rx)

Powder for Injection: 5 mg, 10 mg

PHARMACOKINETICS

Absorption: Well absorbed following SubQ, IM administration. **Metabolism:** Metabolized in liver. **Excretion:** Eliminated in feces via biliary system, excreted in urine. **Half-life:** *IM/SubQ: 3–5 hrs.*

ACTION/*THERAPEUTIC EFFECT*

Stimulates linear growth. Increases number, size of muscle cells, increases red cell mass. Affects carbohydrate metabolism (antagonizes action of insulin), fats (increases mobilization of fats), and proteins (increases cellular protein synthesis).

USES

Long-term treatment of children who have growth failure due to endogenous growth hormone deficiency or associated w/chronic renal insufficiency (Nutropin only). Long-term therapy in adults w/growth hormone deficiency. Long-term treatment of short stature associated w/Turner's syndrome, treatment of AIDS-wasting syndrome.

STORAGE/HANDLING

Refrigerate vials. After reconstitution, stable for 14 days refrigerated. Avoid freezing.

ADMINISTRATION

IM/SubQ:

- *Humatrope:* Reconstitute each 5 mg vial w/1.5–5 ml diluent or sterile water for injection. (If sterile water used, use 1 dose/vial, refrigerate solution if not used immediately, use within 24 hrs, discard unused portion.)
- *Nutropin:* Reconstitute 5 mg vial w/1–5 mg (10 mg w/1–10 ml) bacteriostatic water for injection.
- Do not shake.
- Do not inject if solution is cloudy or contains particulate matter.

INDICATIONS/ROUTES/DOSAGE

Growth hormone deficiency:
IM/SubQ: (Humatrope): Up to 0.06 mg/kg 3 times/wk.

SubQ: Adults: 0.04 mg/kg/wk divided into 6–7 injections. *Maximum:* 0.08 mg/kg/wk.

SubQ: (Nutropin): 0.3 mg/kg/wk.

Chronic renal insufficiency:
SubQ: (Nutropin): 0.35 mg/kg/wk.

Turner's syndrome:
SubQ: 0.375 mg/kg/wk divided into 3–7 equal doses/wk.

AIDS-wasting syndrome:
SubQ: 4–6 mg at bedtime.

CONTRAINDICATIONS

Pts w/closed epiphyses, active neoplasia (intracranial tumors must be inactive and antitumor therapy complete before somat-

S

ropin therapy; discontinue if tumor growth recurs). Do not use supplied diluent when sensitivity to m-cresol or glycerin is known.

CAUTIONS

Diabetes mellitus, hypothyroidism, pts whose growth hormone deficiency is secondary to an intracranial lesion.

INTERACTIONS

DRUG: *Glucocorticoids* (chronic use) may decrease effects. **HERBAL:** None known. **FOOD:** None significant. **ALTERED LAB VALUES:** May increase fatty acid, phosphate concentration. May decrease glucose tolerance, thyroid function tests.

SIDE EFFECTS

FREQUENT: Development of persistent antibodies to growth hormone (generally does not cause failure to respond to somatropin); hypercalciuria during first 2–3 mos of therapy. **OCCASIONAL:** Headache, muscle pain, weakness, mild hyperglycemia, allergic reaction (rash, itching), pain, swelling at injection site, pain in hip or knee.

ADVERSE REACTIONS/TOXIC EFFECTS

Hypothyroidism (must be treated or will interfere w/response to somatropin).

PATIENT CONSIDERATIONS

BASELINE ASSESSMENT

Question sensitivity to m-cresol, glycerin. Establish baseline blood glucose, thyroid function, and bone age determinations.

INTERVENTION/EVALUATION

Monitor blood glucose levels and check for hyperglycemia (polyuria, polydipsia, polyphagia). Assess for developing hypothyroidism: forgetfulness, dry skin and hair, feeling cold, apathy, lethargy, weight gain, bradycardia. During early therapy, be alert to renal calculi associated w/hypercalciuria (flank pain and colic, chills, fever, urinary frequency, hematuria).

PATIENT/FAMILY TEACHING

Somatropin therapy may continue for years, as long as pt is responsive, until mature adult height is reached or epiphyses close. Importance of regular visits to the physician, tests during therapy. Record height, weight as directed by physician. Signs and symptoms of hypothyroidism, hyperglycemia, renal calculi: Report promptly.

sotalol

sew-tah-lol
(Betapace)

CANADIAN AVAILABILITY
Sotacor

PREGNANCY CATEGORY B
(D if used in second or third trimester)

CLASSIFICATION

Beta-adrenergic blocking agent

AVAILABILITY (Rx)

Tablets: 80 mg, 120 mg, 160 mg, 240 mg

PHARMACOKINETICS

Absorption: Well absorbed from GI tract. Widely distributed. **Excretion:** Primarily excreted unchanged in urine. **Half-life:** 12 hrs (increased in elderly, pts w/decreased renal function).

ACTION/*THERAPEUTIC EFFECT*

Prolongs action potential and effective refractory period, QT interval. Decreases heart rate, AV nodal conduction; increases AV nodal refractoriness, *producing antiarrhythmic activity.*

USES/*UNLABELED*

Treatment of documented, life-threatening ventricular arrhythmias. *Treatment of chronic angina pectoris, hypertension, hypertrophic cardiomyopathy, myocardial infarction, pheochromocytoma, tremors, anxiety, thyrotoxicosis, mitral valve prolapse syndrome. Maintenance of normal heart rhythms in chronic or recurring atrial fibrillation or flutter.*

ADMINISTRATION

ORAL:

- May give w/o regard to food.

INDICATIONS/ROUTES/DOSAGE

Antiarrhythmic:

Oral: Adults, elderly: Initially, 80 mg 2 times/day. May increase gradually at 2–3 day intervals. ***Range:*** 240–320 mg/day.
Note: Some pts may require 480–640 mg/day. Dosing more than 2 times/day usually not necessary due to long half-life.

Dosage in renal impairment:

CREATININE CLEARANCE	DOSAGE INTERVAL
30–60 ml/min	24 hrs
10–30 ml/min	36–48 hrs
<10 ml/min	Individualized

CONTRAINDICATIONS

Bronchial asthma, uncontrolled cardiac failure, sinus bradycardia, second- and third-degree heart block, cardiogenic shock, long QT syndrome (unless functioning pacemaker present).

CAUTIONS

Pts w/history of ventricular tachycardia, ventricular fibrillation, cardiomegaly, CHF, diabetes mellitus, excessive prolongation of QT interval, hypokalemia, and hypomagnesium. Severe, prolonged diarrhea. Pts w/sick-sinus syndrome; pts at risk of developing thyrotoxicosis. Avoid abrupt withdrawal.

INTERACTIONS

DRUG: ***Antiarrhythmics, phenothiazine, tricyclic antidepressants, terfenadine, astemizole*** may increase prolonged QT interval. May increase proarrhythmia w/***digoxin. Calcium channel blockers*** may increase effect on AV conduction, B/P. May mask signs of hypoglycemia, prolong effect of ***insulin, oral hypoglycemics.*** May inhibit effects of ***sympathomimetics.*** May potentiate rebound hypertension seen after discontinuing ***clonidine.*** **HERBAL:** None known. **FOOD:** None significant. **ALTERED LAB VALUES:** May increase glucose, alkaline phosphatase, LDH, SGOT (AST), SGPT (ALT), lipoproteins, triglycerides.

SIDE EFFECTS

FREQUENT: Decreased sexual ability, drowsiness, trouble sleeping, unusually tired/weak. **OCCASIONAL:** Bradycardia, difficulty breathing, CHF (swelling of feet, shortness of breath), depression, cold hands/feet, diarrhea, constipation, anxiety, nasal congestion, nausea, vomiting. **RARE:** Altered taste, dry eyes, itching, numbness of fingers, toes, scalp.

ADVERSE REACTIONS/TOXIC EFFECTS

Bradycardia, CHF, hypotension, bronchospasm, hypoglycemia,

prolonged QT interval, torsade de pointes, ventricular tachycardia, premature ventricular complexes.

PATIENT CONSIDERATIONS

Baseline Assessment

Pt must be on continuous cardiac monitoring upon initiation of therapy. Establish baseline B/P and pulse. Do not administer w/o consulting physician if pulse is below 60 beats/min.

Intervention/Evaluation

Monitor B/P for hypotension, pulse for bradycardia. Assess for CHF: dyspnea, peripheral edema, jugular vein distension, increased weight, rales in lungs, decreased urine output.

Patient/Family Teaching

May have lightheadedness; do not drive or perform tasks that require alert response if this occurs. Carry identification bracelet/card. Teach pt/family to correctly take B/P, pulse before dosing; contact physician if below parameters, usually systolic B/P of 90 mm Hg, pulse of 60 beats/min. Change positions slowly to prevent orthostatic hypotension. Do not take OTC cold medications, nasal decongestants. Restrict sodium and alcohol as ordered. Do not stop taking drug suddenly. Report chest pain, fatigue, shortness of breath.

---

sparfloxacin

spar-**flocks**-ah-sin
(Zagam)

PREGNANCY CATEGORY C

CLASSIFICATION

Antibiotic: Fluoroquinolone

AVAILABILITY (Rx)

Tablets: 200 mg

PHARMACOKINETICS

Absorption: Well absorbed following oral administration. Widely distributed. **Metabolism:** Metabolized in the liver. **Excretion:** Excreted primarily in the urine with a lesser amount eliminated in the feces. **Half-life:** 16–30 hrs.

ACTION/*THERAPEUTIC EFFECT*

Inhibits the DNA enzyme, gyrase, in susceptible microorganisms, interfering with bacterial DNA replication and repair, *producing bactericidal activity.*

USES

Treatment of community-acquired pneumonia, acute bacterial exacerbation of chronic bronchitis.

ADMINISTRATION

ORAL:

- May be given w/o regard to meals.
- Do not crush or break film-coated tablets.

INDICATIONS/ROUTES/DOSAGES

Bronchitis, pneumonia:
Oral: Adults ≥18 yrs, elderly: Initially, two 200 mg tablets as a loading dose on the first day. Then one 200 mg tablet q24h for a total of 10 days.

Dosage in renal impairment (creatinine clearance <50 ml/min):
Oral: Adults ≥18 yrs, elderly: Initially, two 200 mg tablets as a loading dose on the first day. Then one 200 mg tablet q48h for a total of 9 days.

CONTRAINDICATIONS

History of hypersensitivity to fluoroquinolone antibiotics, cinoxacin, nalidixic acid.

CAUTIONS

Impaired renal/hepatic function.

INTERACTIONS

DRUG: *Astemizole, cisapride, erythromycin, phenothiazines, tricyclic antidepressants* may cause torsades de pointes. *Antacids, iron preparations, sucralfate* may decrease sparfloxacin serum levels (give sparfloxacin at least 4 hrs after any of these medications). **HERBAL:** St. John's wort may increase risk of photosensitivity. **FOOD:** May give w/o regard to food. **ALTERED LAB VALUES:** May increase SGOT (AST), SGOT (ALT), alkaline phosphatase, WBC count.

SIDE EFFECTS

FREQUENT (4–8%): Photosensitivity, diarrhea, nausea, headache. **RARE (1–2%):** Dyspepsia, dizziness, insomnia, abdominal pain, change in taste.

ADVERSE REACTIONS/TOXIC EFFECTS

Superinfection (particularly enterococcal or fungal overgrowth of nonsusceptible organisms) may occur. Hypersensitivity reactions have occurred in those receiving fluoroquinolone therapy.

PATIENT CONSIDERATIONS

BASELINE ASSESSMENT

Question for hypersensitivity to sparfloxacin or other fluoroquinolones. Obtain specimens for culture and sensitivity test (therapy may begin before results are known).

INTERVENTION/EVALUATION

Report hypersensitivity reaction: skin rash, urticaria, pruritus, photosensitivity promptly. Be alert for superinfection (e.g., genital-anal pruritus, ulceration or changes in oral mucosa, moderate to severe diarrhea, new or increased fever). Provide symptomatic relief for nausea. Evaluate food tolerance, change in taste sensation.

PATIENT/FAMILY TEACHING

Do not take antacids 2 hrs before or after taking medication (reduces/destroys effectiveness). Avoid excessive sunlight/artificial ultraviolet light (reaction may occur up to several weeks after stopping therapy). Continue medication for full length of treatment. Sugarless gum, hard candy may relieve bad taste.

spectinomycin hydrochloride

speck-tin-oh-**my**-sin
(Trobicin)

PREGNANCY CATEGORY B

CLASSIFICATION

Antibiotic

AVAILABILITY (Rx)

Powder for Injection: 400 mg/ml (2 g, 4 g vials)

PHARMACOKINETICS

Absorption: Rapidly, completely absorbed after IM administration. Primarily concentrated in urine. **Excretion:** Excreted in urine. Removed by hemodialysis. **Half-**

life: 1–3 hrs (increased in decreased renal function).

ACTION/*THERAPEUTIC EFFECT*

Inhibits protein synthesis of bacterial cells, *producing bacterial cell death.*

USES/*UNLABELED*

Treatment of acute gonococcal urethritis, proctitis in males, acute gonococcal cervicitis and proctitis in females. *Treatment of disseminated gonorrhea.*

STORAGE/HANDLING

Following reconstitution, stable for 24 hrs at room temperature. Use within 24 hrs.

ADMINISTRATION

IM:

- For IM injection, reconstitute each 2 g vial w/3.2 ml bacteriostatic water for injection containing 0.9% benzyl alcohol (6.2 ml to 4 g vial) to provide concentration of 400 mg/ml.
- Shake vigorously.
- Inject deep IM into upper outer quadrant of gluteal muscle (use 20 gauge needle).
- Do not inject more than 5 ml in one site.
- Observe pt for 1 hr after injection for potential anaphylaxis.

INDICATIONS/ROUTES/DOSAGE

Usual adult dosage:
IM: 2 g once. In areas where antibiotic resistance is known to be prevalent, 4 g (10 ml) divided between 2 injection sites is preferred.

CONTRAINDICATIONS

None significant.

CAUTIONS

History of allergies.

INTERACTIONS

DRUG: None significant. **HERBAL:** None known. **FOOD:** None significant. **ALTERED LAB VALUES:** None significant.

SIDE EFFECTS

FREQUENT: Pain at injection site. **OCCASIONAL:** Dizziness, insomnia. **RARE:** Decreased urine output.

ADVERSE REACTIONS/TOXIC EFFECTS

Hypersensitivity reaction characterized as chills, fever, nausea, vomiting, urticaria.

PATIENT CONSIDERATIONS

BASELINE ASSESSMENT

Question pt for history of allergies, particularly to spectinomycin. Obtain culture and sensitivity test before giving first dose (therapy may begin before results are known). Serologic test for syphilis should be completed before therapy.

INTERVENTION/EVALUATION

Observe pt for 1 hr after injection because of potential for anaphylaxis.

PATIENT/FAMILY TEACHING

May have discomfort at injection site.

spironolactone

spear-own-oh-**lak**-tone.
(Aldactone)

FIXED-COMBINATION(S)
W/hydrochlorothiazide, a thiazide diuretic **(Aldactazide, Spironazide)**

CANADIAN AVAILABILITY
Aldactone, Novospiroton

PREGNANCY CATEGORY D

CLASSIFICATION

Diuretic: Potassium sparing

AVAILABILITY (Rx)

Tablets: 25 mg, 50 mg, 100 mg

PHARMACODYNAMICS

	ONSET	PEAK	DURATION
Oral	24–48 hrs	48–72 hrs	48–72 hrs

PHARMACOKINETICS

Absorption: Well absorbed from GI tract (increased w/food). **Metabolism:** Metabolized in liver to active metabolite. **Excretion:** Primarily excreted in urine. **Half-life:** 9–24 hrs.

ACTION/*THERAPEUTIC EFFECT*

Competitively inhibits action of aldosterone. Interferes w/sodium reabsorption in distal tubule, *increasing potassium retention while promoting sodium and water excretion.*

USES/*UNLABELED*

Treatment of excessive aldosterone production, essential hypertension, CHF, edema due to CHF, cirrhosis of liver/nephrotic syndrome. Adjunct to potassium-losing diuretics or to potentiate action of other diuretics. Diagnosis of hyperaldosteronism. *Treatment of polycystic ovary syndrome, female hirsutism.*

STORAGE/HANDLING

Oral suspension containing crushed tablets in cherry syrup is stable for up to 30 days if refrigerated.

ADMINISTRATION

ORAL:

- Cherry suspension available for pediatric administration.
- Drug absorption enhanced if taken w/food.
- Scored tablets may be crushed.
- Do not crush or break film-coated tablets.

INDICATIONS/ROUTES/DOSAGE

Note: Use loading dose to prevent delay in therapeutic effect (may take up to 3 days).

CHF:
Oral: Adults, elderly: 25 mg/day.

Edema:
Oral: Adults: 25–200 mg daily. Give in single or equally divided doses. *Children:* 3.3 mg/kg daily.

Hypokalemia:
Oral: Adults: 25–100 mg daily.

Hypertension:
Oral: Adults: 50–100 mg daily.

Usual elderly dosage:
Oral: Initially, 25–50 mg/day. May increase by 25–50 mg/day q5days.

Diagnosis of primary aldosteronism:
Oral: Adults: 400 mg daily for 3–4 wks. Increase in potassium and reduction in hypertension point to primary aldosteronism. This dosage may be tried for 4 days w/increase in potassium levels during use as the diagnostic indicator. *Children:* 125–375 mg/m^2 over 24 hrs.

Preop or maintenance therapy for hyperaldosteronism:
Oral: Adults: 100–400 mg daily for preop therapy; 400 mg initial dose followed by lowest therapeutic dose at 100–300 mg/day for maintenance if surgery cannot be done.

CONTRAINDICATIONS

Acute renal insufficiency/impairment, anuria, BUN/creatinine over twice normal values levels, hyperkalemia.

CAUTIONS

Hepatic/renal impairment.

INTERACTIONS

DRUG: May decrease effect of ***anticoagulants, heparin. NSAIDs*** may decrease antihypertensive effect. ***ACE inhibitors (e.g., captopril), potassium-containing medications, potassium supplements*** may increase potassium. May decrease ***lithium*** clearance, increase toxicity. May increase ***digoxin*** half-life. **HERBAL:** Licorice may decrease effects. **FOOD:** None significant. **ALTERED LAB VALUES:** May increase BUN, calcium excretion, creatinine, glucose, magnesium, potassium, uric acid. May decrease sodium.

SIDE EFFECTS

FREQUENT: Hyperkalemia for those on potassium supplements or those w/renal insufficiency; dehydration, hyponatremia, lethargy. **OCCASIONAL:** Nausea, vomiting, anorexia, cramping, diarrhea, headache, ataxia, drowsiness, confusion, fever. ***Male:*** Gynecomastia, impotence, decreased libido. ***Females:*** Menstrual irregularities/amenorrhea, postmenopausal bleeding, breast tenderness. **RARE:** Rash, urticaria, hirsutism. Those w/primary aldosteronism may experience rapid weight loss, severe fatigue during high-dose therapy.

ADVERSE REACTIONS/TOXIC EFFECTS

Severe hyperkalemia may produce arrhythmias, bradycardia, tented T waves, widening QRS, ST depression. These can proceed to cardiac standstill or ventricular fibrillation. Cirrhosis pts at risk for hepatic decompensation if dehydration/hyponatremia occurs.

PATIENT CONSIDERATIONS

Baseline Assessment

Weigh pt; initiate strict I&O. Evaluate hydration status by assessing mucous membranes, skin turgor. Obtain baseline electrolytes, renal/hepatic functions, urinalysis. EKG may be ordered. Assess for edema; note location and extent. Check baseline vital signs, note pulse rate/regularity.

Intervention/Evaluation

Monitor electrolyte values, especially for increased potassium. Monitor B/P levels. Monitor for hyponatremia: mental confusion, thirst, cold/clammy skin, drowsiness, dry mouth. Monitor for hyperkalemia: colic, diarrhea, muscle twitching followed by weakness/paralysis, arrhythmias. Obtain daily weight. Note changes in edema, skin turgor.

Patient/Family Teaching

Expect increase in volume, frequency of urination. Therapeutic effect takes several days to begin and can last for several days when drug is discontinued. This may not apply if pt is on a potassium-losing drug concomitantly (diet and use of supplements should be established by physician). Notify physician for irregular/slow pulse, electrolyte imbalance (signs noted above). Avoid foods high in potassium such as whole grains (cereals), legumes, meat, bananas, apricots, orange juice, potatoes (white, sweet), raisins.

stavudine (d4T)

stah-view-deen
(Zerit)

CANADIAN AVAILABILITY
Zerit

PREGNANCY CATEGORY C

CLASSIFICATION

Antiviral

AVAILABILITY (Rx)

Capsules: 15 mg, 20 mg, 30 mg, 40 mg. **Oral Solution:** 1 mg/ml.

PHARMACOKINETICS

Absorption: Rapidly, completely absorbed following oral administration. Equally distributed into extravascular spaces. **Metabolism:** Undergoes minimal metabolism. **Excretion:** Excreted in urine. **Half-life:** 1.5 hrs (increased in decreased renal function).

ACTION/*THERAPEUTIC EFFECT*

Inhibits HIV reverse transcriptase via viral DNA chain termination. Also inhibits RNA- and DNA-dependent DNA polymerase, an enzyme necessary for viral HIV replication, *slowing HIV replication, reducing progression of HIV infection.*

USES

Treatment of adults w/advanced HIV infection who are intolerant or have experienced deterioration w/other drug therapy. First-line component in treatment of HIV.

ADMINISTRATION

ORAL:

- May give w/o regard to meals.

INDICATIONS/ROUTES/DOSAGE

HIV infection:

Oral: Adults ≥60 kg: 40 mg twice daily. ***Adults <60 kg:*** 30 mg twice daily. If peripheral neuropathy or elevated hepatic transaminases present, stop therapy. If symptoms resolve completely, resume treatment using following schedule: ***Adults ≥60 kg:*** 20 mg twice daily. ***Adults <60 kg:*** 15 mg twice daily.

Children ≥30 kg: Same as adults; ***<30 kg:*** 2 mg/kg/day.

Dosage in renal impairment:
Dose and/or frequency is modified based on creatinine clearance, pt weight.

CREATININE CLEARANCE	≥60 KG	≤60 KG
> 50	40 mg q12h	30 mg q12h
26–50	20 mg q12h	15 mg q12h
10–25	20 mg q24h	15 mg q24h

CONTRAINDICATIONS

None significant.

CAUTIONS

History of peripheral neuropathy.

INTERACTIONS

DRUG: None significant. **HERBAL:** St. John's wort may decrease concentration, effects. **FOOD:** None significant. **ALTERED LAB VALUES:** Commonly increases SGOT (AST), SGPT (ALT). May decrease neutrophil count.

SIDE EFFECTS

FREQUENT: Headache (55%), diarrhea (50%), chills/fever (38%), nausea/vomiting, myalgia (35%), rash (33%), asthenia [loss of strength, energy] (28%), insomnia, abdominal pain (26%), anxiety (22%), arthralgia (18%), back pain (20%), sweating (19%), malaise (17%), depression (14%). **OCCASIONAL:** Anorexia, weight loss, nervousness, dizziness, conjunctivitis, dyspepsia, dyspnea. **RARE:** Constipation, vasodilation, confusion, migraine, urticaria, abnormal vision.

S

ADVERSE REACTIONS/TOXIC EFFECTS

Peripheral neuropathy, characterized by numbness, tingling, or pain in hands or feet, occurs frequently (15%-21%). Ulcerative stomatitis (erythema/ulcers of oral mucosa, glossitis, gingivitis), pneumonia, benign skin neoplasms occur occasionally. Pancreatitis occurs rarely.

PATIENT CONSIDERATIONS

Baseline Assessment

Obtain baseline laboratory testing, especially liver function tests, before beginning stavudine therapy and at periodic intervals during therapy. Offer emotional support. Obtain medication history. Question pt for previous history of peripheral neuropathy.

Intervention/Evaluation

Monitor for peripheral neuropathy (characterized by numbness, tingling, or pain in hands or feet). Symptoms resolve promptly if therapy is discontinued (symptoms may worsen temporarily after drug is withdrawn). If symptoms resolve completely, reduced dosage may be resumed. Assess for headache, nausea, skin rash. Monitor skin for evidence of rash, signs of chills/fever. Determine pattern of bowel activity and stool consistency. Assess for muscle or joint aches, dizziness, sleep pattern. Assess eating pattern; monitor for weight loss. Check eyes for signs of conjunctivitis.

Patient/Family Teaching

Continue therapy for full length of treatment. Doses should be evenly spaced. Do not take any medications, including OTC drugs, w/o consulting physician. Stavudine is not a cure for HIV infection, nor does it reduce risk of transmission to others. Pt may continue to experience illnesses, including opportunistic infections. Do not drive, use machinery, or engage in other activities that require mental acuity if experiencing dizziness.

streptokinase

strep-toe-**kine**-ace
(Kabikinase, Streptase)

CANADIAN AVAILABILITY
Kabikinase, Streptase

PREGNANCY CATEGORY C

CLASSIFICATION

Thrombolytic

AVAILABILITY (Rx)

Powder for Injection: 250,000 IU, 600,000 IU, 750,000 IU, 1.5 million IU

PHARMACOKINETICS

Rapidly cleared from plasma by antibodies, reticuloendothelial system. Route of elimination unknown. Duration of action continues for several hours after discontinuing medication. **Half-life:** 23 min.

ACTION/*THERAPEUTIC EFFECT*

Activates fibrinolytic system by converting plasminogen to plasmin (enzyme that degrades fibrin clots). Acts indirectly by forming complex w/plasminogen, which converts plasminogen to plasmin. *Resultant effect destroys thrombi.* Action occurs within thrombus, on its surface, and in circulating blood.

USES

Management of acute myocardial infarction (lyses thrombi obstructing coronary arteries, decreases infarct size, improves ventricular function after MI, decreases CHF, mortality associated w/AMI). Lysis of diagnosed pulmonary emboli, acute/extensive thrombi of deep veins, and acute arterial thrombi/emboli. Clears totally/partially occluded arteriovenous cannulae.

STORAGE/HANDLING

Store vials at room temperature. Reconstitute vials immediately before use. Solution for direct IV administration may be used within 8 hrs of reconstitution. Discard unused portion.

ADMINISTRATION

Note: Must be administered within 12–14 hrs of clot formation (little effect on older, organized clots).

IV:

- Give by direct IV/IV infusion (via infusion pump). Infuse into selected thrombosed coronary artery, intra-arterially, or by cannula.
- Reconstitute vial w/5 ml 5% dextrose or 0.9% NaCl solution. (Add diluent slowly to side of vial, roll and tilt to avoid foaming. Do not shake vial.)
- Slight flocculation may occur; does not affect safe use of the drug.
- Further dilute w/50–500 ml 5% dextrose or 0.9% NaCl.
- If minor bleeding occurs at puncture sites, apply pressure for 30 min, then apply pressure dressing.
- Monitor B/P during infusion (hypotension may be severe, occurs in 1–10%). Decrease of infusion rate may be necessary.
- If uncontrolled hemorrhage occurs, discontinue infusion immediately (slowing rate of infusion may produce worsening hemorrhage). Do not use dextran to control hemorrhage.

INTRACORONARY:

- Monitor for arrhythmias during and immediately after infusion (atrial/ventricular).

INDICATIONS/ROUTES/DOSAGE

Note: Do not use from 5 days to 6 mos of previous streptokinase treatment of streptococcal infection (pharyngitis, rheumatic fever, acute glomerulonephritis secondary to streptococcal infection).

Acute evolving transmural myocardial infarction (give as soon as possible after symptoms occur):

IV Infusion: Adults, elderly: (1.5 million units diluted to 45 ml): 1.5 million IU infused over 60 min.

Intracoronary Infusion: Adults, elderly: (250,000 units diluted to 125 ml): Initially, 20,000 IU (10 ml) bolus; then, 2,000 IU/min for 60 min. ***Total dose:*** 140,000 IU.

Pulmonary embolism, deep vein thrombosis, arterial thrombosis/embolism (give within 7 days after onset):

IV Infusion: Adults, elderly: (1.5 million units diluted to 90 ml): Initially, 250,000 IU infused over 30 min; then, 100,000 IU/hr for 24–72 hrs for arterial thrombosis/embolism, 24–72 hrs for pulmonary embolism, 72 hrs for deep vein thrombosis.

Intracoronary Infusion: Adults, elderly: (1.5 million units diluted to 45 ml): Initially, 250,000 IU infused over 30 min; then, 100,000 IU/hr for maintenance.

Arteriovenous cannulae occlusion:
Instill 100,000–250,000 IU into each occluded cannula limb; clamp for 2 hrs. Aspirate contents of infused cannula limb; flush w/saline, reconnect cannula.

CONTRAINDICATIONS

Active internal bleeding, recent (within 2 mos) cerebrovascular accident, intracranial/intraspinal surgery, intracranial neoplasm, severe uncontrolled hypertension.

CAUTIONS

Recent (10 days) major surgery/ GI bleeding, obstetrical delivery, organ biopsy, trauma (cardiopulmonary resuscitation); uncontrolled arterial hypertension, left heart thrombus, endocarditis, severe hepatic/renal disease, pregnancy, elderly, cerebrovascular disease, diabetic retinopathy, thrombophlebitis, occluded AV cannula at infected site.

INTERACTIONS

DRUG: *Anticoagulants, heparin* may increase risk of hemorrhage. *Platelet aggregation inhibitors (e.g., aspirin)* may increase risk of bleeding. **HERBAL:** None known. **FOOD:** None significant. **ALTERED LAB VALUES:** Decreases plasminogen and fibrinogen level during infusion, decreasing clotting time (confirms presence of lysis).

SIDE EFFECTS

FREQUENT: Fever, superficial bleeding at puncture sites, decreased blood pressure. **OCCASIONAL:** Allergic reaction (rash, wheezing), bruising. **RARE:** Skin lesions.

ADVERSE REACTIONS/TOXIC EFFECTS

Severe internal hemorrhage may occur. Lysis of coronary thrombi may produce atrial/ventricular arrhythmias.

PATIENT CONSIDERATIONS

Baseline Assessment

Assess Hct, platelet count, thrombin (TT), activated thromboplastin (APTT), prothrombin (PT) time, fibrinogen level, before therapy is instituted. If heparin is component of treatment, discontinue before streptokinase is instituted (TT/APTT should be less than twice normal value before institution of therapy).

Intervention/Evaluation

Monitor EKG continuously. Assess clinical response, vital signs (pulse, temperature, respiratory rate, B/P) q4h or per protocol. Handle pt carefully and as infrequently as possible to prevent bleeding. Do not obtain B/P in lower extremities (possible deep vein thrombi). Monitor TT, PT, APTT, fibrinogen level q4h after initiation of therapy. Check stool for occult blood. Assess for decrease in B/P, increase in pulse rate, complaint of abdominal/ back pain, severe headache (may be evidence of hemorrhage). Question for increase in amount of discharge during menses. Assess area of thromboembolus for color, temperature. Assess peripheral pulses, skin for bruises and petechiae. Check for excessive bleeding from minor cuts, scratches. Assess urine output for hematuria.

---

streptomycin sulfate

(Streptomycin)

See Classification section under: Antibiotics: Aminoglycosides

streptozocin

(Zanosar)

See Classification section under: Cancer chemotherapy

succinylcholine chloride

(Anectine, Quelicin)

See Classification section under: Neuromuscular blockers

sucralfate

sue-kral-fate

(Carafate)

CANADIAN AVAILABILITY

Novo-Sucralate, Sulcrate

PREGNANCY CATEGORY B

CLASSIFICATION

Antiulcer

AVAILABILITY (Rx)

Tablets: 1 g. **Oral Suspension:** 500 mg/5 ml.

PHARMACOKINETICS

Absorption: Minimally absorbed from GI tract. **Excretion:** Eliminated in feces w/small amount excreted in urine.

ACTION/*THERAPEUTIC EFFECT*

Forms adhesive gel that adheres to ulcer site. *Gel protects damaged mucosa from further destruction by absorbing gastric acid, pepsin, bile salts* and reacting w/exudation of proteins.

USES/*UNLABELED*

Short-term treatment (up to 8 wks) of duodenal ulcer. Maintenance therapy of duodenal ulcer after healing of acute ulcers. *Treatment of gastric ulcer, rheumatoid arthritis (relieves GI symptoms associated w/NSAIDs), prevents/treatment of stress-related mucosal damage especially ICU pts, treatment of gastroesophageal reflux.*

ADMINISTRATION

ORAL:

- Administer 1 hr before meals and at bedtime.
- Tablets may be crushed/dissolved in water.
- Avoid antacids ½ hr before or after giving sucralfate.

INDICATIONS/ROUTES/DOSAGE

Note: 1 g = 10 ml suspension.

Duodenal ulcers, active:
Oral: Adults, elderly: 1 g 4 times/day (before meals and at bedtime) for up to 8 wks.

Duodenal ulcers, maintenance:
Oral: Adults, elderly: 1 g 2 times/day.

CONTRAINDICATIONS

None significant.

CAUTIONS

None significant.

INTERACTIONS

DRUG: ***Antacids*** may interfere w/binding (do not give within ½ hr). May decrease absorption of ***digoxin, phenytoin, quinolones (e.g., ciprofloxacin), theophylline*** (do not give within 2–3 hrs of sucralfate). **HERBAL:** None known. **FOOD:** None significant. **ALTERED LAB VALUES:** None significant.

SIDE EFFECTS

FREQUENT (2%): Constipation. **OCCASIONAL (<2%):** Dry mouth, backache, diarrhea, dizziness, drowsiness, nausea, indigestion, skin rash/hives/itching, stomach discomfort.

ADVERSE REACTIONS/TOXIC EFFECTS

None significant.

PATIENT CONSIDERATIONS

INTERVENTION/EVALUATION

Monitor stool consistency and frequency.

PATIENT/FAMILY TEACHING

Take medication on an empty stomach. Antacids may be given as an adjunct but should not be taken for 30 min before or after sucralfate (formation of sucralfate gel is activated by stomach acid). Dry mouth may be relieved by sour hard candy or sips of tepid water.

---

sufentanil citrate

(Sufenta)

See Classification section under: Opioid analgesics

---

sulconazole nitrate

(Exelderm)

See Classification section under: Antifungals: topical

---

sulfacetamide sodium

sul-fah-**see**-tah-mide

(AK-Sulf, Bleph-10, Isopto Cetamide, Ophthacet, Sodium Sulamyd, Sulfair)

FIXED-COMBINATION(S)

W/phenylephrine hydrochloride, a sympathomimetic **(Vasosulf)**; w/prednisolone, a steroid **(Blephamide, Cetapred, Metimyd, Optimyd, Sulphrin, Vasocidin)**

CANADIAN AVAILABILITY

Cetamide, Diosulf, Sodium Sulamyd

PREGNANCY CATEGORY C

CLASSIFICATION

Sulfonamide

AVAILABILITY (Rx)

Ophthalmic Solution: 10%, 15%, 30%. **Ophthalmic Ointment:** 10%. **Topical Lotion:** 10%.

PHARMACOKINETICS

Absorption: Minimal absorption after ophthalmic administration.

ACTION/*THERAPEUTIC EFFECT*

Interferes w/synthesis of folic acid that bacteria require for growth, *preventing further bacterial growth.* Bacteriostatic.

USES/*UNLABELED*

Treatment of corneal ulcers, conjunctivitis and other superficial infections of the eye, prophylaxis after injuries to the eye/removal of foreign bodies, adjunctive therapy for trachoma and inclusion conjunctivitis. ***Topical lotion:*** Seborrheic dermatitis, seborrheic sicca (dandruff), secondary bacterial skin infections. ***Ophthalmic:*** *Treatment of bacterial blepharitis, blepharoconjunctivitis, bacterial keratitis, keratoconjunctivitis.*

STORAGE/HANDLING

Protect from light. May develop a yellow-brown or reddish brown color. Do not use if color change occurs/precipitate forms.

ADMINISTRATION

OPHTHALMIC:

- Place finger on lower eyelid and pull out until a pocket is formed between eye and lower lid.
- Hold dropper above pocket and place correct number of drops ($^1/_4$–$^1/_2$ inch ointment) into pocket. Close eye gently.
- For solution: Apply digital pressure to lacrimal sac for 1–2 min (minimizes drainage into nose and throat, reducing risk of systemic effects). For ointment: Close eye for 1–2 min, rolling eyeball (increases contact area of drug to eye).
- Remove excess solution/ointment around eye w/tissue.

INDICATIONS/ROUTES/DOSAGE

Usual ophthalmic dosage:
Ophthalmic: Adults, elderly: Ointment: Apply small amount in lower conjunctival sac 1–4 times/day and at bedtime. ***Solution:*** 1–3 drops to lower conjunctival sac q2–3h.

Usual topical dosage:
Topical: Adults, elderly: Apply 1–4 times/day.

CONTRAINDICATIONS

Hypersensitivity to sulfonamides or any component of preparation (some products contain sulfite).

CAUTIONS

Extremely dry eye. Application of lotion to large infected, denuded, or debrided areas.

INTERACTIONS

DRUG: *Silver-containing preparations* are incompatible. **HERBAL:** None known. **FOOD:** None significant. **ALTERED LAB VALUES:** None significant.

SIDE EFFECTS

FREQUENT: Transient burning, stinging w/ophthalmic application. **OCCASIONAL:** Headache, local irritation. **RARE:** Hypersensitivity: erythema, rash, itching, swelling. Retarded corneal healing, photosensitivity.

ADVERSE REACTIONS/TOXIC EFFECTS

Superinfection, drug-induced lupus erythematosus, Stevens-Johnson syndrome occur rarely; nephrotoxicity w/high dermatologic concentrations.

PATIENT CONSIDERATIONS

Baseline Assessment

Question for hypersensitivity to sulfonamides, any ingredients of preparation (e.g., sulfite).

Intervention/Evaluation

Withhold medication and notify physician at once of hypersensitivity reaction (redness, itching, urticaria, rash). Assess for fever, joint pain, or sores in mouth—discontinue drug and inform physician immediately.

Patient/Family Teaching

Continue therapy as directed. May have transient burning, stinging upon ophthalmic application; may cause sensitivity to light—wear sunglasses, avoid bright light. Notify physician of *any* new symptom, especially swelling, itching, rash, joint pain, fever. For topical skin/scalp treatment, cleanse (shampoo) area before application to ensure direct contact w/affected areas.

sulfasalazine

sul-fah-**sal**-ah-zeen
(Azulfidine, Azulfidine EN-tabs)

CANADIAN AVAILABILITY
Salazopyrin, SAS-500

PREGNANCY CATEGORY B
(D if given near term)

CLASSIFICATION

Sulfonamide, anti-inflammatory

AVAILABILITY (Rx)

Tablets: 500 mg. **Oral Suspension:** 250 mg/5 ml.

PHARMACOKINETICS

Absorption: Poorly absorbed from GI tract. Cleaved in colon by intestinal bacterial forming sulfapyridine and mesalamine (5-ASA). Absorbed in colon. Widely distributed. **Metabolism:** Metabolized in liver. **Excretion:** Primarily excreted in urine. **Half-life:** sulfapyridine: 6–14 hrs; 5-ASA: 0.6–1.4 hrs.

ACTION / *THERAPEUTIC EFFECT*

Blocks prostaglandin synthesis, *producing anti-inflammatory and antibacterial effect.*

USES / *UNLABELED*

Treatment of ulcerative colitis, inflammatory bowel disease, rheumatoid arthritis. Juvenile rheumatoid arthritis in children 6–16 yrs. *Treatment of ankylosing spondylitis.*

ADMINISTRATION

ORAL:

- Space doses evenly (intervals not to exceed 8 hrs).
- Administer after meals if possible (prolong intestinal passage).
- Swallow enteric-coated tablets whole; do not chew.
- Give w/8 oz water; encourage several glasses of water between meals.

INDICATIONS / ROUTES / DOSAGE

Ulcerative colitis:
Oral: Adults, elderly: Initially, 1–4 g/day in divided doses. ***Maintenance:*** 2 g/day in 4 divided doses. ***Children >2 yrs:*** Initially, 40–60 mg/kg/day in 4–6 divided doses. ***Maintenance:*** 20–30 mg/kg in 4 divided doses. ***Maximum:*** 2 g/day.

Rheumatoid arthritis:
Oral: Adults, elderly: Initially, 0.5–1 g/day for 1 wk. Increase by 0.5 g/wk, up to 3 g/day.

CONTRAINDICATIONS

Hypersensitivity to salicylates, sulfonamides, sulfonylureas, thiazide or loop diuretics, carbonic anhydrase inhibitors, sunscreens containing PABA, local anesthetics, pregnancy at term, severe hepatic/renal dysfunction, porphyria, intestinal/urinary tract obstruction, children <2 yrs.

CAUTIONS

Severe allergies, bronchial asthma, impaired hepatic/renal function, G-6-PD deficiency.

INTERACTIONS

DRUG: May increase effects of ***oral anticoagulants, anticonvulsants, oral hypoglycemics, methotrexate. Hemolytics*** may increase toxicity. ***Hepatotoxic medications*** may increase hepatotoxicity. **HERBAL:** None known. **FOOD:** None significant. **ALTERED LAB VALUES:** None significant.

SIDE EFFECTS

FREQUENT (33%): Anorexia, nausea, vomiting, headache, oligospermia (generally reversed by withdrawal of drug). **OCCASIONAL (1–5%):** Hypersensitivity reaction: rash, urticaria, pruritus, fever, anemia. **RARE (<1%):** Tinnitus, hypoglycemia, diuresis, goiter production, photosensitivity.

ADVERSE REACTIONS/TOXIC EFFECTS

Anaphylaxis, Stevens-Johnson syndrome, hematologic toxicity (leukopenia, agranulocytosis); hepatotoxicity, nephrotoxicity occur rarely.

PATIENT CONSIDERATIONS

Baseline Assessment

Question for hypersensitivity to medications (see Contraindications). Check initial urinalysis, CBC, hepatic and renal function tests.

Intervention/Evaluation

Check I&O, urinalysis, renal function tests; assure adequate hydration (minimum output 1,500 ml/24 hr) to prevent nephrotoxicity. Evaluate food tolerance (distribute doses more evenly or consult physician regarding enteric-coated tablets, reduction of dose). Assess skin for rash (discontinue drug/notify physician at first sign). Check pattern of bowel activity, stool consistency (dosage may need to be increased if diarrhea continues/recurs). Monitor CBC closely; assess for/report immediately hematologic effects: bleeding, bruising, fever, sore throat, pallor, weakness, purpura, jaundice.

Patient/Family Teaching

May cause orange-yellow discoloration of urine, skin. Space doses evenly around the clock. Take after food w/8 oz water; drink several glasses of water between meals. Continue for full length of treatment; may be necessary to take drug even after symptoms relieved. Do not take any other medications (including vitamins) w/o consulting physician. Follow-up, lab tests are essential. In event of dental/other surgery inform dentist/surgeon of sulfasalazine therapy. Notify physician of any new symptom, immediately for fever, sore throat, shortness of breath, rash, any bleeding, ringing in ears. Avoid exposure to sun/ultraviolet light until photosensitivity determined (may last for months after last dose).

S

sulindac

suel-**in**-dak
(Clinoril)

CANADIAN AVAILABILITY
Apo-Sulin, Novo Sundac

PREGNANCY CATEGORY B
(D if used in third trimester or near delivery)

CLASSIFICATION

Nonsteroidal anti-inflammatory

AVAILABILITY (Rx)

Tablets: 150 mg, 200 mg

PHARMACODYNAMICS

	ONSET	PEAK	DURATION
Oral (antirheumatic):	7 days	2–3wks	—

PHARMACOKINETICS

Absorption: Well absorbed from GI tract. **Metabolism:** Metabolized in liver to active metabolite. **Excretion:** Primarily excreted in urine. **Half-life:** 7.8 hrs; metabolite: 16.4 hrs.

ACTION/*THERAPEUTIC EFFECT*

Produces analgesic and anti-inflammatory effect by inhibiting prostaglandin synthesis, *reducing inflammatory response and intensity of pain stimulus reaching sensory nerve endings.*

USES

Treatment of pain of rheumatoid arthritis, osteoarthritis, ankylosing spondylitis, acute painful shoulder, bursitis/tendinitis, acute gouty arthritis.

ADMINISTRATION

ORAL:

- May give w/food, milk, or antacids if GI distress occurs.

INDICATIONS/ROUTES/DOSAGE

Rheumatoid arthritis, osteoarthritis, ankylosing spondylitis:
Oral: Adults, elderly: Initially, 150 mg 2 times/day, up to 400 mg/day.

Acute painful shoulder, gouty arthritis, bursitis, tendinitis:
Oral: Adults, elderly: 200 mg 2 times/day.

CONTRAINDICATIONS

Active peptic ulcer, GI ulceration, chronic inflammation of GI tract, GI bleeding disorders, history of hypersensitivity to aspirin/NSAIDs.

CAUTIONS

Impaired renal/hepatic function, history of GI tract disease, predisposition to fluid retention.

INTERACTIONS

DRUG: May increase effects of ***oral anticoagulants, heparin, thrombolytics.*** May decrease effect of ***antihypertensives, diuretics. Salicylates, aspirin*** may increase risk of GI side effects, bleeding. ***Bone marrow depressants*** may increase risk of hematologic reactions. May increase concentration, toxicity of ***lithium.*** May increase ***methotrexate*** toxicity. ***Probenecid*** may increase concentration. ***Antacids*** may decrease concentration. **HERBAL:** May decrease effects of feverfew. Ginkgo biloba may increase risk of bleeding. **FOOD:** None significant. **ALTERED LAB VALUES:** May increase alkaline phosphatase, liver function tests.

SIDE EFFECTS

Note: Age increases possibility of side effects. **FREQUENT (3–9%):** Diarrhea/constipation, indigestion, nausea, maculopapular rash, dermatitis, dizziness, headache. **OCCASIONAL (1–3%):** Anorexia, GI cramps, flatulence.

ADVERSE REACTIONS/TOXIC EFFECTS

GI bleeding, peptic ulcer occur infrequently. Nephrotoxicity (glomerular nephritis, interstitial nephritis, and nephrotic syndrome) may occur in those w/preexisting impaired renal function. Acute hypersensitivity reaction (fever, chills, joint pain) occurs rarely.

PATIENT CONSIDERATIONS

BASELINE ASSESSMENT

Assess onset, type, location, and duration of pain, fever, or inflammation. Inspect appearance of affected joints for immobility, deformities, and skin condition.

INTERVENTION/EVALUATION

Assist w/ambulation if dizziness occurs. Monitor pattern of daily bowel activity, stool consistency.

Assess for evidence of rash. Evaluate for therapeutic response: relief of pain, stiffness, swelling, increase in joint mobility, reduced joint tenderness, improved grip strength.

PATIENT/FAMILY TEACHING

Therapeutic antiarthritic effect noted 1–3 wks after therapy begins. Avoid aspirin, alcohol during therapy (increases risk of GI bleeding). If GI upset occurs, take w/food, milk.

sumatriptan succinate injection

sue-mah-**trip**-tan
(Imitrex)

CANADIAN AVAILABILITY
Imitrex

PREGNANCY CATEGORY C

CLASSIFICATION

Antimigraine

AVAILABILITY (Rx)

Tablets: 25 mg, 50 mg. **Injection:** 12 mg/ml. **Nasal Spray:** 5 mg, 20 mg.

PHARMACODYNAMICS

	ONSET	PEAK	DURATION
SubQ	<10 min	<2 hrs	—

PHARMACOKINETICS

Absorption: Rapidly absorbed after SubQ administration. Widely distributed, protein binding (10–21%). **Metabolism:** Undergoes first-pass hepatic metabolism. **Excretion:** Excreted in urine. **Half-life:** 2 hrs.

ACTION/*THERAPEUTIC EFFECT*

Binds selectively to vascular receptors producing a vasoconstrictive effect on cranial blood vessels, *producing relief of migraine headache.* Efficiency of relief unaffected by aura, duration of attack, concurrent use of other antimigraine medications (e.g., beta blockers).

USES

Acute treatment of migraine headache w/ or w/o aura; treatment of cluster headaches.

STORAGE/HANDLING

Store at room temperature.

INDICATIONS/ROUTES/DOSAGE

Vascular headache:
SubQ: Adults, elderly: 6 mg. ***Maximum:*** No more than two 6 mg injections within a 24 hr period separated by at least 1 hr between injections.

Oral: Adults, elderly: 50 mg. ***Maximum single dose:*** 100 mg. May repeat no sooner than 2 hrs. ***Maximum:*** 300 mg/24 hrs.

Nasal: Adults, elderly: 5–20 mg; may repeat in 2 hrs. ***Maximum:*** 40 mg/24 hrs.

CONTRAINDICATIONS

IV use, those w/ischemic heart disease (angina pectoris, history of myocardial infarction), silent ischemia, Prinzmetal's angina, uncontrolled hypertension, concurrent ergotamine-containing preparations, hemiplegic or basilar migraine.

CAUTIONS

Hepatic, renal impairment. Pt profile suggesting cardiovascular risks.

INTERACTIONS

DRUG: *Ergotamine-containing drugs* may produce vasospastic reaction. *Monoamine oxidase inhibitors* may increase concentration, half-life. **HERBAL:** None known. **FOOD:** None significant. **ALTERED LAB VALUES:** None significant.

SIDE EFFECTS

FREQUENT: *Oral (5–10%):* Tingling, nasal discomfort. *SubQ (>10%):* Injection site reactions, tingling, warm, hot sensation, dizziness, vertigo. *Nasal (>10%):* Bad, unusual taste, nausea, vomiting. OCCASIONAL: *Oral (1–5%):* Flushing, weakness, visual disturbances. *SubQ (2–10%):* Burning sensation, numbness, chest discomfort, drowsiness, weakness. *Nasal (1–5%):* Discomfort of nasal cavity/throat, dizziness. RARE: *Oral (<1%):* Agitation, eye irritation, dysuria. *SubQ (<2%):* Anxiety, fatigue, sweating, muscle cramps, muscle pain. *Nasal (<1%):* Burning sensation.

ADVERSE REACTIONS/TOXIC EFFECTS

Excessive dosage may produce tremor, redness of extremities, reduced respirations, cyanosis, convulsions, paralysis. Serious arrhythmias occur rarely, but particularly in those w/hypertension, obesity, smokers, diabetics, and those w/strong family history of coronary artery disease.

PATIENT CONSIDERATIONS

Baseline Assessment

Question pt regarding history of peripheral vascular disease, renal/hepatic impairment, or possibility of pregnancy. Question pt regarding onset, location, and duration of migraine and possible precipitating symptoms.

Intervention/Evaluation

Evaluate for relief of migraine headache and resulting photophobia, phonophobia (sound sensitivity), nausea and vomiting.

Patient/Family Teaching

Teach pt proper loading of autoinjector, injection technique, and discarding of syringe. Do not use more than 2 injections during any 24 hr period and allow at least 1 hr between injections. If experience wheezing, heart throbbing, skin rash, swelling of eyelids/face/lips, pain/tightness in chest or throat, contact physician immediately.

tacrine

tay-crin
(Cognex)

PREGNANCY CATEGORY C

CLASSIFICATION

Cholinergic agent

AVAILABILITY (Rx)

Capsules: 10 mg, 20 mg, 30 mg, 40 mg

PHARMACOKINETICS

Absorption: Rapidly absorbed from GI tract. **Metabolism:** Undergoes first-pass metabolism in liver. **Half-life:** 2–4 hrs.

ACTION/*THERAPEUTIC EFFECT*

Elevates acetylcholine concentrations in cerebral cortex by slowing degeneration of acetylcholine released by still intact cholinergic neurons (Alzheimer's disease involves degeneration of cholinergic neuronal pathways). *Resultant effect slows Alzheimer's disease process.*

USES

Symptomatic treatment of pts w/Alzheimer's disease.

ADMINISTRATION

ORAL:

- May give w/o regard to food.

INDICATIONS/ROUTES/DOSAGE

Alzheimer's disease:

Oral: Adults, elderly: Initially, 10 mg 4 times/day for 6 wks; then 20 mg 4 times/day for 6 wks; then 30 mg 4 times/day for 12 wks; then to maximum of 40 mg 4 times/day if needed.

Note: If medication is stopped for >14 days, must retitrate as noted above.

CONTRAINDICATIONS

Known hypersensitivity to cholinergics; current treatment w/other cholinesterase inhibitors; severe, active liver disease; active, untreated gastric/duodenal ulcers; mechanical obstruction of intestine/urinary tract; pregnancy, nursing, or childbearing potential.

CAUTIONS

Known liver dysfunction, asthma, COPD, seizure disorders, bradycardia, hyperthyroidism, cardiac arrhythmias, history of gastric/intestinal ulcers, alcohol abuse.

INTERACTIONS

DRUG: May increase ***theophylline*** concentration; ***cimetidine*** may increase tacrine concentrations; may interfere w/***anticholinergics;*** may increase adverse effects of *NSAIDs.* **HERBAL:** None known. **FOOD:** None significant. **ALTERED LAB VALUES:** Increases SGOT (AST), SGPT (ALT); alters hematocrit, hemoglobin, electrolytes.

SIDE EFFECTS

FREQUENT (>10%): Headache, nausea, vomiting, diarrhea, dizziness. **OCCASIONAL (3–10%):** Fatigue, chest pain, decreased weight, dyspepsia, loss of appetite, abdominal pain, constipation, confusion, ataxia, inability to sleep, rhinitis, cough, rash, muscle pain. **RARE (<3%):** Asthenia, back pain, tremor.

ADVERSE REACTIONS/TOXIC EFFECTS

Overdose can cause cholinergic crises (increased salivation, lacrimation, urination, defecation, bradycardia, hypotension, increased muscle weakness). Treatment aimed at general supportive measures, use of anticholinergics (e.g., atropine).

PATIENT CONSIDERATIONS

BASELINE ASSESSMENT

Assess cognitive, behavioral, and functional deficits of pt. Assess liver function.

INTERVENTION/EVALUATION

Monitor cognitive, behavioral, and functional status of pt. Monitor SGOT (AST), SGPT (ALT). EKG evaluation, periodic rhythm strips in pts w/underlying arrhythmias. Monitor for symptoms of ulcer, GI bleeding.

PATIENT/FAMILY TEACHING

Take at regular intervals, between meals (may take w/meals if GI upset occurs). Do not reduce or stop medication; do not increase dosage w/o physician direction. Report increasing or new symptoms. Do not smoke (reduces plasma concentration of tacrine). Periodic lab tests are essential. Inform family of local chapter of Alzheimer's Disease Association (provides a guide to services for these pts).

tacrolimus

tack-row-**lee**-mus
(Prograf)

CANADIAN AVAILABILITY
Prograf

PREGNANCY CATEGORY C

CLASSIFICATION

Immunosuppressant

AVAILABILITY (Rx)

Capsules: 1 mg, 5 mg. **Injection:** 5 mg/ml.

PHARMACOKINETICS

Absorption: Variably absorbed following oral administration (food reduces absorption). **Metabolism:** Extensively metabolized in the liver. **Excretion:** Excreted in urine. **Half-life:** 11.7 hrs.

ACTION/*THERAPEUTIC EFFECT*

Binds to intracellular protein, forming a complex, inhibiting phosphatase activity. This effect results in inhibition of T-lymphocyte activation, suppressing immunologically mediated inflammatory response. *Assists in prevention of liver transplant rejection.*

USES/*UNLABELED*

Prophylaxis of organ rejection in pts receiving allogeneic liver transplants, kidney transplants. Should be used concurrently w/adrenal corticosteroids. *Bone marrow, cardiac, pancreas, pancreatic island cell, and small-bowel transplantation. Treatment of autoimmune disease, severe recalcitrant psoriasis.*

STORAGE/HANDLING

Store diluted infusion solution in glass or polyethylene containers and discard after 24 hrs. Do not store in a PVC container (decreased stability, potential for extraction).

ADMINISTRATION

IV:

- Dilute w/0.9% NaCl injection or 5% dextrose injection to concentration between 0.004 and 0.02 mg/ml.
- Give as continuous IV infusion.
- Continuously monitor pt for anaphylaxis for at least 30 min following start of infusion. Stop infusion immediately at first sign of hypersensitivity reaction.

INDICATIONS/ROUTES/DOSAGE

Note: In pts unable to take capsules, initiate therapy with IV infusion. Give oral dose 8–12 hrs after discontinuing IV infusion. Titrate dosing based on clinical assessments of rejection and tolerability. In pts w/hepatic/renal function impairment, give lowest IV and oral dosing range (delay dosing up to 48 hrs or longer in pts w/postop oliguria).

Liver transplantation:
IV Infusion: Adults, elderly: 0.05–0.1 mg/kg/day with initial dose given no sooner than 6 hrs after transplant. Give adult pts doses at lower end of dosing range. Give in combination w/adrenal corticosteroids. Transfer to oral therapy when oral tolerance is apparent (usually occurs within 2–3 days).

Oral: Adults: 0.15–0.3 mg/kg/day given in 2 divided daily doses q12h. Give initial dose no sooner than 6 hrs after transplant. Give in combination w/adrenal corticosteroids.

Pediatric dosage (w/o preexisting renal or hepatic dysfunction):
IV Infusion: 0.1 mg/kg/day.

Oral: 0.3 mg/kg/day.

CONTRAINDICATIONS

Hypersensitivity to tacrolimus, hypersensitivity to HCO-60 polyoxyl 60 hydrogenated castor oil (used in vehicle for injection), cyclosporine (increased risk of ototoxicity).

CAUTIONS

Immunosuppressed pts, renal/hepatic function impairment.

INTERACTIONS

DRUG: ***Aminoglycosides, amphotericin B, cisplatin*** increase risk of renal dysfunction. ***Cyclosporine*** increases risk of nephrotoxicity. ***Antifungals, bromocriptine, calcium channel blockers, cimetidine, clarithromycin, cyclosporine, danazol, diltiazem, erythromycin, methylprednisolone, metoclopramide*** increase tacrolimus blood levels. ***Carbamazepine, phenobarbital, phenytoin, rifamycins*** decrease tacrolimus blood levels. Other ***immunosuppressants*** may increase risk of infection or development of lymphomas. ***Live virus vaccines*** may potentiate virus replication, increase vaccine side effects, decrease pt's antibody response to vaccine. **HERBAL:** None known. **FOOD:** None significant. **ALTERED LAB VALUES:** May increase creatinine, BUN, WBCs, glucose. May decrease thrombocytes, RBCs, magnesium. Alters potassium level.

T

SIDE EFFECTS

FREQUENT (>30%): Headache, tremor, insomnia, paresthesia, diarrhea, nausea, constipation, vomiting, abdominal pain, hypertension. **OCCASIONAL (10–30%):** Rash, pruritus, anorexia, asthenia, peripheral edema.

ADVERSE REACTIONS/TOXIC EFFECTS

Nephrotoxicity, pleural effusion occur frequently. Overt nephrotoxicity characterized by increasing serum creatinine, decrease in urine output. Thrombocytopenia, leukocytosis, anemia, atelectasis occur occasionally. Neurotoxicity, including tremor, headache, mental status changes, occur commonly. Sepsis, infection occur occasionally. Significant anemia, thrombocytopenia, leukocytosis may occur.

PATIENT CONSIDERATIONS

BASELINE ASSESSMENT

Assess medical history, especially renal function, drug history, especially other immunosuppressants. Have aqueous solution of epinephrine 1:1,000 available at bedside as well as O_2 before beginning IV infusion. Assess pt continuously for first 30 min following start of infusion and at frequent intervals thereafter.

INTERVENTION/EVALUATION

Closely monitor pts w/impaired renal function. Monitor lab values, especially serum creatinine, serum potassium levels. CBC w/differential, hepatic function tests. Monitor I&O closely. CBC should be performed weekly during first month of therapy, twice monthly during second and third months of treatment, then monthly throughout the first year. Report any major change in assessment of pt. Routinely watch for any change from normal.

PATIENT/FAMILY TEACHING

Contact physician if unusual bleeding or bruising, sore throat, mouth sores, abdominal pain, or fever occurs. Inform pts of need for laboratory tests while taking medication, increased risk of neoplasia.

talc

(Sclerosol)

See Supplement

tamoxifen citrate

(Nolvadex)

See Classification section under: Cancer chemotherapy

tamsulosin hydrochloride

tam-sul-**owe**-sin

(Flomax)

CANADIAN AVAILABILITY

Flomax

PREGNANCY CATEGORY B

CLASSIFICATION

Alpha-1-adrenergic blocker

AVAILABILITY (Rx)

Capsules: 0.4 mg

PHARMACOKINETICS

Absorption: Well absorbed following oral administration. Widely distributed. Protein binding 94–99%. **Metabolism:** Metabolized in the liver. **Excretion:** Primarily excreted in the urine. **Half-life:** 9–13 hrs.

ACTION / *THERAPEUTIC EFFECT*

An alpha-1 antagonist, targets receptors around bladder neck and prostate capsule, *resulting in relaxation of problem organs, improvement in urinary flow, symptoms of prostate hyperplasia.*

USES

Treatment of signs and symptoms of benign prostatic hyperplasia.

ADMINISTRATION

ORAL:

- Give at the same time each day, $\frac{1}{2}$ hr following the same meal.
- Do not crush or open capsule unless directed by physician.

INDICATIONS/ROUTES/DOSAGES

Benign prostatic hypertrophy: ***Oral: Adults:*** 0.4 mg once daily, approximately 30 min after same meal each day. Dosage may be increased to 0.8 mg once daily.

CONTRAINDICATIONS

History of sensitivity to tamsulosin.

CAUTIONS

Renal/hepatic function impairment.

INTERACTIONS

DRUG: Other alpha blocking agents ***(prazosin, terazosin, doxazosin)*** may have additive effect. May alter effects of ***warfarin.*** **HERBAL:** None known. **FOOD:** None significant. **ALTERED LAB VALUES:** None significant.

SIDE EFFECTS

FREQUENT: (5–21%): Headache, dizziness, abnormal ejaculation, asthenia (weakness), back pain, diarrhea, rhinitis. **OCCASIONAL (<5%):** Decreased libido, drowsiness, insomnia, nausea, orthostatic hypotension, chest discomfort.

ADVERSE REACTIONS/TOXIC EFFECTS

None significant.

PATIENT CONSIDERATIONS

Baseline Assessment

Question for sensitivity to tamsulosin, use of other alpha blocking agents, warfarin.

Intervention/Evaluation

Monitor pattern of daily bowel activity and stool consistency. Assist with ambulation if dizziness, lightheadedness occurs. Monitor renal function lab values.

Patient/Family Teaching

Take at the same time each day, 30 min after a meal. Caution when getting up from sitting or lying position. Avoid tasks that require alertness, motor skills until response to drug is established. Nasal congestion may occur. Do not chew, crush, or open capsule.

---

tazarotene

(Tazorac)

See Supplement

---

telmisartan

tell-mih-**sar**-tan

(Micardis)

FIXED-COMBINATION(S)

W/hydrochlorothiazide, a diuretic **(Micardis HCT)**

PREGNANCY CATEGORY C

Third trimester

PREGNANCY CATEGORY D

Second and third trimester

CLASSIFICATION

Antihypertensive

AVAILABILITY (Rx)

Tablets: 40 mg, 80 mg

PHARMACODYNAMICS

	ONSET	PEAK	DURATION
Oral	—	0.5–1 hr	24 hrs

PHARMACOKINETICS

Absorption: Rapidly and completely absorbed following oral administration. Bound to plasma proteins (99%). **Metabolism:** Undergoes hepatic metabolism to inactive metabolite. **Excretion:** Excreted in the feces. Not removed by hemodialysis. **Half-life:** 24 hrs.

T

ACTION/ *THERAPEUTIC EFFECT*

Potent vasodilator. An angiotensin II receptor (type AT_1) antagonist; blocks vasoconstrictor and aldesterone-secreting effects of angiotensin II, inhibiting the binding of angiotensin II to the AT_1 receptors, *producing vasodilation, decreased peripheral resistance, decrease in B/P.*

USES/ *UNLABELED*

Treatment of hypertension alone or in combination with other antihypertensives. *Treatment of heart failure.*

ADMINISTRATION

ORAL:

- Give w/o regard to meals.

INDICATIONS/ROUTES/DOSAGES

Note: May be given concurrently w/other antihypertensives. If B/P is not controlled by telmisartan alone, a diuretic may be added.

Hypertension:
Oral: Adults, elderly: 40 mg once daily. ***Dose range:*** 20–80 mg.

CONTRAINDICATIONS

None significant.

CAUTIONS

Biliary obstructive disorders, hepatic insufficiency.

INTERACTIONS

DRUG: Increases ***digoxin*** plasma concentration. Slightly decreases ***warfarin*** plasma concentration. **HERBAL:** None known. **FOOD:** None significant. **ALTERED LAB VALUES:** May increase in serum creatinine. May decrease Hgb, Hct.

SIDE EFFECTS

OCCASIONAL (3–7%): Upper respiratory tract infection, sinusitis, back/leg pain, diarrhea. **RARE (1%):** Dizziness, headache, fatigue, nausea, heartburn, myalgia, cough, peripheral edema.

ADVERSE REACTIONS/TOXIC EFFECTS

Overdosage may manifest as hypotension and tachycardia; bradycardia occurs less often. Institute supportive measures.

PATIENT CONSIDERATIONS

BASELINE ASSESSMENT

Obtain B/P and apical pulse immediately before each dose, in addition to regular monitoring (be alert to fluctuations). If excessive reduction in B/P occurs, place pt in supine position, feet slightly elevated. Question possibility of pregnancy (see Pregnancy Category). Assess medication history (especially diuretic). Question for history of hepatic/renal impairment, renal artery stenosis. Obtain BUN, serum creatinine, Hgb, and vital signs, particularly B/P, pulse rate.

INTERVENTION/EVALUATION

Maintain hydration (offer fluids frequently). Assess for evidence of upper respiratory infection. Assist with ambulation if dizziness occurs. Monitor all blood serum levels. Assess B/P for hypertension/hypotension.

PATIENT/FAMILY TEACHING

Inform female pt regarding consequences of second- and third-trimester exposure to irbesartan. Report pregnancy to physician as soon as possible. Avoid tasks that require alertness, motor skills (possible dizziness effect). Report any sign of infection (sore throat, fever). Do not stop taking medication. Need for lifelong control.

Caution against exercising during hot weather (risk of dehydration, hypotension).

temazepam

tem-**az**-eh-pam
(Restoril)

CANADIAN AVAILABILITY
Restoril

PREGNANCY CATEGORY X

CLASSIFICATION

Sedative-hypnotic **(Schedule IV)**

AVAILABILITY (Rx)

Capsules: 7.5 mg, 15 mg, 30 mg

PHARMACOKINETICS

Absorption: Well absorbed from GI tract. Widely distributed. Crosses blood-brain barrier. **Metabolism:** Metabolized in liver. **Excretion:** Primarily excreted in urine. **Half-life:** 8–15 hrs.

ACTION/*THERAPEUTIC EFFECT*

Enhances action of inhibitory neurotransmitter gamma-aminobutyric acid (GABA), *producing hypnotic effect due to CNS depression.*

USES

Short-term treatment of insomnia (up to 5 wks). Reduces sleep-induction time, number of nocturnal awakenings; increases length of sleep.

ADMINISTRATION

ORAL:

- Give w/o regard to meals.
- Capsules may be emptied and mixed w/food.

INDICATIONS/ROUTES/DOSAGE

Hypnotic:
Oral: Adults >18 yrs: 15–30 mg at bedtime. ***Elderly/debilitated:*** 7.5–15 mg at bedtime.

CONTRAINDICATIONS

Acute narrow-angle glaucoma, acute alcohol intoxication.

CAUTIONS

Impaired renal/hepatic function.

INTERACTIONS

DRUG: *Alcohol, CNS depressants* may increase CNS depressant effect. **HERBAL:** Kava kava, valerian may increase CNS effects. **FOOD:** None significant. **ALTERED LAB VALUES:** None significant.

SIDE EFFECTS

FREQUENT: Drowsiness, sedation, rebound insomnia (may occur for 1–2 nights after drug is discontinued), dizziness, confusion, euphoria. **OCCASIONAL:** Weakness, anorexia, diarrhea. **RARE:** Paradoxical CNS excitement, restlessness (particularly noted in elderly/debilitated).

ADVERSE REACTION/TOXIC EFFECTS

Abrupt or too rapid withdrawal may result in pronounced restlessness, irritability, insomnia, hand tremors, abdominal/muscle cramps, sweating, vomiting, seizures. Overdosage results in somnolence, confusion, diminished reflexes, coma.

PATIENT CONSIDERATIONS

BASELINE ASSESSMENT

Question for possibility of pregnancy before initiating therapy (Pregnancy Category X). Assess B/P, pulse, respirations immediately before administration. Raise bed rails. Provide environment conducive to sleep (back rub, quiet environment, low lighting).

INTERVENTION/EVALUATION

Assess sleep pattern of pt. Assess elderly/debilitated for paradoxical reaction, particularly during early therapy. Evaluate for therapeutic response: decrease in number of nocturnal awakenings, increase in length of sleep.

PATIENT/FAMILY TEACHING

Do not exceed prescribed dosage. Smoking reduces drug effectiveness. Rebound insomnia may occur when drug is discontinued after short-term therapy. Avoid alcohol and other CNS depressants. Inform physician if you are or are planning to become pregnant.

temozolomide

(Termodar)

See Supplement

tenecteplase

(TNKase)

See Supplement

teniposide

(Vumon)

See Classification section under: Cancer chemotherapy

terazosin hydrochloride

tear-**aye**-zoe-sin

(Hytrin)

CANADIAN AVAILABILITY

Apo-Terazosin, Hytrin

PREGNANCY CATEGORY C

CLASSIFICATION

Antihypertensive

AVAILABILITY (Rx)

Capsules: 1 mg, 2 mg, 5 mg, 10 mg

PHARMACODYNAMICS

	ONSET	PEAK	DURATION
Oral	15 min	1–2 hrs	12–24 hrs

PHARMACOKINETICS

Absorption: Rapid, complete absorption from GI tract. **Metabolism:** Metabolized in liver to active metabolite. **Excretion:** Primarily eliminated in feces via biliary system; excreted in urine. **Half-life:** 12 hrs.

ACTION/*THERAPEUTIC EFFECT*

Blocks alpha-adrenergic receptors. ***Hypertension:*** *Produces vasodilation, decreases peripheral resistance.* ***Benign prostatic hypertrophy:*** *Relaxes smooth muscle in bladder neck and prostate.*

USES

Treatment of mild to moderate hypertension. Used alone or in combination w/other antihypertensives. Treatment of benign prostatic hypertrophy.

ADMINISTRATION

ORAL:

- May give w/o regard to food.
- Tablets may be crushed.
- Administer first dose at bedtime (minimizes risk of fainting due to "first-dose syncope").

INDICATIONS/ROUTES/DOSAGE

Note: If medication is discontinued for several days, retitrate initially using 1 mg dose at bedtime.

Hypertension:
Oral: Adults, elderly: Initially, 1 mg at bedtime. Slowly increase dose to desired levels. ***Range:*** 1–5 mg/day as single or 2 divided doses. ***Maximum:*** 20 mg.

Benign prostatic hypertrophy:
Oral: Adults, elderly: Initially, 1 mg at bedtime. May increase up to 10 mg/day. ***Maximum:*** 20 mg/day.

CONTRAINDICATIONS

None significant.

CAUTIONS

Chronic renal failure, impaired hepatic function.

INTERACTIONS

DRUG: *Estrogen, NSAIDs, sympathomimetics* may decrease effect. *Hypotension-producing medications* may increase antihypertensive effect. **HERBAL:** None known. **FOOD:** None significant. **ALTERED LAB VALUES:** May decrease albumin, total protein, Hgb, Hct, WBC.

SIDE EFFECTS

FREQUENT (>5%): Dizziness, headache, unusually tired. **OCCASIONAL (1–5%):** Shortness of breath, peripheral edema (swelling of legs, feet), orthostatic hypotension, palpitations, tachycardia, back or joint pain, blurred vision, nausea, vomiting, nasal congestion, drowsiness.

ADVERSE REACTIONS/TOXIC EFFECTS

"First-dose syncope" (hypotension w/sudden loss of consciousness) generally occurs 30–90 min after giving initial dose of ≥2 mg, a too rapid increase in dose, or addition of another hypotensive agent to therapy. May be preceded by tachycardia (120–160 beats/min).

PATIENT CONSIDERATIONS

Baseline Assessment

Give first dose at bedtime. If initial dose is given during daytime, pt must remain recumbent for 3–4 hrs. Assess B/P, pulse immediately before each dose, and q15–30min until stabilized (be alert to B/P fluctuations).

Intervention/Evaluation

Monitor pulse diligently ("first-dose syncope" may be preceded by tachycardia). Assist w/ambulation if dizziness occurs. Assess for peripheral edema of hands, feet (usually, first area of low extremity swelling is behind medial malleolus in ambulatory, sacral area in bedridden).

Patient/Family Teaching

Noncola carbonated beverage, unsalted crackers, dry toast may relieve nausea. Nasal congestion may occur. Full therapeutic effect may not occur for 3–4 wks. Use caution driving, performing tasks requiring mental alertness. Use caution rising from sitting position. Report dizziness, palpitation, if bothersome.

terbinafine hydrochloride

tur-**bin**-ah-feen
(Lamisil, Lamisil Derma Gel)

CANADIAN AVAILABILITY
Lamisil

PREGNANCY CATEGORY B

CLASSIFICATION

Antifungal

AVAILABILITY (Rx)

Tablets: 250 mg. **Cream (OTC):** 1%. **Gel, Solution:** 1%.

PHARMACOKINETICS

Absorption: ***Topical:*** Minimal systemic absorption. ***Oral:*** Well absorbed following oral administration (unaffected by food). Distributed to sebum and skin. **Metabolism:** Extensively metabolized. **Excretion:** Eliminated in urine. **Half-life:** 200–400 hrs.

ACTION / *THERAPEUTIC EFFECT*

Fungicidal. Inhibits the enzyme, squalene epoxidase, interfering w/biosynthesis in fungi, *resulting in fungal cell death.*

USES

Systemic: Treatment of onychomycosis (fungal disease of nails due to dermatophytes). ***Topical:*** Treatment of *Tinea cruris* (jock itch), *T. pedis* (athlete's foot), *T. corporis* (ringworm). ***Derma-Gel:*** Treatment of *T. corporis, . T. pedis,* and *T. versicolor.*

ADMINISTRATION

ORAL:

- May give w/o regard to food.

INDICATIONS/ROUTES/DOSAGE

Note: Topical therapy for minimum 1 wk, not to exceed 4 wks.

Tinea pedis:
Topical: Adults, elderly, adolescents: Apply 2 times/day until signs/symptoms significantly improved.

Tinea cruris, T. corporis:
Topical: Adults, elderly, adolescents: Apply 1–2 times/day until signs/symptoms significantly improved.

Onychomycosis:
Oral: Adults, elderly, adolescents: 250 mg/day for 6 wks (fingernails), 12 wks (toenails).

CONTRAINDICATIONS

Hypersensitivity to terbinafine or any component in formulation. ***Oral:*** Preexisting liver disease or renal impairment (creatinine clearance ≤ 50 ml/min). Safety in children <12 yrs not established.

CAUTIONS

None significant.

INTERACTIONS

DRUG: ***Alcohol, other hepatotoxic medications*** may increase risk hepatotoxicity. ***Liver enzyme inhibitors*** may decrease clearance (e.g., ***cimetidine***). ***Liver enzyme inducers*** may increase clearance (e.g., ***rifampin***). **HERBAL:** None known. **FOOD:** None significant. **ALTERED LAB VALUES:** May increase SGPT (ALT), SGOT (AST).

SIDE EFFECTS

FREQUENT: ***Oral:*** Headache (13%). **OCCASIONAL:** ***Oral:*** Diarrhea, rash (6%), dyspepsia (4%), pruritus, taste disturbance, nausea (3%). **RARE:** ***Oral:*** Abdominal pain, flatulence, urticaria, visual disturbance. ***Topical:*** Irritation, burning, itching, dryness.

ADVERSE REACTIONS/TOXIC EFFECTS

Hepatobiliary dysfunction (including cholestatic hepatitis), serious skin reactions, severe neutropenia occur rarely. Ocular lens and retina changes have been noted.

PATIENT CONSIDERATIONS

BASELINE ASSESSMENT

Assure that diagnostic tests have

been completed, (e.g., culture or direct microscopic examination of scrapings from infected tissue). Liver function tests should be obtained in pts receiving treatment for >6 wks. Assess medication history. Obtain medical history, especially alcoholism, liver/renal impairment.

INTERVENTION/EVALUATION

Check for therapeutic response. Discontinue medication, notify physician if local reaction occurs (irritation, redness, swelling, itching, oozing, blistering, burning). Monitor CBC, liver function tests in pts receiving treatment for >6 wks.

PATIENT/FAMILY TEACHING

Complete full course of treatment. Use only as directed for the time indicated. Do not use topical cream for oral or intravaginal use; use externally only. Keep areas clean and dry; wear light clothing to promote ventilation. Separate personal items. Avoid topical cream contact w/eyes, nose, mouth, or other mucous membranes. Rub well into affected, surrounding area. Do not cover w/occlusive dressing or use other preparations w/o consulting physician. Notify physician if skin irritation, diarrhea occurs.

terbutaline sulfate

tur-**byew**-ta-leen

(Brethaire, Brethine, Bricanyl)

CANADIAN AVAILABILITY

Bricanyl

PREGNANCY CATEGORY B

CLASSIFICATION

Sympathomimetic

AVAILABILITY (Rx)

Tablets: 2.5 mg, 5 mg. **Aerosol:** 0.2 mg/activation. **Injection:** 1 mg/ml.

PHARMACODYNAMICS

	ONSET	PEAK	DURATION
Oral			
	30 min	1–3 hrs	4–8 hrs
SubQ			
	15 min	30–60 min	1.5–4 hrs
Inhalation			
	5–30 min	1–2 hrs	3–4 hrs

PHARMACOKINETICS

Absorption: Moderately absorbed from GI tract; well absorbed after SubQ administration. **Metabolism:** Metabolized in liver. **Excretion:** Primarily excreted in urine. **Half-life:** 11–16 hrs.

ACTION/*THERAPEUTIC EFFECT*

Bronchospasm: Stimulates beta$_2$-adrenergic receptors, *relaxes bronchial smooth muscle, relieves bronchospasm, reduces airway resistance.* ***Labor:*** *Relaxes uterine muscle, inhibiting uterine contractions.*

USES

Symptomatic relief of reversible bronchospasm due to bronchial asthma, bronchitis, emphysema. Delays premature labor in pregnancies between 20 and 34 wks.

STORAGE/HANDLING

Store oral, parenteral forms at room temperature. Do not use if solution appears discolored.

ADMINISTRATION

ORAL:

- May give w/o regard to food (take w/food if GI upset occurs).

- Tablets may be crushed.

INHALATION:

- Shake container well, exhale completely. Holding mouthpiece 1 inch away from lips, inhale and hold breath as long as possible before exhaling.
- Wait 1–10 min before inhaling second dose (allows for deeper bronchial penetration).
- Rinse mouth w/water immediately after inhalation (prevents mouth/throat dryness).

SUBQ:

- Inject SubQ into lateral deltoid region.

INDICATIONS/ROUTES/DOSAGE

Bronchospasm:
Oral: Adults, elderly, children >15 yrs: Initially, 2.5 mg 3–4 times/day. *Maintenance:* 2.5–5 mg 3 times/day q6h while awake. *Maximum:* 15 mg/day. *Children 12–15 yrs:* 2.5 mg 3 times/day. *Maximum:* 7.5 mg/day.

Inhalation: Adults, elderly, children >12 yrs: 2 inhalations q4–6h. Allow at least 1 min between inhalations.

SubQ: Adults: Initially, 0.25 mg. Repeat in 15–30 min if substantial improvement does not occur. *Maximum:* No more than 0.5 mg/4 hrs.

Premature labor:
Oral: Adults: 2.5 mg q4–6h until term.

IV Infusion: Adults: Initially, 10 mcg/min, increase by 5 mcg/min q10min up to maximum of 80 mcg/min or until contractions cease. (After contractions cease for $^1/_2$–1 hr, decrease by 5 mcg/min to lowest effective dose).

SubQ: Adults: 0.25 mg q1h until contractions cease.

CONTRAINDICATIONS

History of hypersensitivity to sympathomimetics.

CAUTIONS

Impaired cardiac function, diabetes mellitus, hypertension, hyperthyroidism, history of seizures.

INTERACTIONS

DRUG: *Tricyclic antidepressants* may increase cardiovascular effects. *MAO inhibitors* may increase risk of hypertensive crises. May decrease effects of *beta blockers. Digoxin, sympathomimetics* may increase risk of arrhythmias. HERBAL: None known. FOOD: None significant. ALTERED LAB VALUES: May decrease serum potassium levels.

SIDE EFFECTS

FREQUENT: Shakiness, restlessness, increased heart rate, and mild transient nausea if taken on an empty stomach. Drying or irritation of oropharynx noted w/inhalation therapy.

ADVERSE REACTIONS/TOXIC EFFECTS

Too frequent or excessive use may lead to loss of bronchodilating effectiveness and/or severe, paradoxical bronchoconstriction. Excessive sympathomimetic stimulation may cause palpitations, extrasystoles, tachycardia, chest pain, slight increase in B/P followed by a substantial decrease, chills, sweating, and blanching of skin.

PATIENT CONSIDERATIONS

BASELINE ASSESSMENT

Bronchospasm: Offer emotional support (high incidence of anxiety due to difficulty in breathing and sympathomimetic response to drug). *Preterm labor:* Assess uterine contractions (intensity, frequency, duration).

INTERVENTION/EVALUATION

Bronchospasm: Monitor rate, depth, rhythm, type of respiration; quality and rate of pulse. Assess lung sounds for rhonchi, wheezing, rales. Monitor arterial blood gases. Observe lips, fingernails for blue or dusky color in light-skinned pts; gray in dark-skinned pts. Observe for clavicular retractions, hand tremor. Evaluate for clinical improvement (quieter, slower respirations, relaxed facial expression, cessation of clavicular retractions). *Preterm labor:* Assess maternal heart rate, B/P, blood glucose, fluid status. Determine fetal heart rate.

PATIENT/FAMILY TEACHING

Bronchospasm: Increase fluid intake (decreases lung secretion viscosity). Do not take more than 2 inhalations at any one time (excessive use may produce paradoxical bronchoconstriction, or a decreased bronchodilating effect). Rinsing mouth w/water immediately after inhalation may prevent mouth/throat dryness. Avoid excessive use of caffeine derivatives (chocolate, coffee, tea, cola, cocoa). *Preterm labor:* Contractions may resume while on oral therapy. Contact physician if 4–6 contractions per hour occur.

terconazole

ter-**con**-ah-zole
(Terazol)

CANADIAN AVAILABILITY
Terazol

PREGNANCY CATEGORY C

CLASSIFICATION

Antifungal

AVAILABILITY (Rx)

Vaginal Cream: 0.4%, 0.8%. **Vaginal Suppository:** 80 mg.

PHARMACOKINETICS

Absorption: Systemic absorption minimal following intravaginal administration.

ACTION/*THERAPEUTIC EFFECT*

Disrupts fungal cell membrane permeability, *producing antifungal activity.*

USES

Treatment of vulvovaginal candidiasis (moniliasis).

ADMINISTRATION

INTRAVAGINAL:

- Use disposable gloves; always wash hands thoroughly after application.
- Follow manufacturer's directions for use of applicator.
- Insert suppository, applicator high in vagina.
- Administration at bedtime is preferred.

INDICATIONS/ROUTES/DOSAGE

Vulvovaginal candidiasis:
Intravaginal: Adults, elderly: Tablet: 1 suppository vaginally at bedtime for 3 days. ***Cream* (0.4%):** 1 applicatorful at bedtime for 7 days; **0.8%** for 3 days.

CONTRAINDICATIONS

Hypersensitivity to terconazole or any component of the cream or suppository.

CAUTIONS

Safety and efficacy in children not established.

INTERACTIONS

DRUG: None significant. **HERBAL:** None known. **FOOD:** None significant. **ALTERED LAB VALUES:** None significant.

SIDE EFFECTS

FREQUENT (>10%): Headache, vulvovaginal burning. **OCCASIONAL (1–10%):** Dysmenorrhea, pain in female genitalia, abdominal pain, fever, itching. **RARE (<1%):** Chills.

ADVERSE REACTIONS/TOXIC EFFECTS

None significant.

PATIENT CONSIDERATIONS

Baseline Assessment

Question for hypersensitivity to terconazole or components of preparation. Confirm that a potassium hydroxide (KOH) culture and/or smear were done for accurate diagnosis; therapy may begin before results known. For suppository, inquire about use of vaginal contraceptives (such as diaphragm), because base of suppository interacts w/rubber latex.

Intervention/Evaluation

Monitor temperature at least daily. Assess for therapeutic response or burning, itching, pain, or irritation.

Patient/Family Teaching

Do not interrupt or stop regimen, even during menses. Teach pt proper insertion. Not affected by oral contraception. Notify physician of increased itching, irritation, burning. Consult physician about sexual intercourse, douching, or the use of other vaginal products. Do not use vaginal contraceptive diaphragms, condoms within 72 hrs after treatment. Avoid contact w/eyes. Wash hands thoroughly after application.

---

testolactone

(Teslac)

See Classification section under: Cancer chemotherapy

---

testosterone

tess-**toss**-ter-own

(Andronaq, Histerone)

testosterone cypionate

(Depotest, Depo-Testosterone)

testosterone enanthate

(Delatest)

testosterone propionate

(Testex)

testosterone transdermal

(Androderm, Testoderm, Testoderm TTS)

FIXED-COMBINATION(S)

Testosterone cypionate w/estradiol cypionate, an estrogen **(depAndrogyn, Duratestrin, De-Comberol)**; testosterone enanthate w/estradiol cypionate **(Deladumone)**

CANADIAN AVAILABILITY

Delatestryl

PREGNANCY CATEGORY X

CLASSIFICATION

Androgen

AVAILABILITY (Rx)

Injection: 25 mg/ml, 50 mg/ml, 100 mg/ml. **Transdermal Patch:** 2.5 mg/24 hr, 4 mg/24 hr, 6 mg/24 hr.

Cypionate: Injection: 100 mg/ml, 200 mg/ml

Enanthate: Injection: 100 mg/ml, 200 mg/ml

Propionate: Injection: 100 mg/ml

PHARMACOKINETICS

Absorption: Well absorbed after IM administration. **Metabolism:** Metabolized in liver (undergoes first-pass metabolism). **Excretion:** Primarily excreted in urine. **Half-life:** 10–20 min.

ACTION/*THERAPEUTIC EFFECT*

Stimulates spermatogenesis, development of male secondary sex characteristics, sexual maturation at puberty. Stimulates production of RBCs. *Initiates male puberty, corrects hormonal deficiency, suppresses tumor growth in breast cancer.*

USES

Treatment of delayed puberty; testicular failure due to cryptorchidism, bilateral orchism, orchitis, vanishing testis syndrome, or orchidectomy; hypogonadotropic hypogonadism due to pituitary/hypothalamic injury (tumors, trauma, or radiation), idiopathic gonadotropin or luteinizing hormone releasing hormone deficiency. Palliative therapy in women 1–5 yrs postmenopausal w/advancing, inoperable metastatic breast cancer or premenopausal women who have benefited from oophorectomy and have a hormone-responsive tumor. Prevention of postpartum breast pain and engorgement. In combination w/estrogens for management of moderate to severe vasomotor symptoms associated w/menopause when estrogens alone are not effective.

ADMINISTRATION

IM:

- Give deep in gluteal muscle.
- Do *not* give IV.
- Warming and shaking redissolves crystals that may form in long-acting preparations.
- Wet needle of syringe may cause solution to become cloudy; this does not affect potency.

TRANSDERMAL:

TESTODERM:

- Apply to clean, dry scrotal skin that has been dry-shaved (optimal skin contact).
- Testoderm TTS may be applied to arm, back or upper buttock.

ANDRODERM:

- Apply to clean, dry area on skin on back, abdomen, upper arms, or thighs.
- Do not apply to bony prominences (e.g., shoulder) or oily, damaged, irritated skin. Do not apply to scrotum.
- Rotate application site with 7 day interval to same site.

INDICATIONS/ROUTES/DOSAGE

TESTOSTERONE, TESTOSTERONE PROPIONATE:

Androgen replacement therapy:
IM: Adults: 25–50 mg 2–3 times/wk.

Palliation of mammary cancer:
IM: Adults, elderly: 50–100 mg 3 times/wk.

Postpartum breast engorgement (propionate):
IM: Adults: 25–50 mg/day for 3–4 days (begin at time of delivery).

T

TESTOSTERONE CYPIONATE, TESTOSTERONE ENANTHATE:

Male hypogonadism (replacement therapy):
IM: Adults: 50–400 mg q2–4wks.

Males (delayed puberty):
IM: Adults: 50–200 mg q2–4wks.

Females: (palliation of inoperable breast cancer):
IM: Adults, elderly: 200–400 mg q2–4wks.

TESTOSTERONE TRANSDERMAL:

Males (replacement therapy):
Topical: Adults: 6 mg/day system.

CONTRAINDICATIONS

Hypersensitivity to drug or components of preparation; serious cardiac, renal, or hepatic dysfunction. Do not use for men w/carcinomas of the breast or prostate.

EXTREME CAUTION

In children because of bone maturation effects.

CAUTIONS

Epilepsy, migraine, or other conditions aggravated by fluid retention; metastatic breast cancer or immobility increases risk of hypercalcemia.

INTERACTIONS

DRUG: May increase effect of ***oral anticoagulants. Hepatotoxic medications*** may increase hepatotoxicity. **HERBAL:** None known. **FOOD:** None significant. **ALTERED LAB VALUES:** May increase SGOT (AST), alkaline phosphatase, bilirubin, calcium, potassium, sodium, Hgb, Hct, LDL. May decrease HDL.

SIDE EFFECTS

FREQUENT: Gynecomastia, acne, amenorrhea or other menstrual irregularities. ***Females:*** hirsutism, deepening of voice, clitoral enlargement (may not be reversible when drug discontinued). **OCCASIONAL:** Edema, nausea, insomnia, oligospermia, priapism, male pattern of baldness, bladder irritability, hypercalcemia in immobilized pts or those w/breast cancer, hypercholesterolemia, inflammation and pain at IM injection site. ***Transdermal:*** Itching, erythema, skin irritation. **RARE:** Polycythemia w/high dosage, hypersensitivity.

ADVERSE REACTIONS/TOXIC EFFECTS

Peliosis hepatitis (liver, spleen replaced w/blood-filled cysts), hepatic neoplasms and hepatocellular carcinoma have been associated w/prolonged high-dosage, anaphylactoid reactions.

PATIENT CONSIDERATIONS

BASELINE ASSESSMENT

Question for hypersensitivity to testosterone. Establish baseline weight, B/P, Hgb, and Hct. Check liver function test results, electrolytes, and cholesterol if ordered. Wrist x-rays may be ordered to determine bone maturation in children.

INTERVENTION/EVALUATION

Weigh daily and report weekly gain of more than 5 lbs; evaluate for edema. Monitor I&O. Check B/P at least 2 times/day. Assess electrolytes, cholesterol, Hgb, and Hct (periodically for high dosage), liver function test results. W/breast cancer or immobility, check for hypercalcemia (lethargy, muscle weakness, confusion, irritability). Assure adequate intake of protein, calories. Assess for virilization. Monitor sleep patterns. Check injection site for redness, swelling, or pain.

PATIENT/FAMILY TEACHING

Regular visits to physician and monitoring tests are necessary. Do not take any other medications w/o consulting physician. Teach diet high in protein, calories. Food may be tolerated better in small, frequent feedings. Weigh daily, report 5 lbs/gain/wk. Notify physician if nausea, vomiting, acne, or ankle swelling occurs. *Females:* Promptly report menstrual irregularities, hoarseness, deepening of voice. *Males"* Report frequent erections, difficulty urinating, gynecomastia.

tetracaine

(Pontocaine)

See Classification section under: Anesthetics: local

tetracycline hydrochloride

tet-rah-**sigh**-clean

(Achromycin, Actisite, Panmycin, Robitet, Sumycin, Topicycline)

CANADIAN AVAILABILITY

Apo-Tetra, Novotetra

PREGNANCY CATEGORY D

CLASSIFICATION

Antibiotic: Tetracycline

AVAILABILITY (Rx)

Capsules: 250 mg, 500 mg. **Tablets:** 250 mg, 500 mg. **Topical Solution. Topical Ointment:** 3%.

PHARMACOKINETICS

Absorption: Readily absorbed from GI tract. Widely distributed. **Excretion:** Excreted in urine; eliminated in feces via biliary system. Slowly removed by hemodialysis. **Half-life:** 6–11 hrs (increased in decreased renal function).

ACTION/*THERAPEUTIC EFFECT*

Inhibits protein synthesis by binding to ribosomes, *preventing bacterial cell growth.* Bacteriostatic.

USES/*UNLABELED*

Treatment of uncomplicated gonorrhea, syphilis (when allergic to penicillin), adjunctive therapy for acne, urinary tract infection, Rocky Mountain spotted fever, typhus, Q fever, cholera, psittacosis, brucellosis, yaws, bejel, pinta, anthrax, actinomycosis, Whipple's disease, rat bite fever. Treatment of H. Pylori-associated peptic ulcer disease (w/bismuth subsalicylate/metronidazole). ***Topical:*** Inflammatory acne vulgaris, superficial infections. *Treatment of gonorrhea, malaria.*

STORAGE/HANDLING

Store capsules, oral suspension at room temperature.

ADMINISTRATION

ORAL:

- Give capsules, tablets w/full glass of water 1 hr before or 2 hrs after meals, milk.

TOPICAL:

- Cleanse area gently before application.
- Apply only to affected area.

INDICATIONS/ROUTES/DOSAGE

Note: Space doses evenly around the clock.

Usual dosage:
Oral: Adults, elderly: 1–3 g/day in 2–4 divided doses. ***Children >8 yrs:*** 25–50 mg/kg/day in 2–4 divided doses.

***H. pylori* peptic ulcer:**
Oral: Adults: 500 mg 4 times/day for 14 days (w/bismuth subsalicylate, metronidazole).

Usual topical dosage:
Topical: Adults, elderly: Apply 2 times/day in morning, evening.

CONTRAINDICATIONS

Hypersensitivity to tetracyclines, sulfite, children ≤age 8 yrs.

CAUTIONS

Sun/ultraviolet light exposure (severe photosensitivity reaction).

INTERACTIONS

DRUG: ***Cholestyramine, colestipol*** may decrease absorption. May decrease effect of ***oral contraceptives. Carbamazepine, phenytoin*** may decrease concentrations. **HERBAL:** St. John's wort may increase risk of photosensitivity. **FOOD:** Avoid dairy products 1 hr before or 2 hrs after taking tetracycline. **ALTERED LAB VALUES:** May increase BUN, SGOT (AST), SGPT (ALT), alkaline phosphatase, amylase, bilirubin concentrations.

SIDE EFFECTS

FREQUENT: Dizziness, lightheadedness, diarrhea, nausea, vomiting, stomach cramps, increased sensitivity of skin to sunlight. ***Topical:*** Dry scaly skin, stinging, burning feeling. **OCCASIONAL:** Pigmentation of skin, mucous, membranes, itching in rectal/genital area, sore mouth, tongue. ***Topical:*** Pain, redness, swelling, other skin irritation.

ADVERSE REACTIONS/TOXIC EFFECTS

Superinfection (especially fungal), anaphylaxis, increased intracranial pressure, bulging fontanelles occur rarely in infants.

PATIENT CONSIDERATIONS

BASELINE ASSESSMENT

Question for history of allergies, especially tetracyclines, sulfite. Obtain specimens for culture and sensitivity before giving first dose (therapy may begin before results are known).

INTERVENTION/EVALUATION

Assess skin for rash. Determine pattern of bowel activity and stool consistency. Monitor food intake, tolerance. Be alert for superinfection: diarrhea, ulceration, or changes of oral mucosa, anal/genital pruritus. Monitor B/P and level of consciousness because of potential for increased intracranial pressure.

PATIENT/FAMILY TEACHING

Continue antibiotic for full length of treatment. Space doses evenly. Take oral doses on empty stomach (1 hr before or 2 hrs after food/beverages). Drink full glass of water w/capsules and avoid bedtime doses. Notify physician in event of diarrhea, rash, other new symptom. Protect skin from sun exposure. Consult physician before taking any other medication. *Topical:* Skin may turn yellow w/Topicycline application (washing removes solution); fabrics may be stained by heavy application. Do not apply to deep/open wounds.

tetrahydrozyline hydrochloride

tet-rah-high-**droz**-ah-leen
(Visine, Tyzine)

FIXED-COMBINATION(S)
W/benzalkonium chloride, a wetting agent, and edetate disodium, a chelating agent **(Murine Plus, Visine A.C.)**

PREGNANCY CATEGORY C

CLASSIFICATION

Sympathomimetic

AVAILABILITY (OTC)

Nasal Solution: 0.05%, 0.1%. **Ophthalmic Solution:** 0.05%.

PHARMACODYNAMICS

	ONSET	PEAK	DURATION
Ophthalmic			
	Several minutes	—	4–8 hrs
Intranasal			
	Several minutes	—	4–8 hrs

PHARMACOKINETICS

Absorption: May be systemically absorbed. **Metabolism/excretion:** Metabolic, elimination rates unknown.

ACTION/*THERAPEUTIC EFFECT*

Stimulates alpha-adrenergic receptors in sympathetic nervous system. ***Ophthalmic:*** Constricts arterioles, *reduces redness, irritation.* ***Intranasal:*** Constricts arterioles, *reduces congestion.*

USES

Ophthalmic: Relief of itching, minor irritation and to control hyperemia in pts w/superficial corneal vascularity. Combination solutions relieve discomfort due to minor eye irritations and symptoms related to dry eyes. ***Intranasal:*** Relief of nasal congestion of rhinitis, the common cold, sinusitis, hay fever, or other allergies; reduces swelling and improves visualization for surgery or diagnostic procedures; opens obstructed eustachian ostia in pts w/ear inflammation.

ADMINISTRATION

OPHTHALMIC:

- Instruct pt to tilt head backward and look up.
- Gently pull lower lid down to form pouch and instill medication.
- Do not touch tip of applicator to lids or any surface.
- After releasing lower lid, have pt close eyes w/o squeezing.
- Apply gentle finger pressure to lacrimal sac (bridge of the nose, inside corner of the eye) for 1–2 min.
- Remove excess solution around eye w/tissue. Wash hands immediately to remove medication on hands.

INTRANASAL:

- Drops should be administered w/pt in lateral, head-low position or reclining w/head tilted back as far as possible.
- Pt should maintain same position for 5 min, then drops applied to other nostril.
- Dropper containers should be used by only one person; tips of dispensers or droppers should be rinsed well w/hot water after use.

INDICATIONS/ROUTES/DOSAGE

Usual nasal dosage:
Adults, elderly, children >6 yrs: 2–4 drops (0.1% solution) to each nostril q4–6h (no sooner than

q3h). *Children, 2–6 yrs:* 2–3 drops (0.05% solution) to each nostril q4–6h (no sooner than q3h).

Usual ophthalmic dosage: *Adults, elderly, children:* 1–2 drops (0.05%) 2–4 times/day.

CONTRAINDICATIONS

Known hypersensitivity to tetrahydrozyline or components of preparation; children <2 yrs of age (the 0.1% nasal solution is contraindicated in children <6 yrs of age); pts w/angle closure glaucoma or other serious eye diseases.

CAUTIONS

Some caution should be taken when using w/cardiac disease, hyperthyroidism, hypertension, diabetes mellitus, cerebral arteriosclerosis, bronchial asthma, monoamine oxidase inhibitors.

INTERACTIONS

DRUG: ***Maprotiline, tricyclic antidepressants*** may increase pressor effects. ***MAO inhibitors*** may cause severe hypertensive reaction. **HERBAL:** Ma Huang (Ephedra) may increase CNS effects. **FOOD:** None significant. **ALTERED LAB VALUES:** None significant.

SIDE EFFECTS

OCCASIONAL: ***Intranasal:*** Transient burning, stinging, sneezing, dryness of mucosa. ***Ophthalmic:*** Irritation, blurred vision, mydriasis. Systemic sympathomimetic effects may occur w/either route: headache, hypertension, weakness, sweating, palpitations, tremors. Prolonged use may result in rebound congestion.

ADVERSE REACTIONS/TOXIC EFFECTS

Overdosage may result in CNS depression w/drowsiness, decreased body temperature, bradycardia, hypotension, coma, apnea.

PATIENT CONSIDERATIONS

PATIENT/FAMILY TEACHING

Discard if solution becomes cloudy or discolored. Overuse of vasoconstrictors may produce rebound congestion, hyperemia. Avoid excessive dosage, prolonged or too frequent use. *Ophthalmic:* Do not use w/glaucoma unless under advice and direction of physician. Remove contact lenses before administration. Do not use w/wetting agents for contact lenses. Discontinue and consult physician immediately if ocular pain or visual changes occur, if condition worsens or continues for more than 72 hrs. *Intranasal:* Discontinue and consult physician if rebound congestion occurs.

---

thalidomide

(Thalomid)

See Supplement

---

thiamine hydrochloride (vitamin B_1)

thigh-ah-min

(Betalin)

CANADIAN AVAILABILITY

Betaxin

PREGNANCY CATEGORY A

(C if used in doses above RDA)

CLASSIFICATION

Vitamin: B-complex

AVAILABILITY (OTC)

Tablets: 5 mg, 10 mg, 25 mg, 50 mg, 100 mg, 250 mg, 500 mg. **Injection (Rx):** 100 mg/ml.

PHARMACOKINETICS

Absorption: Readily absorbed from GI tract primarily in duodenum, after IM administration. Widely distributed. **Metabolism:** Metabolized in liver. **Excretion:** Primarily excreted in urine.

ACTION/*THERAPEUTIC EFFECT*

Combines w/adenosine triphosphate (ATP) in liver, kidney, leukocytes to form thiamine diphosphate, which is *necessary for carbohydrate metabolism.*

USES

Prevention/treatment of thiamine deficiency (e.g., beriberi, alcoholic w/altered sensorium).

STORAGE/HANDLING

Store oral, parenteral forms at room temperature.

ADMINISTRATION

Note: IM/IV administration used only in acutely ill or those unresponsive to oral route (GI malabsorption syndrome). IM route preferred to IV use. Give by direct IV, or add to most IV solutions and give as infusion.

INDICATIONS/ROUTES/DOSAGE

Dietary supplement:
Oral: Adults, elderly: 1–2 mg/day. ***Children:*** 0.5–1 mg/day. ***Infants:*** 0.3–0.5 mg/day.

Thiamine deficiency:
Oral: Adults, elderly: 5–30 mg/day, in single or 3 divided doses, for 1 mo. ***Children:*** 10–50 mg/day in 3 divided doses.

Critically ill/malabsorption syndrome:
IM/IV: Adults, elderly: 5–100 mg, 3 times/day. ***Children:*** 10–25 mg/day.

Metabolic disorders:
Oral: Adults, elderly, children: 10–20 mg/day; up to 4 g in divided doses/day.

CONTRAINDICATIONS

None significant.

CAUTIONS

None significant.

INTERACTIONS

DRUG: None significant. **HERBAL:** None known. **FOOD:** None significant. **ALTERED LAB VALUES:** None significant.

SIDE EFFECTS

FREQUENT: Pain, induration, tenderness at IM injection site.

ADVERSE REACTIONS/TOXIC EFFECTS

Rare, severe hypersensitivity reaction w/IV administration may result in feeling of warmth, pruritus, urticaria, weakness, sweating, nausea, restlessness, tightness of throat, angioedema (swelling of face/lips), cyanosis, pulmonary edema, GI tract bleeding, cardiovascular collapse.

PATIENT CONSIDERATIONS

INTERVENTION/EVALUATION

Monitor lab values for erythrocyte activity, EKG readings. Assess for clinical improvement (improved sense of well-being, weight gain). Observe for reversal of deficiency symptoms (*neurologic:* peripheral neuropathy, hyporeflexia, nystagmus, ophthalmoplegia, ataxia, muscle weakness; *cardiac:* venous hypertension, bounding arterial pulse, tachycardia, edema; *mental:* confused state).

PATIENT/FAMILY TEACHING

Discomfort may occur w/IM injection. Foods rich in thiamine include pork, organ meats, whole grain and enriched cereals, legumes, nuts, seeds, yeast, wheat germ, rice bran.

thiethylperazine maleate

thigh-eth-ill-**pear**-ah-zeen
(Torecan)

PREGNANCY CATEGORY C

CLASSIFICATION

Antiemetic

AVAILABILITY (Rx)

Tablets: 10 mg. **Suppository:** 10 mg. **Injection:** 5 mg/ml.

PHARMACODYNAMICS

	ONSET	PEAK	DURATION
Oral	30–60 min	—	4 hrs
IM	30 min	—	4 hrs
Rectal	30–60 min	—	4 hrs

PHARMACOKINETICS

Absorption: Well absorbed after oral, rectal, IM administration. Widely distributed, primarily in CNS. **Metabolism:** Metabolized in liver. **Excretion:** Excreted in urine.

ACTION/*THERAPEUTIC EFFECT*

Acts centrally to block dopamine receptors in chemoreceptor trigger zone (CTZ) in CNS, *relieving nausea and vomiting.*

USES

Control of nausea and vomiting.

STORAGE/HANDLING

Store oral, rectal, parenteral forms at room temperature.

ADMINISTRATION

ORAL:

- Give w/o regard to meals.

IM:

- Give deep IM into large muscle mass, preferably upper outer gluteus maximus.

RECTAL:

- If suppository is too soft, chill for 30 min in refrigerator or run cold water over foil wrapper.
- Moisten suppository w/cold water before inserting well into rectum.

INDICATIONS/ROUTES/DOSAGE

Note: Do not use IV route (produces severe hypotension).

Nausea, vomiting:
Oral, Rectal, IM: Adults, elderly: 10 mg, 1–3 times/day.

CONTRAINDICATIONS

Severe CNS depression, comatose states, hypersensitivity to phenothiazines, pregnancy.

CAUTIONS

Elderly, debilitated, dehydration, electrolyte imbalance, high fever.

INTERACTIONS

DRUG: *Alcohol, CNS depressants* may increase CNS, respiratory depression, increase hypotension. May block alpha-adrenergic effects of ***epinephrine*** (causing hypotension, tachycardia). ***Extra-***

pyramidal symptom (EPS)–producing medications may increase risk of EPS. May inhibit effects of ***levodopa.*** May increase cardiac effects w/***quinidine.*** **HERBAL:** None known. **FOOD:** None significant. **ALTERED LAB VALUES:** None significant.

SIDE EFFECTS

FREQUENT: Drowsiness, dizziness. **OCCASIONAL:** Agranulocytosis (sore throat, fever, unusual bruising/bleeding), cholestatic jaundice, blurred vision, decreased color vision or night vision, fever, headache, orthostatic hypotension, rash, ringing in ears, constipation, dry mouth, decreased sweating, paradoxical reaction (excitement, nervousness, irritability).

ADVERSE REACTIONS/TOXIC EFFECTS

Extrapyramidal symptoms manifested as torticollis (neck muscle spasm), oculogyric crisis (rolling back of eyes), akathisia (motor restlessness, anxiety) occur rarely.

PATIENT CONSIDERATIONS

Baseline Assessment

Assess for dehydration if excessive vomiting occurs (poor skin turgor, dry mucous membranes, longitudinal furrows in tongue).

Intervention Evaluation

Monitor B/P especially before dosing. Assist w/ambulation if dizziness or hypotension occurs. Assess for improvement of dehydration status. Monitor I&O. Monitor for evidence of fever. Assess any vomitus. Be alert for extrapyramidal symptoms.

Patient/Family Teaching

Report visual disturbances, headache. Dry mouth is expected response to medication. Relief from nausea/vomiting generally occurs within 30 min of drug administration. Avoid alcohol and other CNS depressants. Change positions slowly to prevent postural hypotension. Avoid tasks requiring alert response until assured drug does not cause impairment.

---

thioguanine

(Thioguanine)

See Classification section under: Cancer chemotherapy

---

thiopental sodium

(Pentothal)

See Classification section under: Anesthetics: general

---

thioridazine

thigh-oh-**rid**-ah-zeen

(Mellaril-S)

thioridazine hydrochloride

(Mellaril)

CANADIAN AVAILABILITY

Apo-Thioridazine, Mellaril

PREGNANCY CATEGORY C

CLASSIFICATION

Antipsychotic

AVAILABILITY (Rx)

Tablets: 10 mg, 15 mg, 25 mg, 50

mg, 100 mg, 150 mg, 200 mg. **Oral Concentrate:** 30 mg/ml, 100 mg/ml. **Oral Suspension:** 25 mg/5 ml, 100 mg/5 ml.

PHARMACOKINETICS

Absorption: Variably absorbed from GI tract. Widely distributed. **Metabolism:** Metabolized in liver to some active metabolites. **Excretion:** Excreted in urine, eliminated in feces.

ACTION/*THERAPEUTIC EFFECT*

Blocks dopamine at postsynaptic receptor sites, *suppressing behavioral response in psychosis, reducing locomotor activity, aggressiveness, suppressing conditioned responses.* Possesses strong anticholinergic, sedative effects.

USES

Management of psychotic disorders, severe behavioral disturbances in children, including those w/excessive motor activity, conduct disorders. Used in short-term treatment of moderate to marked depression w/variable degrees of anxiety.

ADMINISTRATION

ORAL:

- Dilute oral concentrate solution in water or fruit juice just before administration.
- Do not crush, chew, or break tablets.

INDICATIONS/ROUTES/DOSAGE

Psychotic disorders:
Oral: Adults: 50–100 mg 3 times/day in hospitalized pts. May gradually increase to 800 mg/day maximum. Dosage from 200–800 mg/day should be divided into 2–3 doses. Reduce dose gradually when therapeutic response is achieved.

Depression w/anxiety:
Oral: Adults: 25 mg 3 times/day. *Total dose range/day:* 10 mg 2 times/day to 50 mg 3–4 times/day.

Usual elderly dosage (nonpsychotic):
Oral: Initially, 10–25 mg 12 times/day. May increase by 10–25 mg q4–7 days. *Maximum:* 400 mg/day.

Usual pediatric dosage:
Oral: Children 2–12 yrs: 0.5–3 mg/kg/day.

CONTRAINDICATIONS

Severe CNS depression, comatose states, severe cardiovascular disease, bone marrow depression, subcortical brain damage.

CAUTIONS

Impaired respiratory/hepatic/renal/cardiac function, alcohol withdrawal, history of seizures, urinary retention, glaucoma, prostatic hypertrophy, hypocalcemia (increases susceptibility to dystonias). Prolongs QT interval.

INTERACTIONS

DRUG: *Alcohol, CNS depressants* may increase CNS, respiratory depression, hypotensive effects. *Tricyclic antidepressants, MAO inhibitors* may increase sedative, anticholinergic effects. *Antithyroid agents* may increase risk of agranulocytosis. Extrapyramidal symptoms (EPS) may increase w/*EPS-producing medications. Hypotensives* may increase hypotension. May decrease *levodopa* effects. *Lithium* may decrease absorption, produce adverse neurologic effects. **HERBAL:** None known. **FOOD:** None significant. **ALTERED LAB VALUES:** May cause EKG changes.

SIDE EFFECTS

Generally well tolerated w/only mild and transient effects. **OCCASIONAL:** Drowsiness during early therapy, dry mouth, blurred vision, lethargy, constipation or diarrhea, nasal congestion, peripheral edema, urinary retention. **RARE:** Ocular changes, skin pigmentation (those on high doses for prolonged periods).

ADVERSE REACTIONS/TOXIC EFFECTS

Extrapyramidal symptoms appear dose related (particularly high dosage) and are divided into 3 categories: akathisia (inability to sit still, tapping of feet, urge to move around); parkinsonian symptoms (mask-like face, tremors, shuffling gait, hypersalivation); and acute dystonias: torticollis (neck muscle spasm), opisthotonos (rigidity of back muscles), and oculogyric crisis (rolling back of eyes). Dystonic reaction may also produce profuse sweating, pallor. Tardive dyskinesia (protrusion of tongue, puffing of cheeks, chewing/puckering of the mouth) occurs rarely (may be irreversible). Abrupt withdrawal following long-term therapy may precipitate nausea, vomiting, gastritis, dizziness, tremors. Blood dyscrasias, particularly agranulocytosis, mild leukopenia (sore mouth/gums/throat) may occur. May lower seizure threshold.

PATIENT CONSIDERATIONS

Baseline Assessment

Avoid skin contact w/solution (contact dermatitis). Assess behavior, appearance, emotional status, response to environment, speech pattern, thought content.

Intervention Evaluation

Monitor B/P for hypotension. Assess for extrapyramidal symptoms. Monitor WBC, differential count for blood dyscrasias. Monitor for fine tongue movement (may be early sign of tardive dyskinesia). Supervise suicidal risk pt closely during early therapy (as depression lessens, energy level improves, but suicide potential increases). Assess for therapeutic response (interest in surroundings, improvement in self-care, increased ability to concentrate, relaxed facial expression).

Patient/Family Teaching

Full therapeutic effect may take up to 6 wks. Urine may darken. Do not abruptly withdraw from long-term drug therapy. Report visual disturbances. Sugarless gum, sips of tepid water may relieve dry mouth. Drowsiness generally subsides during continued therapy. Avoid tasks that require alertness, motor skills until response to drug is established.

---

thiotepa

(Thioplex, Thiotepa)

See Classification section under: Cancer chemotherapy

---

thiothixene

thigh-oh-**thicks**-een

(Navane caps)

thiothixene hydrochloride

(Navane solution, injection)

CANADIAN AVAILABILITY
Navane

PREGNANCY CATEGORY C

CLASSIFICATION

Antipsychotic

AVAILABILITY (Rx)

Capsules: 1 mg, 2 mg, 5 mg, 10 mg, 20 mg. **Oral Concentrate:** 5 mg/ml. **Injection:** 2 mg/ml, 5 mg/ml.

PHARMACODYNAMICS

	ONSET	PEAK	DURATION
IM	—	1–6 hrs	—

PHARMACOKINETICS

Absorption: Well absorbed from GI tract, after IM administration. Widely distributed. **Metabolism:** Metabolized in liver. **Excretion:** Primarily excreted in urine. **Half-life:** 34 hrs.

ACTION/*THERAPEUTIC EFFECT*

Blocks postsynaptic dopamine receptor sites in brain. Has alpha-adrenergic blocking effects; depresses release of hypothalamic, hypophyseal hormones. *Suppresses behavioral response in psychosis.*

USES

Symptomatic management of psychotic disorders.

STORAGE/HANDLING

Reconstituted solutions stable for 48 hrs at room temperature.

ADMINISTRATION

ORAL:

- Give w/o regard to meals.
- Avoid skin contact w/oral solution (contact dermatitis).

IM:

- Following parenteral form, pt must remain recumbent for 30–60 min in head-low position w/legs raised, to minimize hypotensive effect.
- For IM injection, reconstitute 10 mg thiothixene hydrochloride w/2.2 ml sterile water for injection, yielding final solution of 5 mg/ml.
- Inject slow, deep IM into upper outer quadrant of gluteus maximus or midlateral thigh.

INDICATIONS/ROUTES/DOSAGE

Note: Reduce dosage gradually to optimum response, then decrease to lowest effective level for maintenance. Replace parenteral therapy w/oral therapy as soon as possible.

Mild to moderate symptoms:
Oral: Adults: 2 mg 3 times/day. May be increased gradually to 15 mg/day.

Severe symptoms:
Oral: Adults: 5 mg 2 times/day. Increase gradually to 60 mg if needed. ***Usual dose range:*** 20–30 mg/day.

IM: Adults: 4 mg 2–4 times/day. May increase to maximum 30 mg/day. ***Usual dose range:*** 16–20 mg/day.

Usual elderly dosage:
Oral: Initially, 1–2 mg 1–2 times/day. May increase by 1–2 mg q4–7days. ***Maximum:*** 30 mg/day.

CONTRAINDICATIONS

Comatose states, circulatory collapse, CNS depression, blood dyscrasias.

EXTREME CAUTION

History of seizures.

CAUTIONS

Severe cardiovascular disorders, alcoholic withdrawal, pt exposure to extreme heat, glaucoma, prostatic hypertrophy.

INTERACTIONS

DRUG: *Alcohol, CNS depressants* may increase CNS, respiratory depression, increase hypotension. *Extrapyramidal symptom (EPS)–producing medications* may increase risk of EPS. May inhibit effects of ***levodopa.*** May increase cardiac effects w/***quinidine.*** **HERBAL:** None known. **FOOD:** None significant. **ALTERED LAB VALUES:** May decrease uric acid.

SIDE EFFECTS

FREQUENT: Constipation, decreased sweating, drowsiness, dry mouth, increased appetite, weight gain, increased sensitivity of skin to sunlight, nasal congestion, orthostatic hypotension. **OCCASIONAL:** Skin rash, blurred vision, skin discoloration, changes in menstrual period, decreased sexual ability, swelling of breasts. **RARE:** Blood dyscrasias, heat stroke.

ADVERSE REACTIONS/TOXIC EFFECTS

Frequently noted extrapyramidal symptom is akathisia (motor restlessness, anxiety). Occurring less frequently is akinesia (rigidity, tremor, salivation, mask-like facial expression, reduced voluntary movements). Infrequently noted are dystonias: torticollis (neck muscle spasm), opisthotonos (rigidity of back muscles), and oculogyric crisis (rolling back of eyes). Tardive dyskinesia (protrusion of tongue, puffing of cheeks, chewing/puckering of mouth) occurs rarely but may be irreversible. Risk is greater in female geriatric pts. Grand mal seizures may occur in epileptic pts (risk higher w/IM administration).

PATIENT CONSIDERATIONS

Baseline Assessment

Assess behavior, appearance, emotional status, response to environment, speech pattern, thought content.

Intervention/Evaluation

Supervise suicidal risk pt closely during early therapy (as depression lessens, energy level improves, increasing suicide potential). Monitor B/P for hypotension. Assess for peripheral edema behind medial malleolus (sacral area in bedridden pts). Assess stools; prevent constipation. Monitor for EPS, tardive dyskinesia (see Adverse Reactions/Toxic Effects) and potentially fatal, rare neuroleptic malignant syndrome: fever, irregular pulse or B/P, muscle rigidity, altered mental status. Assess for therapeutic response (interest in surroundings, improvement in self-care, increased ability to concentrate, relaxed facial expression).

Patient/Family Teaching

Full therapeutic effect may take up to 6 wks. Report visual disturbances. Sugarless gum, sips of tepid water may relieve dry mouth. Drowsiness generally subsides during continued therapy. Avoid tasks that require alertness, motor skills until response to drug is established. Avoid alcohol and other CNS depressants.

---

thyroid

(S-P-T, Thyrar, Armour Thyroid)

See Classification section under: Thyroid

T

tiagabine hydrochloride

tie-**ah**-ga-bean
(Gabitril)

PREGNANCY CATEGORY C

CLASSIFICATION

Anticonvulsant

AVAILABILITY (Rx)

Tablets: 2 mg, 4 mg, 12 mg, 16 mg, 20 mg

PHARMACOKINETICS

Absorption: Rapidly and completely absorbed following oral administration. Bound to plasma proteins (96%), mainly to albumin. **Metabolism:** Metabolized in the liver. **Excretion:** Primarily eliminated in feces. **Half-life:** 4–9 hrs.

ACTION/*THERAPEUTIC EFFECT*

Blocks uptake of gamma aminobutyric acid (GABA), the major inhibitory neurotransmitter in the CNS, into presynaptic neurons and permitting more GABA available on the surfaces of postsynaptic cells, *inhibiting seizure activity.*

USES

Adjunctive therapy for the treatment of partial seizures.

ADMINISTRATION

ORAL:

- Give w/food.

INDICATIONS/ROUTES/DOSAGES

Partial seizures:
Oral: Adults >18 yrs: Initially, 4 mg once daily. May increase by 4–8 mg/day at weekly intervals. ***Maximum:*** 56 mg/day. Give total daily dose in two to four divided doses. ***Children 12–18 yrs:*** Initially, 4 mg once daily. May increase by 4 mg at beginning of week 2. May increase by 4–8 mg/day at weekly intervals. ***Maximum:*** 32 mg/day.

CONTRAINDICATIONS

None significant.

CAUTIONS

Sensitivity to tiagabine, pregnancy, use of other anticonvulsant (especially carbamazepine, phenobarbital, phenytoin, primidone), history of status epilepticus, impaired liver function, abnormal EEG.

INTERACTIONS

DRUG: Clearance is increased with concurrent use of ***carbamazepine, phenobarbital, phenytoin, primidone.*** **HERBAL:** None known. **FOOD:** None significant. **ALTERED LAB VALUES:** None significant.

SIDE EFFECTS

FREQUENT (10–27%): Dizziness, asthenia (weakness), somnolence, nausea, nervousness, rash. **OCCASIONAL (4–9%):** Tremor, diarrhea, vomiting, pharyngitis, abdominal pain, insomnia, difficulty with concentration/attention, muscular incoordination, confusion, paresthesia. **RARE: (2–3%):** Depression, increased appetite, pruritus, vasodilation.

ADVERSE REACTIONS/TOXIC EFFECTS

Overdosage may manifest as severe agitation, impaired consciousness, lethargy, mental depression, severe muscle twitching or jerking, increase in seizures, speech difficulties.

PATIENT CONSIDERATIONS

BASELINE ASSESSMENT

Review history of seizure disorder (intensity, frequency, duration, LOC). Provide safety precautions, quiet, dark environment. Question sensitivity to tiagabine, pregnancy, use of other anticonvulsant medication (especially carbamazepine, phenobarbital, phenytoin, primidone).

INTERVENTION/EVALUATION

Observe frequently for recurrence of seizure activity. Assess for clinical improvement (decrease in intensity/frequency of seizures). Monitor tiagabine plasma concentration. Assist with ambulation if dizziness occurs.

PATIENT/FAMILY TEACHING

Avoid tasks that require alertness, motor skills until response to drug is established (may cause dizziness, drowsiness, impaired thinking). Avoid use of alcohol, other CNS depressants. Do not abruptly discontinue (may precipitate seizures). Strict maintenance of drug therapy is essential for seizure control. Take medication with food. Drowsiness usually diminished with continued therapy.

ticarcillin disodium

(Ticar)

See Classification section under: Antibiotics: penicillins

ticarcillin disodium/clavulanate potassium

tie-car-**sill**-in/klah-view-**lan**-ate
(Timentin)

CANADIAN AVAILABILITY
Timentin

PREGNANCY CATEGORY B

CLASSIFICATION

Antibiotic: Penicillin

AVAILABILITY (Rx)

Powder for Injection: 3.1 g. **Solution for Infusion:** 3.1 g/100 ml.

PHARMACOKINETICS

Widely distributed. **Metabolism:** Minimal metabolism in liver. **Excretion:** Primarily excreted unchanged in urine. Moderately removed by hemodialysis. **Half-life:** 1–1.2 hrs (increased in decreased renal function).

ACTION/*THERAPEUTIC EFFECT*

Ticarcillin: Binds to bacterial cell wall inhibiting bacterial cell wall synthesis, *causing cell lysis, death.* ***Clavulanate:*** Inhibits bacterial beta-lactamase *protecting ticarcillin from enzymatic degradation.* Bactericidal.

USES

Treatment of septicemia, skin/skin structure, bone and joint, lower respiratory, urinary tract infections, endometritis.

STORAGE/HANDLING

Solution appears colorless to pale yellow (if solution darkens, indicates loss of potency). IV infusion (piggyback) stable for 24 hrs at room temperature, 3 days if refrigerated. Discard if precipitate forms.

ADMINISTRATION

IV:

- For IV infusion (piggyback), reconstitute each 3.1 g vial w/13 ml sterile water for injection or 0.9% NaCl injection to provide concentration of 200 mg ticarcillin and 6.7 mg clavulanic acid per ml.
- Shake vial to assist reconstitution.
- Further dilute w/50–100 ml 5% dextrose or 0.9% NaCl. Infuse over 30 min.
- Because of potential for hypersensitivity/anaphylaxis, start initial dose at few drops/min, increase slowly to ordered rate; stay w/pt first 10–15 min, then check q10min.
- Alternating IV sites, use large veins to reduce risk of phlebitis.

INDICATIONS/ROUTES/DOSAGE

Systemic and urinary tract infections:
IV: Adults >60 kg: 3.1 g q4–6h. ***Adults <60 kg, children >12 yrs:*** 200–300 mg/kg/day in divided doses q4–6h.

Gynecologic infections:
IV: Adults >60 kg: 200 mg/kg/day in divided doses q6h up to 300 mg/kg/day in divided doses q4h.

Usual pediatric dosage:
IV: Children <60 kg: 200–300 mg/kg/day. **>60 kg:** 3.1 g q4–6h.

Dosage in renal/hepatic impairment:
Hepatic impairment alone usually requires no change. Renal impairment alone, administer 3.1 g initially, then modify dose and/or frequency based on creatinine clearance and/or severity of infection.

CREATININE CLEARANCE	DOSAGE
30–60 ml/min	2 g IV q4h
10–30 ml/min	2 g q8h
<10 ml/min	2 g q12h
10 ml/min w/liver impairment	2 g q24h

CONTRAINDICATIONS

Hypersensitivity to any penicillin.

CAUTIONS

History of allergies, especially cephalosporins.

INTERACTIONS

DRUG: ***Anticoagulants, heparin, thrombolytics, NSAIDs*** may increase risk of hemorrhage w/high doses of ticarcillin. ***Probenecid*** may increase concentration, risk of toxicity. **HERBAL:** None known. **FOOD:** None significant. **ALTERED LAB VALUES:**: May cause positive Coombs' test. May increase SGOT (AST), SGPT (ALT), alkaline phosphatase, bilirubin, creatinine, LDH, bleeding time. May decrease potassium, sodium, uric acid.

SIDE EFFECTS

FREQUENT: Phlebitis, thrombophlebitis w/IV dose, rash, urticaria, pruritus, taste/smell disturbances. **OCCASIONAL:** Nausea, diarrhea, vomiting, flatulence. **RARE:** Headache, bleeding, hyperkalemia, or hypokalemia.

ADVERSE REACTIONS/TOXIC EFFECTS

Overdosage may produce seizures, neurologic reactions. Superinfections, potentially fatal antibiotic-associated colitis may result from bacterial imbalance. Severe hypersensitivity reactions, including anaphylaxis, occur rarely.

PATIENT CONSIDERATIONS

BASELINE ASSESSMENT

Question for history of allergies, especially penicillins, cephalosporins. Obtain specimen for culture and sensitivity before giving first dose (therapy may begin before results are known).

INTERVENTION/EVALUATION

Hold medication and promptly report rash (hypersensitivity) or diarrhea (w/fever, abdominal pain, mucus and blood in stool may indicate antibiotic-associated colitis). Assess food tolerance. Provide mouth care, sugarless gum or hard candy to offset taste, smell effects. Evaluate IV site for phlebitis (heat, pain, red streaking over vein). Monitor I&O, urinalysis, renal function tests. Assess for bleeding: overt bleeding, bruising or tissue swelling; check hematology reports. Monitor electrolytes, particularly potassium. Be alert for superinfection: increased fever, onset of sore throat, diarrhea, vomiting, ulceration or other oral changes, anal/genital pruritus.

PATIENT/FAMILY TEACHING

Continue antibiotic for full length of treatment. Space doses evenly. Notify physician in event of rash, diarrhea, bleeding, bruising, or other new symptom.

ticlopidine hydrochloride

tie-**clow**-pih-deen
(Ticlid)

CANADIAN AVAILABILITY
Apo-Ticlopidine, Ticlid

PREGNANCY CATEGORY B

CLASSIFICATION

Platelet aggregation inhibitor

AVAILABILITY (Rx)

Tablets: 250 mg

PHARMACOKINETICS

Absorption: Rapidly, well absorbed from GI tract (absorption increases after meals). **Metabolism:** Metabolized in liver to active metabolite. **Excretion:** Primarily excreted in urine. **Half-life:** single dose: 7.9–12.6 hrs; repeated doses: 4–5 days.

ACTION/*THERAPEUTIC EFFECT*

Inhibits release of platelet granule constituents, platelet-platelet interactions, and adhesion to endothelium and atheromatous plaque, *preventing platelet aggregation.*

USES/*UNLABELED*

To reduce risk of stroke in those who have experienced strokelike warnings or those w/history of thrombotic stroke. *Treatment of intermittent claudication, subarachnoid hemorrhage, sickle-cell disease.*

ADMINISTRATION

ORAL:

- Give w/food or just after meals (bioavailability increased, GI discomfort decreased).

INDICATIONS/ROUTES/DOSAGE

Prevention of stroke:
Oral: Adults, elderly: 250 mg 2 times/day.

T

CONTRAINDICATIONS

Hematopoietic disorders (neutropenia, thrombocytopenia), presence of hemostatic disorder, active pathologic bleeding (bleeding peptic ulcer, intracranial bleeding), severe liver impairment.

CAUTIONS

Those at risk of increased bleeding from trauma, surgery, pathologic conditions.

INTERACTIONS

DRUG: May increase risk of bleeding w/***oral anticoagulants, heparin, thrombolytics, aspirin.*** **HERBAL:** Ginkgo biloba may increase risk of bleeding. **FOOD:** None significant. **ALTERED LAB VALUES:** May increase alkaline phosphatase, bilirubin, liver function tests, cholesterol, triglycerides. May prolong bleeding time. May decrease neutrophil, platelet count.

SIDE EFFECTS

FREQUENT (>7%): Skin rash, diarrhea, indigestion, nausea, abdominal pain. **OCCASIONAL (1–7%):** Bloating, vomiting, dizziness, itching, neutropenia, purpura, thrombocytopenia, bleeding, complications, agranulocytosis. **RARE (<1%):** Hepatitis, cholestatic jaundice, hives, tinnitus.

ADVERSE REACTIONS/TOXIC EFFECTS

Thrombotic thrombocytopenic purpura (TTP).

PATIENT CONSIDERATIONS

Baseline Assessment

Drug should be discontinued 10–14 days before surgery if antiplatelet effect is not desired.

Intervention/Evaluation

Assist w/ambulation if dizziness occurs. Monitor heart sounds by auscultation. Assess B/P for hypotension. Assess skin for flushing, rash.

Patient/Family Teaching

If nausea occurs, cola, unsalted crackers, or dry toast may relieve effect. Therapeutic response may not be achieved before 2–3 mos of continuous therapy. Report any unusual bleeding/bruising or rash.

tiludronate sodium

tie-**lew**-droh-nate
(Skelid)

PREGNANCY CATEGORY C

CLASSIFICATION

Bone resorption inhibitor, calcium regulator

AVAILABILITY (Rx)

Tablets: 240 mg (equivalent to 200 mg tiludronic acid)

PHARMACOKINETICS

Absorption: Rapidly absorbed following oral administration and distributed to bone with uptake greatest at sites of active bone turnover. Highly bound to protein, especially albumin. **Half-life:** 150 hrs in those with Paget's disease.

ACTION/*THERAPEUTIC EFFECT*

Inhibits abnormal bone resorption, evidenced by significant decrease in serum alkaline phosphatase (marker of bone formation) and urinary creatinine (marker of bone resorption), *decreasing osteolysis of both axial and appedicular skeleton.*

USES

Treatment of those with Paget's disease of bone having alkaline phosphatase at least two times the upper limit of normal, or those symptomatic or at risk for future complications from Paget's disease.

ADMINISTRATION

ORAL:

- Give with 6–8 ounces plain water only (beverages other than plain water, including mineral water, food, and some medications [indomethacin] reduce drug absorption).
- Do not give within 2 hrs of food ingestion.
- Take antacids at a different time of day than tiludronate ingestion (antacids prevent tiludronate absorption).

INDICATIONS/ROUTES/DOSAGES

Note: Give with 6–8 ounces of plain water only. Do not give within 2 hrs of food, antacids, calcium supplement, salicylates or indomethacin.

Paget's disease:
Oral: Adults: 400 mg once daily for 3 mos.

CONTRAINDICATIONS

GI disease (dysphagia, duodenitis, esophagitis, gastric ulcer), renal function impairment, history of hypersensitivity to biphosphates.

CAUTIONS

Hyperparathyroidism, hypocalcemia, vitamin D deficiency.

INTERACTIONS

DRUG: ***Antacids, calcium supplements, salicylates, indomethacin*** interferes with absorption. Do not give within 2 hrs of tiludronate administration. **HERBAL:** None known. **FOOD:** Effectiveness is decreased when taken within 2 hrs of food ingestion. **ALTERED LAB VALUES:** None significant.

SIDE EFFECTS

OCCASIONAL (4–9%): Diarrhea, nausea, headache, dyspepsia, sinusitis, rhinitis, upper respiratory infection, paresthesia, dizziness, vomiting. **RARE (3%):** Flatulence, arthralgia, conjunctivitis, peripheral edema, rash.

ADVERSE REACTIONS/TOXIC EFFECTS

Glaucoma, cataracts, hyperparathyroidism, vitamin D deficiency occur rarely.

PATIENT CONSIDERATIONS

Baseline Assessment

Hypocalcemia, vitamin D deficiency must be corrected before therapy begins. Obtain baseline alkaline phosphatase, urinary creatinine, serum calcium, phosphates.

Interventions/Evaluation

Monitor electrolytes, especially calcium and alkaline phosphatase serum levels. Monitor stool frequency and consistency (watery, loose, soft, semisolid, solid). Evaluate pain in those with Paget's disease. Monitor serum alkaline phosphatase, urinary creatinine, serum calcium, phosphates.

Patient/Family Teaching

Expected benefits occur only when medication is taken with a full glass (6–8 oz) of plain water only. Separate food ingestion,

other beverages, including mineral water, and other drug administration and tiludronate administration by 2 hrs. Weight-bearing exercise, decrease or modification of cigarette smoking, alcohol consumption is advised. Report nausea, diarrhea, rash.

timolol maleate

tim-oh-lol

(Betimol, Blocadren, Timoptic, Timoptic XE)

FIXED-COMBINATION(S)

W/dorzoloamide, a carbonic anhydrase inhibitor **(CoSopt)**; w/hydrochlorothiazide, a diuretic **(Timolide)**

CANADIAN AVAILABILITY

Apo-Timol, Blocadren, Timoptic

PREGNANCY CATEGORY C

(D if used in second or third trimester)

CLASSIFICATION

Beta-adrenergic blocker

AVAILABILITY (Rx)

Tablets: 5 mg, 10 mg, 20 mg. **Ophthalmic Solution:** 0.25%, 0.5%. **Ophthalmic Gel:** 0.25%, 0.5%.

PHARMACODYNAMICS

	ONSET	PEAK	DURATION
Eye drops			
	30 min	1–2 hrs	12–24 hrs

PHARMACOKINETICS

Absorption: Well absorbed from GI tract. Minimal absorption following ophthalmic administration. **Metabolism:** Metabolized in liver. **Excretion:** Primarily excreted in urine. Not removed by hemodialysis. **Half-life:** 4 hrs. ***Ophthalmic:*** Systemic absorption may occur.

ACTION / *THERAPEUTIC EFFECT*

Nonselective beta-adrenergic blocking agent. Blocks $beta_1$-adrenergic receptors, *slowing sinus heart rate, decreasing cardiac output, decreasing B/P.* Blocks $beta_2$-adrenergic receptors, *increasing airway resistance.* Decreases myocardial ischemia severity by decreasing oxygen requirements. *Reduces intraocular pressure (IOP).*

USES / *UNLABELED*

Management of mild to moderate hypertension. Used alone or in combination w/diuretics, especially thiazide type. Reduces cardiovascular mortality in those w/definite/suspected acute MI. Prophylaxis of migraine headache. ***Ophthalmic:*** Reduces IOP in management of open-angle glaucoma, aphakic glaucoma, ocular hypertension, secondary glaucoma. ***Systemic:*** *Treatment of chronic angina pectoris, cardiac arrhythmias, hypertrophic cardiomyopathy, pheochromocytoma, tremors, anxiety, thyrotoxicosis.* ***Ophthalmic:*** *W/miotics decreases IOP in acute/chronic angle closure glaucoma, treatment of secondary glaucoma, malignant glaucoma, angle closure glaucoma during/after iridectomy. Treatment of migraines.*

STORAGE/HANDLING

Store oral form, ophthalmic solution, gel at room temperature.

ADMINISTRATION

ORAL:

- May be given w/o regard to meals.
- Tablets may be crushed.

OPHTHALMIC:

- **Note:** When using gel, invert container, shake once prior to each use.
- Place finger on lower eyelid and pull out until pocket is formed between eye and lower lid.
- Hold dropper above pocket and place prescribed number of drops into pocket. Instruct pt to close eyes gently so medication will not be squeezed out of sac.
- Apply gentle finger pressure to the lacrimal sac at inner canthus for 1 min following installation (lessens risk of systemic absorption).

INDICATIONS/ROUTES/DOSAGE

Hypertension:
Oral: Adults, elderly: Initially, 10 mg 2 times/day, alone or in combination w/other therapy. Gradually increase at intervals of not less than 1 wk. ***Maintenance:*** 20–60 mg/day in 2 divided doses.

Myocardial infarction:
Oral: Adults, elderly: 10 mg 2 times/day, beginning within 1–4 wks after infarction.

Migraine prophylaxis:
Oral: Adults, elderly: Initially, 10 mg 2 times/day. ***Range:*** 10–30 mg/day.

Glaucoma:
Ophthalmic: Adults, elderly: 1 drop of 0.25% solution in affected eye(s) 2 times/day. May be increased to 1 drop of 0.5% solution in affected eye(s) 2 times/day. When IOP is controlled, dosage may be reduced to 1 drop 1 time/day. If pt is transferred to timolol from another antiglaucoma agent, administer concurrently for 1 day. Discontinue other agent on following day. ***Timoptic XE:*** 1 drop/day.

CONTRAINDICATIONS

Bronchial asthma, COPD, uncontrolled cardiac failure, sinus bradycardia, heart block greater than first degree, cardiogenic shock, CHF unless secondary to tachyarrhythmias, those on MAO inhibitors.

CAUTIONS

Inadequate cardiac function, impaired renal/hepatic function, hyperthyroidism.

INTERACTIONS

DRUG: ***Diuretics, other hypotensives*** may increase hypotensive effect. ***Sympathomimetics, xanthines*** may mutually inhibit effects. May mask symptoms of hypoglycemia, prolong hypoglycemic effect of ***insulin, oral hypoglycemics. NSAIDs*** may decrease antihypertensive effect. **HERBAL:** None known. **FOOD:** None significant. **ALTERED LAB VALUES:** May increase ANA titer, SGOT (AST), SGPT (ALT), alkaline phosphatase, LDH, bilirubin, BUN, creatinine, potassium, uric acid, lipoproteins, triglycerides.

SIDE EFFECTS

FREQUENT: Decreased sexual ability, drowsiness, trouble sleeping, unusually tired/weak. *Ophthalmic:* Eye irritation, visual disturbance. **OCCASIONAL:** Bradycardia, difficulty breathing, CHF (swelling of feet, shortness of breath), depression, cold hands/feet, diarrhea, constipation, anxiety, nasal congestion, nausea, vomiting. **RARE:** Altered taste, dry eyes, itching, numbness of fingers, toes, scalp.

ADVERSE REACTIONS/TOXIC EFFECTS

Oral form may produce profound bradycardia, hypotension, bronchospasm. Abrupt withdrawal may result in sweating, palpitations, headache, tremulousness. May precipitate CHF, myocardial

T

infarction in those w/cardiac disease, thyroid storm in those w/thyrotoxicosis, peripheral ischemia in those w/existing peripheral vascular disease. Hypoglycemia may occur in previously controlled diabetics. Ophthalmic overdosage may produce bradycardia, hypotension, bronchospasm, acute cardiac failure.

PATIENT CONSIDERATIONS

BASELINE ASSESSMENT

Assess B/P, apical pulse immediately before drug is administered (if pulse is 60/min or below, or systolic B/P is below 90 mm Hg, withhold medication, contact physician).

INTERVENTION/EVALUATION

Monitor B/P for hypotension, respiration for shortness of breath. Assess pulse for strength/weakness, irregular rate, bradycardia. Monitor EKG for cardiac arrhythmias, particularly PVCs. Monitor stool frequency and consistency. Assist w/ambulation if dizziness occurs. Assess for evidence of CHF: dyspnea (particularly on exertion or lying down), night cough, peripheral edema, distended neck veins. Monitor I&O (increase in weight, decrease in urine output may indicate CHF). Assess for nausea, diaphoresis, headache, fatigue. *Ophthalmic:* Monitor B/P and pulse regularly.

PATIENT/FAMILY TEACHING

Do not abruptly discontinue medication. Compliance w/therapy regimen is essential to control glaucoma, hypertension, angina, arrhythmias. To avoid hypotensive effect, rise slowly from lying to sitting position, wait momentarily before standing. Avoid tasks that require alertness, motor skills until response to drug is established. Report shortness of breath, excessive fatigue, prolonged dizziness/headache. Do not use nasal decongestants, OTC cold preparations (stimulants) w/o physician approval. Monitor B/P, pulse before taking medication. Restrict salt, alcohol intake. *Ophthalmic:* Teach pt how to instill drops correctly, how to take pulse. Importance of maintaining regimen, of keeping office visits to check IOP. Transient stinging, discomfort may occur upon instillation. Report difficulty breathing immediately.

---

tinzaparin

(Innohep)

See Supplement

---

tioconazole

tie-oh-**con**-ah-zole

(Monistat-1, Vagistat)

CANADIAN AVAILABILITY

Gynecure, Trosyd

PREGNANCY CATEGORY C

CLASSIFICATION

Antifungal

AVAILABILITY (OTC)

Vaginal Ointment: 6.5%

PHARMACOKINETICS

Absorption: Systemic absorption minimal.

ACTION/*THERAPEUTIC EFFECT*

Inhibits synthesis of ergosterol (vital

component of fungal cell formation), *damaging fungal cell membrane. Fungistatic.*

USES

Treatment of vulvovaginal candidiasis (moniliasis).

ADMINISTRATION

INTRAVAGINAL:

- Use disposable gloves; always wash hands thoroughly after application.
- Follow manufacturer's directions for use of applicator.
- Insert applicator high in vagina.
- Administer preferably at bedtime.

INDICATIONS/ROUTES/DOSAGE

Vulvovaginal candidiasis:
Intravaginal: Adults, elderly: 1 applicatorful just before bedtime as a single dose.

CONTRAINDICATIONS

Hypersensitivity to tioconazole, other imidazole antifungal agents, or any component of the cream/suppository.

CAUTIONS

Safety and efficacy in children and diabetic pts not established.

INTERACTIONS

DRUG: None significant. **HERBAL:** None known. **FOOD:** None significant. **ALTERED LAB VALUES:** None significant.

SIDE EFFECTS

FREQUENT: Headache (26% of pts). **OCCASIONAL (1–6%):** Burning, itching. **RARE (<1%):** Irritation, vaginal pain, dysuria, dryness of vaginal secretions, vulvar edema/swelling.

ADVERSE REACTIONS/TOXIC EFFECTS

None significant.

PATIENT CONSIDERATIONS

Baseline Assessment

Question for hypersensitivity to tioconazole, other imidazole antifungal agents, or components of preparation. Confirm that potassium hydroxide culture and/or smears were done for accurate diagnosis; therapy may begin before results known. Inquire about use of rubber/latex contraceptives, because there is interaction between such products and the medication.

Intervention/Evaluation

Assess for therapeutic response or burning, itching, pain, or irritation.

Patient/Family Teaching

Do not interrupt/stop regimen, even during menses. Teach pt proper insertion. Not affected by oral contraception. Notify physician of increased itching, irritation, burning. Consult physician about sexual intercourse, douching, or the use of other vaginal products. Do not use vaginal contraceptive diaphragms, condoms within 72 hrs after treatment. Avoid contact w/eyes. Wash hands thoroughly after application.

tirofiban hydrochloride

turr-**oh**-bih-fan
(Aggrastat)

PREGNANCY CATEGORY B

CLASSIFICATION

Antiplatelet

AVAILABILITY (Rx)

Injection for Solution: 250 mcg/ml; **Injection:** 50 mcg/ml

PHARMACODYNAMICS

	ONSET	PEAK	DURATION
Oral	Immediate	—	Duration of infusion

PHARMACOKINETICS

Absorption: Poorly bound to plasma proteins; unbound fraction in plasma: 35%. **Metabolism:** Limited. **Excretion:** Primarily eliminated in the urine (65%) and to a lesser amount, in the feces. **Half-life:**2 hrs. Clearance is significantly decreased in severe renal impairment (creatinine clearance < 30 ml/min. Removed by hemodialysis.

ACTION/*THERAPEUTIC EFFECT*

Inhibits binding of the platelet glycoprotein (GP) IIb/IIIa receptor (the major platelet surface receptor involved in platelet aggregation), *inhibiting platelet aggregation.* Inhibition persists over the duration of the maintenance infusion and is reversible after infusion is completed.

USES

In combination with heparin, treatment of acute coronary syndrome, including those to be managed medically and those undergoing percutaneous transluminal coronary angioplasty (PTCA) or atherectomy.

STORAGE

Store at room temperature. Discard unused solution within 24 hrs following the start of the infusion.

ADMINISTRATION

IV:

- **Note:** Heparin and tirobifan can be administered through the same IV line.

Injection for solution (250 mcg/ml):

- Withdraw and discard 100 ml from a 500 ml bag 0.9% sodium chloride or 5% dextrose in water and replace this volume with 100 ml of tirobifan (from two 50 ml vials) or withdraw and discard 50 ml from a 250 ml bag and replace with 50 ml of tirobifan (from one 50 ml vial) to achieve a final concentration of 50 mcg/ml.
- Mix well before administration.

Injection (50 mcg/ml) premix in 500 ml *IntraVia* container:

- To open the *IntraVia* container, tear off the dust cover.
- Check for leaks by squeezing the inner bag firmly; if any leak is found or if the solution is not clear, discard the solution.
- Do not add other drugs or remove solution directly from the bag with a syringe. Do not use plastic containers in series connections (may result in air embolism by drawing air from the first container if it is empty of solution).

INDICATIONS/ROUTES/DOSAGES

Inhibition of platelet aggregation: *IV: **Adults, elderly:*** Give at initial rate of 0.4 mcg/kg/min for 30 min and then continue at 0.1 mcg/kg/min. ***Severe renal insufficiency (creatinine clearance < 30 ml/min):*** half the usual rate of infusion.

CONTRAINDICATIONS

Active internal bleeding or history of bleeding within the past 30 days, history of intracranial hemorrhage or neoplasm, arteriovenous malformation or aneurysm, history of thrombocytopenia following prior exposure to tirobifan, history of stroke within 30 days, history of hemorrhagic stroke, major surgical procedure or severe physical trauma within 30 days, history or findings of aortic dissection, severe hypertension (systolic B/P > 180 mm Hg or diastolic B/P > 110 mm Hg), concurrent use of other parenteral GP IIb/IIIa platelet inhibitors, acute pericarditis.

CAUTIONS

Patients with platelet counts <150,000/mm^3, hemorrhagic retinopathy, elderly (increased risk of bleeding complications).

INTERACTIONS

DRUG: ***Warfarin, aspirin, heparin*** increases risk of bleeding. **HERBAL:** Ginkgo biloba may increase risk of bleeding. **FOOD:** None significant. **ALTERED LAB VALUES:** Prolongs bleeding time, decreases Hgb, Hct, APTT.

SIDE EFFECTS

OCCASIONAL (3–6%): Pelvis pain, bradycardia, dizziness, leg pain. **RARE (1–2%):** Edema/swelling, vasovagal reaction, sweating, nausea, fever, headache.

ADVERSE REACTIONS/TOXIC EFFECTS

Overdosage manifested as primarily minor mucocutaneous bleeding and bleeding at the femoral artery access site.

PATIENT CONSIDERATIONS

Baseline Assessment

Assess platelet count, Hgb, Hct prior to treatment, within 6 hrs following the loading dose and at least daily thereafter during therapy. If platelet count <90,000/mm^3, additional platelet counts should be obtained routinely to avoid thrombocytopenia. If thrombocytopenia occurs, drug therapy and heparin should be discontinued.

Intervention/Evaluation

Monitor APTT 6 hrs after the beginning of the heparin infusion. Adjust heparin dosage to maintain APTT at ≈2 times control. Diligently monitor for potential bleeding, particularly at other arterial and venous puncture sites, IM injection site. If possible, urinary catheters, nasogastric tubes should be avoided. Maintain complete bed rest with head of the bed elevated at 30°.

T

tizanidine hydrochloride

tie-**zan**-ih-deen
(Zanaflex)

PREGNANCY CATEGORY C

CLASSIFICATION

Muscle relaxant

AVAILABILITY (Rx)

Tablets: 4 mg

PHARMACODYNAMICS

	ONSET	PEAK	DURATION
Oral	30 min	1–2 hrs	3–6 hrs

PHARMACOKINETICS

Absorption: Completely absorbed following oral administration. 30% bound to plasma proteins. Widely distributed throughout the body. **Metabolism:** Extensive first-pass metabolism in the liver to inactive metabolite. **Excretion:** Eliminated in urine and feces. **Half-life:**2.5 hrs.

ACTION/*THERAPEUTIC EFFECT*

Increases presynaptic inhibition of spinal motor neurons mediated by alpha$_2$-adrenergic agonists, reducing facilitation to postsynaptic motor neurons, *reducing muscle spasticity.*

USES/*UNLABELED*

For acute and intermittent management of increased muscle tone (spasms, stiffness, rigidity) associated with spasticity. *Spasticity associated with multiple sclerosis and spinal cord injury.*

INDICATIONS/ROUTES/DOSAGES

Muscle spasticity:
Oral: Adults, elderly: Initially, 4 mg. May gradually increase in 2–4 mg increments to optimum effect. May repeat dose at 6–8 hr intervals to a maximum of 3 doses per 24 hrs. ***Maximum:*** 36 mg/day.

CONTRAINDICATIONS

History of hypersensitivity to tizanidine.

CAUTIONS

Renal insufficiency, hepatic function impairment, elderly (clearance is decreased 4-fold).

INTERACTIONS

DRUG: *Oral contraceptives*>may reduce tizanidine clearance. May increase serum levels/toxicity of ***phenytoin. Alcohol, CNS depressants*** may increase CNS depressant effects. ***Antihypertensives*** may increase tizandidine's hypotensive potential. **HERBAL:** None known. **FOOD:** May give w/o regard to food. **ALTERED LAB VALUES:** May increase ALT (SGPT), AST (SGOT), alkaline phosphatase.

SIDE EFFECTS

FREQUENT: (41–49%): Dry mouth, somnolence, asthenia (loss of strength, weakness). **OCCASIONAL (4–16%):** Dizziness, urinary tract infection, constipation. **RARE (3%):** Nervousness, amblyopia (dimness of vision), pharyngitis, rhinitis, vomiting, urinary frequency.

ADVERSE REACTIONS/TOXIC EFFECTS

Hypotension with a reduction in either diastolic or systolic B/P and may be associated with bradycardia, orthostatic hypotension and rarely, syncope. As dosage increases, risk of hypotension increases and is noted within 1 hr after dosing.

PATIENT CONSIDERATIONS

BASELINE ASSESSMENT

Record onset, type, location, and duration of muscular spasm. Check for immobility, stiffness, swelling. Obtain baseline liver function tests, alkaline phosphatase, and total bilirubin.

INTERVENTION/EVALUATION

Assist with ambulation at all times. For those on long-term therapy, liver/renal function tests should be performed periodically. Evaluate for therapeutic response (decreased intensity of skeletal muscle pain/tenderness, improved mobility, decrease in spasticity). For those at increased risk of orthostatic hypotension, instruct pt to rise slowly from lying to sitting and from sitting to supine position.

PATIENT/FAMILY TEACHING

Avoid tasks that require alertness, motor skills until response to drug is established. Avoid sudden changes in posture. Avoid alcohol or other CNS depressants while taking medication.

tobramycin sulfate

tow-bra-**my**-sin
(Nebcin, Tobi, Tobrex)

FIXED-COMBINATION(S)
W/dexamethasone, a steroid **(TobraDex)**

CANADIAN AVAILABILITY
Nebcin, Tobrex

PREGNANCY CATEGORY D
Ophthalmic: Pregnancy Category B.

CLASSIFICATION

Antibiotic: Aminoglycoside

AVAILABILITY (Rx)

Injection: 10 mg/ml, 40 mg/ml. **Powder for Injection:** 1.2 g. **Ophthalmic Solution:** 0.3%. **Ophthalmic Ointment:** 3 mg/g. **Inhalation Solution:** 300 mg/5 ml.

PHARMACOKINETICS

Absorption: Rapid, complete absorption after IM administration. Widely distributed (does not cross blood-brain barrier, low concentrations in CSF). **Excretion:** Excreted unchanged in urine. Removed by hemodialysis. **Half-life:** 2–4 hrs (increased in decreased renal function, neonates; decreased in cystic fibrosis, burn or febrile pts).

ACTION/*THERAPEUTIC EFFECT*

Irreversibly binds to protein on bacterial ribosome, *interfering in protein synthesis of susceptible microorganisms.*

USES

Skin/skin structure, bone, joint, respiratory tract infections; postop, burn, intra-abdominal infections, complicated urinary tract infections, septicemia, meningitis. ***Ophthalmic:*** Superficial eye infections: blepharitis, conjunctivitis, keratitis, corneal ulcers. ***Inhalation:*** Bronchopulmonary infections in pts w/cystic fibrosis.

STORAGE/HANDLING

Store vials, ophthalmic ointment, solution at room temperature. Solutions may be discolored by light/air (does not affect potency). Intermittent IV infusion (piggyback) stable for 24 hrs at room temperature. Discard if precipitate forms.

ADMINISTRATION

IM:

- To minimize discomfort, give deep IM slowly. Less painful if injected into gluteus maximus rather than lateral aspect of thigh.

IV:

- Dilute w/50–200 ml 5% dextrose, 0.9% NaCl, or other compatible fluid. Amount of diluent for infants, children depends on individual need.
- Infuse over 20–60 min.
- Alternating IV sites, use large veins to reduce risk of phlebitis.

OPHTHALMIC:

- Place finger on lower eyelid and pull out until a pocket is formed between eye and lower lid.
- Hold dropper above pocket and place correct number of drops ($^1/_4$–$^1/_2$ inch ointment) into pocket. Have pt close eye gently.

- *Solution:* Apply digital pressure to lacrimal sac for 1–2 min (minimizes drainage into nose and throat, reducing risk of systemic effects.) *Ointment:* Close eye for 1–2 min, rolling eyeball (increases contact area of drug to eye).
- Remove excess solution or ointment around eye w/tissue.

INDICATIONS/ROUTES/DOSAGE

Note: Dosage based on ideal body weight. Peak, trough level is determined periodically to maintain desired serum concentrations (minimizes risk of toxicity). *Recommended peak level:* 4–10 mcg/ml; *trough level:* 1–2 mcg/ml.

Moderate to severe infections:
IM/IV: Adults, elderly: 3 mg/kg/day in divided doses q8h.

Life-threatening infections:
IM/IV: Adults, elderly: Up to 5 mg/kg/day in divided doses q6–8h.

Usual dosage for children, infants:
IM/IV: Children, infants: 6–7.5 mg/kg/day in 3–4 divided doses.

Dosage in renal impairment:
Dose and/or frequency is modified based on degree of renal impairment, serum concentration of drug. After loading dose of 1–2 mg/kg, maintenance dose/frequency based on serum creatinine/creatinine clearance.

Usual ophthalmic dosage:
Ophthalmic Ointment: Adults, elderly: Thin strip to conjunctiva q8–12h (q3–4h for severe infections). *Ophthalmic Solution:* Adults, elderly: 1–2 drops q4h (2 drops every hour for severe infections).

Usual inhalation dosage:
Adults, elderly: 80 mg twice daily for 28 days, then off for 28 days.

CONTRAINDICATIONS

Hypersensitivity to tobramycin, other aminoglycosides (cross-sensitivity).

CAUTIONS

Elderly, neonates because of renal insufficiency/immaturity; neuromuscular disorders (potential for respiratory depression), prior hearing loss, vertigo, renal impairment. Cumulative effects may occur w/concurrent ophthalmic and systemic administration.

INTERACTIONS

DRUG: Other ***aminoglycosides, nephrotoxic, ototoxic-producing medications*** may increase toxicity. May increase effects of ***neuromuscular blocking agents.*** **HERBAL:** None known. **FOOD:** None significant. **ALTERED LAB VALUES:** May increase BUN, SGPT (ALT), SGOT (AST), bilirubin, creatinine, LDH concentrations; may decrease serum calcium, magnesium, potassium, sodium concentrations.

SIDE EFFECTS

OCCASIONAL: Pain, induration at IM injection site; phlebitis, thrombophlebitis w/IV administration; hypersensitivity reactions (rash, fever, urticaria, pruritus). *Ophthalmic:* Tearing, itching, redness, swelling of eyelid. **RARE:** Hypotension, nausea, vomiting.

ADVERSE REACTIONS/TOXIC EFFECTS

Nephrotoxicity (evidenced by increased BUN and serum creatinine, decreased creatinine clearance) may be reversible if drug stopped at first sign of symptoms; irreversible ototoxicity (tinnitus, dizziness, ringing/roaring in ears, reduced hearing) and neurotoxicity (headache, dizziness, lethargy, tremors, visual disturbances) occur occasionally. Risk is greater w/higher dosages, prolonged therapy, or if solution is applied directly to mucosa. Superinfections, particularly w/fungi, may result from bacterial imbalance via any route of administration; anaphylaxis.

PATIENT CONSIDERATIONS

Baseline Assessment

Dehydration must be treated before parenteral therapy is begun. Question for history of allergies, especially to aminoglycosides and sulfite (and parabens for topical/ophthalmic routes). Establish baseline for hearing acuity. Obtain specimens for culture, sensitivity before giving first dose (therapy may begin before results are known).

Intervention/Evaluation

Monitor I&O (maintain hydration), urinalysis (casts, RBCs, WBCs, decrease in specific gravity). Monitor results of peak/trough blood tests. Be alert to ototoxic and neurotoxic symptoms (see Adverse Reactions/Toxic Effects). Check IM injection site for pain, induration. Evaluate IV site for phlebitis (heat, pain, red streaking over vein). Assess for rash (*ophthalmic*—assess for redness, swelling, itching, tearing). Be alert for superinfection particularly genital/anal pruritus, changes of oral mucosa, diarrhea. When treating pts w/neuromuscular disorders, assess respiratory response carefully.

Patient/Family Teaching

Continue antibiotic for full length of treatment. Space doses evenly. Discomfort may occur w/IM injection. Notify physician in event of any hearing, visual, balance, urinary problems even after therapy is completed. Do not take other medication w/o consulting physician. Lab tests are an essential part of therapy. *Ophthalmic:* Blurred vision/tearing may occur briefly after application. Contact physician if tearing, redness, or irritation continues.

T

tocainide hydrochloride

toe-**kay**-nied
(Tonocard)

CANADIAN AVAILABILITY
Tonocard

PREGNANCY CATEGORY C

CLASSIFICATION

Antiarrhythmic

AVAILABILITY (Rx)

Tablets: 400 mg, 600 mg

PHARMACOKINETICS

Absorption: Completely absorbed from GI tract. Widely distributed. **Metabolism:** Metabolized in liver. **Excretion:** Primarily excreted in urine. Removed by hemodialysis. **Half-life:** 15 hrs (increased in decreased renal function).

ACTION/*THERAPEUTIC EFFECT*

Shortens action potential duration, decreases effective refractory period, automaticity in His-Purkinje system of myocardium by blocking sodium transport across myocardial cell membranes, *suppressing ventricular arrhythmias.*

USES

Suppression, prevention of ventricular arrhythmias including frequent unifocal/multifocal coupled premature ventricular contractions and paroxysmal ventricular tachycardia.

ADMINISTRATION

ORAL:

- Do not crush or break film-coated tablets.
- May give w/food (decreases GI upset).
- Monitor EKG for cardiac changes, particularly shortening of QT interval. Notify physician of any significant interval changes.

INDICATIONS/ROUTES/DOSAGE

Note: When giving tocainide in those receiving IV lidocaine, give single 600 mg dose 6 hrs before cessation of lidocaine and repeat in 6 hrs. Then give standard tocainide maintenance doses.

Ventricular arrhythmias:

Oral: Adults, elderly: Initially, 400 mg q8h. ***Maintenance:*** 1.2–1.8 g/day in divided doses q8h. ***Maximum:*** 2,400 mg/day.

CONTRAINDICATIONS

Hypersensitivity to local anesthetics, second- or third-degree AV block.

CAUTIONS

CHF, elderly, severe respiratory depression, bradycardia, incomplete heart block.

INTERACTIONS

DRUG: ***Other antiarrhythmics*** may increase risk of adverse cardiac effects. ***Beta-adrenergic blockers*** may increase pulmonary wedge pressure, decrease cardiac index. **HERBAL:** None known. **FOOD:** None significant. **ALTERED LAB VALUES:** None significant.

SIDE EFFECTS

Generally well tolerated. **FREQUENT (3–10%):** Minor, transient lightheadedness, dizziness, nausea, paresthesia, rash, tremor. **OCCASIONAL (1–3%):** Clammy skin, night sweats, joint pain. **RARE (<1%):** Restlessness, nervousness, disorientation, mood changes, ataxia (muscular incoordination), visual disturbances.

ADVERSE REACTIONS/TOXIC EFFECTS

High dosage may produce bradycardia/tachycardia, hypotension, palpitations, increased ventricular arrhythmias, PVCs, chest pain, exacerbation of CHF.

PATIENT CONSIDERATIONS

BASELINE ASSESSMENT

Assess pulse for strength/weakness, irregular rate. Monitor EKG for cardiac changes, particularly shortening of QT interval. Notify physician of any significant interval changes. Monitor fluid and electrolyte serum levels. Assess hand movement for sign of tremor (usually first clinical sign that maximum dose is being reached). Assess sleeping pt for night sweats. Question for tingling/numbness in

hands/feet. Assess skin for rash, clamminess. Observe for CNS disturbances (restlessness, disorientation, mood changes, incoordination). Assist w/ambulation if lightheadedness, dizziness occur. Assess for evidence of CHF: dyspnea (particularly on exertion or lying down), night cough, peripheral edema, distended neck veins. Monitor I&O (increase in weight, decrease in urine output may indicate CHF). Monitor for therapeutic serum level (3–10 mcg/ml).

Patient/Family Teaching

Avoid tasks that require alertness, motor skills until response to drug is established. Side effects generally disappear w/continued therapy. Unsalted crackers, dry toast may relieve nausea.

---

tolazamide

(Tolinase, Tolamide)

See Classification section under: Antidiabetic agents

---

tolazoline hydrochloride

toe-**laze**-oh-lean

(Priscoline)

CLASSIFICATION

Antihypertensive

AVAILABILITY (Rx)

Injection: 25 mg/ml

PHARMACOKINETICS

Absorption: Rapidly, completely absorbed. Concentrated primarily in liver, kidney. **Excretion:** Excreted unchanged in urine. **Half-life:** 3–10 hrs.

ACTION/*THERAPEUTIC EFFECT*

Directly relaxes vascular smooth muscle, *causes vasodilation, decreases peripheral resistance.* Has moderate alpha-adrenergic blocking activity.

USES

Treatment of persistent pulmonary vasoconstriction and hypertension of newborn (persistent fetal circulation). Improves oxygenation.

ADMINISTRATION

IV:

- Monitor B/P diligently for systemic hypotension. If hypotension occurs, place in supine position w/feet elevated, give IV fluids. Do not administer epinephrine. Tolazoline may cause "epinephrine reversal" (further B/P decrease followed by rebound hypertension).

INDICATIONS/ROUTES/DOSAGE

Persistent fetal circulation:
IV: Newborn: Initially, 1–2 mg/kg via scalp vein over 10 min; then, IV infusion of 1–2 mg/kg/hr.

CONTRAINDICATIONS

None significant.

CAUTIONS

Known/suspected mitral stenosis.

INTERACTIONS

DRUG: Antagonizes vasoconstriction caused by ***dopamine.*** Decreases effects of ***metaraminol, ephedrine, phenylephrine.*** **HERBAL:** None known. **FOOD:** None significant. **ALTERED LAB VALUES:** None significant.

SIDE EFFECTS

OCCASIONAL: Nausea, diarrhea, vomiting, increased pilomotor activity (goose bumps), peripheral vasodilation (flushing), tachycardia. RARE: Mydriasis.

ADVERSE REACTIONS/TOXIC EFFECTS

GI hemorrhage, hypochloremic alkalosis, cardiac arrhythmias, hypotension, oliguria, hepatitis, thrombocytopenia, leukopenia may occur.

PATIENT CONSIDERATIONS

Baseline Assessment

Obtain B/P immediately before each dose, in addition to regular monitoring (be alert to fluctuations). If excessive reduction in B/P occurs, place pt in supine position w/feet elevated, give IV fluids.

Intervention/Evaluation

Monitor vital signs, oxygenation, acid-base balance, fluid and electrolytes.

---

tolbutamide

(Orinase, Oramide)

See Classification section under: Antidiabetic agents

---

tolcapone

toll-cah-pone

(Tasmar)

CANADIAN AVAILABILITY

Tasmar

PREGNANCY CATEGORY C

CLASSIFICATION

Antiparkinson agent

AVAILABILITY (Rx)

Tablets: 100 mg, 200 mg

PHARMACOKINETICS

Absorption: Rapidly absorbed following oral administration. Highly bound to plasma protein, mainly albumin (99.9%). **Metabolism:** Metabolized in the liver. **Excretion:** Eliminated primarily in the urine (60%) and to a lesser amount (40%) in the feces. **Half-life:** 2–3 hrs.

ACTION/*THERAPEUTIC EFFECT*

Inhibits the enzyme COMT, sustaining plasma levels and thereby increasing the duration of action of levodopa, resulting in greater effect *relieving signs and symptoms of Parkinson's disease.*

USES

Adjunctive therapy to levodopa and carbidopa for treatment of signs and symptoms of idiopathic Parkinson's disease.

INDICATIONS/ROUTES/DOSAGES

Note: May combine tolcapone with both the immediate and sustained-release form of levodopa/carbidopa.

Parkinson's disease:

Oral: Adults, elderly: Initially, 100–200 mg 3 times/day. ***Maximum:*** 600 mg/day. ***Moderate to severe cirrhosis of liver:*** Do not increase to 200 mg 3 times/day.

CONTRAINDICATIONS

None significant.

CAUTIONS

Sensitivity to tolcapone, severe renal impairment, severe liver impairment, those with history of hallucinations, baseline hypotension, history of orthostatic hypotension.

INTERACTIONS

DRUG: Increases *levodopa* duration of action. **HERBAL:** None known. **FOOD:** Food given 1 hr before or 2 hrs after tolcapone administration decreases bioavailability by 10–20%. **ALTERED LAB VALUES:** May increase AST (SGOT), ALT (SGPT).

SIDE EFFECTS

Note: Frequency of occurrence increases with dosage amount. Following is based on 200 mg dose. **FREQUENT:** Nausea **(35%), (16–25%):** Insomnia, somnolence, anorexia, diarrhea, muscle cramps, orthostatic hypotension, excessive dreaming. **OCCASIONAL (4–11%):** Headache, vomiting, confusion, hallucinations, constipation, increased sweating, urine discoloration (bright yellow), dry eyes, abdominal pain, dizziness, flatulence. **RARE (2–3%):** Dyspepsia, neck pain, hypotension, fatigue, chest discomfort.

ADVERSE REACTIONS/TOXIC EFFECTS

Upper respiratory infection, urinary tract infection occur occasionally (5–7%). Too rapid withdrawal from therapy may produce withdrawal emergent hyperpyrexia characterized by elevated temperature, muscular rigidity, altered consciousness. An increase in dyskinesia (impaired voluntary movement) or dystonia (impaired muscular tone) occur frequently.

PATIENT CONSIDERATIONS

Baseline Assessment

Serum transaminase levels should be monitored every 2 wks for first year, every 4 wks for next 6 mos, and every 8 wks thereafter. Treatment should be discontinued if ALT (SGPT) exceeds 5 times the normal range or if jaundice develops. If hallucination occurs may be eliminated if levodopa dosage is reduced. Hallucinations generally are accompanied by confusion and to a lesser extent, insomnia.

Interventions/Evaluation

Instruct pt to rise from lying to sitting or sitting to standing position slowly to prevent risk of postural hypotension. Assist with ambulation if dizziness occurs. Assess for clinical reversal of symptoms (improvement of tremor of head/hands at rest, mask-like facial expression, shuffling gait, muscular rigidity).

Patient/Family Teaching

If nausea occurs, take medication with food. Drowsiness, dizziness, nausea may be an initial response of drug but diminishes or disappears with continued treatment. Postural hypotension may occur more frequently during initial therapy. Avoid tasks that require alertness, motor skills until response to drug is established. Hallucinations may occur, more so in the elderly than in younger pts with Parkinson's disease and typically within the first 2 wks of therapy. Inform physician if possibility of pregnancy occurs. Urine will change color to a bright yellow.

tolmetin sodium

toll-**meh**-tin
(Tolectin)

CANADIAN AVAILABILITY
Tolectin

PREGNANCY CATEGORY C
(D if used in third trimester or near delivery)

CLASSIFICATION

Nonsteroidal anti-inflammatory

AVAILABILITY (Rx)

Tablets: 200 mg, 600 mg. **Capsules:** 400 mg.

PHARMACODYNAMICS

	ONSET	PEAK	DURATION
Oral (antirheumatic):	7 days	1–2 wks	—

PHARMACOKINETICS

Absorption: Rapidly, completely absorbed from GI tract. **Metabolism:** Metabolized in liver. **Excretion:** Excreted in urine. **Half-life:** 5 hrs.

ACTION / *THERAPEUTIC EFFECT*

Produces analgesic and anti-inflammatory effect by inhibiting prostaglandin synthesis, *reducing inflammatory response and intensity of pain stimulus reaching sensory nerve endings.*

USES / *UNLABELED*

Relief of pain, disability associated w/rheumatoid arthritis, juvenile rheumatoid arthritis, osteoarthritis. *Treatment of ankylosing spondylitis, psoriatic arthritis.*

ADMINISTRATION

ORAL:

- May give w/food, milk, or antacids if GI distress occurs.

INDICATIONS / ROUTES / DOSAGE

Rheumatoid arthritis, osteoarthritis:
Oral: Adults, elderly: Initially, 400 mg 3 times/day (including 1 dose upon arising, 1 dose at bedtime). Adjust dose at 1–2 wk intervals. *Maintenance:* 600–1,800 mg/day in 3–4 divided doses.

Juvenile rheumatoid arthritis:
Oral: Children >2 yrs: Initially, 20 mg/kg/day in 3–4 divided doses. *Maintenance:* 15–30 mg/kg/day in 3–4 divided doses.

CONTRAINDICATIONS

History of hypersensitivity to aspirin or other NSAIDs, those severely incapacitated, bedridden, wheelchair bound.

CAUTIONS

Impaired renal function, impaired cardiac function, coagulation disorders, history of upper GI disease.

INTERACTIONS

DRUG: May increase effects of ***oral anticoagulants, heparin, thrombolytics.*** May decrease effect of ***antihypertensives, diuretics. Salicylates, aspirin*** may increase risk of GI side effects, bleeding. ***Bone marrow depressants*** may increase risk of hematologic reactions. May increase concentration, toxicity of ***lithium.*** May increase ***methotrexate*** toxicity. ***Probenecid*** may increase concentration. ***Antacids*** may decrease concentration. **HERBAL:** May decrease effects of feverfew. Ginkgo biloba may increase risk of bleeding. **FOOD:** None significant. **ALTERED LAB VALUES:** May increase BUN, potassium, liver function tests. May decrease Hgb, Hct. May prolong bleeding time.

SIDE EFFECTS

FREQUENT (3–9%): Increased blood pressure, muscle pain, fluid retention, edema, dizziness, headache, unusually weakness, abdominal pain, diarrhea, nausea, indigestion, vomiting, weight loss. **OCCASIONAL (1–3%):** Chest pain, itching, rash, GI ulceration, blurred or double vision, tinnitus, drowsiness, nervousness, insomnia, constipation. **RARE (<1%):** Unexplained nosebleeds, hives, GI bleeding, dysuria, fever, swollen lymph nodes, stomatitis, glossitis, trouble breathing, decreased appetite.

ADVERSE REACTIONS/TOXIC EFFECTS

Peptic ulcer, GI bleeding, gastritis, severe hepatic reaction (cholestasis, jaundice) occur rarely. Nephrotoxicity (dysuria, hematuria, proteinuria, nephrotic syndrome) and severe hypersensitivity reaction (fever, chills, bronchospasm) occur rarely.

PATIENT CONSIDERATIONS

Baseline Assessment

Assess onset, type, location, and duration of pain/inflammation. Inspect appearance of affected joints for immobility, deformities, and skin condition.

Intervention/Evaluation

Monitor pattern of daily bowel activity, stool consistency. Assist w/ambulation if dizziness occurs. Monitor for evidence of GI distress. Evaluate for therapeutic response (relief of pain, stiffness, swelling; increase in joint mobility, reduced joint tenderness, improved grip strength).

Patient/Family Teaching

Therapeutic effect noted in 1–3 wks. Avoid tasks that require alertness, motor skills until response to drug is established. If GI upset occurs, take w/food, milk. Avoid aspirin, alcohol during therapy (increases risk of GI bleeding). Report headache, GI distress.

tolnaftate

(Tinactin, Aftate)

See Classification section under: Antifungals: topical

tolterodine tartrate

toll-**tear**-oh-deen

(Detrol)

PREGNANCY CATEGORY C

CLASSIFICATION

Urinary tract agent

AVAILABILITY (Rx)

Tablets: 1 mg, 2 mg

PHARMACOKINETICS

Absorption: Rapidly, well absorbed following oral administration. Highly bound to plasma proteins. **Metabolism:** Extensive first-pass hepatic metabolism to active metabolite. **Excretion:** Primarily excreted in the urine. **Half-life:** 1.9–3.7 hrs.

ACTION/*THERAPEUTIC EFFECT*

A muscarinic receptor antagonist, exhibits potent antimuscarinic activity thereby relaxing urinary bladder contraction, *decreasing urinary frequency, urgency.*

USES

Treatment of those with an overactive bladder with symptoms of urinary frequency, urgency or urge incontinence.

INDICATIONS/ROUTES/DOSAGES

Overactive bladder:

Oral: Adults, elderly: 2 mg twice daily.

Severe hepatic impairment: 1 mg twice daily.

CONTRAINDICATIONS

Urinary retention, uncontrolled narrow-angle glaucoma, history of hypersensitivity to tolterodine.

CAUTIONS

Renal function impairment, clinically significant bladder outflow obstruction (risk of urinary retention), GI obstructive disorders, e.g., pyloric stenosis (risk of gastric retention), treated narrow-angle glaucoma.

INTERACTIONS

DRUG: *Clarithromycin, erythromycin, itraconazole, ketoconazole, miconazole* may increase concentration of tolterodine. *Fluoxetine* may inhibit metabolism of tolterodine. **HERBAL:** None known. **FOOD:** None significant. **ALTERED LAB VALUES:** None significant.

SIDE EFFECTS

FREQUENT: (40%): Dry mouth. **OCCASIONAL (4–11%):** Headache, dizziness, abdominal pain, fatigue, constipation, dyspepsia, upper respiratory infection, urinary tract infection, abnormal vision (including accommodation, dry eyes), nausea, diarrhea. **RARE (3%):** Somnolence, chest/back pain, arthralgia, rash, weight gain, dry skin.

ADVERSE REACTIONS/TOXIC EFFECTS

Overdosage can result in severe anticholinergic effects, including GI cramping, feeling of facial warmth, excessive salivation, sweating, lacrimation, pallor, urinary urgency, blurred vision and QT interval prolongation.

PATIENT CONSIDERATIONS

INTERVENTION/EVALUATION

Assist with ambulation if dizziness, lightheadedness occurs. Question for change in vision.

PATIENT/FAMILY TEACHING

Sips of tepid water or sour, hard candy may relieve dry mouth. Report nausea, constipation, and visual abnormalities.

---

topiramate

toe-**pier**-ah-mate
(Topamax)

CANADIAN AVAILABILITY
Topamax

PREGNANCY CATEGORY C

CLASSIFICATION

Anticonvulsant

AVAILABILITY (Rx)

Sprinkle Capsules: 15 mg, 25 mg. **Tablets:** 25 mg, 100 mg, 200 mg.

PHARMACOKINETICS

Absorption: Rapidly absorbed following oral administration. Bound to plasma proteins. **Metabolism:** Not extensively metabolized. **Excretion:** Primarily excreted unchanged in the urine. Cleared by hemodialysis. **Half-life:** 21 hrs.

ACTION/*THERAPEUTIC EFFECT*

Blocks repetitive, sustained firing of neurons by enhancing the ability of gamma aminobutyric acid (GABA) to induce a flux of chloride ions into the neurons, *decreasing seizure frequency.*

USES/*UNLABELED*

Adjunctive therapy for the treatment of partial onset seizures in adults. ***Children 2–16 yrs:*** Treatment of tonic-clonic seizures. *Treatment of migraines.*

ADMINISTRATION

ORAL:

- Do not break tablets (bitter taste).
- Give w/o regard to meals.
- Capsules may be swallowed whole or contents sprinkled on a teaspoon of soft food and swallowed immediately, not chewed.

INDICATIONS/ROUTES/DOSAGES

Partial seizures:
Oral: Adults >18 yrs, elderly: Initially, 50 mg/day followed by weekly increments of 50 mg to total daily dosage of 400 mg/day in 2 divided doses. ***Children (2–16 yrs):*** 5–9 mg/kg/day in 2 divided doses.

CONTRAINDICATIONS

None significant.

CAUTIONS

Sensitivity to topiramate, impaired liver/renal function, predisposition to renal calculi.

INTERACTIONS

DRUG: ***Phenytoin, valproic acid, carbamazepine*** may decrease topiramate concentration. ***Carbonic anhydrase inhibitors*** may increase risk of renal calculi. May decrease effective of ***oral contraceptives. Alcohol, CNS depressants*** may increase CNS depression. **HERBAL:** None known. **FOOD:** None significant. **ALTERED LAB VALUES:** None significant.

SIDE EFFECTS

FREQUENT (10–30%): Somnolence, dizziness, ataxia, nervousness, nystagmus (involuntary eye movement), diplopia (double vision), paresthesia, nausea, tremor. **OCCASIONAL (3–9%):** Confusion, breast pain, dysmenorrhea, dyspepsia, depression, asthenia (loss of strength), pharyngitis, weight loss, anorexia, rash, back/abdominal/leg pain, difficulty with coordination, sinusitis, agitation, flulike symptoms. **RARE: (2–3%):** Mood disturbances (irritability, depression), dry mouth, aggressive reaction.

ADVERSE REACTIONS/TOXIC EFFECTS

Psychomotor slowing, difficulty with concentration, language problems, especially word-finding difficulties, and memory disturbances occur occasionally. These events are generally mild to moderate but may be severe enough to require withdrawal from drug therapy.

PATIENT CONSIDERATIONS

BASELINE ASSESSMENT

Review history of seizure disorder (intensity, frequency, duration, LOC). Provide safety precautions, quiet, dark environment. Question sensitivity to topiramate, pregnancy, use of other anticonvulsant medication (especially carbamazepine, valproic acid, phenytoin, carbonic anhydrase inhibitors). Assess renal function. Instruct pt to use alternative/additional means of contraception (topiramate decreases effectiveness of oral contraceptives).

INTERVENTION/EVALUATION

Observe frequently for recurrence of seizure activity. Assess for clinical improvement (decrease in intensity/frequency of seizures). Monitor renal function tests (BUN, creatinine). Assist with ambulation if dizziness occurs.

PATIENT/FAMILY TEACHING

Avoid tasks that require alertness, motor skills until response to drug is established (may cause dizziness, drowsiness, impaired thinking). Avoid use of alcohol, other CNS depressants. Do not abruptly discontinue (may precipitate seizures). Strict maintenance of drug therapy is essential for seizure control. Drowsiness usually diminished with continued therapy. Do not break tablets (bitter taste). Maintain adequate fluid intake (decreases risk of renal stone formation).

topotecan

(Hycamtin)
See Classification section under: Cancer chemotherapy

toremifene

(Fareston)
See Supplement
See Classification section under: Cancer chemotherapy

torsemide

tore-seh-mide
(Demadex)

CANADIAN AVAILABILITY
Demadex

PREGNANCY CATEGORY B

CLASSIFICATION

Diuretic: Loop

AVAILABILITY (Rx)

Tablets: 5 mg, 10 mg, 20 mg, 100 mg. **Injection:** 10 mg/ml.

PHARMACODYNAMICS

	ONSET	PEAK	DURATION
Oral	1 hr	1–2 hrs	6–8 hrs
IV	20 min	1 hr	6–8 hrs

PHARMACOKINETICS

Absorption: Rapidly, well absorbed from GI tract. **Metabolism:** Metabolized in liver. **Excretion:** Primarily excreted in urine. **Half-life:** 3.3 hrs.

ACTION/*THERAPEUTIC EFFECT*

Diuretic: Enhances excretion of sodium, chloride, potassium, water at ascending limb of loop of Henle, *producing diuretic effect.* ***Antihypertensive:*** Reduces plasma, extracellular fluid volume, *lowering B/P.*

USES

Treatment of hypertension either alone or in combination w/other antihypertensives. Edema associated w/CHF, renal disease, hepatic cirrhosis, chronic renal failure.

STORAGE/HANDLING

Store oral, parenteral forms at room temperature.

ADMINISTRATION

ORAL:

- May take w/o regard to food. Give w/food to avoid GI upset, preferably w/breakfast (prevents nocturia).

IV:

- Give slowly over 2 min or as continuous IV infusion.
- Give high doses slowly (minimizes risk of ototoxicity).

INDICATIONS/ROUTES/DOSAGE

Hypertension:
Oral: Adults, elderly: Initially, 5 mg/day. May increase to 10

mg/day if no response in 4–6 wks. If no response, additional antihypertensive added.

Congestive heart failure:
IV/Oral: Adults, elderly: Initially, 10–20 mg/day. May increase by approximately doubling dose until desired diuretic dose attained. (Dose >200 mg not adequately studied.)

Chronic renal failure:
IV/Oral: Adults, elderly: Initially, 20 mg/day. May increase by approximately doubling dose until desired diuretic dose attained. (Dose >200 mg not adequately studied.)

Hepatic cirrhosis:
IV/Oral: Adults, elderly: Initially, 5 mg/day (w/aldosterone antagonist or potassium-sparing diuretic). May increase by approximately doubling dose until desired diuretic dose attained. (Dose >40 mg not adequately studied.)

CONTRAINDICATIONS

Anuria, hepatic coma, severe electrolyte depletion.

EXTREME CAUTION

Hypersensitivity to sulfonamides.

CAUTIONS

Elderly, cardiac pts, pts w/history of ventricular arrhythmias, pts w/hepatic cirrhosis, ascites. Renal impairment, systemic lupus erythematosus. Safety in children not known.

INTERACTIONS

DRUG: May increase antihypertensive effect of ***other antihypertensives. NSAIDs, probenecid*** may decrease effect. May increase risk of ***digoxin***-induced arrhythmias (due to hypokalemia). ***Amphotericin*** may increase risk nephrotoxicity. Effects of ***anticoagulants, heparin, thrombolytics*** may be decreased, hypokalemia-causing medications may increase risk of hypokalemia; may increase risk of ***lithium*** toxicity. ***Nephrotoxic/ototoxic medications*** may increase nephrotoxicity/ototoxicity. **HERBAL:** None known. **FOOD:** None significant. **ALTERED LAB VALUES:** May increase uric acid, BUN, creatinine. May decrease calcium, chloride, magnesium, potassium, sodium.

SIDE EFFECTS

FREQUENT (3–10%): Headache, dizziness, rhinitis. **OCCASIONAL (1–3%):** Asthenia, insomnia, nervousness, diarrhea, constipation, nausea, dyspepsia, edema, EKG changes, sore throat, cough, arthralgia, myalgia. **RARE (<1%):** Syncope, hypotension, arrhythmias.

T

ADVERSE REACTIONS/TOXIC EFFECTS

Overdosage produces acute, profound water loss, volume and electrolyte depletion, dehydration, decreased blood volume, circulatory collapse. Ototoxicity may occur: High IV doses must be given slowly to minimize ototoxicity.

PATIENT CONSIDERATIONS

BASELINE ASSESSMENT

Assess B/P for hypotension. Check electrolyte levels, especially potassium. Obtain baseline weight; check for edema, rales in lungs.

INTERVENTION/EVALUATION

Monitor B/P, electrolytes (especially potassium), I&O, weight. Notify physician of any hearing abnormality. Note extent of diure-

sis. Assess lungs for rales. Check for signs of edema, particularly of dependent areas. Although less potassium is lost w/torsemide than furosemide, assess for signs of hypokalemia (change of muscle strength, tremor, muscle cramps, change in mental status, cardiac arrhythmias).

PATIENT/FAMILY TEACHING

Take medication in morning to prevent nocturia. Expect increased frequency and volume of urination. Report irregular heartbeats, signs of hypokalemia (see above), muscle weakness, cramps, nausea, or dizziness. Change positions slowly to prevent orthostatic hypotension. Do not take other medications (including OTC drugs) w/o consulting physician. Eat foods high in potassium such as whole grains (cereals), legumes, meat, bananas, apricots, orange juice, potatoes (white, sweet), raisins.

tramadol hydrochloride

tray-mah-doal
(Ultram)

PREGNANCY CATEGORY C

CLASSIFICATION

Analgesic

AVAILABILITY (Rx)

Tablets: 50 mg

PHARMACODYNAMICS

	ONSET	PEAK	DURATION
Oral	<1 hr	2–3 hrs	4–6 hrs

PHARMACOKINETICS

Absorption: Rapidly, almost completely absorbed following oral administration. **Metabolism:** Extensively metabolized in liver to active metabolite (reduced in pts w/advanced cirrhosis). **Excretion:** Primarily excreted in urine. Minimally removed by hemodialysis. **Half-life:** 6–7 hrs.

ACTION/*THERAPEUTIC EFFECT*

Binds to μ-opiate receptors and inhibits reuptake of norepinephrine and serotonin. *Reduces intensity of pain stimuli incoming from sensory nerve endings, altering pain perception and emotional response to pain.*

USES

Management of moderate to moderately severe pain.

ADMINISTRATION

ORAL:

- Give w/o regard to meals.

INDICATIONS/ROUTES/DOSAGE

Moderate to moderately severe pain:
Oral: Adults, elderly: 50–100 mg q4–6h. *Maximum <75 yrs:* 400 mg/day. *Maximum >75 yrs:* 300 mg/day.

Renal function impairment (creatinine clearance <30 ml/min):
Note: Dialysis pts can receive their regular dose on day of dialysis.

Oral: Adults, elderly: Increase dosing interval to 12 hrs. *Maximum daily dose:* 200 mg.

Hepatic function impairment:
Oral: Adults, elderly: 50 mg q12h.

CONTRAINDICATIONS

Hypersensitivity to tramadol, acute

intoxication w/alcohol, hypnotics, centrally acting analgesics, opioids or psychotropic drugs.

EXTREME CAUTION

CNS depression, anoxia, advanced liver cirrhosis, epilepsy, respiratory depression, acute alcoholism, shock.

CAUTIONS

Sensitivity to opioids, increased intracranial pressure, impaired hepatic/renal function, acute abdominal conditions, opioid-dependent pts.

INTERACTIONS

DRUG: ***Alcohol, CNS depressants*** may increase CNS effects or respiratory depression, hypotension. ***MAO inhibitors*** increase tramadol concentration. ***Carbamazepine*** increases tramadol metabolism, decreases concentration. **HERBAL:** None known. **FOOD:** None significant. **ALTERED LAB VALUES:** May increase creatinine, liver enzymes. May decrease hemoglobin, proteinuria.

SIDE EFFECTS

FREQUENT (15–25%): Dizziness/vertigo, nausea, constipation, headache, somnolence. **OCCASIONAL (5–10%):** Vomiting, pruritus, CNS stimulation (nervousness, anxiety, agitation, tremor, euphoria, mood swings, hallucinations), asthenia, sweating, dyspepsia, dry mouth, diarrhea. **RARE (<5%):** Malaise, vasodilation, anorexia, flatulence, rash, visual disturbance, urinary retention/frequency, menopausal symptoms.

ADVERSE REACTIONS/TOXIC EFFECTS

Overdosage results in respiratory depression, skeletal muscle flaccidity, cold clammy skin, cyanosis, extreme somnolence progressing to seizures, stupor, coma. Tolerance to analgesic effect, physical dependence may occur w/repeated use. Prolonged duration of action, cumulative effect may occur in those w/impaired hepatic, renal function.

PATIENT CONSIDERATIONS

BASELINE ASSESSMENT

Assess onset, type, location, and duration of pain. Effect of medication is reduced if full pain recurs before next dose. Assess drug history, especially carbamazepine, CNS depressant medication, MAO inhibitors. Review past medical history, especially epilepsy/seizures. Assess renal/liver function lab values.

INTERVENTION/EVALUATION

Assist w/ambulation if dizziness, vertigo occurs. Dry crackers, cola may relieve nausea. Question bowel activity, frequency. Palpate bladder for urinary retention. Monitor pattern of daily bowel activity and stool consistency. Sips of tepid water may relieve dry mouth. Assess for clinical improvement and record onset of relief of pain. Assess skin for evidence of rash, pruritus.

PATIENT/FAMILY TEACHING

Avoid tasks that require alertness, motor skills until response to drug is established. Tolerance/dependence may occur w/prolonged use of high doses.

trandolapril

tran-**doal**-ah-prill
(Mavik)

FIXED-COMBINATION(S)
W/verapamil, a calcium channel blocker **(Tarka)**

CANADIAN AVAILABILITY
Mavik

PREGNANCY CATEGORY C
First trimester.

PREGNANCY CATEGORY D
Second and third trimesters.

CLASSIFICATION

Angiotensin-converting enzyme (ACE) inhibitor, antihypertensive

AVAILABILITY (Rx)

Tablets: 1 mg, 2 mg, 4 mg

PHARMACOKINETICS

Absorption: Slowly absorbed from GI tract. **Metabolism:** Metabolized in liver, GI mucosa to active metabolite. **Excretion:** Primarily excreted in urine. Minimal removal by hemodialysis. **Half-life:** 6–10 hrs.

ACTION / *THERAPEUTIC EFFECT*

Suppresses renin-angiotensin-aldosterone system (prevents conversion of angiotensin I toangiotensin II, a potent vasoconstrictor; may also inhibit angiotensin II at local vascular and renal sites). Decreases plasma angiotensin II, increases plasma renin activity, decreases aldosterone secretion. *Reduces peripheral arterial resistance, pulmonary capillary wedge pressure; improves cardiac output, exercise tolerance.*

USES

Treatment of hypertension. Used alone or in combination w/other antihypertensives. Treatment of congestive heart failure (CHF).

ADMINISTRATION

ORAL:
- May give w/o regard to meals.
- Tablets may be crushed.

INDICATIONS/ROUTES/DOSAGE

Hypertension (w/o diuretic):
Oral: Adults, elderly: Initially, 1 mg once daily in nonblack pts, 2 mg once daily in black pts. Adjust dose at least at 7 day intervals. ***Maintenance:*** 2–4 mg/day. ***Maximum:*** 8 mg/day.

CHF:
Oral: Adults, elderly: Initially, 0.5–1 mg, titrated to target dose of 4 mg/day.

CONTRAINDICATIONS

History of angioedema w/previous treatment w/ACE inhibitors.

CAUTIONS

Renal impairment, those w/sodium depletion or on diuretic therapy, dialysis, hypovolemia, coronary or cerebrovascular insufficiency.

INTERACTIONS

DRUG: ***Alcohol, diuretics, hypotensive agents*** may increase effects. ***NSAIDs*** may decrease effect. ***Potassium-sparing diuretics, potassium supplements*** may cause hyperkalemia. May increase ***lithium*** concentration, toxicity. **HERBAL:** None known. **FOOD:** None significant. **ALTERED LAB VALUES:** May increase potassium, SGOT (AST), SGPT (ALT), alkaline phosphatase, bilirubin, BUN, creatinine. May decrease sodium. May cause positive ANA titer.

SIDE EFFECTS

FREQUENT (>10%): Hypotension, dizziness, cough. **OCCASIONAL (1–6%):** Headache, fatigue, muscle pain, asthenia (loss of strength). **RARE (<1%):** Chest pain, palpitations, insomnia, numbness in feet, drowsiness, nausea, vomiting, constipation, flushed skin, angioedema.

ADVERSE REACTIONS/TOXIC EFFECTS

Excessive hypotension ("first-dose syncope") may occur in those w/CHF, severely salt/volume depleted. Angioedema (swelling of face/lips), hyperkalemia occur rarely. Agranulocytosis, neutropenia may be noted in those w/impaired renal function or collagen vascular disease (systemic lupus erythematosus, scleroderma). Nephrotic syndrome may be noted in those w/history of renal disease.

PATIENT CONSIDERATIONS

Baseline Assessment

Obtain B/P immediately before each dose, in addition to regular monitoring (be alert to fluctuations). Renal function tests should be performed before therapy begins. In those w/renal impairment, autoimmune disease, or taking drugs that affect leukocytes or immune response, CBC and differential count should be performed before therapy begins and q2wks for 3 mos, then periodically thereafter.

Intervention/Evaluation

If excessive reduction in B/P occurs, place pt in supine position w/legs elevated. Assist w/ambulation if dizziness occurs. Assess for urinary frequency. Auscultate lung sounds for rales, wheezing in those w/CHF. Monitor urinalysis for proteinuria. Monitor serum potassium levels in those on concurrent diuretic therapy. Monitor pattern of daily bowel activity and stool consistency.

Patient/Family Teaching

Report any sign of infection (sore throat, fever). Several weeks may be needed for full therapeutic effect of B/P reduction. Skipping doses or voluntarily discontinuing drug may produce severe, rebound hypertension. To reduce hypotensive effect, rise slowly from lying to sitting position and permit legs to dangle from bed momentarily before standing. Report facial swelling, difficulty swallowing. Avoid potassium supplements/salt substitutes.

T

tranylcypromine sulfate

tran-ill-**sip**-roe-meen
(Parnate)

CANADIAN AVAILABILITY
Parnate

PREGNANCY CATEGORY C

CLASSIFICATION

Antidepressant: MAO inhibitor

AVAILABILITY (Rx)

Tablets: 10 mg

PHARMACOKINETICS

Absorption: Well absorbed from GI tract. **Metabolism:** Metabolized in liver. **Excretion:** Primarily excreted in urine. **Half-life:** 1.5–3 hrs.

ACTION/*THERAPEUTIC EFFECT*

Inhibits MAO enzyme (assists in metabolism of sympathomimetic amines) at CNS storage sites. Levels of epinephrine, norepinephrine, serotonin, dopamine increased at neuron receptor sites, *producing antidepressant effect.*

USES

Symptomatic treatment of severe depression in hospitalized or closely supervised pts who have not responded to other antidepressant therapy, including electroconvulsive therapy.

ADMINISTRATION

ORAL:

- Give w/food if GI distress occurs.

INDICATIONS/ROUTES/DOSAGE

Oral: Adults, elderly: 30 mg/day in divided doses. May increase dose by 10 mg/day at intervals of 1–3 wks. ***Maximum:*** 60 mg/day.

CONTRAINDICATIONS

Pts >60 yrs, debilitated/hypertensive pts, cerebrovascular/cardiovascular disease, foods containing tryptophan/tyramine, within 10 days of elective surgery, pheochromocytoma, congestive heart failure, history of liver disease, abnormal liver function tests, severe renal impairment, history of severe/recurrent headache.

CAUTIONS

Impaired renal function, history of seizures, parkinsonian syndrome, diabetic pts, hyperthyroidism.

INTERACTIONS

DRUG: ***Alcohol, CNS depressants*** may increase CNS depressant effects. ***Tricyclic antidepressants, fluoxetine, trazodone*** may cause serotonin syndrome. May increase effect of ***oral hypoglycemics, insulin.*** B/P may increase w/***buspirone. Caffeine-containing medications*** may increase cardiac arrhythmias, hypertension. May precipitate hypertensive crises w/***carbamazepine, cyclobenzaprine, maprotiline, other MAO inhibitors. Meperidine, other opioid analgesics*** may produce immediate excitation, sweating, rigidity, severe hypertension or hypotension, severe respiratory distress, coma, convulsions, vascular collapse, death. May increase CNS stimulant, vasopressor effects. **HERBAL:** None known. **FOOD:** Tyramine, foods w/pressor amines (e.g., aged cheese) may cause sudden, severe hypertension. **ALTERED LAB VALUES:** None significant.

SIDE EFFECTS

FREQUENT: Postural hypotension, restlessness, GI upset, insomnia, dizziness, lethargy, weakness, dry mouth, peripheral edema. **OCCASIONAL:** Flushing, increased perspiration, rash, urinary frequency, increased appetite, transient impotence. **RARE:** Visual disturbances.

ADVERSE REACTIONS/TOXIC EFFECTS

Hypertensive crisis may be noted by hypertension, occipital headache radiating frontally, neck stiffness/soreness, nausea, vomiting, sweating, fever/chilliness, clammy skin, dilated pupils, palpitations. Tachycardia/bradycardia, constricting chest pain may also be present. Antidote for hypertensive crisis: 5–10 mg phentolamine IV injection.

PATIENT CONSIDERATIONS

Baseline Assessment

Periodic liver function tests should be performed in those requiring high dosage and/or undergoing prolonged therapy. MAO inhibitor therapy should be discontinued for 7–14 days before elective surgery.

Intervention/Evaluation

Assess appearance, behavior, speech pattern, level of interest, mood. Monitor for occipital headache radiating frontally, and/or neck stiffness or soreness (may be first signal of impending hypertensive crisis). Monitor blood pressure diligently for hypertension. Assess skin temperature for fever. Discontinue medication immediately if palpitations or frequent headaches occur.

Patient/Family Teaching

Antidepressant relief may be noted during first week of therapy; maximum benefit noted within 3 wks. Report headache, neck stiffness/soreness immediately. To avoid orthostatic hypotension, change from lying to sitting position slowly and dangle legs momentarily before standing. Avoid tasks that require alertness, motor skills until response to drug is established. Avoid foods that require bacteria/molds for their preparation/preservation or those that contain tyramine, e.g., cheese, sour cream, beer, wine, pickled herring, liver, figs, raisins, bananas, avocados, soy sauce, yeast extracts, yogurt, papaya, broad beans, meat tenderizers, or excessive amounts of caffeine (coffee, tea, chocolate), or OTC preparations for hay fever, colds, weight reduction.

trastuzumab

(Herceptin)
See Classification section under: Cancer chemotherapy

trazodone hydrochloride

tra-zoh-doan
(Desyrel)

CANADIAN AVAILABILITY
Desyrel

PREGNANCY CATEGORY C

CLASSIFICATION

Antidepressant

AVAILABILITY (Rx)

Tablets: 50 mg, 100 mg, 150 mg, 300 mg

PHARMACOKINETICS

Absorption: Well absorbed from GI tract. **Metabolism:** Metabolized in liver. **Excretion:** Primarily excreted in urine. **Half-life:** 5–9 hrs.

ACTION/*THERAPEUTIC EFFECT*

Blocks reuptake of serotonin by CNS presynaptic neuronal membranes, increasing availability at postsynaptic neuronal receptor sites. Resulting enhancement of synaptic activity *produces antidepressant effect.*

USES/*UNLABELED*

Treatment of depression exhibited as persistent, prominent dysphoria (occurring nearly every day for at least 2 wks) manifested by 4 of 8 symptoms: appetite change, sleep pattern change, increased fatigue, impaired concentration, feelings of guilt or worthlessness, loss of interest in usual activities, psychomotor agitation or retardation, suicidal tendencies. *Treatment of neurogenic pain.*

ADMINISTRATION

ORAL:

- Give shortly after snack, meal (reduces risk of dizziness, lightheadedness).
- Tablets may be crushed.

INDICATIONS/ROUTES/DOSAGE

Antidepressant:
Oral: Adults: Initially, 150 mg daily in equally divided doses. Increase by 50 mg/day at 3–4 day intervals until therapeutic response is achieved. Do not exceed 400 mg/day for outpatients, 600 mg/day for hospitalized pts.

Usual elderly dosage:
Oral: Initially, 25–50 mg at bedtime. May increase by 25–50 mg q3–7days. ***Range:*** 75–150 mg/day.

CONTRAINDICATIONS

Recovery phase of MI, surgical pts, electroconvulsive therapy.

CAUTIONS

Cardiovascular disease, MAO inhibitor therapy.

INTERACTIONS

DRUG: *Alcohol, CNS depression–producing medications* may increase CNS depression. May increase effects of ***antihypertensives.*** May increase concentration of ***digoxin, phenytoin.*** **HERBAL:** St. John's wort may increase adverse effects. Ginkgo biloba may increase risk of depression. **FOOD:** None significant. **ALTERED LAB VALUES:** May decrease neutrophil, leukocyte counts.

SIDE EFFECTS

FREQUENT (3–9%): Drowsiness, dry mouth, lightheadedness/dizziness, headache, blurred vision, nausea/vomiting. **OCCASIONAL (1–3%):** Nervousness, fatigue, constipation, generalized aches and pains, mild hypotension.

ADVERSE REACTIONS/TOXIC EFFECTS

Priapism (painful, prolonged penile erection), decreased/increased libido, retrograde ejaculation, impotence have been noted rarely. Appears to be less cardiotoxic than other antidepressants, although arrhythmias may occur in pts w/preexisting cardiac disease.

PATIENT CONSIDERATIONS

BASELINE ASSESSEMENT

For those on long-term therapy, liver/renal function tests, blood counts should be performed periodically.

INTERVENTION/EVALUATION

Supervise suicidal risk pt closely during early therapy (as depression lessens, energy level improves, increasing suicide potential). Assess appearance, behavior, speech pattern, level of interest, mood. Monitor WBC and neutrophil count (drug should be stopped if levels fall below normal). Assist w/ambulation if dizziness or lightheadedness occurs.

PATIENT/FAMILY TEACHING

Immediately discontinue medication and consult physician if priapism occurs. Change positions slowly to avoid hypotensive effect. Tolerance to sedative and anticholinergic effects usually develops during early therapy. Photosensitivity to sun may occur. Dry mouth may be relieved by sugarless gum, sips of tepid water. Report visual disturbances. Do not

abruptly discontinue medication. Avoid tasks that require alertness, motor skills until response to drug is established. Avoid alcohol.

tretinoin

tret-ih-noyn

(Avita, Renova, Retin-A, Retin-A Micro, Vesanoid)

FIXED-COMBINATION(S)

W/octyl methoxycinnamate and oxybenzone, moistures, and SPF-12, a sunscreen **(Retin-A Regimen Kit)**

CANADIAN AVAILABILITY

Retin-A, Stieva-A, Vesanoid, Vitamin A Acid

PREGNANCY CATEGORY C

Topical, oral: Teratogenic, embryotoxic effect. Pregnancy Category D.

CLASSIFICATION

Antiacne, transdermal, antineoplastic

AVAILABILITY (Rx)

Capsules: 10 mg. **Cream:** 0.025%, 0.05%, 0.1%. **Cream (Avita):** 0.025%; **(Renova):** 0.05%. **Gel:** 0.025%, 0.01%; **(Retin-A Micro):** 0.1%. **Liquid:** 0.05%.

PHARMACOKINETICS

Topical: **Absorption:** Minimally absorbed. ***Oral:*** Well absorbed following oral administration. **Excretion:** Primarily excreted in urine. **Half-life:** 0.5–2 hrs.

ACTION/*THERAPEUTIC EFFECT*

Antiacne: Decreases cohesiveness of follicular epithelial cells. Increases turnover of follicular epithelial cells, *causing expulsion of blackheads.* Bacterial skin counts are not altered. ***Transdermal:*** Exerts its effects on growth and differentiation of epithelial cells, *alleviating fine wrinkles, hyperpigmentation.* ***Antineoplastic:*** Induces maturation, decreases proliferation of acute promyelocytic leukemia (APL) cells, *followed by repopulation of bone marrow and blood by normal hematopoietic cells.*

USES/*UNLABELED*

Topical: Treatment of acne vulgaris, especially grades I–III in which blackheads, papules, pustules predominate. ***Transdermal:*** Treatment of fine wrinkles, hyperpigmentation. ***Antineoplastic:*** Induction of remission in pts with acute promyelocytic leukemia (APL). *Treatment of disorders of keratinization, including photoaged skin, liver spots.*

T

ADMINISTRATION

ORAL:

- Do not crush or break capsule.

TOPICAL:

- Thoroughly cleanse area before applying tretinoin.
- Lightly cover only the affected area. Liquid may be applied w/fingertip, gauze, or cotton, taking care to avoid running onto unaffected skin.
- Keep medication away from eyes, mouth, angles of nose, mucous membranes.
- Wash hands immediately after application.

INDICATIONS/ROUTES/DOSAGE

Acne:

Topical: Adults: Apply once daily at bedtime.

Transdermal:

Topical: Adults: Apply to face once daily at bedtime.

Acute promyelocytic leukemia: *Oral: Adults:* 45 mg/m²/day given as two evenly divided doses until complete remission is documented. Discontinue therapy 30 days after complete remission or after 90 days of treatment, whichever comes first.

CONTRAINDICATIONS

Hypersensitivity to any component of the preparation, sensitivity to parabens (used as preservative in gelatin capsule).

EXTREME CAUTION

Topical: Eczema, sun exposure.

CAUTIONS

Topical: Those w/considerable sun exposure in their occupation or hypersensitivity to sun. *Oral:* Elevated cholesterol/triglycerides.

INTERACTIONS

DRUG: *Topical: Keratolytic agents* (e.g., ***sulfur, benzoyl peroxide, salicylic acid),*** medicated soaps, shampoos, astringents, spice or lime cologne, permanent wave solutions, hair depilatories may increase skin irritation. ***Photosensitive medication (thiazides, tetracyclines, fluoroquinolones, phenothiazines, sulfonamides)*** augments phototoxicity. *Oral: Ketoconazole* may increase tretinoin concentration. **HERBAL:** None known. **FOOD:** None significant. **ALTERED LAB VALUES:** *Oral:* Leukocytosis occurs commonly (40%). May elevate liver function tests, cholesterol, triglycerides.

SIDE EFFECTS

Topical: Local inflammatory reactions are to be expected and are reversible w/discontinuation of tretinoin. **FREQUENT (>10%):** Headache, dry skin/oral mucosa, cheilitis (crusting, swelling of lips), nausea, vomiting, bone pain, arthralgia, myalgia, rash, fever, weakness, fatigue. *Topical:* Transient feeling of warmth or stinging, erythema, peeling. **OCCASIONAL (1–10%)** *Oral:* Pruritus, increased sweating visual disturbances, alopecia, skin changes, dizziness, flushing, abdominal pain. *Topical:* Temporary hyperpigmentation, severe erythema, crusting, blistering, edema. **RARE (<1%):** *Topical:* Contact allergy.

ADVERSE REACTIONS/TOXIC EFFECTS

Oral: Retinoic acid syndrome (fever, dyspnea, weight gain, abnormal chest auscultatory findings [pulmonary infiltrates, pleural or pericardial effusions], episodic hypotension) occurs commonly (25%) as does leukocytosis (40%). Syndrome generally occurs during first month of therapy (sometimes occurs following first dose). High-dose steroids (dexamethasone 10 mg IV) at first suspicion of syndrome reduces morbidity, mortality. Pseudo tumor cerebri may be noted, especially in children (headache, nausea, vomiting, visual disturbances). *Topical:* Possible tumorigenic potential when combined w/ultraviolet radiation.

PATIENT CONSIDERATIONS

BASELINE ASSESSMENT

Oral: **Inform women of childbearing potential of risk to fetus if pregnancy occurs. Instruct in need for use of two reliable forms of contraceptives concurrently during therapy and for 1 mo after discontinuation of therapy, even in infertile, premenopausal women. Pregnancy test should be obtained within 1 wk prior to institution of therapy.** Obtain initial liver function tests, cholesterol, triglyceride levels.

INTERVENTION/EVALUATION

Oral: Monitor liver function tests, hematologic, coagulation profiles, cholesterol, triglycerides. Monitor signs/symptoms of pseudo tumor cerebri in children.

PATIENT/FAMILY TEACHING

Topical: Avoid exposure to sunlight or sunbeds; use sunscreens and protective clothing. Affected areas should also be protected from wind, cold. If skin is already sunburned, do not use until fully recovered. Do not use more often than instructed or use larger amount of medication (does not lead to more rapid or better results). Keep tretinoin away from eyes, mouth, angles of nose and mucous membranes. Do not use medicated, drying, or abrasive soaps; wash face no more than 2–3 times/day with bland soap. Avoid use of preparations containing alcohol, menthol, spice, or lime such as shaving lotions, astringents, perfume. Application may cause temporary warmth or stinging feeling. Mild redness, peeling are expected; decrease frequency or discontinue medication if excessive reaction occurs. Nonmedicated cosmetics may be used; however, cosmetics must be removed before tretinoin application. Improvement noted during first 24 wks of therapy. *Antiacne:* Therapeutic results noted in 2–3 wks; optimal results in 6 wks. *Oral:* Explain purpose of medication, adverse effects. Report adverse effects to physician.

triamcinolone

try-am-**sin**-oh-lone
(Aristocort, Kenacort)

triamcinolone diacetate

(Amcort, Aristocort Intralesional, Trilone)

triamcinolone acetonide

(Aristocort, Azmacort, Kenalog, Nasacort AQ)

triamcinolone hexacetonide

(Aristospan)

FIXED-COMBINATION(S)

Triamcinolone acetonide w/nystatin, an antifungal **(Myco-Aricin, Myco II, Myco-Biotic, Mycogen II, Nystolone)**

CANADIAN AVAILABILITY

Aristocort, Azmacort, Kenalog, Triaderm

PREGNANCY CATEGORY C

CLASSIFICATION

Corticosteroid

AVAILABILITY (Rx)

Tablets: 1 mg, 2 mg, 4 mg, 8 mg. **Syrup:** 4 mg/5 ml. **Aerosol (respiratory inhalant), Nasal Spray, Ointment:** 0.025%, 0.1%, 0.5%. **Cream:** 0.025%, 0.1%, 0.5%. **Lotion:** 0.025%, 0.1%.

Acetonide: Injection: 3 mg/ml, 10 mg/ml, 40 mg/ml

Diacetate: Injection: 25 mg/ml, 40 mg/ml

Hexacetone: Injection: 5 mg/ml, 20 mg/ml

PHARMACOKINETICS

Absorption: Rapidly absorbed after inhalation. Completely ab-

T

sorbed after oral administration; well absorbed after IM administration. Widely distributed. **Metabolism:** Metabolized in liver. **Excretion:** Primarily excreted in urine. **Half-life:** 2–5 hrs.

ACTION / *THERAPEUTIC EFFECT*

Inhibits accumulation of inflammatory cells at inflammation sites, phagocytosis, lysosomal enzyme release and synthesis and/or release of mediators of inflammation. *Prevents/suppresses cell-mediated immune reactions. Decreases/prevents tissue response to inflammatory process.*

USES

Substitution therapy in deficiency states: Acute/chronic adrenal insufficiency, congenital adrenal hyperplasia, adrenal insufficiency secondary to pituitary insufficiency. ***Nonendocrine disorders:*** Arthritis, rheumatic carditis, allergic, collagen, intestinal tract, liver, ocular, renal, and skin diseases, bronchial asthma, cerebral edema, malignancies. Allergic rhinitis. ***Inhalation:*** Maintenance prophylaxis of asthma.

ADMINISTRATION

ORAL:

- Give w/food or milk.
- Single doses given before 9 AM; multiple doses at evenly spaced intervals.

IM:

- Do *not* give IV.
- Give deep IM in gluteus maximus.

INHALATION:

- Shake and inhale immediately before use.
- Pt should exhale completely; place mouthpiece 2 fingers' width away from mouth.
- Tilt head back; while activating inhaler, take slow, deep breath for 3–5 sec.
- Pt should hold breath as long as possible (5–10 sec), then exhale slowly.
- Wait 1 min between inhalations when multiple inhalations ordered.
- Following treatment, pt should thoroughly rinse mouth w/water or mouthwash.

TOPICAL:

- Gently cleanse area before application.
- Use occlusive dressings only as ordered.
- Apply sparingly and rub into area thoroughly.

INDICATIONS/ROUTES/DOSAGE

Usual oral dosage:
Oral: Adults, elderly: 4–60 mg/day.

Triamcinolone diacetate:
IM: Adults, elderly: 40 mg/wk.

Intra-articular, Intralesional: Adults, elderly: 5–40 mg.

Triamcinolone acetonide:
IM: Adults, elderly: Initially, 2.5–60 mg/day.

Intra-articular: Adults, elderly: Initially, 2.5–40 mg up to 100 mg.

Triamcinolone hexacetonide:
Intra-articular: Adults, elderly: 2–20 mg.

Control of bronchial asthma:
Inhalation: Adults, elderly: 2 inhalations 3–4 times/day. ***Children 6–12 yrs:*** 1–2 inhalations 3–4 times/day. ***Maximum:*** 12 inhalations/day.

Rhinitis:
Intranasal: Adults, children >6 yrs: 2 sprays each nostril daily.

Usual topical dosage:
Topical: Adults, elderly: Sparingly 2–4 times/day. May give 1–2 times/day or intermittent therapy.

CONTRAINDICATIONS

Hypersensitivity to any corticosteroid or tartrazine, systemic fungal infection, peptic ulcers (except life-threatening situations). IM injection, oral inhalation not for children <6 yrs of age. Avoid immunizations, smallpox vaccination. *Topical:* Marked circulation impairment.

CAUTIONS

History of tuberculosis (may reactivate disease), hypothyroidism, cirrhosis, nonspecific ulcerative colitis, CHF, hypertension, psychosis, renal insufficiency. Prolonged therapy should be discontinued slowly.

INTERACTIONS

DRUG: *Amphotericin* may increase hypokalemia. May decrease effect of ***oral hypoglycemics, insulin, diuretics, potassium supplements.*** May increase ***digoxin*** toxicity (due to hypokalemia). ***Hepatic enzyme inducers*** may decrease effect. ***Live virus vaccines*** may potentiate virus replication, increase vaccine side effects, decrease pt's antibody response to vaccine. **HERBAL:** None known. **FOOD:** None significant. **ALTERED LAB VALUES:** May decrease calcium, potassium, thyroxine. May increase cholesterol, lipids, glucose, sodium, amylase.

SIDE EFFECTS

FREQUENT: Increased appetite, exaggerated sense of well-being, abdominal distension, weight gain, insomnia, mood swings. ***High dose, prolonged therapy:*** Increased susceptibility to infection (signs/symptoms masked); slow wound healing; hypokalemia, hypocalcemia; GI distress. **OCCASIONAL:** Headache, vertigo. **RARE:** Increased blood coagulability, tachycardia, frequency or urgency of urination, psychosis. ***Topical:*** Allergic contact dermatitis.

ADVERSE REACTIONS/TOXIC EFFECTS

Long-term therapy: muscle wasting (especially arms, legs), osteoporosis, spontaneous fractures, amenorrhea, cataracts, glaucoma, peptic ulcer, CHF. ***Abrupt withdrawal following long-term therapy:*** anorexia, nausea, fever, headache, joint pain, rebound inflammation, fatigue, weakness, lethargy, dizziness, orthostatic hypotension. Anaphylaxis w/parenteral administration. Sudden discontinuance may be fatal. Blindness has occurred rarely after intralesional injection around face, head.

PATIENT CONSIDERATIONS

BASELINE ASSESSMENT

Question for hypersensitivity to any of the corticosteroids or tartrazine (Kenacort). Obtain baselines for height, weight, B/P, glucose, electrolytes. Check results of initial tests, (e.g., TB skin test, x-rays, EKG).

INTERVENTION/EVALUATION

Monitor I&O, daily weight; assess for edema. Evaluate food tolerance and bowel activity; promptly report hyperacidity. Check B/P, temperature, pulse, respiration at least 2 times/day. Be alert to infection: sore throat, fever, or vague symptoms. Monitor elec-

T

trolytes. Watch for hypocalcemia (muscle twitching, cramps, positive Trousseau's or Chvostek's signs) or hypokalemia (weakness and muscle cramps, numbness/tingling, especially in lower extremities, nausea and vomiting, irritability, EKG changes). Assess emotional status, ability to sleep. Check lab results for blood coagulability and clinical evidence of thromboembolism. Provide assistance w/ambulation.

PATIENT/FAMILY TEACHING

Take w/food or milk. Carry identification of drug and dose, physician name and phone number. Do not change dose/schedule or stop taking drug, must taper off gradually under medical supervision. Notify physician of fever, sore throat, muscle aches, sudden weight gain/swelling. W/dietician give instructions for prescribed diet (usually sodium restricted w/high vitamin D, protein, and potassium). Maintain careful personal hygiene, avoid exposure to disease or trauma. Severe stress (serious infection, surgery, or trauma) may require increased dosage. Do not take any other medication w/o consulting physician. Follow-up visits, lab tests are necessary; children must be assessed for growth retardation. Inform dentist or other physicians of triamcinolone therapy now or within past 12 mos. Caution against overuse of joints injected for symptomatic relief. Teach proper oral inhalation technique. *Topical:* Apply after shower/bath for best absorption. Do not cover unless physician orders; do not use tight diapers, plastic pants or coverings. Avoid contact w/eyes. Do not expose treated area to sunlight.

triamterene

try-**am**-tur-een
(Dyrenium)

FIXED-COMBINATION(S)
W/hydrochlorothiazide, a thiazide diuretic **(Dyazide, Maxzide)**

CANADIAN AVAILABILITY
Dyrenium

PREGNANCY CATEGORY D

CLASSIFICATION

Diuretic: Potassium sparing

AVAILABILITY (Rx)

Capsules: 50 mg, 100 mg

PHARMACODYNAMICS

	ONSET	PEAK	DURATION
Oral	2–4 hrs	6–8 hrs	12–16 hrs

PHARMACOKINETICS

Absorption: Incompletely absorbed from GI tract. Widely distributed. **Metabolism:** Metabolized in liver. **Excretion:** Primarily eliminated in feces via biliary route. **Half-life:** 1.5–2 hrs (increased in decreased renal function).

ACTION/*THERAPEUTIC EFFECT*

Competitively inhibits action of aldosterone. Interferes w/sodium reabsorption in distal tubule, *increasing potassium retention while promoting sodium and water excretion.*

USES/*UNLABELED*

Treatment of edema associated w/CHF, hepatic cirrhosis, nephrotic syndrome, steroid-induced edema, idiopathic edema, edema due to secondary hyperaldosteronism. May be used alone or w/other diuretics. *Treatment adjunct for hypertension, prophylaxis/treatment of hypokalemia.*

ADMINISTRATION

ORAL:

- May give w/food if GI disturbances occur.
- Do not crush or break capsules.

INDICATIONS/ROUTES/DOSAGE

Note: Fixed-combination medication should not be used for initial therapy but rather for maintenance therapy.

Dyrenium:
Oral: Adults: Initially, 100 mg twice daily after meals. ***Maintenance:*** 100 mg/day or every other day. ***Maximum:*** 300 mg/day. When used concurrently w/other diuretics, decrease dosage of each drug initially; adjust to pt's needs.

Usual elderly dosage:
Oral: Initially, 50 mg/day. ***Maximum:*** 100 mg/day in 1–2 doses.

Dyazide, Maxzide:
Oral: Adults: 1–2 capsules/tablets per day.

CONTRAINDICATIONS

Severe or progressive renal disease, severe hepatic disease, preexisting or drug-induced hyperkalemia.

CAUTIONS

Impaired hepatic or kidney function, history of renal calculi, diabetes mellitus.

INTERACTIONS

DRUG: May decrease effect of ***anticoagulants, heparin. NSAIDs*** may decrease antihypertensive effect. ***ACE inhibitors (e.g., captopril), potassium-containing medications, potassium supplements*** may increase potassium. May decrease ***lithium*** clearance, increase toxicity. **HERBAL:** None known. **FOOD:** None significant. **ALTERED LAB VALUES:** May increase BUN, calcium excretion, creatinine, glucose, magnesium, potassium, uric acid. May decrease sodium.

SIDE EFFECTS

OCCASIONAL: Headache, dizziness, nausea, vomiting, diarrhea, stomach cramps, hyponatremia (drowsiness, dry mouth, increased thirst, lack of energy), increased sensitivity skin to sunlight. **RARE:** Agranulocytosis (fever, chills), allergic reaction (shortness of breath, rash, itching), burning, inflamed, bright red tongue, cracked corners of mouth, nephrolithiasis, thrombocytopenia (unusual bleeding/bruising).

T

ADVERSE REACTIONS/TOXIC EFFECTS

Severe hyperkalemia may produce irritability, anxiety, heaviness of legs, paresthesia, hypotension, bradycardia, tented T waves, widening QRS, ST depression.

PATIENT CONSIDERATIONS

Baseline Assessment

Assess baseline electrolytes, particularly check for low potassium. Assess renal/hepatic functions. Assess edema (note location, extent), skin turgor, mucous membranes for hydration status. Assess muscle strength, mental status. Note skin temperature, moisture. Obtain baseline weight. Initiate strict I&O. Note pulse rate/regularity.

Intervention/Evaluation

Monitor B/P, vital signs, electrolytes (particularly potassium), I&O, weight. Note extent of diuresis. Watch for changes from initial assessment (hyperkalemia may result in muscle strength changes, tremor, muscle cramps), change in mental status (orientation, alertness, confusion), cardiac arrhythmias. Monitor potassium level, particularly during initial therapy. Weigh daily. Assess lung sounds for rhonchi, wheezing.

PATIENT/FAMILY TEACHING

Expect increase in volume and frequency of urination. Therapeutic effect takes several days to begin and can last for several days when drug is discontinued. High-potassium diet/potassium supplements can be dangerous, especially if pt has renal/hepatic problems. Avoid prolonged exposure to sunlight. Report severe or persistent weakness, headache, dry mouth, nausea, vomiting, fever, sore throat, unusual bleeding or bruising.

triazolam

try-**aye**-zoe-lam
(Halcion)

CANADIAN AVAILABILITY
Apo-Triazo, Halcion

PREGNANCY CATEGORY X

CLASSIFICATION

Sedative-hypnotic **(Schedule IV)**

AVAILABILITY (Rx)

Tablets: 0.125 mg, 0.25 mg

PHARMACOKINETICS

Absorption: Well absorbed from GI tract. Widely distributed (crosses blood-brain barrier). **Metabolism:** Metabolized in liver (undergoes first-pass liver extraction). **Excretion:** Primarily excreted in urine. **Half-life:** 1.5–5.5 hrs.

ACTION/*THERAPEUTIC EFFECT*

Enhances action of inhibitory neurotransmitter gamma-aminobutyric acid (GABA), *producing hypnotic effect due to CNS depression.*

USES

Short-term treatment of insomnia (up to 6 wks). Reduces sleep-induction time, number of nocturnal awakenings; increases length of sleep.

ADMINISTRATION

ORAL:
- Give w/o regard to meals.
- Tablets may be crushed.

INDICATIONS/ROUTES/DOSAGE

Hypnotic:
Oral: Adults >18 yrs: 0.125–0.5 mg at bedtime. ***Elderly:*** 0.0625–0.125 mg at bedtime.

CONTRAINDICATIONS

Acute narrow-angle glaucoma, acute alcohol intoxication.

CAUTIONS

Impaired renal/hepatic function.

INTERACTIONS

DRUG: *Alcohol, CNS depressants* may increase CNS depressant effect. **HERBAL:** Kava kava, valerian may increase CNS depression. **FOOD:** Grapefruit juice can alter absorption. **ALTERED LAB VALUES:** None significant.

SIDE EFFECTS

FREQUENT: Drowsiness, sedation, headache, dizziness, nervousness, lightheadedness, incoordination, nausea. **OCCASIONAL:** Euphoria, tachycardia, abdominal cramps, visual disturbances. **RARE:** Paradoxical CNS excitement, restlessness, particularly noted in elderly, debilitated.

ADVERSE REACTIONS/TOXIC EFFECTS

Abrupt or too rapid withdrawal may result in pronounced restlessness, irritability, insomnia, hand tremors, abdominal/muscle cramps, sweating, vomiting, seizures. Overdosage results in somnolence, confusion, diminished reflexes, coma.

PATIENT CONSIDERATIONS

BASELINE ASSESSMENT

Question for possibility of pregnancy before initiating therapy (Pregnancy Category X). Assess B/P, pulse, respirations immediately before administration. Raise bed rails. Provide environment conducive to sleep (backrub, quiet environment, low lighting).

INTERVENTION/EVALUATION

Assess sleep pattern of pt. Assess elderly/debilitated for paradoxical reaction, particularly during early therapy. Evaluate for therapeutic response to insomnia: decrease in number of nocturnal awakenings, increase in length of sleep.

PATIENT/FAMILY TEACHING

Smoking reduces drug effectiveness. Rebound insomnia may occur when drug is discontinued after short-term therapy. Avoid alcohol and other CNS depressants. Inform physician if you are or are planning to become pregnant. May experience disturbed sleep for 1–2 nights after discontinuing triazolam. Avoid concomitant grapefruit juice.

trifluoperazine hydrochloride

try-floo-oh-**pear**-ah-zeen
(Stelazine)

CANADIAN AVAILABILITY
Apo-Trifluoperazine, Stelazine

PREGNANCY CATEGORY C

CLASSIFICATION

Antipsychotic

AVAILABILITY (Rx)

Tablets: 1 mg, 2 mg, 5 mg, 10 mg. **Oral Concentrate:** 10 mg/ml. **Injection:** 2 mg/ml.

PHARMACOKINETICS

Absorption: Variably absorbed after oral administration, well absorbed after IM administration. Widely distributed. **Metabolism:** Metabolized in liver to some active metabolites. **Excretion:** Primarily excreted in urine.

ACTION/*THERAPEUTIC EFFECT*

Blocks dopamine at postsynaptic receptor sites, *suppressing behavioral response in psychosis, reducing locomotor activity/aggressiveness, suppressing conditioned responses.* Has strong extrapyramidal, antiemetic action; weak anticholinergic, sedative effects.

USES

Management of psychotic disorders, nonpsychotic anxiety.

STORAGE/HANDLING

Store oral solutions, parenteral form at room temperature. Slight yellow discoloration of solutions does not affect potency, but discard if markedly discolored or if precipitate forms.

ADMINISTRATION

ORAL:

- Add oral concentrate to 60 ml tomato or fruit juice, milk, carbonated beverages, coffee, tea, water. May also add to semisolid food.

IM:

- Pt must remain recumbent for 30–60 min in head-low position w/legs raised, to minimize hypotensive effect.
- Inject slow, deep IM into upper outer quadrant of gluteus maximus. If irritation occurs, further injections may be diluted w/0.9% NaCl or 2% procaine hydrochloride.

INDICATIONS/ROUTES/DOSAGE

Note: Decrease dosage gradually to optimum response, then decrease to lowest effective level for maintenance. Replace parenteral therapy w/oral therapy as soon as possible.

Psychotic disorders (hospitalized):
Oral: Adults: 2–5 mg twice daily. Gradually increase to average daily dose of 15–20 mg (up to 40 mg may be required in severe cases). ***Children 6–12 yrs:*** 1 mg 1–2 times/day. Gradually increase to maximum daily dose of 15 mg.

IM: Adults: 1–2 mg q4–6h. Do not exceed 6 mg/24 hrs. ***Children 6–12 yrs:*** 1 mg 1–2 times/day.

Psychotic disorders (outpatient):
Oral: Adults: 1–2 mg 2 times/day.

Nonpsychotic anxiety:
Oral/IM: Adults: 1–2 mg 2 times/day.

Usual elderly dosage:
Oral: Initially, 1–5 mg 2 times/day. ***Range:*** 15–20 mg/day. ***Maximum:*** 40 mg/day.

IM: Initially, 1 mg q4–6h as needed. ***Maximum:*** 6 mg/day.

CONTRAINDICATIONS

Severe CNS depression, comatose states, severe cardiovascular disease, bone marrow depression, subcortical brain damage.

CAUTIONS

Impaired respiratory/hepatic/renal/cardiac function, alcohol withdrawal, history of seizures, urinary retention, glaucoma, prostatic hypertrophy, hypocalcemia (increases susceptibility to dystonias).

INTERACTIONS

DRUG: ***Alcohol, CNS depressants*** may increase CNS, respiratory depression, hypotensive effects. ***Tricyclic antidepressants, MAO inhibitors*** may increase sedative, anticholinergic effects. ***Antithyroid agents*** may increase risk of agranulocytosis. Extrapyramidal symptoms (EPS) may increase w/***EPS–producing medications. Hypotensives*** may increase hypotension. May decrease ***levodopa*** effects. ***Lithium*** may decrease absorption, produce adverse neurologic effects. **HERBAL:** None known. **FOOD:** None significant. **ALTERED LAB VALUES:** May cause EKG changes.

SIDE EFFECTS

FREQUENT: Hypotension, dizziness, and fainting occur frequently after first injection, occasionally after subsequent injections, and rarely w/oral dosage. **OCCASIONAL:** Drowsiness during early therapy, dry mouth, blurred vision, lethargy, constipation or diarrhea, nasal congestion, peripheral edema, urinary retention. **RARE:** Ocular changes, skin pigmentation (those on high doses for prolonged periods).

ADVERSE REACTIONS/TOXIC EFFECTS

Extrapyramidal symptoms appear dose related (particularly high dosage) and are divided into 3 categories: akathisia (inability to sit still, tapping of feet, urge to move around); parkinsonian symptoms (mask-like face, tremors, shuffling gait, hypersalivation); and acute dystonias: torticollis (neck muscle spasm), opisthotonos (rigidity of back muscles), and oculogyric crisis (rolling back of eyes). Dystonic reaction may also produce profuse sweating, pallor. Tardive dyskinesia (protrusion of tongue, puffing of cheeks, chewing/puckering of the mouth) occurs rarely (may be irreversible). Abrupt withdrawal following long-term therapy may precipitate nausea, vomiting, gastritis, dizziness, tremors. Blood dyscrasias, particularly agranulocytosis, mild leukopenia (sore mouth/gums/throat) may occur. May lower seizure threshold.

PATIENT CONSIDERATIONS

Baseline Assessment

Avoid skin contact w/solution (contact dermatitis). Assess behavior, appearance, emotional status, response to environment, speech pattern, thought content.

Intervention/Evaluation

Monitor B/P for hypotension. Assess for extrapyramidal symptoms. Monitor WBC, differential count for blood dyscrasias. Monitor for fine tongue movement (may be early sign of tardive dyskinesia). Supervise suicidal risk pt closely during early therapy (as depression lessens, energy level improves, increasing suicide potential). Assess for therapeutic response (interest in surroundings, improvement in self-care, increased ability to concentrate, relaxed facial expression).

Patient/Family Teaching

Maximum therapeutic response occurs in 2–3 wks. Urine may darken. Do not abruptly withdraw from long-term drug therapy. Report visual disturbances. Sugarless gum, sips of tepid water may relieve dry mouth. Drowsiness generally subsides during continued therapy. Avoid tasks that require alertness, motor skills until response to drug is established. Avoid alcohol.

T

trifluridine

try-**fleur**-ih-deen
(Viroptic)

CANADIAN AVAILABILITY
Viroptic

PREGNANCY CATEGORY C

CLASSIFICATION

Antiviral

AVAILABILITY (Rx)

Ophthalmic Solution: 1%

PHARMACOKINETICS

Intraocular penetration occurs after instillation. **Half-life:** 12–18 min.

ACTION/*THERAPEUTIC EFFECT*

Incorporated into DNA causing increased rate of mutation and errors in protein formation, *preventing viral replication.*

USES

Recurrent epithelial keratitis and primary keratoconjunctivitis caused by herpes simplex types I and II. Treatment of epithelial keratitis not responding to idoxuridine or resistant to vidarabine.

STORAGE/HANDLING

Refrigerate ophthalmic solution.

ADMINISTRATION

OPHTHALMIC:

- Instruct pt to lie down or tilt head backward and look up.
- Gently pull lower eyelid down to form pocket between eye and lower lid. Hold dropper above pocket and place prescribed number of drops in pocket (do not touch tip of applicator to any surface).
- Close eye gently. Apply gentle finger pressure to lacrimal sac (bridge of nose, inside corner of eye) for 1–2 min (minimized drainage into nose and throat, reducing risk of systemic effects).
- Remove excess solution around eye w/tissue.
- Tell pt not to close eyes tightly or blink more often than necessary.
- Never rinse dropper.

INDICATIONS/ROUTES/DOSAGE

Usual ophthalmic dosage:
Adults, elderly: 1 drop onto cornea q2h while awake. ***Maximum:*** 9 drops/day. Continue until corneal ulcer has completely reepithelialized; then, 1 drop q4h while awake (minimum: 5 drops/day) for an additional 7 days.

CONTRAINDICATIONS

Hypersensitivity to trifluridine or any component of the preparation.

INTERACTIONS

DRUG: None significant. **HERBAL:** None known. **FOOD:** None significant. **ALTERED LAB VALUES:** None significant.

SIDE EFFECTS

FREQUENT: Transient stinging or burning w/instillation. **OCCASIONAL:** Edema of eyelid. **RARE:** Hypersensitivity reaction: itching, redness, swelling, increased irritation; superficial punctate keratopathy, increased intraocular pressure, keratitis sicca.

ADVERSE REACTIONS/TOXIC EFFECTS

Ocular toxicity may occur if used longer than 21 days.

PATIENT CONSIDERATIONS

Baseline Assessment

Question for hypersensitivity to trifluridine or components of preparation.

Intervention/Evaluation

Evaluate for therapeutic response or burning/stinging, edema of eyelid, hypersensitivity reaction.

Patient/Family Teaching

Use only as directed by physician (assure proper administration); do not stop or increase frequency of doses. Contact physician if no improvement after 7 days or complete healing after 14. Do not continue longer than 21 days. Refrigerate; avoid freezing. Mild, transient burning, stinging may occur when instilled. Promptly report itching, swelling, redness, or any increased irritation. Medication and personal items in contact w/eye should not be shared. Do not use any other products, including makeup, around the eye w/o advice of physician.

trihexyphenidyl hydrochloride

try-**he**x-eh-fen-ih-dill
(Artane)

CANADIAN AVAILABILITY
Apo-Trihex

PREGNANCY CATEGORY C

CLASSIFICATION

Anticholinergic, antiparkinson

AVAILABILITY (Rx)

Tablets: 2 mg, 5 mg. **Capsules (sustained-release):** 5 mg. **Elixir:** 2 mg/5 ml.

PHARMACODYNAMICS

	ONSET	PEAK	DURATION
Oral	1 hr	2–3 hrs	6–12 hrs

PHARMACOKINETICS

Absorption: Well absorbed from GI tract. **Excretion:** Primarily excreted in urine. **Half-life:** 5.6–10.2 hrs.

ACTION/*THERAPEUTIC EFFECT*

Blocks central cholinergic receptors (aids in balancing cholinergic and dopaminergic activity). *Decreases salivation, relaxes smooth muscle.*

USES

Adjunctive treatment for all forms of Parkinson's disease, including postencephalitic, arteriosclerotic, idiopathic types. Controls symptoms of drug-induced extrapyramidal symptoms.

ADMINISTRATION

ORAL:

- May take w/o regard to food; give w/food if GI distress occurs.
- Scored tablets may be crushed; do not crush or break sustained-release capsules.

INDICATIONS/ROUTES/DOSAGE

Parkinsonism:
Note: Do not use sustained-release capsules for initial therapy. Once stabilized, may switch, on mg-for-mg basis, giving a single daily dose after breakfast or 2 divided doses 12 hrs apart.

Oral: Adults, elderly: Initially, 1 mg on first day. May increase by 2 mg/day at 3–5 day intervals up to 6–10 mg/day (12–15 mg/day in pts w/postencephalitic parkinsonism).

Drug-induced extrapyramidal symptoms:
Oral: Adults, elderly: Initially, 1 mg/day. ***Range:*** 5–15 mg/day.

CONTRAINDICATIONS

Angle closure glaucoma, GI obstruction, paralytic ileus, intestinal atony, severe ulcerative colitis, prostatic hypertrophy, myasthenia gravis, megacolon.

CAUTIONS

Treated open-angle glaucoma, autonomic neuropathy, pulmonary disease, esophageal reflux, hiatal hernia, heart disease, hyperthyroidism, hypertension.

INTERACTIONS

DRUG: *Alcohol, CNS depressants* may increase sedative effect. *Amantadine, anticholinergics, MAO inhibitors* may increase anticholinergic effects. *Antacids, antidiarrheals* may decrease absorption, effects. **HERBAL:** None known. **FOOD:** None significant. **ALTERED LAB VALUES:** None significant.

SIDE EFFECTS

Note: Elderly (>60 yrs) tend to develop mental confusion, disorientation, agitation, psychotic-like symptoms. **FREQUENT:** Drowsiness, dizziness, muscular weakness, dry mouth/nose/throat/lips, urinary retention, thickening of bronchial secretions. Sedation, dizziness, hypotension more likely noted in elderly. **OCCASIONAL:** Epigastric distress, flushing, visual disturbances, hearing disturbances, paresthesia, sweating, chills.

ADVERSE REACTIONS/TOXIC EFFECTS

Children may experience dominant paradoxical reaction (restlessness, insomnia, euphoria, nervousness, tremors). Overdosage in children may result in hallucinations, convulsions, death. Hypersensitivity reaction (eczema, pruritus, rash, cardiac disturbances, photosensitivity) may occur. Overdosage may vary from CNS depression (sedation, apnea, cardiovascular collapse, death) to severe paradoxical reaction (hallucinations, tremor, seizures).

PATIENT CONSIDERATIONS

Baseline Assessment

If pt is undergoing allergic reaction, obtain history of recently ingested foods, drugs, environmental exposure, recent emotional stress. Monitor rate, depth, rhythm, type of respiration; quality and rate of pulse. Assess lung sounds for rhonchi, wheezing, rales.

Intervention/Evaluation

Be alert to neurologic effects: headache, lethargy, mental confusion, agitation. Monitor children closely for paradoxical reaction. Assess for clinical reversal of symptoms (improvement of tremor of head/hands at rest, masklike facial expression, shuffling gait, muscular rigidity).

Patient/Family Teaching

Avoid tasks that require alertness, motor skills until response to drug is established. Dry mouth, drowsiness, dizziness may be an expected response of drug. Avoid alcoholic beverages during therapy. Sugarless gum, sips of tepid water may relieve dry mouth. Coffee/tea may help reduce drowsiness.

trimethobenzamide hydrochloride

try-meth-oh-**benz**-ah-mide
(Tigan)

PREGNANCY CATEGORY C

CLASSIFICATION

Antiemetic

AVAILABILITY (Rx)

Capsules: 100 mg, 250 mg. **Suppositories:** 100 mg, 200 mg. **Injection:** 100 mg/ml.

PHARMACODYNAMICS

	ONSET	PEAK	DURATION
Oral	10–40 min	—	3–4 hrs
IM	15–30 min	—	2–3 hrs

PHARMACOKINETICS

Absorption: Partially absorbed from GI tract. Distributed primarily to liver. **Metabolism:** Metabolic fate unknown. **Excretion:** Excreted in urine.

ACTION/*THERAPEUTIC EFFECT*

Acts at the chemoreceptor trigger zone in CNS (medulla oblongata), *relieving nausea and vomiting.*

USES

Control of nausea and vomiting.

STORAGE/HANDLING

Store oral, rectal, parenteral form at room temperature.

ADMINISTRATION

ORAL:
- Give w/o regard to meals.
- Do not crush or break capsule form.

IM:
- Give deep IM into large muscle mass, preferably upper outer gluteus maximus.

RECTAL:
- If suppository is too soft, chill for 30 min in refrigerator or run cold water over foil wrapper.
- Moisten suppository w/cold water before inserting well up into rectum.

INDICATIONS/ROUTES/DOSAGE

Note: Do not use IV route (produces severe hypotension).

Nausea, vomiting:
Oral: Adults, elderly: 250 mg 3–4 times/day. ***Children 30–100 lbs:*** 100–200 mg 3–4 times/day.

IM: Adults, elderly: 200 mg 3–4 times/day.

Rectal: Adults, elderly: 200 mg 3–4 times/day. ***Children 30–100 lbs:*** 100–200 mg 3–4 times/day. ***Children <30 lbs:*** 100 mg 3–4 times/ day. Do not use in premature or newborn infants.

CONTRAINDICATIONS

Hypersensitivity to benzocaine or similar local anesthetics; parenteral form in children, suppositories in premature infants or neonates.

CAUTIONS

Elderly, debilitated, dehydration, electrolyte imbalance, high fever.

INTERACTIONS

DRUG: ***CNS depression-producing medications*** may increase CNS depression. **HERBAL:** None known. **FOOD:** None significant. **ALTERED LAB VALUES:** None significant.

SIDE EFFECTS

Note: Elderly (>60 yrs) tend to develop mental confusion, disorientation, agitation, psychotic-like symptoms. **FREQUENT:** Drowsiness. **OCCASIONAL:** Blurred vision, diarrhea, dizziness, headache, muscle cramps. **RARE:** Skin rash, seizures, depression, episthotonus, Parkinson's syndrome, Reye's syndrome (vomiting, seizures).

ADVERSE REACTIONS/TOXIC EFFECTS

Hypersensitivity reaction manifested as extrapyramidal symptoms (muscle rigidity, allergic skin reactions) occurs rarely. Children may experience dominant paradoxical reaction (restlessness, insomnia, euphoria, nervousness, tremors). Overdosage may vary from CNS depression (sedation, apnea, cardiovascular collapse, death) to severe paradoxical reaction (hallucinations, tremor, seizures).

PATIENT CONSIDERATIONS

Baseline Assessment

Assess for dehydration if excessive vomiting occurs (poor skin turgor, dry mucous membranes, longitudinal furrows in tongue).

Intervention/Evaluation

Check B/P, especially in elderly (increased risk of hypotension). Assess children closely for paradoxical reaction. Monitor serum electrolytes in those with severe vomiting. Assess skin turgor, mucous membranes to evaluate hydration status. Assess for extrapyramidal symptoms (hypersensitivity). Measure I&O and assess any vomitus.

Patient/Family Teaching

Report visual disturbances, headache. Dry mouth is expected response to medication. Relief from nausea/vomiting generally occurs within 30 min of drug administration.

---

trimethoprim

try-**meth**-oh-prim
(Primsol, Proloprim, Trimpex)

FIXED-COMBINATION(S)
W/sulfamethoxazole, a sulfonamide **(Bactrim, Septra)**

CANADIAN AVAILABILITY
Proloprim

PREGNANCY CATEGORY C

CLASSIFICATION

Anti-infective

AVAILABILITY (Rx)

Tablets: 100 mg, 200 mg. **Oral Solution.**

PHARMACOKINETICS

Absorption: Rapidly, completely absorbed from GI tract. Widely distributed including CSF. **Metabolism:** Metabolized in liver. **Excretion:** Primarily excreted in urine. Moderately removed by hemodialysis. **Half-life:** 8–10 hrs (increased in decreased renal function, newborns; decreased in children).

ACTION/*THERAPEUTIC EFFECT*

Blocks bacterial biosynthesis of nucleic acids and proteins by interfering with metabolism of folinic acid, *producing antibacterial activity.*

USES/*UNLABELED*

Treatment of initial acute uncomplicated urinary tract infections (UTIs). *Prophylaxis of bacterial UTI, treatment of pneumonia caused by Pneumocystis carinii.*

ADMINISTRATION

ORAL:

- Space doses evenly to maintain constant level in urine.
- Give w/o regard to meals (if stomach upset occurs, give w/food).

INDICATIONS/ROUTES/DOSAGE

Acute, uncomplicated UTIs:
Oral: Adults, elderly: 100 mg q12h or 200 mg once daily for 10 days.

Dosage in renal impairment:
The dose and/or frequency is modified in response to degree of renal impairment, severity of infection, and serum concentration of drug.

CREATININE CLEARANCE	DOSAGE
>30 ml/min	No change
15–30 ml/min	50 mg q12h

CONTRAINDICATIONS

Hypersensitivity to trimethoprim, infants <2 mos, megaloblastic anemia due to folic acid deficiency.

CAUTIONS

Impaired renal or hepatic function, children who have X chromosome w/mental retardation, pts who have possible folic acid deficiency.

INTERACTIONS

DRUG: *Folate antagonists (e.g., methotrexate)* may increase risk of myeloblastic anemia. **HERBAL:** None known. **FOOD:** None significant. **ALTERED LAB VALUES:** May increase BUN, SGOT (AST), SGPT (ALT), serum bilirubin, creatinine concentration.

SIDE EFFECTS

OCCASIONAL: Nausea, vomiting, diarrhea, decreased appetite, stomach cramps, headache. **RARE:** Hypersensitivity reaction (rash, itching), methemoglobinemia (blue color on fingernails, lips or skin, difficulty breathing, pale skin, sore throat, fever, unusual bleeding or bruising, unusually tired).

ADVERSE REACTIONS/TOXIC EFFECTS

Stevens-Johnson syndrome, erythema multiforme, exfoliative dermatitis, anaphylaxis occur rarely. Hematologic toxicity (thrombocytopenia, neutropenia, leukopenia, megaloblastic anemia) more likely to occur in elderly, debilitated, alcoholics, those w/impaired renal function or receiving prolonged high dosage.

PATIENT CONSIDERATIONS

BASELINE ASSESSMENT

Question for history of hypersensitivity to trimethoprim. Obtain specimens for diagnostic tests before giving first dose (therapy may begin before results are known). Identify hematology baseline reports.

INTERVENTION/EVALUATION

Assess skin for rash. Evaluate food tolerance. Monitor hematology reports, renal, hepatic test results if ordered. Check for developing signs of hematologic toxicity: pallor, fever, sore throat, malaise, bleeding, or bruising.

PATIENT/FAMILY TEACHING

Space doses evenly. Complete full length of therapy (may be 10–14 days). May take on empty stomach or w/food if stomach upset occurs. Avoid sun/ultraviolet light; use sunscreen, wear protective clothing. Immediately report pallor, tiredness, sore throat, bleeding, bruising or discoloration of skin, fever to physician.

trimetrexate glucuronate

try-meh-**trex**-ate
(Neutrexin)

CANADIAN AVAILABILITY
Neutrexin

PREGNANCY CATEGORY D

CLASSIFICATION

Antiprotozoal

AVAILABILITY (Rx)

Powder for Injection: 25 mg

PHARMACOKINETICS

Following IV administration, distributed readily into ascitic fluid. **Metabolism:** Metabolized in liver. **Excretion:** Eliminated in urine. **Half-life:** 11–20 hrs.

ACTION / *THERAPEUTIC EFFECT*

Inhibits the enzyme dihydrofolate reductase (DHFR), *disrupting purine, DNA, RNA, protein synthesis, with consequent cell death.*

USES / *UNLABELED*

Alternative therapy w/concurrent leucovorin administration for treatment of moderate to severe *Pneumocystis carinii pneumonia* (PCP) in immunocompromised pts, including pts w/acquired immunodeficiency syndrome (AIDS), who are intolerant of, or are refractory to, trimethoprim-sulfamethoxazole (TMP/SMZ) therapy or for whom TMP/SMZ is contraindicated. *Treatment of non small cell lung, prostate, and colorectal cancer.*

STORAGE/HANDLING

Store vials for parenteral use at room temperature. After reconstitution, solution is stable under refrigeration or at room temperature for up to 24 hrs. Reconstituted solution appears as pale greenish yellow. Inspect for particulate matter. Discard if cloudiness or precipitate is present. Do not freeze reconstituted solution. Discard unused portion after 24 hrs.

ADMINISTRATION

IV:

- **Note:** If solution comes in contact w/skin or mucosa, wash w/soap and water immediately. Use proper cytoxic disposal technique. Do not reconstitute w/solution containing either chloride ion or leucovorin because precipitate occurs instantly.
- Reconstitute each 25 mg vial w/2 ml 5% dextrose injection or sterile water for injection to provide concentration of 12.5 mg/ml. Complete dissolution should occur within 30 sec.
- Filter the reconstituted solution prior to further dilution.
- Further dilute w/5% dextrose to yield a final concentration of 0.25–2 mg/ml.
- Give diluted solution by IV infusion over 60–90 min.
- Flush IV line thoroughly with at least 10 ml 5% dextrose before and after administering trimetrexate.

INDICATIONS/ROUTES/DOSAGE

Note: Even though trimetrexate and leucovorin are given concurrently, they must be administered separately or precipitate will occur instantly; flush IV line thoroughly with 10 ml 5% dextrose between infusions. Dilute leukovorin according to leukovorin instructions and give over 5–10 min q6h.

PCP:

IV Infusion: Adults: Trimetrexate: 45 mg/m^2 once daily over 60–90 min. ***Leucovorin:*** 20 mg/m^2 over 5–10 min q6h for total daily dose of 80 mg/m^2, or orally as 4 doses of 20 mg/m^2 spaced equally throughout the day. Round up the oral dose to the next higher 25 mg increment. ***Recommended course of therapy:*** 21 days trimetrexate, 24 days leucovorin.

Note: In event of hematologic, renal, hepatic toxicities, doses of trimetrexate and leukovorin should be modified.

CONTRAINDICATIONS

Clinically significant hypersensitivity to trimetrexate, leucovorin, or methotrexate.

CAUTIONS

Fertility impairment, pts w/hematologic, renal, hepatic impairment.

INTERACTIONS

DRUG: ***Erythromycin, rifampin, rifabutin, ketoconazole, fluconazole, acetaminophen*** may alter timetrexate plasma concentration. ***Cimetidine*** reduces trimetrexate metabolism. ***Clotrimazole, ketoconazole, miconazole*** may inhibit trimetrexate metabolism. **HERBAL:** None known. **FOOD:** None significant. **ALTERED LAB VALUES:** May increase SGOT (AST), SGPT (ALT), alkaline phosphatase, bilirubin, BUN, serum creatinine. May decrease Hgb, Hct, leukocytes, platelet counts.

SIDE EFFECTS

OCCASIONAL: Fever, rash, pruritus, nausea, vomiting, confusion. **RARE:** Fatigue.

ADVERSE REACTIONS/TOXIC EFFECTS

Trimetrexate given without concurrent leucovorin may result in serious or fatal hematologic, hepatic, and/or renal complications, including bone marrow suppression, oral and GI mucosal ulceration, and renal and hepatic dysfunction. In event of overdose, stop trimetrexate and give leucovorin 40 mg/m^2 q6h for 3 days. Anaphylaxis occurs rarely.

PATIENT CONSIDERATIONS

Baseline Assessment

Offer emotional support to pt and family. Leucovorin therapy must extend for 72 hrs past the last dose of trimetrexate. Advise women of childbearing potential to avoid pregnancy. Blood tests should be performed twice weekly during therapy. Question for sensitivity to trimetrexate, methotrexate, leucovorin, medication history, particularly bone marrow depressants, hepato/nephrotoxic medication. To allow for full therapeutic effect of trimetrexate to occur, zidovudine treatment should be discontinued during trimetrexate therapy.

Intervention/Evaluation

Closely monitor neutrophil count, platelet count, liver function tests (SGOT, SGPT, alkaline phosphatase), renal values (serum creatinine, BUN) for development of serious toxicities. Carefully assess and treat pts w/nephrotoxic, myelosuppressive, or hepatotoxic drugs given during trimetrexate therapy.

Patient/Family Teaching

Failure to take the recommended dose and duration of leucovorin can lead to fatal toxicity. Use two forms of contraception during therapy. Avoid persons w/bacterial infections. Immediately contact physician if fever, chills, cough or hoarseness, lower back or side pain, or painful urination occurs. Report any unusual bleeding or bruising, black tarry stools, blood in urine or stools, pinpoint red spots on skin.

troglitazone

trow-**glit**-ah-zone
(Rezulin)

PREGNANCY CATEGORY B

CLASSIFICATION

Antidiabetic

AVAILABILITY (Rx)

Tablets: 200 mg, 300 mg, 400 mg

PHARMACOKINETICS

Absorption: Rapidly absorbed following oral administration. Highly protein bound (> 99%), primarily to albumin. Steady-state plasma concentration is reached in 3–5 days. **Metabolism:** Metabolized in the liver. **Excretion:** Excreted mainly in the feces with a lesser amount in the urine. **Half-life:** 16–34 hrs.

ACTION/*THERAPEUTIC EFFECT*

Improves target cell response to insulin without increasing pancreatic insulin secretion. Decreases hepatic glucose output, increases insulin-dependent glucose utilization in skeletal muscle, *lowering blood glucose concentration.*

USES/*UNLABELED*

Adjunct to diet and exercise to lower blood glucose in pts with Type II non-insulin-dependent diabetes mellitus (NIDDM). Used in combination with a sulfonylurea, metformin, or insulin to improve glycemic control. *Treatment of polycystic ovary syndrome and essential hypertension with NIDDM.*

ADMINISTRATION

ORAL:

- Give w/meals (enhances absorption).

INDICATIONS/ROUTES/DOSAGES

Diabetes mellitus, combination therapy:

Oral: Adults, elderly: Insulin: Initially, 200 mg once/day. Continue current insulin dose. May increase dose after 2–4 wks. ***Usual dose:*** 400 mg/day. ***Maximum:*** 600 mg/day. Insulin should be decreased 10–25% when fasting glucose levels decrease to <120 mg/dl.

Sulfonylureas: Initially, 200 mg once/day. If response is not adequate, increase troglitazone at 2–4 wks after initial dosage. ***Maximum:*** 600 mg/day.

Monotherapy: Monotherapy is not to be used if pt is well controlled with a sulfonylurea (it should be added to, not substituted for, a sulfonylurea). Initially, 400 mg once/day. May increase to 600 mg once/day after once month.

CONTRAINDICATIONS

Diabetic ketoacidosis, Type 1 diabetes mellitus, active liver disease or increased serum transaminase levels (ALT (SGPT) > 1.5 times the normal serum level), history of hypersensitivity to troglitazone.

CAUTIONS

Hepatic function impairment, congestive heart failure.

INTERACTIONS

DRUG: *Cholestyramine* may decrease absorption. May alter effects of ***oral contraceptives, astemizole, calcium channel blockers, cisapride, cyclosporine, corticosteroids, tacrolimus, triazolam, trimetrexate, HMG-CoA reductase inhibitors.*** **HERBAL:** None known. **FOOD:** Food enhances extent of troglitazone absorption. **ALTERED LAB VALUES:** May increase ALT (SGPT, AST (SGOT), serum bilirubin, slightly increase HDL, LDL and total cholesterol. May decrease alkaline phosphatase, GGT, triglycerides, Hgb, HCT, neutrophil count slightly.

SIDE EFFECTS

FREQUENT (6–18%): Infection, headache, asthenia (loss of strength), dizziness, back pain, nausea. **OCCASIONAL (5%):** Rhinitis, diarrhea, urinary tract infection, peripheral edema, pharyngitis.

ADVERSE REACTIONS/TOXIC EFFECTS

Hepatocellular injury occurs rarely but in very rare cases may lead to hepatic failure leading to death or liver transplant. Obtain liver function tests at the first sign of hepatic dysfunction (nausea, vomiting, abdominal pain, fatigue, anorexia, dark urine).

PATIENT CONSIDERATIONS

BASELINE ASSESSMENT

Check serum transaminase levels at the start of therapy and monthly thereafter. Discuss lifestyle to determine extent of learning, emotional needs. Assure follow-up instruction if pt/family do not thoroughly understand diabetes management or glucose-testing technique.

INTERVENTIONS/EVALUATION

Check serum transaminase levels monthly for the first 8 mos and then every 2 mos for the first year of therapy, and periodically thereafter. Monitor blood glucose, Hgb, liver function tests, especially SGOT, SGPT. Assess for hypoglycemia (cool wet skin, tremors, dizziness, anxiety, headache, tachycardia, numbness in mouth, hunger, diplopia) or hyperglycemia (polyuria, polyphagia, polydipsia, nausea, vomiting, dim vision, fatigue, deep rapid breathing). Be alert to conditions that alter glucose requirements: fever, increased activity or stress, surgical procedures.

PATIENT/FAMILY TEACHING

Diabetes mellitus requires lifelong control. Prescribed diet and exercise is principal part of treatment; do not skip or delay meals. Wear medical alert identification. Continue to adhere to dietary instructions, a regular exercise program and regular testing of urine or blood glucose. When taking combination drug therapy with a sulfonylurea or insulin, have a source of glucose available to treat symptoms of low blood sugar. Take troglitazone with meals.

trovafloxacin

tro-vah-**flocks**-ah-sin
(Trovan)

PREGNANCY CATEGORY C

CLASSIFICATION

Antibiotic: Fluoroquinolone

AVAILABILITY (Rx)

Tablets: 100 mg, 200 mg. **Solution for Injection:** 5 mg/ml alatrofloxacin mesylate.

PHARMACOKINETICS

Absorption: Well absorbed following oral administration. Widely distributed throughout body tissue. Highly bound to proteins (76%). **Metabolism:** Metabolized in the liver. **Excretion:** Eliminated primarily by biliary excretion. **Half-life:** 9–13 hrs.

ACTION/ *THERAPEUTIC EFFECT*

Inhibits the DNA enzyme, gyrase, in susceptible microorganisms, interfering with bacterial DNA replication and repair, *producing bactericidal activity.*

USES

Treatment of acute bacterial exacerbation of chronic bronchitis, acute sinusitis, pneumonia, intra-abdominal, gynecologic, pelvic, urinary tract, skin/skin structure infections, surgical prophylaxis.

STORAGE

After reconstitution, solution is stable for 7 days if refrigerated, 3 days at room temperature.

ADMINISTRATION

ORAL:

- May give w/o regard to food.
- Do not administer antacids (aluminum, magnesium), sucralfate, iron and multivitamin preparations with zinc within 2 hrs of trovafloxacin administration (significantly reduces absorption).
- Encourage cranberry juice, citrus fruits (acidifies urine).

IV:

- Compatible with 0.45% sodium chloride, 5% dextrose, 5% dextrose/0.45% sodium chloride, 5% dextrose/0.2% sodium chloride, 5% dextrose/lactated Ringer's solution.
- Incompatible w/0.9% NaCl or lactated Ringer's. Note: 0.9% NaCl may be used to flush IV line before or after administration of trovafloxacin.
- After reconstitution, must be diluted to a final concentration of 1 or 2 mg/ml.
- Do not add other medications to trovafloxacin through the same IV line. If the same line is used for other subsequent infusion medications, flush the line before and after trovafloxacin infusion.
- Infuse over 60 min through Y-type IV infusion (piggyback). Avoid a more rapid infusion.

INDICATIONS/ROUTES/DOSAGES

Usual dosage:
Oral/IV: Adults > 18 yrs, elderly: 100–300 mg as a single dose q24h for 7–14 days.

Dosage in chronic hepatitis disease (cirrhosis):

NORMAL HEPATIC DOSE	CHRONIC HEPATITIS DOSE
300 mg IV	200 mg IV
200 mg oral/IV	100 mg oral/IV
100 mg oral	100 mg oral

CONTRAINDICATIONS

History of hypersensitivity to fluoroquinolone antibiotics.

CAUTIONS

Chronic hepatic disease, those with known/suspected CNS disorder (epilepsy, severe cerebral arteriosclerosis).

INTERACTIONS

DRUG: *Aluminum/magnesium containing antacids, sucralfate, iron preparations, morphine,* decreases oral trovafloxacin absorption. **HERBAL:** None known. **FOOD:** None significant. **ALTERED LAB VALUES:** May increase SGOT (AST), SGOT (ALT).

SIDE EFFECTS

FREQUENT (11%): Dizziness. **OCCASIONAL (3–8%):** Nausea, headache, lightheadedness, vomiting. **RARE (≤2%):** Diarrhea, abdominal pain, rash, pruritus, photosensitivity.

ADVERSE REACTIONS/TOXIC EFFECTS

Superinfection (particularly enterococcal or fungal overgrowth of nonsusceptible organisms) may occur. Hypersensitivity reactions have occurred in those receiving fluoroquinolone therapy.

PATIENT CONSIDERATIONS

BASELINE ASSESSMENT

Question for hypersensitivity to trovafloxacin or other fluoroquinolones. Obtain specimens for culture and sensitivity test (therapy may begin before results are known).

INTERVENTION/EVALUATION

Report hypersensitivity reaction: skin rash, urticaria, pruritus, photosensitivity promptly. Be alert for superinfection (e.g., genital-anal pruritus, ulceration or changes in oral mucosa, moderate to severe diarrhea, new or increased fever). Provide symptomatic relief for nausea. Assist with ambulation if dizziness occurs.

PATIENT/FAMILY TEACHING

Do not take antacids 2 hrs before or after taking medication (reduces/destroys effectiveness). Eat/drink high sources of ascorbic acid (cranberry juice, citrus fruits). Avoid excessive sunlight/artificial ultraviolet light (reaction may occur up to several weeks after stopping therapy). Continue medication for full length of treatment.

tubocurarine chloride

(Tubarine)

See Classification section under: Neuromuscular blockers

unoprostone
(Rescula)
See Supplement

urokinase

your-oh-**kine**-ace
(Abbokinase)

CANADIAN AVAILABILITY
Abbokinase

PREGNANCY CATEGORY B

CLASSIFICATION

Thrombolytic

AVAILABILITY (Rx)

Powder for Injection: 250,000 IU/vial; 5,000 IU/ml

PHARMACOKINETICS

Rapidly cleared from circulation by liver. **Excretion:** Small amounts eliminated in urine and via bile. **Half-life:** 20 min.

ACTION/ *THERAPEUTIC EFFECT*

Acts directly on the fibrinolytic system to convert plasminogen to plasmin, an enzyme *that degrades fibrin clots, fibrinogen, and other plasma proteins.*

USES

Lysis of acute pulmonary emboli, pulmonary emboli accompanied by unstable hemodynamics, acute thrombi obstructing coronary arteries associated with evolving transmural myocardial infarction. Restores patency to IV catheters obstructed by clotted blood or fibrin.

STORAGE/HANDLING

Refrigerate vials. Reconstitute immediately before use. After reconstitution, solution is stable for 24 hrs at room temperature or if refrigerated. Solutions are clear, colorless to light straw. Do not use if solution is highly colored; discard unused portions.

ADMINISTRATION

- **Note:** Must be administered within 12–14 hrs of clot formation (little effect on older, organized clots).

IV:

- Give by IV infusion via pump; via coronary catheter into thrombosed coronary artery; or via syringe into occluded IV catheter.
- For IV infusion, reconstitute each 250,000 IU vial with 5 ml sterile water for injection to provide a concentration of 50,000 IU/ml. Further dilute up to 200 ml with 5% dextrose or 0.9% NaCl.
- For intracoronary administration, reconstitute three 250,000 IU vials with 5 ml sterile water for injection for each vial. Further dilute with 500 ml 5% dextrose or 0.9% NaCl to provide a concentration of 1,500 IU/ml.
- Gently roll and tilt vial (minimizes formation of filaments). Do not shake vial.
- Solutions may be filtered through 0.45 micron or smaller filter.
- If minor bleeding occurs at puncture sites, apply pressure for 30 min, then apply pressure dressing.
- If uncontrolled hemorrhage occurs, discontinue infusion immediately (slowing rate of infusion may produce worsening hemorrhage). Do not use dextran to control hemorrhage.
- Avoid undue pressure when drug is injected into catheter (can rupture catheter or expel clot into circulation).

INDICATIONS/ROUTES/DOSAGE

Pulmonary embolism:
IV: Adults, elderly: Initially, 4,400

IU/kg at rate of 90 ml/hr over 10 min; then, 4,400 IU/kg at rate of 15 ml/hr for 12 hrs. Flush tubing. Follow with anticoagulant therapy.

Coronary artery thrombi:
Intracoronary: Adults, elderly: 6,000 IU/min for up to 2 hrs.

Note: Before therapy, give 2,500–10,000 U heparin by IV injection; continue heparin after artery is opened.

Occluded IV catheter:
Disconnect IV tubing from catheter; attach a 1 ml TB syringe with 5,000 U urokinase to catheter; inject urokinase slowly (equal to volume of catheter). Wait 5 min. Connect empty 5 ml syringe; aspirate residual clot. When patency is restored, aspirate 4–5 ml blood. Irrigate with 0.9% NaCl; reconnect IV tubing to catheter.

CONTRAINDICATIONS

Active internal bleeding, recent (within 2 mos) cerebrovascular accident, intracranial/intraspinal surgery, intracranial neoplasm.

CAUTIONS

Recent (within 10 days) major surgery/GI bleeding, OB delivery, organ biopsy, recent trauma (cardiopulmonary resuscitation, uncontrolled arterial hypertension, left ventricular thrombus), endocarditis, severe hepatic/renal disease, pregnancy, elderly, cerebrovascular disease, diabetic retinopathy, thrombophlebitis, occluded AV cannula at infected site.

INTERACTIONS

DRUG: ***Anticoagulants, heparin*** may increase risk of hemorrhage. ***NSAIDs, platelet aggregate*** inhibitors may increase risk of bleeding. ***Antifibrinolytics (e.g., aminocaproic acid)*** may antagonize effects. **HERBAL:** Feverfew, ginkgo may increase risk of bleeding. **FOOD:** None significant. **ALTERED LAB VALUES:** Decreases plasminogen and fibrinogen level during infusion, decreasing clotting time (confirms presence of lysis). Increases APTT, PT, TT.

SIDE EFFECTS

FREQUENT: Superficial or surface bleeding at puncture sites (venous cutdowns, arterial punctures, surgical sites, IM sites, retroperitoneal/intracerebral sites); internal bleeding (GI/GU tract, vaginal). **RARE:** Mild allergic reaction (rash, wheezing).

ADVERSE REACTIONS/TOXIC EFFECTS

Severe internal hemorrhage may occur. Lysis of coronary thrombi may produce atrial/ventricular arrhythmias.

U

PATIENT CONSIDERATIONS

BASELINE ASSESSMENT

Avoid arterial invasive technique before and during treatment. If arterial puncture is necessary, use upper extremity vessels. Assess Hct, platelet count, thrombin (TT), activated thromboplastin (APTT), prothrombin time (PT), fibrinogen level before therapy is instituted.

INTERVENTION/EVALUATION

Handle pt as carefully and infrequently as possible to prevent bleeding. Never give urokinase via IM injection route. Monitor clinical response, vital signs (pulse, temperature, respiratory rate, B/P) q4h. Do not obtain B/P in lower extremities (possible deep vein thrombi). Monitor TT, PT, APTT, fibrinogen level q4h or per protocol after initiation of therapy, stool culture for occult blood. Assess for decrease in B/P, increase in pulse rate, complaint of abdominal/back pain, severe headache (may be evidence of hemorrhage). Question for increase in amount of discharge during menses. Assess peripheral pulses; assess skin for bruises, petechiae. Check for excessive bleeding from minor cuts, scratches. Assess urine for hematuria.

ursodiol (ursodeoxycholic acid)

er-**sew**-dee-ol
(Actigall, Urso)

CANADIAN AVAILABILITY
Ursofalk

PREGNANCY CATEGORY B

CLASSIFICATION

Gallstone solubilizing agent

AVAILABILITY (Rx)

Capsules: 300 mg

PHARMACOKINETICS

Absorption: Readily absorbed from small bowel. Undergoes first-pass hepatic extraction. Distributed primarily in liver, bile, intestinal lumen. Protein binding: high. **Metabolism:** Metabolized in liver. **Excretion:** Excreted into bile and eliminated in feces.

ACTION/*THERAPEUTIC EFFECT*

Suppresses hepatic synthesis, secretion of cholesterol and inhibits intestinal absorption of cholesterol. *Changes the bile of pts with gallstones from cholesterol precipitating (capable of forming crystals) to cholesterol solubilizing (capable of being dissolved).*

USES/*UNLABELED*

Dissolution of radiolucent, noncalcified gallstones when cholecystectomy is an unacceptable method of treatment. Treatment of biliary cirrhosis. Prevention of gallstones. *Treatment of biliary atresia, sclerosing cholangitis, alcoholic cirrhosis, chronic hepatitis; prophylaxis of liver transplant rejection, gallstone formation.*

INDICATIONS/ROUTES/DOSAGE

Usual dosage:

Oral: Adults, elderly: 8–10 mg/kg/day in 2–3 divided doses. Treatment may require months of therapy. Obtain ultrasound image of gallbladder at 6 mo intervals for first year. If dissolved, continue therapy and repeat ultrasound within 1–3 mos.

Prevention of gallstones:

Oral: Adults, elderly: 300 mg 2 times/day.

CONTRAINDICATIONS

Calcified cholesterol stones, radiopaque stones, radiolucent bile pigment stones, allergy to bile acids, chronic liver disease.

CAUTIONS

None significant.

INTERACTIONS

DRUG: ***Aluminum-containing antacids, cholestyramine, colestipol*** may decrease absorption, effects. ***Estrogens, oral contraceptives*** may decrease effect. **HERBAL:** None known. **FOOD:** None significant. **ALTERED LAB VALUES:** May alter liver function tests.

SIDE EFFECTS

OCCASIONAL: Diarrhea.

ADVERSE REACTIONS/TOXIC EFFECTS

None significant.

PATIENT CONSIDERATIONS

Baseline Assessment

SGOT (AST) and SGPT (ALT) liver function tests should be obtained before therapy begins, after 1 and 3 mos of therapy, and q6mos thereafter. Those w/significant liver test abnormalities should be monitored more frequently.

Intervention/Evaluation

Monitor liver function tests in those w/impaired liver function (metabolic acidosis may occur during infusion).

Patient/Family Teaching

Treatment requires months of therapy.

valacyclovir

val-ah-**sigh**-klo-veer
(Valtrex)

CANADIAN AVAILABILITY
Valtrex

PREGNANCY CATEGORY B

CLASSIFICATION

Antiviral

AVAILABILITY (Rx)

Tablets: 500 mg

PHARMACOKINETICS

Absorption: Rapidly absorbed following oral administration. **Metabolism:** Rapidly converted by hydrolysis to active compound, acyclovir. Widely distributed to tissues/body fluids (including CSF). **Excretion:** Primarily eliminated in urine. **Half-life:** 2.5–3.3 hrs (increased in reduced renal function).

ACTION/*THERAPEUTIC EFFECT*

Converted to acyclovir triphosphate, becoming part of DNA chain, *interfering w/DNA synthesis and viral replication of herpes simplex and varicella zoster virus.* Virustatic.

USES

Treatment of herpes zoster (shingles) in immunocompetent adults. Episodic treatment of recurrent genital herpes in immunocompetent adults. Prevention of recurrent genital herpes. Treatment of initial genital herpes.

V

ADMINISTRATION

ORAL:

- Give w/o regard to meals.
- Do not crush or break tablets.

INDICATIONS/ROUTES/DOSAGE

Note: Therapy should be initiated at first sign of shingles (most effective within 48 hrs of onset of zoster rash).

Herpes zoster (shingles):
Oral: Adults, elderly: 1 g 3 times daily for 7 days.

Recurrent genital herpes:
Oral: Adults, elderly: 500 mg twice daily for 5 days.

Prevention of herpes:
Oral: Adults, elderly: 500–1,000 mg/day.

Initial treatment of genital herpes:
Oral: Adults, elderly: 1 g twice daily for 10 days.

Dosage in renal impairment:

CREATININE CLEARANCE	HERPES ZOSTER	GENITAL HERPES
≥ 50	1 g q8h	500 mg q12h
30–49	1 g q12h	500 mg q12h
10–29	1 g q24h	500 mg q24h
<10	500 mg q24h	500 mg q24h

CONTRAINDICATIONS

Hypersensitivity or intolerance to valacyclovir, acyclovir, or components of formulation.

CAUTIONS

Bone marrow or renal transplantation, advanced HIV infections, renal or hepatic impairment, dehydration, fluid/electrolyte imbalance, concurrent use of nephrotoxic agents, neurologic abnormalities.

INTERACTIONS

DRUG: *Probenecid, cimetidine* may increase acyclovir concentration. **HERBAL:** None known. **FOOD:** None significant. **ALTERED LAB VALUES:** None significant.

SIDE EFFECTS

Herpes zoster: FREQUENT (>10%): Nausea, headache. **OCCASIONAL (3–10%):** Vomiting, diarrhea, constipation (≥50 yrs), asthenia, dizziness (≥50 yrs). **RARE (1–3%):** Abdominal pain, anorexia.

Genital herpes: FREQUENT (>10%): Headache. **OCCASIONAL (3–10%):** Nausea, diarrhea, dizziness. **RARE (1–3%):** Asthenia, abdominal pain.

ADVERSE REACTION/TOXIC EFFECTS

None significant.

PATIENT CONSIDERATIONS

Baseline Assessment

Question history of allergies, particularly to valacyclovir, acyclovir. Tissue cultures for herpes zoster and herpes simplex should be done before giving first dose (therapy may proceed before results are known). Assess medical history, especially advanced HIV infection, bone marrow/renal transplantation, hepatic/renal function.

Intervention/Evaluation

Evaluate cutaneous lesions. Manage herpes zoster with strict isolation. Provide analgesics and comfort measures for herpes zoster; especially exhausting to elderly. Encourage fluids. Keep pt's fingernails short, hands clean.

Patient/Family Teaching

Drink adequate fluids. Do not touch lesions with fingers to avoid spreading infection to new site. *Genital herpes:* Continue therapy for full length of treatment. Space doses evenly. Avoid sexual intercourse during duration of lesions to prevent infecting partner. Valacyclovir does not cure herpes. Notify physician if lesions do not improve or recur. Pap smears should be done at least annually due to increased risk of cancer of cervix in women w/genital herpes. Initiate treatment at first sign of a recurrent episode of genital herpes or herpes zoster (early treatment, that is, within first 24–48 hrs, is imperative for therapeutic results).

valproic acid

val-**pro**-ick
(Depakene)

valproate sodium

(Depakene syrup)

divalproex sodium

(Depacon, Depakote)

CANADIAN AVAILABILITY

Divalproex sodium **(Epival)**, valproic acid **(Depakene)**

PREGNANCY CATEGORY D

CLASSIFICATION

Anticonvulsant

AVAILABILITY (Rx)

Capsules: 250 mg (valproic acid). **Syrup:** 250 mg/5 ml (valproic acid). **Tablets (delayed-release):** 125 mg, 250 mg, 500 mg (divalproex). **Capsules (sprinkle):** 125 mg (divalproex). **Injection.**

PHARMACOKINETICS

Absorption: Well absorbed from GI tract. **Metabolism:** Metabolized in liver. **Excretion:** Primarily excreted in urine. **Half-life:** 6–16 hrs (may be increased in decreased liver function, elderly, children <18 mos).

ACTION/*THERAPEUTIC EFFECT*

Directly increases concentration of the inhibitory neurotransmitter gamma-aminobutyric acid (GABA), *producing anticonvulsant effect.*

USES/*UNLABELED*

Prophylaxis of absence seizures (petit mal), myoclonic, tonic-clonic seizure control. Used principally as adjunct w/other anticonvulsant agents. Treatment of manic episodes w/bipolar disorders, complex partial seizures. Prophylaxis of migraine headaches. *Treatment of myoclonic, simple partial, tonic-clonic seizures, migraines.*

ADMINISTRATION

ORAL:

- Give w/food if GI distress occurs.
- Do not crush, chew, or break enteric-coated tablets.
- Do not mix solution w/carbonated drinks (may produce local mouth irritation, unpleasant taste).

INDICATIONS/ROUTES/DOSAGE

Anticonvulsant:

Oral: Adults, elderly, children: Initially, 15 mg/kg daily (if dosage exceeds 250 mg daily, give in two or more equally divided doses). Increase at 1 wk intervals by 5–10 mg/kg daily until seizures are controlled or unacceptable effects occur. ***Maximum daily dose:*** 60 mg/kg.

Manic episodes:

Oral: Adults, elderly: Initially, 750 mg/day in divided doses. ***Maximum:*** 60 mg/kg/day.

Migraines:

Oral: Adults: 250 mg 2 times/day.

CONTRAINDICATIONS

Hepatic disease.

CAUTIONS

History of hepatic disease, bleeding abnormalities, pancreatitis.

INTERACTIONS

DRUG: ***Alcohol, CNS depressants*** may increase CNS depressant effects. May increase risk of bleeding w/***anticoagulants, heparin, thrombolytics, platelet aggregation inhibitors.*** May increase concentration of ***amitriptyline, primidone. Carbamazepine*** may decrease concentration. ***Hepatotoxic medications*** may increase risk of hepatotoxicity. May alter ***phenytoin*** protein binding, increasing toxicity. ***Phenytoin*** may decrease effect.

V

HERBAL: None known. **FOOD:** None significant. **ALTERED LAB VALUES:** May increase SGOT (AST), SGPT (ALT), LDH, bilirubin.

SIDE EFFECTS

FREQUENT: Abdominal or stomach pain, loss of appetite, changes in menstrual period, diarrhea, alopecia, indigestion, nausea, vomiting, trembling in arms or hands, change in weight. **OCCASIONAL:** Constipation, dizziness, drowsiness, headache, skin rash, unusual excitement, restlessness. **RARE:** Changes in mood, double vision, nystagmus, spots before eyes, unusual bruising or bleeding.

ADVERSE REACTIONS/TOXIC EFFECTS

Hepatotoxicity may occur, particularly in the first 6 mos of therapy. May not be preceded by abnormal liver function tests, but may be noted as loss of seizure control, malaise, weakness, lethargy, anorexia, and vomiting. Blood dyscrasias may occur.

PATIENT CONSIDERATIONS

Baseline Assessment

Review history of seizure disorder (intensity, frequency, duration, level of consciousness). Initiate safety measures, quiet dark environment. CBC, platelet count should be performed before and 2 wks after therapy begins, then 2 wks after maintenance dose is given.

Intervention/Evaluation

Observe frequently for recurrence of seizure activity. Monitor liver function, CBC, platelet count. Assess skin for bruising, petechiae. Monitor for clinical improvement (decrease in intensity or frequency of seizures).

Patient/Family Teaching

Do not abruptly withdraw medication following long-term use (may precipitate seizures). Strict maintenance of drug therapy is essential for seizure control. Drowsiness usually disappears during continued therapy. Avoid tasks that require alertness, motor skills until response to drug is established. Avoid alcohol. Carry identification card/bracelet to note anticonvulsant therapy. Teach pts about their seizure condition and role in its management. If noncompliance is an issue in causing acute seizures, discuss reasons for noncompliance and address them.

---

valrubicin

(Valstar)

See Classification section under: Cancer chemotherapy

---

valsartan

val-**sar**-tan

(Diovan)

FIXED-COMBINATION(S)

W/hydrochlorothiazide, a diuretic **(Diovan HCT)**

CANADIAN AVAILABILITY

Diovan

PREGNANCY CATEGORY C

Third trimester

PREGNANCY CATEGORY D

Second and third trimester

CLASSIFICATION

Antihypertensive

AVAILABILITY (Rx)

Capsules: 80 mg, 160 mg

PHARMACOKINETICS

Absorption: Poorly absorbed following oral administration. Food decreases peak plasma concentration. Highly bound to plasma proteins (95%). **Metabolism:** Metabolized in the liver. **Excretion:** Recovered primarily in feces and to a lesser extent, in urine. **Half-life:** 6 hrs.

ACTION/*THERAPEUTIC EFFECT*

Potent vasodilator. An angiotensin II receptor (type AT_1) antagonist; blocks vasoconstrictor and aldesterone-secreting effects of angiotensin II, inhibiting the binding of angiotensin II to the AT_1 receptors, *producing vasodilation, decreased peripheral resistance, decrease in B/P.*

USES/*UNLABELED*

Treatment of hypertension alone or in combination with other antihypertensives. *Treatment of heart failure.*

ADMINISTRATION

ORAL:

- Give w/o regard to meals.

INDICATIONS/ROUTES/DOSAGES

Note: May be given concurrently w/other antihypertensives. If B/P is not controlled by valsartan alone, a diuretic may be added.

Hypertension:

Oral: Adults, elderly, mildly impaired renal or hepatic function: 80 mg once daily in pts who are not volume depleted. ***Dose range:*** 80–320 mg once daily.

CONTRAINDICATIONS

None significant.

CAUTIONS

Renal/hepatic function impairment, renal arterial stenosis, severe CHF, dehydration.

INTERACTIONS

DRUG: *Diuretics* produces additive hypotensive effects. **HERBAL:** None known. **FOOD:** Food slows absorption but not bioavailability. **ALTERED LAB VALUES:** May increase liver enzymes, bilirubin, creatinine, potassium. May decrease Hgb, Hct.

SIDE EFFECTS

RARE: **(1–2%):** Insomnia, fatigue, heartburn, abdominal pain, dizziness, headache, diarrhea, nausea, vomiting, arthralgia, edema.

ADVERSE REACTIONS/TOXIC EFFECTS

Overdosage may manifest as hypotension and tachycardia; bradycardia occurs less often. Institute supportive measures. Viral infection, upper respiratory infection (cough, pharyngitis, sinusitis, rhinitis) occur rarely.

PATIENT CONSIDERATIONS

BASELINE ASSESSMENT

Obtain B/P and apical pulse immediately before each dose, in addition to regular monitoring (be alert to fluctuations). If excessive reduction in B/P occurs, place pt in supine position, feet slightly elevated. Question possibility of pregnancy (see Pregnancy Category). Assess medication history (especially diuretic). Question for history of hepatic/renal impairment, renal artery stenosis, history of severe CHF. Obtain BUN, serum creatinine, SGOT (AST), SGPT (ALT), alkaline phosphatase, bilirubin, Hgb, Hct, and vital signs, particularly B/P, pulse rate.

INTERVENTION/EVALUATION

Maintain hydration (offer fluids frequently). Assess for evidence of upper respiratory infection. Monitor all blood serum levels. Assess B/P for hypertension/hypotension.

V

PATIENT/FAMILY TEACHING

Inform female pt regarding consequences of second- and third-trimester exposure to valsartan. Report pregnancy to physician as soon as possible. Report any sign of infection (sore throat, fever). Do not stop taking medication. Need for lifelong control. Caution against exercising during hot weather (risk of dehydration, hypotension).

vancomycin hydrochloride

van-koe-**my**-sin

(Vancocin, Vancoled)

CANADIAN AVAILABILITY
Vancocin

PREGNANCY CATEGORY C

CLASSIFICATION

Antibiotic

AVAILABILITY (Rx)

Capsules: 125 mg, 250 mg. **Powder for Oral Solution:** 1 g, 10 g. **Powder for Injection:** 500 mg, 1 g.

PHARMACOKINETICS

Oral: **Absorption:** Poorly absorbed from GI tract. **Excretion:** Primarily eliminated in feces. ***Parenteral:*** Widely distributed. **Excretion:** Primarily excreted unchanged in urine. Not removed by hemodialysis. **Half-life:** 4–11 hrs (increased in decreased renal function).

ACTION/*THERAPEUTIC EFFECT*

Inhibits cell wall synthesis by binding to bacterial cell wall, altering cell membrane permeability, inhibiting RNA synthesis, *producing bacterial cell death.* Bactericidal.

USES/*UNLABELED*

Systemic: Treatment of respiratory tract, bone, skin/soft tissue infections, endocarditis, peritonitis, septicemia. Given prophylactically to those at risk for bacterial endocarditis (if penicillin contraindicated) when undergoing dental, respiratory, GI, GU, biliary surgery/invasive procedures. ***Oral:*** Treatment of antibiotic colitis, pseudomembranous colitis, antibiotic-associated diarrhea, staphylococcal enterocolitis. *Treatment of brain abscess, staphylococcal/streptococcal meningitis, perioperative infections.*

STORAGE/HANDLING

Store capsules at room temperature. Oral solutions stable for 2 wks if refrigerated. IV infusion (piggyback) stable for 24 hrs at room temperature, 96 hrs if refrigerated. Discard if precipitate forms.

ADMINISTRATION

ORAL:

- Generally not given for systemic infections because of poor absorption from GI tract; however, some pts w/colitis may have effective absorption.
- Powder for oral solution may be reconstituted, given by mouth or nasogastric tube.
- Do not use powder for oral solution for IV administration.

IV:

- **Note:** Give by intermittent IV infusion (piggyback), continuous IV infusion. Do not give IV push (may result in exaggerated hypotension).
- For intermittent IV infusion

(piggyback), reconstitute each 500 mg vial w/10 ml sterile water for injection (20 ml for 1 g vial) to provide concentration of 50 mg/ml.

- Further dilute each 500 mg w/at least 100 ml 5% dextrose, 0.9% NaCl, or other compatible IV fluid. Infuse over at least 1 hr.
- For IV infusion, add 1–2 g reconstituted vancomycin to sufficient amount 5% dextrose or 0.9% NaCl to infuse over 24 hrs.
- Monitor B/P closely during IV infusion.
- ADD-Vantage vials should not be used in neonates, infants, children requiring less than 500 mg dose.
- Alternating IV sites, use large veins q2–3 days to reduce risk of phlebitis.

INDICATIONS/ROUTES/DOSAGE

Usual parenteral dosage:
IV: Adults, elderly: 500 mg q6h or 1 g q12h. *Children >1 mo:* 40 mg/kg/day in divided doses. *Maximum:* 2 g/day. *Neonates:* 15 mg/kg initially, then 10 mg/kg q8–12h.

Dosage in renal impairment:
After a loading dose, subsequent dose and/or frequency is modified based on degree of renal impairment, severity of infection, serum concentration of drug.

Staphylococcal enterocolitis, antibiotic-associated pseudomembranous colitis caused by *Clostridium difficile*:
Oral: Adults, elderly: 0.5–2 g/day in 3–4 divided doses for 7–10 days. *Children:* 40 mg/kg/day in 3–4 divided doses for 7–10 days. *Maximum:* 2 g/day.

CONTRAINDICATIONS

None significant.

CAUTIONS

Renal dysfunction, preexisting hearing impairment, concurrent therapy w/other ototoxic/nephrotoxic medications.

INTERACTIONS

DRUG: *Oral: Cholestyramine, colestipol* may decrease effect. *Parenteral: Aminoglycosides, amphotericin, aspirin, bumetanide, carmustine, cisplatin, cyclosporine, ethacrynic acid, furosemide, streptozocin* may increase ototoxicity and/or nephrotoxicity. **HERBAL:** None known. **FOOD:** None signficant. **ALTERED LAB VALUES:** May increase BUN.

SIDE EFFECTS

FREQUENT: *Oral:* Bitter/unpleasant taste, nausea, vomiting, mouth irritation (oral solution). **RARE:** *Systemic:* Phlebitis, thrombophlebitis, pain at IV site. Necrosis may occur w/extravasation. Dizziness, vertigo, tinnitus, chills, fever, rash. *Oral:* Skin rash.

V

ADVERSE REACTIONS/TOXIC EFFECTS

Nephrotoxicity (change in amount/frequency of urination, nausea, vomiting, increased thirst, anorexia); ototoxicity (deafness due to damage to auditory branch of eighth cranial nerve); red-neck syndrome (too rapid injection): chills, fever, fast heartbeat, nausea, vomiting, itching, rash, redness on face/neck/arms/back; unpleasant taste.

PATIENT CONSIDERATIONS

BASELINE ASSESSMENT

Question pt for history of allergy to vancomycin. Avoid other ototoxic and nephrotoxic medications if possible. Obtain culture and sensitivity test before giving

first dose (therapy may begin before results are known).

INTERVENTION/EVALUATION

Evaluate IV site for phlebitis (heat, pain, red streaking over vein). Monitor renal function tests, I&O. Assess skin for rash. Check hearing acuity, balance. Monitor B/P carefully during infusion.

PATIENT/FAMILY TEACHING

Continue therapy for full length of treatment. Doses should be evenly spaced. Notify physician in event of tinnitus, rash, other new symptom. Lab tests are important part of total therapy.

vasopressin

vay-sew-**press**-in
(Pitressin)

CANADIAN AVAILABILITY
Pressyn

PREGNANCY CATEGORY B

CLASSIFICATION

Vasopressor, antidiuretic

AVAILABILITY (Rx)

Injection: 20 units/ml

PHARMACODYNAMICS

	ONSET	PEAK	DURATION
IM/SubQ	—	—	2–8 hrs
IV	—	—	0.5–1 hr

PHARMACOKINETICS

Distributed throughout extracellular fluid. **Metabolism:** Metabolized in liver, kidney. **Excretion:** Primarily excreted in urine. **Half-life:** 10–20 min.

ACTION/*THERAPEUTIC EFFECT*

Increases reabsorption of water by the renal tubules *resulting in decreased urinary flow rate,* increased urine osmolality. Urea is also reabsorbed by the collecting ducts. Directly stimulates contraction of smooth muscle, *preventing abdominal distension, intestinal paresis.* Causes vasoconstriction w/reduced blood flow in coronary, peripheral, cerebral, and pulmonary vessels, but particularly in portal and splanchnic vessels. In large doses, may cause mild uterine contractions.

USES/*UNLABELED*

Treatment of adult shock-refractory ventricular fibrillation (Class IIb). Prevents/controls polydipsia, polyuria, dehydration in pts w/neurogenic diabetes insipidus. Stimulates peristalsis in the prevention or treatment of postop abdominal distension, intestinal paresis. *Adjunct in treatment of acute, massive hemorrhage.*

ADMINISTRATION

SubQ/IM:

- Give 1–2 glasses of water at time of administration to reduce side effects.

IV INFUSION:

- Dilute w/5% dextrose in water or 0.9% NaCl to concentration of 0.1–1 units/ml.

INDICATIONS/ROUTES/DOSAGE

Cardiac arrest:
IV: Adults, elderly: 40 units as a one-time dose.

Diabetes insipidus:
Note: May administer intranasally on cotton pledgets, by nasal spray; individualize dosage.

IM/SubQ: Adults, elderly: 5–10 units, 2–4 times/day. ***Range:*** 5–60 units/day. ***Children:*** 2.5–10 units, 2–4 times/day.

Abdominal distension:
IM: Adults, elderly: Initially, 5 units. Subsequent doses of 10 units q3–4h.

GI hemorrhage:
IV Infusion: Adults, elderly: Initially, 0.2–0.4 units/min progressively increased to 0.9 units/min.

CONTRAINDICATIONS

Anaphylaxis or hypersensitivity to vasopressin or components, chronic nephritis w/nitrogen retention.

CAUTIONS

Migraine, epilepsy, heart failure, asthma, or any condition in which rapid addition of extracellular water may be a risk. Extreme caution in pts w/vascular disease, especially coronary artery disease.

INTERACTIONS

DRUG: *Carbamazepine, chlorpropamide, clofibrate* may increase effects. *Demeclocycline, lithium, norepinephrine* may decrease effect. **HERBAL:** None known. **FOOD:** None significant. **ALTERED LAB VALUES:** None significant.

SIDE EFFECTS

FREQUENT: Pain at injection site w/vasopressin tannate. **OCCASIONAL:** Stomach cramps, nausea, vomiting, diarrhea, dizziness, diaphoresis, paleness, circumoral pallor, trembling, "pounding" in head, eructation, and flatulence. **RARE:** Chest pain, confusion. ***Allergic reactions:*** Rash or hives, pruritus, wheezing or difficulty breathing, swelling of mouth, face, feet, hands. Sterile abscess w/vasopressin tannate.

ADVERSE REACTIONS/TOXIC EFFECTS

Anaphylaxis, myocardial infarction, and water intoxication have occurred. Elderly and very young at higher risk for water intoxication.

PATIENT CONSIDERATIONS

Baseline Assessment

Question for hypersensitivity to vasopressin, components. Establish baselines for weight, B/P, pulse, electrolytes, urine specific gravity.

Intervention/Evaluation

Monitor I&O closely, restrict intake as necessary to prevent water intoxication. Weigh daily if indicated. Check B/P and pulse 2 times/day. Monitor electrolytes, urine specific gravity. Evaluate injection site for erythema, pain, abscess. Report side effects to physician for dose reduction. Be alert for early signs of water intoxication (drowsiness, listlessness, headache). Hold medication and report immediately any chest pain/allergic symptoms.

Patient/Family Teaching

Promptly report headache, chest pain, shortness of breath, or other symptom. Stress importance of I&O.

---

varicella vaccine

(Varivax)
See Classification section under: Immunizations

---

vecuronium bromide

(Norcuron)
See Classification section under: Neuromuscular blockers

---

venlafaxine

ven-lah-**facks**-een
(Effexor, Effexor XR)

CANADIAN AVAILABILITY
Effexor

PREGNANCY CATEGORY C

CLASSIFICATION

Antidepressant

AVAILABILITY (Rx)

Tablets: 25 mg, 37.5 mg, 50 mg, 75 mg, 100 mg. **Effexor XR:** 37.5 mg, 75 mg, 150 mg.

PHARMACOKINETICS

Absorption: Well absorbed from GI tract. **Metabolism:** Metabolized in liver to active metabolite. **Excretion:** Primarily excreted in urine. **Half-life:** 3–7 hrs; metabolite: 9–13 hrs (increased in pts w/liver and/or renal disease).

ACTION/*THERAPEUTIC EFFECT*

Potentiates CNS neurotransmitter activity. Inhibits reuptake of serotonin, norepinephrine (weakly inhibits dopamine reuptake), *producing antidepressant activity.*

USES

Treatment of depression exhibited as persistent, prominent dysphoria (occurring nearly every day for at least 2 wks) manifested by 4 of 8 symptoms: change in appetite, change in sleep pattern, increased fatigue, impaired concentration, feelings of guilt or worthlessness, loss of interest in usual activities, psychomotor agitation or retardation, or suicidal tendencies. Psychotherapy augments therapeutic result. Treatment of anxiety (extended-release formulation).

ADMINISTRATION

ORAL:

- May give w/o regard to food. Give w/food or milk if GI distress occurs.
- Scored tablet may be crushed.
- Do not crush extended-release capsules.

INDICATIONS/ROUTES/DOSAGE

Note: Decrease dose by 50% in pts w/moderate liver impairment; 25% in mild to moderate renal impairment (50% in pts on dialysis, withholding dose until completion of dialysis). When discontinuing the medication, taper slowly over 2 wks.

Depression, anxiety (extended-release):

Oral: Adults, elderly: Initially, 75 mg/day in 2–3 divided doses w/food. May increase by 75 mg/day no sooner than 4 day intervals. ***Maximum:*** 375 mg/day in 3 divided doses. ***Extended-Release:*** 75 mg/day as single dose. May increase by 75 mg/day at intervals of at least 4 days. ***Maximum:*** 225 mg/day.

CONTRAINDICATIONS

Hypersensitivity to venlafaxine. Children <18 yrs of age (safety unknown). Pts currently receiving MAO inhibitors (see Drug Interactions).

CAUTIONS

Renal, hepatic impairment. History of mania, seizures, those w/metabolic or hemodynamic disease, hypertension, history of drug abuse.

INTERACTIONS

DRUG: ***MAO inhibitors (MAOIs)*** may cause hyperthermia, rigidity, myoclonus, autonomic instability (including rapid fluctuations of vital signs), mental status changes, coma, extreme agitation. May cause neuroleptic malignant syndrome (wait 14 days after discontinuing MAOIs to start or wait 7 days after discontinuing venlafaxine before starting MAOIs). **HERBAL:** St. John's wort may increase risk of adverse effects. **FOOD:** None significant. **ALTERED LAB VALUES:** May increase serum cholesterol, uric acid, alkaline phosphatase, SGOT (AST), SGPT (ALT), bilirubin, BUN. May decrease sodium, phosphate. May alter glucose, potassium.

SIDE EFFECTS

FREQUENT (>20%): Nausea, somnolence, headache, dry mouth. **OCCASIONAL (10–20%):** Dizziness, insomnia, constipation, sweating, nervousness, asthenia (loss of strength, energy), ejaculatory disturbance, anorexia. **RARE (10%):** Anxiety, blurred vision, diarrhea, vomiting, tremor, abnormal dreams, impotence.

ADVERSE REACTIONS/TOXIC EFFECTS

Sustained increase in diastolic B/P (10–15 mm Hg) occurs occasionally.

PATIENT CONSIDERATIONS

Baseline Assessment

Obtain initial weight and B/P. Assess appearance, behavior, speech pattern, level of interest, mood.

Intervention/Evaluation

Check B/P regularly for hypertension. Monitor weight and encourage small, frequent meals of favorite foods to prevent weight loss, especially in underweight pts. Assess sleep pattern for insomnia. Check during waking hours for somnolence or dizziness and anxiety; provide assistance as necessary. Supervise suicidal risk pt closely during early therapy (as depression lessens, energy level improves, increasing suicide potential). Assess appearance, behavior, speech pattern, level of interest, mood for therapeutic response.

Patient/Family Teaching

Take w/food. Do not increase, decrease, or suddenly stop medication. Venlafaxine may decrease appetite and cause weight loss. Do not drive or perform tasks that require alert response until certain drug does not cause impairment. Inform physician if breast feeding, pregnant or planning to become pregnant. Avoid alcohol. Do not take any other medication including OTC preparations w/o consulting physician. Report rash, hives, or other allergic responses promptly.

verapamil hydrochloride

ver-**ap**-ah-mill

(Calan, Covera-HS, Isoptin, Verelan, Verelan PM)

FIXED-COMBINATION(S)

W/trandolapril, an angiotensin inhibitor **(Tarka)**

CANADIAN AVAILABILITY

Apo-Verap, Chronovera, Isoptin, Novoveramil, Verelan

PREGNANCY CATEGORY C

CLASSIFICATION

Calcium channel blocker

AVAILABILITY (Rx)

Tablets: 40 mg, 80 mg, 120 mg. **Tablets (sustained-release):** 120 mg, 180 mg, 240 mg. **Capsules (sustained-release):** 120 mg, 180 mg, 240 mg, 360 mg. **Verelan PM:** 100 mg, 200 mg, 300 mg. **Injection:** 5 mg/2 ml.

V

PHARMACODYNAMICS

	ONSET	PEAK	DURATION
Oral			
	30 min	1–2 hrs	6–8 hrs
Extended-release			
	30 min	—	—
IV			
	1–2 min	3–5 min	10–60 min

PHARMACOKINETICS

Absorption: Well absorbed from GI tract. **Metabolism:** Undergoes first-pass metabolism in liver. Metabolized in liver to active metabolite. **Excretion:** Primarily excreted in urine. Not removed by hemodialysis. **Half-life:** ***oral:*** 2.8–7.4 hrs; ***IV:*** 2–5 hrs.

ACTION/*THERAPEUTIC EFFECT*

Inhibits calcium ion entry across cell membranes of cardiac and vascular smooth muscle (dilates coronary arteries, peripheral arteries, arterioles). *Decreases heart rate, myocardial contractility, slows SA and AV conduction. Decreases total peripheral vascular resistance by vasodilation.*

USES/*UNLABELED*

Parenteral: Management of supraventricular tachyarrhythmias, temporary control of rapid ventricular rate in atrial flutter/fibrillation. ***Oral:*** Management of spastic (Prinzmetal's variant) angina, unstable (crescendo, preinfarction) angina, chronic stable angina (effort-associated angina), hypertension, prevention of recurrent PSVT, and (w/digoxin) control of ventricular resting rate in those w/atrial flutter and/or fibrillation. *Treatment of hypertrophic cardiomyopathy, vascular headaches, migraines.*

ADMINISTRATION

ORAL:

- Give sustained-release tablets w/food. Verelan may be taken w/o regard to food.
- Do not crush or break sustained-released tablets. Do not break capsules.
- Verelan may be opened and sprinkled on food.

IV:

- Administer direct IV >2 min for adults, children (administer >3 min for elderly).
- Continuous EKG monitoring during IV injection is required for children, recommended for adults.
- Monitor EKG for rapid ventricular rates, extreme bradycardia, heart block, asystole, prolongation of PR interval. Notify physician of any significant changes.
- Monitor B/P q5–10min.
- Pt should remain recumbent for at least 1 hr following IV administration.

INDICATIONS/ROUTES/DOSAGE

Supraventricular tachyarrhythmias:
IV: Adults, elderly: Initially, 5–10 mg, repeat in 30 min w/10 mg dose. ***Children 1–15 yrs:*** 2–5 mg, repeat in 30 min up to 10 mg. ***Children <1 yr:*** 0.75–2 mg, repeat after 30 min. ***Maximum single dose:*** 10 mg.

Arrhythmias:
Oral: Adults, elderly: 240–480 mg/day in 3–4 divided doses.

Angina:
Oral: Adults, elderly: Initially, 80–120 mg 3 times/day (40 mg in elderly, pts w/liver dysfunction). Titrate to optimal dose. ***Maintenance:*** 240–480 mg/day in

3–4 divided doses. *Covera-HS:* 180–480 mg/day at bedtime.

Hypertension:
Oral: Adults, elderly: Initially, 40–80 mg 3 times/day. *Maintenance:* Up to 480 mg/day. *Covera-HS:* 180–480 mg/day at bedtime. *Verelan PM:* 100–300 mg/day.

Extended-Release Tablets: 120–240 mg/day up to 480 mg/day in 2 divided doses.

CONTRAINDICATIONS

Sick-sinus syndrome/second- or third-degree AV block (except in presence of pacemaker), cardiogenic shock, severe hypotension (<90 mm Hg, systolic), severe CHF (unless secondary to supraventricular tachycardia).

CAUTIONS

Impaired renal, hepatic function.

INTERACTIONS

DRUG: *Beta blockers* may have additive effect. May increase ***digoxin*** concentration. ***Procainamide, quinidine*** may increase risk of QT interval prolongation. ***Carbamazepine, quinidine, theophylline*** may increase concentration, toxicity. ***Disopyramide*** may increase negative inotropic effect. **HERBAL:** None known. **FOOD:** Grapefruit juice may increase concentration. **ALTERED LAB VALUES:** PR interval may be increased.

SIDE EFFECTS

FREQUENT (5–10%): Constipation. OCCASIONAL (1–5%): Dizziness, lightheadedness, headache, asthenia, nausea, peripheral edema, hypotension, bradycardia, CHF, rash, shortness of breath. RARE (<1%): Altered sleep, blurred vision, confusion, diarrhea, abdominal discomfort, dry mouth, palpitations, itching, alopecia, muscle pain.

ADVERSE REACTIONS/TOXIC EFFECTS

Rapid ventricular rate in atrial flutter/fibrillation, marked hypotension, extreme bradycardia, CHF, asystole, and second- and third-degree AV block occur rarely.

PATIENT CONSIDERATIONS

Baseline Assessment

Concurrent therapy of sublingual nitroglycerin may be used for relief of anginal pain. Record onset, type (sharp, dull, squeezing), radiation, location, intensity, and duration of anginal pain and precipitating factors (exertion, emotional stress). Check B/P for hypotension, pulse for bradycardia immediately before giving medication.

V

Intervention/Evaluation

Assess pulse for strength/weakness, irregular rate. Monitor EKG for cardiac changes, particularly prolongation of PR interval. Notify physician of any significant interval changes. Assist w/ambulation if dizziness occurs. Assess for peripheral edema behind medial malleolus (sacral area in bedridden pts). For those taking oral form, check stool consistency, frequency. Monitor for therapeutic serum level (0.1–0.3 mcg/ml).

Patient/Family Teaching

Do not abruptly discontinue medication. Compliance w/therapy regimen is essential to control anginal pain. To avoid hypotensive effect, rise slowly from lying to sitting position, wait momentarily

before standing. Avoid tasks that require alertness, motor skills until response to drug is established. Contact physician/nurse if irregular heartbeat, shortness of breath, pronounced dizziness, nausea, or constipation occurs. Avoid concomitant grapefruit juice.

vidarabine

vy-**dare**-ah-been
(Ara-A, Vira-A)

PREGNANCY CATEGORY C

CLASSIFICATION

Antiviral

AVAILABILITY (Rx)

Ophthalmic Ointment: 3%

PHARMACOKINETICS

Trace amounts in aqueous humor only if there is an epithelial defect in cornea.

ACTION/*THERAPEUTIC EFFECT*

Appears to interfere w/viral DNA synthesis, *regenerating corneal epithelium.*

USES

Treatment of keratitis, keratoconjunctivitis caused by herpes simplex virus, types 1 and 2.

STORAGE/HANDLING

Store at room temperature.

ADMINISTRATION

OPHTHALMIC:

- Place finger on lower eyelid and pull out until a pocket is formed between eye and lower lid.
- Place $\frac{1}{4}$–$\frac{1}{2}$ inch ointment into pocket.
- Have pt close eye for 1–2 min, rolling eyeball (increases contact area of drug to eye).
- Remove excess ointment around eye w/tissue.

INDICATIONS/ROUTES/DOSAGE

Usual ophthalmic dosage:
Ophthalmic: Adults, elderly: 0.5 inch into lower conjunctival sac 5 times/day at 3 hr intervals. After reepithelialization, treat additional 7 days at dosage of 2 times/day.

CONTRAINDICATIONS

Hypersensitivity to vidarabine, components of preparation.

INTERACTIONS

DRUG: None significant. **HERBAL:** None known. **FOOD:** None significant. **ALTERED LAB VALUES:** None significant.

SIDE EFFECTS

FREQUENT: Burning, itching, irritation. **OCCASIONAL:** Foreign body sensation, tearing, sensitivity, pain, photophobia.

ADVERSE REACTIONS/TOXIC EFFECTS

None significant.

PATIENT CONSIDERATIONS

BASELINE ASSESSMENT

Question history of allergy to vidarabine, components of preparation.

INTERVENTION/EVALUATION

Assess for irritation, itching, burning.

PATIENT/FAMILY TEACHING

Assure proper administration. Notify physician if there is no improvement in 7 days or if burning, irritation, pain devel-

ops. Do not stop or increase doses. Ointment should be continued for 5–7 days after infection is gone to prevent recurrence of infection. A temporary haze may occur after application to eye; sunglasses will decrease sensitivity to light. Use other eye products, including makeup, only w/advice of physician. Refrigerate, avoid freezing; if using another eye ointment, wait at least 10 min between dosing.

vigabatrin

(Sabril)

See Supplement

See Classification section under: Anticonvulsants

vinblastine sulfate

(Velban, Velsar)

See Classification section under: Cancer chemotherapy

vincristine sulfate

(Oncovin, Vincasar PFS)

See Classification section under: Cancer chemotherapy

vinorelbine

(Navelbine)

See Classification section under: Cancer chemotherapy

vitamin A

(Aquasol A)

PREGNANCY CATEGORY A

(X if used in doses above RDA)

CLASSIFICATION

Fat-soluble vitamin

AVAILABILITY (OTC)

Tablets: 5,000 IU. **Capsules:** 10,000 IU, 25,000 IU **(Rx),** 50,000 IU **(Rx). Drops:** 5,000 IU/0.1 ml. **Injection:** 50,000 IU/ml **(Rx).**

PHARMACOKINETICS

Absorption: Absorption dependent on bile salts, pancreatic lipase, dietary fat. Transported in blood to liver, stored in parenchymal liver cells, then transported in plasma as retinol, as needed. **Metabolism:** Metabolized in liver. **Excretion:** Excreted in bile and to a lesser amount in urine.

ACTION / *THERAPEUTIC EFFECT*

May be a cofactor in biochemical reactions. *Essential for normal function of retina. Necessary for visual adaptation to darkness, bone growth, testicular and ovarian function, embryonic development.*

V

USES

Treatment of vitamin A deficiency (biliary tract or pancreatic disease, sprue, colitis, hepatic cirrhosis, celiac disease, regional enteritis, extreme dietary inadequacy, partial gastrectomy, cystic fibrosis).

STORAGE/HANDLING

Store oral forms at room temperature. Refrigerate vials.

ADMINISTRATION

Note: IM administration used only in acutely ill or those unresponsive to oral route (GI malabsorption syndrome).

ORAL:

- Do not crush or break capsule form.

- May take w/o regard to food.

INDICATIONS/ROUTES/DOSAGE

Severe deficiency (Xerophthalmia): *Oral: Adults, elderly:* 25–50,000 IU/day. *Children >1 yr:* 200,000 IU as single dose; repeat following day and 4 wks later. 6 mos-1 yr: 100,000 IU as single dose; repeat following day and 4 wks later.

IM: Adults, elderly, children >8 yrs: 50–100,000IU/day for 3 days, then 50,000 IU daily for 2 wks. *Children 1–8 yrs:* 5–15,000 IU/day for 10 days. <1 yr: 5–10,000 IU/day for 10 days.

Dietary supplement:
Oral: Adults, elderly: 4,000–5,000 IU/day. *Children 7–10 yrs:* 3,300–3,500 IU/day. *Children 4–6 yrs:* 2,500 IU/day. *Children 6 mos–3 yrs:* 1,500–2,000 IU/day. *Neonates to 6 mos:* 1,500 IU/day.

CONTRAINDICATIONS

Hypervitaminosis A, oral use in malabsorption syndrome.

CAUTIONS

Renal impairment.

INTERACTIONS

DRUG: *Cholestyramine, colestipol, mineral oil* may decrease absorption. *Isotretinoin* may increase toxicity. **HERBAL:** None known. **FOOD:** None significant. **ALTERED LAB VALUES:** May increase BUN, calcium, cholesterol, triglycerides. May decrease erythrocyte, leukocyte counts.

SIDE EFFECTS

None significant.

ADVERSE REACTIONS/TOXIC EFFECTS

Chronic overdosage produces malaise, nausea, vomiting, drying/cracking of skin/lips, inflammation of tongue/gums, irritability, loss of hair, night sweats. Bulging fontanelles in infants noted.

PATIENT CONSIDERATIONS

INTERVENTION/EVALUATION

Closely supervise for overdosage symptoms during prolonged daily administration over 25,000 IU. Monitor for therapeutic serum vitamin A levels (80–300 IU/ml).

PATIENT/FAMILY TEACHING

Foods rich in vitamin A include cod, halibut, tuna, shark (naturally occurring vitamin A found only in animal sources). Avoid taking mineral oil, cholestyramine (Questran) while taking vitamin A.

vitamin D calcifediol
(Calderol)

calcitriol
(Calcijex, Rocaltrol)

dihydrotachysterol
(DHT, Hytakerol)

ergocalciferol
(Calciferol, Deltalin, Drisdol)

CANADIAN AVAILABILITY
Calciferol, Calcijex, Drisdol, Hytakerol, Rocaltrol

PREGNANCY CATEGORY A
(D if used in doses above RDA)

CLASSIFICATION

Fat-soluble vitamin

AVAILABILITY (Rx)

Calcifediol: Capsules: 20 mcg, 50 mcg.

Calcitriol: Capsules: 0.25 mcg, 0.5 mcg. **Injection:** 1 mcg/ml, 2 mcg/ml.

Dihydrotachysterol: Tablets: 0.125 mg, 0.2 mg, 0.4 mg. **Capsules:** 0.125 mg. **Oral Solution:** 0.2 mg/ml, 0.25 mg/ml.

Ergocalciferol: Liquid (OTC): 8,000 IU/ml. **Capsules:** 50,000 IU. **Tablets:** 50,000 IU. **Injection:** 500,000 IU/ml.

PHARMACOKINETICS

Absorption: Readily absorbed from small intestine. Concentrated primarily in liver, fat depots. **Metabolism:** Activated in liver, kidney. **Excretion:** Eliminated via biliary system; excreted in urine. **Half-life:** ***calcifediol:*** 10–22 days; ***calcitrol:*** 3–6 hrs; ***ergocalciferol:*** 19–48 hrs.

ACTION/*THERAPEUTIC EFFECT*

Essential for absorption and utilization of calcium and phosphate, normal calcification of bone, regulation of serum calcium concentration (w/parathyroid, calcitonin).

USES

Prevention/treatment of rickets or osteomalacia; management of hypocalcemia associated w/hypoparathyroidism.

ADMINISTRATION

ORAL:

- May take w/o regard to food.
- Swallow whole; do not crush/chew.

INDICATIONS/ROUTES/DOSAGE

CALCIFEDIOL:

Metabolic bone disease, hypocalcemia (dialysis pts):
Oral: Adults, elderly: Initially, 300–350 mcg/wk given daily or every other day. May increase at 4 wk intervals. ***Maintenance:*** 50–100 mcg/day or 100 and 200 mcg on alternate days.

CALCITRIOL:

Hypocalcemia (dialysis pts):
Oral: Adults, elderly: Initially, 0.25 mcg/day. May increase by 0.25 mcg/day q4–8wks. ***Range:*** 0.25–1 mcg/day.

Hypoparathyroidism:
Oral: Adults, elderly, children: Initially, 0.25 mcg/day. May increase at 2–4 wk intervals. ***Maintenance: Adults, children ≥6 yrs:*** 0.5–2 mcg/day. ***Children 1–5 yrs:*** 0.25–0.75 mcg/day.

CHOLECALCIFEROL:

Dietary supplement, deficiency:
Oral: Adults, elderly: 400–1,000 IU/day.

DIHYDROTACHYSTEROL:

Postop tetany, idiopathic tetany, hypoparathyroidism:
Oral: Adults, elderly: Initially, 0.8–2.4 mg/day for several days. ***Maintenance:*** 0.2–1 mg/day.

ERGOCALCIFEROL:

Familial hypophosphatemia:
Oral: Adults, elderly: 10,000–80,000 IU/day plus 1–2 g/day elemental phosphorus.

Hypoparathyroidism:
Oral: Adults, elderly: 50,000–200,000 IU/day plus 500 mg elemental calcium 6 times/day.

Refractory rickets:
Oral: Adults, elderly: 12,000–500,000 IU/day.

CONTRAINDICATIONS

Hypercalcemia, vitamin D toxicity, malabsorption syndrome, hypervitaminosis D, decreased renal function, abnormal sensitivity to vitamin D effects (those w/idiopathic hypercalcemia).

CAUTIONS

Those w/kidney stones, coronary disease, renal function impairment, arteriosclerosis, hypoparathyroidism, those w/tartrazine sensitivity.

INTERACTIONS

DRUG: *Aluminum-containing antacid (long-term use)* may increase aluminum concentration, aluminum bone toxicity. *Magnesium-containing antacids* may increase magnesium concentration. *Calcium-containing preparations, thiazide diuretics* may increase risk of hypercalcemia. **HERBAL:** None known. **FOOD:** None significant. **ALTERED LAB VALUES:** Alkaline phosphatase.

SIDE EFFECTS

None significant.

ADVERSE REACTIONS/TOXIC EFFECTS

Early signs of overdosage manifested as weakness, headache, somnolence, nausea, vomiting, dry mouth, constipation, muscle and bone pain, metallic taste sensation. Later signs of overdosage evidenced by polyuria, polydipsia, anorexia, weight loss, nocturia, photophobia, rhinorrhea, pruritus, disorientation, hallucinations, hyperthermia, hypertension, cardiac arrhythmias.

PATIENT CONSIDERATIONS

BASELINE ASSESSMENT

Therapy should begin at lowest possible dose.

INTERVENTION/EVALUATION

Monitor serum calcium and urinary calcium levels, serum phosphate, magnesium, creatinine, alkaline phosphatases and BUN determinations (therapeutic serum calcium level: 9–10 mg/dl). Estimate daily dietary calcium intake. Encourage adequate fluid intake.

PATIENT/FAMILY TEACHING

Foods rich in vitamin D include vegetable oils, vegetable shortening, margarine, leafy vegetables, milk, eggs, meats. Do not take mineral oil while on vitamin D therapy. If on chronic renal dialysis, do not take magnesium-containing antacids during vitamin D therapy. Drink plenty of liquids.

vitamin E

(Aquasol E)

CANADIAN AVAILABILITY
Aquasol E

PREGNANCY CATEGORY A
(C if used in doses above RDA)

CLASSIFICATION

Fat-soluble vitamin

AVAILABILITY (OTC)

Tablets: 200 IU, 400 IU. **Capsules:** 100 IU, 200 IU, 400 IU, 500 IU, 600 IU, 1,000 IU. **Drops:** 50 mg/ml.

PHARMACOKINETICS

Absorption: Variably absorbed

from GI tract (requires bile salts, dietary fat, normal pancreatic function). Primarily concentrated in adipose tissue. **Metabolism:** Metabolized in liver. **Excretion:** Primarily eliminated via biliary system.

ACTION/*THERAPEUTIC EFFECT*

Essential nutritional element. An antioxidant, *protects cells from oxidation. Protects red blood cells against hemolysis.* May act as cofactor in enzyme systems.

USES/*UNLABELED*

Treatment of vitamin E deficiency. *Decreases severity of tardive dyskinesia.*

ADMINISTRATION

ORAL:

- Do not crush or break tablets/capsules.
- May take w/o regard to food.

INDICATIONS/ROUTES/DOSAGE

Vitamin E deficiency:
Oral: Adults, elderly, children: Individualized.

CONTRAINDICATIONS

None significant.

CAUTIONS

None significant.

INTERACTIONS

DRUG: May impair hematologic response in pts w/iron deficiency anemia. ***Iron*** (large doses) may increase vitamin E requirements. ***Cholestyramine, colestipol, mineral oil*** may decrease absorption. **HERBAL:** None known. **FOOD:** None significant. **ALTERED LAB VALUES:** None significant.

SIDE EFFECTS

None significant.

ADVERSE/TOXIC EFFECTS

Chronic overdosage produces fatigue, weakness, nausea, headache, blurred vision, flatulence, diarrhea.

PATIENT CONSIDERATIONS

PATIENT/FAMILY TEACHING

Foods rich in vitamin E include vegetable oils, vegetable shortening, margarine, leafy vegetables, milk, eggs, meats.

vitamin K phytonadione (vitamin K_1)

fy-toe-na-**dye**-own
(AquaMEPHYTON, Konakion, Mephyton)

PREGNANCY CATEGORY C

CLASSIFICATION

Nutritional supplement, antidote (drug-induced hypoprothrombinemia), antihemorrhagic

AVAILABILITY (Rx)

Tablets: 5 mg. **Injection:** 2 mg/ml, 10 mg/ml.

PHARMACOKINETICS

Absorption: Readily absorbed from GI tract (duodenum), after IM, SubQ administration. **Metabolism:** Metabolized in liver. **Excretion:** Excreted in urine, eliminated via biliary system. ***Parenteral:*** Controls hemorrhage within 3–6

V

hrs, normal prothrombin time in 12–14 hrs. ***Oral:*** Effect in 6–10 hrs.

ACTION/*THERAPEUTIC EFFECT*

Necessary for hepatic formation of coagulation factors II, VII, IX, and X, *which are essential for normal clotting of blood.*

USES

Prevention, treatment of hemorrhagic states in neonates; antidote for hemorrhage induced by oral anticoagulants, hypoprothombinemic states due to vitamin K deficiency. Will not counteract anticoagulation effect of heparin.

ADMINISTRATION

ORAL:

- Scored tablets may be crushed.

SUBQ/IM:

- Inject into anterolateral aspect of thigh/deltoid region.

IV:

- **Note:** Restrict to emergency use only.
- May dilute w/preservative-free NaCl or 5% dextrose immediately before use. Do not use other diluents. Discard unused portions.
- Administer slow IV at rate of 1 mg/min.
- Monitor continuously for hypersensitivity, anaphylactic reaction during and immediately following IV administration.

INDICATIONS/ROUTES/DOSAGE

Anticoagulant-induced hypoprothrombinemia:
Oral/IM/SubQ/IV: Adults, elderly: 2.5–10 mg up to 25 mg. Subsequent dosage based on pt condition, prothrombin time.

Hemorrhagic disease of newborn:
IM: Infants: 0.5–1 mg in first hour of birth.

CONTRAINDICATIONS

Last few weeks of pregnancy or neonates.

CAUTIONS

Those w/asthma, impaired hepatic function.

INTERACTIONS

DRUG: ***Broad-spectrum antibiotics, high-dose salicylates*** may increase vitamin K requirements. May decrease effect of ***oral anticoagulants. Cholestyramine, colestipol, mineral oil, sucralfate*** may decrease absorption. **HERBAL:** None known. **FOOD:** None significant. **ALTERED LAB VALUES:** None significant.

SIDE EFFECTS

Note: Oral or SubQ administration less likely to produce side effects than IM or IV route. **OCCASIONAL:** Pain, soreness, swelling at IM injection site; repeated injections: pruritic erythema; flushed face, unusual taste.

ADVERSE REACTIONS/TOXIC EFFECTS

May produce hyperbilirubinemia in newborn (especially premature infants). Rarely, severe reaction occurs immediately following IV administration (cramp-like pain, chest pain, dyspnea, facial flushing, dizziness, rapid/weak pulse, rash, profuse sweating, hypotension; may progress to shock, cardiac arrest).

PATIENT CONSIDERATIONS

INTERVENTION/EVALUATION

Monitor prothrombin time routinely

in those taking anticoagulants. Assess skin for bruises, petechiae. Assess gums for gingival bleeding, erythema. Monitor urine output for hematuria. Assess hematocrit, platelet count, urine/stool culture for occult blood. Assess for decrease in B/P, increase in pulse rate, complaint of abdominal or back pain, severe headache (may be evidence of hemorrhage). Question for increase in amount of discharge during menses. Assess peripheral pulses, skin for bruises, petechiae. Check for excessive bleeding from minor cuts, scratches. Assess urine output for hematuria.

PATIENT/FAMILY TEACHING

Discomfort may occur w/parenteral administration. *Adults:* Use electric razor, soft toothbrush to prevent bleeding. Report any sign of red or dark urine, black or red stool, coffee-ground vomitus, red-speckled mucus from cough. Do not use any OTC medication w/o physician approval (may interfere w/platelet aggregation). Foods rich in vitamin K_1 include leafy green vegetables, meat, cow's milk, vegetable oil, egg yolks, tomatoes.

warfarin sodium

war-fair-in

(Coumadin, Panwarfin, Sofarin)

CANADIAN AVAILABILITY

Coumadin, Warfilone

PREGNANCY CATEGORY D

CLASSIFICATION

Anticoagulant

AVAILABILITY (Rx)

Tablets: 1 mg, 2 mg, 2.5 mg, 3 mg, 5 mg, 6 mg, 7.5 mg, 10 mg. **Injection:** 5 mg vials.

PHARMACODYNAMICS

	ONSET	PEAK	DURATION
Oral	—	1.5–3 days	2–5 days

PHARMACOKINETICS

Absorption: Well absorbed from GI tract. **Metabolism:** Metabolized in liver. **Excretion:** Primarily excreted in urine. **Half-life:** 1.5–2.5 days.

ACTION/*THERAPEUTIC EFFECT*

Interferes w/hepatic synthesis of vitamin K–dependent clotting factors, resulting in depletion of coagulation factors II, VII, IX, X. *Prevents further extension of formed existing clot; prevents new clot formation or secondary thromboembolic complications.*

USES/*UNLABELED*

Prophylaxis, treatment of venous thrombosis, pulmonary embolism. Treatment of thromboembolism associated w/chronic atrial fibrillation. Adjunct in treatment of coronary occlusion. Prophylaxis/treatment of thromboembolic complications associated w/cardiac valve replacement. Reduces risk of death, recurrent MI, stroke, embolization after myocardial infarction. *Prophylaxis vs. recurrence cerebral embolism, myocardial reinfarction, treatment adjunct in transient ischemic attacks.*

ADMINISTRATION

ORAL:

- Scored tablets may be crushed.
- May give w/o regard to food. If GI upset occurs, give w/food.

INDICATIONS/ROUTES/DOSAGE

Note: Dosage highly individualized, based on prothrombin time (PT), INR.

Oral/IV: Adults: Initially, 5–15 mg, then adjust dose. *Maintenance:* 2–10 mg/day based on prothrombin determinations.

Usual elderly dosage:
Oral/IV: 2–5 mg/day (maintenance).

CONTRAINDICATIONS

Bleeding abnormalities, hemophilia, thrombocytopenia, brain/spinal cord surgery, spinal anesthesia, eye surgery; bleeding from GI, respiratory, or GU tract; threatened abortion, aneurysm, ascorbic acid deficiency, acute nephritis, cerebrovascular hemorrhage, eclampsia, pre-eclampsia, blood dyscrasias, hypertension, severe hepatic disease, pericardial effusion, bacterial endocarditis, visceral carcinoma, following spinal puncture, IUD insertion, or any potential for bleeding abnormalities.

CAUTIONS

Factors increasing risk of hemorrhage, active tuberculosis, severe diabetes, GI tract ulcer disease, during menstruation, postpartum period.

INTERACTIONS

DRUG: *Increased effect with:* ***Acetaminophen (regular use), allopurinol, amiodarone, anabolic steroids, androgens, aspirin, cefamandole, cefoperazone, chloral hydrate, chloramphenicol, cimetidine, clofibrate, danazol, dextrothyroxine, diflunisal, disulfiram, erythromycin, fenoprofen, gemfibrozil, indomethacin, methimazole, metronidazole, oral hypoglycemics, phenytoin, plicamycin, PTU, quinidine, salicylates, sulfinpyrazone, sulfonamides, sulindac, troglitazone.*** *Decreased effect with:* ***Barbiturates, carbamazepine, cholestyramine, colestipol, estramustine, estrogens, griseofulvin, primidone, rifampin, vitamin K.*** **HERBAL:** Garlic, ginger, ginkgo, feverfew may increase effect; ginseng may decrease effect. **FOOD:** None significant. **ALTERED LAB VALUES:** None significant.

SIDE EFFECTS

OCCASIONAL: GI distress (nausea, anorexia, abdominal cramps, diarrhea). **RARE:** Hypersensitivity reaction (dermatitis, urticaria, especially in those sensitive to aspirin).

ADVERSE REACTIONS/TOXIC EFFECTS

Bleeding complications ranging from local ecchymoses to major hemorrhage. Drug should be discontinued immediately and vitamin K (phytonadione) administered. Mild hemorrhage: 2.5–10 mg PO/IM/IV. Severe hemorrhage: 10–15 mg IV and repeated q4h, as necessary. Hepatotoxicity, blood dyscrasias, necrosis, vasculitis, local thrombosis occur rarely.

PATIENT CONSIDERATIONS

BASELINE ASSESSMENT

Cross-check dose w/co-worker. Determine INR before administration and daily after therapy initiation. When stabilized, follow w/INR determination q4–6wks.

INTERVENTION/EVALUATION

Monitor INR reports diligently. Assess Hct, platelet count, urine/stool culture for occult blood, SGOT (AST), SGPT (ALT), regardless of route of administration. Be alert to complaints of abdominal back pain, severe headache (may be signs of hemorrhage). Decrease in B/P, increase in pulse rate may also be sign of hemorrhage. Question for increase in amount of discharge during menses. Assess area of thromboembolus for color, temperature. Assess peripheral pulses, skin for bruises, petechiae. Check for excessive bleeding from minor cuts, scratches. Assess gums for erythema, gingival bleeding. Assess urine output for hematuria.

PATIENT/FAMILY TEACHING

Take medication exactly as prescribed. Do not take or discontinue any other medication except on advice of physician. Avoid alcohol, salicylates, or drastic dietary changes. Do not change from one brand to another. Consult w/physician before surgery or dental work. Urine may become red orange. Notify physician if bleeding, bruising, red or brown urine, black stools occur. Use electric razor, soft toothbrush to prevent bleeding. Report any sign of red or dark urine, black or red stool, coffee-ground vomitus, red-speckled mucus from cough. Do not use any OTC medication w/o physician approval (may interfere w/platelet aggregation).

zafirlukast

zay-**fur**-leu-cast
(Accolate)

CANADIAN AVAILABILITY
Accolate

PREGNANCY CATEGORY B

CLASSIFICATION

Leukotriene receptor antagonist

AVAILABILITY (Rx)

Tablets: 10 mg, 20 mg

PHARMACOKINETICS

Absorption: Rapidly absorbed following oral administration (food reduces absorption). **Metabolism:** Extensively metabolized in liver. **Excretion:** Primarily excreted in feces. **Half-life:** 10 hrs.

ACTION/*THERAPEUTIC EFFECT*

Binds to leukotriene receptors. Inhibits bronchoconstriction due to sulfur dioxide, cold air, specific antigens (grass, cat dander, ragweed) *reducing airway edema, smooth muscle constriction, altered cellular activity associated w/inflammatory process.*

USES

Prophylaxis, chronic treatment of bronchial asthma.

ADMINISTRATION

ORAL:

- Give 1 hr before or 2 hrs after meals.
- Do not crush or break tablets.

INDICATIONS/ROUTES/DOSAGE

Bronchial asthma:
Oral: Adults, elderly, children >12 yrs: 20 mg twice daily. ***Children 7–12 yrs:*** 10 mg twice daily.

CONTRAINDICATIONS

Hypersensitivity to zafirlukast.

CAUTIONS

Impaired hepatic function.

INTERACTIONS

DRUG: *Aspirin* increases concentration. Coadministration of ***warfarin*** increases prothrombin time (PT). ***Erythromycin, terfenadine, theophylline*** decrease concentration.

HERBAL: None known. **FOOD:** None significant. **ALTERED LAB VALUES:** May increase SGPT (ALT).

SIDE EFFECTS

FREQUENT: Headache **(13%)**. **OCCASIONAL (<3%):** Nausea, diarrhea **(3%)**. **RARE:** Generalized pain, asthenia, myalgia, fever, dyspepsia, vomiting, dizziness.

ADVERSE REACTIONS/TOXIC EFFECTS

Coadministration of inhaled corticosteroids increase risks of upper respiratory infection.

PATIENT CONSIDERATIONS

Baseline Assessment

Obtain medication history. Assess liver function lab values.

Intervention/Evaluation

Monitor rate, depth, rhythm, type of respiration; quality and rate of pulse. Assess lung sounds for rhonchi, wheezing, rales. Observe lips, fingernails for blue or dusky color in light-skinned pts; gray in dark-skinned pts. Monitor liver function tests.

Patient/Family Teaching

Increase fluid intake (decreases lung secretion viscosity). Take as prescribed, even during symptom-free periods. Do not use for acute asthma episodes. Do not alter/stop other asthma medications. Nursing mothers should not breast-feed. Report nausea, jaundice, abdominal pain, flulike symptoms, or worsening of asthma.

---

zalcitabine

zal-**site**-ah-bean
(Hivid)

CANADIAN AVAILABILITY

Hivid

PREGNANCY CATEGORY C

CLASSIFICATION

Antiviral

AVAILABILITY (RX)

Tablets: 0.375 mg, 0.75 mg

PHARMACOKINETICS

Absorption: Readily absorbed from GI tract (food decreases absorption). **Metabolism:** Undergoes phosphorylation intracellularly to the active metabolite. **Excretion:** Primarily excreted in urine. Unknown whether removed by hemodialysis. **Half-life:** 1–3 hrs; metabolite: 2.6–10 hrs (increased in decreased renal function).

ACTION/*THERAPEUTIC EFFECT*

Intracellularly converted to active metabolite. Inhibits viral DNA synthesis, *preventing replication of human immunodeficiency virus (HIV-1).*

USES

Management of adult pts w/advanced HIV disease who are either intolerant to zidovudine or have disease progression while receiving zidovudine.

ADMINISTRATION

ORAL:

- Best taken on empty stomach (food decreases absorption).
- May take w/food to decrease GI distress.
- Space doses evenly around the clock.

INDICATIONS/ROUTES/DOSAGE

HIV infection:
Oral: Adults: 0.75 mg q8h (may be given w/zidovudine).

Dosage in renal impairment:
Based on creatinine clearance.

CREATININE CLEARANCE	DOSE
10–40 ml/min	0.75 mg q12h
<10 ml/min	0.75 mg q24h

CONTRAINDICATIONS

Hypersensitivity to zalcitabine or components of preparation. Pts w/moderate/severe peripheral neuropathy. Children <13 yrs (safety not known).

EXTREME CAUTION

Those w/low CD4 cell counts (risk of peripheral neuropathy is greater), preexisting neuropathy.

CAUTIONS

Pts w/history of pancreatitis or increased amylase, history of ethanol abuse. History of CHF, baseline cardiomyopathy, decreased renal function, liver disease.

INTERACTIONS

DRUG: Medications associated w/peripheral neuropathy may increase risk (e.g., ***cisplatin, disulfiram, phenytoin, vincristine***). Medications causing pancreatitis may increase risk (e.g., ***IV pentamidine***). **HERBAL:** None known. **FOOD:** None significant. **ALTERED LAB VALUES:** May increase SGOT (AST), SGPT (ALT), alkaline phosphatase, amylase, lipase, triglyceride concentrations. May cause leukopenia, neutropenia, eosinophilia, thrombocytopenia.

SIDE EFFECTS

OCCASIONAL (1–4%): Arthralgia (joint pain), fever, skin rash, muscle pain, ulcerations of mouth or throat, nausea, diarrhea, abdominal pain., headache. **RARE (<1%):** Liver toxicity, leukopenia, neutropenia (fever, sore throat), pancreatitis.

ADVERSE REACTIONS/TOXIC EFFECTS

Peripheral neuropathy occurs commonly (17–31%), characterized by numbness, tingling, burning, and pain of lower extremities. May be followed by sharp shooting pain and progress to severe continuous burning pain that may be irreversible if the drug is not discontinued in time. Pancreatitis occurs rarely.

PATIENT CONSIDERATIONS

BASELINE ASSESSMENT

Offer emotional support to pt and family. Monitor CBC, triglycerides, and serum amylase levels before and during therapy.

INTERVENTION/EVALUATION

Stop medication and notify physician immediately if signs and symptoms of peripheral neuropathy develop: numbness, tingling, burning, or shooting pains of extremities, loss of vibratory sense or ankle reflex. Although rare, be alert to impending potentially fatal pancreatitis: increasing serum amylase, rising triglycerides, nausea, vomiting, abdominal pain (withhold medication and notify physician). Assess for therapeutic response: weight gain, increased energy, decreased fatigue.

PATIENT/FAMILY TEACHING

Not a cure for HIV; may continue to contract illnesses associated w/advanced HIV infection. Does not preclude the need to continue practices to prevent transmission of HIV. Report promptly any signs and symptoms of peripheral neuropathy or pancreatitis (see Adverse Reactions/Toxic Effects). Women of childbearing age should use contraception.

zaleplon

(Sonata)
See Supplement

zanamivir

(Relenza)
See Supplement

zidovudine

zye-**dough**-view-deen
(AZT, Retrovir)

FIXED-COMBINATION(S)

W/lamivudine, an antiviral **(Combivir)**; w/abacavir, lamivudine, an antiviral **(Trizivir)**

CANADIAN AVAILABILITY

Apo-Zidovudine, Novo-AZT, Retrovir

PREGNANCY CATEGORY C

CLASSIFICATION

Antiviral

AVAILABILITY (Rx)

Capsules: 100 mg, 300 mg. **Syrup:** 50 mg/5 ml. **Injection:** 10 mg/ml.

PHARMACOKINETICS

Absorption: Rapidly, completely absorbed from GI tract. **Metabolism:** Undergoes first-pass metabolism in liver. Widely distributed. Crosses blood-brain barrier, CSF. **Excretion:** Primarily excreted in urine. Minimal removal by hemodialysis. **Half-life:** 0.8–1.2 hrs (increased in decreased renal function).

ACTION/*THERAPEUTIC EFFECT*

Interferes w/viral RNA-dependent DNA polymerase, an enzyme necessary for viral HIV replication, *slowing HIV replication, reducing progression of HIV infection.*

USES/*UNLABELED*

IV: Management of select adult pts w/symptomatic HIV infection (AIDS, advanced HIV disease). *Oral:* Management of pts w/HIV infection having evidence of impaired immunity. HIV-infected children (>3 mos) who have HIV-related symptoms or asymptomatic w/abnormal lab values showing significant HIV-related immunosuppression. Prevents maternal–fetal HIV transmission. *Prophylaxis in occupational exposure at risk of acquiring HIV.*

STORAGE/HANDLING

Keep capsules in cool, dry place. Protect from light. After dilution, IV solution stable for 24 hrs at room temperature; 48 hrs if refrigerated. Recommend use within 8 hrs if stored at room temperature; 24 hrs if refrigerated. Do not use if particulate matter present or discoloration occurs.

ADMINISTRATION

ORAL:

- Food, milk do not affect GI absorption.
- Space doses evenly around the clock.

IV:

- Must dilute before administration.
- Calculated dose added to D_5W to provide a concentration no greater than 4 mg/ml.
- Infuse over 1 hr.

INDICATIONS/ROUTES/DOSAGE

HIV infection:

Oral: Adults: 200 mg q8h or 300 mg q12h.

Usual dose for children:
Oral: Children >3 mos: Initially, 180 mg/mm^3 q6h up to 200 mg q6h.

Usual parenteral dosage:
IV: Adults, elderly: 1–2 mg/kg q4h around the clock.

Dosage adjustment:
Significant anemia w/o granulocytopenia may necessitate dose interruption until some evidence of bone marrow recovery observed.

CONTRAINDICATIONS

Life-threatening allergies to zidovudine or components of preparation.

CAUTIONS

Bone marrow compromise, renal and hepatic dysfunction, decreased hepatic blood flow.

INTERACTIONS

DRUG: *Bone marrow depressants, ganciclovir* may increase myelosuppression. *Clarithromycin* may decrease concentrations. *Probenecid* may increase concentrations, risk of toxicity. **HERBAL:** None known. **FOOD:** None significant. **ALTERED LAB VALUES:** May increase mean corpuscular volume.

SIDE EFFECTS

FREQUENT: Headache, nausea, malaise, anorexia, dizziness. **OCCASIONAL:** Myopathy, diarrhea, abdominal pain, asthenia (loss of strength and energy), rash. **RARE:** Insomnia, constipation, paresthesia, dyspnea.

ADVERSE REACTIONS/TOXIC EFFECTS

Anemia (occurring most commonly after 4–6 wks of therapy) and granulocytopenia, particularly significant in those w/pretherapy low baselines, occur rarely. Nausea, vomiting, neurotoxicity (ataxia, fatigue, lethargy, nystagmus), seizures.

PATIENT CONSIDERATIONS

Baseline Assessment

Question history of allergy to zidovudine or components of preparation. Avoid drugs that are nephrotoxic, cytotoxic, or myelosuppressive—may increase risk of toxicity. Obtain specimens for viral diagnostic tests before starting therapy (therapy may begin before results are obtained). Check hematology reports for accurate baseline.

Intervention/Evaluation

Monitor hematology reports for anemia and granulocytopenia; check for bleeding. Assess for headache, dizziness. Determine pattern of bowel activity. Evaluate skin for acne or rash. Be alert to development of opportunistic infections (e.g., fever, chills, cough, myalgia). Assess food tolerance. Monitor I&O, renal and liver function tests. Check for insomnia.

Patient/Family Teaching

Continue therapy for full length of treatment. Doses should be evenly spaced around the clock. Zidovudine does not cure AIDS or HIV disease, acts to reduce symptomatology and slow/arrest progress of disease. Avoid sexual activity; do not share needles (zidovudine does not prevent spread of infection). Do not take any medications w/o physician approval; even acetaminophen/aspirin may have serious consequence. Bleeding from gums, nose, or rectum may occur and should be reported to physician immediately. Blood counts

are essential because of bleeding potential. Dental work should be done before therapy or after blood counts return to normal (often weeks after therapy has stopped). Report any new symptoms to physician.

zileuton

zye-**lew**-ton
(Zyflo)

PREGNANCY CATEGORY C

CLASSIFICATION

Anti-asthmatic

AVAILABILITY (Rx)

Tablets: 600 mg

PHARMACODYNAMICS

	ONSET	PEAK	DURATION
Oral	—	2 hrs	—

PHARMACOKINETICS

Absorption: Rapidly, completely absorbed following oral administration. Highly bound to plasma proteins, especially albumin (93%). **Metabolism:** Metabolized in the liver. **Excretion:** Eliminated in the feces. Not removed by dialysis. **Half-life:** 2.5 hrs.

ACTION / *THERAPEUTIC EFFECT*

Inhibits the enzyme responsible for producing inflammatory response. Prevents formation of leukotrienes (leukotrienes induce bronchoconstricton response, enhances vascular permeability, stimulates mucus secretion) *Prevents airway edema, smooth muscle contraction, and the inflammatory process, relieving signs and symptoms of bronchial asthma.*

USES

Prophylaxis and chronic treatment of asthma. Not for use in reversal of bronchospasm in acute asthma attacks, status asthmaticus, exercise-induced bronchospasm.

ADMINISTRATION

ORAL:

- May give w/o regard to food.

INDICATIONS/ROUTES/DOSAGES

Bronchial asthma:

Oral: Adults, elderly: One 600 mg tablet 4 times/day. ***Total daily dosage:*** 2,400 mg.

CONTRAINDICATIONS

Active liver disease, impaired liver function.

CAUTIONS

History of hypersensitivity to zileuton, alcoholism.

INTERACTIONS

DRUG: May increase concentration/toxicity of ***astemizole, cisapride, cyclosporine, calcium channel blockers, (i.e., nifedipine), theophylline.*** Increases PT in those receiving ***warfarin.*** May increase effects of ***beta blockers (propranolol).*** May decrease effects of ***terfenadine.*** **HERBAL:** None known. **FOOD:** None significant. **ALTERED LAB VALUES:** May increase liver transaminase, SGOT (ALT).

SIDE EFFECTS

FREQUENT (25%): Headache. **OCCASIONAL (3–8%):** Dyspepsia, nausea, abdominal pain, asthenia (loss of strength), myalgia. **RARE (1%):** Conjunctivitis, constipation, dizziness, flatulence, insomnia.

ADVERSE REACTIONS/TOXIC EFFECTS

Liver dysfunction occurs rarely and may be manifested as right upper quadrant pain, nausea, fatigue, lethargy, pruritus, jaundice or flulike symptoms.

PATIENT CONSIDERATIONS

BASELINE ASSESSMENT

Obtain baseline hepatic transaminase level, ALT (SGOT) before therapy begins. Monitor transaminase levels routinely thereafter. Monitor ALT (SGOT) monthly for the first 3 mos and every 2–3 mos for the remainder of the first year and periodically thereafter during long-term therapy.

INTERVENTION/EVALUATION

Monitor rate, depth, rhythm, type of respirations, quality and rate of pulse. Assess lung sounds for rhonchi, wheezing, rales. Observe lips, fingernails for blue or dusky color in light-skinned pts, gray in dark-skinned pts. Monitor liver function test results.

PATIENT/FAMILY TEACHING

Increase fluid intake (decreases lung secretion viscosity). Take as prescribed, even during symptom-free periods as well as during worsening asthma. Do not alter/stop other asthma medications. Drug is not for the treatment of acute asthma attacks.

zinc acetate

(Galzin)

See Supplement

zolmitriptan

zoll-mih-**trip**-tan

(Zomig)

PREGNANCY CATEGORY C

CLASSIFICATION

Antimigraine

AVAILABILITY (Rx)

Tablets: 2.5 mg, 5 mg

PHARMACOKINETICS

Absorption: Rapidly but incompletely absorbed following oral administration. **Metabolism:** Undergoes first-pass metabolism in the liver to active metabolite. **Excretion:** Eliminated primarily in the urine (60%) with lesser amount excreted in the feces (30%). **Half-life:** 3 hrs.

ACTION/*THERAPEUTIC EFFECT*

Binds selectively to vascular receptors producing a vasoconstrictive effect on cranial blood vessels, *producing relief of migraine headache.*

USES

Treatment of acute migraine attack w/ or w/o aura.

ADMINISTRATION

- May give w/o regard to food.

INDICATIONS/ROUTES/DOSAGES

Migraine:

Oral: Adults >18 yrs: Initially, 2.5 mg or less. If headache returns, may repeat dose in 2 hrs. *Maximum:* 10 mg/24 hrs.

CONTRAINDICATIONS

Coronary artery disease, uncontrolled hypertension, ischemic heart disease (angina pectoris, history of

MI, silent ischemia), Prinzmetal's angina, concurrent use (or within 24 hrs) of ergotamine-containing preparations, concurrent (or within 2 wks) of MAO therapy, hemiplegic or basilar migraine, within 24 hrs of another serotonin receptor agonist, Wolff-Parkinson-White syndrome, arrhythmias associated with cardiac conduction pathways disorders.

CAUTIONS

Mild-to-moderate renal/hepatic impairment, pt profile suggesting cardiovascular risks, controlled hypertension, history of CVA.

INTERACTIONS

DRUG: *Ergotamine*-containing drugs may produce vasospastic reaction. ***MAO inhibitors*** may dramatically increase plasma concentration of zolmitriptan. Combined use of ***fluoxetine, fluvoxamine, paroxetine, sertraline*** may produce weakness, hyperreflexia, incoordination. ***Oral contraceptives*** reduce zolmitriptan's clearance, volume of distribution. **HERBAL:** None known. **FOOD:** None significant. **ALTERED LAB VALUES:** None significant.

SIDE EFFECTS

FREQUENT (6–8%): Dizziness, tingling, neck/throat/jaw pressure, somnolence. **OCCASIONAL (3–5%):** Sensation of warm/hot, weakness, chest pressure. **RARE (1–2%):** Sweating, myalgia, paresthesia.

ADVERSE REACTIONS/TOXIC EFFECTS

Cardiac events (ischemia, coronary artery vasospasm, MI), noncardiac vasospasm-related reactions (hemorrhage, stroke) occur rarely but particularly in those with hypertension, obesity, smokers, diabetes, strong family history of coronary artery disease, male > 40 yrs, postmenopausal women.

PATIENT CONSIDERATIONS

BASELINE ASSESSMENT

Question regarding history of peripheral vascular disease or coronary artery disease, renal/hepatic impairment, use of MAO inhibitors. Question pt regarding onset, location, and duration of migraine and possible precipitating symptoms.

INTERVENTIONS/EVALUATION

Monitor for evidence of dizziness. Monitor B/P, especially in those with liver impairment. Assess for relief of migraine headache and migraine potential for photophobia, phonophobia (sound sensitivity, light sensitivity, nausea, vomiting).

PATIENT/FAMILY TEACHING

Take a single dose as soon as symptoms of an actual migraine attack appear. Medication is intended to relieve migraine, not to prevent or reduce number of attacks. Lie down in quiet dark room for additional benefit after taking medication. Avoid tasks that require alertness, motor skills until response to drug is established. If heart throbbing, pain/tightness in chest or throat, or pain or weakness of extremities occurs, contact physician immediately.

zolpidem tartrate

zole-pih-dem
(Ambien)

PREGNANCY CATEGORY B

CLASSIFICATION

Sedative-hypnotic (**Schedule IV**)

AVAILABILITY (Rx)

Tablets: 5 mg, 10 mg

PHARMACOKINETICS

Absorption: Rapidly absorbed from GI tract. **Metabolism:** Metabolized in liver. **Excretion:** Primarily excreted in urine. **Half-life:** 1.4–4.5 hrs (increased in decreased liver function).

ACTION/*THERAPEUTIC EFFECT*

Enhances action of inhibitory neurotransmitter gamma-aminobutyric acid (GABA), *producing hypnotic effect due to CNS depression.* Interacts with GABA receptor, inducing sleep w/fewer nightly awakenings, improvement of sleep quality.

USES

Short-term treatment of insomnia. Reduces sleep-induction time, number of nocturnal awakenings; increases length of sleep, improvement of sleep quality.

ADMINISTRATION

ORAL:

- For faster sleep onset, do not give w/or immediately after a meal.

INDICATIONS/ROUTES/DOSAGE

Hypnotic:
Oral: Adults: 10 mg at bedtime. *Elderly, debilitated:* 5 mg at bedtime.

CONTRAINDICATIONS

None significant.

CAUTIONS

Impaired hepatic function.

INTERACTIONS

DRUG: Potentiated effects when used w/other *CNS depressants.* **HERBAL:** None known. **FOOD:** None significant. **ALTERED LAB VALUES:** None significant.

SIDE EFFECTS

OCCASIONAL: Headache (7%). **RARE (<2%):** Drowsiness, dizziness, nausea, diarrhea, muscle pain.

ADVERSE REACTIONS/TOXIC EFFECTS

Overdosage may produce severe ataxia (clumsiness, unsteadiness), slow heartbeat, diplopia, altered vision, severe drowsiness, nausea, vomiting, difficulty breathing, unconsciousness. Abrupt withdrawal of drug after long-term use may produce weakness, facial flushing, sweating, vomiting, tremor. Tolerance/dependence may occur w/prolonged use of high doses.

PATIENT CONSIDERATIONS

Baseline Assessment

Assess B/P, pulse, respirations. Raise bed rails, provide call light. Provide environment conducive to sleep (back rub, quiet environment, low lighting).

Intervention/Evaluation

Assess sleep pattern of pt. Evaluate for therapeutic response to insomnia: decrease in number of nocturnal awakenings, increase in length of sleep.

Patient/Family Teaching

Do not abruptly withdraw medication following long-term use. Avoid alcohol, tasks that require alertness, motor skills until response to drug is established. Tolerance/dependence may occur w/prolonged use of high doses.

Drug Classification Contents

anesthetics: general

ACTION

Produces loss of consciousness and loss of response to all sensations including pain, touch, taste, temperature. General anesthetics can be classified as inhalation anesthetics and IV anesthetics. Inhalation anesthetics are further classified as gases and volatile liquids. IV anesthetics can be used alone or to supplement inhalation anesthetics. They decrease dosage of inhalation anesthetics and produce effects not achieved by inhalation anesthetics.

Ideally, an inhalation general anesthetic would produce unconsciousness, analgesia, muscle relaxation, and amnesia w/o side effects. Because no agent possesses all of these properties, medications are combined to achieve what inhalation anesthetics can't do alone and to reduce side effects. These medications include short-acting barbiturates (induce anesthesia), neuromuscular blocking agents (cause muscle relaxation), opioid analgesics, and nitrous oxide (provides analgesia).

Adjuncts to anesthesia are combined to enhance beneficial effects of inhalation anesthetics, reduce side effects and include:

Benzodiazepines: Reduce anxiety, enhance amnesia.
Barbiturates: Decrease anxiety, induce sedation.
Opioids: Relieve pain both preop and postop.
Anticholinergics: Decrease risk of bradycardia.
Antiemetics: Reduce nausea, vomiting.
Neuromuscular blocking agents: Cause skeletal muscle relaxation.

SIDE EFFECTS

Inhalation anesthetics: Respiratory cardiac depression (most pts require mechanical ventilation support). May increase sensitivity of heart to catecholamine stimulation (may cause dysrhythmias). Malignant hyperthermia (muscle rigidity, profound temperature increase). Aspiration of gastric fluid (may cause bronchospasm, pneumonia—prevented by use of endotracheal tube).

INTERACTIONS

Opioid analgesics may decrease the dose of inhalation anesthetic. CNS depressants may cause additive CNS depression. CNS stimulants may increase the dose of inhalation anesthetic.

PATIENT CONSIDERATIONS

Preop:

BASELINE ASSESSMENT: Obtain thorough history of drug use (drugs affecting cardiovascular, respiratory system may affect response to

anesthetics; accurate drug history may decrease risk of possible drug interactions), history of any disease of cardiovascular, respiratory system. Obtain baseline B/P, heart rate, respiratory rate. Ensure preop medications are administered 30–60 min before surgery.

Postop:
BASELINE ASSESSMENT: Obtain information about all medications pt received during surgery (anesthetics/adjunctive medication), which assists in anticipated time of emergence from anesthesia. EVALUATION/INTERVENTION: Position pt on side or w/head to side (decreases risk of aspiration). Monitor vital signs (B/P, pulse rate, respiratory rate) until recovery complete. Observe for cardiovascular, respiratory distress. Employ side rails or straps to prevent accidental falls. Assist in ambulation. Monitor bowel function, urine output. Assess need for opioid analgesics in management of postop pain. Assistance w/ambulation; another driver necessary upon discharge.

ANESTHETICS: GENERAL

Generic Name	Brand Name(s)	Class	Type
desflurane	Suprane	Inhalation anesthetic	Volatile liquid
enflurane	Ethrane	Inhalation anesthetic	Volatile liquid
etomidate	Amidate	IV anesthetic	Hypnotic
halothane	Fluothane	Inhalation anesthetic	Volatile liquid
isoflurane	Forane	Inhalation anesthetic	Volatile liquid
ketamine	Ketalar	IV anesthetic	Miscellaneous
methohexital	Brevital	IV anesthetic	Barbiturate
methoxyflurane	Penthrane	Inhalation anesthetic	Volatile liquid
midazolam	Versed	IV anesthetic	Benzodiazepine
nitrous oxide	—	Inhalation anesthetic	Gas
propofol	Diprivan	IV anesthetic	Sedative-hypnotic
thiamylal	Surital	IV anesthetic	Barbiturate
thiopental	Pentothal	IV anesthetic	Barbiturate

anesthetics: local

ACTION

Blocks initiation and conduction of nerve impulses (decreases membrane permeability to sodium) that inhibit depolarization and action potential w/conduction blockade (occurs only in neurons located near site of administration). May also cause CNS depression and/or stimulation. May depress cardiac conduction, excitability and cause peripheral vasodilation. Does not cause generalized depression.

Local anesthetics can be classified based on their structure: esters or amides. Amide type have a lower incidence of allergic reaction and are metabolized by liver enzymes; esters are metabolized by enzymes in plasma.

USES

May be given topically (surface anesthesia) and by injection (local infiltration, peripheral nerve block [axillary], IV regional [Bier block], epidural, and spinal anesthesia).

Topical:
Applied to skin to relieve pain, itching, soreness to mucous membranes of nose, mouth, pharynx, larynx, trachea, bronchi, vagina, urethra.

Injection:
Local infiltration: Inject directly into tissue to be incised or stimulated mechanically.
Peripheral nerve block (axillary): Inject into/near nerves supplying surgical field, but at a site distant from surgical field.

LOCAL ANESTHETICS

Generic Name	Brand Name(s)	Type	Uses	Onset	Peak	Duration
benzocaine	Many	Ester	Top: skin, mucous membrane	—	1 min	30–60 min
bupivacaine	Marcaine Sensorcaine	Amide	Infiltration Epidural Nerve block Spinal	5 min	—	2–4 hrs
butamben	Butesin	Ester	Top: skin	—	—	—
chloroprocaine	Nesacaine	Ester	Nerve block Epidural	6–12 min	—	15–30 min
cocaine		Ester	Top: mucous membrane	—	2–5 min	30–120 min
dibucaine	Nupercainal	Amide	Top: skin	—	<15 min	3–4 hrs
lidocaine	Xylocaine	Amide	Top: skin, mucous membrane Infiltration Nerve block	—	2–5 min	30–60 min
			IV regional Epidural Spinal	0.5–1 min	—	30–60 min
mepivacaine	Carbocaine Polocaine	Amide Infiltration	Nerve block Epidural	3–5 min	—	45–90 min
procaine	Novocain	Ester	Infiltration Nerve block	2–5 min	—	15–30 min
ropivacaine	Naropin	Amide	Epidural Nerve block Infiltration	10 min	—	2–4 hrs
tetracaine	Pontocaine	Ester	Top: skin	—	3–8 min	30–60 min
			Spinal	≤15 min	—	2–3 hrs

Top = topical.

IV regional (Bier block): Used to anesthetize limbs, injecting into distal vein of area or leg. Before administration, blood is removed from vein (apply Esmarch bandage) and tourniquet applied to limb, preventing anesthetic from entering general circulation. After administration, anesthetic diffuses from vasculature, becoming evenly distributed to all areas of occluded limb. After loosening of tourniquet, about 15–30% anesthetic is released into systemic circulation.

Epidural: Inject into epidural space (within spinal column outside dura mater). Diffusion across dura into subarachnoid space produces anesthesia of nerve roots and spinal cord.

Spinal: Inject into subarachnoid space (lumbar region below the termination of the cord).

PRECAUTIONS

CONTRAINDICATIONS: Hypersensitivity to local anesthetics. Pts w/complete heart block, severe hemorrhage, severe hypotension, shock. Local infection at site of lumbar puncture, septicemia. **CAUTIONS:** Pts w/cardiovascular function impairment, drug sensitivity. Inflammation and/or infection in region of injection. CNS disease, coagulation defects caused by anticoagulant therapy or hematologic disorders. With preparations containing a vasoconstrictor; pts w/cardiac disease, arrhythmias, hyperthyroidism, hypertension, or peripheral vascular disease.

INTERACTIONS

CNS depression–producing medications may cause additive depressant effect. Use vasoconstrictors (e.g., epinephrine) cautiously (if at all) when anesthetizing areas w/end arteries (e.g., toes, fingers).

SIDE EFFECTS

Allergic reactions ranging from dermatitis to anaphylaxis are more likely w/ester type. No cross-sensitivity between esters and amides. Cardiac depression (bradycardia, AV heart block, decreased contractility, and possibly cardiac arrest), peripheral vasodilation (may cause hypotension) can occur. CNS toxicity (stimulation followed by depression). Stimulation may cause convulsions. Depression may result in drowsiness, unconsciousness, even respiratory depression.

PATIENT CONSIDERATIONS

BASELINE ASSESSMENT: Resuscitative medication and equipment should be readily available. Inform pts they may experience temporary loss of sensation. INTERVENTION/EVALUATION: Monitor cardiovascular status, respirations, and state of consciousness closely during and after drug is administered. If ECG shows arrhythmias, prolongation of PR interval, QRS complex, inform physician immediately. Assess pulse for irregular rate, strength/weakness, bradycardia. Assess B/P for evidence of hypotension. PATIENT/FAMILY TEACHING: If medication used for dental procedure, avoid chewing solid foods or testing anesthetized site by biting or probing. Caution against activities that might cause unintentional harm.

angiotensin-converting enzyme (ACE) inhibitors

ACTION

Suppresses renin-angiotensin-aldosterone system (prevents conversion of angiotensin I to angiotensin II, a potent vasoconstrictor).

Hypertension: Inhibits activity of angiotensin I converting enzyme. Decreases conversion of angiotensin I to angiotensin II, a potent vasoconstrictor. Results in increase in plasma renin activity and decreased aldosterone secretion. Reduces peripheral vascular resistance.

CHF: Decreases peripheral vascular resistance (afterload), pulmonary capillary wedge pressure (preload), pulmonary vascular resistance. Increases cardiac output, exercise tolerance.

USES

Treatment of hypertension alone or in combination w/other antihypertensives. Adjunctive therapy for CHF (in combination w/cardiac glycosides, diuretics).

PRECAUTIONS

CONTRAINDICATIONS: History of angioedema w/previous treatment w/ACE inhibitors. **CAUTIONS:** Renal impairment, those w/sodium depletion or on diuretic therapy, dialysis, hypovolemia, coronary or cerebrovascular insufficiency. Safety in pregnancy/lactation not established.

INTERACTIONS

May increase lithium concentrations, toxicity. Hyperkalemia may occur w/potassium-sparing diuretics, potassium supplements, or potassium-containing salt substitutes. Alcohol, diuretics, hypotensive agents may increase antihypertensive effect. NSAIDs, aspirin may decrease hypotensive effect.

SIDE EFFECTS

Rash and/or urticaria, change or decrease in sense of taste, orthostatic hypotension during initial therapy. Urinary frequency. Cough, proteinuria (mostly occurs in those w/history of renal disease), dry mouth, GI distress, headache, dizziness.

TOXIC EFFECTS/ADVERSE REACTIONS

Excessive hypotension ("first-dose syncope") may occur in those w/CHF, severely salt/volume depleted. Angioedema (swelling of face/lips), hyperkalemia occur rarely. Agranulocytosis, neutropenia may be noted in those w/impaired renal function or collagen vascular disease (systemic lupus erythematosus, scleroderma). Nephrotic syndrome may be noted in those w/history of renal disease.

PATIENT CONSIDERATIONS

GENERAL: Use cardiac monitor for IV administration and preferably for initiation of oral therapy. BASELINE ASSESSMENT: Initial B/P, apical pulse. INTERVENTION/EVALUATION: Monitor B/P and apical pulse before giving drug and p.r.n.; notify physician before administration if B/P or pulse is not within agreed parameters. If excessive hypotension, place pt in supine position w/legs elevated. Assess extremities for edema; weigh daily; check lungs for rales. Monitor I&O. Check lab results, esp. electrolytes and drug levels. Monitor frequency, consistency of stools; prevent constipation. PATIENT/FAMILY TEACHING: Teach how to take B/P, pulse correctly. Change position slowly to prevent orthostatic hypotension. Do not take OTC cold preparations, nasal decongestants w/o consulting physician. Restrict sodium and alcohol as ordered. Do not skip dose or stop taking medication; rebound hypertension may occur.

ACE INHIBITORS

Generic Name	Brand Name(s)	Use	Decrease B/P: Onset (hrs)	Decrease B/P: Duration (hrs)	Rte Adm	Dosage Range (mg/day)
benazepril	Lotensin	Hypertension	1	24	PO	20–80
captopril	Capoten	Hypertension	0.25	(dose	PO	50–450
		CHF		related)		12.5–450
enalapril	Vasotec	Hypertension	1	24	PO	10–40
		CHF			IV	5–20
					PO	5–20
fosinopril	Monopril	Hypertension	1	24	PO	20–80
		CHF			PO	5–40
lisinopril	Prinivil	Hypertension	1	24	PO	20–40
	Zestril	CHF			PO	5–20
moexipril	Univasc	Hypertension	1	24	PO	7.5–30
quinapril	Accupril	Hypertension	1	24	PO	20–80
		CHF				
ramipril	Altace	Hypertension	1	24	PO	2.5–20
		CHF			PO	1.25–5
trandolapril	Mavik	Hypertension	1	24	PO	1–4

antacids

ACTION

Act primarily in stomach to neutralize gastric acid (increase pH). The ability to increase pH depends on dose, dosage form used, presence or absence of food in stomach, and acid neutralizing capacity (ANC). ANC is the number of mEq of hydrochloric acid that can be neutralized by a particular weight or volume of antacid. There are 4 major groups of antacids: (1) aluminum compounds, (2) magnesium compounds, (3) sodium compounds, and (4) calcium compounds.

USES

Symptomatic relief of heartburn, acid indigestion; treatment of peptic ulcer disease, prevention of aspiration pneumonia before anesthesia, prophylaxis vs. stress ulceration; symptomatic relief of gastroesophageal reflux disease (GERD), gastritis, hiatal hernia. In addition, aluminum carbonate used for hyperphosphatemia; calcium carbonate for calcium deficiency states; and magnesium oxide for magnesium deficiency states.

PRECAUTIONS

CONTRAINDICATIONS: Sensitivity to any components, first trimester of pregnancy, renal dysfunction, young children. **CAUTIONS:** Specific selection of antacid should consider preexisting bowel status, components (e.g., sodium) in relation to other medical conditions. Administer with care in elderly.

INTERACTIONS

Antacids may interact with medication by increasing gastric pH (affects absorption), absorbing or binding to medications, or increasing urinary pH (affects rate of elimination). Interactions may be prevented by avoiding concurrent use and taking antacids 2 hrs before or after ingestion of other medications.

SIDE EFFECTS

Diarrhea or constipation, depending on specific drug administered.

TOXIC EFFECTS/ADVERSE REACTIONS

Aluminum compounds in large amounts may cause severe constipation, hypophosphatemia, and osteomalacia. Magnesium compounds may cause hypermagnesemia and profound diarrhea. Calcium antacids may cause acid rebound, alkalosis, and renal calculi. W/sodium compounds, risk of systemic alkalosis, sodium overload with retention, and rebound hypersecretion.

PATIENT CONSIDERATIONS

GENERAL: Avoid sodium-based compounds for pts on low sodium diets; calcium or magnesium compounds for pts with renal impairment. Do not give other oral medication within 1–2 hrs of antacid administration. INTERVENTION/EVALUATION: Monitor stools for diarrhea or constipation. Assess for relief of gastric distress. PATIENT/FAMILY TEACHING: For best results, take 1–3 hrs after meals. Chewable tablets should be chewed thoroughly before swallowing (may be followed by water or milk). Maintain adequate fluid intake. Eat small, frequent meals free of coffee and other caffeine products. Avoid alcohol.

ANTACIDS

Brand Name	Active Ingredient: $Al(OH)_2$ (mg)	$Mg(OH)_2$ (mg)	$CaCO_3$ (mg)	Other	Sodium Content (mEq/5 ml)	ANC
Amphojel	320	—	—	—	<2.3	10
Alternagel	600	—	—	Simethicone	<2.5	16
Dialume	500	—	—	—	<1.2	10
Gelusil	200	200	—	Simethicone	0.7	12
Maalox	225	200	—	—	1.4	13.3
Maalox TC	600	300	—	Sorbitol	0.8	27.2
Mag-Ox 400	—	400	—	—	—	—
MOM	—	390	—	—	0.12	14
Mylanta	200	200	—	Simethicone	0.68	12.7
Mylanta II	400	400	—	Simethicone	1.14	25.4
Riopan Plus	—	—	—	Magaldrate Simethicone	<0.1	15
Tums	—	—	500	—	<2.0	10

ANC = acid neutralizing capacity.

antianxiety

ACTION

Benzodiazepines are the largest and most frequently prescribed group of antianxiety agents. Exact mechanism unknown; may increase the inhibiting effect of gamma-aminobutyric acid (GABA) (inhibiting nerve impulse transmission) as well as other inhibitory transmitters by binding to specific benzodiazepine receptors in various areas of the CNS.

USES

Treatment of anxiety. Additionally, some benzodiazepines are used as hypnotics, anticonvulsants to prevent delirium tremors during alcohol withdrawal and as adjunctive therapy for relaxation of skeletal muscle spasms. Midazolam, a short-acting injectable form, is used for preop sedation, relieving anxiety for short diagnostic endoscopic procedures.

PRECAUTIONS

CONTRAINDICATIONS: Hypersensitivity, renal or hepatic dysfunction, CNS depression, history of drug abuse, pregnancy, glaucoma, lactation, young children, within 14 days of MAO inhibitors, myasthenia gravis. **CAUTION:** Elderly or debilitated, pts w/COPD. Drugs should be withdrawn slowly.

INTERACTIONS

CNS depressants (e.g., alcohol, barbiturates, narcotics) may increase CNS effects of benzodiazepines (e.g., sedation).

ANTIANXIETY

GENERIC NAME	BRAND NAME(S)	USES	DOSAGE RANGE (MG/DAY)
alprazolam	Xanax	Anxiety Panic disorder	PO: 0.75–4
chlordiazepoxide	Librium Libritabs	Anxiety Alcohol withdrawal Preop	PO: 15–100
clonazepam	Klonopin	Anticonvulsant	PO: 1.5–20
clorazepate	Tranxene	Anxiety Alcohol withdrawal	PO: 15–60
diazepam	Valium	Anxiety Alcohol withdrawal Anticonvulsant Muscle relaxant	PO: 4–40
lorazepam	Ativan	Anxiety Preanesthetic	PO: 2–4
oxazepam	Serax	Anxiety	PO: 30–120

Dosage: oral.

SIDE EFFECTS

Drowsiness is the most common side effect; usually disappears w/continued use. Dizziness, hypotension occur frequently.

TOXIC EFFECTS/ADVERSE REACTIONS

Incidence of toxicity is very low when antianxiety drugs are taken alone. Confusion, hypersensitivity reactions, headache, stupor, paradoxical excitement, nausea and vomiting, blood dyscrasias, jaundice (hepatic dysfunction) are rare effects. These vary according to individual drug. IV administration may cause respiratory depression, apnea.

PATIENT CONSIDERATIONS

GENERAL: Provide restful environment and measures for comfort. Comply w/federal narcotic laws regarding Schedule IV drugs. Consider potential for abuse/dependence. For IV administration, have respiratory equipment available; keep pt recumbent. Most antianxiety drugs should not be mixed w/other drugs in a syringe. INTERVENTION/EVALUATION: Monitor B/P. Assess for therapeutic response (according to reason for use, e.g., seizure activity, anxiety, alcohol withdrawal) or paradoxical reaction. Take safety precautions for drowsiness, dizziness. PATIENT/FAMILY TEACHING: Avoid smoking; may interfere w/drug action. Do not drive or perform tasks requiring mental acuity until response to medication is controlled. Consult physician before taking other medications. Do not take alcohol. Medication must not be stopped abruptly. Inform other physicians, dentist of drug therapy.

antiarrhythmics

ACTION

Antiarrhythmics are classified according to electrophysiologic effects they produce and/or their presumed mechanism of action.

Class IA: Inhibit inward sodium current, depress phase 0 depolarization, slow conduction velocity in myocardial Purkinje fibers.

Class IB: Inhibit inward sodium current, slight change phase 0 depolarization/slows conduction velocity in Purkinje system. Effects markedly intensified when membrane depolarized or frequency of excitation is increased. Hastens repolarization.

Class IC: Marked depression phase 0, slowing impulse conduction, suppressing inward sodium current and spontaneous ventricular premature complexes.

Class II: Depress phase IV depolarization; block excessive sympathetic activity.

Class III: Prolong action potential duration and refractoriness in Purkinje and ventricular muscle fibers.

Class IV: Depress Ca^{+2}-dependent action potentials, slow conduction in AV node.

Digoxin: Decreases maximal diastolic potential and action potential duration.

Adenosine: Slows conduction time through AV node; may interrupt reentry pathways through AV node.

USES

Prevention and treatment of cardiac arrhythmias, such as premature ventricular contractions, ventricular tachycardia, premature atrial contractions, paroxysmal atrial tachycardia, atrial fibrillation and flutter.

PRECAUTIONS

CONTRAINDICATIONS: Hypersensitivity, pregnancy, lactation, children, severe bradycardia, second- or third-degree AV block, severe CHF, aortic stenosis, hypotension, cardiogenic shock, hepatic or renal dysfunction. **CAUTIONS:** Elderly generally require lowered dosage. Administer w/caution to pts w/diabetes mellitus, acute myocardial infarctions, and liver dysfunction. Have emergency cart readily available when administering agents through IV.

INTERACTIONS

Interactions are specific to each agent, which should be noted before administration. Refer to individual monographs.

SIDE EFFECTS

Hypotension, bradycardia, drowsiness, lightheadedness. Other side effects are specific to individual drug.

ANTIARRHYTHMICS

GENERIC NAME	BRAND NAME(S)	CLASS	ONSET	DURATION	DOSAGE RANGE
acebutolol*	Sectral	II	—	24–30 hrs	600–1,200 mg/day
adenosine	Adenocard		34 sec	1–2 min	IV: 6 mg, MR w/12 mg at 1–2 min intervals
amiodarone	Cordarone	III	1–3 wks	—	Initial: 800–1,600 mg/day for 1–3 wks Maintenance: 600–800 mg/day
bretylium	Bretylol	III	—	6–8 hrs	IV: 1–2 mg/min
digoxin*	Lanoxin		0.5–2 hrs	>24 hrs	0.125–0.375 mg/day
disopyramide	Norpace Norpace SR	IA	0.5 hr	6–7 hrs	400–800 mg/day
esmolol*	Brevibloc	II	<5 min	Short	IV: 50–200 mcg/kg/min
flecainide	Tambocor	IC	—	—	200–400 mg/day
ibutilide	Corvert	III	—	—	IV: >60 kg: 1 mg over 10 min <60 kg: 0.01 mg/kg
lidocaine	Xylocaine	IB	—	0.25 hr	IV: 50–100 mg bolus, 1–4 mg/min infusion
mexiletine	Mexitil	IB	0.5–2 hrs	8–12 hrs	600–1,200 mg/day
moricizine	Ethmozine	IA	2 hrs	10–24 hrs	600–900 mg/day
phenytoin*	Dilantin	1B	0.5–1 hr	>24 hrs	IV: 100–1,000 mg PO: 100 mg q6–12h
procainamide	Pronestyl Procan SR	IA	0.5 hr	>3 hrs 6 hrs	PO: 250–500 mg q3h SR: 250–750 mg q6h
propafenone	Rhythmol	IC	—	—	450–900 mg/day
propranolol*	Inderal	II	0.5 hr	3–5 hrs	10–30 mg 3–4×/day
quinidine	Cardioquin Quinaglute Quinidex	IA	0.5 hr —	6–8 hrs 8–12 hrs	PO: 200–600 mg q2–4h SR: 300–600 mg q8h
sotalol*	Betapace	III	—	—	160–640 mg/day
tocainide	Tonocard	IB	1–2 hrs	8–12 hrs	1,200–1,800 mg/day
verapamil*	Calan Isoptin	IV	0.5 hr	6 hrs	IV: 5–10 mg

*These agents are also discussed w/other classifications.

TOXIC EFFECTS/ADVERSE REACTIONS

Visual disturbances, tinnitus or difficulty hearing, vomiting, constipation or diarrhea, headache, confusion, diaphoresis, anginal attack, rapid rhythm, cardiac arrest. Other signs specific to each drug.

PATIENT CONSIDERATIONS

GENERAL: Use cardiac monitor for IV administration and preferably for initiation of oral therapy. BASELINE ASSESSMENT: Initial B/P, apical pulse. INTERVENTION/EVALUATION: Monitor B/P and apical pulse before giving drug and p.r.n.; notify physician before administration if B/P or pulse is not within agreed parameters. Assess extremities for edema; weigh daily; check lungs for rales. Monitor I&O. Check lab results, esp. electrolytes and drug levels. Monitor frequency, consistency of stools; prevent constipation. PATIENT/FAMILY TEACHING: Teach how to take pulse correctly. Change position slowly to prevent ortho-

static hypotension. Do not take other medications, including OTC, w/o consulting physician. Restrict sodium and alcohol as ordered.

antibiotics

ACTION

Antibiotics (antimicrobial agents) are natural or synthetic compounds that have the ability to kill or suppress the growth of microorganisms. Narrow-spectrum agents are effective against few microorganisms, whereas broad-spectrum agents are effective against a wide variety. Antimicrobial agents may also be classified based on their mechanism of action.

- Agents that inhibit cell wall synthesis or activate enzymes that disrupt cell wall, causing a weakening in the cell wall, cell lysis, and death. Includes penicillins, cephalosporins, vancomycin, and imidazole antifungal agents.
- Agents that act directly on cell wall, affecting permeability of cell membranes, causing leakage of intracellular substances. Includes antifungal agents amphotericin and nystatin, polymixin, and colistin.
- Agents that bind to ribosomal subunits, altering protein synthesis and eventually causing cell death. Includes aminoglycosides.
- Agents that affect bacterial ribosome function, altering protein synthesis and causing slow microbial growth. Does not cause cell death. Includes chloramphenicol, clindamycin, erythromycin, tetracyclines.
- Agents that inhibit nucleic acid metabolism by binding to nucleic acid or interacting with enzymes necessary for nucleic acid synthesis. Inhibits DNA or RNA synthesis. Includes rifampin, metronidazole, quinolones (e.g., ciprofloxacin).
- Agents that inhibit specific metabolic steps necessary for microorganisms, causing a decrease in essential cell components or synthesis of nonfunctional analogues of normal metabolites. Includes trimethoprim and sulfonamides.
- Agents that inhibit viral DNA synthesis by binding to viral enzymes necessary for DNA synthesis, preventing viral replication. Includes acyclovir, vidarabine.

SELECTION OF ANTIMICROBIAL AGENTS

Goal of therapy is to produce a favorable therapeutic result by achieving antimicrobial action at the site of infection sufficient to inhibit the growth of the microorganism. The agent selected should be the most active against the most likely infecting organism, least likely to cause toxicity or allergic reaction. Factors to consider in selection of an antimicrobial agent include:

- Sensitivity pattern of the infecting microorganism.
- Location and severity of infection (may determine the route of administration).

- Pt's ability to eliminate the drug (status of renal and liver function).
- Pt's defense mechanisms (includes both cellular and humoral immunity).
- Pt's age, pregnancy, genetic factors, allergy, disorder of CNS, preexisting medical problems.

USES

Treatment of wide range of gram-positive or gram-negative bacterial infections; suppression of intestinal flora before surgery; control of acne; prophylactically to prevent rheumatic fever; prophylactically in high-risk situations (e.g., some surgical procedures or medical states) to prevent bacterial infection.

PRECAUTIONS

CONTRAINDICATIONS: Hypersensitivity to prescribed antibiotics, others in its family, or components of the drug. Some antibiotics are contraindicated in infants and children (e.g., tetracyclines, quinolones). **EXTREME CAUTION:** Pregnancy and lactation (avoid unless benefits clearly outweigh risks). **CAUTIONS:** Renal or hepatic dysfunction. Elderly and very young may be more sensitive to effects of these drugs and may require adjusted dosage. Extra care w/gastrointestinal diseases and bleeding disorders.

INTERACTIONS

Concurrent use w/other antibiotics or drugs that add to or potentiate toxic effects is to be avoided. Alcohol should not be taken w/antibiotics; several may interact w/alcohol to produce a disulfiram reaction. Antacids should be administered 2 hrs before or after oral antibiotics to prevent interference w/absorption. Refer to specific classification pages or individual monographs.

SIDE EFFECTS

Side effects most commonly associated w/antibiotics are anorexia, nausea, vomiting, and diarrhea. Some, such as tetracyclines, produce photosensitivity. Refer to individual monographs.

TOXIC EFFECTS/ADVERSE REACTIONS

Skin rash, seen most often w/penicillins and cephalosporins, is a sign of hypersensitivity. Sensitivity reactions may range from mild rash to anaphylaxis. Superinfections may result from alteration of bacterial environment. Ototoxicity and nephrotoxicity are potential adverse reactions of a number of antibiotics, esp. the aminoglycosides. Tetracyclines combine w/calcium in forming teeth and may produce discoloration. Severe diarrhea, antibiotic-associated colitis have occurred from several of the antimicrobials (clindamycin has a particular risk for this reaction).

PATIENT CONSIDERATIONS

GENERAL: Administer drugs on schedule to maintain blood levels. Initiate IV solutions slowly w/close observation for sensitivity re-

sponse. BASELINE ASSESSMENT: Question for history of previous drug reaction. Culture/sensitivity must be done before first dose (may give before results are obtained). Assess WBC results, temperature, pulse, respiration. INTERVENTION/EVALUATION: Monitor lab results, particularly WBC and culture/sensitivity reports. Assess for adverse reactions. PATIENT/FAMILY TEACHING: Space doses evenly. Continue therapy for full duration. Avoid alcohol, antacids, or other medication w/o consulting physician. Notify physician of diarrhea, rash, or other new symptom.

antibiotic: aminoglycosides

ACTION

Bactericidal. Transported across bacterial cell membrane, irreversibly binds to specific receptor proteins of bacterial ribosomes. Interferes w/protein synthesis, preventing cell reproduction and eventually causing cell death.

USES

Treatment of serious infections when other, less toxic agents are not effective, are contraindicated, or require adjunctive therapy (e.g., w/penicillins or cephalosporins). Used primarily in the treatment of infections caused by gram-negative microorganisms, such as those caused by *Proteus, Klebsiella, Pseudomonas, Escherichia coli, Serratia,* and *Enterobacter.* Inactive against most gram-positive microorganisms. Not well absorbed systemically from GI tract (must be administered parenterally for systemic infections). Oral agents are given to suppress intestinal bacteria.

PRECAUTIONS

CONTRAINDICATIONS: Hypersensitivity to any of the aminoglycosides; pregnancy/lactation. Not to be given orally to pts w/bowel obstruction. **CAUTIONS:** Elderly, infants, and children. Those w/dehydration or renal dysfunction must be monitored very closely. Use for pts w/Parkinson's disease or myasthenia gravis may result in further muscle weakness.

INTERACTIONS

Other aminoglycosides, nephrotoxic, ototoxic-producing medications may increase toxicity. May increase effects of neuromuscular blocking agents.

SIDE EFFECTS

Nausea or diarrhea w/oral administration. Headache, increased salivation, anorexia. Photosensitivity when administered topically.

AMINOGLYCOSIDES

Generic Name	Brand Name(s)	Rte Adm	Blood Levels Peak (mcg/ml)	Blood Levels Trough (mcg/ml)	Dosage Range*
amikacin	Amikin	IM, IV	15–30	5–10	Adults: 15 mg/kg/day Children: 15 mg/kg/day
gentamicin	Garamycin Jenamicin	IM, IV, Topical Ophthalmic	4–10	1–2	Adults: 3–5 mg/kg/day Children: 6–7.5 mg/kg/day
kanamycin	Kantrex Klebcil	PO, Irrigation	—	—	PO: 8–12 g/day
neomycin	Mycifradin Neobiotic	PO, Topical Ophthalmic			PO: 1 g × 3 dose preop
netilmicin	Netromycin	IM, IV	6–12	0.5–2	Adults: 3–6.5 mg/kg/day Children: 5.5–8 mg/kg/day
streptomycin	Streptomycin	IM	—	—	Adults: 15 mg/kg/day; maximum: 1 g Children: 20–40 mg/kg/day; maximum: 1 g
tobramycin	Nebcin	IM, IV, Ophthalmic	4–10	1–2	Adults: 3–5 mg/kg/day Children: 6–7.5 mg/kg/day

*Dosage, interval based on serum drug concentration.

TOXIC EFFECTS/ADVERSE REACTIONS

Serious toxicity, primarily ototoxicity and nephrotoxicity, is a major factor in limiting the usefulness of the aminoglycosides. Ototoxicity is suggested by dizziness, vertigo, tinnitus, hearing loss. Nephrotoxicity may be signaled by proteinuria, increased BUN, oliguria. Neuromuscular blockade can occur w/high doses, resulting in weakness, shortness of breath, and even respiratory paralysis. Hypersensitivity reactions may occur. Note also that systemic effects may result from wound irrigation or topical application.

PATIENT CONSIDERATIONS

GENERAL: Administer on schedule to maintain blood levels. Initiate IV solutions slowly at first w/close observation for sensitivity response. BASELINE ASSESSMENT: Inquire about previous reactions to aminoglycosides. Culture/sensitivity must be done before first dose (may give before results are known). Assess WBC results, temperature, pulse, respiration. INTERVENTION/EVALUATION: Maintain good hydration and I&O. Monitor plasma concentration levels (peak and trough values) to determine continued dosage. Check WBC and culture/sensitivity results. Assess temperature, pulse, respiration, esp. rate, depth, and ease of respirations. Be alert for adverse reactions: ototoxicity, nephrotoxicity, neuromuscular blockade, allergic reaction. PATIENT/FAMILY TEACHING: Space doses evenly. Continue therapy for full duration. Avoid taking even OTC medications w/o physician direction. Notify physician in event of any hearing, visual, balance, urinary problems even after therapy is completed.

antibiotic: cephalosporins

ACTION

Cephalosporins inhibit cell wall synthesis or activate enzymes that disrupt cell wall, causing a weakening in the cell wall, cell lysis, and cell death. May be bacteriostatic or bactericidal. Most effective against rapidly dividing cells.

USES

Broad-spectrum antibiotics, which, like penicillins, may be used in a number of diseases including respiratory diseases, skin and soft tissue infection, bone/joint infections, genitourinary infections, prophylactically in some surgical procedures.

First generation cephalosporins have good activity against gram-positive organisms and moderate activity against gram-negative organisms including *Escherichia coli, Klebsiella pneumoniae, Proteus mirabilis.*

Second generation cephalosporins have increased activity against gram-negative organisms.

Third generation cephalosporins are less active against gram-positive organisms but more active against the Enterobacteriaceae w/some activity against *Pseudomonas aeruginosa.*

Fourth generation cephalosporins have good activity against gram-positive organisms (e.g., *Staphylococcus aureus*) and gram-negative organisms (e.g., *Pseudomonas aeruginosa*).

PRECAUTIONS

CONTRAINDICATIONS: Hypersensitivity to cephalosporins or penicillins. **CAUTION:** Careful monitoring is essential in bleeding disorders, gastrointestinal disease, renal and hepatic dysfunction. See individual monographs for pregnancy/lactation precautions.

INTERACTIONS

Interaction between alcohol and some of the cephalosporins (e.g., cefamandole, cefoperazone, cefotetan) may cause buildup of acetaldehyde in the blood w/disulfiramlike reaction: headache, palpitations, chest pain, hypotension, nausea, vomiting, and abdominal pain. Alcohol in any form is to be avoided up to 72 hours after drug administration. Bacteriostatic drugs may decrease effects of cephalosporins. Probenecid increases blood levels; aminoglycosides and several diuretics may increase risk of renal toxicity. Cefamandole, cefoperazone, cefotetan may increase hypoprothrombinemic effect of oral anticoagulants.

CEPHALOSPORINS

GENERIC NAME	BRAND NAME(S)	GENERATION	RTE ADMIN	DOSAGE RANGE
cefaclor	Ceclor	Second	PO	Adults: 250–500 mg q8h Children: 20–40 mg/kg/day
cefadroxil	Duricef Ultracef	First	PO	Adults: 1–2 g/day Children: 30 mg/kg/day
cefamandole	Mandol	Second	IM, IV	Adults: 1.5–12 g/day Children: 50–150 mg/kg/day
cefazolin	Ancef Kefzol Zolicef	First	IM, IV	Adults: 0.75–6 g/day Children: 25–100 mg/kg/day
cefdinir	Omnicef	Third	PO	Adults: 600 mg/day Children: 14 mg/kg/day
cefepime	Maxipime	Fourth	IM, IV	Adults: 1–6 g/day
cefixime	Suprax	Third	PO	Adults: 400 mg/day Children: 8 mg/kg/day
cefmetazole	Zefazone	Second	IM, IV	Adults: 4–8 g/day
cefoperazone	Cefobid	Third	IM, IV	Adults: 2–12 g/day
cefotaxime	Claforan	Third	IM, IV	Adults: 2–12 g/day Children: 100–200 mg/kg/day
cefotetan	Cefotan	Second	IM, IV	Adults: 1–6 g/day
cefoxitin	Mefoxin	Second	IM, IV	Adults: 3–12 g/day Children: 80–160 mg/kg/day
cefpodoxime	Vantin	Second	PO	Adults: 200–800 mg/day Children: 10 mg/kg/day
cefprozil	Cefzil	Second	PO	Adults: 0.5–1 g/day Children: 30 mg/kg/day
ceftazidime	Fortaz Tazicef Tazidime	Third	IM, IV	Adults: 0.5–6 g/day Children: 90–150 mg/kg/day
ceftibuten	Cedax	Third	PO	Adults: 400 mg/day Children: 9 mg/kg/day
ceftizoxime	Cefizox	Third	IM, IV	Adults: 1–12 g/day Children: 150–200 mg/kg/day
ceftriaxone	Rocephin	Third	IM, IV	Adults: 1–4 g/day Children: 50–100 mg/kg/day
cefuroxime	Ceftin Kefurox Zinacef	Second	PO, IM, IV	Adults(PO): 0.25–1 g/day Adults (IM, IV): 2.25–9 g/day Children (PO): 250–500 mg/day Children (IM, IV): 50–100 mg/kg/day
cephalexin	Keftab Keflet	First	PO	Adults: 1–4 g/day Children: 25–100 mg/kg/day
cephalothin	Keflin Seffin	First	IM, IV	Adults: 2–12 g/day Children: 80–160 mg/kg/day
loracarbef	Lorabid	Second	PO	Adults: 200–800 mg/day Children: 15–30 mg/kg/day

SIDE EFFECTS

Mild nausea, vomiting, or diarrhea, esp. w/oral administration.

TOXIC EFFECTS/ADVERSE REACTIONS

Hypersensitivity reactions, particularly skin rash, may progress to anaphylaxis; superinfections, including antibiotic-associated colitis. Hypoprothrombinemia and thrombocytopenia may occur w/potential for hemorrhage. Nephrotoxicity may occur, esp. w/high dosages.

PATIENT CONSIDERATIONS

GENERAL: Administer on schedule to maintain blood levels. Initiate IV solutions slowly at first w/close observation for sensitivity response. BASELINE ASSESSMENT: Inquire about previous reactions to cephalosporins, penicillins. W/history of penicillin allergy, have emergency equipment, medications available. Culture/sensitivity must be done before first dose (may give before results are known). Assess WBC results, temperature, pulse, respiration. INTERVENTION/ASSESSMENT: Monitor WBC results, temperature, pulse, respiration. Assess for adverse reactions, esp. allergic reaction, superinfections including antibiotic-associated colitis. PATIENT/FAMILY TEACHING: Space doses evenly. Continue therapy for full duration. Avoid alcohol, antacids, or other medications w/o consulting physician. Notify physician promptly of rash or diarrhea.

---

antibiotic: fluoroquinolones

The fluoroquinolones include ciprofloxacin, enoxacin, levofloxacin, lomefloxacin, norfloxacin, ofloxacin, and sparfloxacin.

ACTION

Bactericidal. Inhibits DNA gyrase in susceptible microorganisms, interfering w/bacterial DNA replication and repair.

USES

Fluoroquinolones have activity against a wide range of gram-negative and gram-positive organisms. Ciprofloxacin, levofloxacin, ofloxacin, and sparfloxacin are used primarily in the treatment of lower respiratory infections, skin/skin structure, UTIs, and sexually transmitted diseases; enoxacin, lomefloxacin, and norfloxacin are used primarily in the treatment of UTIs. Ciprofloxacin, norfloxacin, and ofloxacin are also available in ophthalmic forms for treating ophthalmic infections.

CLASSIFICATION

PRECAUTIONS

CONTRAINDICATIONS: Hypersensitivity to fluoroquinolones or quinolone group of antibacterial agents. Do not use in children <18 yrs of age. *Ophthalmic:* vaccinia, varicella, epithelial herpes simplex, keratitis, mycobacterial infection, fungal disease of ocular structure. **CAUTIONS:** Concurrent theophylline or caffeine use. Pts w/CNS disorder or other factors that increase risk of seizures. Renal impairment (alterations in dosage is necessary).

INTERACTIONS

Antacids, iron preparations, sucralfate may decrease absorption. Decreases clearance, may increase concentration, toxicity of theophylline. May increase effects of oral anticoagulants.

SIDE EFFECTS

FREQUENT: *Systemic:* Dizziness, lightheadedness, headache, insomnia/drowsiness, nausea, vomiting, diarrhea, stomach pain or discomfort. *Ophthalmic:* Burning, crusting in corner of eye. **OCCASIONAL:** *Systemic:* Increased sensitivity of skin to sunlight. *Ophthalmic:* Bad taste, sense of something in eye, redness of eyelids, itching eye. **RARE:** *Systemic:* Confusion, tremors, hallucinations, hypersensitivity reaction, interstitial nephritis, pain at injection site. May cause inflamed/ruptured tendons. *Ophthalmic:* Swelling of eyelid, increased sensitivity of eye to light, tearing.

TOXIC EFFECTS/ADVERSE REACTIONS

Superinfection, severe hypersensitivity reaction occur rarely. Arthropathy (joint disease w/swelling, pain, clubbing of fingers and toes, degeneration of stress-bearing portion of a joint) may occur if given to children <18 yrs. *Ophthalmic:* Sensitization may contraindicate later systemic use of fluoroquinolones.

ANTIBIOTIC: FLUOROQUINOLONES

Generic Name	Brand Name(s)	Usual Daily Dosage
ciprofloxacin	Cipro	PO: Adults, elderly: 250–750 mg q12h IV: Adults, elderly: 200–400 mg q12h
	Ciloxan	Ophthalmic: Adults, elderly: 1–2 drops 4–6 times/day
enoxacin	Penetrex	PO: Adults, elderly: 200–400 mg q12h
grepafloxacin	Raxar	PO: Adults, elderly: 400–600 mg/day
levofloxacin	Levaquin	PO: Adults, elderly: 250–750 mg as single daily dose IV: Adults, elderly: 250–750 mg as single daily dose
lomefloxacin	Maxaquin	PO: Adults, elderly: 400 mg q24h
norfloxacin	Noroxin	PO: Adults, elderly: 400 mg q12h
	Chibroxin	Ophthalmic: Adults, elderly: 1–2 drops 4 times/day
ofloxacin	Floxin	PO: Adults, elderly: 200–400 mg q12h IV: Adults, elderly: 200–400 mg q12h
	Ocuflox	Ophthalmic: Adults, elderly: 1–2 drops 4–6 times/day
sparfloxacin	Zagam	PO: Adults, elderly: 400 mg once, then 200 mg daily

PATIENT CONSIDERATIONS

GENERAL: Administer on schedule to maintain blood levels. Initiate IV solutions slowly at first w/close observation for sensitivity response. BASELINE ASSESSMENT: Inquire about previous reactions to fluoroquinolones. Culture/sensitivity must be done before first dose (may give before results are known). Assess WBC results, temperature, pulse, respiration. INTERVENTION/EVALUATION: Maintain good hydration and I&O. Check WBC and culture/sensitivity results. Assess temperature, pulse, respirations esp. rate, depth, and ease of respirations. Be alert for adverse reaction: allergic reactions, superinfections. Check for therapeutic response, side effects. PATIENT/FAMILY TEACHING: Space

doses evenly. Continue therapy for full course. Avoid taking OTC medication w/o physician direction. Promptly notify physician of rash or diarrhea. Drink fluids liberally. Do not take antacids containing magnesium or aluminum or products containing iron or zinc simultaneously or within 4 hrs prior to or 2 hrs after dosing. Avoid excessive sunlight/artificial ultraviolet light; wear sunscreen, protective clothing. Avoid tasks requiring alertness, motor skills until response to drug is established. Notify physician of inflammation or tendon pain.

antibiotic: macrolides

The macrolides include azithromycin, clarithromycin, dirithromycin, and erythromycin.

ACTION

Bacteriostatic or bactericidal. Reversibly binds to the P site of the 50S ribosomal subunit of susceptible organisms, inhibiting RNA-dependent protein synthesis.

USES

Macrolides have activity primarily vs. gram-positive microorganisms and gram-negative cocci. Azithromycin and clarithromycin appear to be more potent than erythromycin. Macrolides are used in the treatment of pharyngitis/tonsillitis, sinusitis, chronic bronchitis, pneumonia, uncomplicated skin/skin structure infections.

PRECAUTIONS

CONTRAINDICATIONS: Hypersensitivity to any macrolide antibiotic. *Clarithromycin:* Pts receiving terfenadine or astemizole having preexisting cardiac abnormalities or electrolyte disturbances. **Note:** Caution with other macrolides. *Erythromycin estolate:* Preexisting liver disease. **CAUTIONS:** Hepatic and renal dysfunction.

INTERACTIONS

Azithromycin: May increase serum concentrations of carbamazepine, cyclosporine, theophylline, warfarin. Aluminum/magnesium-containing antacids may decrease concentration (give 1 hr before or 2 hrs after antacid).

Clarithromycin: May increase concentration, toxicity of astemizole, carbamazepine, cisapride, digoxin, terfenadine, theophylline. May decrease concentration of zidovudine. May increase warfarin effects. Rifampin may decrease clarithromycin concentrations.

Dirithromycin: None significant.

Erythromycin: May inhibit metabolism of carbamazepine. May decrease effects of chloramphenicol, clindamycin. May increase concentration, toxicity of cyclosporine, felodipine, lovastatin, simvastatin. Hepatotoxic medications may increase hepatotoxicity. May increase risk of cardiotoxicity w/cisapride, terfenadine. May increase risk of toxicity w/theophylline. May increase effect of warfarin.

SIDE EFFECTS

Azithromycin:
Occasional: Abdominal pain, nausea, vomiting, diarrhea. **Rare:** Headache, dizziness, allergic reaction, acute interstitial nephritis.

Clarithromycin:
Occasional: Abnormal taste, nausea, vomiting, diarrhea, abdominal pain, headache. **Rare:** Liver toxicity, hypersensitivity reaction, thrombycytopenia.

Dirithromycin:
Occasional: Abdominal pain, headache, nausea, diarrhea, vomiting, dyspepsia, nonspecific pain, asthenia. **RARE:** Rash, flatulence, dyspnea, pruritus, urticaria, insomnia.

Erythromycin:
Frequent: Nausea, vomiting, diarrhea, abdominal discomfort. **Occasional:** Liver toxicity, hypersensitivity reaction (skin rash, redness, itching, oral or vaginal candidiasis). **Rare:** Cardiotoxicity (QT prolongation), reversible hearing loss, pancreatitis.

TOXIC EFFECTS/ADVERSE REACTIONS

Superinfection esp. antibiotic-associated colitis may result from altered bacterial balance.

ANTIBIOTIC: MACROLIDES

Generic Name	Brand Name(s)	Usual Daily Dosage
azithromycin	Zithromax	PO: Adults, elderly: 500 mg on day 1, 250 mg on days 2–5. Children: 10 mg/kg on day 1, 5 mg/kg on days 2–5.
clarithromycin	Biaxin	PO: Adults, elderly: 250–500 mg q12h. Children: 7.5 mg/kg q12h.
dirithromycin	Dynabec	PO: Adults, elderly, children >12 yrs: 500 mg/day as a single dose.
erythromycin	E-Mycin, Erytab, Eryc, PCE, Ilotycin, Ilosone, EES, Pediamycin, Eryped, Erythrocin	PO: Adults, elderly: 250–500 mg q6h. Children: 30–50 mg/kg/day. IV: Adults, elderly, children: 15–20 mg/kg/day. Maximum: 4 g/day.

PATIENT CONSIDERATIONS

GENERAL: Administer on schedule to maintain blood levels. Initiate IV solution slowly w/close observation for sensitivity response. BASELINE ASSESSMENT: Inquire about previous reactions to macrolides. Culture/sensitivity must be done before first dose (may give before results are known). Assess WBC results, temperature, pulse, respiration. INTERVENTION/EVALUATION: Maintain good hydration and I&O. Check WBC and culture/sensitivity results. Assess

temperature, pulse, respirations esp. rate, depth, and ease of respirations. Be alert for adverse reaction: allergic reactions, superinfections. Check for therapeutic response, side effects. PATIENT/FAMILY TEACHING: Space doses evenly. Continue therapy for full course. Avoid taking OTC medication w/o physician direction. Promptly notify physician of rash or diarrhea. Drink fluids liberally.

Azithromycin: Take at least 1 hr prior to or 2 hrs after a meal. Avoid giving w/food. Avoid simultaneous administration of magnesium or aluminum-containing antacids.

Clarithromycin: May take w/o regard to meals, may take w/milk. Shake suspension well; do not refrigerate.

Dirithromycin: Take w/food or within 1 hr of eating. Do not cut, chew, crush tablets.

Erythromycin: May take w/o regard to meals.

antibiotic: penicillins

ACTION

Penicillins inhibit cell wall synthesis or activate enzymes, which disrupt cell wall, causing a weakening in the cell wall, cell lysis, and cell death. May be bacteriostatic or bactericidal. Most effective against rapidly dividing cells.

USES

Penicillins may be used to treat a large number of infections including pneumonia and other respiratory diseases, urinary tract infections, septicemia, meningitis, intra-abdominal infections, gonorrhea and syphilis, bone/joint infection.

PRECAUTIONS

CONTRAINDICATIONS: Hypersensitivity to penicillin, cephalosporins, or components. **CAUTIONS:** Extreme caution w/history of allergies, asthma; gastrointestinal disease; renal dysfunction; bleeding disorders; and (for some penicillins) hepatic dysfunction.

INTERACTIONS

Bacteriostatic antibiotics (e.g., tetracyclines) may decrease bactericidal effects of penicillins. Concurrent use w/allopurinol and ampicillin increases risk of skin rash. Pts should be advised that estrogen contraceptives may have decreased effectiveness when given w/penicillin. Anticoagulants may increase potential for bleeding w/high-dose penicillin therapy. Probenecid increases effects by interfering w/excretion.

SIDE EFFECTS

Mild nausea, vomiting, or diarrhea; sore tongue or mouth.

PENICILLINS

Generic Name	Brand Name(s)	Rte Admin	Type	Dosage Range
amoxicillin	Amoxil Polymox Trimox Wymox	Broad spectrum	PO	Adults: 0.75–1.5 g/day Children: 20–40 mg/kg/day
amoxicillin/ clavulanate	Augmentin	Broad spectrum	PO	Adults: 0.75–1.5 g/day Children: 20–40 mg/kg/day
ampicillin	Omnipen Polycillin Principen	Broad spectrum	PO, IM, IV	Adults: 1–12 g/day Children: 50–200 mg/kg/day
ampicillin/ sulbactam	Unasyn	Broad spectrum	IM, IV	Adults: 6–12 g/day
bacampicillin	Spectrobid	Broad spectrum	PO	Adults: 800–1,600 mg/day Children: 25–50 mg/kg/day
carbenicillin	Geocillin	Extended spectrum	PO	Adults: 382–764 mg 4×/day
cloxacillin	Cloxapen Tegopen	Penicillinase resistant	PO	Adults: 1–2 g/day Children: 50–100 mg/kg/day
dicloxacillin	Dynapen Pathocil	Pencillinase resistant	PO	Adults: 1–2 g/day Children: 12.5–25 mg/kg/day
methicillin	Staphcillin	Penicillinase resistant	IM, IV	Adults: 4–12 g/day Children: 100–300 mg/kg/day
mezlocillin	Mezlin	Extended spectrum	IM, IV	Adults: 6–18 g/day Children: 150–300 mg/kg/day
nafcillin	Nafcil Unipen	Penicillinase resistant	PO, IM, IV	Adults (PO): 1–6 g/day Adults (IM, IV): 2–6 g/day Children (PO): 25 50 mg/kg/day Children (IM, IV): 50 mg/kg/day
oxacillin	Bactocill Prostaphlin	Penicillinase resistant	PO, IM, IV	Adults (PO): 2–6 g/day Adults (IM, IV): 2–6 g/day Children (PO): 50 100 mg/ kg/day Children (IM, IV): 50–100 mg/ kg/day
penicillin G benzathine	Bicillin Permapen	Natural	IM	Adults: 1.2 million units/day Children: 0.3–1.2 million units/ day
penicillin G postassium	Pentids Pfizerpen	Natural	IM, IV	Adults: 2–24 million units/day Children: 100,000– 250,000 units/kg/day
penicillin G procaine	Crysticillin A.S. Wycillin	Natural	IM	Adults: 0.6–1.2 million units/day Children: 0.6–1.2 million units/ day
penicillin V potassium	Pen-Vee K V-Cillin K Veetids	Natural	PO	Adults: 0.5–2 g/day Children: 25–50 mg/kg/day
piperacillin	Pipracil	Extended spectrum	IM, IV	Adults: 6–18 g/day Children: 200–300 mg/kg/day
piperacillin tazobactam	Zosyn	Extended spectrum	IV	Adults: 3.375 g q6h
ticarcillin	Ticar	Extended spectrum	IM, IV	Adults: 12–24 g/day Children: 50–300 mg/kg/day
ticarcillin clavulanate	Timentin	Extended spectrum	IM, IV	Adults: 3.1 g q4–6h

Natural penicillins are very active against gram-positive cocci but ineffective against most strains of *Staphylococcus aureus* (inactivated by enzyme penicillinase).

Penicillinase-resistant penicillins are effective against penicillinase-producing *Staphylococcus aureus* but are less effective against gram-positive cocci than the natural penicillins.

Broad-spectrum penicillins are effective against gram-positive cocci and some gram-negative bacteria (e.g., *Hemophilus influenzae, Escherichia coli, Proteus mirabilis*).

Extended-spectrum penicillins are effective against *Pseudomonas aeruginosa, Enterobacter, Proteus* species, *Klebsiella,* and some other gram-negative microorganisms.

TOXIC EFFECTS/ADVERSE REACTIONS

Hypersensitivity/allergic reactions ranging from skin rashes, urticaria, itching to full anaphylaxis. Superinfections, including antibiotic-associated colitis. Neurotoxicity, hematologic effects may occur in select drugs.

PATIENT CONSIDERATIONS

GENERAL: Administer drugs on proper schedule to maintain blood levels. Initiate IV solutions slowly at first w/close observation for sensitivity response. BASELINE ASSESSMENT: Question for history of hypersensitivity to penicillin or cephalosporins. W/history of cephalosporin reaction, have emergency equipment, medications available. Culture/sensitivity must be done before first dose (may give before results are obtained). Assess WBC results, temperature, pulse, respiration. INTERVENTION/EVALUATION: Monitor temperature, lab results, particularly WBC and culture/sensitivity reports. Assess for adverse reactions, esp. allergic reactions, superinfection. PATIENT/FAMILY TEACHING: Space doses evenly. Continue therapy for full duration, usually 7–10 days. Avoid alcohol, antacids, or other medications w/o consulting physician. Promptly notify physician of rash or diarrhea.

anticholinergics

ACTION

These agents are known as anticholinergics, antimuscarinics, or parasympatholytics. Competitively block muscarinic receptors. Inhibit action of acetylcholine. Prevent stimulation of receptors by muscarinic agonists. Areas affected include:

Eye: Cause mydriasis (pupil dilation), cycloplegia (paralysis of ciliary muscle).

Heart: Increase heart rate.

Gastrointestinal: Decrease salivary secretion, gastric secretion; decrease tone and motility of gastrointestinal tract.

Respiratory: Decrease secretion of nose, mouth, pharynx, bronchi; cause relaxation of bronchi.

Urinary tract: Decrease tone, contraction of ureter and urinary bladder.

USES

Management of peptic ulcer, ophthalmic administration (produce mydriasis/cycloplegia), asthma (induce bronchodilation), antagonize reflex vagal-mediated bradycardia, Parkinson's disease, administered before general anesthetic to decrease excessive salivation/secretion of respiratory tract, spastic disorders of biliary tract, antidote/antagonize effects of anticholinesterase agents; antidote for mushroom poisoning.

PRECAUTIONS

CONTRAINDICATIONS: Hypersensitivity, glaucoma, hepatic or renal dysfunction, tachycardia, ulcerative colitis, intestinal obstruction, paralytic ileus, bladder neck obstruction, myasthenia gravis, asthma. **CAUTIONS:** Pts w/cardiac disease, elderly, infants, and young children (who are particularly susceptible to toxic effects) should be monitored closely. Drugs cross placenta and are excreted in breast milk. May inhibit lactation.

INTERACTIONS

Antacids, antidiarrheals may decrease absorption. Anticholinergics may increase effects. May decrease absorption of ketoconazole. May increase severity of gastrointestinal lesions w/potassium chloride (wax matrix).

SIDE EFFECTS

Antisalivary (dry mouth), blurred vision, urinary hesitation/retention, constipation, flushing, lightheadedness, mild tachycardia.

TOXIC EFFECTS/ADVERSE REACTIONS

CNS excitation, nausea and vomiting, hypertension, increased intraocular pressure, rash, elevated temperature, thick respiratory secretions and respiratory difficulties, impotence.

ANTICHOLINERGICS

Generic Name	Brand Name(s)	Rte Adm	Dosage Range
atropine	Atropine	IM, IV, SubQ	Adults: 0.3–1.2 mg Children: 0.01 mg/kg
dicyclomine	Bentyl	PO, IM	Adults: PO: 80–160 mg/day; IM: 80 mg/day
glycopyrrolate	Robinul	PO, IM, IV	Adults: PO: 2–6 mg/day; IM, IV: 0.1–0.2 mg
scopolamine	Scopolamine	IM, IV, SubQ	Adults: 0.3–0.65 mg Children: 0.006 mg/kg
	Transderm Scop	Topical	Adults: 1.5 mg

PATIENT CONSIDERATIONS

GENERAL: For long-term therapy, change medication gradually. BASELINE ASSESSMENT: Check B/P, pulse, respirations. INTERVENTION/EVALUATION: Assess bowel activity, abdominal distention, bowel sounds. Monitor I&O, check for urination, palpate for distended bladder. Check B/P, pulse, respirations, EKG. Assess for adverse reactions, esp. in geriatric pts and those w/chronic lung conditions. PATIENT/FAMILY TEACHING: Mouthwash, cold drinks, hard candy or gum (if permitted) may be used for dry mouth. Take safety precautions w/drowsiness, blurred vision, or lightheadedness; do not drive or perform activities requiring mental acuity. Increased fluid intake to decrease viscosity of secretions, aid in bowel elimination. *Ophthalmic:* Protect eyes from light; wear sunglasses.

anticoagulants/antiplatelets/thrombolytics

ACTION

Anticoagulants: Inhibit blood coagulation by preventing the formation of new clots and extension of existing ones. *Do not dissolve formed clots.* Anticoagulants are subdivided into two common classes: *Heparin:* Directly interferes w/blood coagulation by blocking the conversion of prothrombin to thrombin and fibrinogen to fibrin. *Coumarin:* Acts indirectly to prevent synthesis in the liver of vitamin K–dependent clotting factors.

Antiplatelets: Interfere w/platelet aggregation. Effects are irreversible for life of platelet.

Thrombolytics: Act directly or indirectly on fibrinolytic system to dissolve clots (converting plasminogen to plasmin, an enzyme that digests fibrin clot).

USES

Anticoagulants: Primarily decrease risk of venous thromboembolism.

Antiplatelets: Primarily decrease risk of arterial thromboembolism.

Thrombolytics: Lyse existing clots.

Treatment and prevention of venous thromboembolism, acute myocardial infarction, acute cerebral embolism; reduces risk of acute myocardial infarction, total mortality in pts w/unstable angina; occlusion of saphenous grafts following open heart surgery; embolism in select pts w/atrial fibrillation, prosthetic heart valves, valvular heart disease, cardiomyopathy. Heparin also used for acute/chronic consumption coagulopathies (disseminated intravascular coagulation).

PRECAUTIONS

CONTRAINDICATIONS: Hypersensitivity, active bleeding, blood dyscrasias and bleeding tendencies, pregnancy. **CAUTIONS:** Renal, hepatic dysfunction; alcoholism; history of allergy.

ANTICOAGULANTS/ANTIPLATELETS/THROMBOLYTICS

Generic Name	Brand Name(s)	Class	Dosage Range
alteplase	Activase	Thrombolytic	Adults: IV infusion: 100 mg over 3 hrs (2 hrs for pulmonary embolism)
anagrelide	Agrylin	Antiplatelet	Adults: PO: 2–10 mg/day
anistreplase	Eminase	Thrombolytic	Adults: IV push: 30 units over 2–5 min
ardeparin	Normiflo	Anticoagulant	Adults: SubQ: 50 U/kg q12 h
aspirin	—	Antiplatelet	Adults: 81–325 mg/day
clopidogrel	Plavix	Antiplatelet	Adults: PO: 75 mg once daily
dalteparin	Fragmin	Anticoagulant	Adults: SubQ: 200 IU/kg once daily or 100 IU/kg q12h
danaparoid	Organan	Anticoagulant	Adults: SubQ: 750 units q12h
dipyridamole	Persantine	Antiplatelet	Adults: 75–100 mg 4 times/day
enoxaparin	Lovenox	Anticoagulant	Adults: 30 mg q12h
heparin	—	Anticoagulant	Adults: IV bolus: 5,000 units then IV infusion of 20,000–40,000 units/day Children: IV bolus: 50 units/kg then IV infusion of 20,000 units/m²/24 hrs
reteplase	Retavase	Thrombolytic	Adults: IV: 10 units q30min × 2 doses
streptokinase	Kabikinase Streptase	Thrombolytic	Adults: (AMI) 1.5 million units over 60 min
tenecteplase	TNKase	Thrombolytic	Adults: IV: up to 50 mg (based on patient weight)
ticlopidine	Ticlid	Antiplatelet	Adults: 250 mg 2 times/day
tinzaparin	Innohep	Anticoagulant	Adults: SubQ: 175 IU/kg once daily
urokinase	Abbokinase	Thrombolytic	Adults: IV: 4,400 IU/kg over 10 min, then 4,400 IU/kg/min for 12–24 hrs
warfarin	Coumadin	Anticoagulant	Adults: Initially, 5–10 mg/day, then 2–10 mg/day

INTERACTIONS

Anticoagulants interact with many drugs and foods. Pts should be cautioned against smoking, alcohol consumption, and use of OTC drugs. Aspirin, many NSAIDs, antihistamines, diuretics, antibiotics, estrogen contraceptives are among the drugs that affect anticoagulant action. Any medication taken with an anticoagulant should be checked for interaction. Prothrombin time (PT) may be shortened by high-fat diet or sudden increase in foods rich in vitamin K. Antidote for heparin: protamine sulfate; for coumarins: vitamin K.

SIDE EFFECTS

Not common. Local reactions w/parenteral administration. Nausea, vomiting, anorexia, and diarrhea w/oral administration.

TOXIC EFFECTS/ADVERSE REACTIONS

Minor bleeding to major hemorrhage. Thrombocytopenia and alopecia are transient and reversible. Jaundice, hepatitis, increased serum transaminase levels w/coumarin therapy. Hypersensitivity reactions are rare: fever, chills, urticaria.

PATIENT CONSIDERATIONS

GENERAL: Do not discontinue abruptly. Monitor coagulation test results before administration: for heparin therapy, the activated partial thromboplastin time (APTT); for coumarin therapy, the PT. Consult physician for targeted coagulation range for individual pt (generally, dosage is adjusted to keep results about 1.5–2 times control value for APTT, 1.5 times control value for PT). INTERVENTION/EVALUATION: Assess for bleeding: vital signs, bruises, overt bleeding, and blood in sputum, urine, and feces. Check for headache, abdominal or back pain. PATIENT/FAMILY TEACHING: Importance of taking drug as directed and periodic lab tests to determine response to medication. Explain how to check for bleeding signs. Carry identification indicating anticoagulant therapy. Avoid large quantities of vitamin K–rich food, such as green leafy vegetables, liver, fish, bananas, cauliflower, tomatoes (decrease effects of oral anticoagulants). Consult physician before taking other medications (including aspirin). Avoid alcohol. Avoid activities w/high risk of injury. Inform physician, dentist of anticoagulant therapy before surgical/dental procedures.

anticonvulsants

ACTION

Seizures consist of abnormal and excessive discharges from the brain. Anticonvulsants can prevent or reduce excessive discharge of neurons w/seizure foci or decrease the spread of excitation from seizure foci to normal neurons. Exact mechanism unknown. Anticonvulsants include the hydantoins, barbiturates, succinimides, oxazolidinediones, benzodiazepines, and several miscellaneous agents.

USES

Anticonvulsants are generally effective in the treatment of *absence (petit mal) seizures* (brief, abrupt loss of consciousness, some clonic motor activity ranging from eyelid blinking to jerking of entire body); *tonic-clonic (grand mal) seizures* (major convulsions, usually beginning w/spasm of all body musculature, then clonic jerking, followed by depression of all central function); and *complex partial seizures* (confused behavior, impaired consciousness, bizarre generalized EEG activity). Other types of seizures generally respond poorly to anticonvulsant therapy.

PRECAUTIONS

CONTRAINDICATIONS: Hypersensitivity, hepatic, renal, or thyroid dysfunction, alcoholism, blood dyscrasias; diabetes mellitus, cardiac disease/impairment, lactation. **CAUTIONS:** Pregnancy—risk/benefit must be weighed in relation to congenital abnormalities. Elderly, children, and debilitated.

INTERACTIONS

Drug interactions are extensive; any other medication administered should be carefully checked for interaction w/anticonvulsants. Teach pts never to take medication w/o consulting physician. Effects are increased by CNS depressants; decreased w/tricyclic antidepressants, phenothiazine antipsychotics, antacids. Refer to individual monographs.

SIDE EFFECTS

Drowsiness, sedation, mild dizziness, gingival hyperplasia, anorexia, nausea, vomiting, hyperglycemia, and glycosuria.

TOXIC EFFECTS/ADVERSE REACTIONS

Visual disturbances, unusual excitement, confusion, skin disorders. Stevens-Johnson syndrome (headache, arthralgia, skin lesions w/other symptoms), liver damage, hirsutism, blood dyscrasias, enlarged lymph glands in neck and under arms.

PATIENT CONSIDERATIONS

GENERAL: Status epilepticus is a life-threatening emergency that requires immediate IV medication (diazepam is the drug of choice). Never mix parenteral solutions w/other drugs or IV fluids—should be administered via slow IV push. When discontinued, gradual reduction is recommended. Provide protection against injury. INTERVENTION/EVALUATION: Monitor B/P, pulse, respirations, serum drug levels. Assess neurologic status. Identify characteristics of seizures if they occur. PATIENT/FAMILY TEACHING: Therapy is usually several years to life. Take w/food or fluids to minimize GI irritation. Important to take as directed. Do not take other medications w/o consulting physician. Avoid alcohol. Do not drive or engage in activities requiring mental acuity until physician approves (seizures and response to drug are controlled). Carry identification card/bracelet indicating anticonvulsant therapy.

ANTICONVULSANTS

Generic Name	Brand Name(s)	Class	Uses	Dosage Range
carbamazepine	Tegretol	Miscellaneous	Complex partial, tonic-clonic, mixed seizures, trigeminal neuralgia	Adults: 800–1,200 mg/day Children: 400–800 mg/day
clonazepam	Klonopin	Benzodiazepine	Petit mal, akinetic, myoclonic, absence	Adults: 1.5–20 mg/day Children: 0.01–0.2 mg/kg/day
clorazepate	Tranxene	Benzodiazepine	Partial seizures	Adults: 7.5–90 mg/day Children: 7.5–60 mg/day
diazepam	Valium	Benzodiazepine	Adjunctive therapy status epilepticus	Adults: PO: 4–40 mg/day; IM/IV: 5–30 mg Children: PO: 3–10 mg/day; IM/IV: 1–10 mg
ethosuximide	Zarontin	Succinimide	Absence seizures	Children: 20 mg/kg/day
felbamate	Felbatol	Miscellaneous	Partial seizures, Lennox-Gustaut syndrome	Adults: 1,200–3,600 mg/day Children ≥14 yrs: 1,200–3,600 mg/day

ANTICONVULSANTS *(continued)*

Generic Name	Brand Name(s)	Class	Uses	Dosage Range
fosphenytoin	Cerebyx	Hydantoin	Tonic-clonic, complex partial, autonomic seizures, status epilepticus	Status epilepticus: IV: 15–20 mg PE/kg Nonemergent: IM/IV: Initially, 10–20 mg PE/kg; then 4–6 mg PE/kg/day
gabapentum	Neurontin	Miscellaneous	Partial seizures	Adults: 900–1,800 mg/day Children >12 yrs: 900–1,800 mg/day
lamotrigine	Lamictal	Miscellaneous	Partial seizures	Adults: 100–500 mg/day
oxcarbazepine	Trileptal	Miscellaneous	Partial seizures	Initially, 600 mg/day up to 2,400 mg/day
phenobarbital	Luminal	Barbiturate	Tonic-clonic, partial, status epilepticus	Adults: PO: 100–300 mg/day; IM/IV: 200–600 mg Children: PO: 3–5 mg/kg/day; IM/IV: 100–400 mg
phenytoin	Dilantin	Hydantoin	Tonic-clonic, complex partial, autonomic seizures, status epilepticus	Adults: PO: 300–600 mg/day; IV: 150–250 mg Status epilepticus: 15–18 mg/kg Children: PO: 4–8 mg/kg/day Status epilepticus: 10–15 mg/kg
primidone	Mysoline	Miscellaneous	Complex partial, partial, akinetic, tonic-clonic	Adults: 0.75–2 g/day Children: 10–25 mg/kg/day
tiagabine	Gabitril	Miscellaneous	Partial seizures	Adults: Initially, 4 mg; maximum: 56 mg Children: Initially, 4 mg; maximum: 32 mg
topiramate	Topamax	Miscellaneous	Partial seizures	Adults: PO: 50–400 mg/day
valproic acid	Depakene Depakote	Miscellaneous	Absence, multiple seizure types	Adults, children: 15–60 mg/kg/day
vigabatrin	Sabril	Miscellaneous	Partial seizures	Adults: 1–4 g/day
zonisamide	Zonegran	Miscellaneous	Partial seizures	Adults: 500 mg/day

antidepressants

ACTION

Antidepressants are classified as tricyclic, monoamine oxidase (MAO) inhibitors, or miscellaneous. Depression may be due to reduced functioning of monoamine neurotransmitters in the CNS (decreased amount and/or decreased effects at receptor sites).

Antidepressants block metabolism, increase amount/effects of monoamine neurotransmitters (e.g., norepinephrine, serotonin [5-HT]), and act at receptor sites (change responsiveness/sensitivities of both pre- and postsynaptic receptor sites).

Miscellaneous, Tricyclics: Block reuptake of neurotransmitter at presynaptic nerve endings. Potency/selectivity varies w/these agents.

MAO inhibitors: Inhibit enzyme MAO, thus interfering w/degradation of monoamine neurotransmitters.

USES

Used primarily for the treatment of depression. Imipramine is also used for childhood enuresis. Clomipramine is used only for obsessive-compulsive disorder (OCD). MAO inhibitors are rarely used as initial therapy except for pts unresponsive to other therapy or when other therapy is contraindicated.

PRECAUTIONS

CONTRAINDICATIONS: Pregnancy, lactation, children <16 yrs of age (exception: imipramine to treat enuresis in children >6 yrs of age), hypersensitivity, liver dysfunction, renal dysfunction, glaucoma, elderly, CHF. **CAUTIONS:** Never use MAO inhibitors and tricyclic antidepressants together—can result in death. Effects of antidepressants can last 2–3 wks after discontinuation.

INTERACTIONS

Tricyclic antidepressants: Alcohol, CNS depressants may increase CNS, respiratory depression, hypotensive effects. Antithyroid agents may increase risk of agranulocytosis. Phenothiazines may increase sedative, anticholinergic effects. Cimetidine may increase concentration, toxicity. May decrease effects of clonidine, guanadrel. May increase cardiac effects w/sympathomimetics. May increase risk of hypertensive crisis, hyperpyretic, convulsion w/MAO inhibitors.

MAO inhibitors: Alcohol, CNS depressants may increase CNS depressant effects. Tricyclic antidepressants, fluoxetine, trazodone may cause serotonin syndrome. May increase effect of oral hypoglycemics, insulin. B/P may increase w/buspirone. Caffeine-containing medications may increase cardiac arrhythmias, hypertension. May precipitate hypertensive crises w/carbamazepine, cyclobenzaprine, maprotiline, other MAO inhibitors. Meperidine, other opioid analgesics may produce immediate excitation, sweating, rigidity, severe hypertension or hypotension, severe respiratory distress, coma, convulsions, vascular collapse, death. May increase CNS stimulant, vasopressor effects. Tyramine, foods w/pressor amines (e.g., aged cheese) may cause sudden, severe hypertension.

ANTIDEPRESSANTS

Generic Name	Brand Name(s)	Type	Amine Uptake Blockage	Dosage Range (mg/day)
amitriptyline	Elavil Endep	Tricyclic	Norepinephrine Serotonin	PO: 40–300
amoxapine	Asendin	Tricyclic	Norepinephrine Serotonin	PO: 100–600
bupropion	Wellbutrin	Miscellaneous	—	PO: 200–450

ANTIDEPRESSANTS *(continued)*

Generic Name	Brand Name(s)	Type	Amine Uptake Blockage	Dosage Range (mg/day)
citalopram	Celexa	Miscellaneous	Serotonin	PO: 20–40
clomipramine	Anafranil	Tricyclic	Norepinephrine Serotonin	PO: 25–250
desipramine	Norpramin Pertofrane	Tricyclic	Norepinephrine Serotonin	PO: 25–100
doxepin	Adapin Sinequan	Tricyclic	Norepinephrine Serotonin	PO: 75–300
fluoxetine	Prozac	Miscellaneous	Serotonin	PO: 20–80
fluvoxamine	Luvox	Miscellaneous	Serotonin	PO: 100–300
imipramine	Janimine Tofranil	Tricyclic	Norepinephrine Serotonin	PO: 30–300
maprotiline	Ludiomil	Miscellaneous	Norepinephrine	PO: 25–225
mirtazapine	Remeron	Miscellaneous	Norepinephrine Serotonin	PO: 5–30
nefazodone	Serzone	Miscellaneous	Serotonin Serotonin receptor	PO: 200–600
nortriptyline	Aventyl Pamelor	Tricyclic	Norepinephrine Serotonin	PO: 25–100
paroxetine	Paxil	Miscellaneous	Serotonin	PO: 20–50
phenelzine	Nardil	MAO inhibitor	—	PO: 15–90
protriptyline	Vivactil	Tricyclic	Norepinephrine Serotonin	PO: 15–60
sertraline	Zoloft	Miscellaneous	Serotonin	PO: 50–200
tranylcypromine	Parnate	MAO inhibitor	—	PO: 30–60
trazodone	Desyrel	Miscellaneous	Serotonin	PO: 50–600
venlafaxine	Effexor	Miscellaneous	Norepinephrine Serotonin	PO: 75–375

SIDE EFFECTS

Tricyclic antidepressants: Dizziness, drowsiness, dry mouth, headache, weight gain, photosensitivity. *MAO inhibitors:* Dizziness and orthostatic hypotension, blurred vision, constipation, difficulty w/urination, mild headache, weight gain, insomnia.

TOXIC EFFECTS/ADVERSE REACTIONS

Tricyclic antidepressants: Severe drowsiness, confusion, hallucinations, seizures, tachycardia or bradycardia, difficulty breathing. *MAO inhibitors:* Severe drowsiness or dizziness, hypertension or hypotension, tachycardia, difficulty sleeping, hallucinations, respiratory depression.

PATIENT CONSIDERATIONS

GENERAL: Closely supervise pts (potential for suicide increases when emerging from depression). Elderly should be observed carefully for increased response; small doses are usually indicated. BASELINE ASSESSMENT: Determine initial B/P. Assess pt and environment for support needed. INTERVENTION/EVALUATION: Monitor B/P. Assess mental status. Check bowel activity; avoid constipation. PA-

CLASSIFICATION

TIENT/FAMILY TEACHING: Change positions slowly to avoid orthostatic hypotension. Take medication as ordered; do not stop taking or increase dosage. Avoid driving or performing tasks that require mental acuity until response to drug controlled. Extremely important to refrain from alcohol and other medications during therapy and for 2–3 wks thereafter. Omit foods rich in tyramine, such as products containing yeast, beer/wine, aged cheese (list of foods to avoid should be given); ingestion of such foods and antidepressant may cause hypertensive crisis. Inform other physicians or dentist of antidepressant therapy. Use protection from sunlight w/specific drugs. To the extent possible, drugs that cause drowsiness should be taken at bedtime, those causing insomnia should be taken in the morning.

antidiabetics

Five major groups of medication are currently available in the treatment of diabetes mellitus: insulin, sulfonylureas, alpha-glucosidase inhibitors, biguanides, and thiazolinediones.

ACTION

Insulin: A hormone synthesized and secreted by beta cells of Langerhans' islet in the pancreas. Controls storage and utilization of glucose, amino acids, and fatty acids by activated transport systems/enzymes. Inhibits breakdown of glycogen, fat, protein. Insulin lowers blood glucose by inhibiting glycogenolysis and gluconeogenesis in liver; stimulates glucose uptake by muscle, adipose tissue. Activity of insulin is initiated by binding to cell surface receptors.

Sulfonylureas: Stimulate release of insulin from beta cells; increases sensitivity of insulin to peripheral tissue. Endogenous insulin must be present for oral hypoglycemics to be effective.

Alpha-glucosidase inhibitors: Work locally in small intestine slowing carbohydrate breakdown and glucose absorption.

Biguanides: Decrease hepatic glucose output, enhances peripheral glucose uptake.

Thiazolinediones: Decrease insulin resistance.

USES

Insulin: Treatment of insulin-dependent diabetes (type I) and noninsulin-dependent diabetes (type II). Also used in acute situations such as ketoacidosis, severe infections, major surgery in otherwise noninsulin-dependent diabetics. Administered to pts receiving parenteral nutrition. Drug of choice during pregnancy.

Sulfonylureas: Controls hyperglycemia in type II diabetes not controlled by weight and diet alone. Chlorpropamide also used in adjunctive treatment of neurogenic diabetes insipidus.

Alpha-glucosidase inhibitors: Adjunct to diet to lower blood glucose in pts with noninsulin-dependent diabetes mellitus (NIDDM) whose hyperglycemia cannot be managed by diet alone.

Biguanides: Adjunct to diet to lower blood glucose in pts with noninsulin-dependent diabetes mellitus (NIDDM) whose hyperglycemia cannot be managed by diet alone.

Thiazolinediones: Adjunct in pts with NIDDM currently on insulin therapy.

INSULIN

		Hypoglycemic Effect		
	Brand Name(s)	**Onset (hrs)**	**Peak (hrs)**	**Duration (hrs)**
RAPID ACTING				
regular insulin	Humulin R Novolin R Velosulin	0.5–0.75	2–4	3–6
insulin aspart	Novolog	0.25	1–3	3–5
insulin lispro	Humalog	0.15–0.25	0.75–1	2–4
INTERMEDIATE ACTING				
lente insulin	Humulin L Novolin L	1–2.5	7–15	24
NPH	Humulin N Novolin N	1–1.5	4–12	24
LONG ACTING				
ultralente	Ultralente Humulin U	4–8	10–30	>36
insulin glarging	Lantus	1.1	5	24

PRECAUTIONS

CONTRAINDICATIONS: *Insulin:* Hypersensitivity to animal proteins (human insulin available). Hypoglycemia. *Sulfonylureas:* Hypersensitivity to sulfonamides, pregnancy, severe stress or infection, before surgical procedures, in type I insulin-dependent diabetes; hepatic or renal dysfunction; hypoglycemia; lactation. *Alpha-glucosidase inhibitors:* Hypersensitivity to drug, diabetic ketoacidosis, cirrhosis, inflammatory bowel disease, colonic ulceration, partial intestinal obstruction, chronic intestinal disease associated w/disorders of digestion or absorption. *Biguanides:* Renal disease/dysfunction, hypersensitivity to drug, acute or chronic metabolic acidosis. **CAUTION:** Elderly or debilitated pts. Renal or hepatic impairment; alcoholics; cardiac impairment.

INTERACTION

Insulin: Glucocorticoids, thiazide diuretics may increase blood glucose. Alcohol may increase insulin effect. Beta-adrenergic blockers may increase risk of hypo/hyperglycemia, mask signs of hypoglycemia, prolong period of hypoglycemia.

Sulfonylureas: May increase effects of oral anticoagulants. Chloramphenicol, MAO inhibitors, salicylates, sulfonamides may increase effects. Beta blockers may increase hypoglycemic effect, may mask signs of hypoglycemia.

Alpha-glucosidase inhibitors: Digestive enzymes, intestinal absorbents (e.g., charcoal) may decrease effect.

Biguanides: Alcohol potentiates effect on lactate metabolism. Cimetidine, furosemide, nifedipine may increase concentration. Iodinated contrast material may lead to acute renal failure, associated w/lactic acidosis.

ORAL ANTIDIABETIC AGENTS

Generic Name	Brand Name(s)	Type	Usual Daily Dosage: Initially	Usual Daily Dosage: Average Range
acarbose	Precose	Alpha-glucosidase inhibitor	75 mg	150–300 mg
acetohexamide	Dymelor	Sulfonylurea	250 mg	250–1,500 mg
chlorpropamide	Diabinese	Sulfonylurea	100 mg	100–750 mg
glimepiride	Amaryl	Sulfonylurea	1–2 mg	1–4 mg
glipizide	Glucotrol	Sulfonylurea	2.5–5 mg	2.5–40 mg
glyburide	Diabeta Micronase Glynase	Sulfonylurea	1.25–5mg	1.25–20 mg
metformin	Glucophage	Biguanide	500 mg	500–2,550 mg
miglitol	Glyset	Alpha-glucosidase inhibitor	75 mg	75–300 mg
nateglinide	Starlix	Miscellaneous	N/A	N/A
repaglinide	Prandin	Miscellaneous	—	1–16 mg/day
tolazamide	Tolinase	Sulfonylurea	100 mg	100–1,000 mg
tolbutamide	Orinase	Sulfonylurea	500 mg	500–3,000 mg

SIDE EFFECTS

Insulin: Hypoglycemia, local redness, swelling, itching at injection site.

Sulfonylureas: Hypoglycemia, nausea, heartburn, epigastric fullness, pruritus.

Alpha-glucosidase inhibitors: Abdominal pain, diarrhea, flatulence.

Biguanides: Watery diarrhea, abdominal pain, nausea, dyspepsia, anorexia, metallic taste.

Thiazolinedione: Infection, headache, pain, asthenia.

TOXIC EFFECTS/ADVERSE REACTIONS

Severe hypoglycemia (due to hyperinsulinism) may occur in overdose of insulin, decrease or delay of food intake, excessive exercise, or those w/brittle diabetes. *Sulfonylureas:* Urticaria or rash; mild anemia, thrombocytopenia, hepatic impairment. Diabetic ketoacidosis may result from stress, illness, omission of insulin dose, or long-term poor insulin control.

PATIENT CONSIDERATIONS

GENERAL: Administer per schedule; rotate insulin injection sites. Recognize peak action times (see grid) as hypoglycemic reactions may occur at these times. Provide meals on time. INTERVENTION/EVALUATION: Monitor blood glucose levels, food consumption.

Check for hypoglycemia: cool, wet skin; tremors; dizziness; headache; anxiety; tachycardia; numbness in mouth; hunger; diplopia; restlessness, diaphoresis in sleeping pt. Check for hyperglycemia: polyuria, polyphagia, polydipsia, nausea and vomiting, dim vision, fatigue, deep rapid breathing. PATIENT/FAMILY TEACHING: Diabetes mellitus requires lifelong control. Prescribed diet is essential part of treatment; do not skip or delay meals. Weight control, exercise, hygiene (including foot care), and nonsmoking are integral part of therapy. Significance of illness, stress, and exercise on regime. Teach how to handle, administer insulin. Oral hypoglycemics should be taken 15–30 min before meal. Carry candy, sugar packets, or other sugar supplements for immediate response to hypoglycemia. Wear, carry medical alert identification. Avoid alcohol; do not take other medication w/o consulting physician. Protect skin; limit sun exposure. Select clothing, positions that do not restrict blood flow. Avoid injuries, exposure to infections. Inform dentist, physician of this medication before any treatment.

antidiarrheals

ACTION

Systemic agents: Act at smooth muscle receptors (enteric) disrupting peristaltic movements, decreasing GI motility, increasing transit time of intestinal contents.

Local agents: Adsorb toxic substances and fluids to large surface areas of particles in the preparation. Some of these agents coat and protect irritated intestinal walls. May have local anti-inflammatory action.

USES

Acute diarrhea, chronic diarrhea of inflammatory bowel disease, reduction of fluid from ileostomies.

PRECAUTIONS

CONTRAINDICATIONS: Children <2 years of age, hypersensitivity to any component. Safety not established in pregnancy, lactation. **CAUTIONS:** Young children, elderly. Not for antibiotic-associated colitis or ulcerative colitis.

INTERACTIONS

Vary according to components of individual agents. CNS depressants, anticholinergics, antihistamines increase effects of antidiarrheals.

SIDE EFFECTS

Constipation, drowsiness w/systemic agents (nausea and dry mouth w/diphenoxylate hydrochloride w/atropine sulfate).

ANTIDIARRHEALS

GENERIC NAME	BRAND NAME(S)	TYPE	FORMS	DOSAGE RANGE
bismuth subsalicylate	Pepto-Bismol	Local	Suspension Tablets	Adults: 2 tablets or 30 ml Children 9–12 yrs: 1 tablet or 15 ml Children 6–9 yrs: ⅔ tablet or 10 ml Children 3–6 yrs: ⅓ tablet or 5 ml
diphenoxylate (w/atropine)	Lomotil	Systemic	Liquid Tablets	Adults: 5 mg 4×/day Children: (liquid only): 0.3–0.4 mg/kg/day in 4 divided doses
kaolin (w/pectin)	Kaopectate	Local	Suspension	Adults: 60–120 ml after each BM Children 6–12 yrs: 30–60 ml Children 3–6 yrs: 15–30 ml
loperamide	Imodium	Systemic	Capsules Liquid	Adults: Initially, 4 mg; maximum: 16 mg/day Children 8–12 yrs: 2 mg 3×/day Children 5–8 yrs: 2 mg 2×/day Children 2–5 yrs: 1 mg 3×/day (liquid)

TOXIC EFFECTS/ADVERSE REACTIONS

Adverse reactions are infrequent w/proper dosage. Abdominal distention and cramps, dizziness, nausea and vomiting, drug dependence w/long-term use (atropine side effects w/diphenoxylate w/atropine).

PATIENT CONSIDERATIONS

GENERAL: Discontinue medication when diarrhea controlled or if abdominal distention occurs. Maintain hydration (offer 2,000–3,000 ml of fluid/day to adults). INTERVENTION/EVALUATION: Monitor stool frequency and consistency (watery, loose, soft, semisolid, solid). Check I&O and assess hydration, esp. in very young and old. PATIENT/FAMILY TEACHING: Avoid tasks that require alertness, motor skills until response to drug is established. Do not ingest alcohol or barbiturates, esp. w/drugs containing atropine. Contact physician for diarrhea that persists more than 2 days, high fever, blood in stool, or abdominal distention.

antifungals: topical

ACTION

Exact mechanism unknown. May deplete essential intracellular components by inhibiting transport of potassium, other ions into cells; alter membrane permeability resulting in loss of potassium, other cellular components.

USES

Treatment of tinea infections, cutaneous candidiasis (moniliasis) due to *Candida albicans.* Natamycin: treatment of fungal blepharitis, conjunctivitis, and keratitis.

PRECAUTIONS

CONTRAINDICATIONS: Hypersensitivity to the medication, any component of preparation. **CAUTIONS:** For external/topical use only. Avoid contact w/eyes (except natamycin). May irritate sensitized skin; discontinue if it occurs.

INTERACTIONS

None significant.

SIDE EFFECTS

Occasional: Burning, itching, stinging, erythema, pruritic rash, irritation.

TOXIC EFFECTS/ADVERSE REACTIONS

None significant.

ANTIFUNGALS: TOPICAL

Generic Name	Brand Name(s)	Availability
ciclopirox	Loprox	Cream Lotion
clioquinol	Vioform	Cream Ointment
clotrimazole	Lotrimin Mycelex	Cream Lotion Solution
econazole	Spectazole	Cream
miconazole	Micatin Monistat	Cream Powder Spray
natamycin	Natacyn	Ophthalmic suspension
tolnaftate	NP-27 Tinactin	Cream Gel Solution
triacetin	Fungoid	Cream Solution
undecylenic acid	Desenex	Cream Ointment Powder

PATIENT CONSIDERATIONS

BASELINE ASSESSMENT: Assess area of infection. Question pt as to hypersensitivity history to medication. INTERVENTION/EVALUATION: Assess improvement or increased irritation, burning, itching, swelling, oozing, redness of affected area. PATIENT/FAMILY TEACHING: For external use only, avoid contact in eyes (Exception: natamycin). Cleanse skin with soap/water and dry thoroughly. If condition persists/worsens or if irritation occurs, contact physician. Use for full treatment term, even if symptoms improve. Notify physician if no improvement seen. Avoid use of occlusive dressings unless otherwise directed.

antiglaucoma agents

Glaucoma is a condition of the eye in which an elevation of intraocular pressure (IOP) leads to damage of the optic nerve and loss of visual fields, and ultimately blindness. Increased IOP results from decreased outflow of aqueous humor through the trabecular network. The most common type of glaucoma is primary open-angle glaucoma. Treatment is accomplished by medical, laser, or surgical management.

ACTION

Currently, seven groups of agents are used in the therapy of primary open-angle glaucoma. The goal of therapy is to reduce elevated IOP, which may be accomplished by (1) decreasing the rate of aqueous humor production, and (2) increasing the rate of outflow of aqueous humor through the trabecular meshwork or uveoscleral route.

Parasympathomimetic: Miotic: direct acting: Directly stimulates smooth muscle receptors in the eye (contracts ciliary muscle, widening the trabecular meshwork; increases aqueous fluid outflow). *Miotic: indirect (anticholinesterase inhibitor):* Inhibits enzyme cholinesterase, potentiating the action of acetylcholine. Directly stimulates smooth muscle receptors in the eye (contracts ciliary muscle, widening the trabecular meshwork; increases aqueous fluid outflow).

Sympathomimetic: Alpha/beta agonists: Stimulate both alpha and beta adrenergic receptors: increases both uveoscleral and trabecular meshwork outflow of aqueous humor. *Alpha-2 agonists:* Decrease aqueous humor production and increase uveoscleral outflow of aqueous humor.

Beta blockers: Decrease production of aqueous humor, may increase aqueous outflow.

Carbonic anhydrase inhibitors: Inhibit enzyme carbonic anhydrase (decreases formation of aqueous fluid).

Prostaglandin: Increases outflow of aqueous fluid through the uveoscleral route.

USES

Reduction of elevated IOP in pts w/open-angle glaucoma and ocular hypertension.

PRECAUTIONS

CONTRAINDICATIONS: Hypersensitivity to medication or any component of the formulation. *Sympathomimetic:* Narrow-angle or shallow-angle glaucoma. *Beta blockers:* Bronchial asthma, history of bronchial asthma, severe COPD, sinus bradycardia, second- or third-degree AV block, CHF. *Miotic: direct acting:* Conditions where constriction is undesirable (e.g., acute iritis/uveitis, some forms of secondary glaucoma). *Miotic: indirect:* Active uveal inflammation, any inflammatory disease of iris or ciliary body, glaucoma associated w/iridocyclitis. **CAUTIONS:** *Sympathomimetic:* History of hypertension, diabetes, hyperthyroidism, heart disease, cerebral arteriosclerosis, bronchial asthma. *Beta blockers:* History of diabetes, hyperthyroidism, cerebral vascular insufficiency. *Miotic: direct acting:* History of acute cardiac failure, bronchial asthma, peptic ulcer, hyperthyroidism, GI spasm, urinary tract obstruction, Parkinson's disease, recent myocardial infarction, hyper/hypotension. *Miotic: indirect:* Myasthenia gravis, narrow-angle glaucoma, bronchial asthma, GI spasm, peptic ulcer, recent myocardial infarction, epilepsy, Parkinson's disease. *Carbonic anhydrase inhibitors:* Pts w/renal or hepatic impairment.

INTERACTIONS

Sympathomimetic: Tricyclic antidepressants may increase cardiovascular effects, may decrease effects of beta blockers; digoxin, other sympathomimetics may increase risk of arrhythmias. *Beta blockers:* Systemic beta blockers may increase effects on systemic blockade; quinidine, verapamil may cause sinus bradycardia. *Miotic: direct acting:* Topical NSAIDs may decrease effect. *Miotic: indirect:* W/succinylcholine during general anesthesia, may cause respiratory and cardiovascular collapse. *Carbonic anhydrase inhibitors:* None significant. *Prostaglandin:* Eye drops containing thimerosal may cause precipitate (give w/interval of at least 5 min).

SIDE EFFECTS

Parasympathomimetic: Direct acting: Decreased vision/dark adaptation, pupil constriction, difficulty driving at night, brow ache, increased perspiration/salivation/bronchial secretions. *Indirect acting:* Same as direct acting. Additionally: cataracts, iris cysts, cystoid macular edema, corneal toxicity.

Sympathomimetic: Alpha/beta: Conjunctival pigment deposit, stinging/burning, pupil dilation, macular edema, corneal endothelium damage, hypertension, increased heart rate, arrhythmias, headache, nervousness. *Alpha-2 agonist:* Hyperemia, pruritus, lid edema, dry eye, conjunctival blanching, mydriasis, fatigue, dry mouth/nose.

Beta blockers: Burning, stinging, ocular irritation, conjunctivitis, blepharitis, keratitis, visual disturbances, brow ache.

Carbonic anhydrase inhibitors: Stinging, bitter taste, paresthesias, GI upset, altered taste, lethargy, depression, diuresis.

Prostaglandin: Redness, conjunctival irritation, iris pigmentation.

TOXIC EFFECTS/ADVERSE REACTIONS

None significant.

ANTIGLAUCOMA AGENTS

GENERIC NAME	BRAND NAME(S)	AVAILABILITY	USUAL DOSAGE
PARASYMPATHOMIMETIC			
Direct Acting			
carbachol	Isopto Carbachol	Solution: 0.75%, 1.5%, 2.25%, 3%	1 drop 2 times/day
pilocarpine	Isopto Carpine	Solution: 0.25%, 0.5%, 1%, 2%, 3%, 4%, 5%, 6%, 8%, 10%	1–2 drops 3–4 times/day
		Gel: 4%	0.5 inch at bedtime
	Ocusert	Insert: 20 mcg/hr, 40 mcg/hr	One insert weekly
Indirect Acting			
echothiophate	Phospholine Iodide	Solution: 0.03%, 0.06%, 0.125%, 0.25%	1 drop 2 times/day
physostigmine	Eserine	Ointment: 0.25%	Apply up to 3 times/day
demecarium	Humorsol	Solution: 0.125%, 0.25%	1–2 drops 2 times/day up to 2 times/wk
SYMPATHOMIMETIC			
Alpha/Beta			
epinephrine	Epifrin, Epinal, Glaucon	Solution: 0.5%, 1%, 2%	1 drop 1–2 times/day
dipivefrin	Propine	Solution: 0.1%	1 drop q12h
Alpha-2 agonist			
apraclonidine	Iopidine	Solution: 0.5%	1–2 drops 3 times/day
brimonidine	Alphagan	Solution: 0.2%	1–2 drops 2–3 times/day
BETA BLOCKERS			
betaxolol	Betoptic	Suspension: 0.25%	1–2 drops 2 times/day
		Solution: 0.5%	1–2 drops 2 times/day
carteolol	Ocupress	Solution: 1%	1 drop 2 times/day
levobunolol	Betagan	Solution: 0.25%, 0.5%	1 drop 1–2 times/day
metipranolol	Optipranolol	Solution: 0.3%	1 drop 2 times/day
timolol	Betimol, Timoptic	Solution: 0.25%, 0.5%	1 drop 2 times/day
	Timoptic XE	Gel: 0.25%, 0.5%	1 drop daily
CARBONIC ANHYDRASE INHIBITORS			
dorzolamide	Trusopt	Solution: 2%	1 drop 2–3 times/day
brinzolamide	Azopt	Suspension: 1%	1 drop 3 times/day
acetazolamide	Diamox	Tablets: 125 mg, 250 mg Capsules: 500 mg	250 mg to 1 g/day
methazolamide	Neptazine	Tablets: 25 mg, 50 mg	50–100 mg 2–3 times/day
dichlorphenamide	Daranide	Tablets: 50 mg	25–50 mg 1–3 times/day
PROSTAGLANDIN			
latanoprost	Xalatan	Solution: 0.005%	1 drop daily in evening
unoprostone	Rescula	Solution: 0.15%	1 drop 2 times/day

PATIENT CONSIDERATIONS

BASELINE ASSESSMENT: Question for hypersensitivity to medication or any component of formulation. Obtain baseline pulse, B/P. Assess physical appearance of eye and pt's perception of vision. EVALUA-

TION/INTERVENTION: Evaluate therapeutic response. Assess for systemic effects. Check B/P, pulse, respirations. PATIENT/FAMILY TEACHING: Teach proper administration of ophthalmic medication. To avoid contamination, do not touch container to any surface. Replace cap after using. Report any decrease in visual acuity, any ocular reaction. Slight stinging/burning may occur on initial instillation. Avoid allowing tip of container to contact eye or surrounding structures. If more than one topical ophthalmic drug is being used, administer at least 5 min apart.

antihistamines

ACTION

Antihistamines (H_1 antagonists) inhibit vasoconstrictor effects and vasodilator effects on endothelial cells of histamine. They block increased capillary permeability, formation of edema/wheal caused by histamine. Many antihistamines can bind to receptors in CNS causing primarily depression (decreased alertness, slowed reaction times, somnolence) but also stimulation (restless, nervousness, inability to sleep). Some may counter motion sickness.

USES

Symptomatic relief of upper respiratory allergic disorders. Allergic reactions associated w/other drugs respond to antihistamines, as do blood transfusion reactions. Used as a second-choice drug in the treatment of angioneurotic edema. Effective in treatment of acute urticaria and other dermatologic conditions. May also be used for preop sedation. Parkinson's disease and motion sickness.

PRECAUTIONS

CONTRAINDICATIONS: Hypersensitivity-cross sensitivity, infants, asthma, narrow-angle glaucoma, prostatic hypertrophy, bladder neck obstruction, CNS depression, hypertension, third trimester of pregnancy, lactation. **CAUTIONS:** Young children, elderly experience exaggerated results: Children, paradoxical excitement; elderly, heavy sedation. Care should be exercised w/cardiovascular disease, hyperthyroidism, and convulsive disorders. Safety during first and second trimester of pregnancy not established.

INTERACTIONS

Alcohol, CNS depressants may increase CNS depressant effects. Anticholinergics may increase anticholinergic effects. MAO inhibitors may increase anticholinergic, CNS depressant effects. Erythromycin, ketoconazole may increase risk of cardiotoxic effect w/astemizole, terfenadine.

ANTIHISTAMINES

GENERIC NAME	BRAND NAME(S)	DOSAGE RANGE
brompheniramine	Dimetane	Adults: 4 mg q4–6h Children 6–12 yrs: 2 mg q4–6h
cetirizine	Zyrtec	Adults: 5–20 mg/day
chlorpheniramine	Chlor-Trimeton	Adults, children >12 yrs: 4 mg q4–6h Children 6–12 yrs: 2 mg q4–6h
clemastine	Tavist	Adults, children >12 yrs: 1.34 mg 2x/day up to 2.68 mg 3x/day
cyproheptadine	Periactin	Adults: 4–20 mg/day Children 7–14 yrs: 4 mg 2–3x/day Children 2–7 yrs: 2 mg 2–3x/day
dexchlorpheniramine	Polaramine	Adults: 2 mg q4–6h Children 6–11 yrs: 1 mg q4–6h
dimenhydrinate	Dramamine	Adults, children >12 yrs: 50–100 mg q4–6h Children 6–12 yrs: 25–50 mg q6–8h Children 2–6 yrs: Up to 12.5–25 mg q6–8h
diphenhydramine	Benadryl	Adults: 25–50 mg q6–8h Children >10 kg: 12.5–25 mg 3–4x/day
loratidine	Claritin	Adults: 10 mg/day Children >12 yrs: 10 mg/day
promethazine	Phenergan	Adults: 25 mg at bedtime or 12.5 mg 3–4x/day Children: 25 mg at hs or 6.25 12.5 mg 3–4x/day

SIDE EFFECTS

Sedation, headache, dizziness, nervousness, restlessness, irritability, loss of appetite, palpitations, urinary retention, constipation.

TOXIC EFFECTS/ADVERSE REACTIONS

Convulsions, hallucinations, tight chest w/shortness of breath, incoordination, flushing of face, hyperthermia, CNS may demonstrate overstimulation or depression. Children are particularly susceptible to overdosage.

PATIENT CONSIDERATIONS

GENERAL: Take safety precautions when given concurrently w/narcotic analgesics (use side rails; assist w/ambulation). BASELINE ASSESSMENT: Determine initial B/P, temperature, pulse, respiration. INTERVENTION/EVALUATION: Monitor B/P, temperature, pulse, respiration. Assess therapeutic response to medication; be alert to adverse reactions. Check lung sounds. Maintain I&O; assess for urinary retention. Monitor bowel activity; avoid constipation. PATIENT/FAMILY TEACHING: Take oral doses w/meals. Drink 8 or more glasses of fluid/day to decrease viscosity of secretions and help prevent constipation. Do not drive or engage in activities that may be affected by sedative effects. For motion sickness, take ½ to 1 hour before traveling. Avoid alcohol and other medications unless physician approves. Explain adverse reactions, need to report immediately.

antihyperlipidemics

ACTION

Hyperlipidemias are conditions in which the concentration of cholesterol or triglycerides carrying lipoprotein exceeds normal limits. These elevations can accelerate development of atherosclerosis and may lead to thrombosis or myocardial infarction. Cholesterol and triglycerides are transported in lipoproteins including chylomicrons, very low-density lipoprotein (VLDL), which transport triglycerides, low-density lipoproteins (LDL) and high-density lipoproteins (HDL), which transport cholesterol. Agents used in the treatment of hyperlipidemia include:

HMG CoA reductase inhibitors: Block synthesis of cholesterol in liver. Produce a dose-related decrease in the concentration of LDL cholesterol; decrease triglyceride concentration; increase HDL cholesterol.

Fibric acids: Reduce plasma triglycerides by decreasing concentration of VLDL. Primary effect is to increase lipoprotein lipase (promotes VLDL catabolism). May decrease hepatic synthesis/secretion of VLDL.

Bile acid sequestrants: Decrease concentration of cholesterol by lowering LDL levels. Bind bile acids in intestine causing increased fecal excretion, which causes increased production of bile acids from cholesterol.

USES

HMG CoA reductase inhibitors: Adjunctive therapy for reducing elevated total and LDL cholesterol in pts w/primary hypercholesterolemia (types IIa and IIb). *Fibric acids:* Treatment of hypertriglyceridemia in pts w/type IV and V hyperlipidemia. *Bile acid sequestrants:* Adjunctive therapy for reducing elevated serum cholesterol in pts w/primary hypercholesterolemia (types IIa and IIb).

PRECAUTIONS

CONTRAINDICATIONS: Pregnancy, lactation, hypersensitivity to drug or components, liver disease, biliary cirrhosis or obstruction, severe renal dysfunction. **CAUTIONS:** History of liver disease, substantial alcohol consumption. Safety and efficacy in children not established.

INTERACTIONS

HMG CoA reductase inhibitor: Increased risk of rhabdomyolysis, acute renal failure w/cyclosporine, erythromycin, gemfibrozil, niacin, other immunosuppressants.
Fibric acid: May increase effects of oral anticoagulants, hypoglycemics.
Bile acid sequestrants: May increase effects of anticoagulants by decreasing vitamin K. May decrease warfarin absorption. May bind, decrease absorption of digoxin, thiazides, penicillins, propranolol, tetracyclines, folic acid, thyroid hormones, other medications. Bind, decrease effect of oral vancomycin.

SIDE EFFECTS

GI effects usually lessen or disappear w/continued therapy: constipation, hemorrhoid irritation, diarrhea, abdominal distention, belching, nausea, vomiting. Headache, urticaria, rash. *HMG CoA reductase inhibitors:* Myalgia. Blurred vision w/lovastatin and gemfibrozil.

ANTIHYPERLIPIDEMICS

Generic Name	Brand Name(s)	Type	Dosage Range
atorvastatin	Lipitor	HMG CoA reductase inhibitor	10–80 mg/day
cerivastatin	Baycol	HMG CoA reductase inhibitor	0.2–0.3 mg/day
cholestyramine	Colybar Questran	Bile acid sequestrant	4–24 g/day
colesevelam	Welchol	Bile acid sequestrant	6–7 tablets/day
colestipol	Colestid	Bile acid sequestrant	5–30 g/day
clofibrate	Atromid-S	Fibric acid	2 g/day
fenofibrate	Tricor	Fibric acid	67–201 mg/day
fluvastatin	Lescol	HMG CoA reductase inhibitor	20–40 mg/day
gemfibrozil	Lopid	Fibric acid	1,200 mg/day
lovastatin	Mevacor	HMG CoA reductase inhibitor	20–80 mg/day
pravastatin	Pravachol	HMG CoA reductase inhibitor	10–40 mg/day
simvastatin	Zocor	HMG CoA reductase inhibitor	5–40 mg/day

TOXIC EFFECTS/ADVERSE REACTIONS

Severe constipation w/fecal impaction, GI bleeding, cholelithiasis, acute appendicitis. Angina and cardiac arrhythmias have occurred w/some drugs.

PATIENT CONSIDERATIONS

GENERAL: Dietary corrections should be attempted before initiating drug therapy. BASELINE ASSESSMENT: Determine serum cholesterol and triglyceride levels. INTERVENTION/EVALUATION: Monitor GI effects, esp. constipation or diarrhea. Check serum cholesterol and triglyceride levels periodically. PATIENT/FAMILY TEACHING: Complete full course; do not omit or change doses. Importance of diet in therapy: Reduce fats, sugars, and cholesterol. Eat high-fiber foods (whole grain cereals, fruits, vegetables) to reduce potential for constipation. Drink several glasses of water between meals. Promptly report bleeding, constipation, or muscle pain/tenderness (esp. w/fever or malaise).

antihypertensives

ACTION

Many groups of medications are used in the treatment of hypertension. In addition to the alpha-adrenergic central agonists and peripheral antagonists and vasodilators discussed below, refer to the classifications of diuretics, beta-adrenergic blockers, calcium channel blockers, and ACE inhibitors, or individual monographs of drugs.

Alpha agonists (central action): Stimulate alpha$_2$-adrenergic receptors in cardiovascular centers of CNS, reducing sympathetic outflow and producing antihypertensive effect.

Alpha antagonists (peripheral action): Block alpha$_1$-adrenergic receptors in arterioles, veins inhibiting vasoconstriction, decreasing peripheral vascular resistance, causing a fall in B/P.

Vasodilators: Directly relax arteriolar smooth muscle, decreasing vascular resistance. Exact mechanism unknown.

USES

Treatment of mild to severe hypertension, depending on agent selected.

PRECAUTIONS

CONTRAINDICATIONS: Hypersensitivity; severe hepatic dysfunction; pheochromocytoma; advanced renal disease; rheumatic heart disease; systemic lupus erythematosus. **CAUTIONS:** Renal impairment, children, pregnancy, lactation, elderly, angina or ischemic heart disease, after myocardial infarction.

INTERACTIONS

Diuretics, other antihypertensive agents, alcohol increase hypotensive effects. Sympathomimetics may decrease hypotensive effect. Refer to individual monographs for additional information.

SIDE EFFECTS

Specific reactions vary according to the agent given. Weakness, postural hypotension, headache, fatigue, drowsiness, nausea are common.

ANTIHYPERTENSIVES

		Antihypertensive Effect			
Generic Name	Brand Name(s)	Onset (hrs)	Peak (hrs)	Duration (hrs)	Dosage Range
CENTRAL ACTION					
clonidine	Catapres Catapres-TTS	0.5–1	2–4	12–24	PO: 0.2–0.8 mg/day Topical: 0.1–0.6 mg/wk
guanabenz	Wytensin	1	2–4	6–12	PO: 8–32 mg/day
guanfacine	Tenex	—	1–4	24	PO: 1–3 mg/day
methyldopa	Aldomet	2	4–6	12–24	PO: 0.5–3 g/day
PERIPHERAL ACTION					
doxazosin	Cardura	—	—	—	PO: 2–16 mg/day
guanadrel	Hylorel	0.5–2	4–6	9–14	PO: 20–75 mg/day
prazosin	Minipress	2	1–3	6–12	PO: 6–20 mg/day
terazosin	Hytrin	0.25	1–2	12–24	PO: 1–20 mg/day
VASODILATORS					
hydralazine	Apresoline	0.75	0.5–2	6–8	PO: 40–300 mg/day
minoxidil	Loniten	0.5	2–3	24–72	PO: 10–40 mg/day

TOXIC EFFECTS/ADVERSE REACTIONS

Bradycardia and tachycardia; palpitations; hypersensitivity reactions; nausea, vomiting, diarrhea or constipation, arthralgia, reduced hemoglobin, leukopenia, edema. Other reactions per specific agent.

PATIENT CONSIDERATIONS

GENERAL: For IV administration, monitor pt carefully; place on cardiac monitor and prevent extravasation. BASELINE ASSESSMENT: Determine initial B/P and apical pulse. INTERVENTION/EVALUATION: Monitor apical pulse and B/P; check w/physician for B/P or pulse below parameters set for that pt. Check for edema of hands, feet. PATIENT/FAMILY TEACHING: Teach pt and/or family how to take B/P and pulse. Make position changes slowly (decreases orthostatic hypotension). Follow diet and control weight. Restrict sodium as indicated. Avoid alcohol. Cease smoking. Do not take other medications w/o consulting physician. Do not stop taking medication. Need for lifelong control.

antipsychotics

ACTION

Effects of these agents occur at all levels of the CNS. Antipsychotic mechanism unknown, but may antagonize dopamine action as a neurotransmitter in basal ganglia and limbic system. Antipsychotics may block postsynaptic dopamine receptors, inhibit dopamine release, increase dopamine turnover. These medications can be divided into the phenothiazines and nonphenothiazines (miscellaneous). In addition to their use in symptomatic treatment of psychiatric illness, some have antiemetic, antinausea, antihistamine, anticholinergic, and/or sedative effects.

USES

Antipsychotics are primarily used in managing psychotic illness (esp. those w/increased psychomotor activity). They are also used to treat manic phase of bipolar disorder, behavioral problems in children, nausea and vomiting, intractable hiccups, anxiety and agitation, as adjunct in treatment of tetanus, and to potentiate effects of narcotics.

PRECAUTIONS

CONTRAINDICATIONS: Alcoholism or other CNS depression, hepatic dysfunction, bone marrow depression, hypotension, glaucoma, cardiovascular disease, peptic ulcer, young children, hypersensitivity to any of the phenothiazines, pregnancy, lactation. **CAUTIONS:** Administer cautiously to elderly and debilitated pts; this group is more sensitive to effects and requires lower dosage. Drug should be withdrawn slowly; should be discontinued at least 48 hrs before surgery.

INTERACTIONS

Alcohol, CNS depressants may increase CNS, respiratory depression, hypotensive effects. Tricyclic antidepressants, MAO inhibitors may increase sedative, anticholinergic effects. Antithyroid agents may increase risk of agranulocytosis. Extrapyramidal symptoms (EPS) may increase w/EPS-producing medications. Hypotensives may increase hypotension. May decrease levodopa effects. Lithium may decrease absorption, produce adverse neurologic effects.

ANTIPSYCHOTICS

		Side Effects				
Generic Name	Brand Name(s)	Sedation	Hypotension	Anticholinergic	EPS	Dosage (mg/day)
chlorpromazine	Thorazine	High	High	Moderate	Moderate	30–800
clozapine	Clozaril	High	High	High	Low	25–900
fluphenazine	Prolixin	Low	Low	Low	High	0.5–50
haloperidol	Haldol	Low	Low	Low	High	1–100
loxapine	Loxitane	Moderate	Moderate	Low	High	20–250
mesoridazine	Serentil	High	Moderate	High	Low	30–400
molindone	Moban	Low	Low	Low	High	50–225
olanzapine	Zyprexa	Moderate	Low	Moderate	Low	5–20
perphenazine	Trilafon	Low	Low	Low	High	12–64
pimozide	Orap	Moderate	Low	Moderate	High	1–10
quetiapine	Seroquel	Moderate	Moderate	Moderate	Low	150–750
risperidone	Risperdal	Low	Low	Low	Moderate	4–6
thioridazine	Mellaril	High	High	High	Low	150–800
thiothixene	Navane	Low	Low	Low	High	6–60
trifluoperazine	Stelazine	Low	Low	Low	High	4–40

EPS = extrapyramidal symptoms.

SIDE EFFECTS

Orthostatic hypotension, drowsiness, blurred vision, constipation, nasal congestion, photosensitivity.

TOXIC EFFECTS/ADVERSE REACTIONS

Hyperpyrexia, depression, insomnia, convulsions, hypertension, adynamic ileus, laryngospasm, bronchospasm, urticaria, menstrual irregularities, impotence, urinary retention, blood dyscrasias, systemic lupus-like reaction, extrapyramidal reactions.

PATIENT CONSIDERATIONS

GENERAL: Do not mix parenteral solution w/other drugs in the same syringe; give deep IM injections. Have pt remain recumbent for at least 30 min; following parenteral dose, arise slowly and w/assistance. Avoid skin contact w/solutions (contact dermatitis). BASELINE ASSESSMENT: Determine initial B/P, pulse, respirations. Assess pt and environment for necessary supports. INTERVENTION/EVALUATION: Monitor B/P. Assess mental status, response to surroundings.

Be alert to suicide potential as energy increases. Assure that oral medication is swallowed. Check bowel activity; avoid constipation. Promptly notify physician of extrapyramidal reactions (usually dose related; more frequent in female geriatric pts). PATIENT/FAMILY TEACHING: Take medication as ordered; do not stop taking or increase dosage. Do not drive or perform activities requiring motor skills until response has been controlled. Side effects usually subside after approximately 2 wks of therapy or can be eliminated/minimized by dosage adjustment. Avoid temperature extremes. Avoid alcohol, other medications. Inform other physicians, dentist of drug therapy. Change positions slowly to prevent orthostatic hypotension.

antivirals

Antiviral medications have recently expanded in number due primarily to the increased number of anti-retroviral agents available for treating patients with HIV infection and its complications. Many of the antivirals are directed toward disrupting one of the many steps in viral infection and replication. Viruses consist of either a single- or double-stranded DNA or RNA enclosed in a protein coat (capsid). Some viruses also have a lipoprotein envelope that may also contain antigenic proteins; other viruses contain enzymes that initiate viral replication inside a host cell. Viruses reproduce or replicate within cells of the host depending on metabolic processes of the host cell. They cannot reproduce independent of a host cell because viruses have no metabolic machinery of their own.

Stages of viral replication include cell entry (attachment, penetration); uncoating (release of viral genome); transcription of viral genome (transcription of viral mRNA, replication of viral genome); translation of viral proteins; post-translational modifications; assembly of virion components; release (budding). Replication cycle begins when a virion (viral particle) binds to a receptor site on the plasma membrane of a host cell. Once bound, the virus releases enzymes weakening the plasma membrane, allowing penetration of the virus. Inside the host cell, the outer coat of the virus dissolves releasing viral genetic material (viral genome), which regulates metabolic activity of the host cell by directing its own replication (synthesis of new messenger RNA [mRNA]) using host ribosomes and viral proteins. After viral nucleic acids/proteins (virion compound) are assembled to form a mature virus, it is released from the host cell (budding) for transmission to other host cells, spreading viral infection.

Viruses are DNA or RNA. DNA viruses include herpesvirus (chicken pox, shingles, herpes) and adenoviruses (conjunctivitis, sore throat). Usually DNA viruses enter the host cell nucleus where viral DNA is transcribed into mRNA of host cell by host cell mRNA polymerase; mRNA is then translated into virus-specific protein following the usual host cell mechanisms. RNA viruses include rubella (German measles), orthomyxoviruses (influenza), and paramyxoviruses (measles, mumps). RNA virus replication in the host cell relies on enzymes in the virion to synthesize its mRNA or on the viral RNA serving as its own mRNA. The mRNA is then translated into various viral proteins, including RNA polymerase that directs the synthesis of more viral mRNA. Most RNA viruses do not involve the host cell in viral replication.

One special group of RNA viruses, known as retroviruses, are responsible for diseases such as AIDS and T-cell leukemias. Retroviruses contain a reverse transcriptase enzyme activity that makes a DNA copy of the viral RNA template. This DNA copy is then integrated into the host genome and transcribed into both genome RNA and mRNA for translation into viral proteins, giving rise to new virus particles.

ACTION

Effective antivirals must inhibit virus-specific nucleic acid/protein synthesis. Possible mechanisms of action of antivirals used for non-HIV infection may include interfering with viral DNA synthesis and viral replication, inactivation of viral DNA polymerases, incorporation and termination of the growing viral DNA chain, prevention of release of viral nucleic acid into the host cell, or interference with viral penetration into cells.

Currently three classes of agents are available for the treatment of HIV infection: nucleoside analogues (reverse transcriptase inhibitors), protease inhibitors, and non-nucleoside reverse transcriptase inhibitors (NNRT).

Nucleoside analogues inhibit viral enzyme reverse transcriptase, reducing replication of cell-included HIV virus.

Protease inhibitors suppress viral replication by inhibiting protease, an enzyme responsible for cleaving viral precursor polypeptides with mature/infective virions.

NNRT inhibits catalytic reaction of reverse transcriptase that is independent of nucleoside binding.

USES

Treatment of HIV infection. Treatment of CMV retinitis in patients with AIDS, acute herpes zoster (shingles), genital herpes (recurrent), mucosal and cutaneous herpes simplex virus, chicken pox, and influenza A viral illness.

ANTIVIRALS

Generic Name	Brand Name(s)	Labeled Uses
abacavir	Ziagen	HIV infection
acyclovir	Zovirax	*Parenteral:* Mucosal/cutaneous HSV-1 and HSV-2 Varicella zoster (shingles) Genital herpes Herpes simplex encephalitis

(continued)

ANTIVIRALS *Continued*

GENERIC NAME	BRAND NAME(S)	LABELED USES
		Oral: Genital herpes Herpes zoster (shingles) Chicken pox (varicella)
amantadine	Symmetrel	Influenza A virus respiratory tract illness
cidofovir	Vistide	CMV retinitis in pts w/AIDS
delavirdine	Rescriptor	HIV infection
didanosine	Videx	HIV infection
efavirenz	Sustiva	HIV infection
famciclovir	Famvir	Acute herpes zoster (shingles) Genital herpes (recurrent)
fomivirsen	Vitravene	CMV retinitis
foscarnet	Foscavir	CMV retinitis HSV infections in immunocompromised pts
ganciclovir	Cytovene	CMV retinitis, CMV disease
indinavir	Crixivan	HIV infection
lamivudine	Epivir	HIV infection
lopinavir/ritonavir	Kaletra	HIV infection
nelfinavir	Viracept	HIV infection
nevirapine	Viramune	HIV infection
penciclovir	Denavir	Cold sores
ramantadine	Flumadine	Influenza A virus
ribavirin	Virazole	Lower respiratory infection in infants, children due to respiratory syncytial virus (RSV)
ritonavir	Norvir	HIV infection
saquinavir	Invirase	HIV infection
stavudine	Zerit	HIV infection
valacyclovir	Valtrex	Herpes zoster (shingles) Genital herpes (recurrent)
zalcitabine	Hivid	HIV infection
zidovudine	Retrovir	HIV infection

PRECAUTIONS

CONTRAINDICATIONS: Hypersensitivity to any component of the product.

Note: Because of the diversity of the antivirals, refer to individual monographs for further information on cautions, side effects, adverse/toxic effects, drug interactions, etc.

PATIENT CONSIDERATIONS

BASELINE ASSESSMENT: Assess health history (past medical, drug history, lifestyle, type/severity of symptoms). Ask about fatigue, chills, sweating, skin color changes. Note any localized swelling, pain, tenderness in lymph node regions. Assess for pregnancy/lactation. INTERVENTION/EVALUATION: Monitor renal function, fluid status, I/O, sleep and rest patterns, altered nutrition related to nausea produced by the antivirals. Observe for therapeutic effect, signs/symptoms of improvement. Monitor for undesired clinical response/toxicity associated w/ antivirals. Review results assessing renal/hepatic function and integrity

of hemopoietic system. Inspect IV infusion site carefully. PATIENT/FAMILY TEACHING: Inform pt of importance of immunization and maintaining immunization against viral infections for small children and adults at high risk of acquiring influenza. Inform pt of importance of adequate fluid intake. Call physician if condition worsens or pt experiences any toxicity with the medication. Inform of ways to control spread/recurrence of viral infections. Drug therapy for AIDS/genital herpes does not prevent transmission to others or prevent opportunistic infections.

beta-adrenergic blockers

ACTION

Beta-adrenergic blockers competitively block $beta_1$-adrenergic receptors, located primarily in myocardium, and $beta_2$-adrenergic receptors, located primarily in bronchial and vascular smooth muscle. By occupying beta-receptor sites, these agents prevent naturally occurring or administered epinephrine/norepinephrine from exerting their effects. The results are basically opposite to that of sympathetic stimulation.

Effect of $beta_1$-blockade includes slowing heart rate, decreasing cardiac output and contractility; effect of $beta_2$-blockade includes bronchoconstriction, increased airway resistance in those w/asthma or COPD. Beta blockers can affect cardiac rhythm/automaticity (decrease sinus rate, SA, AV conduction; increase refractory period in AV node). Decrease systolic and diastolic B/P; exact mechanism unknown but may block peripheral receptors, decrease sympathetic outflow from CNS, or decrease renin release from kidney. All beta blockers mask tachycardia that occurs w/hypoglycemia. When applied to the eye, reduces intraocular pressure and aqueous production.

USES

Management of hypertension, angina pectoris, arrhythmias, hypertrophic subaortic stenosis, migraine headaches, myocardial infarction (prevention), glaucoma.

PRECAUTIONS

CONTRAINDICATIONS: Severe renal or hepatic disease, history of allergy, hyperthyroidism, asthma, emphysema, CHF, cerebrovascular accident, hypotension, sinus bradycardia, pregnancy. Safety in lactation not established. **CAUTIONS:** Diabetes mellitus, elderly, peptic ulcer.

INTERACTIONS

Diuretics, other hypotensives may increase hypotensive effect. Sympathomimetics, xanthines may mutually inhibit effects. May mask symptoms of hypoglycemia, prolong hypoglycemic effect of insulin, oral hypoglycemics. NSAIDs may decrease antihypertensive effect. Cimetidine may increase concentration.

BETA BLOCKERS

GENERIC NAME	BRAND NAME(S)	SELECTIVITY	USES	DOSAGE RANGE
acebutolol	Sectral	$Beta_1$	HTN, arrhythmias	HTN: 200–1,200 mg/day Arrhythmias: 600–1,200 mg/day
atenolol	Tenormin	$Beta_1$	HTN, angina, MI	HTN: 50–100 mg/day Angina: 50–200 mg/day MI: 50–100 mg/day
betaxolol	Kerlone Betoptic	$Beta_1$	HTN, ocular HTN, glaucoma	HTN: 10–20 mg/day Ophth: 1 drop 2×/day
bisoprolol	Zebeta	$Beta_1$	HTN	HTN: 2.5–20 mg/day
carteolol	Cartrol	$Beta_1$, $beta_2$	HTN	HTN: 2.5–10 mg/day
carvedilol	Coreg	Beta, $beta_2$, $alpha_1$	HTN	HTN: 12.5–50 mg/day
esmolol	Brevibloc	$Beta_1$	Arrhythmias	Arrhythmias: 50–200 mcg/kg/min
labetalol	Normodyne Trandate	$Beta_1$, $beta_2$ $Alpha_1$	Hypertension	HTN: 200–400 mg/day
levobunolol	Betagan	$Beta_1$, $beta_2$	Ocular HTN, glaucoma	Ophth: 1 drop 1–2×/day
metipranolol	OptiPranolol	$Beta_1$, $beta_2$	Ocular HTN, glaucoma	Ophth: 1 drop 2×/day
metoprolol	Lopressor	$Beta_1$	HTN, angina MI	HTN: 100–450 mg/day Angina: 100–400 mg/day MI: 50 mg q6h
nadolol	Corgard	$Beta_1$, $beta_2$	HTN, angina	HTN: 40–320 mg/day Angina: 40–240 mg/day
penbutolol	Levotol	$Beta_1$, $beta_2$	HTN	HTN: 10–40 mg/day
pindolol	Visken	$Beta_1$, $beta_2$	HTN	HTN: 10–60 mg/day
propranolol	Inderal	$Beta_1$, $beta_2$	HTN, angina, arrhythmias, MI, migraine, tremors	HTN: 120–640 mg/day Angina: 80–320 mg/day Arrhythmias: 10–30 mg 3–4×/day MI: 180–240 mg/day
sotalol	Betapace	$Beta_1$, $beta_2$	Arrhythmias	Arrhythmias: 160–640 mg/day
timolol	Blocadren Timoptic	$Beta_1$, $beta_2$	HTN, MI, migraine, glaucoma	HTN: 10–60 mg/day MI: 10 mg 2×/day Ophth: 1 drop 1–2×/day

HTN = hypertension; MI = myocardial infarction.

SIDE EFFECTS

Postural hypotension, lightheadedness, fatigue, weakness, reflex tachycardia.

TOXIC EFFECTS/ADVERSE REACTIONS

Severe hypotension, nausea and vomiting, bradycardia, heart block, circulatory failure.

PATIENT CONSIDERATIONS

GENERAL: Use cardiac monitor for IV administration and preferably for initiation of oral therapy. BASELINE ASSESSMENT: Initial B/P, apical pulse. INTERVENTION/EVALUATION: Monitor B/P and apical pulse before giving drug; notify physician before administration if B/P or pulse

are not within agreed parameters. Assess for CHF (dyspnea, peripheral edema, jugular venous distension, increased weight, rales in lungs, decreased urine output). Assess extremities for peripheral circulation (warmth, color, quality of pulses). PATIENT/FAMILY TEACHING: Teach how to take B/P, pulse correctly. Change position slowly to prevent orthostatic hypotension. Do not take OTC cold medications, nasal decongestants. Restrict sodium and alcohol as ordered. Do not stop taking drug suddenly. Report chest pain, fatigue, shortness of breath.

bronchodilators

ACTION

Asthma (reversible airway obstruction) is the most common breathing disorder.

Methylxanthines: Directly relax smooth muscle of bronchial airway, pulmonary blood vessels (relieve bronchospasm, increase vital capacity). Increase cyclic 3,5-adenosine monophosphate.

Beta$_2$-adrenergic agonists: Stimulate beta receptors in lung, relax bronchial smooth muscle, increase vital capacity, decrease airway resistance.

Anticholinergics: Inhibit cholinergic receptors on bronchial smooth muscle (block acetylcholine action).

Leukotriene receptor antagonist: Blocks effects of leukotriene (bronchoconstriction, inflammation, edema).

Antileukotriene: Inhibits enzyme 5-lipoxygenase, reducing production of leukotriene, a bronchoconstrictor.

USES

Relief of bronchospasm occurring during anesthesia; in bronchial asthma, bronchitis, or emphysema.

PRECAUTIONS

CONTRAINDICATIONS: Hypersensitivity to that agent or intolerance to others in the classification, components of preparation. Severe renal or hepatic dysfunction. **CAUTIONS:** Pregnancy, lactation, elderly, hepatic disease, CHF, or other cardiac conditions that would be adversely affected by cardiac stimulation.

INTERACTIONS

Methylxanthines: Glucocorticoids may produce hypernatremia. Phenytoin, primidone, rifampin may increase metabolism. Beta blockers may decrease effects. Cimetidine, ciprofloxacin, erythromycin, norfloxacin may increase concentration, toxicity. Smoking may decrease concentration.

Beta$_2$-adrenergic agonists: General anesthetics may increase risk of arrhythmias. Tricyclic antidepressants, maprotiline may increase cardiovascular effects. May have mutually inhibitory effects w/beta-adrenergic blockers. May increase risk of arrhythmias w/digoxin.
Anticholinergics: None significant.

BRONCHODILATORS

GENERIC NAME	BRAND NAME(S)	ROUTE OF ADMINISTRATION	TYPE
albuterol	Proventil Ventolin	Inhalation Oral	Beta$_2$ agonist
aminophylline	—	Oral Intravenous	Methylxanthine
bitolterol	Tornalate	Inhalation	Beta$_2$ agonist
epinephrine	Adrenalin	SubQ Intravenous	Beta$_2$ agonist
ipratropium	Atrovent	Inhalation	Anticholinergic
isoetharine	Bronkosol	Inhalation	Beta$_2$ agonist
isoproterenol	Isuprel	Inhalation	Beta$_2$ agonist
levalbuterol	Xopenex	Inhalation	Beta$_2$ agonist
metaproterenol	Alupent	Inhalation	Beta$_2$ agonist
montelukast	Singulair	Oral	Leukotriene receptor antagonist
salmeterol	Serevent	Inhalation	Beta$_2$ agonist
terbutaline	Brethine Bricanyl	Inhalation Oral SubQ	Beta$_2$ agonist
theophylline	Aerolate Slo-Bid Slo-Phyllin Theo-24 Theo-Dur Theolair Uniphyl	Oral	Methylxanthine
zafirlukast	Accolate	Oral	Leukotriene receptor antagonist
zileuton	Zyflo	Oral	Antileukotriene

SIDE EFFECTS

Nausea, increased pulse rate, nervousness, weakness, trembling, insomnia.

TOXIC EFFECTS/ADVERSE REACTIONS

Tachycardia, irregular heartbeat, headache, nausea and vomiting, severe weakness, increased B/P.

PATIENT CONSIDERATIONS

GENERAL: Administer oral agents on regular schedule. Assist pt in identifying what triggered an acute bronchospasm attack. INTERVENTION/EVALUATION: Monitor arterial blood gases, serum levels for aminophylline, theophylline. Assess lung sounds, B/P, pulse, respirations. Encourage fluid intake to decrease viscosity of secretions. PATIENT/FAMILY TEACHING: Demonstrate correct use of inhalers. Drink 8 or more glasses of fluid/day. Avoid caffeine-containing products, e.g., coffee, tea, colas, chocolate (cause further CNS stimulation). Do not smoke. Use other medications only after consulting physician. Teach effective deep breathing and coughing. Notify physician if symptoms are not relieved or worsen. Report adverse reactions.

calcium channel blockers

ACTION

Calcium channel blockers inhibit the flow of extracellular Ca^{+2} ions across cell membrane of cardiac cells, vascular tissue. Calcium channel blockers relax arterial smooth muscle, depress the rate of sinus node pacemaker, slow AV conduction, decrease heart rate, produce negative inotropic effect (rarely seen clinically due to reflex response). All calcium channel blockers decrease coronary vascular resistance, increase coronary blood flow, reduce myocardial oxygen demand. Degree of action varies w/individual agent.

CALCIUM CHANNEL BLOCKERS

Generic Name	Brand Name(s)	Onset Action	Uses	Rte Admin	Dosage Range
amlodipine	Norvasc	—	Angina	PO	2.5–10 mg/day
			Hypertension		
bepridil	Vascor	1 hr	Angina	PO	200–400 mg/day
diltiazem	Cardizem	30–60 min	Angina	PO, IV	PO: 120–360 mg/day
	Cardizem CD		Hypertension		IV: 20–25 mg
			Arrhythmias		IV bolus; 5–15 mg/hr
					IV infusion
felodipine	Plendil	2–5 hrs	Hypertension	PO	5–10 mg/day
isradipine	DynaCirc	2 hrs	Hypertension	PO	5–20 mg/day
mibefradil	Posicor	—	Hypertension	PO	50–100 mg/day
			Angina	PO	50–100 mg/day
nicardipine	Cardene	20 min	Angina	PO	60–120 mg/day
			Hypertension		
nifedipine	Adalat	20 min	Angina	SL, PO	PO: 30–120 mg/day
	Procardia	Hypertension			XL: 30–60 mg/day
nimodipine	Nimotop	—	Subarachnoid hemorrhage	PO	60 mg q4h × 21 days
nisoldipine	Sular	—	Hypertension	PO	20–60 mg/day
verapamil	Calan	30 min	Angina	PO, IV	PO: 120–480 mg/day
	Isoptin		Hypertension		
	Verelan		Arrhythmias		IV: 5–10 mg, max: 10 mg/dose

SL = sublingual; XL = sustained-release.

USES

Treatment of essential hypertension, treatment and prophylaxis of angina pectoris (including vasospastic, chronic stable, unstable), prevent/control supraventricular tachyarrhythmias, prevent neurologic damage due to subarachnoid hemorrhage.

PRECAUTIONS

CONTRAINDICATIONS: Renal or hepatic dysfunction, heart block, hypotension, extreme bradycardia, aortic stenosis, sick-sinus syndrome, severe left ventricular dysfunction, pregnancy, lactation. **CAUTIONS:** Administer cautiously to elderly because half-life may be increased. Liver enzymes should be monitored periodically.

INTERACTIONS

Beta-adrenergic blockers may have additive effect. May increase digoxin concentration. Procainamide, quinidine may increase risk of QT interval prolongation. Carbamazepine, quinidine, theophylline may increase concentration, toxicity.

SIDE EFFECTS

Headache, nausea, dizziness or lightheadedness, hypotension, constipation.

TOXIC EFFECTS/ADVERSE REACTIONS

Peripheral edema, palpitations, bradycardia, dyspnea, wheezing w/possible pulmonary edema, severe hypotension, second- or third-degree heart block (rare). Administered IV for tachyarrhythmias, verapamil, nicardipine, diltiazem have the greatest potential for severe reactions.

PATIENT CONSIDERATIONS

GENERAL: Parenteral administration requires close cardiac monitoring w/emergency equipment close by. Discontinuation should be gradual. Be alert to potential for hypotension, esp. when pt is taking other antihypertensive drugs or beta-adrenergic blockers. BASELINE ASSESSMENT: Assess initial B/P and apical pulse. INTERVENTION/EVALUATION: Monitor B/P and apical pulse before administration; notify physician before giving dose if not within agreed parameters. Check frequency, consistency of stools; avoid constipation. Assess lungs for rales, extremities for peripheral edema. Check I&O. PATIENT/FAMILY TEACHING: Teach how to take B/P and pulse correctly. Change position slowly to avoid orthostatic hypotension. Restrict sodium as ordered. Avoid alcohol, other medications w/o consulting physician. Do not overexert when anginal pain relieved. Do not stop taking medication. Report irregular heartbeat, dizziness, shortness of breath. Angina can occur if medication is stopped abruptly.

cancer chemotherapy

ACTION

Most antineoplastics inhibit cell replication by interfering w/supply of nutrients or genetic components of the cell (DNA or RNA). Some antineoplastics, referred to as cell cycle-specific (CCS), are particularly effective during a specific phase of cell reproduction (e.g., antimetabolites and plant alkaloids). Other antineoplastics, referred to as cell cycle-nonspecific, act independently of a specific phase of cell division (e.g., alkylating agents and antibiotics). Some hormones are also classified as antineoplastics. Although not cytotoxic, they act to depress cancer growth by altering the hormone environment. In addition, there are a number of miscellaneous agents acting through different mechanisms.

Alkylating agents: Highly reactive compounds forming a bond or cross-link w/DNA, and then damaging cells, likely causing cell death.

Antimetabolites: Capable of inhibiting enzymes necessary for synthesis of essential cellular components or being incorporated into DNA, disrupting DNA function.

Antibiotics: Interact w/DNA, inhibits DNA synthesis, DNA-dependent RNA synthesis; delay or inhibit mitosis.

Hormones: Noncytotoxic, inhibit proliferation by interfering at cellular membrane. May suppress lymphocytes in leukemias/lymphomas, altering hormonal balance in malignancies related to these hormones (e.g., tumors of breast).

Mitotic inhibitors: Act specifically during M (mitosis) phase of cell cycle, preventing cell division.

CANCER CHEMOTHERAPY

Generic Name	Brand Name(s)	Type	Cell Cycle-Specific	Uses
aldesleukin	Proleukin	Miscellaneous	No	Metastatic renal cell carcinoma
altretamine	Hexalen	Miscellaneous	No	Ovarian cancer
anastrozole	Arimidex	Miscellaneous	No	Advanced breast cancer
arsenic trioxide	Trisenox	Miscellaneous	No	Acute promyelocytic leukemia
asparaginase	Elspar	Miscellaneous	No	Acute lymphocytic leukemia
BCG	Pacis TheraCys TICE BCG	Miscellaneous	No	Carcinoma in situ of urinary bladder
bicalutamide	Casodex	Hormone	No	Metastatic prostate cancer
bleomycin	Blenoxane	Antibiotic	Yes	Squamous cell carcinoma, lymphomas, testicular carcinoma
busulfan	Myleran	Alkylating	No	Chronic myelogenous leukemia
capecitabine	Xeloda	Antimetabolite	No	Metastatic breast cancer
carboplatin	Paraplatin	Alkylating	No	Ovarian carcinoma
carmustine	BCNU	Alkylating	No	Brain tumors, multiple myeloma, Hodgkin's, non-Hodgkin's lymphomas
chlorambucil	Leukeran	Alkylating	No	Chronic lymphocytic leukemia, malignant lymphomas
cisplatin	Platinol	Alkylating	No	Metastatic testicular, ovarian tumors, advanced bladder cancer
cladribine	Leustatin	Miscellaneous	No	Hairy cell leukemia
cyclophosphamide	Cytoxan	Alkylating	No	Adenocarcinoma of ovary, breast cancer, malignant lymphomas, retinoblastoma, multiple myeloma, leukemias, mycosis fungoides, neuroblastoma

(continued)

CANCER CHEMOTHERAPY *Continued*

GENERIC NAME	BRAND NAME(S)	TYPE	CELL CYCLE-SPECIFIC	USES
cytarabine	Cytosar	Antimetabolite	Yes	Acute, chronic myelocytic leukemia, acute lymphocytic leukemia
dacarbazine	DTIC	Miscellaneous	No	Metastatic malignant melanoma, Hodgkin's disease
dactinomycin	Cosmegen	Antibiotic	No	Wilms' tumor, rhabdomyosarcoma, choriocarcinoma, testicular carcinoma, Ewing's sarcoma
daunorubicin	Cerubidine	Antibiotic	No	Acute lymphocytic, nonlymphocytic leukemia
diethyl-stilbestrol	Diethyl-stilbestrol	Hormone	No	Breast cancer, prostatic carcinoma
docetaxel	Taxotere	Miscellaneous	No	Breast cancer (local advanced/metastatic)
doxorubicin	Adriamycin Rubex	Antibiotic	No	Acute lymphoblastic leukemia, acute myeloblastic leukemia, Wilms' tumor, neuroblastoma, soft tissue and bone sarcomas, breast, ovarian carcinoma, transitional cell bladder carcinoma, thyroid carcinoma, Hodgkin's, non-Hodgkin's lymphomas, bronchogenic carcinoma, gastric carcinoma
estramustine	Emcyt	Hormone	No	Carcinoma of prostate
etoposide	VePesid	Mitotic inhibitor	Yes	Refractory testicular tumor, small cell lung cancer
floxuridine	FUDR	Antimetabolite	No	GI adenocarcinoma metastatic to liver
fludarabine	Fludara	Antimetabolite	No	Chronic lymphocytic leukemia
fluorouracil	Adrucil Efudex	Antimetabolite	No	Cancer of colon, rectum, breast, stomach, and pancreas
flutamide	Eulexin	Hormone	No	Metastatic prostatic carcinoma
gemcitabine	Gemzar	Miscellaneous	No	Pancreatic cancer
gemtuzumab	Mylotarg	Miscellaneous	No	Acute myeloid leukemia
goserelin	Zoladex	Hormone	No	Carcinoma of prostate
hydroxy urea	Hydrea	Miscellaneous	No	Melanoma, chronic myelocytic leukemia, carcinoma of ovary
idarubicin	Idamycin	Antibiotic	No	Acute myeloid leukemia
ifosfamide	Ifex	Alkylating	No	Germ cell testicular cancer
interferon alfa-2a	Roferon-A	Miscellaneous	No	Hairy cell leukemia, AIDS-related Kaposi's sarcoma
interferon alfa-2b	Intron A	Miscellaneous	No	Hairy cell leukemia, condylomata acuminata, AIDS-related Kaposi's sarcoma
interferon alfa-n3	Alferon N	Miscellaneous	No	Condylomata acuminata
irenotecan	Camptosar	Miscellaneous	No	Metastatic cancer of colon/rectum
letrozole	Femara	Miscellaneous	No	Advanced breast cancer
leuprolide	Lupron	Hormone	No	Advanced prostatic cancer, endometriosis
levamisole	Ergamisol	Miscellaneous	No	Duke's stage C colon cancer
lomustine	CeeNu	Alkylating	No	Brain tumors, Hodgkin's disease
mechlor-ethamine	Mustargen	Alkylating	No	Polycythemia vera, mycosis fungoides, Hodgkin's disease, lymphosarcoma, chronic myelocytic/lymphocytic leukemia bronchogenic cancer
medroxy-progesterone	Depo-Provera	Hormone	No	Endometrial, renal carcinoma
megestrol	Megace	Hormone	No	Breast, endometrial carcinoma

CANCER CHEMOTHERAPY *Continued*

GENERIC NAME	BRAND NAME(S)	TYPE	CELL CYCLE-SPECIFIC	USES
melphalan	Alkeran	Alkylating	No	Multiple myeloma, ovarian carcinoma
mercaptopurine	Purinethol	Antimetabolite	Yes	Acute lymphatic myelogenous leukemia
methotrexate	Folex	Antimetabolite	Yes	Gestational choriocarcinoma, choriocarcinoma destruens, hydatiform mole, acute lymphocytic leukemia
mitomycin	Mutamycin	Antibiotic	No	Disseminated adenocarcinoma of stomach, pancreas
mitotane	Lysodren	Miscellaneous	No	Adrenal cortical carcinoma
mitoxantrone	Novantrone	Antibiotic	No	Acute nonlymphocytic leukemia
nilutamide	Nilandron	Hormone	No	Metastatic prostatic carcinoma
paclitaxol	Taxol	Miscellaneous	No	Metastatic carcinoma of ovary
pegaspargase	Oncaspar	Miscellaneous	Yes	Acute lymphoblastic leukemia
pentostatin	Nipent	Antibiotic	No	Hairy cell leukemia
plicamycin	Mithracin	Antibiotic	No	Malignant testicular tumors
porfimer	Photofrin	Miscellaneous	No	Esophageal cancer
procarbazine	Matulane	Miscellaneous	No	Hodgkin's disease
streptozocin	Zanosar	Alkylating	No	Metastatic islet cell cancer of pancreas
tamoxifen	Nolvadex	Hormone	No	Metastatic breast cancer
teniposide	Vumen	Mitotic inhibitor	Yes	Refractory acute lymphoblastic leukemia (ALL)
testolactone	Teslac	Hormone	No	Breast carcinoma
thioguanine	Thioguanine	Antimetabolite	Yes	Acute nonlymphocytic leukemia
thiotepa	Thiotepa	Alkylating	No	Adenocarcinoma of breast, ovary; papillary cancer of urinary bladder
topotecan	Hycamtin	Miscellaneous	No	Ovarian cancer
toremifene	Fareston	Hormone	No	Advanced breast cancer
trastuzumab	Herceptin	Miscellaneous	No	Breast cancer
tretinoin	Vesanoid	Miscellaneous	No	Acute promyelocytic leukemia
triptorelin	Trelstar	Miscellaneous	No	Prostate cancer
valrubicin	Valstar	Antibiotic	Yes	Bladder cancer
vinblastine	Velban	Mitotic inhibitor	Yes	Hodgkin's disease, lymphocytic lymphoma, histiocytic lymphoma, mycosis fungoides, advanced testicular carcinoma, Kaposi's sarcoma, breast cancer
vincristine	Oncovin	Mitotic inhibitor	Yes	Acute leukemia, Hodgkin's disease, non-Hodgkin's malignant lymphoma, rhabdomyosarcoma, neuroblastoma, Wilms' tumor
vinorelbine	Navelbine	Mitotic inhibitor	Yes	Metastatic breast cancer, non small cell lung cancer, ovarian cancer, Hodgkin's disease

USES

Treatment of a wide variety of cancers; may be palliative or curative. Treatment of choice in hematologic cancers. Frequently used as adjunctive therapy, e.g., w/surgery or irradiation; most effective when tumor mass has been removed or reduced by radiation. Often used in combinations to increase therapeutic results, decrease toxic effects. Certain agents may be used in nonmalignant conditions; polycythemia vera, psoriasis, rheumatoid arthritis, or immunosuppression in organ transplantation (used only in select cases that are severe and unresponsive to other forms of therapy). Refer to individual monographs.

PRECAUTIONS

CONTRAINDICATIONS: Known hypersensitivity, hepatic or renal insufficiency, severe leukopenia, thrombocytopenia, anemia, pregnancy, lactation (other per individual drug). **CAUTION:** Elderly or very young, infection, radiation therapy, use of other antineoplastics.

INTERACTIONS

Highly complex agents; therefore, check the interactions of each carefully. Anticoagulants and other bone marrow depressants (including other antineoplastics) may increase the risk of myelosuppression effects. Refer to specific monographs.

SIDE EFFECTS

Stomatitis, nausea and vomiting, diarrhea, alopecia w/several drugs, myelosuppression (see Toxic Effects/Adverse Reactions), hyperuricemia effects on reproduction or local tissue injury.

TOXIC EFFECTS/ADVERSE REACTIONS

Narrow margin of safety between therapeutic and toxic response. Generally proportional to dosage and length of therapy. Myelosuppression (reduction in leukocytes, lymphocytes, thrombocytes, and erythrocytes) may precipitate life-threatening hemorrhage, infection, or anemia. Extravasation at IV site. Toxicity often a major factor in continuing therapy.

PATIENT CONSIDERATIONS

GENERAL: Take special precautions in handling agents to protect self and others (these drugs are highly toxic and may be inhaled or absorbed through skin; also cause local tissue damage upon contact): (1) Wear gloves, perhaps gown/mask/eye protectors (NIH guidelines). (2) Avoid contaminating articles w/agents. (3) Dispose of all contaminated materials in specifically identified containers. Administer precisely according to schedule. Use strict asepsis and protect pt from infection. When platelet count drops, avoid even the slightest trauma (such as injection or rectal temperature). BASELINE ASSESSMENT: Baseline lab values for RBC/WBC, platelets, vital signs are essential. INTERVENTION/EVALUATION: Monitor laboratory results, esp. RBC, WBC, and platelet counts; promptly report significant changes. Assess for bleeding, signs of infection, anemia. Infuse IV solutions, medications carefully to prevent extravasation. Extravasation is an *emergency* (standing orders and antidote kits must be available before administration). Monitor I&O. Assess response to medication; provide interventions, e.g., mouth care to relieve stomatitis; small, frequent meals of preferred foods/antiemetics for nausea and vomiting. PATIENT/FAMILY TEACHING: Individualized nature of therapy and need for lab tests.

Explain that alopecia is reversible, but new hair may have different color, texture. Assist in supporting body image. Despite possible infertility from drug, need for appropriate contraception due to risk of fetal abnormalities; inform physician immediately if pregnancy is suspected. Avoid crowds, persons w/known infections; report signs of infection at once (fever, malaise, flulike symptoms, etc.). Avoid contact w/anyone who recently received live virus vaccine; do not receive vaccinations. Promptly notify physician of bleeding, bruising, unexplained swelling.

cardiac glycosides

ACTION

Direct action on myocardium causes increased force of contraction, resulting in increased stroke volume and cardiac output. Depression of SA node, decreased conduction time through AV node, and decreased electrical impulses due to vagal stimulation slow heart rate. Improved myocardial contractility is probably due to improved transport of calcium, sodium, and potassium ions across cell membranes.

USES

CHF, atrial fibrillation, atrial flutter, paroxysmal atrial tachycardia, and treatment of cardiogenic shock w/pulmonary edema.

PRECAUTIONS

CONTRAINDICATIONS: History of hypersensitivity, digitalis toxicity, ventricular fibrillation, ventricular tachycardia (unless due to CHF), severe myocarditis. **CAUTIONS:** Renal insufficiency, hypokalemia, incomplete AV block, infants and children, elderly and debilitated pts. Safety in pregnancy, lactation not established.

INTERACTIONS

Glucocorticoids, amphotericin, potassium-depleting diuretics may increase toxicity (due to hypokalemia). Amiodarone may increase concentration, toxicity; additive effect on SA, AV nodes. Antiarrhythmics, parenteral calcium, sympathomimetics may increase risk of arrhythmias. Antidiarrheals, cholestyramine, colestipol may decrease absorption. Diltiazem, verapamil, quinidine may increase concentrations. Parenteral magnesium may cause conduction changes, heart block.

SIDE EFFECTS

The margin of safety between a therapeutic and a toxic dose is very narrow.

TOXIC EFFECTS/ADVERSE REACTIONS

Anorexia, nausea and vomiting, abdominal pain, and diarrhea occur commonly. Arrhythmias, such as premature ventricular contractions (PVCs) and bradycardia, also may signal overdosage. CNS effects are most common in elderly pts; headache, drowsiness, confusion, and visual disturbances such as halos around objects, altered color perception, blurring and flickering dots. In children arrhythmias are the most reliable sign; other effects are rarely seen.

PATIENT CONSIDERATIONS

GENERAL: Parenteral administration requires close cardiac monitoring. BASELINE ASSESSMENT: Establish initial B/P and apical pulse. INTERVENTION/EVALUATION: Assess apical pulse before giving each dose; withhold and notify physician if pulse below 60 or above 100 for adults. Measure I&O; weigh daily. Check for dependent edema; auscultate lungs for rales. Monitor potassium. PATIENT/FAMILY TEACHING: Take as prescribed; do not miss dose or take extra dose. Teach pt/family to take pulse and report pulse outside parameters determined by physician. Restrict sodium and alcohol as ordered. Cease smoking. Avoid OTC cold preparations, nasal decongestants, coffee, tea, colas, chocolates (stimulants).

cholinergic agonists/anticholinesterase

ACTION

CHOLINERGIC AGONISTS: Referred to as muscarinics or parasympathetics and consist of two basic drug groups: choline esters and cholinomimetic alkaloids. Primary action mimics actions of acetylcholine at postganglionic parasympathetic nerves. Primary properties include the following: *Cardiovascular system:* Vasodilation, decreased cardiac rate, decreased conduction in SA, AV nodes, decreased force of myocardial contraction. *Gastrointestinal:* Increased tone, motility of GI smooth muscle, increased secretory activity of GI tract. *Urinary tract:* Increased contraction of detrusor muscle of urinary bladder, resulting in micturition. *Eye:* Miosis, contraction of ciliary muscle.

ANTICHOLINESTERASE (anti-ChE), also known as cholinesterase inhibitors: Inactivates cholinesterase, which prevents acetylcholine breakdown causing acetylcholine to accumulate at cholinergic receptor sites. These agents can be considered indirect-acting cholinergic agonists. Primary properties include action of cholinergic agonists just noted. *Skeletal neuromuscular junction:* Effects are dose dependent. At therapeutic doses, increases force of skeletal muscle contraction; at toxic doses, reduces muscle strength.

USES

Paralytic ileus and atony of urinary bladder. Treatment of primary, and some secondary, glaucoma. Myasthenia gravis (weakness, marked fatigue of skeletal muscle). Terminates, reverses effects of neuromuscular blocking agents.

PRECAUTIONS

CONTRAINDICATIONS: Intestinal or urinary tract obstructions, known hypersensitivity, pregnancy, lactation, acute peptic ulcer, hyperthyroidism, peritonitis, bronchial asthma. **CAUTIONS:** Have atropine readily available in case of cholinergic crisis.

INTERACTIONS

Given with other cholinergics—increased effects w/greater potential for toxicity. Ganglionic blocking agents, used concurrently with cholinergics, may produce significant fall in B/P. Anticholinergics antagonize effects of cholinergics.

SIDE EFFECTS

Increased urinary frequency, salivation, belching, nausea, dizziness. Side effects infrequent, more likely w/subcutaneous injection or high doses.

TOXIC EFFECTS/ADVERSE REACTIONS

Overdose (cholinergic crisis): Abdominal cramps, diarrhea, excessive salivation, diaphoresis, muscle weakness, respiratory difficulty. Requires immediate treatment.

CHOLINERGIC AGONISTS

Generic Name	Brand Name(s)	Type	Use	Dosage Range
acetylcholine	Miochol	Cholinergic	Miotic	Ophth: 0.5–2 ml
bethanechol	Urecholine	Cholinergic	Nonobstructive urinary retention	PO: 10–50 mg 3–4x/day SubQ: 2.5–5 mg 3–4x/day
carbachol	Carbachol	Cholinergic	Miotic Glaucoma	Ophth: 0.5 ml Ophth: 1–2 drops up to 4x/day
demecarium	Humorsol	Anti-ChE	Glaucoma	Ophth: 1–2 drops 2x/day to 2 drops/wk
echothiophate	Phospholine	Anti-ChE	Glaucoma	Ophth: 1 drop qOd to 2x/day
edrophonium	Tensilon	Anti-ChE	Dx, myasthenia gravis Reverse tubocurarine	IV: 10 mg in 30–45 secs; max: 40 mg
isoflurophate	Floropryl	Anti-ChE	Glaucoma	Ophth ointment: q8–72h
neostigmine	Prostigmin	Anti-ChE	Dx/tx, myasthenia gravis Antidote Neuromuscular blocker	PO: 15–375 mg/day SubQ, IM: 0.5 mg; 0.01–0.04 mg/kg IV: 0.5–2 mg
physostigmine	Eserine	Anti-ChE	Glaucoma Antidote	Ophth: 1–2 drops up to 4x/day IM, IV: 0.5–2 mg
pilocarpine	Isopto Carpine Ocusert	Cholinergic	Glaucoma	Ophth: 1–2 drops up to 6x/day Every 7 days
pyridostigmine	Mestinon	Anti-ChE	Tx, myasthenia gravis Reverse tubocurarine	PO: 60–1,500 mg/day IM: 0.5–1.5 mg/kg IV: 0.1–0.25 mg/kg

PATIENT CONSIDERATIONS

GENERAL: Have atropine readily available in case of cholinergic crisis. BASELINE ASSESSMENT: Check pulse, respirations. INTERVENTION/EVALUATION: Monitor pulse, respiration; be alert for signs/symptoms of cholinergic crisis. Assess for therapeutic results: (1) In abdominal distention or paralytic ileus, listen for bowel sounds, check passing of flatus or stool, measure abdomen for decreased distention. (2) For urinary retention, palpate bladder and check for urination. Implement measures that support urination, e.g., running water, pouring warm water over perineum, privacy. If urination does not occur, determine whether catheterization is needed. Determine cause of urinary retention, e.g., trauma from surgical manipulation or narcotics given for pain. (3) For myasthenia gravis, observe for improved muscle tone and subsequently greater activity, less fatigue. PATIENT/FAMILY TEACHING: Explain purpose of medication. Increased salivation is to be expected. Call for assistance to bathroom after subcutaneous injection.

corticosteroids

ACTION

Synthesized by adrenal cortex, the corticosteroids can be divided into glucocorticoids (hepatic glycogen deposition) and mineralocorticoids (sodium retention). Corticosteroids have numerous effects including the following: *Carbohydrate, protein metabolism:* Increase glucose formation, decrease peripheral utilization, enhance glycogen storage, increase gluconeogenesis (transformation of protein to glucose). *Lipid metabolism:* Redistribute body fat, lipolysis of triglyceride of adipose tissue. *Electrolyte/water balance:* Enhance sodium reabsorption, potassium excretion, increase extracellular volume. *Formed elements:* Increase hemoglobin, red blood cell count, decrease number of lymphocytes, eosinophils, monocytes, basophils, increase polymorphonuclear leukocytes. *Anti-inflammatory:* Inhibit anti-inflammatory process (edema, capillary dilatation, migration of leukocytes into inflamed area, phagocytic activity). *Immunosuppression:* Inhibit early steps in immunity.

USES

Replacement therapy in adrenal insufficiency, including Addison's disease. Symptomatic treatment of multiorgan disease/conditions. Rheumatoid and osteo arthritis, severe psoriasis, ulcerative colitis, lupus erythematosus, anaphylactic shock, status asthmaticus, organ transplant.

PRECAUTIONS

CONTRAINDICATIONS: Hypersensitivity; peptic ulcer, tuberculosis, or any suspected infection; blood clotting disorders; severe renal or hepatic impairment; CHF or hypertension, lactation. **CAUTIONS:** Cautious administration in children, geriatric, and postmenopausal pts. Safe use during pregnancy has not been established.

INTERACTIONS

Amphotericin may increase hypokalemia. May decrease effect of oral hypoglycemics, insulin, diuretics, potassium supplements. May increase digoxin toxicity (due to hypokalemia). Hepatic enzyme inducers may decrease effect. Live virus vaccines may potentiate virus replication, increase vaccine side effects, decrease pt's antibody response to vaccine.

CORTICOSTEROIDS

GENERIC NAME	BRAND NAME(S)	RTE ADMIN
alclometasone	Aclovate	Topical
amcinonide	Cyclocort	Topical
beclomethasone	Beclovent, Vanceril Beconase, Vancenase	Inhalation, intranasal
betamethasone	Celestone, Diprosone Uticort, Valisone	Topical, oral, IV, intralesional, intra-articular
budesonide	Rhinocort	Intranasal
clobetasol	Temovate	Topical
cortisone	Cortone	Topical, oral
desonide	Tridesilone	Topical
desoximetasone	Topicort	Topical
dexamethasone	Decadron	Topical, oral, IM, IV, ophthalmic, intranasal, inhalation
fludrocortisone	Florinef	Oral
flunisolide	Aerobid, Nasalide	Inhalation, intranasal
fluocinolone	Synalar, Synemol	Topical
fluorometholone	FML	Ophthalmic
flurandrenolide	Cordran	Topical
fluticasone	Cutivate, Flonase	Topical, intranasal
halcinonide	Halog	Topical
halobetasol	Ultravate	Topical
hydrocortisone	Cort-Dome, Cortef, Hydrocortone, Solu-Cortef	Topical, oral, IM, IV, SubQ, rectal
methylprednisolone	Medrol, Solu-Medrol	Oral, IM, IV
mometasone	Elocon	Topical
prednicarbate	Dermatop	Topical
prednisolone	Delta-Cortef, Hydeltra, Hydeltrasol	Oral, IM, IV, intralesional, intra-articular
prednisone	Deltasone, Meticorten, Orasone	Oral
rimexolone	Vexol	Ophthalmic
triamcinolone	Azmacort, Kenalog, Nasacort	Oral, inhalation, intranasal

SIDE EFFECTS

Rarely cause side effects w/short-term high dose or replacement therapy. Sodium/water retention, increased appetite.

TOXIC EFFECTS/ADVERSE REACTIONS

Long-term therapy causes numerous adverse reactions; peptic ulcer and steroid diabetes are the most serious. Osteoporosis, petechiae, hirsutism, acne, menstrual irregularities. Cushing-like symptoms (moon face, excess fat deposits of trunk, neck, and shoulders w/buffalo hump, wasting of arms and legs). Edema, hypertension. May have depression, personality change, and insomnia; cataracts or glaucoma, delayed healing, suppressed immune response.

PATIENT CONSIDERATIONS

GENERAL: Take precautions to avoid infection; recognize that these agents mask signs and symptoms of developing illness. Administer oral drugs w/food or milk in early morning in a single dose. Withdraw medication slowly. BASELINE ASSESSMENT: Determine initial B/P, temperature, pulse, respiration, weight, blood glucose, electrolytes, EKG and TB skin test results. INTERVENTION/EVALUATION: Monitor B/P, temperature, pulse, respiration, daily weight, I&O, blood glucose, and electrolytes (esp. potassium and calcium). Be alert for signs and symptoms of hypokalemia, hypocalcemia. Check dependent areas for edema. Assess for mood, personality change. PATIENT/FAMILY TEACHING: Follow-up visits and lab tests are essential. Carry identification of drug and dose, physician name and phone number. Do not change dose/schedule or stop taking drug; must taper off gradually under medical supervision. Report severe symptoms (visual disturbances or severe gastric distress) to physician immediately. Promptly report sudden weight gain or swelling, sore throat, fever, or other signs of infection. Wounds may heal slowly. Avoid crowds, persons w/known infections. Do not receive vaccinations. Do not take aspirin or any other medication w/o consulting physician. Give instructions for diet (usually sodium restricted w/high vitamin D, protein, and potassium). Inform dentist or other physicians of glucocorticoid therapy now or within past 12 mos. Do not overuse joint that was injected for symptomatic relief. For topical application, apply after shower for best absorption; do not cover; avoid sunlight on treated area.

corticosteroids: topical

ACTION

Diffuses across cell membranes, forms complexes w/cytoplasm. Complexes stimulate protein synthesis of inhibitory enzymes responsible for anti-inflammatory effects (e.g., inhibit edema, erythema, pruritus, capillary dilation, phagocytic activity).

Topical corticosteroids can be classified based on potency:

Low: Modest anti-inflammatory effect, safest for chronic application, facial and intertriginous application, w/occlusion, for infants/young children.

Medium: For moderate inflammatory conditions (e.g., chronic eczematous dermatoses). May use for facial and intertriginous application for only limited time.

High: For more severe inflammatory conditions (e.g., lichen simplex chronicus, psoriasis). May use for facial and intertriginous application for short time only. Used in areas of thickened skin due to chronic conditions.

Very high: Alternative to systemic therapy for local effect (e.g., chronic lesions caused by psoriasis). Increased risk of skin atrophy. Used for short periods on small areas. Avoid occlusive dressings.

CORTICOSTEROIDS: TOPICAL

GENERIC NAME	BRAND NAME(S)	POTENCY	DOSAGE FORMS
alclometasone	Aclovate	Low	Cream, ointment
amcinonide	Cyclocort	High	Cream, ointment, lotion
betamethasone benzoate	Uticort	Medium	Cream, lotion, gel
betamethasone dipropionate	Diprosone Maxivate	High	Ointment, cream, lotion, aerosol
betamethasone dipropionate (augmented)	Diprolene	Very high	Ointment, cream, gel, lotion
betamethasone valerate	Valisone	High	Ointment, cream, lotion
clobetasol	Temovate	Very high	Ointment, cream
desonide	Tridesilon	Low	Ointment, cream, lotion
desoximetasone	Topicort	High	Ointment, cream, gel
dexamethasone	Decadron	Medium	Cream
flucinonide	Lidex	High	Cream, ointment, solution, gel
fluocinolone	Synalar	High	Ointment, cream, solution
flurandrenolide	Cordran	Medium	Ointment, cream, lotion
fluticasone	Cutivate	Medium	Ointment, cream
halcinonide	Halog	High	Ointment, cream, solution
halobetasol	Ultravate	Very high	Ointment, cream
hydrocortisone	Cort-Dome Hytone	Medium	Ointment, cream, lotion, gel
mometasone	Elocon	Medium	Ointment, cream, lotion
prednicarbate	Dermatop	—	Cream
triamcinolone	Aristocort Kenalog	Medium	Ointment, cream, lotion

USES

Provides relief of inflammation/pruritus associated w/corticosteroid-responsive disorders: e.g., contact dermatitis, eczema, insect bite reactions, first- and second-degree localized burns/sunburn.

PRECAUTIONS

CONTRAINDICATIONS: Hypersensitivity to corticosteroids. Do not use on preexisting skin atrophy, infection at treatment site w/o antibiotics, herpes simplex. Treatment of rosacea, perioral dermatitis or acne. Prolonged use (may cause glaucoma, cataracts). **CAUTIONS:** Use smallest therapeutic dose for children (chronic use may interfere w/growth and development). Local irritation: discontinue. Skin infection: treat w/appropriate antifungal or antibacterial agent.

INTERACTIONS

None significant.

SIDE EFFECTS

Contact dermatitis (burning/itching of skin). Painful, red, itchy, pus-containing blisters; thinning of skin w/easy bruising. Dryness, irritation, skin redness or scaling of skin lesions, skin rash.

TOXIC EFFECTS/ADVERSE REACTIONS

None significant.

PATIENT CONSIDERATIONS

BASELINE ASSESSMENT: Question for hypersensitivity to corticosteroid. Establish baseline assessment of skin disorder. INTERVENTION/EVALUATION: Assess involved area for therapeutic response or irritation. PATIENT/FAMILY TEACHING: Apply after shower or bath for best absorption; rub thin film gently into affected area. Do not cover; do not use tight diapers, plastic pants, or coverings. Do not apply to weepy, denuded areas. Do not expose treated areas to sunlight (severe sunburn may occur). Use only for prescribed area and no longer than ordered. Report adverse local reactions. Avoid contact w/eyes.

---

diuretics

ACTION

Diuretics act to increase the excretion of water/sodium and other electrolytes via the kidneys. Exact mechanism of antihypertensive effect unknown; may be due to reduced plasma volume or decreased peripheral vascular resistance. Subclassifications of diuretics are based on their mechanism and site of action.

Thiazides: Act at the cortical diluting segment of nephron, block reabsorption of Na, Cl, and water; promote excretion of Na, Cl, K, and water.

Loop: Act primarily at the thick ascending limb of Henle's loop to inhibit Na, Cl, and water absorption.

Potassium-sparing: Spironolactone blocks aldosterone action on distal nephron (causes K retention, Na excretion). Triamterene, amiloride act on distal nephron, decreasing Na reuptake, reducing K secretion.

Osmotic: Elevate osmolarity of glomerular filtrate preventing reabsorption of water, increased excretion of Na, Cl.

USES

Thiazides: Management of edema resulting from a number of causes (e.g., CHF, hepatic cirrhosis); hypertension either alone or in combination w/other antihypertensives.

Loop: Management of edema associated w/CHF, cirrhosis of liver, and renal disease. Furosemide used in treatment of hypertension alone or in combination w/other antihypertensives.

Potassium-sparing: Adjunctive treatment w/thiazides, loop diuretics in treatment of CHF and hypertension.

Osmotics: Reduction of intraocular pressure for ophthalmic surgery, edema, elevated intracranial pressure, and facilitating excretion of toxic substances.

DIURETICS

GENERIC NAME	BRAND NAME(S)	TYPE	DIURETIC EFFECT: ONSET	PEAK	DURATION	DOSAGE RANGE
amiloride	Midamor	K-sparing	2 hrs	6–10 hrs	24 hrs	HTN: 5–20 mg/day Edema: 5–20 mg/day
bumetanide	Bumex	Loop	0.5–1 hr	1–2 hrs	4–6 hrs	Edema: 0.5–10 mg/day
chlorothiazide	Diuril	Thiazide	1–2 hrs	4 hrs	6–12 hrs	HTN: 0.5–2 g/day Edema: 0.5–2 g 1–2x/day
chlorthalidone	Hygroton	Thiazide	2 hrs	2–6 hrs	24–72 hrs	HTN: 25–100 mg/day Edema: 50–200 mg/day
ethacrynic acid	Edecrin	Loop	0.5 hrs	2 hrs	6–8 hrs	Edema: 50–200 mg/day
furosemide	Lasix	Loop	1 hr	1–2 hrs	6–8 hrs	HTN: 40 mg 2x/day Edema: up to 600 mg/day
glycerin	Glycerin	Osmotic	10–30 min	1–1.5 hrs	4–5 hrs	Edema: 1–1.5 g/kg
hydrochlorothiazide	Esidrix Hydro-Diuril Oretic	Thiazide	2 hrs	4–6 hrs	6–12 hrs	HTN: 25–100 mg/day Edema: 25–200 mg/day
indapamide	Lozol	Thiazide	1–2 hrs	2 hrs	Up to 36 hrs	HTN: 2.5–5 mg/day Edema: 2.5–5 mg/day
mannitol	Mannitol	Osmotic	0.5–1 hr	1 hr	6–8 hrs	Edema: 50–200 g/day
metolazone	Diulo Zaroxolyn	Thiazide	1 hr	2 hrs	12–24 hrs	HTN: 2.5–5 mg/day Edema: 5–20 mg/day
spironolactone	Aldactone	K-sparing	24–48 hrs	48–72 hrs	48–72 hrs	HTN: 50–100 mg/day Edema: 25–200 mg/day
torsemide	Demadex	Loop	10–60 min	1–2 hrs	6–8 hrs	HTN: 5–10 mg/day Edema: 10–200 mg/day
triamterene	Dyrenium	K-sparing	2–4 hrs	6–8 hrs	12–16 hrs	HTN: up to 300 mg/day Edema: up to 300 mg/day

HTN = hypertension.

PRECAUTIONS

CONTRAINDICATIONS: Severe hepatic or renal dysfunction. Hypersensitivity to the drug (sensitivity to sulfonamides when giving thiazides). Potassium-sparing diuretics should not be given in hyperkalemia; osmotics are contraindicated in intracranial bleeding. Dehydration, pregnancy, infants and children, lactation. **CAUTIONS:** Administer cautiously to elderly, pts w/diabetes mellitus, gout or hyperuricemia, history of lupus erythematosus (may cause exacerbation).

INTERACTIONS

Thiazides: Cholestyramine, colestipol may decrease absorption, effects. May increase digoxin toxicity (due to hypokalemia). May increase lithium toxicity.

Loop: Amphotericin, ototoxic, nephrotoxic agents may increase toxicity. May decrease effect of anticoagulants, heparin. Hypokalemia-causing agents may increase hypokalemia. May increase risk of lithium toxicity.

Potassium-sparing: May decrease anticoagulants, heparin effects. NSAIDs may decrease antihypertensive effect. ACE inhibitors (e.g., captopril), potassium-containing medications, potassium supplements may increase potassium. May increase digoxin, lithium toxicity.

SIDE EFFECTS

Orthostatic hypotension, dizziness, anorexia or nausea, headache, lethargy.

TOXIC EFFECTS/ADVERSE REACTIONS

Unusual weakness, heaviness of legs, weak pulse indicate electrolyte (potassium) imbalance. Dehydration; hyperkalemia w/potassium-sparing diuretics; tinnitus and hearing loss w/loop diuretics; hypotension. Hypersensitivity reactions rarely. Impotence, GI bleeding.

PATIENT CONSIDERATIONS

GENERAL: If possible, administer dose in morning to avoid disturbing sleep w/urination. Provide assistance to bathroom, if needed; be sure pts confined to bed have call light handy. INTERVENTION/EVALUATION: Monitor I&O, weight. Check B/P and apical pulse, potassium levels. Assess for edema of dependent areas. Auscultate lungs for rales. PATIENT/FAMILY TEACHING: Medication will cause increased urination. Consult physician regarding alcohol and other medications. Eat foods high in potassium such as whole grains (cereals), legumes, meat, bananas, apricots, orange juice, potatoes (white, sweet), raisins (except w/potassium-sparing diuretics).

fertility agents

Infertility is defined as a decreased ability to reproduce as opposed to sterility, the inability to reproduce. Infertility may be due to reproduction dysfunction of the male, female, or both. In order to make an accurate diagnosis of the cause of infertility, a variety of tests may be performed: semen analysis, determining basal body temperature patterns, measuring estrogen and progesterone levels, endometrial biopsy and fallopian tube patency. The more accurate the diagnosis, the better chance of treating infertility successfully.

FEMALE INFERTILITY

Female infertility can be due to disruption of any phase of the reproductive process. The most critical phases include follicular maturation, ovulation, transport of the ovum through the fallopian tubes, fertilization of the ovum, nidation and growth/development of the conceptus. Causes of infertility include the following:

Anovulation, failure of follicular maturation: Absence of adequate hormonal stimulation; ovarian follicles do not ripen and ovulation will not occur.

Unfavorable cervical mucus: Normally the cervical glands secrete large volumes of thin, watery mucus, but if the mucus is unfavorable (scant or thick or sticky), sperm is unable to pass through to the uterus.

Hyperprolactinemia: Excessive prolactin secretion may cause amenorrhea, galactorrhea, and infertility.

Luteal phase defect: Progesterone secretion by the corpus luteum is insufficient to maintain endometrial integrity.

Endometriosis: Endometrial tissue is implanted in abnormal locations (e.g., uterine wall, ovary, extragenital sites).

Androgen excess: May decrease fertility (the most common condition is polycystic ovary).

MALE INFERTILITY

Male infertility is due to decreased density or motility of sperm or semen of abnormal volume or quality. The most obvious manifestation of male infertility is impotence (inability to achieve erection). Whereas in female infertility, an identifiable endocrine disorder can be found, most cases of male infertility are not associated with an identifiable endocrine disorder.

MEDICATIONS TREATING INFERTILITY

The majority of medications used in treating infertility are directed at improving female reproductive function. These medications can improve maturation of ovarian follicles, ovulation, produce a favorable cervical mucus, control endometriosis, and reduce excessive prolactin levels.

Clomiphene (Clomid, Serophene)

Action: Blocks receptors for estrogen. The hypothalamus stimulates the anterior pituitary to increase secretion of luteinizing hormone (LH) and follicle-stimulating hormone (FSH), which then stimulate the ovary, promoting follicular maturation and ovulation.

Uses: Promotes follicular maturation and ovulation in selected infertile women.

Adverse Effects: Hot flushes, nausea, abdominal discomfort, bloating, breast engorgement. Multiple births occur in 8–10% of pregnancies. Excessive stimulation may produce ovarian enlargement. May induce luteal phase defect.

Menotropins (Humegon, Pergonal)

Action: Gonadotropic agent w/follicle-stimulating hormone (FSH) and luteinizing hormone (LH) actions. Promotes ovarian follicular growth and maturation in women; stimulates spermatogenesis in men.

Uses: Treatment of infertility: in conjunction w/chorionic gonadotropin (HCG) to stimulate ovulation and pregnancy in women w/secondary ovarian dysfunction and to stimulate spermatogenesis in men w/primary or secondary hypogonadotropic hypogonadism.

Adverse Effects: Pain, rash, swelling, irritation at injection site. Mild to moderate ovarian enlargement w/abdominal distention and pain. Ovarian enlargement occurring rapidly may be accompanied by ascites, pleural effusion, and pain. Additionally, menotropins may produce spontaneous abortion and multiple births (20% of pregnancies).

DRUGS FOR INFERTILITY

Generic Name	Brand Name	Dosage
bromocriptine	Parlodel	PO: Initially 0.5–2.5 mg/day increased by 2.5 mg every 3–7 days. Range: 2.5–15 mg/day.
Cetrorelix	Cetrotide	SubQ: 0.25 mg daily on day 5 or 6; continue until HCG administered OR 3 mg once on day 7 (range 5–9)
clomiphene	Clomid Serophene	PO: Initially, 50 mg/day for 5 days (start any time in patients who have had no recent uterine bleeding). If progestin-induced bleeding is planned, or spontaneous uterine bleeding occurs prior to therapy, start on or about the 5th day of cycle. If ovulation has not occurred, administer a 2nd course at 100 mg/day for 5 days starting as early as 30 days after the previous course. Three courses are an adequate therapeutic trial.
danazol	Danocrine	PO: 200–300 mg 2 ×/day
follitropin	Gonal-F	SC: 75–150 IU/day
gonadorelin	Lutrepulse	Pump via indwelling catheter 5 mcg q90 min SC/IV: 100 mcg as single injection
human chorionic gonadotropin	Pergonal Profasai	IM: 5,000–10,000 units 24 hrs after last dose of menotropins
menotropins	Pergonal	IM: 75 IU FSH/75 IU LH daily for 7–12 days. Follow with 10,000 HCG 1 day after last dose of menotropins (if estrogen levels >150 mcg/24 hrs, not advised to give HCG). May repeat course at least twice. If no response, increase FSH/LH to 150 IU daily. May repeat twice.
nafarelin	Synarel	Intranasal: 200 mcg (one spray) in morning and evening alternating nostrils
urofollitropin	Fertinex	SC: 75–150 IU/day

Gonadorelin (Factrel, Lutrepulse)

Action: Stimulates synthesis, release of luteinizing hormone (LH) and follicle-stimulating hormone (FSH) from the anterior pituitary. Stimulates release of gonadotropin-releasing hormone from the hypothalamus.

Uses: Induction of ovulation in women with primary hypothalamic amenorrhea; promotes follicular maturation and ovulation.

Adverse Effects: Ovarian hyperstimulation. Inflammation, infection, mild phlebitis, hematoma at catheter site (if administration via an indwelling IV catheter). Multiple births (12% of pregnancies).

Human Chorionic Gonadotropin (HCG) (APL, Pregnyl, Profasai HP)
Action: Similar in structure and identical in action to luteinizing hormone (LH). Stimulates production of progesterone by the corpus luteum causing maturation of the corpus luteum and triggers ovulation in women with normally functioning ovaries.

Uses: Induction of ovulation and pregnancy in women with secondary anovulation (after pretreatment with menotropin).

Adverse Effects: Ovarian hyperstimulation. May provoke rupture of ovarian cysts. Multiple births may be induced. Edema, pain at injection site, and CNS effects (headache, irritability, restlessness, fatigue).

Bromocriptine (Parlodel)
Action: Directly inhibits prolactin release from the anterior pituitary. Stimulates presynaptic and postsynaptic dopamine receptors.

Uses: Treatment of hyperprolactinemia conditions (amenorrhea with or without galactorrhea, prolactin secreting adenomas, infertility).

Adverse Effects: Nausea, headache, dizziness, fatigue, abdominal cramps.

Danazol (Danocrine)
Action: Inhibits several enzymes required for synthesis of ovarian hormones, suppresses secretion of LH and FSH, and acts directly on the implant to block ovarian hormone receptors. Atrophies ectopic endometrial tissue.

Uses: Treatment of endometriosis and associated infertility.

Adverse Effects: May induce virilization (acne, deepening of the voice, growth of facial hair). May cause edema, liver dysfunction.

Nafarelin (Synarel)
Action: Indirectly suppresses ovarian hormone production (LH and FSH).

Uses: Management of endometriosis, including pain relief and reduction of endometriotic lesions.

Adverse Effects: Hot flushes, vaginal dryness, decreased libido, mood changes, headache, nasal irritation, decreased bone density.

H_2 antagonists

ACTION

Inhibit gastric acid secretion by interfering w/histamine at the histamine H_2 receptors in parietal cells. Also inhibits acid secretion caused by gastrin. Inhibition occurs w/basal (fasting), nocturnal, food-stimulated, or fundic distention secretion. H_2 antagonists decrease both the volume and H_2 concentration of gastric juices.

USES

Short-term treatment of duodenal ulcer, active benign gastric ulcer; maintenance therapy of duodenal ulcer; pathologic hypersecretory conditions (e.g., Zollinger-Ellison syndrome); gastroesophageal reflux disease; and prevention of upper GI bleeding in critically ill pts.

PRECAUTIONS

CONTRAINDICATIONS: Cross-sensitivity. Pregnancy and lactation; children. **CAUTIONS:** Elderly pts and those w/reduced renal or hepatic function.

INTERACTIONS

Note: Interactions more likely to occur w/cimetidine.
Antacids may decrease absorption (avoid use within ½–1 hr). May decrease ketoconazole absorption (give at least 2 hrs after). May decrease metabolism, increase concentration of oral anticoagulants, tricyclic antidepressants, oral hypoglycemics, metoprolol, metronidazole, phenytoin, propranolol, theophylline, calcium channel blockers, cyclosporine, lidocaine.

H_2 ANTAGONISTS

Generic Name	Brand Name(s)	Rte Admin	Use: Dosage
cimetidine	Tagamet	PO, IM, IV, IV infusion	Tx duodenal ulcer: 800 mg/hs, 400 mg 2×/day, 300 mg 4×/day Maintenance duodenal ulcer: 400 mg/hs Tx gastric ulcer: 800 mg/hs; 300 mg 4×/day GERD: 1,600 mg/day Hypersecretory conditions: 1,200–2,400 mg/day Prevents upper GI bleeding: 50 mg/hr as IV infusion
famotidine	Pepcid	PO, IV	Tx duodenal ulcer: 40 mg/day Maintenance duodenal ulcer: 20 mg/day Tx gastric ulcer: 40 mg/day GERD: 40–80 mg/day Hypersecretory conditions: 80–640 mg/day
nizatidine	Axid	PO	Tx duodenal ulcer: 300 mg/day Maintenance duodenal ulcer: 150 mg/day
ranitidine	Zantac	PO, IM, IV, IV infusion	Tx duodenal ulcer: 300 mg/day Maintenance duodenal ulcer: 150 mg/day Tx gastric ulcer: 300 mg/day GERD: 300 mg/day Hypersecretory conditions: 0.3–6 g/day
roxatidine	Roxin	PO	Tx duodenal ulcer: 150 mg/day Prevention duodenal/gastric ulcer: 75 mg/day

GERD = gastroesophageal reflux disease; Tx = treatment; hs = bedtime.

SIDE EFFECTS

Dizziness, headache, muscle cramps, rash, diarrhea or constipation. Confusion, esp. in elderly, debilitated, those w/renal or hepatic dysfunction.

TOXIC EFFECTS/ADVERSE REACTIONS

Unusual weakness or tiredness (may suggest blood dyscrasias), bradycardia or tachycardia, unusual bleeding; decreased sexual ability—esp. w/Zollinger-Ellison syndrome.

PATIENT CONSIDERATIONS

GENERAL: Administer oral agents w/meals and at bedtime for maximal effects. Antacids should not be taken within 1 hr of histamine receptor antagonists. Infuse IV solution slowly. BASELINE ASSESSMENT: Determine baselines for B/P, pulse. INTERVENTION/EVALUATION: Assess for abdominal pain, discomfort. Monitor B/P, pulse (esp. w/IV route). Check stools and emesis for blood. Assess for confusion, esp. in elderly, debilitated, and those w/renal or hepatic dysfunction. PATIENT/FAMILY TEACHING: Avoid alcohol, aspirin, spicy foods, and other foods known to cause distress. Need to cease smoking. Importance of completing therapy. Notify physician of abdominal or epigastric pain, blood in stool or emesis, dark tarry stools.

hematinic preparations

ACTION

Iron supplements are provided to assure adequate supplies for the formation of hemoglobin, which is needed for erythropoiesis and O_2 transport.

USES

Prevention or treatment of iron deficiency resulting from improper diet, pregnancy, impairment of absorption, or prolonged blood loss.

PRECAUTIONS

CONTRAINDICATIONS: Peptic ulcers, anemias caused by other factors, multiple blood transfusions, ulcerative colitis, cirrhosis, hypersensitivity to agent, hepatitis. **CAUTIONS:** Pts w/allergy, rheumatoid arthritis.

IRON PREPARATIONS

Generic Name	Brand Name(s)	Iron (%)	Dose Providing 100 mg Iron
ferrous fumarate	Feostat	33	300
ferrous gluconate	Fergon	11.6	860
ferrous sulfate	Mol-Iron Fer-In-Sol liquid Feosol liquid	20	500
ferrous sulfate exsiccated	Fer-In-Sol caps Feosol tabs/caps Slow FE	30	330

INTERACTIONS

Antacids, cimetidine, tetracycline may decrease iron absorption; iron may decrease absorption of methyldopa, quinolones, tetracycline.

SIDE EFFECTS

Nausea, vomiting, diarrhea or constipation, heartburn, hypersensitivity reactions: rash, urticaria, pruritus.

TOXIC EFFECTS/ADVERSE REACTIONS

Severe gastrointestinal effects, anaphylactic reactions, fever, chills, arthralgia, hypotension, local abscess at IM injection site.

PATIENT CONSIDERATIONS

GENERAL: Give oral iron on empty stomach, w/food to reduce gastrointestinal symptoms. Provide straw w/oral liquid form to avoid tooth discoloration. INTERVENTION/EVALUATION: Laboratory results (hemoglobin, blood counts). Assess skin color, esp. at nail beds, earlobes, sublingual areas. Check for fatigue, increased respirations (low hemoglobin may cause hypoxia). PATIENT/FAMILY TEACHING: Stools will be discolored (dark green or black). Importance of balanced diet; identify foods high in iron: egg yolks, dried fruits, meats (esp. organ meats), whole grains, and dark green leafy vegetables.

hormones

Functions of the body are regulated by two major control systems: the nervous system and endocrine (hormone) system. Together, they maintain homeostasis and control different metabolic functions in the body.

Hormones are concerned with control of different metabolic functions in the body (e.g., rates of chemical reactions in cells, transporting substances through cell membranes, cellular metabolism [growth/secretions]). By definition, a hormone is a chemical substance secreted into body fluids by cells and has control over other cells in the body. Hormones can be local or general. *Local hormones* have specific local effects (e.g., acetylcholine, which is secreted at parasympathetic and skeletal nerve endings). *General hormones* are mostly secreted by specific endocrine glands (e.g., epinephrine/norepinephrine are secreted by the adrenal medulla in response to sympathetic stimulation), transported in the blood to all parts of the body causing many different reactions. Some general hormones affect all or almost all cells of the body (e.g., thyroid hormone from the thyroid gland increases the rate of most chemical reactions in almost all cells of the body); other general hormones affect only specific tissue (e.g., ovarian hormones are specific to female sex organs and secondary sexual characteristics of the female).

ACTION

Endocrine hormones almost never directly act intracellularly affecting chemical reactions. They first combine with hormone receptors either on the cell surface or inside the cell (cell cytoplasm or nucleus). The combination of hormone and receptors alters the function of the receptor, and the receptor is the direct cause of the hormone effects. Altered receptor function may include the following: *Altered cell permeability,* which causes a change in protein structure of the receptor usually opening or closing a channel for one or more ions. The movement of these ions causes the effect of the hormone. *Activation of intracellular enzymes* immediately inside the cell membrane: e.g., hormone combines with receptor that then becomes the activated enzyme adenyl cyclase, which causes formation of cAMP. **Note:** Camp has effects inside the cell. It is not the hormone but cAMP causing these effects.

Regulation of hormone secretion is controlled by internal control system, the negative feedback system:

Endocrine gland oversecretes
Hormone exerts more and more of its effect
Target organ performs its function
Too much function in turn feeds back to endocrine gland to decrease secretory rate

The endocrine system contains many glands and hormones. A summary of the important glands and their hormones secreted are as follows:

The pituitary gland (hypophysis) is a small gland found in the sella turcica at the base of the brain. The pituitary is divided into two portions physiologically: the anterior pituitary (adenohypophysis) and the posterior pituitary (neurohypophysis). Six important hormones are secreted from the anterior pituitary and two from the posterior pituitary.

Anterior pituitary hormones:
- Growth hormone
- Adrenocorticotropin (corticotropin)
- Thyroid-stimulating hormone (thyrotropin)
- Follicle-stimulating hormone (FSH)
- Luteinizing hormone (LH)
- Prolactin

Posterior pituitary hormones:
- Antidiuretic hormone (vasopressin)
- Oxytocin

Almost all secretions of the pituitary hormones are controlled by hormonal or nervous signals from the hypothalamus. The hypothalamus is a center of information concerned with the well-being of the body, which in turn is used to control secretions of the important pituitary hormones just listed. Secretions from the posterior pituitary are controlled by nerve signals originating in the hypothalamus; anterior pituitary hormones are controlled by hormones secreted within the hypothalamus. These hormones are as follows:

Thyrotropin releasing hormone (TRH) releasing thyroid-stimulating hormone
Corticotropin-releasing hormone (CRH) releasing adrenocorticotropin
Growth hormone–releasing hormone (GHRH) releasing growth hormone and growth hormone inhibitory hormone (GHIH) (also same as somatostatin)
Gonadotropin-releasing hormone (GnRH) releasing the two gonadotropic hormones LH and FSH
Prolactin inhibitory factor (PIF) causing inhibition of prolactin and prolactin-releasing factor

ANTERIOR PITUITARY HORMONES

All anterior pituitary hormones (except growth hormone) have as their principal effect stimulating target glands.

GROWTH HORMONE (GH)

Growth hormone affects almost all tissues of the body. GH (somatopropin) causes growth in almost all tissues of the body (increases cell size, increases mitosis with increased number of cells, and differentiates certain types of cells). Metabolic effects include increased rate of protein synthesis, mobilization of fatty acids from adipose tissue, decreased rate of glucose utilization.

THYROID-STIMULATING HORMONE (TSH)

Thyroid-stimulating hormone controls secretion of the thyroid hormones. The thyroid gland is located immediately below the larynx on either side of and anterior to the trachea and secretes two significant hormones, thyroxine (T4) and tri-iodothyroxine (T3), which have a profound effect on increasing the metabolic rate of the body. The thyroid gland also secretes calcitonin, an important hormone for calcium metabolism. Calcitonin promotes deposition of calcium in the bones, which decreases calcium concentration in the extracellular fluid.

ADRENOCORTICOTROPIN

Adrenocorticotropin causes the adrenal cortex to secrete adrenocortical hormones. The adrenal glands lie at the superior poles of the two kidneys. Each gland is composed of two distinct parts, the adrenal medulla and cortex. The adrenal medulla, related to the sympathetic nervous system, secretes the hormones epinephrine and norepinephrine. When stimulated, they cause constriction of blood vessels, increased activity of the heart, inhibitory effects on the GI tract, and dilation of the pupils. The adrenal cortex secretes corticosteroids, of which there are two major types: mineralocorticoids and glucocorticoids. Aldosterone, the principal mineralocorticoid, primarily affects electrolytes of the extracellular fluids. Cortisol, the principal glucocorticoid, affects glucose, protein, and fat metabolism.

LUTEINIZING HORMONE (LH)

Luteinizing hormone plays an important role in ovulation and causes secretion of female sex hormones by the ovaries and testosterone by the testes.

FOLLICLE-STIMULATING HORMONE (FSH)

Follicle-stimulating hormone causes growth of follicles in the ovaries prior to ovulation and promotes formation of sperm in the testes.

Ovarian sex hormones are estrogens and progestins. Estradiol is the most important estrogen; progesterone, the most important progestin.

Estrogens mainly promote proliferation and growth of specific cells in the body and are responsible for development of most of the secondary sex characteristics. Primarily cause cellular proliferation and growth of tissues of sex organs/other tissue related to reproduction. Ovaries, fallopian tubes, uterus, vagina increase in size. Estrogen initiates growth of breast and milk-producing apparatus, external appearance.

Progesterone stimulates secretion of the uterine endometrium during the latter half of the female sexual cycle, preparing the uterus for implantation of the fertilized ovum. Decreases the frequency of uterine contractions (helps prevent expulsion of the implanted ovum). Progesterone promotes development of breasts, causing alveolar cells to proliferate, enlarge, and become secretory in nature.

Testosterone is secreted by the testes and formed by the interstitial cells of Leydig. Testosterone production increases under the stimulus of the anterior pituitary gonadotropic hormones. It is responsible for distinguishing characteristics of the masculine body (stimulates the growth of male sex organs and promotes the development of male secondary sex characteristics: e.g., distribution of body hair, effect on voice, protein formation, and muscular development).

PROLACTIN

Prolactin promotes the development of breasts and secretion of milk.

POSTERIOR PITUITARY HORMONES

ANTIDIURETIC HORMONE (ADH) (VASOPRESSIN)

Antidiuretic hormone can cause antidiuresis (decreased excretion of water by the kidneys). In the presence of ADH the permeability of the renal collecting ducts and tubules to water increases, which allows water to be absorbed, conserving water in the body. ADH in higher concentrations is a very potent vasoconstrictor, constricting arterioles everywhere in the body, increasing B/P.

OXYTOCIN

Oxytocin contracts the uterus during the birthing process, esp. toward the end of the pregnancy, helping to expel the baby. Oxytocin also contracts myoepithelial cells in the breasts, causing milk to be expressed from the alveoli into the ducts so the baby can obtain it by suckling.

PANCREAS

The pancreas is composed of two tissue types: (1) acini (secretes digestive juices in the duodenum) and (2) islets of Langerhans (secrete insulin/glucagon directly into the blood). The islets of Langerhans contain three cells: alpha, beta, delta. Alpha cells secrete glucagon, beta cells secrete insulin, and delta cells secrete somatostatin.

Insulin promotes glucose entry into most cells, thus controlling the rate of metabolism of most carbohydrates. Also insulin affects fat metabolism.

Glucagon effects are opposite insulin, the most important of which is increasing blood glucose concentration by releasing it from the liver into the circulating body fluids.

Somatostatin (same chemical as secreted by the hypothalamus) has multiple inhibitory effects: depresses secretion of insulin and glucagon, decreases GI motility, decreases secretions/absorption of the GI tract.

human immunodeficiency virus (HIV) infection

Acquired immunodeficiency syndrome (AIDS) was first recognized in 1981. Initially described in healthy, young homosexual men. AIDS was characterized by profound immunologic deficits, multiple opportunistic infections, and malignant neoplasms.

AIDS is caused by a retrovirus, human immunodeficiency virus (HIV). There are two types of HIV: HIV-1 and HIV-2, with HIV-1 the most common in the United States. Infection with HIV causes progressive deterioration in cell-mediated immunity, the most severe form resulting in AIDS. Although there is no cure for HIV infection, many advances in our understanding of the replication cycles of the HIV virus, therapies designed to inhibit this retrovirus, and therapies to overcome the many opportunistic infections associated with this virus have given renewed hope that controlling the progression of HIV may be possible and AIDS may be treated as a chronic disease.

HIV is a retrovirus primarily infecting CD4+ T-helper cells. After binding to a CD4 receptor protein, the virus enters the cell, is uncoated, and with the help of the enzyme reverse transcriptase (RT), the viral RNA is transcribed into a complementary DNA, which in turn is incorporated into the genome (complete gene complement) of the CD4+ T-cell. HIV replication is a continuous process without a period of latency.

HIV infection causes a wide range of immunologic abnormalities; the most important is a decrease in the number of CD4+ T cells. By definition, AIDS includes all HIV-infected adolescents and adults having a CD4 count below 200/mm^3 (normal: CD4 >1,000 cells/mm^3) regardless of symptoms or one of the AIDS-related opportunistic infections, regardless of CD4 count.

TRANSMISSION/GOALS OF THERAPY

HIV infection occurs through contact with infected blood and contaminated body fluids. Contact may occur through sexual intercourse (hetero- and homosexual), sharing blood-contaminated needles by injection drug users, infection of infants through pregnancy and during delivery and by breast feeding, via a needle stick injury or splashing of skin or mucous membranes, and through receipt of infected blood products or organs.

The goal in managing HIV/AIDS is to delay disease progression and to minimize associated opportunistic infections and malignancies. Therapy should prolong survival and improve quality of life. This is undertaken by initiating antiretroviral therapy, being aggressive in offering prophylaxis/treatment of opportunistic infections, and intensive nutritional therapy/supportive care.

ANTIRETROVIRAL AGENTS

Antiretroviral agents are classified as nucleoside analogues, non-nucleoside analogues, and protease inhibitors. Nucleoside and non-nucleoside analogues act by inhibiting HIV RT, which is responsible for viral replication early in the virus life cycle. Protease inhibitors block protease, an enzyme required for viral replication late in the virus life cycle.

Usually combinations of these agents may be most effective in suppressing viral replication. Several different combinations are currently being used, but the most effective combination is still unclear at this time. For more information about these agents, refer to the individual monographs.

ANTIRETROVIRAL AGENTS FOR TREATMENT OF HIV INFECTION

GENERIC NAME	BRAND NAME(S)	AVAILABILITY	DOSAGE
NUCLEOSIDE ANALOGUES			
abacavir	Ziagen	—	300 mg 2 times/day
didanosine (ddI)	Videx	Tablets Oral soln	Tablets: (>60 kg): 200 mg 2 times/day (<60 kg): 125 mg 2 times/day Oral Solution: (>60 kg): 250 mg 2 times/day (<60 kg): 167 mg 2 times/day
lamivudine (3TC)	Epivir	Tablets Oral soln	Adults: 150 mg 2 times/day Children (3 mos–12 yrs): 4 mg/kg 2 times/day
stavudine (d4T)	Zerit	Capsules	(>60 kg): 40 mg 2 times/day (20 mg 2 times/day if peripheral neuropathy occurs)
zalcitabine (ddC)	Hivid	Tablets	(>60 kg): 0.75 mg 3 times/day (<60 kg): 0.375 mg 3 times/day
zidovudine (ZDV)	Retrovir	Capsules Tablets	500–600 mg/day (100 mg 5 times/day or 200 mg 3 times/day or 300 mg 2 times/day (Decrease to 100 mg 3 times/day if anemia, headache, nausea, insomnia)
NON-NUCLEOSIDE ANALOGUES			
delavirdine (DLV)	Rescriptor	Tablets	200 mg 3 times/day for 14 days, then 400 mg 3 times/day if no rash
efavirenz	Sustiva	Capsules	Adults: 600 mg/day Children: 10–15 kg: 200 mg; 15–20 kg: 250 mg; 20–25 kg: 300 mg; 25–32.5 kg: 350 mg; 32.5–40 kg: 400 mg; > 40 kg: 600 mg
nevirapine (NVP)	Viramune	Tablets	200 mg daily for 14 days, then 200 mg 2 times/day if no rash
PROTEASE INHIBITORS			
indinavir	Crixivan	Capsules	800 mg every 8 hrs (adjust dosage in liver disease)
lopinavir/ritonavir	Kaletra	Capsules Oral solution	Adults, children > 12 yrs 400 mg 2 times/day Children 6 months–12 yrs 7–15 kg; 12 mg/kg 2 times/day 15–40 kg; 10 mg/kg 2 times/day; >40 kg: 400 mg 2 times/day
nelfinavir	Viracept	Tablets Oral powder	Adults: 750 mg q8h Children: 20–25 mg/kg q8h
ritonavir	Norvir	Capsules Oral soln	300 mg 2 times/day for 1 day, then 400 mg 2 times/day for 2 days, then 500 mg 2 times/day for 1 day, then 600 mg 2 times/day
saquinavir	Invirase	Capsules	600 mg 3 times/day

OPPORTUNISTIC INFECTIONS AND NEOPLASMS

Once the CD4 count drops to <200/mm^3, many opportunistic infections develop. The lower the CD4 count, the greater the risk and number of infections. In most instances, with all the microorganisms, there is breakthrough and progression. There are no cures, and lifelong treatment is required to prevent recurrence of infections.

CLASSIFICATION

Candida: Fungal infection. Symptoms: patches of inflammation with or without ulceration. May cause difficulty swallowing, nausea, sternal pain. Women: thick vaginal discharge/pruritus. Diagnosis by KOH-scraping from mucous membranes.

Cryptococcus: Fungal infection. Symptoms: fever, malaise, headache, cough, GI disturbances. May localize in CNS (meningitis, encephalitis), memory loss, confusion. Diagnosis by culture of cerebrospinal fluid (CSF).

Cytomegalovirus: Symptoms: painless, progressive loss of vision, sometimes complicated by retinal detachment. In the GI tract, causes nausea, vomiting, weight loss. Diagnosis by fundoscopic examination.

Herpes Simplex: HSV-1 and HSV-2. Symptoms: orolabial, genital, anorectal (pain, itching, painful defecation), mucocutaneous lesions, esophagitis; less common: encephalitis. Diagnosis by viral culture.

Histoplasma: Fungal infection. Symptoms: often asymptomatic, may cause flulike symptoms, high fever, weight loss, liver and spleen enlargement. Diagnosis by fungal cultures.

Kaposi's Sarcoma: Symptoms: red-blue blotches or nodules ranging in size from a few millimeters to several centimeters in diameter. The lesion may bleed. Nodules may appear in the mouth or in the viscera. Diagnosis by biopsy.

Mycobacterium avium complex (MAC): Symptoms: high spiking fevers, diarrhea, night sweats, malaise, weight loss, anemia, neutropenia. Diagnosis by blood cultures or biopsy of liver, bone marrow, and lymph nodes.

Pneumocystis carnii pneumonia (PCP): Symptoms: fever, dyspnea, tachypnea with or without rales or rhonchi, and nonproductive or mildly productive cough, chills, sweats. Diagnosis by special stains of bronchial washings or open lung biopsy.

THERAPIES FOR COMMON OPPORTUNISTIC INFECTIONS

Clinical Disease	Prophylactic Agents	Agents for Acute Infection	
Candida	clotrimazole troches fluconazole ketoconazole nystatin	Oral: Esophageal:	clotrimazole nystatin fluconazole ketoconazole
Cryptococcus	fluconazole	amphotericin w/or w/o flucytosine, followed by fluconazole	
Cytomegalovirus	oral ganciclovir	ganciclovir (IV) foscarnet	
Herpes simplex	oral acyclovir	oral acyclovir	
Histoplasma	—	amphotericin itraconazole	
Kaposi's sarcoma	—	individualized:	bleomycin doxorubicin etoposide interferon a vinblastine vincristine
Mycobacterium avium complex	azithromycin clarithromycin rifabutin	clarithromycin + ethambutol (may add rifampin) clofazime ciprofloxacin	

THERAPIES FOR COMMON OPPORTUNISTIC INFECTIONS Continued)

CLINICAL DISEASE	PROPHYLACTIC AGENTS	AGENTS FOR ACUTE INFECTION
Pneumocystic carnii pneumonia	trimethoprim-sulfamethoxazole dapsone pentamidine (aerosol)	trimethoprim-sulfamethoxazole pentamidine IV atovaquone (mild cases)
Salmonella	—	ciprofloxacin trimethoprim-sulfamethoxazole
Toxoplasma gondii	trimethoprim-sulfamethoxazole dapsone + pyrimethamine	pyrimethamine + sulfadiazine + folinic acid
Tuberculosis	isoniazid rifampin	isoniazid + rifampin + pyrazinamide + ethambutol or streptomycin

Salmonella: Symptoms: fever, chills, night sweats. Diagnosis by blood cultures.

Toxoplasma gondii: Primarily infects the brain and eye. Symptoms: fever, headache, seizures, focal neurologic abnormalities and mental status changes. Diagnosis is presumptive or based on CT or MRI.

Tuberculosis (mycobacterium): Symptoms: Cough, fever, sweating, malaise, fatigue, weight loss, nonpleuritic chest pain, dyspnea. Diagnosis by TB smear, culture.

immunizations

DIPHTHERIA AND TETANUS TOXOID, PERTUSSIS VACCINE (DTP)

INDICATIONS

Immunization vs. diphtheria, tetanus, and pertussis (whooping cough).

DOSAGE

Note: Diphtheria and tetanus toxoid for pediatric use (DT) indicated for immunization of infants and children 6 wks up to 7 yrs when there is a contraindication to pertussis vaccine (acute infection or febrile illness, occurrence of any neurologic symptoms following administration of DPT for use, history of seizures, any evolving or changing disorder affecting the CNS). If no contraindication, diphtheria/tetanus/pertussis is preferred.

IM: Children >2 mos and <7 yrs: 0.5 ml at 2, 4, and 6 mos. The fourth dose of DTP may be administered as early as 12 mos, provided at least 6 mos have elapsed since the 3rd dose. Combined DTP-Hib products may be used when administered simultaneously. Diphtheria and tetanus toxoids and acellular pertussis vaccine (DTaP) can be used for the 4th and/or 5th dose of DTP in children 15 mos. If 4th dose given after 4th birthday, a booster (5th) dose is not necessary.

CLASSIFICATION

CONTRAINDICATIONS

Evolving or changing CNS disorders, progressive encephalopathy, uncontrolled epilepsy, severe febrile illness.

ADVERSE EFFECTS

Mild to moderate swelling, tenderness, redness, pain or lump at injection site. Fever 100.4–102.2° F.

DIPHTHERIA AND TETANUS TOXOID

INDICATIONS

Immunization against diphtheria and tetanus.

DOSAGE

Note: Diphtheria and tetanus toxoid for pediatric use (DT) indicated for immunization of infants and children 6 wks up to 7 yrs when there is a contraindication to pertussis vaccine (acute infection or febrile illness, occurrence of any neurologic symptoms following administration of DPT for use, history of seizures, any evolving or changing disorder affecting the CNS). If no contraindication, diphtheria/tetanus/pertussis is preferred.

IM: Children >6 wks to 1 yr: 0.5 ml at 4–8 wk intervals for a total of 3 doses. A 4th dose of 0.5 ml given 6–12 mos after 3rd dose. A booster (5th) dose given at 4–6 yrs of age.

IM: Children 1–7 yrs: 0.5 ml followed by 0.5 ml 4–8 wks later. A 3rd 0.5 ml dose given 6–12 mos after the 2nd dose. A booster (4th) dose given at 4–6 yrs unless the 3rd dose given after the 4th birthday; then the 4th dose is not necessary.

IM: Adults, adolescents: (Note: Use DT for adult use): 0.5 ml followed by 0.5 ml 4–8 wks later. A 3rd dose of 0.5 ml given 6–12 mos after the 2nd. A booster dose of 0.5 ml given every 10 yrs thereafter.

CONTRAINDICATIONS

Acute infection, febrile illness, tetanus infection, sensitivity to tetanus/diphtheria.

ADVERSE EFFECTS

Redness, hard lump at injection site, induration. *Adults:* Axillary lymphadenopathy, chills, headache, hypotension, muscle aches. *Pediatrics:* Fever under 103° F, swelling/pain/tenderness at injection site, anorexia, drowsiness, vomiting, persistent crying.

HAEMOPHILUS INFLUENZAE TYPE B CONJUGATE VACCINE

INDICATIONS

Routine immunization of children against invasive disease caused by *H. influenzae* type b (bacterial meningitis, epiglottis, sepsis, septic arthritis, osteomyelitis, pericarditis, pneumonia).

DOSAGE

Note: Three haemophilus b conjugate vaccines are available for use in infants: (1) Hib oligosaccaride conjugate vaccine (HbOC) HibTITER, (2) Hib polysaccharide conjugate vaccine (PRP-T) ActHIB and OmniHIB, and (3) Hib polysaccharide conjugate vaccine (PRP-OMP) PedvaxHIB. Children who have received PRP-OMP at 2 and 4 mos do not require a dose at 6 mos. Following the primary infant Hib conjugate vaccine series, any Hib conjugate vaccine may be administered as a booster dose at age 12–15 mos. PRP-D (ProHIBit) is licensed only for use >15 mos.

IM: Infants: 0.5 ml at 2, 4 and 6 mos, booster at age 12–15 mos.

CONTRAINDICATIONS

Acute or febrile illness.

ADVERSE EFFECTS

Erythema at injection site, induration, fever, diarrhea, vomiting, irritability, lethargy, anorexia.

HEPATITIS B VACCINE

INDICATIONS

Immunization against infection caused by all known subtypes hepatitis B virus for persons of all ages esp. those at increased risk of infection (e.g., health-care workers who may be exposed via blood or pts' specimens, household and sexual contacts of hepatitis B carriers, dialysis, renal failure pts, hematology/oncology units, infants born of HBsAg-positive mothers whether HBsAg positive or negative, military personnel, persons at increased risk due to sexual practices).

DOSAGE

Children of HBsAg-negative mothers:
IM: Recombivax HB: 2.5 mcg, Engerix-B: 10 mcg: Birth, 2nd dose between 1–4 mos (provided at least 1 mo elapsed since receiving the first dose); 3rd dose between 6 and 18 mos.

Children of HBsAg-positive mothers:
Note: Hepatitis B immune globulin (HBIG) given within 12 hrs of birth.
IM: Recombivax HB: 5 mcg, Engerix-B: 10 mcg: Birth, 2nd dose 1–2 mos, and 3rd dose at 6 mos.

Children of HbsAg status unknown:
IM: Recombivax HB: 5 mcg, Engerix-B: 10 mcg: Birth, 2nd dose at 1 mo, and 3rd dose at 6 mos.

Note: Adolescents who have not received 3 doses of hepatitis B should initiate or complete series at 11–12 yrs, the 2nd dose at least 1 mo after the 1st dose, the 3rd dose at least 4 mos after the 1st and 2 mos after the 2nd dose.

Adolescents, adults:
Recombivax HB:
IM: 11–19 yrs: 0.5 ml (5 mcg) initially, 1 and 6 mos after initial dose; **20 yrs or greater:** 1 ml (10 mcg) initially, then 1 and 6 mos after initial dose.

Engerix-B:
IM: >11 yrs: 1 ml (20 mcg) initially, then 1 and 6 mos after initial dose.

CONTRAINDICATIONS

Sensitivity to hepatitis B vaccine, allergy to yeast, severely compromised cardiopulmonary status, moderate to severe illness w/ or w/o fever, immune deficiency conditions.

ADVERSE EFFECTS

Soreness at injection site, fatigue, fever, headache, vertigo, induration, redness, swelling, pain, itching, ecchymoses, tenderness at injection site.

HEPATITIS B IMMUNE GLOBULIN (HBIG)

INDICATIONS

Postexposure prophylaxis for hepatitis B infection. Provides passive immunization following exposure to hepatitis B virus and for infants born to mothers who are hepatitis B surface antigen positive (HBsAg-positive).

DOSAGE

Infants of HBsAg-positive mothers:
IM: 0.5 ml within 12 hrs of birth.

Postexposure prophylaxis:
IM: Adults: 0.06 ml/kg (usually 3–5 ml) within 24 hrs if possible after exposure. Begin hepatitis B vaccine as soon as possible but within 7 days of exposure.

ADVERSE REACTIONS

Local pain, tenderness, urticaria.

INFLUENZAE VIRUS VACCINE

INDICATIONS

Annual vaccination for adults w/chronic cardiovascular/pulmonary diseases, metabolic disease, nursing home residents, health-care workers dealing w/high-risk pts, healthy adults >65 yrs, children w/chronic metabolic or cardiopulmonary disease.

DOSAGE

IM: Adults, elderly, children >9 yrs: 0.5 ml as single dose. **Children 3–9 yrs:** 0.5 ml one or two times (1 mo apart). **Children 6–35 mos:** 0.25 ml one or two times (1 mo apart). **Note:** Give two doses to children <9 yrs when receiving vaccine for first time.

CONTRAINDICATIONS

History of allergy to eggs. Defer immunization in presence of acute respiratory disease or other active infection or febrile illness.

ADVERSE EFFECTS

Tenderness, redness, induration at injection site, low-grade fever, malaise.

MEASLES VACCINE, LIVE

INDICATIONS

Active immunization against measles (rubeola) in persons 15 mos or older, infants 12–15 mos in high-risk areas or traveling outside the United States. A second dose is recommended.

DOSAGE

SubQ: Adults, children ≥15 mos: 0.5 ml into outer aspect of upper arm. Usually given as MMR (Measles, Mumps, Rubella) for most vaccinations at age 15 mos.

Note: The second dose of MMR vaccine may be given at any time provided 1 mo has elapsed since the first dose. Monovalent measles vaccine may be given as early as 6 mos but two doses of trivalent vaccine still to be given w/first at age 15 mos.

CONTRAINDICATIONS

Immunosuppressed pts, pregnant women, history of egg allergy, hypersensitivity to neomycin (contained in product). Any febrile respiratory infection or other active febrile infection. Active untreated TB. Pts w/blood dyscrasias, leukemia, lymphomas, malignant neoplasms affecting bone marrow or lymphatic system.

ADVERSE EFFECTS

Febrile reaction (rarely above 39.4° C), transient rash, burning, stinging at injection site.

MUMPS VIRUS VACCINE, LIVE

INDICATIONS

Active immunity against mumps in persons ≥12 mos of age.

DOSAGE

SubQ: Adults, children >12 mos: 0.5 ml into outer aspect of upper arm. Usually given as MMR for most vaccinations at age 15 mos.

Note: The second dose of MMR may be given at any time provided at least 1 mo has elapsed since the first dose. Those born after 1/1/57 should receive two trivalent doses (MMR).

CONTRAINDICATIONS

Immunosuppressed pts, pregnant women, history of egg allergy, hypersensitivity to neomycin (contained in product). Any febrile respiratory infection or other active febrile infection. Active untreated TB. Pts w/blood dyscrasias, leukemia, lymphomas, malignant neoplasms affecting bone marrow or lymphatic system.

ADVERSE EFFECTS

Febrile reaction (rarely above 39.4° C), transient rash, burning, stinging at injection site.

PERTUSSIS

See Diphtheria and Tetanus Toxoid, Pertussis Vaccine (DTP)

PNEUMOCOCCAL VACCINE, POLYVALENT

INDICATIONS

Immunization against pneumococcal pneumonia/bacteremia caused by types of pneumococci in vaccine. Indicated in pts at increased risk of pneumococcal disease: immunocompromised (e.g., Hodgkin's disease, renal failure, HIV infection), pts w/splenic dysfunction or anatomic asplenia, chronic cardiovascular or pulmonary disease, alcoholism, elderly (esp. institutionalized).

DOSAGE

IM/SubQ: Adults, children ≥2 yrs: 0.5 ml as single dose.

CONTRAINDICATION

Hypersensitivity, previous immunization w/any polyvalent pneumococcal vaccine.

ADVERSE EFFECTS

Erythema, hard lump, swelling, soreness at injection site, swollen glands, arthralgia, myalgia, asthenia, fever, skin rash.

POLIO VACCINE, LIVE, ORAL

INDICATIONS

Prevention of poliomyelitis caused by poliovirus 1, 2, 3. Immunization recommended for all children and young adults up to 18 yrs.

DOSAGE

Note: Polio vaccine live oral (OPV) is recommended for routine childhood vaccination. Inactivated poliovirus vaccine (IPV) is recommended for individuals with altered immunocompetence. For primary immunization, IPV should be given w/minimum interval of 4 wks between 1st and 2nd doses and 6 mos between 2nd and 3rd doses.

PO: Infants: Three doses of 0.5 ml. First dose at 6–12 wks of age, 2nd dose 8 wks after 1st dose, 3rd dose 8–12 mos after 2nd dose. **Older children:** First 2 doses 8 wks apart, 3rd dose 6–12 mos following the 2nd dose. Fourth dose given upon entering elementary school (not required if 3rd dose given on or after 4th birthday).

CONTRAINDICATIONS

Pts or household members w/immunosuppression (e.g., leukemia, lymphoma, lowered resistance to infection from steroid therapy). Defer in presence of any acute illness, vomiting, diarrhea, and in pts w/advanced debilitated disease (inactivated poliovirus vaccine recommended).

ADVERSE EFFECTS

No immediate effect seen with oral administration.

RECOMMENDATIONS FOR IMMUNIZATION OF INFANTS/CHILDREN

	Birth	1 Mo	2 Mos	4 Mos	6 Mos	12 Mos	15 Mos	18 Mos	4–6 Yrs
Diphtheria[1,2]			x	x	x			x	x
Tetanus[1,2]			x	x	x			x	x
Pertussis[1,2]			x	x	x			x	x
Measles[3]							x		x
Mumps[3]							x		x
Rubella[3]							x		x
Haemophilus[4]			x	x	x		x		
HibTITER									
ProHIBit							x		
PedvaxHIB			x	x		x			
Hepatitis B	x	x			x				
HBsAg-negative[5] mothers									
HBsAg-positive mothers	x	x			x				
Poliovirus			x	x				x	x
varicella						x			

[1]Usually given as diphtheria and tetanus toxoid combined w/pertussis vaccine.

[2]Booster given at 10 yr intervals to maintain immunity.

[3]Usually given as combined measles, mumps, rubella (MMR) vaccine.

[4]Dosage schedule dependent on vaccine formulation and manufacturer used.

[5]See monograph for alternate schedule.

RH$_O$(D) IMMUNE GLOBULIN (RDIG)

INDICATIONS

Suppresses immune response of nonsensitized Rh_o(D) negative pts who receive Rh_o(D) positive blood due to fetomaternal hemorrhage, abdominal trauma, amniocentesis, abortion, or full-term delivery. RDIG prevents future chance of erythroblastosis fetalis in subsequent pregnancies with an Rh_o(D) positive fetus.

DOSAGE

Term delivery:
IM: 300 mcg within 72 hrs.

After amniocentesis, miscarriage, abortion, ectopic pregnancy >13 wks:
IM: 300 mcg one time.

Before delivery:
IM: 300 mcg at 28 wks, 300 mcg within 72 hrs of delivery.

Transfusion accident:
IM: Dependent on volume of packed red cells or whole blood transfused.

Termination of pregnancy (<13 wks):
IM: 50 mcg within 72 hrs.

Note: Do not give to individuals that are positive Rh_o(D) and Du antigens or those w/anti-Rh_o(D) antibodies.

ADVERSE EFFECTS

Fever, injection site tenderness.

RUBELLA VIRUS VACCINE, LIVE (GERMAN MEASLES)

INDICATIONS

Active immunization against rubella (German measles). Intended to reduce occurrence of congenital rubella syndrome among offspring or women contracting rubella during pregnancy. Indicated for children ≥12 mos w/o evidence of wild virus infection, women of childbearing potential for whom serologic testing unavailable (up to 45 yrs of age), those at substantial risk for exposure.

DOSAGE

SubQ: Adults, children at age 15 mos: 0.5 ml into outer aspect of upper arm. Usually given as MMR for most vaccinations at 15 mos.

Note: Second dose of MMR may be given at any time provided at least 1 mo has elapsed since the first dose.

CONTRAINDICATIONS

Immunosuppressed pts, pregnant women, history of egg allergy, hypersensitivity to neomycin (contained in product). Any febrile respiratory infection or other active febrile infection. Active untreated TB. Pts w/blood dyscrasias, leukemia, lymphomas, malignant neoplasms affecting bone marrow or lymphatic system.

ADVERSE EFFECTS

Increase w/age of pt. Lymphadenopathy, skin rash, urticaria, fever, malaise, sore throat, headache, myalgia, paresthesia of extremities.

TETANUS TOXOID ADSORBED (TTA)

INDICATION

Active immunity against tetanus (esp. military personnel, farm/utility workers, those working w/horses, firefighters, occupations that render liable to even minor lacerations/abrasions).

DOSAGE

Also see Diphtheria/Tetanus/Pertussis and Diphtheria/Tetanus.

IM: Adults, adolescents: 0.5 ml at initial visit, 2nd dose 4–8 wks after 1st dose, 3rd dose 6–12 mos after 2nd dose. Booster dose every 10 yrs.

CONTRAINDICATIONS

Acute respiratory infection or other active infection except for emergency booster doses.

ADVERSE EFFECTS

Local reactions at injection site (warmth, redness, induration, hard lump, pain, tenderness, itching, swelling), chills, fever, skin rash.

VARICELLA VIRUS VACCINE

INDICATIONS

Vaccination against varicella (chicken pox).

DOSAGE

SubQ: Adults, children >12 yrs: 1st dose 0.5 ml, then 2nd dose 4–8 wks later. **Children (1–12 yrs):** Single 0.5 ml dose at any time after 12 mos of age.

CONTRAINDICATIONS

Hypersensitivity to any component of vaccine. History of allergy to neomycin. Pts w/blood dyscrasias, leukemia, lymphoma, other malignant neoplasms affecting bone marrow or lymphatic system. Pts immunosuppressed, active untreated tuberculosis, any febrile respiratory illness or active febrile infection, pregnancy.

ADVERSE EFFECTS

Pain, redness at injection site, rash, fever.

laxatives

ACTION

Laxatives ease or stimulate defecation. Mechanisms by which this is accomplished include (1) attracting, retaining fluid in colonic contents due to hydrophilic or osmotic properties; (2) acting directly or indirectly on mucosa to decrease absorption of water and NaCl; or (3) increasing intestinal motility, decreasing absorption of water and NaCl by virtue of decreased transit time.

Bulk-forming: Acts primarily in small/large intestine. Retains water in stool, may bind water, ions in colonic lumen (soften feces, increase bulk); may increase colonic bacteria growth (increases fecal mass). Produces soft stool in 1–3 days.

LAXATIVES

Generic Name	Brand Name(s)	Type	Dosage Range
bisacodyl	Dulcolax	Stimulant	Adults (PO): 10–15 mg; (Rectal): 10 mg Children >6 yrs (PO): 5–10 mg Children <2 yrs (Rectal): 5 mg
cascara	Cascara	Stimulant	Adults: 1 tablet or 5 ml
castor oil	Castor Oil	Stimulant	Adults: 15–60 ml Children (6–12 yrs): 5–15 ml
docusate CA	Surfak	Surfactant	Adults: 240 mg/day Children >6 yrs: 50–150 mg/day
docusate K	Dialose	Surfactant	Adults: 100–300 mg/day Children >6 yrs: 100 mg at hs
docusate Na	Colace	Surfactant	Adults: 50–500 mg/day Children (6–12 yrs): 40–120 mg; (3–6 yrs): 20–60 mg; (<3 yrs): 10–40 mg
lactulose	Cephulac	Osmotic	Adults: 30–45 ml 3–4×/day Children: 40–90 ml/day in divided doses Infants: 2.5–10 ml/day in divided doses
magnesium citrate	Citro-Nesia	Saline	Adults: 240 ml as needed Children: 120 ml as needed
magnesium hydroxide	MOM	Saline	Adults: 30–60 ml/day Children: 5–30 ml/day
magnesium sulfate	Epsom Salt	Saline	Adults: 10–15 g in glass water Children: 5–10 g in glass water
methylcellulose	Citrucel	Bulk-forming	Adults: 5–20 ml liquid 3×/day or 1 tablespoonful 1–3×/day (mix w/water, other fluid)
mineral oil	Mineral Oil	Lubricant	Adults: 5–45 ml Children: 5–20 ml
phenolpthalein	Modane	Stimulant	Adults: 60–194 mg at hs
poycarbophil	Mitrolan	Bulk-forming	Adults: 1 g 4×/day; maximum: 6 g/day Children (6–12 yrs): 500 mg 1–3×/day; maximum: 3 g/day Children (3–6 yrs): 500 mg 2×/day; maximum: 2 g/day
psyllium	Metamucil	Bulk-forming	Adults: 1 tsp 1–3×/day (mix w/water, other fluid)
senna	Senokot	Stimulant	Adults: 2–8 tablets/day Children: 1–4 tablets/day

hs = bedtime.

Castor oil: Acts in small intestine. Reduces absorption of fluid, electrolytes; stimulates intestinal peristalsis. Produces watery stool in 2–6 hrs. *Lactulose:* Acts in colon. Similar to saline laxatives. Osmotic action may be enhanced in distal ileum/colon by bacterial metabolism to lactate, other organic acids. This decrease in pH increases motility, secretion. Produces soft stool in 1–3 days.

Saline: Acts in small/large intestine, colon (sodium phosphate). Poorly, slowly absorbed, causes hormone cholecystokinin release from duodenum (stimulates fluid secretion, motility), possesses osmotic properties, produces watery stool in 2–6 hrs (low doses produce semifluid stool in 6–12 hrs).

Stimulant: Acts in colon. Enhances accumulation of water/electrolytes in colonic lumen, enhances intestinal motility. May act directly on intestinal mucosa. Produces semifluid stool in 6–12 hrs (**Note:** Bisacodyl suppository acts in 15–60 min).

Surfactants: Act in small and large intestines. Hydrate and soften stools by their surfactant action facilitating penetration of fat and water into stool. Produce soft stool in 1–3 days.

USES

Short-term treatment of constipation; evacuate colon before rectal/bowel examination; prevent straining (e.g., after anorectal surgery, myocardial infarction); reduce painful elimination (e.g., episiotomy, hemorrhoids, anorectal lesions); modify effluent from ileostomy, colostomy; prevent fecal impaction; remove ingested poisons.

PRECAUTIONS

CONTRAINDICATIONS: Acute surgical abdomen, abdominal pain, intestinal obstruction or perforation, fecal impaction, undiagnosed rectal bleeding, young children. **CAUTIONS:** Select laxative carefully for diabetics and pts on sodium-restricted diet. (No saline laxative.) Avoid overuse/abuse.

INTERACTIONS

Cholinergics increase effects; anticholinergics and CNS depressants decrease effects. Mineral oil impairs absorption of vitamins A, D, E, and K. Antacids decrease laxative action of bisacodyl tablets. Laxative may decrease absorption of other drugs by increasing rate of passage.

SIDE EFFECTS

Cramping, frequent liquid stools, nausea, weakness, perianal irritation.

TOXIC EFFECTS/ADVERSE REACTIONS

Incidence rare. Severe diarrhea may cause dehydration and electrolyte imbalance. Fluid retention with saline laxative may cause edema and electrolyte imbalance. *Bulk-forming laxative:* Allergic reaction, impaction.

PATIENT CONSIDERATIONS

GENERAL: Give w/at least 8 oz of water and provide 6–8 glasses of water that day (unless pt on water restriction). Most laxatives should be given on an empty stomach at bedtime to provide morning evacuation. Provide call light and assistance as indicated. BASELINE ASSESSMENT: Results of laxative. PATIENT/FAMILY TEACHING: Avoid chronic use. Stress value of high-fiber diet, fluid intake, exercise, and regular bowel habits.

neuromuscular blockers

ACTION

Interrupt nerve impulse transmission at skeletal neuromuscular junction and/or autonomic ganglia (these receptors are called "nicotinic-cholinergic"). Further classified by whether or not they cause depolarization of motor end plate (nondepolarizing vs. depolarizing). Combine w/nicotinic-cholinergic receptor at postjunctional membrane blocking competitive transmitter action of acetylcholine. When administered, motor weakness gives way to total flaccid paralysis. Cause relaxation of skeletal muscle. Can produce decreased B/P due to release of histamine and to partial ganglionic blockade. Lack CNS effects—do not diminish consciousness or pain perception.

USES

Adjuvant in surgical anesthesia to obtain relaxation of skeletal muscle (esp. abdominal wall) for surgery (allows lighter level of anesthesia, valuable in orthopedic procedures). Neuromuscular blocking agents of short duration often used to facilitate intubation w/endotracheal tube; facilitates laryngoscopy, bronchoscopy, and esophagoscopy in combination w/general anesthetics. Provide muscle relaxation in pts undergoing mechanical ventilation, muscle relaxation in diagnosis of myasthenia gravis. Prevent convulsive movements during electroconvulsive therapy.

PRECAUTIONS

CONTRAINDICATIONS: Contraindicated during pregnancy, lactation, hypersensitivity to drug or components, pts who have own or family history of malignant hyperthermia. Use w/extreme caution, if at all, in pts w/myasthenia gravis. **CAUTIONS:** During cesarean delivery (potential respiratory depression in neonate); caution and reduced dosage during delivery when magnesium sulfate has been administered to pregnant woman (potentiates effects). Cautious use in pts w/hepatic, renal, or pulmonary impairment; respiratory depression; geriatric or debilitated pts.

INTERACTIONS

General anesthetics, antibiotics (esp. aminoglycosides) may increase effects. Anticholinesterase inhibitors (e.g., neostigmine) may decrease effects.

SIDE EFFECTS

Prolonged apnea, residual muscle weakness, hypersensitivity reactions. Many drugs also cause hypotension, wheezing and bronchospasm, cardiac disturbances, flushing, urticaria, pruritus.

TOXIC EFFECTS/ADVERSE REACTIONS

Malignant hyperthermia is rare, but often fatal (esp. w/halothane or succinylcholine). Severely compromised respiratory function; respiratory paralysis.

NEUROMUSCULAR BLOCKING AGENTS

Generic Name	Brand Name(s)	Type	Uses
atracurium	Tracrium	Nondepolarizing	Endotracheal intubation Surgery Mechanical ventilation
cisatracurium	Nimbex	Nondepolarizing	Endotracheal intubation Mechanical ventilation Surgery
doxacurium	Nuromax	Nondepolarizing	Endotracheal intubation Surgery
mivacurium	Mivacron	Nondepolarizing	Surgery Mechanical ventilation Endotracheal intubation
pancuronium	Pavulon	Nondepolarizing	Surgery Mechanical ventilation
pipecuronium	Arduan	Nondepolarizing	Endotracheal intubation Surgery
rocuronium	Zemuron	Nondepolarizing	Endotracheal intubation Surgery Mechanical ventilation
succinylcholine	Anectine Quelicin	Depolarizing	Endotracheal intubation Surgery Mechanical ventilation ECT
tubocurarine	Tubocurarine	Nondepolarizing	Surgery Mechanical ventilation ECT Dx: Myasthenia gravis
vecuronium	Norcuron	Nondepolarizing	Endotracheal intubation Surgery Mechanical ventilation

ECT = electroconvulsive therapy; Dx = diagnosis.

PATIENT CONSIDERATIONS

GENERAL: Have equipment and personnel immediately available to intubate pt and provide mechanical ventilation, including use of positive pressure oxygen. Have anticholinesterase reversal agents immediately available. Drugs do not alter consciousness; pt may be conscious but unable to move, breathe. INTERVENTION/EVALUATION: Continuously monitor B/P, pulse, EKG. PATIENT/FAMILY TEACHING: Explain to conscious pt, family that muscle tone will return. Provide emotional support and monitor respirations carefully during recovery period.

nitrates

ACTION

Relax most smooth muscles, including arteries and veins. Effect is primarily on veins (decrease left/right ventricular end-diastolic pressure).

In angina, nitrates decrease myocardial work and O_2 requirements (decrease preload by venodilation and afterload by arteriodilation). Nitrates also appear to redistribute blood flow to ischemic myocardial areas improving perfusion w/o increase in coronary blood flow.

NITRATES

Generic Name	Rte Admin	Brand Name(s)	Cardiovascular Effect		Dosage Range
			Onset	Duration	
erythrityl	PO	Cardilate	5–30 min	3–6 hrs	5–10 mg before event, up to 100 mg/day
isosorbide	SL	Isordil Sorbitrate	2–5 min	1–3 hrs	2.5–10 mg q2–3h
	PO	Isordil Sorbitrate	20–40 min	4–6 hrs	10–40 mg q6h
	SR	Dilatrate-SR Isordil Sorbitrate	up to 4 hrs	6–8 hrs	40–80 mg q8–12 h
nitroglycerin	SL	Nitrostat	1–3 min	30–60 min	0.3–0.6 mg to 3×/ 15 min
	SR	Nitrobid Nitroglyn	20–45 min	3–8 hrs	2.5 mg 3–4×/day up to 26 mg 3–4×/day
	Trans	Minitran Nitro-Dur Nitrodisc Transderm Nitro	30–60 min	Up to 24 hrs	0.2–0.4 mg/hr up to 0.8 mg/hr
	Top	Nitrol	30–60 min	2–12 hrs	1–2 in q8h up to 4–5 in q4h
pentaerythritol	PO	Duotrate Peritrate	PO: 20–60 min SR: 30 min	5 hrs up to 12 hrs	PO: 10–20 mg 3–4×/ day up to 40 mg 4×/day SR: 1 cap/tab q12h

SL = sublingual; SR = sustained release; Trans = transdermal; Top = topical.

USES

Sublingual: Acute relief of angina pectoris.

Oral, topical: Long-term prophylactic treatment of angina pectoris.

Intravenous: Adjunctive treatment in CHF associated w/acute myocardial infarction. Produces controlled hypotension during surgical procedures; controls B/P in perioperative hypertension, angina unresponsive to organic nitrates or beta blockers.

PRECAUTIONS

CONTRAINDICATIONS: Hypersensitivity, hypotension, severe anemia, head trauma or cerebral hemorrhage, renal or hepatic dysfunction, closed-angle glaucoma, pregnancy, lactation. **CAUTIONS:** Acute MI, hepatic or renal dysfunction, blood volume decrease from diuretics, systolic B/P below 90 mm Hg. Chronic administration may lead to tolerance.

INTERACTIONS

Alcohol, antihypertensives, vasodilators may increase risk of orthostatic hypotension.

SIDE EFFECTS

Headache, hypotension, dizziness, palpitations, skin or mucous membrane sensitivity to nitrites/nitrates.

TOXIC EFFECTS/ADVERSE REACTIONS

Severe headache, significant hypotension, difficulty breathing, chest pain, hypersensitivity reactions.

PATIENT CONSIDERATIONS

GENERAL: IV infusion of nitroglycerin requires special administration set and precise flow rate. BASELINE ASSESSMENT: Record onset, type (sharp, dull, squeezing), radiation, location, intensity, and duration of anginal pain and precipitating factors (exertion, emotional stress). Obtain baseline B/P and apical pulse. INTERVENTION/EVALUATION: Monitor B/P and apical pulse (withhold and notify physician if systolic B/P below 90 mm Hg). Continuous cardiac monitoring is indicated for unrelieved, acute episodes. Assess for relief of anginal pain. Check for local irritation when given dermally or sublingually. PATIENT/FAMILY TEACHING: Avoid high-caffeine foods/fluids, such as coffee, colas, chocolate, tea (increased risk of anginal attacks). Do not take alcohol (can cause hypotensive, shocklike state) or other drugs w/o physician approval. Identify precipitating factors. Take sublingual tablets sitting or lying down for anginal relief; may repeat every 5 min, up to 3 tablets in 15 min. If no relief, have ambulance transport to hospital. Do not change brands; discard expired drugs. Notify physician of severe or persistent headache.

nonsteroidal anti-inflammatory drugs (NSAIDs)

ACTION

Exact mechanism for anti-inflammatory, analgesic, antipyretic effects unknown. Inhibition of enzyme cyclooxygenase, the enzyme responsible for prostaglandin synthesis, appears to be a major mechanism of action. May inhibit other mediators of inflammation (e.g., leukotrienes). Direct action on hypothalamus heat-regulating center may contribute to antipyretic effect.

NSAIDS

GENERIC NAME	BRAND NAME(S)	USE: DOSAGE RANGE
aspirin	many	Aches/pains: 325–650 mg q4h prn Arthritis: 3.2–6 g/day Juvenile rheumatoid arthritis: 60–110 mg/kg/day Acute rheumatic fever: Adults: 5–8 g/day; Children: 100 mg/kg/day x14 days; then, 75 mg/kg/day ×4–6 wks Transient ischemic attacks: 1,300 mg/day Myocardial infarction prophylaxis: 81–325 mg/day Analgesic/antipyretic (children): up to 60–80 mg/kg/day or 10–15 mg/kg/dose q4h
choline salicylate	Arthropan	Arthritis/pain/fever: 870 mg (5 ml) q3–4h up to 6×/day
diclofenac	Voltaren	Arthritis: 100–200 mg/day
diflunisal	Dolobid	Arthritis: 0.5–1 g/day Pain: 1 g, then 0.5 g q8–12h
etodolac	Lodine	Arthritis: 600–800 mg/day Pain: 200–400 mg q6–8h; max: 1200 mg/day
fenoprofen	Nalfon	Arthritis: 300–600 mg 3–4×/day Pain: 200 mg q4–6h prn
flurbiprofen	Ansaid	Arthritis: 200–300 mg/day
ibuprofen	Motrin	Arthritis: 1.2–3.2 g/day Pain: 400 mg q4–6h prn Fever: 200 mg q4–6h prn Primary dysmenorrhea: 400 mg q4h prn Juvenile arthritis: 30–40 mg/kg/day
indomethacin	Indocin	Arthritis: 50–200 mg/day Bursitis/tendonitis: 75–150 mg/day Gouty arthritis: 150 mg/day
ketoprofen	Orudis	Arthritis: 150–300 mg/day Pain/primary dysmenorrhea: 25–50 mg q6–8h as needed
ketorolac	Toradol	Pain: PO: 10 mg q4–6h prn; max: 40 mg/day; IM/IV: 60–120 mg/day
magnesium salicylate	Magan	Arthritis/pain/fever: 3.6–4.8 g/day in 3–4 divided doses
meclofenamate	Meclomen	Arthritis: 200–400 mg/day Pain: 50 mg q4–6h prn Primary dysmenorrhea: 100 mg 3×/day
meloxicam	Mobic	Osteoarthritis: 7.5–15 mg/day
nabumetone	Relafen	Arthritis: 1–2 g/day
naproxen	Anaprox	Arthritis: 250–550 mg/day
	Naprosyn	Pain/1° dysmenorrhea/bursitis/tendonitis: 500 mg, then 250 mg q6–8h Juvenile arthritis: 10 mg/kg in 2 divided doses Gouty arthritis: 750 mg, then 250 mg q8h
oxaprozin	Daypro	Arthritis: 600–1,800 mg/day
piroxicam	Feldene	Arthritis: 20 mg/day
sodium salicylate	Sodium Salicylate	Arthritis/pain/fever: 325–650 mg q4h prn
sulindac	Clinoril	Arthritis: 300 mg/day Acute gouty arthritis/painful shoulder: 400 mg/day
tolmetin	Tolectin	Arthritis: 600–1,800 mg/day Juvenile arthritis: 15–30 mg/kg/day

1° = primary; prn= as circumstances may require.

USES

Provides symptomatic relief from *pain/inflammation* in the treatment of musculoskeletal disorders (e.g., rheumatoid arthritis, osteoarthritis, ankylosing spondylitis); *analgesic* for low to moderate pain; *reduces fever* (many agents not suited for routine/prolonged therapy due to toxicity). By virtue of its action on platelet function, aspirin is used in treatment or prophylaxis of diseases associated w/hypercoagulability (reduces risk of stroke/heart attack).

PRECAUTIONS

CONTRAINDICATIONS: Aspirin sensitivity or allergy to other components; pregnancy; lactation; children <14 yrs of age, gastrointestinal disorders. **CAUTIONS:** Renal or hepatic dysfunctions, cardiac or hypertensive disorders, severe infections, elderly, coagulation defects, otic disease.

INTERACTIONS

Salicylates: Antacids, NSAIDs may increase risk of GI effects (e.g., ulceration). Urinary alkalinizers, antacids increase excretion. Anticoagulants, heparin, thrombolytics increase risk of bleeding. Large doses may increase insulin, oral hypoglycemic effects. Valproic acid, platelet aggregation inhibitors may increase risk of bleeding. May increase toxicity of methotrexate, zidovudine. Ototoxic medications, vancomycin may increase ototoxicity. May decrease effect of probenecid, sulfinpyrazone.

NSAIDs: May increase effects of oral anticoagulants, heparin, thrombolytics. May decrease effect of antihypertensives, diuretics. Salicylates, aspirin may increase risk of GI side effects, bleeding. Bone marrow depressants may increase risk of hematologic reactions. May increase methotrexate toxicity. Probenecid may increase concentration.

SIDE EFFECTS

Gastrointestinal upset, dizziness, headache, constipation or diarrhea. *Ophthalmic:* Burning, stinging on instillation, keratitis, elevated intraocular pressure.

TOXIC EFFECTS/ADVERSE REACTIONS

Hypersensitivity reactions, including skin rash or urticaria. Renal or hepatic toxicity, bone marrow suppression, bleeding, esp. of gastrointestinal tract. Tinnitus and hearing disturbances. Reactions vary by individual drug.

PATIENT CONSIDERATIONS

GENERAL: Check for aspirin sensitivity (cross-sensitivity). Administer on schedule to maintain blood levels. Provide rest, positioning, and other comfort measures for pain relief. BASELINE ASSESSMENT: Assess pain (type, location, intensity). Check temperature, pulse, respirations. INTERVENTION/EVALUATION: Assess pain, therapeutic response (decreased temperature, pain relief, improved mobility). PATIENT/FAMILY TEACHING: Take w/meals or on empty stomach, as indicated by individual drug; however, all drugs may be taken w/food,

if necessary, to reduce GI side effects. Avoid alcohol and consult physician about other medications. Refrain from driving or other activities requiring motor response until certain no dizziness present. Inform other physicians or dentist of drug therapy.

nutrition: enteral

Enteral nutrition (EN), also known as tube feedings, provides food/nutrients via GI tract using special formulas, techniques of delivery, and equipment. All routes of enteral nutrition consist of placement of a tube through which liquid formula is infused.

INDICATIONS

Tube feedings are used in pts w/major trauma, burns, undergoing radiation and/or chemotherapy, w/liver failure, severe renal impairment, w/physical or neurologic impairment, preop and postop to promote anabolism, prevent cachexia, malnutrition.

ROUTES OF ENTERAL NUTRITION DELIVERY

Nasogastric (NG):
INDICATIONS: Most common for short-term feeding in pts unable or unwilling to consume adequate nutrition by mouth. Requires at least partially functioning GI tract. **ADVANTAGES:** Does not require surgical intervention and is fairly easily inserted. Allows full use of digestive tract. Decreases chance hyperosmolar solutions may cause distention, nausea, vomiting. **DISADVANTAGES:** Temporary. May be easily pulled out during routine nursing care. Has potential for pulmonary aspiration of gastric contents, risk of reflux esophagitis, regurgitation.

Nasoduodenal (ND), nasojejunal (NJ):
INDICATIONS: Pts unable or unwilling to consume adequate nutrition by mouth. Requires at least partially functioning GI tract. **ADVANTAGES:** Does not require surgical intervention and is fairly easily inserted. Preferred for pts at risk of aspiration. Valuable for pts w/gastroparesis. **DISADVANTAGES:** Temporary. May be pulled out during routine nursing care. May be dislodged by coughing, vomiting. Small lumen size increases risk of clogging when medication is given through them, more susceptible to rupturing when using infusion device. Must be radiographed for placement, frequently extubated.

Gastrostomy:
INDICATIONS: Pts w/esophageal obstruction or impaired swallowing, pts in whom NG, ND, or NJ not feasible, or when long-term feeding indicated. **ADVANTAGES:** Permanent feeding access. Tubing has larger bore allowing noncontinuous (bolus) feeding (300–400 ml over 30–60 min q3–6h). May be inserted endoscopically using local anesthetic (procedure called percutaneous endoscopic gastrostomy [PEG]).

ENTERAL FORMULAS

PRODUCT	DESCRIPTION	CAL/ML	OSMOLALITY (MOSM/KG)	PROTEIN G/L	CHO G/L	FAT G/L
Advera	HIV infection AIDS	1.3	—	60	216	22.8
Alitrag	Metabolic stress Impaired GI function	1.0	575	52.5	165	15.5
Compleat	Tube feeding	1.1	450	43	130	43
Ensure Plus	Nutrient-dense oral supplement	1.5	690	54.9	199	53.2
Glucerna	Glucose intolerance	1.0	375	41.8	93.7	55.7
Isocal HN	Low residue	1.06	—	43.9	122	45.2
Jevity	Tube feeding w/fiber	1.06	310	44.4	151	36.7
Nepro	Renal dialysis	2.0	635	69.9	212	94.4
Osmolite HN	Low residue	1.06	300	44.4	139	36.7
Pediasure	Children 1–6 yrs	1.0	310	30.0	110	49.9
Perative	Metabolic stress	1.3	425	66.6	176	36.9
Pulmocare	Pulmonary	1.5	465	62.6	106	92
Suplena	Predialysis	2.0	615	30.0	254	95.4
Sustacal	Complete balanced nutrition	1.0	650	61.2	139	23.2
Traumacal	Multiple trauma, major burns	1.5	490	82.3	144	68.4
Travasorb HN	Elemental diet	—	560	15.0	58.3	4.5
Twocal HN	Nutrient dense oral supplement	2.0	690	83.7	216	90.3
Vital HN	Elemental diet	1.0	500	41.7	185	10.8

DISADVANTAGES: Requires surgery, may be inserted in conjunction w/other surgery or endoscopically (see Advantages). Stoma care required. Tube may be inadvertently dislodged. Risk of aspiration, peritonitis, cellulitis, leakage of gastric contents.

Jejunostomy:
INDICATIONS: Pts w/stomach or duodenal obstruction, impaired gastric motility, pts in whom NG, ND, or NJ not feasible, or when long-term feeding indicated. **ADVANTAGES:** Allows early postop feeding (small-bowel function is least affected by surgery). Risk of aspiration reduced. Rarely pulled out inadvertently. **DISADVANTAGES:** Requires surgery (laparotomy). Stoma care required. Risk of intraperitoneal leakage. Can be dislodged easily.

CLASSIFICATION

INITIATING ENTERAL NUTRITION

With continuous feeding, initiation of isotonic (about 300 mOsm/L) or moderately hypertonic feeding (up to 495 mOsm/L) can be given full strength usually at a slow rate (30–50 ml/hr) and gradually increased (25 ml/hr q6–24h). Formulas w/osmolality of >500 mOsm/L are generally started at half strength and gradually increased in rate, then concentration. Tolerance increased if the rate and concentration are not increased simultaneously.

SELECTION OF FORMULAS

Protein: Has many important physiologic roles and is the primary source of nitrogen in the body. Provides 4 kcal/g protein. Sources of protein in enteral feedings: sodium caseinate, calcium caseinate, soy protein, dipeptides.

Carbohydrate (CHO): Provides energy for the body and heat to maintain body temperature. Provides 3.4 kcal/g carbohydrate. Sources of carbohydrate (CHO) in enteral feedings: corn syrup, cornstarch, maltodextrin, lactose, sucrose, glucose.

Fat: Provides concentrated source of energy. Referred to as "kilocalorie dense" or "protein sparing." Provides 9 kcal/g fat. Sources of fat in enteral feedings: corn oil, safflower oil, medium chain triglycerides.

Electrolytes, vitamins, trace elements: Contained in formulas (not found in specialized products for renal and hepatic insufficiency).

All products containing protein, fat, carbohydrate, vitamin, electrolytes, trace elements are nutritionally complete and designed to be used by pts for long periods.

COMPLICATIONS

MECHANICAL: Usually associated w/some aspect of the feeding tube.

Aspiration pneumonia: Caused by delayed gastric emptying, gastroparesis, gastroesophageal reflux, or decreased gag reflex. May be prevented or treated by reducing infusion rate, using lower fat formula, feeding beyond pylorus, checking residuals, using small-bore feeding tubes, elevating head of bed 30–45° during and for 30–60 min after intermittent feeding, and regularly checking tube placement.

Esophageal, mucosal, pharyngeal irritation, otitis: Caused by using large-bore NG tube. Prevented by use of small bore whenever possible.

Irritation, leakage at ostomy site: Caused by drainage of digestive juices from site. Prevented by close attention to skin/stoma care.

Tube, lumen obstruction: Caused by thickened formula residue, formation of formula-medication complexes. Prevented by frequently irrigating tube w/clear water (also before and after giving formulas/medication), avoiding instilling medication if possible.

GASTROINTESTINAL: Usually associated w/formula, rate of delivery, unsanitary handling of solutions or delivery system.

Diarrhea: Caused by low-residue formulas, rapid delivery, use of hyperosmolar formula, hypoalbuminemia, malabsorption, microbial contamination, or rapid GI transit time. Prevented by using fiber-supplemented formulas, decreasing rate of delivery, using dilute formula and gradually increasing strength.

Cramping, gas, abdominal distention: Caused by nutrient malabsorption, rapid delivery of refrigerated formula. Prevented by delivering formula by continuous methods, giving formulas at room temperature, decreasing rate of delivery.

Nausea, vomiting: Caused by rapid delivery of formula, gastric retention. Prevented by reducing rate of delivery, using dilute formulas, selecting low-fat formulas.

Constipation: Caused by inadequate fluid intake, reduced bulk, inactivity. Prevented by supplementing fluid intake, using fiber-supplemented formula, encouraging ambulation.

METABOLIC: Fluid/electrolyte status should be monitored. Refer to monitoring section. Additionally, the very young and very old are at greater risk in developing complications such as dehydration or overhydration.

MONITORING

Daily: Estimate nutrient intake, fluid intake/output, weight of pt, clinical observations.

Weekly: Electrolytes (potassium, sodium, magnesium, calcium, phosphorus), blood glucose, BUN, creatinine, liver function tests (e.g., SGOT [AST], alkaline phosphatase), 24 hour urea and creatinine excretion, total iron binding capacity (TIBC) or serum transferrin, triglycerides, cholesterol.

Monthly: Serum albumin.

Other: Urine glucose, acetone (when blood glucose >250), vital signs (temperature, respirations, pulse, B/P) q8h.

nutrition: parenteral

Parenteral nutrition (PN), also known as total parenteral nutrition (TPN) or hyperalimentation (HAL), provides required nutrients to pts by IV route of administration. The goal of PN is to maintain or restore nutritional status caused by disease, injury, or inability to consume nutrients by other means.

INDICATIONS

Conditions when pt is unable to use alimentary tract via oral, gastrostomy, or jejunostomy routes. Impaired absorption of protein caused by obstruction, inflammation, or antineoplastic therapy. Bowel rest necessary because of GI surgery or ileus, fistulas, or anastomotic leaks. Conditions w/increased metabolic requirements (e.g., burns, infection, trauma). Preserve tissue reserves as in acute renal failure. Inadequate nutrition from tube feeding methods.

COMPONENTS OF PN

In order to meet IV nutritional requirements six essential categories in PN are needed for tissue synthesis and energy balance.

Protein: In the form of crystalline amino acids (CAA), primarily used for protein synthesis. Several products are designed to meet specific needs for pts w/renal failure (e.g., NephrAmine), liver disease (e.g., HepatAmine), stress/trauma (e.g., Aminosyn HBC), use in neonates and pediatrics (e.g., Aminosyn PF, TrophAmine). Calories: 4 kcal/g protein.

Energy: In the form of dextrose, available in concentrations of 5–70%. Dextrose <10% may be given peripherally; concentrations >10% must be given centrally. Calories: 3.4 kcal/g dextrose.

IV fat emulsion: Available in the form of 10 or 20% concentrations. Provides a concentrated source of energy/calories (9 kcal/g fat) and is a source of essential fatty acids. May be administered peripherally or centrally.

Electrolytes: Major electrolytes (calcium, magnesium, potassium, sodium; also acetate, chloride, phosphate). Doses of electrolytes are individualized, based on many factors (e.g., kidney and/or liver function, fluid status).

Vitamins: Essential components in maintaining metabolism and cellular function; widely used in PN.

Trace elements: Necessary in long-term PN administration. Trace elements include zinc, copper, chromium, manganese, selenium, molybdenum, and iodine.

Miscellaneous: Additives include insulin, albumin, heparin, and histamine$_2$ blockers (e.g., cimetidine, rantidine, famotidine). Other medication may be included, but compatibility for admixture should be checked on an individual basis.

ROUTE OF ADMINISTRATION

PN is administered via either peripheral or central vein.
Peripheral: Usually involves 2–3 L/day of 5–10% dextrose w/3–5% amino acid solution along w/IV fat emulsion. Electrolytes, vitamins, trace elements added according to pt needs. Peripheral solutions provide about 2,000 kcal/day and 60–90 g protein/day. **ADVANTAGES:** Lower risks vs. central mode of administration. **DISADVANTAGES:** Peripheral veins may not be suitable (esp. in pts w/illness of long duration); more susceptible to phlebitis (due to osmolalities >600 mOsm/L); veins may be viable only 1–2 wks; large volumes of fluid are needed to meet nutritional requirements, which may be contraindicated in many pts.

Central: Usually utilizes hypertonic dextrose (concentration range of 15–35%) and amino acid solution of 3–7% w/IV fat emulsion. Electrolytes, vitamins, trace elements added according to pt needs. Central solutions provide 2,000–4,000 kcal/day. Must be given through large central vein w/high blood flow allowing rapid dilution avoiding phlebitis/thrombosis (usually through percutaneous insertion of catheter into subclavian vein then advancement of catheter to superior vena cava). **ADVANTAGES:** Allows more alternatives/flexibility in establishing regimens; allows ability to provide full nutritional requirements w/o need of daily fat emulsion; useful in pts who are fluid restricted (increased concentration), pts needing large nutritional requirements (e.g., trauma, malignancy), or for whom PN indicated >7–10 days. **DISADVANTAGES:** Risk w/insertion, use, maintenance of central line; increased risk of infection, catheter-induced trauma, and metabolic changes.

MONITORING

May vary slightly from institution to institution.

Baseline: CBC, platelet count, prothrombin time, weight, body length/head circumference (in infants), electrolytes, glucose, BUN, creatinine, uric acid, total protein, cholesterol, triglycerides, bilirubin, alkaline phosphatase, LDH, SGOT (AST), albumin, other tests as needed.

Daily: Weight, vital signs (TPR), nutritional intake (kcal, protein, fat), electrolytes (potassium, sodium chloride), glucose (serum, urine), acetone, BUN, osmolarity, other tests as needed.

2–3 times/week: CBC, coagulation studies (PT, PTT), creatinine, calcium, magnesium, phosphorus, acid-base status, other tests as needed.

Weekly: Nitrogen balance, total protein, albumin, prealbumin, transferrin, liver function tests (SGOT [AST], SGPT [ALT]), alkaline phosphatase, LDH, bilirubin, Hgb, uric acid, cholesterol, triglycerides, other tests as needed.

COMPLICATIONS

Mechanical: Malfunction in system for IV delivery (e.g., pump failure, problems w/lines, tubing, administration sets, catheter). Pneumothorax, catheter misdirection, arterial puncture, bleeding, hematoma formation may occur w/catheter placement.

Infectious: Infections (pts often more susceptible to infections), catheter sepsis (e.g., fever, shaking chills, glucose intolerance) where no other site of infection identified.

Metabolic: Includes hyperglycemia, elevated cholesterol and triglycerides, abnormal liver function tests.

Fluid, electrolyte, acid-base disturbances: May alter potassium, sodium, phosphate, magnesium levels.

Nutritional: Clinical effects seen may be due to lack of adequate vitamins, trace elements, essential fatty acids.

opioid analgesics

ACTION

Opioids refer to all drugs, natural and synthetic, having actions similar to morphine and to receptors combining w/these agents. Three opioid receptors have been identified: mu, kappa, and delta. Morphinelike opioid agonists act primarily at mu receptors; and opioids w/mixed action are agonists at some receptors, antagonists/weak agonists at other receptors.

Morphinelike: Major effects are on the CNS (produce analgesia, drowsiness, mood changes, mental clouding, analgesia w/o loss of consciousness, nausea and vomiting) and gastrointestinal tract (decrease HCl secretion, diminish biliary, pancreatic, and intestinal secretions; diminish propulsive peristalsis). Also affects respiration (depressed) and cardiovascular system (peripheral vasodilation, decrease peripheral resistance, inhibit baroreceptor reflexes).

Opioids w/mixed action: After binding to receptor, may produce no effect or only limited action. Produce analgesia, euphoria, respiratory and physical depression, have lower abuse potential, may produce withdrawal symptoms in pts w/opioid dependence.

USES

Relief of moderate to severe pain associated w/surgical procedures, myocardial infarction, burns, cancer, or other conditions. May be used as an adjunct to anesthesia, either as a preop medication or intraoperatively as a supplement to anesthesia. Also used for obstetrical analgesia. Codeine and hydrocodone have an antitussive effect. Opium tinctures, such as paregoric, are used for severe diarrhea. Methadone relieves severe pain but is used primarily as part of heroin detoxification.

OPIOID ANALGESICS

Generic (Brand) Names	Equianalgesic to 10 mg IM Morphine	Type	Analgesic Effect: Onset	Analgesic Effect: Peak	Analgesic Effect: Duration	Dosage Range
Alfentanil (Alfenta)	—	Agonist	Immediate	—	—	—
buprenorphine (Buprenex)	IM: 0.3 mg	Mixed	15 min	1 hr	6 hrs	IM, IV: 0.3 mg q6h prn
butorphanol (Stadol)	IM: 2 mg	Mixed	<10 min	0.5–1 hr	2–4 hrs	IM: 2 mg q3–4h prn IV: 1 mg q3–4h prn
codeine	PO: 200 mg IM: 120 mg	Agonist	10–30 min	0.5–1 hr	4–6 hrs	PO, SubQ, IM: Adults: 15–60 mg q4–6h prn Children: 0.5 mg/kg q4–6h prn
dezocine (Dalgan)	IM: 10 mg	Mixed	15–30 min	30–150 min	2–4 hrs	IM: 5–20 mg q3–6h prn IV: 2.5–10 mg q2–4h prn
fentanyl (Sublimaze)	IM: 0.1 mg	Agonist	7–8 min	—	1–2 hrs	—
hydrocodone	—	Agonist	—	—	4–8 hrs	—
hydromorphone (Dilaudid)	PO: 7.5 mg IM: 1.5 mg	Agonist	15–30 min	0.5–1 hr	4–5 hrs	PO: 2 mg q4–6h prn SubQ, IM: 1–2 mg q4–6h prn Rectal: 3 mg q6–8h prn
levorphanol (Levo-dromoran)	IM: 2 mg	Agonist	0.5–1.5 hrs	0.5–1 hr	6–8 hrs	SubQ: 2–3 mg q4h prn

OPIOID ANALGESICS *Continued*

GENERIC (BRAND) NAMES	EQUIANALGESIC TO 10 MG IM MORPHINE	TYPE	ANALGESIC EFFECT ONSET	PEAK	DURATION	DOSAGE RANGE
meperidine (Demerol)	PO: 300 mg IM: 75 mg	Agonist	10–45 min	0.5–1 hr	2–4 hrs	PO, IM, SubQ: Adults: 50–150 mg q3–4h prn Children: 1–1.8 mg/kg q3–4h prn
methadone (Dolophine)	PO: 20 mg IM: 10 mg	Agonist	30–60 min	0.5–1 hr	4–6 hrs	IM, SubQ, PO: 2.5–10 mg q4h prn
morphine (Roxanol, MS Contin)	PO: 60 mg	Agonist	15–60 min	0.5–1 hr	3–7 hrs	PO: 10–30 mg q4h prn IM: 5–20 mg q4h prn
nalbuphine (Nubain)	IM: 10 mg	Mixed	2–15 min	0.5–1 hr	3–6 hrs	SubQ, IM, IV: 10 mg q3–6h prn
oxycodone (Roxicodone)	PO: 30 mg	Agonist	15–30 min	1 hr	4–6 hrs	PO: 5 mg or 5 ml q6h prn
oxymorphone (Numorphan)	IM: 1 mg RTL: 10 mg	Agonist	5–10 min	0.5–1 hr	3–6 hrs	SubQ, IM: 1–1.5 mg q4h prn Rectal: 5 mg q4h prn
pentazocine (Talwin)	PO: 180 mg IM: 60 mg	Mixed	PO: 15–30 min	1–3 hrs	3 hrs	PO: 50–100 mg q3–4h prn
			IM: 15–20 min	15–60 min	3 hrs	IM, SubQ, IV: 30 mg q3–4 h prn
			IV: 2–3 min	—	3 hrs	
propoxyphene (Darvon)	—	Agonist	30–60 min	2–2.5 hrs	4–6 hrs	PO: 100 mg q4h prn
remifentanil (Ultiva)	—	Agonist	<1 min	2–3 min	5 min	IV infusion: 0.025–0.2 mcg/kg/min
sufentanil (Sufenta)	IM: 0.02 mg	Agonist	1.3–3 hrs	—	—	IV: 1–2 mcg/kg

PRECAUTIONS

CONTRAINDICATIONS: Hypersensitivity, pregnancy or lactation, infants, diarrhea caused by poisoning, respiratory depression, asthma, emphysema, convulsive disorders, severe renal or hepatic dysfunction, prostatic hypertrophy, acute ulcerative colitis, increased intracranial pressure. **CAUTIONS:** Pediatric, geriatric, and debilitated pts may be more susceptible to effects. Caution when using for obstetrical analgesia to prevent respiratory depression in neonate. Respiratory depression is a concern in the severely obese. Care when administered to pts in shock or w/reduced blood volume.

INTERACTIONS

Any of the CNS depressants, including alcohol, potentiate effects. Combination w/MAO inhibitors or administration within 14 days of MAO inhibitors may potentiate effects of either agent. Death has resulted from interactions of the above. There is increased muscle relaxation and respiratory depression w/skeletal muscle relaxants. A few of the narcotics have both agonist and antagonist actions; when administered to pts who have been receiving or abusing narcotics, withdrawal symptoms may develop. Narcotic antagonists are given to reverse respiratory depression of narcotic analgesics.

SIDE EFFECTS

Lightheadedness, dizziness, orthostatic hypotension, drowsiness, constipation.

TOXIC EFFECTS/ADVERSE REACTIONS

Respiratory depression, which can lead to respiratory arrest; bradycardia; hypotension; urinary retention/oliguria; CNS depression w/slurred speech, dulled mental responses, or stupor. May have converse excitation reaction w/euphoria and tremors. Hypersensitivity may be evidenced by rash, itching, sneezing. Tolerance, physical and/or psychological dependence may develop.

PATIENT CONSIDERATIONS

GENERAL: When administering intravenously, dilute and give slowly to prevent severe CNS depression and possible cardiac arrest. Give narcotic before pain is intense to break the pain cycle. Maintain appropriate records (most of these are schedule II drugs). BASELINE ASSESSMENT: Determine initial B/P, pulse, respirations. Assess pain for type, location, intensity. INTERVENTION/EVALUATION: Assess response to pain medication. Monitor B/P, pulse, respirations. Maintain I&O; be alert to decreased urination. Avoid constipation. PATIENT/FAMILY TEACHING: Do not smoke (may cause hypoxemia, respiratory depression). Physical and/or mental abilities may be impaired. Do not ambulate w/o assistance; do not drive or engage in activities requiring mental acuity. Refrain from alcohol or other medications. Drug dependence is not likely for short-term medical purposes.

opioid antagonists

ACTION

Prevents/reverses effects of mu receptor opioid agonists (e.g., increases respiration, reverses sedative effect).

USES

Primarily used to reverse respiratory depression induced by narcotic overdosage. Naloxone is the drug of choice for reversal of respiratory depression.

PRECAUTIONS

CONTRAINDICATIONS: Respiratory depression due to other than narcotic analgesics, hypersensitivity, narcotic dependency, pregnancy, lactation, severe hepatic dysfunction. **CAUTION:** Obstetric and surgical pts should be monitored carefully for bleeding. Care in pts w/cardiac irritability.

INTERACTIONS

Reverses opioid effects. Causes withdrawal symptoms in narcotic-dependent pts.

OPIOID ANTAGONISTS

Generic Name	Brand Name(s)	Usual Dosage
nalmefene	Revex	IV/IM/SC: titrated individually
naloxone	Narcan	IV/IM/SC: Adults: 0.4–2 mg Children: 0.01 mg/kg
naltrexone	ReVia	PO: 50 mg/day or 100 mg qOd

SIDE EFFECTS

Reduces or eliminates analgesia. Nausea, vomiting, increase in sweating.

TOXIC EFFECTS/ADVERSE REACTIONS

Hypertension, tachycardia. Withdrawal symptoms when administered to pts dependent on narcotics; general achiness, runny nose, restlessness and irritability, insomnia, anorexia, nausea, and vomiting.

PATIENT CONSIDERATIONS

GENERAL: Have resuscitative equipment immediately available, as well as the antagonist agent. INTERVENTION/EVALUATION: Monitor respirations carefully after antagonist is given (naloxone is not as long acting as some narcotics and dose may have to be repeated). Check B/P and pulse. Be alert to return of pain when narcotic action is reversed. May cause withdrawal symptoms in narcotic-dependent pts.

oral contraceptives

ACTION

Oral contraceptives include estrogen-progestin combinations and progestin-only products. The combinations in turn may be monophasic, biphasic, or triphasic.

Progestin only: Exact mechanism of pregnancy prevention is unknown but may alter cervical mucus, exert a progestational effect on the endometrium rendering the endometrium hostile to implantation by a fertilized ovum, and suppress ovulation.

Estrogen-progestin combination: Suppresses the gonadotropins, follicle-stimulating hormone (FSH) and luteinizing hormone (LH), also alters the genital tract (cervical mucus inhibiting sperm penetration and endometrium reducing likelihood of implantation).

USES

Prevention of pregnancy.

PRECAUTIONS

CONTRAINDICATIONS: Thrombophlebitis, thromboembolic disorders, or a history of deep vein thrombophlebitis, cerebral vascular disease, myocardial infarction, coronary artery disease, known or suspected breast carcinoma or estrogen-dependent neoplasms, carcinoma of endometrium, hepatic adenomas/carcinoma; past/present angina pectoris; undiagnosed abnormal genital bleeding; known or suspected pregnancy; cholestatic jaundice of pregnancy/jaundice w/prior pill use. **CAUTIONS:** History of cigarette smoking (increased risk of cardiovascular side effects from oral contraceptives), lipidemias, history of depression, convulsive disorders, migraine syndrome, asthma, cardiac, liver, or renal impairment, obesity, diabetes mellitus, hypertension.

INTERACTIONS

May increase therapeutic effect, concentration, or toxicity w/tricyclic antidepressants, benzodiazepines, beta-blocking agents, corticosteroids, theophylline. May decrease therapeutic effect of salicylates (increases clearance). Griseofulvin, penicillins, tetracyclines may decrease effect of oral contraceptives. Barbiturates, hydantoins, rifampin may increase hepatic metabolism, decrease oral contraceptive effect.

SIDE EFFECTS

FREQUENT: Breakthrough bleeding, nausea, vomiting. **OCCASIONAL:** Spotting, altered menstrual flow, amenorrhea, vaginal candidiasis, breast tenderness, enlargement, abdominal cramps, bloating, rash, edema, weight change, cholestatic jaundice, migraines, mental depression.

TOXIC EFFECTS/ADVERSE REACTIONS

Thrombophlebitis, venous thrombosis, pulmonary embolism, coronary thrombosis, myocardial infarction, cerebral hemorrhage, hypertension, cerebral thrombosis, arterial thromboembolism, congenital anomalies.

ORAL CONTRACEPTIVES

MONOPHASIC

Brand Name(s)	Estrogen (mcg)	Progestin (mg)
Genora 1/50 Nelova 1/50M Norethin 1/50M Norinyl 1+ 50 Ortho-Novum 1/50	50 mestranol	1 norethindrone
Ovcon-50	50 ethinyl estradiol	1 norethindrone
Demulen 1/50	50 ethinyl estradiol	1 ethynodiol diacetate
Ovral	50 ethinyl estradiol	0.5 norgestrel
Genora 1/35 Nelova 1/35E Norethin 1/35E Norinyl 1+35 Ortho-Novum 1/35	35 ethinyl estradiol	1 norethindrone

ORAL CONTRACEPTIVES *Continued*

MONOPHASIC

BRAND NAME(S)	ESTROGEN (MCG)	PROGESTIN (MG)
Brevicon Genora 0.5/35 Modicon Nelova 0.5/35E	35 ethinyl estradiol	0.5 norethindrone
Ovcon-35	35 ethinyl estradiol	0.4 norethindrone
Ortho-Cyclen	35 ethinyl estradiol	0.25 norgeestimate
Demulen 1/35	35 ethinyl estradial	1 ethynodiol diacetate
Loestrin 21 1.5/30 Loestrin Fe 1.5/30	30 ethinyl estradio	1.5 norethindrone acetate
Lo/Ovral	30 ethinyl estradiol	0.3 norgestrel
Desogen Ortho-Cept	30 ethinyl estradiol	0.15 desogestrel
Levlen Levora Nordette	30 ethinyl estradiol	0.15 levonorgestrel
Loestrin 21 1/20	20 ethinyl estradiol	1 norethindrone acetate

BIPHASIC

	PHASE 1	PHASE 2
Jenest-28	0.5 mg norethindrone 35 mcg ethinyl estradiol	1 mg norethindrone 35 mcg ethinyl estradiol
Nelova 10/11	0.5 mg norethindrone 35 mcg ethinyl estradiol	1 mg norethindrone 35 mcg ethinyl estradiol
Ortho-Novum 10/11	0.5 mg norethindrone 35 mcg ethinyl estradiol	1 mg norethindrone 35 mcg ethinyl estradiol

TRIPHASIC

	PHASE 1	PHASE 2	PHASE 3
Estrastep	1 mg norethindrone 20 mcg ethinyl estradiol	1 mg norethindrone 30 mcg ethinyl estradiol	1 mg norethindrone 35 mcg ethinyl estradiol
Tri-Norinyl	0.5 mg norethindrone 35 mcg ethinyl estradiol	1 mg norethindrone 35 mcg ethinyl estradiol	0.5 mg norethindrone 35 mcg ethinyl estradiol
OrthoNovum 7/7/7	0.5 mg norethindrone 35 mcg ethinyl estradiol	0.75 mg norethindrone 35 mcg ethinyl estradiol	1 mg norethindrone 35 mcg ethinyl estradiol
Tri-Levlen Triphasil	0.05 mg levonorgestrel 30 mcg ethinyl estradiol	0.075 mg levonor-gestrel 40 mcg ethinyl estradiol	0.125 mg levonorgestrel 30 mcg ethinyl estradiol
Ortho Tri-Cyclen	0.18 mg norgestimate 35 mcg ethinyl estradiol	0.215 mg norg-estimate 35 mcg ethinyl estradiol	0.25 mg norgestimate 35 mcg ethinyl estradiol

PROGESTIN ONLY

Micronor Nor Q D	0.35 mg norethindrone
Ovrette	0.075 mg norgestrel

PATIENT CONSIDERATIONS

BASELINE ASSESSMENT: Take complete medical and family history before initiating therapy. B/P, exam of breasts, abdomen and pelvic organs, PAP smear. Assess total and HDL cholesterol. INTERVENTION/EVALUATION: Monitor B/P, total and HDL cholesterol, breast, abdomen, and pelvic organ exams. Be alert to earliest symptoms of thromboembolic and thrombotic disorders. PATIENT/FAMILY TEACHING: Patient package insert available w/product. Take as directed at intervals not exceeding 24 hrs (take at same time each day) w/meals or at bedtime. May cause breakthrough bleeding/spotting; notify physician if bleeding occurs in more than one cycle or lasts longer than a few days. Oral contraceptive do not protect against HIV and other sexually transmitted diseases. Use additional birth control method until after the first week of administration in initial cycle or entire cycle if vomiting/diarrhea occurs.

oxytocics

ACTION

Oxytocics (Pitocin, Syntocinon) stimulate frequency/force of contraction of uterine smooth muscle. Responsiveness of uterus increases closer to term. Stimulates breast (contracting of myoepithelial cells surrounding mammary gland) to release milk.

USES

To induce, augment labor when maternal or fetal medical need exists; control of postpartum hemorrhage; cause uterine contraction after cesarean section or during other uterine surgery; induce therapeutic abortion.

PRECAUTIONS

CONTRAINDICATIONS: Hypersensitivity, cephalopelvic disproportions, unfavorable fetal position, fetal distress when delivery is not immediate, prolapsed cord or indication for surgical intervention. Methylergonovine should not be given to hypertensive pts or in toxemia or pregnancy. Ergonovine is used for postpartum hemorrhage and is contraindicated for labor induction. **CAUTIONS:** Pts >35 yrs of age; heart disease, hypertension; renal or hepatic dysfunction; sepsis.

INTERACTIONS

Caudal block anesthetics, vasopressors may increase pressor effects. Other oxytocics may cause uterine hypertonus, uterine rupture, or cervical lacerations.

SIDE EFFECTS

Nausea or vomiting.

TOXIC EFFECTS/ADVERSE REACTIONS

Arrhythmias, increased bleeding, uterine hypertonicity, hypotension, water intoxication, anaphylactic reaction. Fetus may develop bradycardia, hypoxia and experience trauma from too rapid birth. Peripheral ischemia, severe hypertension w/ergonovine, methylergonovine.

PATIENT CONSIDERATIONS

GENERAL: Regulate infusions precisely. BASELINE ASSESSMENT: Determine initial maternal B/P, pulse, fetal heart rate. INTERVENTION/EVALUATION: Monitor fetal heart rate, maternal B/P and pulse, uterine contractions (duration, strength, frequency) every 15 min. Notify physician of contractions that exceed 1 min, occur more frequently than every 2 min, or stop. Maintain careful I&O; be alert to potential water intoxication. For postpartum hemorrhage: Check uterus for firmness, amount of vaginal bleeding, vital signs. Evaluate extremities for warmth, color, movement, pain. PATIENT/FAMILY TEACHING: Keep pt, family informed of labor progress. Postpartum: Avoid smoking (added vasoconstriction).

sedative-hypnotics

ACTION

Sedatives decrease activity, moderate excitement, and have calming effects. Hypnotics produce drowsiness, enhance onset/maintenance of sleep (resembling natural sleep). Benzodiazepines are the most widely used agents (largely replace barbiturates): greater safety, lower incidence of drug dependence. Benzodiazepines potentiate gamma-aminobutyric acid, which inhibits impulse transmission in the CNS reticular formation in brain. Benzodiazepines decrease sleep latency, number of awakenings, and time spent in awake stage of sleep; increase total sleep time. Schedule IV drugs. See individual monographs for barbiturates.

USES

Treatment of insomnia, e.g., difficulty falling asleep initially, frequent awakening, awakening too early. For preop sedation.

PRECAUTIONS

CONTRAINDICATIONS: Hypersensitivity. Respiratory depression; respiratory diseases, porphyria, severe renal or hepatic dysfunction, history of alcohol or drug abuse, pregnancy, lactation, children. **CAUTIONS:** Elderly are more sensitive to adverse effects.

INTERACTIONS

Alcohol, narcotic analgesics, and other CNS depressants cause further CNS depressive effects. Combination w/CNS depressants should be avoided when possible.

SIDE EFFECTS

Drowsiness, dizziness, hangover, rebound insomnia due to altered REM, non-REM sleep stages.

TOXIC EFFECTS/ADVERSE REACTIONS

Hypersensitivity reactions: rash, urticaria. Confusion, extreme drowsiness, diarrhea. Paradoxical excitation may occur, particularly in the elderly. Overdose: respiratory depression, pulmonary edema, tachycardia and palpitations, marked hypotension, renal and hepatic damage, anoxia, cardiac collapse may proceed to coma and death. Potential for drug abuse and dependence, esp. w/barbiturates.

PATIENT CONSIDERATIONS

GENERAL: Provide environment conducive to sleep and pain relief. Put side rails up, lower bed, and put call light within reach. Assist in identifying cause of insomnia and encourage pt not to depend on medication. Comply w/federal narcotic laws regarding schedule IV drugs. Consider potential for abuse, dependence. Narcotics may need to be reduced when given w/hypnotics. BASELINE ASSESSMENT: Determine initial B/P, pulse, respirations, and sleep pattern. INTERVENTION/EVALUATION: Assure that pt has swallowed oral medication. Assess response to medication, sleep pattern. Monitor B/P, pulse, and respirations. PATIENT/FAMILY TEACHING: Instruct pt not to smoke or get up alone after taking hypnotic. Drowsiness may continue into next day; avoid driving or activities requiring mental acuity until response to drug controlled. Avoid alcohol. Consult physician before taking other medications. Take only as directed; do not increase dosage or abruptly discontinue (possible rebound insomnia).

HYPNOTICS

Generic Name	Brand Name(s)	Dosage Range
estazolam	ProSom	Adults: 1–2 mg before bedtime Elderly, debilitated: 0.5–1 mg at bedtime
flurazepam	Dalmane	Adults: 15–30 mg before bedtime Elderly, debilitated: Initially, 15 mg, then based on pt response
quazepam	Doral	Adults: Initially, 15 mg, may decrease to 7.5 mg in some pts Elderly, debilitated: Initially, 15 mg, then attempt to decrease dose after 1–2 nights
temazepam	Restoril	Adults: 15–30 mg before bedtime Elderly, debilitated: Initially, 15 mg, then based on pt response
triazolam	Halcion	Adults: 0.125–0.5 mg before bedtime Elderly, debilitated: Initially, 0.125 mg until response determined. Range: 0.125–0.25 mg
zolpidem	Ambien	Adults: 10 mg immediately before bedtime Elderly: 5 mg immediately before bedtime.

skeletal muscle relaxants

ACTION

Centrally acting muscle relaxants: Exact mechanism unknown. May act in

CNS at various levels to depress polysynaptic reflexes; sedative effect may be responsible for relaxation of muscle spasm.

Baclofen and diazepam: May mimic actions of gamma-aminobutyric acid on spinal neurons; do not directly affect skeletal muscles.

Dantrolene: Acts directly on skeletal muscle relieving spasticity.

SKELETAL MUSCLE RELAXANTS

Generic Name	Brand Name(s)	Dosage Range
baclofen	Lioresal	Adults: 40–80 mg/day
carisoprodol	Rela Soma	Adults: 350 mg 4×/day
chlorzoxazone	Parafon Forte DSC	Adults: 250–750 mg 3–4×/day Children: 125–500 mg 3–4×/day
cyclobenzaprine	Flexeril	Adults: 10 mg 3×/day
dantrolene	Dantrium	Adults: 25 mg/day initially; gradually increase to 400 mg/day or less
diazepam	Valium	Adults: 2–10 mg 3–4×/day Elderly: 2–2.5 mg initially; gradually increase Children: 1–2.5 mg 3–4×/day
methocarbamol	Robaxin	Adults: 500–1,000 mg 4×/day
orphenadrine	Norflex	Adults: 100 mg morning and evening

USES

Central acting muscle relaxants: Adjunct to rest, physical therapy for relief of discomfort associated w/acute, painful musculoskeletal disorders, i.e., local spasms from muscle injury.

Baclofen, dantrolene, diazepam: Treatment of spasticity characterized by heightened muscle tone, spasm, loss of dexterity caused by multiple sclerosis, cerebral palsy, spinal cord lesions, stroke.

PRECAUTIONS

CONTRAINDICATIONS: Pregnancy, lactation, cross-sensitivity, CNS depression, renal or hepatic dysfunction, children <12 yrs of age. According to specific drug. **CAUTIONS:** Cautious use in pts w/cardiac disease; history of allergy, epilepsy.

INTERACTIONS

Alcohol, narcotic analgesics, sedatives, hypnotics, and other CNS depressants may increase CNS effects (e.g., drowsiness, dizziness, fatigue).

SIDE EFFECTS

Drowsiness, orthostatic hypotension, w/dizziness and lightheadedness, nausea or vomiting, stomach cramps, headache, constipation, blurred vision.

TOXIC EFFECTS/ADVERSE REACTIONS

Hypersensitivity reactions. Severe hypotension, tachycardia, blood dyscrasias, GI bleeding, unusual muscle weakness, hepatotoxicity.

PATIENT CONSIDERATIONS

Provide supportive measures, e.g., bed rest, positioning, exercise, moist heat as indicated. Withdraw drugs slowly. BASELINE ASSESSMENT: Determine degree of immobility. Assess pain (type, location, intensity). INTERVENTION/EVALUATION: Monitor B/P, pulse, respirations. Assess for therapeutic response (increased mobility and decreased pain). PATIENT/FAMILY TEACHING: Administer on schedule to maintain blood levels. Avoid alcohol and consult physician before taking other medications. Do not drive or engage in activities requiring mental acuity (drowsiness, dizziness). Prolonged use may cause dependence.

sympathomimetics

ACTION

Sympathetic nervous system (SNS) is involved in maintaining homeostasis (involved in regulation of heart rate, force of cardiac contractions, B/P, bronchial airway tone, carbohydrate, fatty acid metabolism). The SNS is mediated by neurotransmitters (primarily norepinephrine, epinephrine, and dopamine), which act on adrenergic receptors. These receptors include beta$_1$, beta$_2$, alpha$_1$, alpha$_2$, and dopaminergic. Sympathomimetics differ widely in their actions based on their specificity to affect these receptors. Actions expected by stimulating these receptors include the following:

Alpha$_1$: Mydriasis, constriction of arterioles, veins.

Alpha$_2$: Inhibits transmitter release.

Beta$_1$: Increases rate, force of contraction, conduction velocity of heart, releases renin from kidney.

Beta$_2$: Dilates arterioles, bronchi, relaxes uterus.

Dopamine: Dilates kidney vasculature.

USES

Stimulation of alpha$_1$-receptors: Induces vasoconstriction primarily in skin and mucous membranes; nasal decongestion; combines w/local anesthetics to delay anesthetic absorption; increases B/P in certain hypotensive states; produces mydriasis, facilitating eye exams, ocular surgery.

Stimulation of alpha$_2$-receptors: No therapeutic use.

Stimulation of beta$_1$-receptors: Treatment of cardiac arrest (not primary); treatment of heart failure, shock, AV block (temporary only).

Stimulation of beta$_2$-receptors: Treatment of asthma; delays premature labor.

Stimulation of dopamine receptors: Treatment of shock.

PRECAUTIONS

CONTRAINDICATIONS: Hyperthyroidism, hypertension, cardiovascular disease, narrow-angle glaucoma, Parkinson's disease, psychoneuroses, hypersensitivity. **CAUTIONS:** Diabetes mellitus, urinary tract obstructions, elderly, debilitated, infants and children. See individual monograph for pregnancy, lactation precautions.

SYMPATHOMIMETICS

Generic Name	Brand Name(s)	Receptor Specificity	Primary Clinical Use
albuterol	Proventil Ventolin	$Beta_2$	Bronchodilator
bitolterol	Tornalate	$Beta_2$	Bronchodilator
dobutamine	Dobutrex	$Beta_1$ $Beta_2$ $Alpha_1$	Inotropic support in pts w/cardiac decompensation
dopamine	Intropin	$Beta_1$ $Alpha_1$ Dopaminergic	Cardiogenic, septic shock Pressor agent
epinephrine	Adrenalin Sus-phrine	$Beta_1$ $Beta_2$ $Alpha_1$	Allergic reaction Bronchodilator Local vasoconstriction (w/anesthetics)
isoetharine	Bronkosol	$Beta_2$	Bronchodilator
isoproterenol	Isuprel	$Beta_1$ $Beta_2$	Heart rate stimulator in bradycardia, heart block Vasopressor in shock Bronchodilator
metaproterenol	Alupent	$Beta_2$	Bronchodilator
metaraminol	Aramine	$Beta_1$ $Alpha_1$	Pressor in acute hypotensive states
norepinephrine	Levophed	$Beta_1$ $Alpha_1$	Pressor in acute hypotensive states
phenylephrine	Neo-synephrine	$Alpha_1$	Arterial vasoconstrictor Nasal decongestant Mydriatic
ritodrine	Yutopar	$Beta_2$	Arrest premature labor
terbutaline	Brethine Bricanyl	$Beta_2$	Bronchodilator

INTERACTIONS

Monoamine oxidase (MAO) inhibitors are contraindicated; in combination w/adrenergics, potentiated effects can cause hypertensive crisis, intracranial hemorrhage, and death. Effects of MAO inhibitors may last 3 wks after discontinuation. General anesthetics may increase risk of arrhythmias. Tricyclic antidepressants, maprotiline may increase cardiovascular effects. Norepinephrine may decrease effect of methyldopa. May have mutually inhibitory effects w/beta-adrenergic blockers. May increase risk of arrhythmias w/digoxin. Ergonovine, oxytocin may increase vasoconstriction. Numerous agents interact with adrenergics; review each monograph individually.

SIDE EFFECTS

Palpitations, nervousness, restlessness, sweating, difficulty urinating, headache.

TOXIC EFFECTS/ADVERSE REACTIONS

Nausea and vomiting, tachycardia, pale/cold skin, difficulty breathing, significant increase or decrease in B/P. *Rare:* Chest pain and irregular heartbeat.

PATIENT CONSIDERATIONS

GENERAL: Immediately obtain IV access in cardiac arrest or other emergency. When infusions indicated, pt should be in intensive care unit w/cardiac monitor. Infuse titrate carefully; use infusion pumps for accurate delivery. INTERVENTION/EVALUATION: Monitor vital signs frequently, blood gases, electrolytes, renal and hepatic function results. Assess multiorgan response. PATIENT/FAMILY TEACHING: Measures to prevent recurrence when given for asthma, COPD such as avoidance of respiratory infection, prevention of allergen exposure, increased hydration.

thyroid

ACTION

Thyroid hormone (T_4 [thyroxine] and T_3 [triiodothyroxine]) are essential for normal growth, development, and energy metabolism. *Promotes growth/development:* Controls DNA transcription and protein synthesis. Necessary in development of nervous system. *Stimulates energy use:* Increases basal metabolic rate (increases O_2 consumption, heat production). *Cardiovascular:* Stimulates heart by increased rate, force of contraction, cardiac output.

USES

Treatment of primary or secondary hypothyroidism, myxedema, cretinism, or simple goiter.

PRECAUTIONS

CONTRAINDICATIONS: Hyperthyroidism, myocardial infarction, thyrotoxicosis, nephrosis, hypoadrenalism. **CAUTIONS:** Use with care in pts who have hypertension, cardiac disease, renal insufficiency, diabetes mellitus, or are on anticoagulant therapy.

THYROID

Generic Name	Brand Name(s)	T_4:T_3 Ratio	Dosage Equivalent
levothyroxine	Synthroid	T_4 only	50–60 mcg
liothyronine	Cytomel	T_3 only	15–37.7 mcg
liotrix	Thyrolar	4:1	50–60 mcg T_4 12.5–15 mcg T_3
thyroid	Thyroid	2.5:1	65 mg

INTERACTIONS

May alter oral anticoagulant effects. Cholestyramine, colestipol may decrease absorption. Sympathomimetics may increase effects, coronary insufficiency.

SIDE EFFECTS

Most reactions are due to excessive dosage w/signs, symptoms of hyperthyroidism: weight loss, palpitations, increased appetite, tremors, nervousness, tachycardia, increased B/P, headache, insomnia, menstrual irregularities.

TOXIC EFFECTS/ADVERSE REACTIONS

Hypersensitivity reactions; cardiac arrhythmias, possibly death due to cardiac failure.

PATIENT CONSIDERATIONS

Children need very close monitoring; dosage needs to be higher for growing child. BASELINE ASSESSMENT: Check B/P and pulse, weight. INTERVENTION/EVALUATION: Monitor pulse for rate, rhythm; notify physician of pulse above 100/min or irregular. Check weight daily; assess food intake. Observe for tremors, nervousness, insomnia. PATIENT/FAMILY TEACHING: Do not stop taking medication; generally lifelong therapy. Take medication at the same time each day, preferably in the morning. Teach correct method of taking pulse; check pulse before taking medication, esp. when dosage adjusted. Notify physician of resting pulse that is markedly increased, irregular, 100/min or above. Important to remain under medical supervision, have periodic lab tests. Children may have reversible hair loss, increased aggressiveness during first few months of therapy. Do not take other medications w/o consulting physician. Notify physician promptly of chest pain, weight loss, tremors, insomnia.

vitamins

Vitamins are organic substances required for growth, reproduction, and maintaining health and are obtained from food or supplementation in small quantities (vitamins cannot be synthesized by the body or the rate of synthesis is too slow/inadequate to meet metabolic needs). Vitamins are essential for energy transformation and regulation of metabolic processes. They are catalysts for all reactions using proteins, fats, carbohydrates for energy, growth, and cell maintenance.

Vitamins are divided into two major groups: water soluble and fat soluble. Water-soluble vitamins include vitamin C (ascorbic acid), B-1 (thiamine), B-2 (riboflavin), niacin, B-6 (pyridoxine), folic acid, B-12 (cyanocobalamin). Water-soluble vitamins act as co-enzymes for almost every cellular reaction in the body. B-complex vitamins differ from one another in both structure and function but are grouped together because they first were isolated from the same source (yeast and liver). Fat-soluble vitamins include vitamin A, D, E, and K. They are soluble in lipids and are usually absorbed into the lymphatic system of the small intestine and then into the general circulation. Absorption is facilitated by bile. These vitamins are stored in the body tissue when excessive quantities are consumed. May be toxic when taken in large doses (see sections on individual vitamins).

WATER-SOLUBLE VITAMINS

Ascorbic Acid (Vitamin C)

Function: Co-factor in a number of reactions by transferring electrons to enzymes that provide reducing equivalents (collagen synthesis, conversion of folic acid to folinic acid, microsomal drug metabolism); promotes absorption of iron. At tissue level, required for collagen production, other compounds that compose the intercellular matrix that binds cells together. *Symptoms of Deficiency:* Scurvy: loosening of teeth, gingivitis, anemia, poor wound healing, hemorrhage into muscle/joints, ecchymosis, faulty bone/teeth development, malaise, weakness.

Food Source: Citrus fruits and juices (esp. orange and lemon), tomatoes, potatoes, strawberries, cabbage greens, green/red peppers, broccoli, spinach.

Thiamine (Vitamin B-1)

Function: Co-enzyme for metabolism of carbohydrate, important biochemical conversion cycles.

Symptoms of Deficiency: Nervous system (dry beriberi): peripheral neuritis, gradual loss of muscle strength, personality disturbances, depression, lack of initiative, poor memory, wrist-foot drop. Cardiovascular (wet beriberi): dyspnea on exertion, palpitations, tachycardia, abnormal EKG, high output cardiac failure, fluid accumulation in legs.

Food Source: Pork, peanuts, asparagus, whole grain cereal, beef, beans, fresh peas.

Riboflavin (Vitamin B-2)

Function: Consists of two co-enzymes that are involved in the metabolism of a wide variety of respiratory flavoproteins.

Symptoms of Deficiency: Sore throat, angular stomatitis (cracks in skin at corners of mouth), glossitis, cheilosis (red denuded lips), seborrheic dermatitis of face, dermatitis over trunk/extremities, anemia, neuropathy, corneal vasculization, cataract formation, eyes become light sensitive, easily fatigued, blurred vision, itching.

Food Sources: Meats, chicken, eggs, milk, fish, grain, cereal, broccoli, asparagus, spinach.

Niacin (Nicotinic Acid)

Function: Active form of niacin is nicotinic acid, a constituent of co-enzymes

NAD and NADP, which are vital in metabolism for a wide variety of proteins that catalyze oxidation-reduction reactions essential for tissue respiration.

Symptoms of Deficiency: Pellagra. Symptoms include dermatitis (erythematous eruptions similar to sunburn appearing on back of hands then forehead, feet, and head), digestive tract (stomatitis, enteritis, diarrhea), and CNS (headache, dizziness, insomnia, depression, impaired memory, delusions, hallucinations, dementia).

Food Source: Liver, chicken, yeast, peanuts, cereal bran, fish, cold cereals, whole grains, green vegetables.

PYRIDOXINE (VITAMIN B-6)

Function: Co-enzyme (active form pyridoxal phosphate) in metabolism of amino acids and proteins. A co-factor for more than 60 enzymes.

Symptoms of Deficiency: Skin: seborrheic-like skin lesions about the eyes, nose, mouth with glossitis and stomatitis. Nervous system: convulsive seizures, peripheral neuritis, dulling of mentation.

Food Source: Milk, soybeans, whole grain cereals, meats, bananas, avocados, potatoes, nuts, lentils.

FOLIC ACID

Function: Co-enzyme with important role in synthesis of purine and pyrimidine bases in RNA and DNA; maintenance of normal levels of mature red cells.

Symptoms of Deficiency: Megaloblastic anemia, glossitis, diarrhea, poor growth, frequent infections, depression, mental confusion, irritability, forgetfulness.

Food Source: Green leafy vegetables, liver, lean beef, fish, legumes, whole grains, veal, eggs.

CYANOCOBALAMIN (VITAMIN B-12)

Function: Active co-enzyme essential for cell growth and replication. Essential factor in synthesis of DNA. Involved in fat, protein, carbohydrate metabolism. Primarily active in bone marrow, CNS, and GI tract.

Symptoms of Deficiency: Pernicious or megaloblastic anemia, peripheral neuropathy (tingling/numbness of hands/feet), unsteadiness, decreased deep tendon reflexes, confusion, moodiness, loss of memory, loss of central vision, delusions, hallucinations, glossitis, dementia, mental confusion.
Source: Primary source are certain microorganisms that synthesize B-12. Found in animal protein (meats, oysters, clams) and small amounts in root nodules of legumes and selected vegetables/fruit.

FAT-SOLUBLE VITAMINS

VITAMIN A (RETINOIDS/CAROTENOIDS)

Function: Essential role in the function of the retina. Necessary for growth and differentiation of epithelial tissue. Required for growth of bone, reproduction, and embryonic development. Enhances immune function, may protect against development of certain malignancies.

Symptoms of Deficiency: Skin lesion, night blindness, keratomalacia (desiccation, ulceration, xerosis of cornea), increased respiratory infections, keratinization and drying of epidermis, urinary calculi, impairment of spermatogenesis, degeneration of testes, abortion, diarrhea, impaired taste/smell/hearing.

Toxicity: Dry, pruritic skin, skin desquamation, dermatitis, loss of body hair, fissures of lips, pain/tenderness of bone, hyperostosis, throbbing headache, peripheral edema, fatigue, irritability, increased intracranial pressure, bulging fontanelles, brittle nails, night sweats, insomnia, restlessness.

Food Source: Liver, butter, cheese, whole milk, egg yolk, fish, yellow or green fruits/vegetables.

Vitamin D (calciferol)

Function: Positive regulator of calcium and phosphate homeostasis (facilitates absorption by small intestine, interacts w/parathyroid to enhance mobilization from bone, decrease excretion by kidney). Necessary for proper formation of skeleton and mineral homeostasis.

Symptoms of Deficiency: Children: Rickets: failure to mineralize newly formed bone and cartilage matrix causing a defect in growing, weight bearing causing deformities. *Adults:* Osteomalacia: extreme bone pain/tenderness, muscle weakness.

Toxicity: Anorexia, nausea, vomiting, diarrhea, polyuria, muscle weakness, headache, irreversible renal failure, soft tissue calcification, hypercalcemia, weight loss, hypertension, constipation, vague aches/stiffness.

Food Source: Milk, margarine, liver, butter, egg yolk. Synthesized in skin from endogenous or dietary cholesterol on exposure to sunlight.

Vitamin E (tocopherol)

Function: Antioxidant (may protect essential cell components from oxidation); protects red blood cells from hemolysis. High dose *may* protect against heart disease.

Symptoms of Deficiency: Red blood cell hemolysis, abnormal fat deposits; may cause hemolytic anemia in infants (edema, reticulocytosis, thrombocytosis).

Toxicity: May cause increased serum lipids and cholesterol, erythrocyte hemolysis.

Food Source: Fresh greens, vegetable oil, nuts, whole grains, margarine (made from plant oils), wheat germ.

Vitamin K (menadione, phytonadione)

Function: Necessary for synthesis of several factors required for clotting of blood: prothrombin, and factors VII, IX, X.

VITAMIN-DIETARY ALLOWANCES

	FAT SOLUBLE				WATER SOLUBLE						
Age (yrs)	**A MCG**	**D MCG**	**E MG**	**K MCG**	**C MG**	**B-1 MG**	**B-2 MG**	**Niacin MG**	**B-6 MG**	**Folic Acid MCG**	**B-12 MCG**
0.0–0.5	375	7.5	3	5	30	0.3	0.4	5	0.3	25	0.3
0.5–1.0	375	10	4	10	35	0.4	0.5	6	0.6	35	0.5
1–3	400	10	6	15	40	0.7	0.8	9	1.0	50	0.7
4–6	500	10	7	20	45	0.9	1.1	12	1.1	75	1.0
7–10	700	10	7	30	45	1.0	1.2	13	1.4	100	1.4
Males:											
11–14	1,000	10	10	45	50	1.3	1.5	17	1.7	150	2.0
15–18	1,000	10	10	65	60	1.5	1.8	20	2.0	200	2.0
19–24	1,000	10	10	70	60	1.5	1.7	19	2.0	200	2.0
25–50	1,000	5	10	80	60	1.5	1.7	19	2.0	200	2.0
51+	1,000	5	10	80	60	1.2	1.4	15	2.0	200	2.0
Females:											
11–14	800	10	8	45	50	1.1	1.3	15	1.4	150	2.0
15–18	800	10	8	55	60	1.1	1.3	15	1.5	180	2.0
19–24	800	10	8	60	60	1.1	1.3	15	1.6	180	2.0
25–50	800	5	8	65	60	1.0	1.3	15	1.6	180	2.0
51+	800	5	8	65	60	1.0	1.2	13	1.6	180	2.0
Pregnant	800	10	10	65	70	1.5	1.6	17	2.2	400	2.2
Breast-feeding:											
1st 6 mos	1,300	10	12	65	95	1.6	1.8	20	2.1	280	2.6
2nd 6 mos	1,200	10	11	65	90	1.6	1.7	20	2.1	260	2.6

Symptoms of Deficiency: Increased tendency to bleed (ecchymosis, epistaxis, hematuria, GI bleeding, postop hemorrhage).

Toxicity: Hypersensitivity reaction: flushing, dyspnea, chest pain, cardiovascular collapse. Produces hemolytic anemia, hyperbilirubinemia, kernicterus in newborn.

Food Source: Green leafy vegetables, cauliflower, cabbage, egg yolk, liver.

Appendixes

Appendix A
(POISON) ANTIDOTE CHART

POISON/DRUG	INDICATIONS	ANTIDOTE	DOSAGE
acetaminophen	Treatment of acetaminophen overdose to protect against hepatotoxicity.	N-acetylcysteine (Mucomyst)	Dilute to 5% solution with carbonated beverage, fruit juice, or water and administer orally. **Loading:** 140 mg/kg for one dose. **Maintenance:** 70 mg/kg for 17 doses, starting 4 hrs after loading dose and given every 4 hrs.
atropine, anticholinergic agents, antihistamines, plants containing anticholinergic plants	Reverse toxic effects on the central nervous system (CNS) caused by drugs and plants capable of producing anticholinergic poisoning in clinical or toxic dosages (including tricyclic antidepressants).	physostigmine (Antilirium)	***Children:*** 0.02 mg/kg IM or slow IV injection (0.5 mg/min). May repeat at 5–10 min intervals until therapeutic response or maximum dose of 2 mg is attained. ***Adults:*** Slow IV push (1 mg/min): 0.5–2 mg; may repeat if life-threatening signs, including arrhythmias, convulsions, coma, occur.
cyanide, nitroprusside	Begin treatment at first sign of toxicity if exposure is known or strongly suspected.	amyl nitrite, sodium nitrite, sodium thiosulfate (Cyanide Antidote Kit)	First, crush amyl nitrite pearls in gauze and allow patient to inhale for 15 seconds, then remove for 15 seconds. Use a fresh pearl every 3 min. Continue until injection of 10 ml of 3% (300 mg) sodium nitrite in adults. Inject over 2–5 min. Pediatric dose based on hemoglobin level; if normal hemoglobin assumed, then 0.15–0.33 ml/kg sodium nitrite up to 10 ml may be used. After sodium nitrite immediately inject 50 ml of 25% sodium thiosulfate (12.5 g), slow IV, over 10 min. Use 7 g/m^2, maximum of 12.5 g, in children.

POISON/DRUG	INDICATIONS	ANTIDOTE	DOSAGE
digoxin	Treatment of potentially life-threatening digoxin intoxication.	digoxin-immune Fab (Digibind)	Dose in number of vials = steady-state digoxin level in mg/ml × patient weight in kg divided by 100. 4–6 vials adequate to treat 90–95% of patients with chronic digoxin toxicity. If ingested amount is unknown, give 10–20 vials (400–800 mg). Administer IV over 30 min through a 0.22 micron filter. A bolus injection can be given if cardiac arrest is imminent.
ethylene glycol	Ethylene glycol blood levels >20 mg/dl. Blood levels not readily available and suspected ingestion of toxic amounts. Any symptomatic patient with a history of ethylene glycol ingestion.	fomepizole (Antizol)	**Loading:** 15 mg/kg IV over 30 min followed by 10 mg/kg every 12 hrs for 4 doses, then 15 mg/kg every 12 hrs until ethylene glycol levels are below 20 mg/dl.
hydrofluoric acid (HF), fluoride salts	Calcium gluconate 2.5% gel for dermal exposure to HF <20% concentration. SC injections of calcium gluconate for dermal exposures of HF in >20% concentration or failure to respond to calcium gluconate gel. IV calcium gluconate 10% for serious systemic toxicity following dermal exposure, or ingestion of fluoride salts.	calcium gluconate	Massage 2.5% gel into exposed area for 15 min, repeating as necessary for pain. Infiltrate each cm^2 of exposed area with 0.5 ml 10% calcium gluconate SC, using a 30-gauge needle. Give 0.1–0.2 ml/kg IV 10% calcium gluconate slowly up to 10 ml. Repeat dose if necessary.
iron	Acute iron intoxication. Chronic iron overload.	deferoxamine (Desferal)	**Acute iron intoxication:** IM: 1 g, then 0.5 g q4h × 2 doses, then 0.5 g q4–12h. May give IV infusion 10–15 mg/kg/hr Do not exceed 6 g in 24 hrs. **Chronic iron overload:** IM: 0.5–1 g daily.

(continued)

POISON/DRUG	INDICATIONS	ANTIDOTE	DOSAGE
iron *(continued)*			SubQ: 1–2 g/day (20–40 mg/kg/day) over 8–24 hrs. ***Children:*** Maximum of 6 g/24 hrs or 2 g/dose.
organophosphate insecticides	Synergistic adjunct to atropine therapy. Reverses nicotinic effects such as profound muscle weakness, respiratory depression, and muscle twitching. Organophosphate poisoning. Anticholinesterase drug overdose.	pralidoxim (2-PAM) (Protopam)	***Children: IV:*** 25–50 mg/kg up to 1 g in 250 ml NaCl over 30 min. ***Adults: IV:*** 1–2 g in 100 ml NaCl over 15–30 min. If pulmonary edema present, may give as a 5% solution slow IV push over not less than 5 min. Dosage may be repeated in 1 hr followed by every 8 hrs if indicated.
opiates, alpha2 agonists (e.g., clonidine)	1. Opiate overdose 2. Coma or respiratory depression of unknown origin.	naloxone (Narcan) nalmefene (Revex)	**Naloxone: *Adults:*** Give 0.4–2 mg IV bolus. Doses may be repeated every 2–5 min up to 10 mg if no response. ***Children:*** 0.01 mg/kg. May repeat with 0.1 mg/kg. **Note:** AAP recommends initial dose of 0.1 mg/kg for infants and children up to 5 yrs and weighing <20 kg. ***Children >5 yrs or >20 kg:*** Recommended initial dose is 2 mg. **Nalmefene:** 0.5–1 mg IV every 2 min as needed to a total of 2 mg.
benzodiazepines	Complete or partial reversal of sedative effects of benzodiazepines when general anesthesia has been induced and/or maintained with benzodiazepines, when sedation has been produced with benzodiazepines for diagnostic and therapeutic procedures, management of benzodiazepine overdosage.	flumazenil (Romazicon)	***IV: Adults, elderly:*** Initially, 0.2 mg (2 ml) over 30 seconds; may repeat after 30 seconds with 0.3 mg (3 ml) over 30 seconds if desired level of consciousness not achieved. Further doses of 0.5 mg (5 ml) over 30 seconds may be administered at 60-second intervals. **Maximum:** 3 mg (30 ml) total dose.

POISON/DRUG	INDICATIONS	ANTIDOTE	DOSAGE
benzodiazepines *(continued)*			**Note:** If resedation occurs, repeat dose at 20-min intervals. **Maximum:** 1 mg (given as 0.5 mg/min) at any one time, 3 mg in any 1 hr.
miscellaneous medications	Treatment of drug overdose.	ipecac	***Children (<1 yr):*** 5–10 ml, then ½–1 glass water. ***Children (>1 yr to 12 yrs):*** 15 ml followed by 1–2 glasses water. ***Adults:*** 15–30 ml followed by 3–4 glasses water. **Note:** Repeat dose (15 ml) once in those older than 1 yr if vomiting does not occur within 20–30 min. Perform gastric lavage if vomiting does not occur within 30–45 min after second dose.
miscellaneous medication poisoning	Treatment of drug poisoning.	charcoal, activated	***Adults:*** 25–100 g (or 1 g/kg or approximately 10 times the amount of poison ingested) as a suspension (4–8 oz water). Multiple doses may be used in severe poisoning to prevent desorption from the charcoal; also increases GI clearance and rate of elimination of drugs that undergo an enteral recirculation pattern.

Appendix B
COMMONLY USED ABBREVIATIONS

ac—before meals
ACE—angiotensin-converting enzyme
ANC—absolute neutrophil count
bid—twice daily
B/P—blood pressure
BSA—body surface area
CBC—complete blood count
Ccr—creatinine clearance
CHF—congestive heart failure
Cl—chloride
CNS—central nervous system
CO—cardiac output
COPD—chronic obstructive pulmonary disease
dl—deciliter
DNA—deoxyribonucleic acid
EEG—electroencephalogram
EKG—electrocardiogram
e.g.—example
esp.—especially
g—gram
GI—gastrointestinal
gtt—drop
GU—genitourinary
h or **hrs**—hour(s)
Hct—hematocrit
Hgb—hemoglobin
hs—bedtime
HTN—hypertension
Hx—history
ID—intradermal
IM—intramuscular
I&O—intake and output
IOP—intraocular pressure
IU—international unit
IV—intravenous
K—potassium
kg—kilogram
L—liter
lbs—pounds
LOC—level of consciousness
m^2—meter squared
MAO—monoamine oxidase
mcg—microgram
mEq—milliequivalent
mg—milligram
MI—myocardial infarction
min—minute(s)
ml—milliliter
mm^3—millimeter cubed
mo(s)—month(s)
Na—sodium
NaCl—sodium chloride
NSAIDs—nonsteroidal anti-inflammatory drugs
OD—right eye
OS—left eye
OTC—over the counter
OU—both eyes
oz—ounce
pc—after meals
PO—orally, by mouth
prn—as needed
pt—patient
q—every
qd—daily
qid—four times daily
qOd—every other day
REM—rapid eye movements
RBC—red blood cell count
RNA—ribonucleic acid
Rx—prescription
sec(s)—second(s)
SL—sublingual
SubQ—subcutaneous
tbs—tablespoon
tid—three times daily
TPR—temperature, pulse, respirations
tsp—teaspoonful
w/—with
w/o—without
WBC—white blood cell count
wk(s)—week(s)
yr(s)—year(s)

Appendix C
CONTROLLED DRUGS (UNITED STATES)

Schedule I: Medications having no legal medical use. These substances may be used for research purposes with proper registration (e.g., heroin, LSD).

Schedule II: Medications having a legitimate medical use but are characterized by a very high abuse potential and/or potential for severe physical and psychic dependency. Emergency telephone orders for limited quantities of these drugs are authorized, but the prescriber must provide a written, signed prescription order (e.g., morphine, amphetamines).

Schedule III: Medications having significant abuse potential (less than Schedule II). Telephone orders are permitted (e.g., opiates in combination with other substances such as acetaminophen).

Schedule IV: Medications having a low abuse potential. Telephone orders are permitted (e.g., benzodiazepines, propoxyphene).

Schedule V: Medications having the lowest abuse potential of the controlled substances. Some Schedule V products may be available without a prescription (e.g., certain cough preparations containing limited amounts of an opiate).

Appendix D
DRUGS OF ABUSE

NAME (BRAND)	CLASS	SIGNS AND SYMPTOMS	TREATMENT
Acid (see LSD)			
Adam (see MDMA)			
Amphetamine (Adderall, Dexedrine)	Stimulant	Tachycardia, hypertension, diaphoresis, agitation, headache, seizures, dehydration, hypokalemia, lactic acidosis. Severe overdose: hyperthermia, dysrhythmia, shock, rhabdomyolysis, liver necrosis, acute renal failure.	Control agitation, reverse hyperthermia, support hemodynamic function. **Antidote:** No specific antidote.
Angel dust (see phencyclidine)			
Apache (see fentanyl)			
Barbiturates (Nembutal, Seconal)	Depressant	Hypotension, hypothermia, apnea, nystagmus, ataxia, hyporeflexia, somnolence, stupor, coma.	Airway management, decontamination, supportive care. **Antidote:** No specific antidote.
Barbs (see barbiturates)			
Benzodiazepines (Xanax, Valium, Librium, Halcion)	Depressant	Respiratory depression, hypothermia, hypotension, nystagmus, miosis, diplopia, bradycardia, nausea, vomiting, impaired speech and coordination, amnesia, ataxia, somnolence, confusion, depressed deep tendon reflexes.	**Antidote:** Flumazenil (Romazicon) is a specific antidote.
Black tar (see heroin)			
Horse (see heroin)			
Boomers (see LSD)			
Buttons (see mescaline)			
Cactus (see mescaline)			
Candy (see benzodiazepines)			
China girl (see fentanyl)			
China white (see heroin)			
Cocaine	Stimulant	Hypertension, tachycardia, mild hyperthermia, mydriasis, pallor, diaphoresis, psychosis, paranoid delusions, mania, agitation, seizures.	Control agitation, seizures, hyperthermia, support hemodynamic function. **Antidote:** No specific antidote.

Name (Brand)	Class	Signs and Symptoms	Treatment
Codeine	Opioid	Miosis, respiratory depression, decreased mental status, hypotension, cardiac dysrhythmia, hypoxia, bronchoconstriciton, constipation, decreased intestinal motility, ileus, lethargy, coma.	Airway management, hemodynamic support. **Antidote:** Naloxone, nalmefene.
Coke (see cocaine)			
Crank (see amphetamine)			
Crank (see heroin)			
Crystal (see amphetamine)			
Crystal meth (see methamphetamine)			
Cubes (see LSD)			
Downers (see benzodiapepines)			
Ecstasy (see MDMA)			
Fentanyl (Sublimaze)	Opioid	Miosis, respiratory depression, decreased mental status, hypotension, cardiac dysrhythmia, hypoxia, bronchoconstriction, constipation, decreased intestinal motility, ileus, lethargy, coma.	Airway management, hemodynamic support. **Antidote:** Naloxone, nalmefene.
Flunitrazepam (Rohypnol)	Depressant	Drowsiness, slurred speech, impaired judgment and motor skills, hypothermia, hypotension, bradycardia, diplopia, blurred vision, nystagmus, respiratory depression, nausea, constipation, depression, lethargy, headache, ataxia, coma, amnesia, incoordination, tremors, vertigo.	Supportive care, airway control. **Antidote:** Flumazenil (Romazicon)
Forget me pill (see flunitrazepam)			
Goodfellas (see fentanyl)			
Grass (see marijuana)			
Hashish (see marijuana)			
Heroin	Opioid	Miosis, coma, apnea, pulmonary edema, bradycardia, hypotension, pinpoint pupils, CNS depression, seizures.	Airway management. **Antidote:** Naloxone, nalmefene.
Ice (see amphetamine)			

(continued)

NAME (BRAND)	CLASS	SIGNS AND SYMPTOMS	TREATMENT
LSD	Hallucinogen	Diaphoresis, mydriasis, dizziness, twitching, flushing, hyperreflexia, hypertension, psychosis, behavioral changes, emotional lability, euphoria or dysphoria, paranoia, vomiting, diarrhea, anorexia, restlessness, incoordination, tremors, ataxia.	Airway management, control activity associated with hallucinations, psychosis, panic reaction. **Antidote:** No specific antidote.
Ludes (see methaqualone)			
Magic mushroom (see psilocybin)			
Marijuana	Cannabinoid	Increasd appetite, reduced motility, constipation, urinary retention, seizures, euphoria, somnolence, heightened awareness, relaxation, altered time perception, short-term memory loss, poor concentration, mood alterations, disorientation, decreased strength, ataxia, slurred speech, respiratory depression, coma.	Airway management, supportive care. **Antidote:** No specific antidote.
MDMA Methylenedioxymethamphetamine	Stimulant	Euphoria, intimacy, closeness to others, loss of appetite, tachycardia, jaw tension, bruxism, sweating.	**Antidote:** No specific antidote.
Mescoline	Hallucinogen	Diaphoresis, mydriasis, dizziness, twitching, flushing, hyperreflexia, hypertension, psychosis, behavioral changes, emotional lability, euphoria or dysphoria, paranoia, vomiting, diarrhea, anorexia, restlessness, incoordination, tremors, ataxia.	Airway management, control activity associated with hallucinations,psychosis, panic reaction. **Antidote:** No specific antidote.
Meth (see methamphetamine)			
Methamphetamine (Desoxyn)	Stimulant	Hypertension, hyperthermia, hyperpyrexia, agitation, hyperactivity, fasciculation, seizures, coma, tachycardia, dysrhythmias, pale skin, diaphoresis, restlessness, talkativeness, insomnia, headache, coma, delusions, paranoia, aggressive behavior, visual, tactile, or auditory hallucinations.	Airway control, hyperthermia, seizures, dysrhythmias. **Antidote:** No specific antidote.

NAME (BRAND)	CLASS	SIGNS AND SYMPTOMS	TREATMENT
Methaqualone (Quaalude)	Depressant	Slurred speech, impaired judgment and motor skills, hypothermia, hypotension, bradycardia, diplopia, blurred vision, nystagmus, mydriasis, respiratory depression, depression, lethargy, headache, ataxia, coma, amnesia, incoordination, hypertonicity, myoclonus, tremors, vertigo.	Airway management, supportive care. **Antidote:** No specific antidote.
Methylphenidate (Ritalin)	Stimulant	Agitation, hypertension, tachycardia, hyperthermia, mydriasis, dry mouth, nausea, vomiting, anorexia, abdominal pain, agitation, hyperactivity, insomnia, euphoria, dizziness, paranoid ideation, social withdrawal, delirium, hallucinations, psychosis, tremors, seizures.	Control agitation, hyperthermia, seizures, support hemodynamic function. **Antidote:** No specific antidote.
Miss Emma (see morphine)			
Mister blue (see morphine)			
Morphine (MS-Contin, Roxanol)	Opioid	Miosis, respiratory depression, decreased mental status, hypotension, cardiac dysrhythmia, hypoxia, bronchoconstriction, constipation, decreased intestinal motility, ileus, lethargy, coma.	Airway management, hemodynamic support. **Antidote:** Naloxone, nalmefene.
Oxy (see oxycodone)			
Oxycodone (Oxycontin)	Opioid	Miosis, respiratory depression, decreased mental status, hypotension, cardiac dysrhythmia, hypoxia, bronchoconstriciton, constipation, decreased intestinal motility, ileus, lethargy, coma.	Airway management, hemodynamic support. **Antidote:** Naloxone, nalmefene.
Oxycotton (see oxycodone)			
Peace pill (see phencyclidine)			
Phencyclidine (PCP)	Hallucinogen	Nystagmus, hypertension, tachycardia, agitation, hallucinations, violent behavior, impaired judgment, delusions, psychosis.	Support blood pressure, manage airway, control agitation. **Antidote:** No specific antidote.

(continued)

NAME (BRAND)	CLASS	SIGNS AND SYMPTOMS	TREATMENT
Phennies (see barbiturates)			
Pot (see marijuana)			
Propoxyphene (Darvon)	Depressant	Respiratory depression, seizures, cardiac toxicity, miosis, dysrhythmias, nausea, vomiting, anorexia, abdominal pain, constipation, drowsiness, coma, confusion, hallucinations.	Maintain airway, seizures, cardiac toxicity. **Antidote:** Naloxone.
Psilocybin	Hallucinogen	Diaphoresis, mydriasis, dizziness, twitching, flushing, hyperreflexia, hypertension, psychosis, behavioral changes, emotional lability, euphoria or dysphoria, paranoia, vomiting, diarrhea, anorexia, restlessness, incoordination, tremors, ataxia.	Manage airway, control activity associated with hallucinations, psychosis, panic reaction. **Antidote:** No specific antidote.
Purple passion (see psilocybin)			
Quay (see methaqualone)			
Reefer (see marijuana)			
Rock (see cocaine)			
Rocket fuel (see phencyclidine)			
Roofies (see flunitrazepam)			
Rope (see flunitrazepam)			
Rophies (see flunitrazepam)			
Schoolboy (see codeine)			
Snow (see cocaine)			
Speed (see amphetamine)			
STP (see MDMA)			
Tranks (see benzodiazepines)			
Uppers (see amphetamine)			
White girl (see cocaine)			
Yellow jackets (see barbiturates)			
Yellow sunshine (see LSD)			

Appendix E
EMERGENCY MEDICATION GUIDE

Note: Changes in ACLS guidelines were recently published. The most significant changes include:

- Amiodarone and procainamide are now ahead of lidocaine and adenosine for treatment of hemodynamically stable wide complex tachycardia.
- Amiodarone and sotalol are now included as Class IIa agents for treatment of stable VT.
- Bretyllium is no longer used.
- Lidocaine is no longer the first antiarrhythmic treatment choice for refractory VF or pulseless VT; amiodarone is the first antiarrhythmic drug.
- Magnesium is used only for hypomagnesemia and torsades.
- Add a one-time dose of vasopressin to your choices for treatment of VF and pulseless VT.
- High-dose epinephrine is no longer recommended.

NAME/INDICATIONS	DOSAGE/ROUTES	SIDE EFFECTS
activated charcoal Emergency antidote in treatment of poisoning	***Adults:*** 25–100 g (or 1 g/kg or approximately 10 times the amount of poison ingested) as a suspension (4–8 oz water). Multiple doses may be used in severe poisoning to prevent desorption from the charcoal; also increases GI clearance and rate of elimination of drugs that undergo an enteral recirculation pattern.	Diarrhea, GI discomfort, intestinal gas
adenosine (Adenocard) Conversion of paroxysmal supraventricular tachycardia (PSVT) to regular sinus rhythm	***Adults:*** 6 mg rapid IVP immediately followed by 20 ml normal saline. ***Repeat dose:*** 12 mg. Use proximal IV; administer in port closest to the pt. ***Children:*** 0.1 mg/kg followed by 10 ml normal saline flush.	Dysrhythmias, facial flushing, dyspnea, decreased blood pressure, chest pressure/pain, headache, dizziness
albuterol (Proventil, Ventolin) Asthma, bronchospasm associated with COPD	***Nebulizer:*** 0.5 ml (2.5 mg) in 2–3 ml sodium chloride over 5–10 min. May repeat.	Anxiety, tremors, nervousness, tachycardia, increased blood pressure, palpitations, dizziness, chest pain, headache, vomiting
alteplase (Activase) Management of acute myocardial infarction (AMI)	**Note:** For acute MI or PE, institute or reinstitute heparin near end or immedi-	Superficial bleeding at puncture site, gingival bleeding, decreased B/P

(continued)

NAME/INDICATIONS	DOSAGE/ROUTES	SIDE EFFECTS
for lysis of thrombi obstructing coronary arteries and management of acute massive pulmonary embolus for lysis of acute pulmonary emboli. Treatment of acute ischemic stroke (within 3 hrs of symptoms)	ately after infusion (when PTT or thrombin time returns to twice normal or less). *Acute myocardial infarction:* *IV Infusion:* ***Adults:*** 100 mg over 90 min ***(>67 kg):*** 15 mg bolus given over 1–2 min; then, 50 mg over 30 min; then, 35 mg over 60 min. ***(<67 kg):*** 15 mg bolus, then 0.75 mg/kg over next 30 min (*maximum:* 50 mg), then 0.5 mg/kg over 60 min (*maximum:* 35 mg). *Acute pulmonary emboli:* *IV Infusion:* ***Adults:*** 100 mg over 2 hrs. *Acute ischemic stroke:* *IV Infusion:* ***Adults:*** 0.9 mg/kg over 60 min (10% total dose as initial IV bolus over 1 min). Do not exceed 90 mg total dose.	
amiodarone (Cordarone) Treatment of refractory VF or pulseless VT	Give bolus of 300 mg IV push. If VT/VF recurs or is refractory, a second bolus of 150 mg may be given. *Maximum:* 2.2 g over 24 hrs. After reappearance of circulation, amiodarone can be infused at 1 mg/min for 6 hrs, then 0.5 mg/min.	Hypotension, nausea, fever, bradycardia
amyl nitrite (Vaporole) Treatment of cyanide poisoning. Treatment of angina	1 or 2 ampules containing 0.3 ml of amyl nitrite. Crush and inhale for 15–30 sec. Repeat every 60–90 sec. Administer oxygen between doses.	Hypotension, tachycardia, headache, palpitations, dizziness, nausea, vomiting
atropine sulfate Treatment of bradycardia in advanced cardiac life support	**Note:** Give *rapidly* (prevents paradoxical slowing of heart rate). *IV:* ***Adults, elderly:*** 0.4–1 mg. Repeat at 1–2 hr intervals until desired rate achieved. *Maximum:* 2 mg total dose. ***Children (3 kg):*** 0.1 mg; ***(7–9 kg):*** 0.2 mg; ***(12–16 kg):*** 0.3 mg.	Overdosage produces tachycardia, palpitations, increased respirations, nausea, vomiting

NAME/INDICATIONS	DOSAGE/ROUTES	SIDE EFFECTS
aspirin (ASA) Onset of recent chest pain suggestive of MI, signs and symptoms of recent CVA	160–325 mg (use of chewable tablets recommended).	Nausea, vomiting, heartburn, bronchospasm, dizziness, occult bleeding
bumetanide (Bumex) Treatment of edema associated w/CHF, chronic renal failure including nephrotic syndrome, hepatic cirrhosis w/ascites; treatment of acute pulmonary edema	*IM/IV:* 0.5–1 mg as single dose. May be repeated at 2–3 hr intervals.	Increase in urine frequency/volume. Orthostatic hypotension, dizziness. Blurred vision, diarrhea, headache, anorexia, premature ejaculation, impotence, GI upset
calcium chloride calcium gluconate Acute hypocalcemia (e.g., neonatal hypocalcemic tetany, alkalosis), electrolyte depletion, cardiac arrest (strengthens myocardial contractions), hyperkalemia (reverses EKG, cardiac depression), hypermagnesemia (aids in reversing CNS depression)	***Emergency increase of calcium:*** ***IV: Adults, elderly:*** 7–14 mEq. ***Children:*** 1–7 mEq. ***Infants:*** <1 mEq. May repeat dose q1–3 days. ***Hypocalcemic tetany:*** ***IV: Adults, elderly:*** 4.5–16 mEq. May repeat until therapeutic response. ***Children:*** 0.5–0.7 mEq/kg 3–4 times/day. ***Neonates:*** 2.4 mEq/kg/day in divided doses. ***Cardiopulmonary resuscitation:*** ***IV: Adults, elderly:*** *Calcium gluconate:* 2.3–3.7 mEq. May repeat as needed. *Calcium chloride:* 2.7 mEq. May repeat as needed. ***Children:*** *Calcium chloride:* 0.27 mEq/kg. May repeat in 10 min if needed. ***Hyperkalemia:*** ***IV: Adults, elderly:*** 2.25–14 mEq. Monitor EKG. May repeat after 1–2 min if needed. ***Magnesium intoxication:*** ***IV: Adults, elderly:*** 7 mEq. May repeat based on pt response.	Hypotension, flushing, feeling of warmth, nausea, vomiting; pain, rash, redness, burning at injection site; sweating, decreased B/P
dextrose Hypoglycemia	***Adults, children >8 yrs:*** 50% 25g IVP slowly over 2–3 min. ***Children 1–8 yrs:*** 25% 2 ml/kg slow IVP. ***Children<1 yr:*** 12.5% 2 ml/kg slow IVP.	Local venous irritation, tissue necrosis, diuresis. May cause severe neuro signs and symptoms in alcoholics. Intracranial hemorrhage and venous sclerosis in neonates if not diluted

(continued)

NAME/INDICATIONS	DOSAGE/ROUTES	SIDE EFFECTS
diazepam (Valium) Relief of acute alcohol withdrawal. Adjunct for relief of acute musculoskeletal conditions, treatment of seizures (IV route used for termination of status epilepticus)	***Alcohol withdrawal: IM/IV: Adults, elderly:*** Initially, 10 mg, followed by 5–10 mg q3–4h. ***Musculoskeletal spasm: IM/IV: Adults:*** 5–10 mg q3–4h. ***Seizures: IM/IV: Adults:*** 5–10 mg, repeated at 10–15 min intervals to total of 30 mg. ***Elderly, debilitated:*** 2–5 mg; increase gradually as needed. ***Children:*** 0.5–2 mg.	Drowsiness, sedation, amnesia, ataxia, respiratory depression, respiratory arrest, decreaed blood pressure
diltiazem (Cardizem) Temporary control of rapid ventricular rate in atrial fibrillation/flutter. Rapid conversion of PSVT to normal sinus rhythm	Initially, 0.25 mg/kg actual body weight over 2 min. May repeat in 15 min at dose of 0.35 mg/kg actual body weight. Subsequent doses individualized. After initial bolus injection, 5–10 mg/ hr, may increase at 5 mg/hr up to 15 mg/hr. Maintain over 24 hrs. **Note:** Refer to manufacturer's information for dose concentration/infusion rates.	Peripheral edema, dizziness, lightheadedness, headache, bradycardia, asthenia (loss of strength, weakness). Nausea, constipation, flushing, altered EKG
diphenhydramine (Benadryl) Adjunct to epinephrine in treating severe allergic reactions, including anaphylactic shock. May be used alone in mild to moderate allergic reactions	***IM/IV: Adults:*** 10–50 mg. ***Maximum daily dose:*** 400 mg. ***Children >20 lbs:*** 5 mg/kg/24 hrs 4 times/day.	Drowsiness, headache, confusion, wheezing, palpitations, tachycardia, hypotension, nausea, vomiting
dobutamine (Dobutrex) Short-term management of CHF and cardiogenic shock	***IV Infusion: Adults, elderly:*** 2.5–10 mcg/kg/min. Rarely, infusion rate up to 40 mcg/kg/min to increase cardiac output.	Increased heart rate, blood pressure. Pain at injection site. Nausea, headache, anginal pain, shortness of breath, fever
dopamine (Intropin) Prophylaxis/treatment of acute hypotension, shock (associated w/myocardial infarction, trauma, renal failure, cardiac decompensation, open heart surgery), treatment of low cardiac output, CHF	***IV: Adults, elderly:*** Begin with rate of 1–5 mcg/kg/min in pts likely to respond to minimal treatment. May be gradually increased in 1–4 mcg/kg/min increments at 10–30 min intervals until optimum response achieved. Most pts are maintained on dose of 20 mcq/kg/min or less.	Headache, ectopic beats, tachycardia, anginal pain, palpitations, vasoconstriction, hypotension, nausea, vomiting, dyspnea. Piloerection (goose bumps), bradycardia, widening of QRS complex

NAME/INDICATIONS	DOSAGE/ROUTES	SIDE EFFECTS
epinephrine 1:10,000 Cardiac arrest, profoundly symptomatic bradycardia, anaphylactic shock	***Cardiac arrest:*** 1 mg every 3–5 min. ***Anaphylaxis:*** 0.1–0.5 mg by slow IV infusion. ***Children:*** 0.01 mg/kg.	In noncardiac pts, palpitations, angina, arrhythmias, nausea, vomiting, headache, dizziness
epinephrine 1:1000 Anaphylactic shock, severe allergic reactions, acute bronchial asthma, exacerbation of COPD	***SubQ: Adults:*** 0.3–0.5 mg.	In noncardiac pts, palpitations, angina, arrhythmias, nausea, vomiting, headache, dizziness
etomidate (Amidate) Used for rapid sequence induction of anesthesia prior to intubation. To supplement low-potency agents such as nitrous oxide	***IV: Adults, children >10 yrs:*** 0.2–0.6 mg/kg, administered over 30–60 sec.	Nausea, vomiting, involuntary muscle movements, pain at injection site
fentanyl (Sublimaze)	***IV: Adults, elderly:*** 50–100 mcg q1–2h, as needed.	Confusion, blurred vision, chills, orthostatic hypotension, constipation, difficulty urinating. Too rapid IV results in severe respiratory depression, skeletal and thoracic muscle rigidity resulting in apnea, laryngospasm, bronchospasm, cold and clammy skin, cyanosis, coma
furosemide (Lasix) Treatment of edema associated w/CHF, chronic renal failure including nephrotic syndrome, hepatic cirrhosis, acute pulmonary edema	***IV:*** 1 mg/kg. ***Maximum:*** 2 mg/kg.	Postural hypotension, hypokalemia, dehydration, muscle cramps, weakness, blurred vision, nausea, vomiting, diarrhea
glucagons Hypoglycemia, relax smooth muscle in cases of food obstruction in the esophagus, fecal impaction	***Hypoglycemia, relax smooth muscle:*** ***SubQ/IM/IV: Adults, elderly:*** 0.5–1 mg (0.5–1 unit). May repeat 1–2 additional doses if response delayed. ***Fecal impaction:*** ***IV: Adults, elderly:*** 1 mg.	Nausea, vomiting, allergic reaction (urticaria, respiratory distress, hypotension)
hydrocortisone (Solu-Cortef) Adjunct to epinephrine in anaphylaxis	100–250 mg by IV bolus.	Headache, dizziness, euphoria, nausea, vomiting, edema

(continued)

NAME/INDICATIONS	DOSAGE/ROUTES	SIDE EFFECTS
ipratropium bromide (Atrovent) Adjunctive therapy with albuterol in acute exacerbation of asthma	***Inhalation: Adults, elderly:*** 500 mcg dose. May repeat 1–2 times.	Cough, dry mouth, headache, nausea
insulin Treatment of diabetic ketoacidosis, severely elevated blood glucose levels	Individualized. Use protocol.	Itching, swelling, headache, tachycardia, nausea, hypoglycemia, allergic reactions
ipecac Treatment of poisoning or drug overdose by inducing vomiting in the conscious and alert pt	***Children (<1 yr):*** 5–10 ml, then ½–1 glass water. ***Children (>1 yr to 12 yrs):*** 15 ml followed by 1–2 glasses water. ***Adults:*** 15–30 ml followed by 3–4 glasses water. **Note:** Repeat dose (15 ml) once in pts older than 1 yr if vomiting does not occur within 20–30 min. Perform gastric lavage if vomiting does not occur within 30–45 min after second dose.	Arrhythmias, bradycardia, hypotension, depression, diarrhea
ketamine (Ketalar) For rapid sequence induction of anesthesia prior to intubation. To supplement low-potency agents (e.g., nitrous oxide).	***Direct IV Push: Adults, elderly:*** Initially, 1–4.5 mg/kg to produce 5–10 min anesthesia. ***Children:*** 0.25–1.0 mg/kg	Increase in B/P, pulse. Emergency reaction occurs frequently (12%), resulting in dreamlike state, vivid imagery, hallucination, delirium, occasionally with confusion, excitement, irrational behavior. Lasts from few hours to 24 hrs after administration
labetalol Treatment of severe hypertension, hypertensive emergency	***IV: Adults:*** Initially, 20 mg. Additional doses of 20–80 mg may be given at 10 min intervals, up to total dose of 300 mg.	Drowsiness, dizziness. May precipitate or aggravate CHF (due to decreased myocardial stimulation)
lidocaine (Xylocaine) Ventricular fibrillation, ventricular tachycardia, suppress PVCs, wide-complex tachycardias, wide complex PSVT	***Ventricular arrhythmias: IM: Adults, elderly:*** 300 mg (or 4.3 mg/kg). May repeat in 60–90 min. ***IV: Adults, elderly:*** Initially, 50–100 mg (1 mg/kg) IV bolus at rate of 25–50 mg/min. May repeat in 5 min. Give no more than 200–300 mg in 1 hr. ***Maintenance:*** 20–50 mcg/kg/min	Anxiety, seizures, nausea, vomiting, drowsiness, widening QRS complex

NAME/INDICATIONS	DOSAGE/ROUTES	SIDE EFFECTS
	(1–4 mg/min) as IV infusion. ***Children, infants:*** Initially, 0.5–1 mg/kg IV bolus; may repeat, but total dose not to exceed 3–5 mg/kg. ***Maintenance:*** 10–50 mcg/kg/min as IV infusion.	
magnesium Refractory ventricular fibrillation, cardiac arrest associated with torsades de pointes, preeclampsia, eclampsia, life-threatening arrhythmias caused by digoxin toxicity, torsades de pointes	*IV:* 1–2 g in 10 ml sodium chloride slow IVP over 1–2 min. *Eclampsia:* 1–4 g.	Drowsiness, bradycardia, dysrhythmia, decreased B/P, rash, hypothermia
methylprednisolone (Solu-Medrol) Treatment of asthma, status asthmaticus	*IV:* ***Adults, elderly:*** Initially, 40–125 mg q4–6h. ***Children:*** I mg/kg.	Insomnia, heartburn, nervousness, abdominal distension, increased sweating, acne, mood swings, increased appetite, facial flushing, GI distress, delayed wound healing, increased susceptibility to infection, diarrhea/constipation
midazolam (Versed) Sedation (w/o loss of consciousness) to relieve anxiety; produces anterograde amnesia for short diagnostic, endoscopic procedures, intubated/ mechanical ventilator pts	Initially, 1–2.5 mg; may repeat in 1 mg increments if needed. Total dose not to exceed 0.1 mg/kg.	Decreased respiratory rate, tenderness at IM/IV injection site, pain during injection, desaturation, hiccups, hypotension, paradoxical reaction, nausea, vomiting, headache, coughing
morphine Relief of severe, acute, chronic pain, preop sedation, anesthesia supplement, analgesia during labor. Drug of choice for pain due to myocardial infarction, dyspnea from pulmonary edema not resulting from chemical respiratory irritant	***Pain:*** *IV:* ***Adults, elderly:*** 4–10 mg, given very slowly. ***Myocardial infarction pain, keep SBP>90:*** *IV:* ***Adults, elderly:*** 2–4 mg prn pain.	Sedation, decreased B/P, increased sweating, flushed face, constipation, dizziness, drowsiness, nausea, vomiting, respiratory depression
naloxone (Narcan) Diagnosis and treatment of opioid toxicity, treatment of opioid-induced	***Opioid toxicity (IV route preferred):*** *IM/IV/SubQ:* ***Adults:*** 0.4–2 mg as single dose. May re-	Too rapid reversal of narcotic depression may result in nausea, vomiting, tremulousness, sweating,

(continued)

NAME/INDICATIONS	DOSAGE/ROUTES	SIDE EFFECTS
respiratory depression, and other effects (e.g., sedation, coma, convulsions). Used in neonates to reverse respiratory depression caused by opioids given mother during labor and delivery. Adjunctive therapy to treat hypotension in management of septic shock	peat at 2–3 min intervals. ***Children:*** 0.01 mg/kg. May repeat w/0.1 mg/kg. **Note:** AAP recommends initial dose of 0.1 mg/kg for infants and children up to 5 yrs and weighing <20 kg. Children >5 yrs or >20 kg recommended initial dose is 2 mg. ***Opioid respiratory depression:*** ***IV: Adults:*** 0.1–0.2 mg q2–3 min until adequate ventilation and alertness w/o pain are obtained. May repeat dose at 1–2 hr intervals. ***Children:*** 5–10 mcg (0.005–0.01 mg) q2–3 min. ***Neonates:*** 10 mcg (0.01 mg)/kg. May repeat q2–3 min. ***Septic shock:*** ***IV: Adults:*** 0.03–0.2 mg/kg initially, then IV infusion of 0.03–0.3 mg/kg/hr for 1–20 hrs.	increased B/P, tachycardia. Hypotension or hypertension, ventricular tachycardia and fibrillation, pulmonary edema may occur in pts w/cardiovascular disease
nitroglycerin Acute ischemic coronary syndrome, angina, acute MI	***Sublingual: Adults:*** 0.4 mg. May repeat every 5 min as long as BP>90	Headache (may be severe) occurs mostly in early therapy, diminishes rapidly in intensity, usually disappears during continued treatment; transient flushing of face and neck, dizziness (esp. if pt is standing immobile or is in a warm environment), weakness, postural hypotension. Burning, tingling sensation at oral point of dissolution
nitrous oxide Pain relief from musculoskeletal trauma, burns, kidney stones, severe anxiety	50% nitrous oxide and 50% oxygen; self-administered by mask.	Dizziness, lightheadedness, drowsiness, bizarre behavior, slurred speech, numbness/tingling in face, headache, nausea, vomiting
procainamide (Pronestyl) Refractory ventricular fibrillation, ventricular tachycardia with a pulse, wide complex tachycardia,	30 mg/min, maximum total dose 17 mg/kg. ***Maintenance Infusion:*** 1–4 mg/min.	Confusion, dizziness, hypotension, conduction changes (50% widening of QRS complex, frequent ventricular premature contractions, ventricular tachycar-

NAME/INDICATIONS	DOSAGE/ROUTES	SIDE EFFECTS
paroxysmal supraventricular tachycardia (PSVT)		dia, complete AV block). Prolonged PR and QT intervals, flattened T waves occur less frequently
sodium bicarbonate Prolonged cardiac arrest after defibrillation and cardiac medications, severe acidotic states, hyperkalemia, crush syndrome	***Cardiac arrest:*** ***IV: Adults, elderly:*** Initially, 1 mEq/kg (as 7.5–8.4% solution). May repeat w/0.5 mEq/kg every 10 min during continued arrest. Postresuscitation phase based on arterial blood pH, $PaCO_2$ base deficit. ***Children, infants:*** Initially, 1 mEq/kg. ***Metabolic acidosis (less severe):*** ***IV Infusion: Adults, elderly, older children:*** 2–5 mEq/kg over 4–8 hrs. May repeat based on laboratory values.	CHF, alkalosis, cramps, fluid retention, tissue necrosis with infiltration at IV site
succinylcholine (Anectine) To facilitate rapid endotracheal intubation	***IV: Adults, elderly: IV Bolus:*** 1–2 mg; may repeat once if needed. ***Children:*** 1–1.5 mg/kg; may repeat once if needed.	Hypotension, bradycardia, prolonged respiratory depression, bronchospasm, increased intraocular pressure
tenecteplase (TNKase) Management of acute myocardial infarction (AMI) for lysis of thrombi-obstructing coronary arteries	**Note:** Give as a single IV bolus over 5 sec. ***IV: Adults:*** Dosage based on weight of pt. Treatment to be initiated as soon as possible after onset of AMI symptoms.	Superficial bleeding at puncture sites, gingival bleeding, decreased B/P
terbutaline Treatment of bronchospasm secondary to COPD. Prevention of labor contractions in pts w/prolapsed cord.	***Bronchospasm:*** ***SubQ: Adults:*** Initially, 0.25 mg. Repeat in 15–30 min if substantial improvement does not occur. ***Maximum:*** No more than 0.5 mg/4hrs. ***Prevention of labor contractions:*** ***SubQ: Adults:*** 0.25 mg q1h until contractions cease.	Nervousness, tremors, shakiness, headache, hypertension, tachycardia, nausea, vomiting
thiamine Alcoholism with hypoglycemia, delirium tremens	***IV:*** 100 mg over 2–5 min.	Rare; pain, induration, tenderness at IM injection site

(continued)

NAME/INDICATIONS	DOSAGE/ROUTES	SIDE EFFECTS
vasopressin (Pitressin) Pressor agent for promoting return of spontaneous circulation in cardiac arrest	*IV:* 40 units as a one-time dose	Stomach cramps, nausea, vomiting, diarrhea, dizziness, diaphoresis, paleness, circumoral pallor, trembling, pounding in head, eructation, flatulence
vecruonium (Norcuron) To facilitate rapid endotracheal intubation	***IV Bolus: Adults, elderly:*** 0.08–0.1 mg/kg; may repeat every 20–30 min.	Prolonged paralysis
verapamil (Isoptin) Management of supraventricular tachyarrhythmias, temporary control of rapid ventricular rate in atrial flutter/fibrillation	**Note:** Give slowly over 2–5 min. *IV:* **Adults, elderly:** Initially, 5–10 mg, repeat in 30 min w/10 mg dose. ***Children 1–15 yrs:*** 2–5 mg, repeat in 30 min up to 10 mg. ***Children <1 yr:*** 0.75–2 mg, repeat after 30 min. *Maximum single dose:* 10 mg.	Rapid ventricular rate in atrial flutter/fibrillation, marked hypotension, extreme bradycardia, CHF, asystole, and second- and third-degree AV block occur rarely; dizziness, lightheadedness, headache

Appendix F
GUIDELINES FOR EMERGENCY TREATMENT OF ACUTE CORONARY SYNDROMES (CHEST PAIN)

Initial Assessment and General Treatment of Pt w/Acute Coronary Syndrome

PREHOSPITAL	EMERGENCY DEPARTMENT
Initial Assessment (Goal: Targeted Clinical Exam and 12-lead ECG within 10 min)	
• Obtain brief, targeted Hx/physical exam (determine age, gender; S/S, pain presentation, including location of pain, duration, quality, relation to effort, time of symptom onset; Hx CAD, CAD risk factors present?) Hx of Viagra use? • Assess vital signs, determine oxygen saturation If above consistent w/possible or definite ACS: • Use checklist (yes–no); focus on eligibility for reperfusion therapy; evaluate contraindications to aspirin and heparin • Establish IV access, ECG monitoring • Administer aspirin 162–325 mg (chewed) if no reason for exclusion • Obtain 12-lead ECG (machine interpretation or transmission of ECG to physician) • Draw blood for initial serum cardiac marker levels (to lab on arrival in Emergency Department) Consider triage to facility capable of angiography and revascularization, if any of the following are present: • Signs of shock • Pulmonary edema (rales > halfway up) • Heart rate ≥ 100 beats/min and SBP ≤ 100 mm Hg	**RN triage for rapid care** • Targeted Hx—determine age, gender, S/S, pain presentation, including location of pain, duration, quality, relation to effort, time of symptom onset; Hx CAD, CAD risk factors present? Hx of Viagra use? • Assess vital signs; determine oxygen saturation • Establish IV access, ECG monitoring • Obtain 12-lead ECG (present to physician for review) **Physician evaluation** If above consistent w/possible or definite ACS: • Brief, targeted Hx/physical exam • Evaluate eligibility for reperfusion therapy and contraindications to aspirin and heparin • Administer aspirin 162–325 mg (chewed) if no reason for exclusion • Administer nitroglycerin as indicated • Evaluate 12-lead ECG—categorize pt into 1 of 3 groups: ST-elevation or new or presumably new LBBB; ST-depression/transient ST-segment/T wave changes; normal or nondiagnostic ECG • Obtain serial ECGs in pts w/Hx suggesting MI and nondiagnostic ECG • Obtain baseline serum cardiac marker levels (CK-MB, Troponin T or I, myoglobin) • Obtain lab specimens (CBC, lipid profile, electrolytes, coagulation studies) • Obtain portable chest x-ray • Evaluate results
Routine Measures	
• Oxygen 4 L/min by nasal cannula for first 2–3 hrs (Class IIa) • Oxygen 4 L/min by cannula, titrate if pulmonary congestion, SaO_2 < 90% (Class I) • Aspirin 162–325 mg—chewed (if hypersensitivity exists, ticlopidine); may administer via rectal suppository (325 mg) if nausea, vomiting, upper GI disorder present • NTG SL or spray (ensure IV access, SBP > 90 mm Hg, HR > 50 beats/min, no RV infarction) • Morphine 2–4 mg IV if pain not relieved w/NTG; may repeat every 5 min (ensure SBP > 90 mm Hg)	

Management of ST-Segment Elevation MI[1,2]

ST-segment elevation ≥ 1 mm in two or more anatomically contiguous leads or new, or presumably new, LBBB

↓

Confirm diagnosis by signs/symptoms, ECG, serum cardiac markers

All pts w/ST-segment elevation MI should receive (if no contraindications):

- Antiplatelet therapy—aspirin 162–325 mg (chewed)
- Anti-ischemia therapy (beta-blockers, NTG IV if ongoing ischemia or uncorrected hypertension)
- Antithrombin therapy—heparin (if using fibrin-specific lytics)
- ACE inhibitors (after 6 hrs or when stable)—esp. w/large or anterior MI, heart failure w/o hypotension (SBP > 100 mm Hg), previous MI

<table>
<tr><th colspan="5">Symptom Onset ≤ 12 hours?</th><th colspan="2">Symptom Onset > 12 hours?</th></tr>
<tr><td colspan="5">Pt Eligible for Reperfusion?
Goals
• Fibrinolytics: Door-to-drug time < 30 min
• Primary PCI: Door-to-dilation time 90 ± 30 min</td><td>Persistent Symptoms
↓</td><td>Resolution of Symptoms
↓</td></tr>
<tr><td colspan="3">Yes ↓</td><td colspan="2">No ↓</td><td>Consider reperfusion</td><td rowspan="2">Medical management</td></tr>
<tr><td colspan="3">Signs of cardiogenic shock or contraindications to fibrinolytics?</td><td colspan="2">Persistent or stuttering symptoms or ECG changes?</td><td>Medical management</td></tr>
<tr><td>Yes ↓</td><td colspan="2">No ↓</td><td>Yes ↓</td><td>No ↓</td><td></td><td></td></tr>
<tr><td>PCI
Medical management</td><td colspan="2">Can cath lab be mobilized within 60 min?</td><td>Cardiac cath, medical management</td><td>Medical management</td><td></td><td></td></tr>
<tr><td></td><td>Yes ↓</td><td>No ↓</td><td></td><td></td><td></td><td></td></tr>
<tr><td></td><td>PCI</td><td>Fibrinolysis (alteplase, reteplase, streptokinase, anistreplase, or tenecteplase)</td><td></td><td></td><td></td><td></td></tr>
</table>

Note: PCI = percutaneous coronary intervention (angioplasty ± stent).

[1]Ryan TJ, Antman EM, Brooks NH, Califf RM, Hillis LD, Hiratzka LF, Rapaport E, Riegel B, Russell RO, Smith EE III, Weaver WD. ACC/AHA guidelines for the management of patients with acute myocardial infarction: 1999 update: a report of the American College of Cardiology/American Heart Association Task Force on Practice Guidelines (Committee on Management of Acute Myocardial Infarction).

[2]The American Heart Association in Collaboration with the International Liaison Committee on Resuscitation (ILCOR). Part 7: Era of Reperfusion Section 1: Acute Coronary Syndromes (Acute Myocardial Infarction): A Consensus on Science. *Circulation* 2000; 102 (suppl I):I-178–192.

Management of Unstable Angina/Non-ST-Segment Elevation MI[1,2,3]

ECG changes in 2 or more anatomically contiguous leads:
ST-segment depression > 1 mm or T-wave inversion > 1 mm or
Transient (< 30 min) ST-segment/T-wave changes > 1 mm with discomfort

↓

Confirm diagnosis by signs/symptoms, ECG, serum cardiac markers

↓

- Aspirin 162–325 mg (chewed) if not already administered (and no contraindications) (antiplatelet therapy)
- Heparin IV (antithrombin therapy)

↓

If high-risk patient give:
- Aspirin + glycoprotein IIb/IIIa inhibitors (i.e., Integrilin, Aggrastat, ReoPro) + IV heparin **or**
- Aspirin + glycoprotein IIb/IIIa inhibitors + SC low molecular weight heparin

High-risk criteria
- Persistent ("stuttering") symptoms/recurrent ischemia; left ventricular (LV) dysfunction, CHF; widespread ECG changes; prior MI, positive troponin or CK-MB

↓

Anti-ischemic therapy
- Beta-blockers—if pt not previously on beta-blockers or inadequately treated on current dose of beta-blocker (if no contraindications)
- NTG sublingual tablet or spray, followed by IV NTG if symptoms persist despite sublingual NTG therapy and initiation of beta-blocker therapy (and SBP > 90 mm Hg)
- Morphine 2–4 mg IV (if discomfort is not relieved or symptoms recur despite anti-ischemic therapy)—may repeat every 5 min (ensure SBP > 90 mm Hg)

↓

Assess Clinical Status: Is Pt Clinically Stable?

YES	NO
• Continue in-hospital observation • Consider stress testing	Cardiac cath • If anatomy suitable for revascularization—PCI, CABG • If anatomy unsuitable—medical management

[1]Goldman L, Braunwald E: Primary cardiology, Philadelphia, 1998, W.B. Saunders Company.

[2]Braunwald E, Antman EM, Beasley JW, Califf RM, Cheitlin MD, Hochman JS, Jones RH, Kereiakes D, Kupersmith J, Levin TN, Pepine CJ, Schaeffer JW, Smith EE III, Steward DE, Theroux P. ACC/AHA guidelines for the management of patients with unstable angina and non—ST-segment elevation myocardial infarction: a report of the American College of Cardiology/American Heart Association Task Force on Practice Guidelines (Committee on the Management of Patients with Unstable Angina). J Am Coll Cardiol 2000:36:970–1062.

[3]The American Heart Association in Collaboration with the International Liaison Committee on Resuscitation (ILCOR). Part 7: Era of Reperfusion Section 1: Acute Coronary Syndromes (Acute Myocardial Infarction): A Consensus on Science. *Circulation* 2000; 102 (suppl I):I-178–192.

Management of Pt w/Suspected Acute Coronary Syndrome and Nondiagnostic/Normal ECG

Nondiagnostic or Normal ECG

↓

Evaluate signs/symptoms, serial ECGs, serum cardiac markers

↓

Aspirin + other therapy as appropriate

↓

- Assess pt's clinical risk of death/nonfatal MI
- Hx/physical exam
- Obtain follow-up serum cardiac marker levels, serial ECG monitoring
- Continue evaluation and treatment in Emergency Department chest pain unit or monitored bed
- Consider radionuclide, echocardiography

From Aehlert, B. *ACLS Quick Review Study Guide* (2002). St. Louis, Mosby.

APPENDIX G
HERBAL THERAPIES

The use of herbal therapies is on the increase in the United States. In 1990, an estimated 1 in 3 Americans used at least one form of alternative medicine (of which herbal therapy is part). By 1997, over $12 billion was spent in the United States for vitamins and minerals, herbals, sports supplements or specialty supplements (e.g., glucosamine).

Because of the rise in the use of herbal therapy in the United States, the following is presented to provide some basic information on some of the more popular herbs. Please note this is not an all-inclusive list, which is beyond the scope of this handbook.

NAME	PURPORTED BENEFIT	INTERACTIONS	PRECAUTIONS
Black cohosh	Manage symptoms of menopause, hypercholesterolemia, peripheral arterial disease, anti-inflammatory and sedative effects.	May further reduce lipids and/or blood pressure when combined with prescription medications.	Side effects: nausea, dizziness, visual changes, migraine.
Chamomile	Antispasmodic, sedative, anti-inflammatory, astringent, antibacterial.	May increase bleeding with anticoagulants May increase sedative effect with benzodiazepines.	Anaphylactic reaction if allergic, avoid use if allergic; avoid use if allergic to chrysanthemums, ragweed, and/or asters; delays absorption of medications.
DHEA	Slows aging, boosts energy, controls weight.	None	Side effects: May increase risk of breast/ prostate cancer. Women may develop acne, hair growth on face/body.
Dong quai	Uterine stimulant, anti-inflammatory, vasodilator, CNS stimulant, immunosuppressant, analgesic, antipyretic.	May increase effects of warfarin.	Diarrhea, photosensitivity, skin cancer; avoid in pregnancy/ lactation; essential oil may contain the carcinogen safrole.
Echinacea	Prevents/treats colds, flu, bacterial and fungal infections. An immune system stimulator. Aid to wound healing.	May interfere with immunosuppressive therapy.	Not to be used with weakened immune system (e.g., HIV/AIDS, tuberculosis, multiple sclerosis). Habitual or continued use may cause immune system suppression (should only be taken for 2–3 mos or alternating schedule of q2–3wks).

(continued)

NAME	PURPORTED BENEFIT	INTERACTIONS	PRECAUTIONS
Feverfew	Relieves migraine. Treatment of fever, headache, menstrual irregularities.	May increase bleeding time with aspirin, dipyridamole, warfarin.	Side effects: headache, mouth ulcers. Should be avoided in pregnancy (stimulates menstruation), nursing mother, infants <2 yrs of age.
Garlic	Reduces cholesterol, LDL, triglycerides, increases HDL, lowers B/P, inhibits platelet aggregation. May also possess antibacterial, antiviral, antithrombotic activity.	May increase bleeding time with aspirin, dipyridamole, warfarin.	Side effects: taste, offensive odor. Large doses may cause heartburn, flatulence, other GI distress.
Ginger	Relieves nausea, effective treatment for motion sickness, anti-inflammatory for arthritis, nausea/vomiting associated with pregnancy. Possesses ability to lower platelet aggregation; antithrombotic properties.	None	Avoid during pregnancy when bleeding is a concern. Large overdose could potentially depress the CNS, cause cardiac arrhythmias.
Ginko	Boosts mental prowess by improving memory. Sharpens concentration, pt may think more clearly. Overcomes sexual dysfunction occurring with SSRI antidepressants. May be able to slow progress of Alzheimer's, improve intermittent claudication.	May increase bleeding time with aspirin, dipyridamole, warfarin.	Avoid in pt taking blood thinners or those hypersensitive to poison ivy, cashews, mangos. Side effects: GI disturbances, headache, dizziness, vertigo.
Ginseng	Boosts energy, sexual stamina; decreases stress, effects of aging.	May affect platelet adhesiveness/blood coagulation. Use caution with anticoagulants. May increase hypoglycemia with insulin.	Avoid in pts receiving anticoagulants, medica-tions that increase B/P. Side effects: breast tenderness, nervousness, headache, increased B/P, abnormal vaginal bleeding.
Glucosamine and chondroitin	Osteoarthritis	No known interactions but monitor anticoagulant effects.	None known.
Kava kava	Reduces stress, muscle relaxant, relieves anxiety, induces sleep and counters fatigue.	Increases CNS depression with alcohol, sedatives.	Side effects: GI disturbances, temporary discoloration of skin, hair, nails. Do not use in pregnancy, lactation, endogenous depression.

NAME	PURPORTED BENEFIT	INTERACTIONS	PRECAUTIONS
Kava kava *(continued)*			High doses cause muscle weakness. Chronic use may cause scaly skin resembling psoriasis (reversible). Causes pupil dilation affecting vision (avoid driving, operating heavy machinery).
Ma Huang (Ephedra)	Controls weight, boosts energy. Treatment of colds, allergies, appetite suppressant.	Increases toxicity with beta blockers, MAOIs, caffeine, theophylline, decongestants, St. John's wort.	Linked to high B/P, headache, seizures. Can cause confusion, insomnia, dizziness, sweating, fever, nausea, vomiting.
Melatonin	Aids sleep, prevents jet lag.	Decreases effects of antidepressants.	Side effects: headache, confusion, fatigue. Does not lengthen total sleep time.
Saw Palmetto	Eases symptoms of large prostate (frequency, dysuria, nocturia).	None	Side effects: upset stomach, headache, erectile dysfunction. Does not reduce size of enlarged prostate. Obtain baseline PSA levels before initiating. High doses can cause diarrhea.
St. John's wort	Relieves mild to moderate depression, heals wounds.	May cause "seratonin syndrome" (confusion, agitation, chills, fever, sweating, diarrhea, nausea, muscle spasms or twitching), hyperreflexia, tremor with antidepressants, yohimbe.	Store in cool, dry place (excess heat/light will alter contents). Side effects: dizziness, dry mouth, increased sensitivity to sunlight. Report symptoms of "serotonin syndrome."
Valerian	Aids sleep, relieves restlessness and nervousness. Does not decrease night awakenings.	None	Side effects: heart palpitations, upset stomach, headache, excitability, uneasiness. May cause increased morning drowsiness.
Yohimbe	Male aphrodisiac. Used to treat impotence, erectile dysfunction, orthostatic hypotension.	Decreases effects of antidepressants, antihypertensives, St. John's wort.	High doses linked to weakness, paralysis.

Appendix H
NORMAL LABORATORY VALUES

HEMATOLOGY/COAGULATION

Test	Specimen	Normal Range
Activated partial thromboplastin time (APTT)	Whole blood	25–35 secs
Erythrocyte count (RBC count)	Whole blood	M: 4.3–5.7 million cells/mm^3 F: 3.8–5.1 million cells/mm^3
Hematocrit (HCT, Hct)	Whole blood	M: 39–49% F: 35–45%
Hemoglobin (Hb, Hgb)	Whole blood	M: 13.5–17.5 g/dl F: 12.0–16.0 g/dl
Leucocyte count (WBC count)	Whole blood	4.5–11.0 thousand cells/mm^3
Leucocyte differential count	Whole blood	
Basophils		0–0.75%
Eosinophils		1–3%
Lymphocytes		23–33%
Monocytes		3–7%
Neutrophils—bands		3–5%
Neutrophils—segmented		54–62%
Mean corpuscular hemoglobin (MCH)	Whole blood	26–34 pg/cell
Mean corpuscular hemoglobin concentration (MCHC)	Whole blood	31–37% Hb/cell
Mean corpuscular volume (MCV)	Whole blood	80–100 fL
Partial thromboplastin time (PTT)	Whole blood	60–85 secs
Platelet count (thrombocyte count)	Whole blood	150–450 thousand/mm^3
Prothrombin time (PT)	Whole blood	11–13.5 secs
RBC count (see Erythrocyte count)		

SERUM/URINE VALUES

Test	Specimen	Normal Range
Alanine aminotransferase (ALT, SGPT)	Serum	0–55 units/L
Albumin	Serum	3.5–5 g/dl
Alkaline phosphatase	Serum	M: 53–128 units/L F: 42–98 units/L
Anion gap	Plasma or serum	5–14 mEq/L
Aspartate aminotransferase (AST, SGOT)	Serum	0–50 units/L

TEST	SPECIMEN	NORMAL RANGE
Bilirubin (conjugated direct)	Serum	0–0.4 mg/dl
Bilirubin (total)	Serum	0.2–1.2 mg/dl
Calcium (total)	Serum	8.4–10.2 mg/dl
Carbon dioxide (CO_2) total	Plasma or serum	20–34 mEq/L
Chloride	Plasma or serum	96–112 mEq/L
Cholesterol (total)	Plasma or serum	<200 mg/dl
C-Reactive protein	Serum	68–8200 ng/ml
Creatine kinase (CK)	Serum	M: 38–174 units/L F: 26–140 units/L
Creatine kinase isoenzymes	Serum	Fraction of total: <0.04–0.06
Creatinine	Plasma or serum	M: 0.7–1.3 mg/dl F: 0.6–1.1 mg/dl
Creatinine clearance	Plasma or serum and urine	M: 90–139 ml/min/1.73m^2 F: 80–125 ml/min/1.73m^2
Free thyroxine index (FTI)	Serum	1.1–4.8
Glucose	Serum	Adults: 70–105 mg/dl >60 yrs: 80–115 mg/dl
Hemoglobin A_{1c}	Whole blood	5.6–7.5% of total Hgb
Homovanillic acid (HVA)	Urine, 24 hr	1.4–8.8 mg/day
17-Hydroxycorticosteroids (17-OHCS)	Urine, 24 hr	M: 3–10 mg/day F: 2–8 mg/day
Iron	Serum	M: 65–175 mcg/dl F: 50–170 mcg/dl
Iron binding capacity, total (TIBC)	Serum	250–450 mcg/dl
Lactate dehydrogenase (LDH)	Serum	0–250 units/L
Magnesium	Serum	1.3–2.3 mg/dl
Oxygen (PO_2)	Whole blood, arterial	83–100 mm Hg
Oxygen saturation	Whole blood, arterial	95–98%
pH	Whole blood, arterial	7.35–7.45
Phosphorus, inorganic	Serum	2.7–4.5 mg/dl
Potassium	Serum	3.5–5.1 mEq/L
Protein (total)	Serum	6–8.5 g/dl
Sodium	Plasma or serum	136–146 mEq/L
Specific gravity	Urine	1.002–1.030
Thyrotropin (hTSH)	Plasma or serum	2–10 mcgU/ml
Thyroxine (T_4) total	Serum	5–12 mcg/dl
Triglycerides (TG)	Serum, after 12 hr fast	20–190 mg/dl
Triiodothyronine resin uptake test (T_3RU)	Serum	22–37%
Urea nitrogen	Plasma or serum	7–25 mg/dl
Urea nitrogen/creatinine ratio	Serum	12/1–20/1
Uric acid	Serum	M: 3.5–7.2 mg/dl F: 2.6–6 mg/dl
Vanillylmandelic acid (VMA)	Urine, 24 hr	2–7 mg/day

Appendix 1
FDA PREGNANCY CATEGORIES

Note: Medications should be used during pregnancy only if clearly needed.

A: Adequate and well-controlled studies have failed to show a risk to the fetus in the first trimester of pregnancy (also, no evidence of risk has been seen in later trimesters).

B: Animal reproduction studies have failed to show a risk to the fetus, and there are no adequate/well-controlled studies in pregnant women.

C: Animal reproduction studies have shown an adverse effect on the fetus, and there are no adequate/well-controlled studies in humans. However, the benefits may warrant use of the drug in pregnant women despite potential risks.

D: There is positive evidence of human fetal risk based on data from investigational or marketing experience or from studies in humans, but the potential benefits may warrant use of the drug despite potential risks (e.g., use in life-threatening situations in which other medications cannot be used or are ineffective).

X: Animal or human studies have shown fetal abnormalities, and/or there is evidence of human fetal risk based on adverse reaction data from investigational or marketing experience where the risks in using the medication clearly outweigh potential benefits.

APPENDIX J
TECHNIQUES OF MEDICATION ADMINISTRATION

Ophthalmic:

EYE DROPS:

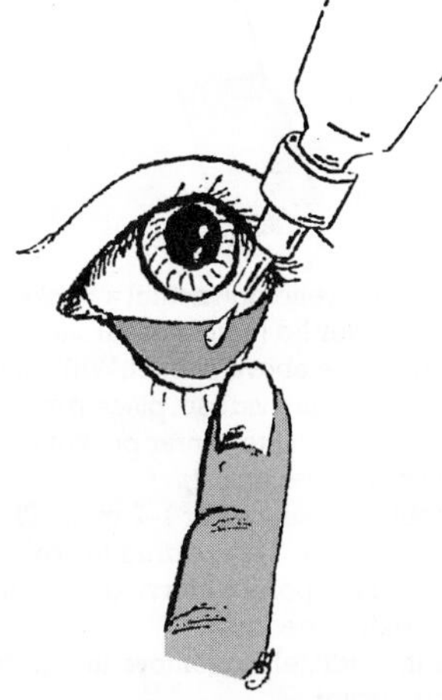

1. Wash hands.
2. Instruct patient to lie down or tilt head backward and look up.
3. Gently pull lower eyelid down until a pocket (pouch) is formed between eye and lower lid (conjunctival sac).
4. Hold dropper above pocket. Without touching tip of eye dropper to eyelid or conjunctival sac, place prescribed number of drops into the center pocket *(placing drops directly onto eye may cause a sudden squeezing of eyelid, with subsequent loss of solution).* Continue to hold the eyelid for a moment after the drops are applied *(allows medication to distribute along entire conjunctival sac).*
5. Instruct patient to close eyes gently so medication will not be squeezed out of sac.
6. Apply gentle finger pressure to the lacrimal sac at the inner canthus (bridge of the nose, inside corner of the eye) for 1–2 min *(promotes absorption, minimizes drainage into nose and throat, lessens risk of systemic absorption).*
7. Remove excess solution around eye with a tissue.
8. Wash hands immediately to remove medication on hands. Never rinse eye dropper.

EYE OINTMENT:

1. Wash hands.
2. Instruct patient to lie down or tilt head backward and look up.

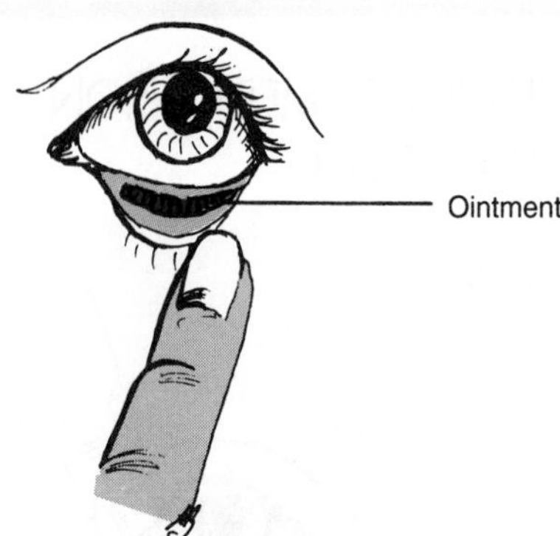

3. Gently pull lower eyelid down until a pocket (pouch) is formed between eye and lower lid (conjunctival sac).
4. Hold applicator tube above pocket. Without touching the applicator tip to eyelid or conjunctival sac, place prescribed amount of ointment (¼–½ inch) into the center pocket *(placing ointment directly onto eye may cause discomfort).*
5. Instruct patient to close eye for 1–2 min, rolling eyeball in all directions *(increases contact area of drug to eye).*
6. Inform patient of temporary blurring of vision. If possible, apply ointment just before bedtime.
7. Wash hands immediately to remove medication on hands. Never rinse tube applicator.

Otic:

1. Ear drops should be at body temperature (wrap hand around bottle to warm contents). *Body temperature instillation prevents startling of patient.*
2. Instruct patient to lie down with head turned so affected ear is upright *(allows medication to drip into ear).*
3. Instill prescribed number of drops toward the canal wall, not directly on eardrum.

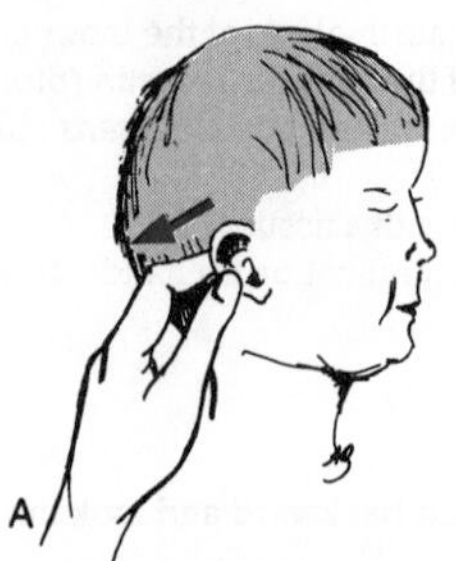

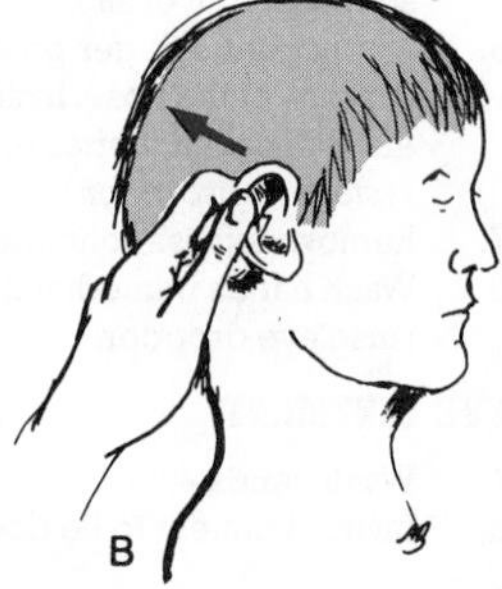

4. To promote correct placement of ear drops, pull the auricle down and posterior in children (A) and pull the auricle up and posterior in adults (B).

Nasal:

NOSE DROPS AND SPRAYS:

1. Instruct patient to blow nose to clear nasal passages as much as possible.
2. Tilt head slightly forward if instilling nasal spray, slightly backward if instilling nasal drops.
3. Insert spray tip into 1 nostril, pointing toward inflamed nasal passages, away from nasal septum.
4. Spray or drop medication into 1 nostril while holding other nostril closed and concurrently inspire through nose to permit medication as high into nasal passages as possible.
5. Discard unused nasal solution after 3 mos.

Inhalation:

AEROSOL (MULTIDOSE INHALERS):

1. Shake container well before each use.
2. Exhale slowly and as completely as possible through the mouth.
3. Place mouthpiece fully into mouth, holding inhaler upright, and close lips fully around mouthpiece.
4. Inhale deeply and slowly through the mouth while depressing the top of the canister with the middle finger.
5. Hold breath as long as possible before exhaling slowly and gently.
6. When two puffs are prescribed, wait 2 min and shake container again before inhaling a second puff *(allows for deeper bronchial penetration).*
7. Rinse mouth w/water immediately after inhalation *(prevents mouth and throat dryness).*

Sublingual:

1. Administer while seated.
2. Dissolve sublingual tablet under tongue (do not chew or swallow tablet).
3. Do not swallow saliva until tablet is dissolved.

Topical:

1. Gently cleanse area prior to application.
2. Use occlusive dressings only as ordered.
3. Without touching applicator tip to skin, apply sparingly; gently rub into area thoroughly unless ordered otherwise.

4. When using aerosol, spray area for 3 secs from 15 cm distance; avoid inhalation.

Transdermal:

1. Apply transdermal patch to clean, dry, hairless skin on upper arm or body (not below knee or elbow).
2. Rotate sites *(prevents skin irritation).*
3. Do not trim patch to adjust dose.

Rectal:

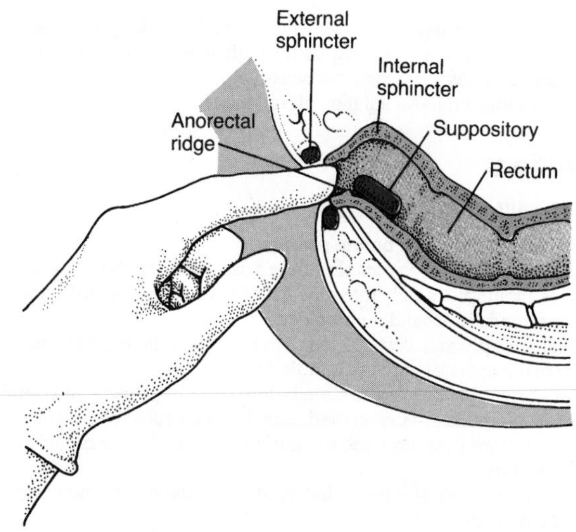

1. Instruct patient to lie in left lateral Sims' position.
2. Moisten suppository with cold water or water-soluble lubricant.
3. Instruct patient to slowly exhale *(relaxes anal sphincter)* while inserting suppository well up into rectum.
4. Inform patient as to length of time (20–30 min) before desire for defecation occurs or <60 min for systemic absorption to occur, depending on purpose for suppository.

SubQ:

1. Use 25–27 gauge, ½–⅝ inch needle; 1–3 ml. Angle of insertion depends on body size: 90° if patient is obese. If patient is very thin, gather the skin at the area of needle insertion and administer also

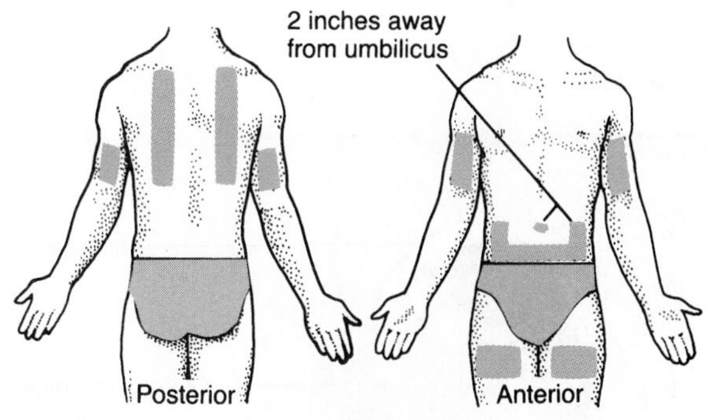

SubQ injection sites

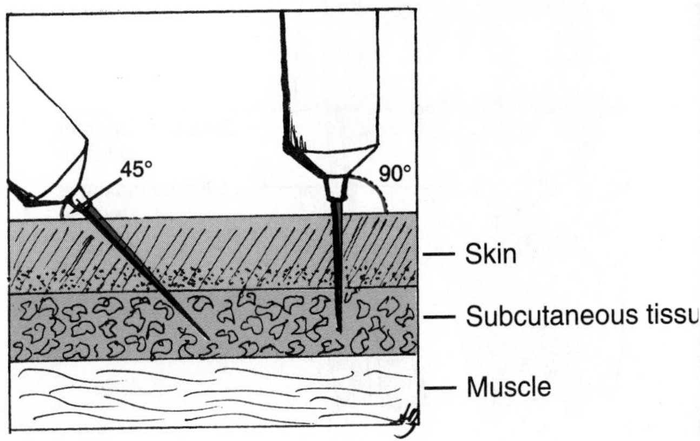

at a 90° angle. A 45° angle may be used in a patient with average weight.

2. Cleanse area to be injected with circular motion.
3. Avoid areas of bony prominence, major nerves, blood vessels.
4. Aspirate syringe before injecting *(to avoid intra-arterial administration),* except insulin, heparin.
5. Inject slowly; remove needle quickly.

IM:

INJECTION SITES:

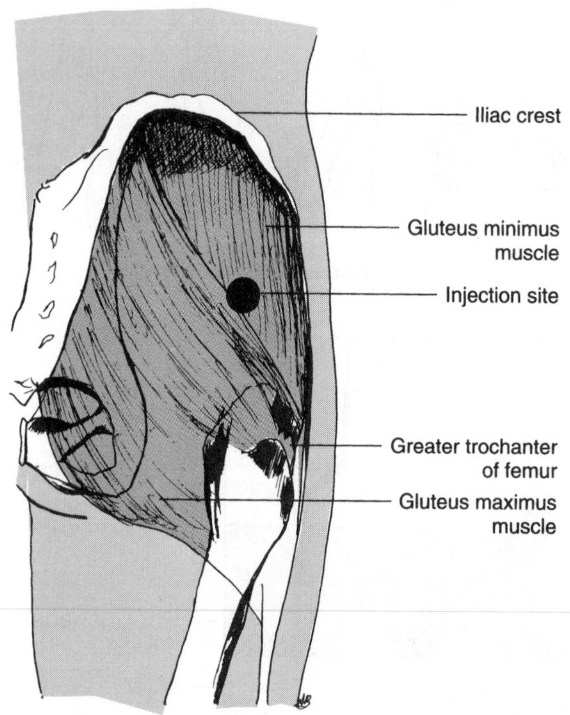

Dorsogluteal (upper outer quadrant)

1. Use this site if volume to be injected is 1–3 ml. Use 18–23 gauge, 1.25–3 in needle. Needle should be long enough to reach the middle of the muscle.
2. Do not use this site in children <2 yrs old or in those who are emaciated. Patient should be in prone position.
3. Using 90° angle, flatten the skin area using the middle and index finger and inject between them.

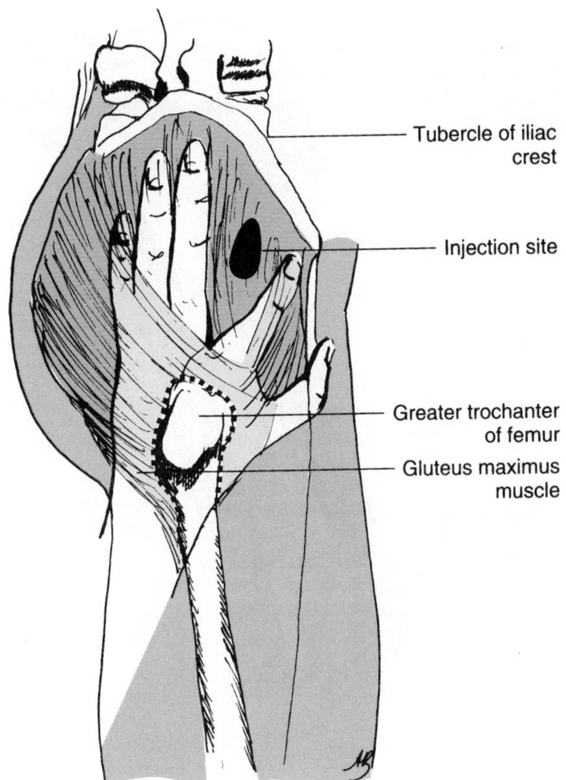

Ventrogluteal

1. Use this site if volume to be injected is 1–5 ml. Use 20–23 gauge, 1.25–2.5 in needle. Needle should be long enough to reach the middle of the muscle.
2. Preferred site for adults, children >7 mos. Patient should be in supine lateral position.
3. Using 90° angle, flatten the skin area using the middle and index finger and inject between them.

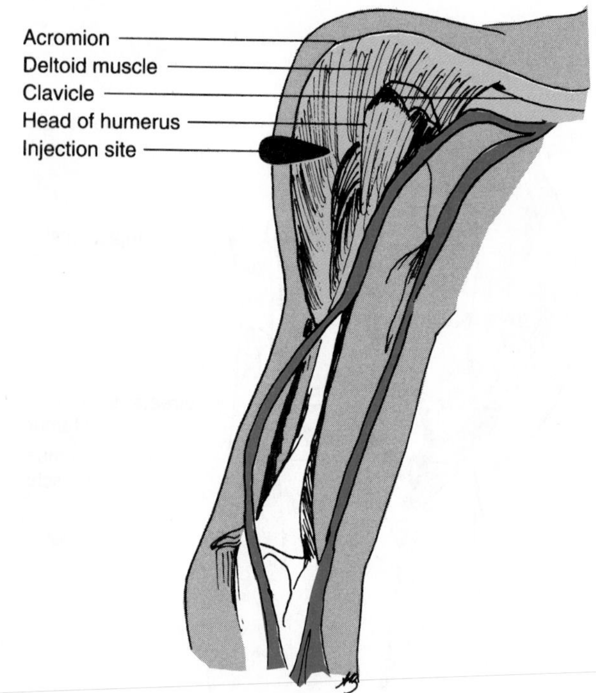

Deltoid

1. Use this site if volume to be injected is 0.5–1 ml. Use 23–25 gauge, $\frac{1}{8}$–1$\frac{1}{2}$ in needle. Needle should be long enough to reach the middle of the muscle.
2. Patient may be in prone, sitting, supine, or standing position.
3. Using 90° angle or angled slightly toward acromion, flatten the skin area using the thumb and index finger and inject between them.

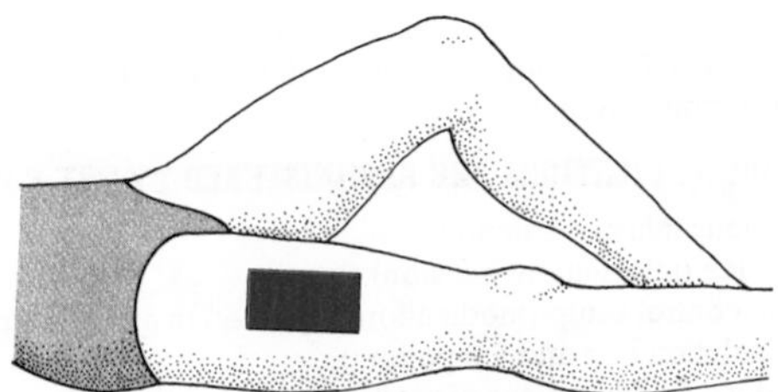

Anterolateral thigh

1. Anterolateral thigh is site of choice for infants and children <7 mos. Use 22–25 gauge, $\frac{5}{8}$–1 in needle.
2. Patient may be in supine or sitting position. Using 90° angle, flatten the skin area using the thumb and index finger and inject between them.

Z-Track Technique:

1. Draw up medication with one needle, and use new needle for injection *(minimizes skin staining)*.
2. Administer deep IM in upper outer quadrant of buttock only (dorsogluteal site).
3. Displace the skin lateral to the injection site before inserting the needle.
4. Withdraw the needle before releasing the skin.

IV:

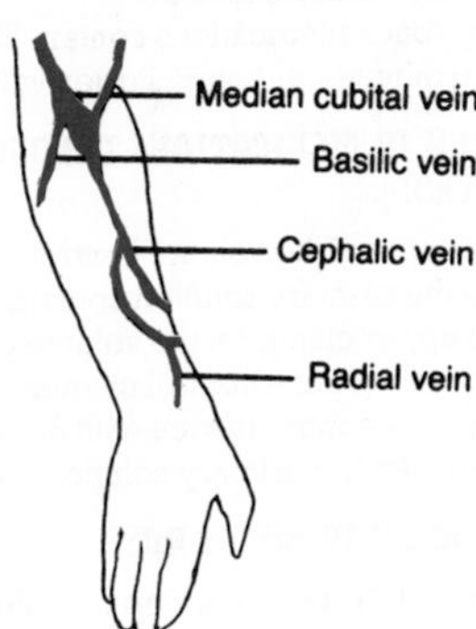

1. Medication may be given as direct IV, intermittent (piggyback), or continuous infusion.
2. Ensure that medication is compatible with solution being infused (see IV compatibility chart in this drug handbook).

3. Do not use if precipitate is present or discoloration occurs.
4. Check IV site frequently for correct infusion rate, evidence of infiltration, extravasation.

INTRAVENOUS MEDICATIONS ARE ADMINISTERED BY THE FOLLOWING:

1. Continuous infusing solution.
2. Piggyback (intermittent infusion).
3. Volume control setup (medication contained in a chamber between the IV solution bag and the patient).
4. Bolus dose (a single dose of medication given through an infusion line or heparin lock). Sometimes this is referred to as an IV push.

ADDING MEDICATION TO A NEWLY PRESCRIBED IV BAG:

1. Remove the plastic cover from the IV bag.
2. Cleanse rubber port with an alcohol swab.
3. Insert the needle into the center of the rubber port.
4. Inject the medication.
5. Withdraw the syringe from the port.
6. Gently rotate the container to mix the solution.
7. Label the IV including the date, time, medication, and dosage. It should be placed so it is easily read when hanging.
8. Spike the IV tubing and prime the tubing.

HANGING AN IV PIGGYBACK (IVPB):

1. When using the piggyback method, lower the primary bag at least 6 inches below the piggyback bag.
2. Set the pump as a secondary infusion when entering the rate of infusion and volume to be infused.
3. Most piggyback medications contain 50–100 cc and usually infuse in 20 to 60 minutes, although larger-volume bags will take longer.

ADMINISTERING IV MEDICATIONS THROUGH A VOLUME CONTROL SETUP (BURETROL):

1. Insert the spike of the volume control set (Buretrol, Soluset, Pediatrol) into the primary solution container.
2. Open the upper clamp on the volume control set and allow sufficient fluid into volume control chamber.
3. Fill the volume control device with 30 cc of fluid by opening the clamp between the primary solution and the volume control device.

ADMINISTERING AN IV BOLUS DOSE:

1. If an existing IV is infusing, stop the infusion by pinching the tubing above the port.
2. Insert the needle into the port and aspirate to observe for a blood return.
3. If the IV is infusing properly with no signs of infiltration or inflammation, it should be patent.
4. Blood indicates that the intravenous line is in the vein.
5. Inject the medication at the prescribed rate.
6. Remove the needle and regulate the IV as prescribed.

Appendix K
TREATMENT OF ARTHRITIS

Rheumatoid Arthritis (RA)

RA is an autoimmune disease of unknown etiology, characterized by chronic inflammation of the synovial tissues lining the joint capsule that may be accompanied by extra-articular involvement. These manifestations may include rheumatoid nodules, vasculitis, neuropathies, xerostomia, pleural effusions, and pericarditis.

MANAGEMENT:

Goals of treatment are:

- Relieve pain
- Inhibit disease progression
- Maintain activities of daily living
- Improve quality of life

Nonpharmacologic treatment:

- Physical and occupational therapy
- Weight loss
- Surgery for most severe cases

Pharmacologic treatment:

- Nonsteroidal anti-inflammatory drugs (NSAIDs)
- Corticosteroids
- Disease-modifying antirheumatic drugs (DMARDs)

Aspirin, traditional nonsteroidal anti-inflammatory drugs (NSAIDs), cyclooxygenase-2 (COX-2) inhibitors and corticosteroids provide symptomatic relief. These medications will reduce pain, stiffness, swelling, and tenderness and will improve mobility and strength, but they will not stop disease progression; gastrointestinal irritation limits their use.

Disease-modifying antirheumatic drugs (DMARDs) alter the course of RA, although they do not prevent bone erosion. The DMARDs are usually started after a clinical progression of inflammation is apparent and before irreversible mechanical damage becomes evident.

Among the newest therapies for RA are the biologic-response modifiers. These agents target TNF, which is thought to play a role in causing inflammation and joint damage.

Disease-Modifying Antirheumatic Drugs (DMARDs)

Generic Name	Brand Name	Dosage	Side Effects
auranofin	Ridaura	***PO:* Adults, elderly:** 6 mg/day in 1 or 2 divided doses. May increase to 9 mg/day (in 3 divided doses) if no response in 6 mos. If response still inadequate, discontinue.	Diarrhea, rash, pruritus, stomatitis, nausea, abdominal pain.
aurothioglucose	Solganal	***IM:* Adults, elderly:** Initially, 10 mg, then 25 mg for 2 doses, then 50 mg/wk thereafter until total dose of 0.8–1 g given. If pt improves and no signs of toxicity, give 50 mg at 3–4 wk intervals for many mos.	Diarrhea, rash, stomatitis, preteinuria, nausea, vomiting, anorexia, abdominal cramps.
azathioprine	Imuran	**Adults:** Initially, 1 mg/kg/day. May increase by 0.5 mg/kg/day after 6–8 wks at 4 wk intervals up to maximum dose of 2.5 mg/kg/day.	Nausea, vomiting, anorexia, rash.
cyclosporine	Neoral	**Adults:** 2.5 mg/kg/day in 2 divided doses.	Mild to moderate hypertension (26%), increased hair growth [hirsutism] (21%), tremor (12%), acne, cramping, gingival hyperplasia (bleeding, tender gums), paresthesia, diarrhea, nausea, vomiting, headache.
gold sodium thiomalate	Myochrysine	***IM:* Adults, elderly:** Initially, 10 mg, then 25 mg for second dose. Follow w/25 mg/wk until improvement noted or total of 1 g administered. **Maintenance:** 25–50 mg q2wks for 2–20 wks; if stable, may increase to q3–4wk intervals. **Children:** Initially, 10 mg, then 1 mg/kg/wk. **Maximum single dose:** 50 mg.	Diarrhea/loose stools, rash, pruritus, abdominal pain, nausea. **OCCASIONAL:** Vomiting, anorexia, flatulence, dyspepsia, conjunctivitis, photosensitivity.

Generic Name	Brand Name	Dosage	Side Effects
hydroxy-chloroquine	Plaquenil	**Adults:** Initially, 400–600 mg (310–465 mg base) daily for 5–10 days; gradually increase dose to optimum response level. Maintenance (usually within 4–12 wks). Decrease dose by 50%, continue at level of 200–400 mg/day. Maximum effect may not be seen for several months.	Mild transient headache, anorexia, nausea, vomiting. Visual disturbances (blurring and difficulty focusing); nervousness; fatigue; pruritus (esp. palms, soles, scalp); bleaching of hair; irritability, personality changes, diarrhea, skin eruptions
leflunomide	Arava	**Adults, elderly:** Initially, 100 mg/day for 3 days, then 10–20 mg/day.	Diarrhea, respiratory tract infection, hair loss, rash, nausea.
methotrexate	Rheumatrex	**Adults:** Initially, 7.5 mg/wk as single dose or 2.5 mg q12h in 3 doses. Adjust dose gradually to achieve optimal response, usually not >20 mg/wk. **Usual elderly dose:** Initially, 5 mg/wk as single or divided doses. May increase up to 7.5 mg/wk. **Maximum:** 20 mg/wk.	Nausea, vomiting, stomatitis. In psoriatic pts, burning, erythema at psoriatic site. Diarrhea, rash, dermatitis, pruritis, alopecia, dizziness, anorexia, malaise, headache, drowsiness, blurred vision.
penicillamine	Cuprimine, Depen	**Adults, elderly:** Initially, 125–250 mg/day. May increase by 125–250 mg/day at 1–3 mo intervals. **Maintenance:** 500–750 mg/day. After 2–3 mos w/no improvement or toxicity, may increase by 250 mg/day at 2–3 mo intervals until remission or toxicity. **Maximum:** 1 g up to 1.5 g/day.	Rash (pruritic, erythematous, maculopapular, morbilliform), reduced/altered sense of taste (hypogeusia), GI disturbances (anorexia, epigastric pain, nausea, vomiting, diarrhea), oral ulcers, glossitis. Proteinuria, hematuria, hot flashes, drug fever.
sulfasalazine	Azulfidine	**Adults, elderly:** Initially, 0.5–1 g/day for 1 wk. Increase by 0.5 g/wk up to 3 g/day.	Hypersensitivity reaction: rash, urticaria, pruritus, fever, anemia. Anorexia, nausea, vomiting, headache, oligospermia (generally reversed by withdrawal of drug).

Biologic-Response Modifiers

Generic Name	Brand Name	Dosage	Side Effects
etanercept	Enbrel	***SubQ:* Adults, elderly:** 25 mg 2 times/wk. **Children (4–17 yrs):** 0.4 mg/kg (**maximum:** 25 mg dose) 2 times/wk.	Injection site reaction (erythema, itching, pain, swelling). Incidence of abdominal pain. Vomiting is higher in children than in adults. Headache, rhinitis, dizziness, pharyngitis, cough, asthenia, abdominal pain, dyspepsia.
infliximab	Remicade	***IV:* Adults:** 3 mg/kg at wks 2 and 6, and q8wks therafter (in combination with methotrexate).	Headache, nausea, fatigue, fever. Fever/chills during infusion, pharyngitis, vomiting, pain, dizziness, bronchitis, rash, rhinitis, coughing, pruritus, sinusitis, myalgia, back pain.

Osteoarthritis

Osteoarthritis (OA) is a noninflammatory degenerative joint disease characterized by degeneration of articular cartilage, hypertrophy of bone at the margins, and changes in the synovial membrane. OA is the leading cause of disability in the United States. Diagnosis of OA is based upon signs and symptoms, history, and physical examination. The most common symptoms of OA are joint stiffness and pain; backache; increase in symptoms in cold, damp weather; limited movement and stiffness in affected joints. OA is most common in weight-bearing joints, hands, spine, toes, and fingers.

Drug therapy for OA includes acetaminophen as first-line therapy, aspirin, traditional NSAIDs, COX-2 inhibitors, topical therapy, and various adjunct treatment.

NSAIDs:

Diclofenac (Cataflam, Voltaren)
Ibuprofen (Motrin, Advil)
Ketoprofen (Orudis)
Nabumetone (Relafen)
Naproxen/naproxen sodium (Anaprox, Naprosyn)
Sulindac (Clinoril)

COX-2 INHIBITORS:

Celecoxib (Celebrex)
Rofecoxib (Vioxx)

ALTERNATIVE THERAPY:

Capsaicin (Zostrix)
Glucosamine and chondroitin
Sodium hyaluronate (Synvisc)

INDEX

Generic names appear in lower case boldface type. U.S. trade names are in regular type, Canadian trade names appear in capital letters, and classifications are in lower case italics.

New Drug Supplement

abacavir
Abreva (see docosanol)
Aceon (see perindopril)
Aciphex (see rabeprazole)
Acova (see argatroban)
Acthrel (see corticorelin)
Actos (see pioglitazone)
adapalene
Agenerase (see amprenavir)
Alamast (see pemirolast)
albendazole
Albenza (see albendazole)
Aldara (see imiquimod)
alitretinoin
Alphagan (see brimonidine)
amprenavir
Angiomax (see bivalirudin)
apraclonidine
argatroban
Aromasin (see exemestane)
Astelin
Avandia (see rosiglitazone)
Avelox (see moxifloxacin)
azelastine
balsalazide
bexarotene
bivalirudin
brimonidine
butenafine
cabergoline
Cerezyme (see imiglucerase)
cetrorelix
Cetrotide (see cetrorelix)
cevimeline
Colazzal (see balsalazide)
colesevelam
Comtan (see entacapone)
Condylox (see podofilox)
corticorelin
Curosurf (see poractant)
Cystagon (see cysteamine bitartrate)
cysteamine bitartrate
Dermatop (see prednicarbate)
dexmedetomidine
Differin (see adapalene)
docosanol
doftilide
dorzolamide
Dostinex (see cabergoline)
Elmiron (see pentosan)
entacapone
eptifibatide
Evoxac (see cevimeline)
Exelon (see rivastigmine)
exemestane
Fareston (see toremifene)
Femara (see letrozole)
Ferrlecit (see sodium ferric gluconate)
gatifloxacin
Geref (see sermorelin)

Havrix (see hepatitis A vaccine)
hepatitis A vaccine
Herceptin (see trastuzumab)
imiglucerase
imiquimod
Innohep (see tinzaparin)
Integrilin (see eptifibatide)
Iopidine (see apraclonidine)
ivermectin
Kaletra (see lopinavir/ritonavir)
Keppra (see levetiracetam)
ketotifen
letrozole
levetiracetam
linezolid
lopinavir/ritonavir
meloxicam
Mentax (see butenafine)
Mifeprex (see mifepristone)
mifepristone
Mobic (see meloxicam)
moxifloxacin
nateglinide
oseltamivir
oxcarbazepine
Panretin (see alitretinoin)
pantoprazole
pemirolast
pentosan
perindopril
pioglitazone
podofilox
poractant
Precedex (see dexmedetomidine)
prednicarbate
Protonix (see pantoprazole)
rabeprazole
Rapamune (see sirolimus)
Relenza (see zanamivir)
Renagel (see sevelamer)
Rescula (see unoprostone)
Respigam (see respiratory syncytial immune globulin)
respiratory syncytial immune globulin
Rho(d) immune globulin IV (human)
Rituxan (see rituximab)
rituximab
rivastigmine
rofecoxib
rosiglitazone
sacrosidase
Sclerosol (see talc)
scopolamine
sermorelin
sevelamer
sirolimus
sodium ferric gluconate
Sonata (see zaleplon)
Starlix (see nateglinide)
Stromectol (see ivermectin)
Sucraid (see sacrosidase)

abacavir

ah-bah-**kay**-veer
(Ziagen)

CLASSIFICATION

Antiviral

AVAILABILITY (Rx)

Tablets: 300 mg. **Oral Solution:** 20 mg/ml.

ACTION/*THERAPEUTIC EFFECT*

Inhibits HIV reverse transcriptase via viral DNA chain termination. Also inhibits RNA and DNA-dependent DNA polymerase, an enzyme necessary for viral HIV replication, *slowing HIV replication and reducing progression of HIV infection.*

USES

Treatment of HIV infection in adults and children >3 mos.

INDICATIONS/DOSAGE/ROUTES

HIV infection:
Oral: Adults: 300 mg 2 times/day. ***Children (3 mos–16 yrs):*** 8 mg/kg twice daily. ***Maximum:***.300 mg twice daily.

SIDE EFFECTS

OCCASIONAL: Hypersensitivity reaction (fever, GI symptoms, malaise, rash). **RARE:** Hypotension, respiratory distress.

adapalene

ah-**dap**-ah-leen
(Differin)

CLASSIFICATION

Antiacne

AVAILABILITY (Rx)

Gel: 0.1%

ACTION/*THERAPEUTIC EFFECT*

Binds to retinoic acid receptors in cell nuclei modulating cell differentiation, keratinization. Possesses anti-inflammatory, comedolytic properties. *Normalizes differentiation of follicular epithelial cells, reduces microcomedome formation.*

USES

Topical treatment of acne vulgaris.

INDICATIONS/DOSAGE/ROUTES

Acne vulgaris:
Topical: Adults, children >12 yrs: Apply to affected area once daily at bedtime after washing.

SIDE EFFECTS

FREQUENT (10–40%): Erythema, scaling, dryness, pruritus, burning. **OCCASIONAL (1–5%):** Skin irritation, stinging, sunburn, acne flares.

albendazole

all-**ben**-dah-zole
(Albenza)

CLASSIFICATION

Anthelmintic

AVAILABILITY (Rx)

Tablets: 200 mg

ACTION/*THERAPEUTIC EFFECT*

Vermicidal. Degrades parasite cytoplasmic microtubules, irreversibly blocks cholinesterase secretion, glucose uptake in helminth and larvae (depletes glycogen, decreases ATP production, depletes energy). *Immobilizes and kills worms.*

USES

Treatment of parenchymal neurocysticercosis caused by active lesions caused by larval forms of pork tapeworm, *Taenia solium.* Treatment of cystic hydatid disease of liver, lung, and peritoneum caused by larval form of dog tapeworm, *Echinococcus granulosus.*

INDICATIONS/DOSAGE/ROUTES

Neurocysticercosis:
Oral: Adults, elderly, >60 kg: 400 mg 2 times/day; ***<60 kg:*** 15 mg/kg/day. Continue for 28 days, rest 14 days, repeat cycle 3 times.

Cystic hydatid:
Oral: Adults, elderly, >60 kg: 400 mg 2 times/day; ***<60 kg:*** 15 mg/kg/day. Continue for 8–30 days.

SIDE EFFECTS

FREQUENT (3–10%): *Neurocysticercosis:* Nausea, vomiting, headache. *Hydatid:* Abnormal liver function tests, abdominal pain, nausea, vomiting. **OCCASIONAL (1–3%):** *Neurocysticercosis:* Increased intracranial pressure, meningeal signs. *Hydatid:* Headache, dizziness, alopecia, fever.

alitretinoin

al-**lee**-tret-ih-nown
(Panretin)

CLASSIFICATION

Antineoplastic: retinoid

AVAILABILITY (Rx)

Gel: 0.1%

ACTION/*THERAPEUTIC EFFECT*

Binds to and activates all known retinoid receptors. Once activated, receptors act as transcription factors, regulating expression of genes that control cellular differentiation, proliferation. *Inhibits growth of Kaposi's sarcoma cells.*

USES/*UNLABELED*

Topical treatment of cutaneous lesions in pts with AIDS-related Kaposi's sarcoma. *Breast, cervical, ovarian, prostatic carcinomas, myelodysplastic syndrome, psoriasis.*

INDICATIONS/DOSAGE/ROUTES

Kaposi's sarcoma:
Topical: Adults: Initially, apply 2 times/day to lesions. May increase to 3–4 times/day. Allow gel to dry 3–5 min before covering with clothing.

SIDE EFFECTS

FREQUENT (>5%): Rash (erythema, scaling, irritation, redness, dermatitis), burning pain, itching, exfoliative dermatitis (flaking, peeling, desquamation, exfoliation), stinging, tingling, swelling, inflammation.

amprenavir

am-**prenn**-ah-veer
(Agenerase)

CLASSIFICATION

Antiviral: protease inhibitor

AVAILABILITY (Rx)

Capsules: 50 mg, 150 mg. **Oral Solution:** 15 mg/ml.

ACTION/*THERAPEUTIC EFFECT*

Inhibits HIV-1 protease by binding to active site of HIV-1 protease. Prevents processing of viral precursors. *Forms immature noninfectious viral particles. Impairs HIV viral replication and proliferation.*

USES

Treatment of HIV-1 infection in combination with other antiretroviral agents.

INDICATIONS/DOSAGE/ROUTES

HIV-1 infection:
Oral: Adults, children 13–16 yrs: Capsules: 1,200 mg 2 times/day. ***Children 4–12 yrs, 13–16 yrs <50 kg:*** 20 mg/kg 2 times/day or 15 mg/kg 3 times/day. ***Maximum:*** 2,400 mg/day. ***Oral Solution: Children 4–12 yrs, 13–16 yrs <50 kg:*** 22.5 mg/day (1.5 ml/kg) 2 times/day or 17 mg/kg (1.1 ml/kg) 3 times/day. ***Maximum:*** 2,800 mg/day.

SIDE EFFECTS

FREQUENT: Nausea (73%), vomiting (29%), diarrhea (33%), oral paresthesia (26%), depression (15%), rash (25%). **OCCASIONAL (5–10%):** Paresthesia (peripheral), taste disorders.

---

apraclonidine

aye-prah-**clon**-ih-deen
(Iopidine)

CLASSIFICATION

Antiglaucoma

AVAILABILITY (Rx)

Ophthalmic Solution: 0.5%, 1%

ACTION/*THERAPEUTIC EFFECT*

Stimulates alpha-adrenergic system reducing formation of aqueous humor. *Reduces elevated intraocular pressure (IOP).*

USES

At 0.5% strength: Short-term adjunctive therapy in glaucoma to decrease IOP. *At 1%:* Controls/prevents postsurgical increased IOP following trabeculoplasty or iridotomy.

INDICATIONS/DOSAGE/ROUTES

Glaucoma:
Ophthalmic: Adults, elderly: 1–2 drops 3 times/day.

SIDE EFFECTS

FREQUENT (4–13%): Hyperemia, pruritus, tearing, lid edema, foreign body sensation, blurred vision, dry eye. **OCCASIONAL (1–3%):** Dry mouth, asthenia, headache, dry nose, altered taste.

---

argatroban

our-ga-**trow**-ban
(Acova)

CLASSIFICATION

Anticoagulant

AVAILABILITY (Rx)

Injection: 100 mg/ml

ACTION/*THERAPEUTIC EFFECT*

A direct thrombin inhibitor that reversibly binds to thrombin active site. Exerts its effect by inhibiting thrombin catalyzed or induced reactions, *producing anticoagulation.*

USES

Prophylaxis or treatment of thrombosis in heparin-induced thrombocytopenia (HIT).

INDICATIONS/DOSAGE/ROUTES

HIT:
IV Infusion: Adults, elderly: Initially, 2 mcg/kg/min administered as continuous infusion. ***Liver impairment:*** Initially, 0.5 mcg/kg/min. After initial dose, may be adjusted until steady-state APTT is 1.5–3 times initial baseline value, not to exceed 100 sec.

SIDE EFFECTS

FREQUENT (3–8%): Dyspnea, hypotension, fever, diarrhea, nausea, ventricular tachycardia, pain, vomiting, infection, atrial fibrillation. OCCASIONAL (1–3%): Cough, abdominal pain, cerebrovascular disorder.

azelastine

aye-zeh-**las**-teen
(Astelin)

CLASSIFICATION

Antihistamine

AVAILABILITY (Rx)

Nasal Spray

ACTION/*THERAPEUTIC EFFECT*

Prevents activation of basophils, mast cells, eosinophils, macrophages, and monocytes; blocks synthesis, release, or target receptors of several mediators of immediate inflammatory response (e.g., histamine); regulates late-phase allergic responses by inhibition of leukotriene-mediated and T-cell responses. *Relieves rhinitis.*

USES

Treatment of symptoms of seasonal allergic rhinitis (e.g., rhinorrhea, sneezing, nasal pruritus).

INDICATIONS/DOSAGE/ROUTES

Seasonal allergic rhinitis:
Intranasal: Adults, elderly, children >12 yrs: 1–2 sprays to each nostril 2 times/day.

SIDE EFFECTS

FREQUENT: Headache (20%), bitter taste (15%), somnolence (11.5%). OCCASIONAL: Nasal burning, pharyngitis, dry mouth, paroxysmal sneezing, nausea, rhinitis, fatigue, dizziness, epistaxis.

balsalazide

ball-**sall**-ah-zide
(Colazal)

CLASSIFICATION

GI anti-inflammatory agent

AVAILABILITY (Rx)

Capsules: 750 mg

ACTION/*THERAPEUTIC EFFECT*

Must be converted to 5-aminosalicylic acid to be effective. Action may include changes in intestinal microflora, altered prostaglandin production, inhibition of function of natural killer cells, mast cells, neutrophils, macrophages, *diminishing inflammatory effect in colon.*

USES

Treatment of ulcerative colitis.

INDICATIONS/DOSAGE/ROUTES

Ulcerative colitis:
Oral: Adults, elderly: 2.25 g 3 times/day.

SIDE EFFECTS

OCCASIONAL: Nausea, headache, diarrhea, abdominal pain, flatus, constipation.

bexarotene

becks-**aye**-row-teen
(Targretin)

CLASSIFICATION

Antineoplastic

AVAILABILITY (Rx)

Capsules. Soft gelatin: 75 mg.

ACTION/*THERAPEUTIC EFFECT*

A selective agonist at retinoid X receptors, which are involved in process of apoptosis (natural process in which body rids itself of unwanted cells). *Shown to inhibit some tumor cell lines of hematopoietic and squamous cell origin.*

USES/*UNLABELED*

Treatment of cutaneous T-cell lymphoma (CTCL) in pts refractory to at least one prior systemic therapy. *Treatment of diabetes mellitus, head, neck, lung, renal cell carcinomas, Kaposi's sarcoma.*

INDICATIONS/DOSAGE/ROUTES

CTCL:
Oral: Adults: 300 mg/m²/day. If no response and initial dose well tolerated, may increase to 400 mg/m²/day.

SIDE EFFECTS

FREQUENT: Lipid abnormalities (79%), hypothyroidism (29%), leukopenia (17%). **OCCASIONAL (<10%):** Diarrhea, fatigue, headache, abnormal liver function tests, rash, itching, pancreatitis.

bivalirudin

bye-val-ih-**rue**-din
(Angiomax)

CLASSIFICATION

Reversible direct thrombin inhibitor. Anticoagulant.

AVAILABILITY (Rx)

Injection: 250 mg vials.

ACTION/*THERAPEUTIC EFFECT*

Directly inhibits thrombin by specifically binding both to the catalytic site and to the anion-binding exosite of circulating and clot-bound thrombin. Thrombin plays central role in thrombotic process, acting to cleave fibrinogen into fibrin monomers and to activate factors XIII, V, and VIII, promoting further thrombin generation. Activates platelets, stimulating aggregation. *Produces immediate anticoagulant effect, w/coagulation times returning to baseline approximately 1 hr following cessation of bivalirudin administration.*

USES

Anticoagulant in pts w/unstable angina undergoing percutaneous transluminal coronary angioplasty (PTCA) in combination w/aspirin.

INDICATIONS/DOSAGE/ROUTES

IV: Adults, elderly: IV bolus 1 mg/kg followed by IV infusion of 2.5 mg/kg/hr over 4 hrs. An additional IV infusion may be initiated at 0.2 mg/kg/hr up to 20 hrs, if needed. Bivalirudin intended for use w/aspirin (300–325 mg daily).

SIDE EFFECTS

FREQUENT (>10%): Back pain, nausea, headache, hypotension. **OCCASIONAL (5–10%):** Hypertension, bradycardia, vomiting, dyspepsia, injection site pain, insomnia, pelvic pain, anxiety, major hemorrhage (3.7%), abdominal pain, fever, nervousness. **RARE (<1%):** Fever, infection, sepsis, syncope, ventricular fibrillation, cerebral ischemia, confusion, facial paralysis, lung edema, kidney failure, oliguria.

brimonidine

bri-**moe**-nih-deen
(Alphagan)

CLASSIFICATION

Antiglaucoma

AVAILABILITY (Rx)

Ophthalmic Solution: 0.2%

ACTION/*THERAPEUTIC EFFECT*

Alpha-2 adrenergic agonist that reduces aqueous humor and increases uveoscleral outflow. *Reduces intraocular pressure (IOP).*

USES

Lowers IOP in pts w/open-angle glaucoma or ocular hypertension.

INDICATIONS/DOSAGE/ROUTES

Usual ophthalmic dosage:
Ophthalmic: Adults, elderly: 1 drop to affected eye(s) 3 times/day (approximately 8 hrs apart).

SIDE EFFECTS

FREQUENT (10–30%): Oral dryness, ocular hyperemia, burning, stinging, headache, fatigue, foreign body sensation, ocular pruritus/allergic reaction. **OCCASIONAL (3–9%):** Corneal staining, photophobia, eyelid erythema, ocular pain/dryness, tearing, eyelid edema, dizziness, asthenia, conjunctival blanching, muscular pain, abnormal vision. **RARE (1–3%):** Lid crusting, conjunctival hemorrhage/discharge, nasal dryness, abnormal taste.

butenafine

beu-**ten**-ah-feen
(Mentax)

CLASSIFICATION

Antifungal: topical

AVAILABILITY (Rx)

Cream: 1%

ACTION/*THERAPEUTIC EFFECT*

Inhibits epoxidation of squalene, blocking biosynthesis of ergosterol, essential for fungal cell membranes. Fungicidal. *Relieves athlete's foot.*

USES

Treatment of interdigital tinea pedis (athlete's foot) due to *E. Floccosum, T. Mentagrophytes,* or *T. Rubrum.*

INDICATIONS/DOSAGE/ROUTES

Tinea pedis:
Topical: Adults, elderly, children >12 yrs: Apply to affected area and immediately surrounding skin daily for 4 wks.

SIDE EFFECTS

OCCASIONAL (2%): Contact dermatitis, burning/stinging, worsening of the condition. **RARE (<2%):** Erythema, irritation, itching.

cabergoline

cab-**err**-go-leen
(Dostinex)

CLASSIFICATION

Antihyperprolactemic

AVAILABILITY (Rx)

Tablets: 0.5 mg

ACTION / *THERAPEUTIC EFFECT*

Agonist at dopamine D2 receptors suppressing prolactin secretion. *Shrinks prolactinomas, restores gonadal function.*

USES

Treatment of hyperprolactemic disorders, either idiopathic or due to pituitary adenomas.

INDICATIONS/DOSAGE/ROUTES

Hyperprolactemia:
Oral: Adults, elderly: 0.5 mg 2 times/week.

SIDE EFFECTS

FREQUENT: Nausea (29%). **OCCASIONAL (5–20%):** Headache, vomiting, vertigo, dizziness, dyspepsia, orthostatic hypotension, constipation.

cetrorelix

see-tro-**ree**-licks
(Cetrotide)

CLASSIFICATION

Sex hormone

AVAILABILITY (Rx)

Injection: 0.25 mg, 3 mg vials.

ACTION / *THERAPEUTIC EFFECT*

A peptide with gonadotropin-releasing hormone (GnRH) antagonistic activity. GnRH induces production and release of LH and FSH from pituitary. Cetrorelix competes with natural GnRH for binding to membrane receptors on pituitary cells, thus *controling release of LH, FSH.*

USES

Inhibition of premature luteinizing hormone (LH) surges in women undergoing controlled ovarian stimulation for treatment of infertility.

INDICATIONS/DOSAGE/ROUTES

Infertility:
SubQ: Adults: Single-dose regimen: 3 mg when serum estradiol level indicates appropriate stimulation, usually day 7. If human chorionic gonadotropin (hCG) has not been given within 4 days after the 3 mg injection, then give 0.25 mg once daily until day of hCG administration. *Multiple-dose regimen:* 0.25 mg day 5 (morning or evening) or day 6 (morning) and continued daily until day of hCG administration.

SIDE EFFECTS

OCCASIONAL: Moderate or severe ovarian stimulation (3.5%). **RARE (<2%):** Nausea, headache, local site reactions (e.g., redness, erythema, bruising, itching, swelling, pruritus).

cevimeline

sev-ee-**me**-line
(Evoxac)

CLASSIFICATION

Cholinergic agonist

AVAILABILITY (Rx)

Capsules: 30 mg.

ACTION/*THERAPEUTIC EFFECT*

Binds to muscarinic receptors, *increasing secretion of exocrine glands (e.g., salivary glands).*

USES

Treatment of dry mouth symptoms in pts w/Sjogren's syndrome.
Note: Contraindicated in pts w/uncontrolled asthma, acute iritis, narrow-angle glaucoma.

INDICATIONS/DOSAGE/ROUTES

Dry mouth:
Oral: Adults: 30 mg 3 times/day.

SIDE EFFECTS

FREQUENT (10–20%): Excessive sweating, headache, nausea, rhinitis, upper respiratory tract infections, diarrhea, sinusitis. **OCCASIONAL (3–10%):** Dyspepsia, abdominal pain, coughing, urinary tract infection, vomiting, back pain, rash, dizziness, fatigue.

colesevelam

ko-leh-**sev**-eh-lam
(Welchol)

CLASSIFICATION

Bile acid sequestrant; anti-hyperlipidemic agent

AVAILABILITY (Rx)

Tablets: 625 mg.

ACTION/*THERAPEUTIC EFFECT*

A nonsystemic polymer that binds with bile acids in the intestine, preventing their reabsorption and removing them from the body, thereby *decreasing LDL cholesterol.*

USES

Adjunctive therapy to diet and exercise used either alone or in combination w/an HMG-CoA reductase inhibitor (e.g., simvastatin) to decrease elevated LDL cholesterol in pts w/primary hypercholesterolemia (Fredrickson type IIa). **Note:** Do not use in pts w/bowel obstruction.

INDICATIONS/DOSAGE/ROUTES

Cholesterol lowering:
Oral: Adults, elderly: 3 tablets w/meals 2 times/day or 6 tablets once daily w/meal. May increase daily dose to 7 tablets/day.

SIDE EFFECTS

FREQUENT (8–12%): Flatulence, constipation, infection, dyspepsia.

corticorelin

core-tih-co-**ree**-lynn
(Acthrel)

CLASSIFICATION

Diagnostic aid

AVAILABILITY (Rx)

Injection: 100 mcg lyophylized cake

ACTION/*THERAPEUTIC EFFECT*

Unknown.

USES

Differentiates pituitary and ectopic production of adrenocorticotropin hormone (ACTH) in patients w/ACTH-dependent Cushing's syndrome.

INDICATIONS/DOSAGE/ROUTES

Differential Dx Cushing syndrome:
IV Infusion: Adults: 1 mcg/kg over 30–60 seconds.

SIDE EFFECTS

OCCASIONAL (16%): Flushing of face, neck, upper chest.

cysteamine bitartrate

sis-**tea**-ah-mean
(Cystagon)

CLASSIFICATION

Urinary tract: Cystine depletor

AVAILABILITY (RX)

Capsules: 50 mg, 150 mg

ACTION/*THERAPEUTIC EFFECT*

Cystine-depleting agent, *lowering cystine content of cells in pts w/cystinosis (an autosomal recessive inborn error of metabolism:* abnormal transport of cystine out of lysosomes). Nephropathic form (accumulation of cystine, crystal formation) may lead to organ damage (esp. kidney, producing end stage renal failure).

USES

Management of nephropathic cystinosis in adults and children.

INDICATIONS/DOSAGE/ROUTES

Nephropathic cystinosis:
Oral: Adults, elderly, children: Initially: maintenance dose gradually increased over 4–6 wks. ***Maintenance: Adults, children >12 yrs, >49.5 kg:*** 2 g/day in 4 divided doses. ***Children (up to 12 yrs):*** 1.3 g/m^2/day given in 4 divided doses. **Note:** Do not give intact capsule to children 6 yrs or less. Sprinkle capsule over food.

SIDE EFFECTS

FREQUENT (5–35%): Vomiting, anorexia, fever, diarrhea, lethargy, rash. **OCCASIONAL (1–5%):** Nausea, abdominal pain, dyspepsia, ataxia, confusion, dizziness, nervousness.

dexmedetomidine

decks-mead-eh-**tome**-ih-deen
(Precedex)

CLASSIFICATION

Sedative

AVAILABILITY (Rx)

Injection: 100 mcg/ml

ACTION/*THERAPEUTIC EFFECT*

Selective alpha-2 adrenoceptor agonist.

USES

Sedation of initially intubated and mechanically ventilated adults during treatment in intensive care setting.

INDICATIONS/DOSAGE/ROUTES

Sedation:
IV Infusion: Adults: Loading dose

of 1 mcg/kg over 10 min followed by maintenance dose of 0.2–0.7 mcg/kg/hr. Can be continuously infused in mechanically ventilated pt before, during, and after extubation. **Note:** Must be diluted w/0.9% NaCl.

SIDE EFFECTS

FREQUENT: Hypotension (30%), nausea (11%). **OCCASIONAL (<10%):** Bradycardia, atrial fibrillation, hypoxia, anemia, pain, pleural effusion, pulmonary edema, leukocytosis.

docosanol

dough-**coe**-san-all
(Abreva)

CLASSIFICATION

Antiviral

AVAILABILITY (OTC)

Cream: 10%.

ACTION/*THERAPEUTIC EFFECT*

Interferes with one or more of the common pathways for viral entry into target cell and subsequent migration to cell nucleus. Inhibits fusion between plasma membrane and herpes simplex virus (HSV) envelope, *reducing duration of symptoms attributed to cold sores, fever blisters.*

USES

Treatment of cold sores or fever blisters due to either herpes simplex virus type 1 or type 2.

INDICATIONS/DOSAGE/ROUTES

Cold sores, fever blisters:
Topical: Adults, elderly: Apply to lesions 5 times/day beginning at the onset of symptoms, continuing until lesions are healed, up to a maximum of 10 days.

SIDE EFFECTS

OCCASIONAL: Headache, skin irritation.

doftilide

doe-**fet**-ill-ide
(Tikosyn)

CLASSIFICATION

Antiarrhythmic: Class III

AVAILABILITY (Rx)

Capsules: 125 mcg, 250 mcg, 500 mcg

ACTION/*THERAPEUTIC EFFECT*

A selective potassium-channel blocker; prolongs repolarization without affecting conduction velocity by blocking one or more time-dependent potassium currents. No effect on sodium channels, adrenergic alpha, beta receptors. *Terminates re-entrant tachyarrhythmias, preventing reinduction.*

USES

Maintenance and conversion of normal sinus rhythm (NSR) in pts with highly symptomatic atrial fibrillation/atrial flutter.

INDICATIONS/DOSAGE/ROUTES

Anti-arrhythmias:
Oral: Adults, elderly: Individualized using a 7-step dosing algorithm dependent upon calculated creatinine clearance and QT measurements.

SIDE EFFECTS

OCCASIONAL (<5%): Increased flatulence, loose stools, mild headaches, ventricular tachycardia, most notably torsade de pointes.

dorzolamide

door-**zoll**-ah-mide
(Trusopt)

CLASSIFICATION

Carbonic anhydrase inhibitor

AVAILABILITY (Rx)

Ophthalmic Solution: 2%

ACTION/*THERAPEUTIC EFFECT*

Inhibits carbonic anhydrase in ciliary processes of eye, decreasing secretion of aqueous humor. Exact mechanism unknown. May slow formation of bicarbonate ions, reducing sodium and fluid transport. *Decreases intraocular pressure (IOP).*

USES

Treatment of elevated IOP in pts with ocular hypertension or open-angle glaucoma.

INDICATIONS/DOSAGE/ROUTES

Reduction of IOP:
Ophthalmic: Adults, elderly: 1 drop in affected eye 3 times/day.

SIDE EFFECTS

FREQUENT (10–33%): Ocular burning, stinging, discomfort immediately after administration; bitter taste; superficial punctate keratitis; ocular allergic reactions. OCCASIONAL (10%): Blurred vision, tearing, dryness, photophobia, headache, nausea, asthenia/fatigue.

entacapone

en-tah-cah-**pone**
(Comtan)

CLASSIFICATION

Anti-Parkinson agent

AVAILABILITY (Rx)

Tablets: 200 mg

ACTION/*THERAPEUTIC EFFECT*

Inhibits enzyme COMT, potentiating dopamine activity. *Increases duration of action of levodopa doses,* decreasing daily levodopa requirements.

USES

In conjunction with levodopa, improves quality of life in pts with Parkinson's disease.

INDICATIONS/DOSAGE/ROUTES

Parkinson's disease:
Oral: Adults, elderly: 200 mg w/each dose of levodopa/carbidopa. *Maximum:* 8 times/day or 1,600 mg/day.

SIDE EFFECTS

FREQUENT: Dyskinesia, hyperkinesia, nausea, urine discoloration (dark yellow or orange), diarrhea, abdominal pain, vomiting, dizziness, orthostatic hypotension, falls, shortness of breath, ataxia, fatigue, constipation, hallucinations.

eptifibatide

ep-tih-**fye**-bah-tide
(Integrilin)

CLASSIFICATION

Antiplatelet, antithrombotic

AVAILABILITY (Rx)

Injection: 0.75 mg/ml, 2 mg/ml

ACTION/*THERAPEUTIC EFFECT*

Produces rapid inhibition of platelet aggregation by preventing binding of fibrinogen to receptor sites on platelets. *Prevents closure of treated coronary arteries. Prevents acute cardiac ischemic complications.*

USES

Treatment of pts w/acute coronary syndrome (ACS), including those managed medically and those undergoing percutaneous coronary intervention (PCI).

INDICATIONS/DOSAGE/ROUTES

Adjunct PCI:
IV Bolus/IV Infusion: Adults, elderly: 135 mcg/kg bolus over 1–2 min, then infusion of 0.5 mcg/kg/min for 20–24 hrs.

ACS:
IV Bolus/IV Infusion: Adults, elderly: 180 mcg/kg bolus then 2 mcg/kg/min until discharge or CABG, up to 72 hrs.

SIDE EFFECTS

FREQUENT (>5%): Bleeding, GI bleeding, hematuria, hematemesis. **OCCASIONAL (1–5%):** Hypotension. **RARE (<1%):** Stroke, anaphylactic shock.

---

exemestane

x-eh-**mess**-tane
(Aromasin)

CLASSIFICATION

Antineoplastic: Hormone

AVAILABILITY (Rx)

Tablets: 25 mg

ACTION/*THERAPEUTIC EFFECT*

An irreversible, steroidal aromatase inactivator (aromatase is the principal enzyme that converts androgens to estrogens in both pre-and postmenopausal women); acts as false substrate for aromatase enzyme; binds irreversibly to active site of enzyme, causing its inactivation. *Significantly lowers circulating estrogen concentration in postmenopausal women.*

USES/*UNLABELED*

Treatment of advanced breast cancer in postmenopausal women whose disease has progressed following tamoxifen therapy. *Prevention of prostate cancer.*

INDICATIONS/DOSAGE/ROUTES

Breast cancer:
Oral: Adults, elderly: 25 mg once daily after a meal.

SIDE EFFECTS

FREQUENT (10–25%): Depression, insomnia, anxiety, nausea, dyspnea, fatigue, hot flashes, pain. **OCCASIONAL (2–10%):** Headache, dizziness, vomiting, constipation, anorexia, diarrhea, increased appetite, cough, edema, flulike symptoms, fever, weakness, confusion, arthralgia, pain (abdominal, back, skeletal), infection, dyspepsia, pharyngitis, rhinitis, alopecia.

---

gatifloxacin

gat-ih-flocks-ah-sin
(Tequin)

CLASSIFICATION

Anti-infective: Quinolone

AVAILABILITY (Rx)

Tablets: 200 mg, 400 mg. **Injection:** 200 mg, 400 mg vials.

ACTION/*THERAPEUTIC EFFECT*

Inhibits DNA enzyme in susceptible micro-organisms, *interfering with bacterial DNA replication.* Bactericidal.

USES

Treatment of community-acquired pneumonia (CAP), sinusitis, acute bacterial exacerbation of chronic bronchitis, urinary tract infections (UTI), gonorrhea.

INDICATIONS/DOSAGE/ROUTES

CAP:
Oral/IV: Adults, elderly: 400 mg/day for 7–14 days.

Acute bacterial exacerbation of chronic bronchitis:
Oral/IV: Adults, elderly: 400 mg/day for 7–10 days.

Sinusitis:
Oral/IV: Adults, elderly: 400 mg/day for 10 days.

UTI:
Oral/IV: Adults, elderly: 200 mg 2 times/day for 7 days.

Gonorrhea:
Oral: Adults: 400 mg as single dose.

SIDE EFFECTS

FREQUENT (5–10%): Nausea. OCCASIONAL (1–5%): Diarrhea, headache, dizziness, vaginitis.

hepatitis A vaccine

(Havrix, Vaqta)

USES

Active immunization of persons >2yrs against disease caused by hepatitis A virus.

DOSAGE

IM: Adults (>18 yrs): Havrix: 1440 ELU, Vaqta: 50 U. ***Children (2–18 yrs):*** Havrix: 720 ELU, Vaqta: 25 U. Booster shot varies from 6 to 18 months (provides persistent antibody concentration).

CONTRAINDICATIONS

Hypersensitivity to any component of the vaccine.

SIDE EFFECTS

OCCASIONAL (1–10%): Injection site soreness, pain, tenderness, induration, redness, swelling, fatigue, fever, malaise, nausea, anorexia, headache.

imiglucerase

im-ih-**gloo**-sir-ace
(Cerezyme)

CLASSIFICATION

Enzyme

AVAILABILITY (Rx)

Powder for Injection: 200 units

ACTION/*THERAPEUTIC EFFECT*

Analogue of enzyme beta-glucocerebrosidase, which catalyzes hydrolysis of glycolipid glucocerebroside to glucose and ceramide. *Minimizes conditions (e.g., anemia, bone disease) associated w/Gaucher's disease.*

USES

Treatment of Gaucher's disease

(characterized by deficiency of beta-glucocerebrosidase activity) results in accumulation of glucocerebrosidase in tissue macrophages becoming engorged. Secondary hematologic sequelae include severe anemia, thrombocytopenia, progressive hepatosplenomegaly, skeletal complications.

INDICATIONS/DOSAGE/ROUTES

Gaucher's disease:
IV Infusion (over 1–2 hrs): ***Adults, elderly, children:*** Initially, 2.5 units/kg 3 times/wk up to 60 units/kg/wk. ***Maintenance:*** Progressive reduction in dosage while monitoring pt response.

SIDE EFFECTS

FREQUENT (3%): Headache. **OCCASIONAL (1–3%):** Nausea, abdominal discomfort, dizziness, pruritus, rash, small decrease in B/P or urinary frequency.

imiquimod

im-**ee**-kwee-mod
(Aldara)

CLASSIFICATION

Immune response modifier

AVAILABILITY (Rx)

Cream: 5%

ACTION/*THERAPEUTIC EFFECT*

Mechanism unknown.

USES

Treatment of external genital and perianal warts/condyloma acuminata in adults.

INDICATIONS/DOSAGE/ROUTES

Warts/condyloma acuminata:
Oral: Adults: Apply 3 times/wk before normal sleeping hours; leave on skin 6–10 hrs. Remove following treatment period. Continue therapy for maximum of 16 weeks.

SIDE EFFECTS

FREQUENT: Local skin reactions: erythema (61%), itching (32%), burning (26%), erosion (30%), excoriation /flaking (20%), fungal infections (women) 11%. **OCCASIONAL (3–8%):** Pain, induration, ulceration, scabbing, soreness, headache, flulike symptoms.

ivermectin

eye-ver-**meck**-tin
(Stromectol)

CLASSIFICATION

Antihelmintic

AVAILABILITY (Rx)

Tablets: 6 mg.

ACTION/*THERAPEUTIC EFFECT*

Selectively binds to chloride ion channels in invertebrate nerve/muscle cells, increasing permeability to chloride ions. *Causes paralysis/death of parasite.*

USES

Treatment of intestinal strongyloidiasis and onchoceriasis.

INDICATIONS/DOSAGE/ROUTES

Strongyloidiasis:
Oral: Adults: 200 mcg/kg as a single dose.

Onchoceriasis:
Oral: Adults: 150 mcg/kg as single dose at 3–12 month intervals.

SIDE EFFECTS

OCCASIONAL: *(strongyloidiasis):* Dizziness (2.8%), pruritus (2.8%), diarrhea (1.8%); nausea (1.8%). *(onchoceriasis):* Tachycardia (3.5%), peripheral edema (3.2%), facial edema (1.2%), orthostatic hypotension (1.1%).

ketotifen

key-**tow**-tih-fen
(Zaditor)

CLASSIFICATION

Antiallergic

AVAILABILITY (Rx)

Ophthalmic Solution: 0.025%

ACTION/*THERAPEUTIC EFFECT*

Selective histamine H^1-antagonist and mast cell stabilizer; suppresses release of mediators from cells involved in hypersensitivity reactions, decreases chemotoxis and activation of eosinophils. *Reduces symptoms of allergic conjuctivitis.*

USES

Temporary relief of itching of eyes due to allergic conjunctivitis.

INDICATIONS/DOSAGE/ROUTES

Allergic conjunctivitis:
Ophthalmic: Adults, elderly, children >3 yrs: 1 drop in affected eye q8–12 hrs.

SIDE EFFECTS

FREQUENT (10–25%): Conjunctival infection, headache, rhinitis.

OCCASIONAL (1–5%): Allergic reaction, burning, stinging, eyelid disorder, flulike syndrome, keratitis, mydriasis, ocular discharge/pain, pharyngitis, photophobia, rash, xerophthalmia.

letrozole

leh-troe-zoll
(Femara)

CLASSIFICATION

Aromatase inhibitor

AVAILABILITY (Rx)

Tablets: 2.5 mg

ACTION/*THERAPEUTIC EFFECT*

Suppresses estrogen biosynthesis in peripheral tissue and cancer tissue by inhibiting enzyme aromatase.

USES

Treatment of advanced breast cancer in postmenopausal women whose disease progressed after antiestrogen therapy.

INDICATIONS/DOSAGE/ROUTES

Breast cancer:
Oral: Adults, elderly: 2.5 mg daily. Continue until tumor progression is evident.

SIDE EFFECTS

FREQUENT: Musculoskeletal effects: skeletal pain, back, arm, leg pain (21%); nausea (13%), headache (9%), fatigue (8%), constipation (8%), arthralgia (8%), vomiting (7%), dyspnea (7%).

levetiracetam

leave-ty-rah-**see**-tam
(Keppra)

CLASSIFICATION

Anticonvulsant

AVAILABILITY (Rx)

Tablets: 250 mg, 500 mg, 750 mg

ACTION/*THERAPEUTIC EFFECT*

Exact mechanism unknown at time of writing. Unrelated to other anticonvulsants.

USES

Adjunctive therapy in treatment of partial onset seizures in adults with epilepsy.

INDICATIONS/DOSAGE/ROUTES

Partial onset seizures:
Oral: Adults, elderly: Initially, 500 mg q12hrs. May increase by 1,000 mg/day every 2 wks. ***Maximum:*** 3,000 mg/day.

Dosage in renal impairment:

CREATININE CLEARANCE	DOSAGE (ML/MIN)
80	500–1,500 mg q12h
50–80	500–1,000 mg q12h
30–50	250–750 mg q12h
<30	250–500 mg q12h

ESRD using dialysis:
500–1,000 mg q12h. (Following dialysis, a 250–500 mg supplemental dose recommended.)

SIDE EFFECTS

FREQUENT (10–15%): Somnolence, asthenia, headache, infection. **OCCASIONAL (3–10%):** Dizziness, pharyngitis, pain, depression, nervousness, vertigo, rhinitis, anorexia. **RARE (<3%):** Amnesia, anxiety, emotional lability, increased cough, sinusitis, anorexia, diplopia.

linezolid

lyn-eh-**zoe**-lid
(Zyvox)

CLASSIFICATION

Antibiotic

AVAILABILITY (Rx)

Tablets: 400 mg, 600 mg. **Powder for Reconstitution (Oral):** 100 mg/5 ml. **Injection:** 2 mg/ml in 100 ml, 200 ml, 300 ml bags.

ACTION/*THERAPEUTIC EFFECT*

Binds to a site on bacterial 23S ribosomal RNA, preventing formation of complex, which is an essential component of bacterial translation process. *Bacteriostatic against enterococci and staphylococci, bactericidal against streptococci.*

USES

Treatment of vancomycin-resistant *Enterococcus faecium* (VRE) infections, nosocomial pneumonia, uncomplicated/complicated skin/skin structure infections, community-acquired pneumonia (CAP).

INDICATIONS/DOSAGE/ROUTES

VRE:
IV/Oral: Adults: 600 mg q12h for 14–28 days.

Nosocomial pneumonia, CAP, complicated skin infections:
IV/Oral: Adults: 600 mg q12h for 10–14 days.

Uncomplicated skin infections:
IV/Oral: Adults: 400 mg q12h for 10–14 days.

SIDE EFFECTS

OCCASIONAL (2–5%): Diarrhea, nausea, headache. **RARE (<2%):** Taste alteration, vaginal candidiasis (itching, discharge), fungal infection, dizziness, tongue discoloration.

lopinavir/ritonavir

low-**pin**-ah-veer/rih-**ton**-ah-veer
(Kaletra)

CLASSIFICATION

Protease inhibitor combination, antiretroviral

AVAILABILITY (Rx)

Capsules: 133.3 mg lopinavir/33.3 mg ritonavir. **Oral Solution:** 80 mg lopinavir/20 mg ritonavir per ml.

ACTION/*THERAPEUTIC EFFECT*

Lopinavir prevents cleavage of a polyprotein, *resulting in production of immature, noninfectious viral particles.* Ritonavir inhibits metabolism of lopinvir, providing increased lopinavir plasma levels.

USES

In combination with other antiretroviral agents for the treatment of HIV infection.

INDICATIONS/DOSAGE/ROUTES

HIV:
PO: Adults: 400/100 mg of lopinavir/ritonavir (3 capsules or 5 ml) twice daily. Increase to 533/133 mg (4 capsules or 6.5 ml) when taken w/efavirenz or nevirapine. ***Children 7–<15 kg w/o efavirenz or nevirapine:*** 12 mg/kg 2 times/day. ***15–40 kg:*** 10 mg/kg 2 times/day. ***Children 7–<15 kg w/efavirenz or nevirapine:*** 13 mg/kg 2 times/day. ***15–50 kg:*** 11 mg/kg 2 times/day.

SIDE EFFECTS

FREQUENT (14%): Diarrhea (mild to moderate severity). **OCCASIONAL (2–6%):** Nausea, asthenia (loss of strength, energy), abdominal pain, headache, vomiting. **RARE (<2%):** Insomnia, rash.

meloxicam

meh-**locks**-ih-cam
(Mobic)

CLASSIFICATION

Nonsteroidal anti-inflammatory; analgesic

AVAILABILITY (Rx)

Tablets: 7.5 mg

ACTION/*THERAPEUTIC EFFECT*

Produces analgesic and anti-inflammatory effect by inhibiting prostaglandin synthesis, *reducing inflammatory response and intensity of pain stimulus reaching sensory nerve endings.*

USES

Relief of signs and symptoms of osteoarthritis.

INDICATIONS/DOSAGE/ROUTES

Osteoarthritis:
PO: Adults: Initially, 7.5 mg/day. ***Maximum:*** 15 mg/day.

SIDE EFFECTS

FREQUENT (7–9%): Dyspepsia (heartburn, indigestion, epigastric pain), headache, diarrhea, nausea. **OCCASIONAL: (3–4%):** Dizziness, insomnia, rash, pruritus, flatulence, constipation, vomiting.

RARE (<2%): Somnolence/drowsiness, urticaria, photosensitivity

mifepristone

my-fih-**priss**-tone
(Mifeprex)

CLASSIFICATION

Abortifacient

AVAILABILITY (Rx)

Tablets: 200 mg.

ACTION / *THERAPEUTIC EFFECT*

Has antiprogestational activity resulting from competitive interaction with progesterone; inhibits activity of endogenous or exogenous progesterone. Also has antiglucocorticoid and weak antiandrogenic activity. *Terminates pregnancy.*

USES / *UNLABELED*

Termination of intrauterine pregnancy. *Postcoital contraception/contragestation; intrauterine fetal death/nonviable early pregnancy, unresectable meningioma, endometriosis, Cushng's syndrome.*

INDICATIONS/DOSAGE/ROUTES

Note: Treatment with mifepristone and misoprostil requires 3 office visits.

Termination of pregnancy:
PO: Adults: *Day 1:* 600 mg as single dose. *Day 3:* 400 mcg misoprostil. *Day 14:* Post-treatment examination.

SIDE EFFECTS

FREQUENT (>10%): Headache, dizziness, abdominal pain, nausea, vomiting, diarrhea, fatigue. **OCCASIONAL (3–10%):** Uterine hemorrhage, back pain, insomnia, vaginitis, dyspepsia, back pain, fever, viral infections, rigors (chills/shaking). **RARE: 1–2%):** Anxiety, syncope, anemia, asthenia, leg pain, sinusitis.

moxifloxacin

mock-ih-**flocks**-ah-sin
(Avelox)

CLASSIFICATION

Anti-infective: Quinolone

AVAILABILITY (Rx)

Tablets: 400 mg

ACTION / *THERAPEUTIC EFFECT*

Inhibits DNA enzyme in susceptible micro-organisms, *interfering with bacterial DNA replication.* Bactericidal.

USES

Treatment of community-acquired pneumonia (CAP), sinusitis, acute bacterial exacerbation of chronic bronchitis.

INDICATIONS/DOSAGE/ROUTES

Sinusitis, CAP:
Oral: Adults, elderly: 400 mg/day for 10 days.

Chronic bronchitis:
Oral: Adults, elderly: 400 mg/day for 5 days.

SIDE EFFECTS

FREQUENT (5–10%): Nausea, diarrhea. **OCCASIONAL (1–5%):** Dizziness, headache, abdominal pain, vomiting, altered taste, dyspepsia.

nateglinide

nay-tih-**glin**-ide
(Starlix)

CLASSIFICATION

Antidiabetic agent, antihyperglycemic

AVAILABILITY (Rx)

Tablets: 60 mg, 120 mg.

ACTION/*THERAPEUTIC EFFECT*

Stimulates release of insulin from beta cells of pancreas by depolarizing beta cells, leading to opening of potassium channels, *thereby lowering glucose concentration.*

USES

Adjunct to diet and exercise to lower blood glucose in pts w/type 2 diabetes mellitus. Used as monotherapy or in combination w/metformin (Glucophage).

INDICATIONS/DOSAGE/ROUTES

Diabetes mellitu:
PO: Adults, elderly: 60 mg 3 times/day. ***Maximum:*** 540 mg/day.

SIDE EFFECTS

FREQUENT (60%): Upper respiratory infection, headache, rhinitis, bronchitis, back pain, hypoglycemia.

oseltamivir

oh-sell-**tam**-ih-veer
(Tamiflu)

CLASSIFICATION

Antiviral

AVAILABILITY (Rx)

Capsules: 75 mg

ACTION/*THERAPEUTIC EFFECT*

Pro-drug hydrolyzed to active ingredient. Selective inhibitor of influenza virus neuraminidase, an enzyme essential for viral replication. Acts against both influenza A and B viruses. *Suppresses spread of infection within respiratory system, reduces duration of clinical symptoms.*

USES

Symptomatic treatment of uncomplicated acute illness caused by influenza A or B virus in adults symptomatic no longer than 2 days.

INDICATIONS/DOSAGE/ROUTES

Influenza:
Oral: Adults, elderly: 75 mg 2 times/day for 5 days.

SIDE EFFECTS

OCCASIONAL (>1%): Nausea, vomiting, bronchitis, insomnia, vertigo.

oxcarbazepine

ox-car-**bay**-zeh-peen
(Trileptal)

CLASSIFICATION

Anticonvulsant

AVAILABILITY (Rx)

Tablets: 150 mg, 300 mg, 600 mg.

ACTION/*THERAPEUTIC EFFECT*

Exact mechanism unknown. Activity primarily through metabolite. Produces blockade of sodium channels, which results in stabilization of hyperexcited neurol membranes, inhibition of repetitive neuronal firing, diminished propagation of synaptic impulses, *preventing seizure spread in intact brain.*

USES / *UNLABELED*

Monotherapy and adjunctive therapy in adults and adjunctive therapy in children 4–16 yrs in treatment of partial seizures. *Atypical panic disorder.*

INDICATIONS/DOSAGE/ROUTES

Note: Give all doses in a twice daily regimen.

Adjunctive therapy:
Oral: Adults, elderly: Initially, 600 mg/day in 2 divided doses. May increase to a maximum of 600 mg/day at weekly intervals. ***Maximum:*** 2,400 mg/day. ***Children 4–16 yrs:*** 8–10 mg/kg. ***Maximum:*** 600 mg/day. Achieve maintenance dose over 2 wks based on pt weight. ***20–29 kg:*** 900 mg/day; ***29.1–39 kg:*** 1,200 mg/day; ***>39 kg:*** 1,800 mg/day.

Conversion to monotherapy:
Oral: Adults, elderly: 600 mg/day in 2 divided doses (while decreasing concomitant anti-epilepsy drug over 3–6 wks), increasing up to 2,400 mg/day over 2–4 wks (see above for guideline to increasing dosage).

Initiation of monotherapy:
Oral: Adults, elderly: 600 mg/day in 2 divided doses. May increase by 300 mg/day every 3 days up to 1,200 mg/day.

SIDE EFFECTS

FREQUENT (>10%): Headache, dizziness, somnolence, ataxia, abnormal gait, nausea, vomiting, abdominal pain, diplopia, abnormal vision, fatigue. **OCCASIONAL (5–10%):** Tremor, diarrhea, dyspepsia, rhinitis.

pantoprazole

pan-tow-**pray**-zoll
(Protonix)

CLASSIFICATION

Gastric acid pump inhibitor

AVAILABILITY (Rx)

Tablets: 40 mg. **Injection:** 40 mg.

ACTION / *THERAPEUTIC EFFECT*

Converted to active metabolite that irreversibly binds to and inhibits H+/K+ ATPase (enzyme on surface of gastric parietal cells). Inhibits hydrogen ion transport into gastric lumen. *Increases gastric pH, reducing gastric acid production.*

USES

Treatment of gastric, duodenal ulcers, gastro-esophageal reflux disease (GERD), *H. pylori* (in combination with antibacterial agents).

INDICATIONS/DOSAGE/ROUTES

Gastric, duodenal ulcers, GERD, *H. pylori:*
Oral/IV: Adults, elderly: 40 mg/day.

SIDE EFFECTS

OCCASIONAL (<2%): Diarrhea, headache, dizziness, pruritus, skin rash.

pemirolast

pem-ee-**row**-last
(Alamast)

CLASSIFICATION

Antiallergic

AVAILABILITY (Rx)

Ophthalmic Solution: 0.1%

ACTION/*THERAPEUTIC EFFECT*

Prevents activation, release of mediators of inflammation (e.g., mast cells). *Reduces symptoms of allergic conjunctivitis.*

USES

Prevention of itchy eyes due to allergic conjuntivitis.

INDICATIONS/DOSAGE/ROUTES

Allergic conjunctivitis:
Ophthalmic: Adults, elderly: 1–2 drops 3–4 times/day.

SIDE EFFECTS

FREQUENT: Transient stinging, burning, instillation discomfort. **OCCASIONAL:** Ocular itching, blurred vision, tearing, headache.

pentosan

pen-toe-san
(Elmiron)

CLASSIFICATION

Urinary tract analgesic

AVAILABILITY (Rx)

Capsules: 100 mg

ACTION/*THERAPEUTIC EFFECT*

Appears to adhere to bladder wall mucosal membrane, may act as a buffering agent to control cell permeability preventing irritating solutes in the urine. Has anticoagulant/fibrinolytic effects. *Relieves bladder pain.*

USES

Relief of bladder pain/discomfort associated with interstitial cystitis.

INDICATIONS/DOSAGE/ROUTES

Interstitial cystitis:
Oral: Adults, elderly: 100 mg 3 times/day.

SIDE EFFECTS

FREQUENT (3–5%): Alopecia, diarrhea, nausea, headache, rash, abdominal pain, dyspepsia. **OCCASIONAL (1–2%):** Dizziness, depression, increased liver function tests.

perindopril

per-**inn**-doe-prill
(Aceon)

CLASSIFICATION

Angiotensin-converting enzyme (ACE) inhibitor

AVAILABILITY (Rx)

Tablets: 2 mg, 4 mg, 8 mg

ACTION/*THERAPEUTIC EFFECT*

Suppresses renin-angiotensin-aldosterone system (prevents conversion of angiotensin I to angiotensin II, a potent vasoconstrictor; may also inhibit angiotensin II at local vascular and renal sites). *Reduces peripheral arterial resistance, B/P.*

USES/*UNLABELED*

Management of hypertension (HTN) alone or in combination with other classes of antihypertensives (e.g., thiazides). *Management of heart failure.*

INDICATIONS/DOSAGE/ROUTES

HTN:
Oral: Adults, elderly: 2–8 mg/day

as single dose or in 2 divided doses. *Maximum:* 16 mg/day.

SIDE EFFECTS

OCCASIONAL (1–5%): Cough, back pain, sinusitus, viral infection, upper extremity pain, dyspepsia, fever, proteinuria, palpitations, hyperkalemia, angioneurotic edema, hypotension, dizziness, fatigue, syncope, azotemia.

pioglitazone

pie-oh-**glit**-ah-zone
(Actos)

CLASSIFICATION

Antidiabetic

AVAILABILITY (Rx)

Tablets: 15 mg, 30 mg, 45 mg

ACTION/*THERAPEUTIC EFFECT*

Increases glucose consumption, facilitates glucose entry to target cells, reduces glucose production by improving insulin sensitivity in pts with insulin resistance. *Reduces plasma glucose, triglycerides, insulin levels in pts with hyperinsulinemia; improves fasting, postprandial hyperglycemia, hyperinsulinemia.*

USES

Monotherapy or in combination with sulfonylurea, metformin, or insulin as adjunct to diet and exercise in pts with type 2 diabetes mellitus.

INDICATIONS/DOSAGE/ROUTES

Diabetes mellitus, monotherapy:
Oral: Adults, elderly: 15–30 mg/day. *Maximum:* 45 mg/day.

Diabetes mellitus, combination:
Oral: Adults, elderly: 15–30 mg/day.

SIDE EFFECTS

FREQUENT (5–15%): Headache, myalgia, pharyngitis, sinusitis, tooth disorder, upper respiratory tract infection, sore throat, increased weight, edema, anemia.

podofilox

poe-doe-**fie**-locks
(Condylox)

CLASSIFICATION

Antimitotic

AVAILABILITY (Rx)

Topical Gel: 0.5%. **Topical Solution:** 0.5%.

ACTION/*THERAPEUTIC EFFECT*

Exact mechanism of action unknown. *Causes necrosis of visible wart tissue.*

USES

Gel: Treatment of anogenital warts. *Solution:* Treatment of external warts.

INDICATIONS/DOSAGE/ROUTES

Anogenital warts:
Topical: Adults: Apply twice daily to warts w/applicator tip or finger.

External warts:
Topical: Adults: Apply morning and evening (q12 hrs) w/cotton-tipped applicator.

SIDE EFFECTS

FREQUENT (50–80%): Burning, pain, inflammation, erosion, itching.

poractant

pour-**act**-tant
(Curosurf)

CLASSIFICATION

Lung surfactant

AVAILABILITY (Rx)

Intratracheal Suspension: 1.5 ml, 3 ml

ACTION/*THERAPEUTIC EFFECT*

Endogenous surfactant reduces surface tension of alvioli during ventilation, stabilizes alveoli against collapse at resting pressure. Deficiency of surfactant results in respiratory distress syndrome (RDS). Poractant compensates for surfactant deficiency, *restoring surface activity to lungs of infants.*

USES/*UNLABELED*

Treatment (rescue) of RDS in premature infants. *Prophylaxis for RDS, adult RDS due to viral pneumonia, following near-drowning, HIV-infected infants with PCP.*

INDICATIONS/DOSAGE/ROUTES

RDS:
Endotracheal: Infants: Initially, 2.5 ml/kg birth weight (BW). Up to 2 subsequent doses of 1.25 ml/kg BW at 12 hr intervals. ***Maximum:*** 5 ml/kg.

SIDE EFFECTS

FREQUENT: Pneumonia (17%), septicemia (14%), bronchopulmonary dysplasia (18%), intracranial hemorrhage (51%), patent ductus arteriosus (60%), pneumothorax (21%), pulmonary interstitial emphysema (21%).

prednicarbate

pred-nih-**car**-bate
(Dermatop)

CLASSIFICATION

Corticosteroid: Topical

AVAILABILITY (Rx)

Cream: 0.1%

ACTION/*THERAPEUTIC EFFECT*

Diffuses across cell membranes forming complexes w/cytoplasm. Complexes stimulate protein synthesis of inhibitory enzymes responsible for anti-inflammatory effects. *Inhibits edema, erythema, pruritus, capillary dilation, phagocytic activity.*

USES

Provides relief of inflammation/pruritus associated w/corticosteroid-responsive disorders.

INDICATIONS/DOSAGE/ROUTES

Usual topical dosage:
Adults, elderly: Apply sparingly 2–4 times/day.

SIDE EFFECTS

FREQUENT: Contact dermatitis (burning/itching of skin); painful, red, itchy, pus-containing blisters; thinning of skin w/easy bruising; dryness, irritation, skin redness or scaling of skin lesions, skin rash.

rabeprazole

ray-beh-**pray**-zoll
(Aciphex)

CLASSIFICATION

Gastric acid pump inhibitor

AVAILABILITY (Rx)

Tablets: 20 mg.

ACTION/ ***THERAPEUTIC EFFECT***

Converted to active metabolite that binds to and inhibits H+/K+ ATPase (enzyme on surface of gastric parietal cells). This action is partially reversible. Inhibits hydrogen ion transport into gastric lumen. *Increases gastric pH, reducing gastric acid production.*

USES

Treatment of duodenal ulcers, gastro-esophageal reflux disease (GERD), hypersecretory syndromes.

INDICATIONS/DOSAGE/ROUTES

Duodenal ulcers, GERD:
Oral: Adults, elderly: 20 mg/day.

Hypersecretory syndromes:
Oral: Adults, elderly: Initially, 60 mg/day. May increase up to 60 mg 2 times/day.

SIDE EFFECTS

OCCASIONAL (<3%): Headache, nausea, dizziness, rash, diarrhea, malaise, skin eruptions.

respiratory syncytial immune globulin

(Respigam)

CLASSIFICATION

Immune serum

AVAILABILITY (Rx)

Injection: 2,500 mcg RSV immune globulin

ACTION/ ***THERAPEUTIC EFFECT***

High concentration of neutralizing and protective antibodies specific for respiratory syncytial virus (RSV).

USES

Prevents serious lower respiratory tract infections caused by RSV in children <24 months w/bronchopulmonary dysplasia or history of premature birth.

INDICATIONS/DOSAGE/ROUTES

RSV:
IV Infusion: Children (<24 months): 750 mg/kg (15 ml/kg). Initially, 1.5 ml/kg/hr for first 15 min; increase to 3 ml/kg/hr for next 15 min, then 6 ml/kg/hr for remainder of infusion. Administer monthly for total of 5 doses beginning in September or October.

SIDE EFFECTS

OCCASIONAL: Fever (6%), respiratory distress (2%), vomiting (2%), wheezing (2%). **RARE (<1%):** Diarrhea, rales, fluid overload, rash, tachycardia, hypertension, hypoxia, gastroenteritis, injection site inflammation.

Rho(D) immune globulin IV (human)

(WinRho SD)

CLASSIFICATION

Immune serum

AVAILABILITY (Rx)

Injection: 600 IU (120 mcg), 1,500 IU (300 mcg)

ACTION/*THERAPEUTIC EFFECT*

Gamma globulin (IgG) fraction containing antibodies to Rho(D) antigen negative individuals. *Increases platelets in idiopathic thrombocytopenic purpura (ITP).* Exact mechanism unknown.

USES

Pregnancy/other obstetric conditions: Suppresses Rh isoimmunization in nonsensitized Rho(D) antigen-negative women, reduces hemolytic disease in Rho(D)-positive fetus in present and future pregnancies. *Transfusion:* Suppresses isoimmunization transfusion w/Rho(D) antigen-positive RBCs or blood components containing Rho(D)-positive RBCs. Treatment of nonsplenectomized Rho(D) antigen-positive children w/chronic or acute ITP, adults w/chronic ITP, or children and adults w/ITP secondary to HIV infection in clinical conditions to prevent excessive hemorrhage.

INDICATIONS/DOSAGE/ROUTES

Pregnancy:
IV/IM: Adults: 1,500 IU (300 mcg) at 28 wks gestation. Give at 12 wk intervals if administered early in pregnancy, 600 IU (120 mcg) as soon as possible after delivery of confirmed Rh_o(D) antigen-positive baby, and within 72 hrs of delivery.

Other obstetric conditions:
IV/IM: Adults: 600 IU (120 mcg) immediately after abortion, amniocentesis, or other manipulations late in pregnancy (after 34 wks gestation) associated w/increased risk of Rh isoimmunization. Give within 72 hrs after the event. Administer 1,500 IU (300 mcg) immediately after amniocentesis before 34 wks gestation or after chorionic villus sampling. Repeat every 12 wks during the pregnancy. In case of threatened abortion, give as soon as possible.

Transfusion:
Note: Within 72 hrs after exposure of incompatible blood transfusion or massive fetal hemorrhage.
IV: Adults: 3,000 IU (600 mcg) q8h until total dose given.
IM: Adults: 6,000 IU (1,200 mcg) q12h until total dose given.

ITP:
IV/IM: Adults, children: Initially, 250 IU (50 mcg)/kg. If Hgb <10 g/dl, give 125–200 IU (25–40 mcg)/kg. Additional doses give 125–300 IU (25–60 mcg)/kg.

SIDE EFFECTS

OCCASIONAL (1–7%): *Rh isoimmunization suppression:* Discomfort, slight swelling at injection site, slight elevation of temperature. *ITP:* Headache, chills, fever.

---

rituximab

rye-**tucks**-ih-mab
(Rituxan)

CLASSIFICATION

Monoclonal antibody

AVAILABILITY (Rx)

Injection: 10 mg/ml

ACTION/*THERAPEUTIC EFFECT*

Binds to malignant cells, allowing immune system to recognize and eliminate these cells. *Reduces tumor size.*

USES

Treatment of relapsed or refractory low-grade or follicular B-cell non-Hodgkins' lymphoma.

INDICATIONS/DOSAGE/ROUTES

Non-Hodgkins' lymphoma:
IV Infusion: Adults: 375 mg/m^2 given once weekly for 4 weeks.

SIDE EFFECTS

FREQUENT: Fever (49%), chills (32%), headache (14%), asthenia (16%), angioedema (13%), hypotension (10%), nausea (18%), rash/pruritus (10%). **OCCASIONAL (<10%):** Myalgia, dizziness, abdominal pain, throat irritation, vomiting, neutropenia, rhinitis, bronchospasm, urticaria.

rivastigmine

rye-vah-**stig**-meen
(Exelon)

CLASSIFICATION

Cholinesterase inhibitor, anti-Alzheimer's dementia agent

AVAILABILITY (Rx)

Capsules: 1.5 mg, 3 mg, 4.5 mg, 6 mg. **Oral Solution:** 2 mg/ml.

ACTION/*THERAPEUTIC EFFECT*

Exact mechanism unknown. *Enhances cholinergic function* by increasing concentration of acetylcholine through reversible inhibition of its hydrolysis by cholinesterase.

USES

Treatment of mild to moderate dementia of the Alzhemier's type.

INDICATIONS/DOSAGE/ROUTES

Alzheimer's disease:
Oral: Adults, elderly: Initially, 1.5 mg twice daily. May increase after minimum of 2 wks to 3 mg twice daily. Subsequent increases to 4.5 mg and 6 mg twice daily may be made after a minimum of 2 wks at previous dose. ***Maximum:*** 6 mg twice daily.

SIDE EFFECTS

FREQUENT (>10%): Dizziness, headache, nausea, vomiting, diarrhea, anorexia, abdominal pain. **OCCASIONAL (3–10%):** Insomnia, confusion, depression, anxiety, hallucinations, tremor, aggressive reaction, dyspepsia, constipation, flatulence, fatigue, urinary tract infection, asthenia, malaise, rhinitis, increased sweating, hypertension, flulike symptoms, decreased weight.

rofecoxib

row-feh-**cox**-ib
(Vioxx)

CLASSIFICATION

Cyclo-O_2ase-2 inhibitor

AVAILABILITY (Rx)

Tablets: 12.5 mg, 25 mg, 50 mg. **Oral Suspension:** 12.5 mg/5 ml, 25 mg/5 ml.

ACTION/*THERAPEUTIC EFFECT*

Selectively inhibits cyclo-O_2ase-2 (required for synthesis of prostaglandins and thromboxane that cause pain and inflammation). *Produces anti-inflammatory and analgesic effects.*

USES

Relief of signs/symptoms of osteoarthritis, management of acute pain in adults, treatment of primary dysmenorrhea.

INDICATIONS/DOSAGE/ROUTES

Osteoarthritis:
Oral: Adults, elderly: 12.5–25 mg/day as single dose.

Acute pain, dysmenorrhea:
Oral: Adults, elderly: 50 mg/day as single dose.

SIDE EFFECTS

FREQUENT (5–10%): Upper respiratory tract infection, diarrhea, nausea. **OCCASIONAL (1–5%):** Abdominal pain, fatigue, dizziness, flulike symptoms, edema, hypertension, dyspepsia, heartburn, sinusitus, headache, urinary tract infection, bronchitis.

rosiglitazone

row-see-**glit**-ah-zone
(Avandia)

CLASSIFICATION

Antidiabetic

AVAILABILITY (Rx)

Tablets: 2 mg, 4 mg, 8 mg

ACTION/*THERAPEUTIC EFFECT*

Increases glucose consumption, facilitates glucose entry to target cells, reduces glucose production by improving insulin sensitivity in pts with insulin resistance. *Reduces plasma glucose, triglycerides, insulin levels in pts with hyperinsulinemia; improves fasting, postprandial hyperglycemia, hyperinsulinemia.*

USES

Monotherapy or in combination with metformin as adjunct to diet and exercise in pts with type 2 diabetes mellitus.

INDICATIONS/DOSAGE/ROUTES

Diabetes mellitus, monotherapy, combination therapy:
Oral: Adults, elderly: Initially, 4 mg/day as single or divided doses. May increase to 8 mg/day.

SIDE EFFECTS

FREQUENT (>5%): Headache, upper respiratory tract infection. **OCCASIONAL (1–5%):** Anemia, diarrhea, back pain, edema, fatigue, sinusitis.

sacrosidase

sack-row-**sigh**-daze
(Sucraid)

CLASSIFICATION

Enzyme

AVAILABILITY (Rx)

Oral Solution: 8,500 IU/ml. **Oral Powder.**

ACTION/*THERAPEUTIC EFFECT*

Hydrolyzes sucrose into glucose and fructose (w/o enzymes, sucrose cannot be absorbed; and its persistence in intestinal lumen leads to osmotic retention of water, resulting in loose stools). Unabsorbed sucrose produces increased amounts of hydrogen, methane, water causing excessive gas, bloating, abdominal cramps, nausea, vomiting. *Allows pt to thrive, maintain expected growth/development curves.*

USES

Oral replacement therapy for genetically determined sucrase deficiency (part of congenital-isomaltase deficiency).

INDICATIONS/DOSAGE/ROUTES

Sucrase deficiency:
Oral: Infants: 1–2 ml (or 1–2 scoops of powder) diluted in 2–4 oz water, milk, or infant formula taken w/each meal or snack. ***Do not heat solutions containing sacrosidase.*** Discard bottles of sacrosidase 4 wks after opening due to bacterial growth potential.

SIDE EFFECTS

FREQUENT (5–10%): Abdominal pain, vomiting. **OCCASIONAL (1–5%):** Diarrhea.

scopolamine

sko-**poll**-ah-meen
(Trans-Derm Scop)

CLASSIFICATION

Anticholinergic

AVAILABILITY (Rx)

Tablets: 0.4 mg. **Transdermal System:** 1.5 mg.

ACTION/*THERAPEUTIC EFFECT*

Reduces excitability of labyrinthine receptors, depressing conduction in vestibular cerebellar pathway, *preventing nausea/vomiting induced by motion.*

INDICATIONS/DOSAGE/ROUTES

Prevention of motion sickness:
Oral: Adults: 1–2 tablets an hour before travel provide effect for several hours.
Transdermal: Adults: 1 system q72 hrs.

SIDE EFFECTS

FREQUENT (>15%): Dry mouth, drowsiness, blurred vision. **RARE (1–5%):** Dizziness, restlessness, hallucinations, confusion, difficulty urinating, rash.

sermorelin

sir-moe-**real**-inn
(Geref)

CLASSIFICATION

Growth hormone

AVAILABILITY (Rx)

Powder for Injection: 50 mcg.

ACTION/*THERAPEUTIC EFFECT*

Directly stimulates pituitary gland to release growth hormone, *increasing plasma growth hormone concentration.*

USES

Treatment of idiopathic growth hormone deficiency in children w/growth failure. Diagnostic aid to evaluate pituitary gland's ability to secrete growth hormone.

INDICATIONS/DOSAGE/ROUTES

Growth hormone deficiency:
SC: Children: 0.03 mg/kg once daily at bedtime. Discontinue when epiphyses are fused.

SIDE EFFECTS

OCCASIONAL: Pain, swelling, redness at injection site, facial flushing, nausea, headache, vomiting, altered taste, chest tightness.

sevelamer

seh-**vell**-ah-mur
(Renagel)

CLASSIFICATION

Urinary tract agent

AVAILABILITY (Rx)

Capsules: 403 mg

ACTION/*THERAPEUTIC EFFECT*

Binds/removes dietary phosphorus in GI tract and eliminates phosphorus through normal digestive process. *Decreases incidence of hypercalcemic episodes in pts receiving calcium acetate treatment.*

USES

Reduction of serum phosphorous in pts w/end-stage renal disease (ESRD).

INDICATIONS/DOSAGE/ROUTES

Hyperphosphatemia:
Oral: Adults, elderly: 2–4 capsules w/each meal depending on severity of hyperphosphatemia.

SIDE EFFECTS

FREQUENT (11–20%): Infection, pain, hypotension, diarrhea, dyspepsia, vomiting. **OCCASIONAL (1–10%):** Headache, hypertension, thrombosis, increased cough.

sirolimus

sigh-row-**lie**-mus
(Rapamune)

CLASSIFICATION

Immunosuppressant

AVAILABILITY (Rx)

Oral Solution: 1 mg/ml

ACTION/*THERAPEUTIC EFFECT*

Inhibits T-lymphocyte proliferation induced by stimulation of cell surface receptors, mitogens, alloantigens, lymphokines. Prevents activation of enzyme TOR, a key regulatory kinase in cell cycle progression. *Inhibits T and B cell proliferation (essential components of immune response).*

USES

Prophylaxis of organ rejection after renal transplants in combination with cyclosporine and corticosteroids.

INDICATIONS/DOSAGE/ROUTES

Prophylaxis of organ rejection:
Oral: Adults: Loading dose: 6 mg. ***Maintenance:*** 2 mg/day.
Children 13 yrs <40 kg: 3 mg/m^2 loading dose; then 1 mg/m^2/day.

SIDE EFFECTS

OCCASIONAL: Hypercholesterolemia, hyperlipidemia, hypertension, rash. (**High dose:** 5 mg/day): Anemia, arthralgia, diarrhea, hypokalemia, thrombocytopenia.

sodium ferric gluconate complex

(Ferrlecit)

CLASSIFICATION

Hematinic

AVAILABILITY (Rx)

Ampules: 12.5 mg/ml elemental iron

ACTION/ *THERAPEUTIC EFFECT*

Repletes total body content of iron.

USES

Treatment of iron-deficiency anemia in pts undergoing chronic hemodialysis who are receiving supplemental erythropoietin therapy.

INDICATIONS/DOSAGE/ROUTES

Note: Initially, a 25 mg test dose is diluted in 50 ml 0.9% NaCl and given over 60 min.
IV Infusion: Adults, elderly: 125 mg in 100 ml 0.9% NaCl infused over 1 hr. Minimum cumulative dose 1 g elemental iron over 8 sessions at sequential dialysis treatment. (May be given during dialysis session itself.)

SIDE EFFECTS

FREQUENT (>3%): Flushing, hypotension, hypersensitivity reaction. **OCCASIONAL (1–3%):** Injection site reaction, pain, headache, abdominal pain, chills, flulike syndrome, dizziness, leg cramps, dyspnea, nausea, vomiting, diarrhea, myalgia, pruritus, edema.

talc

(Sclerosol)

AVAILABILITY (Rx)

Aerosol Spray Intrapleural: 4 g

ACTION/ *THERAPEUTIC EFFECT*

Obliterates the pleural space and prevents reaccumulation of pleural fluid through induction of an inflammatory reaction.

USES

Remedy for cancer pts suffering from pleural effusions.

INDICATIONS/DOSAGE/ROUTES

Pleural effusions:
Aerosol: Adults: 8 g as single treatment.

SIDE EFFECTS

No side effects reported.

tazarotene

tay-zah-**row**-teen
(Tazorac)

CLASSIFICATION

Antipsoriatic

AVAILABILITY (Rx)

Gel: 0.05%, 0.1%

ACTION/ *THERAPEUTIC EFFECT*

Modulates differentiation and proliferation of epithelial tissue; binds selectively to retinoic acid receptors. *Restores normal differentiation of the epidermis and reduction in epidermal inflammation.*

USES

Treatment of stable plaque psoriasis in pts with at least 20% body surface area involvement. Treatment of mild to moderate facial acne.

INDICATIONS/DOSAGE/ROUTES

Psoriasis:
Topical: Adults: Thin film applied once daily in the evening; only cover the lesions, and area should be dry before application.

Acne:
Topical: Adults: Thin film applied

to affected areas once daily in the evening, after face is gently cleansed and dried.

SIDE EFFECTS

FREQUENT (10–30%): *Acne:* Desquamation, burning or stinging, dry skin, itching, erythema. *Psoriasis:* Itching, burning or stinging, erythema, worsening of psoriasis, irritation, skin pain. **OCCASIONAL (1–10%):** *Acne:* Irritation, skin pain, fissuring, localized edema, skin discoloration. *Psoriasis:* Rash, desquamation, contact dermatitis, skin inflammation, fissuring, bleeding, dry skin.

tenecteplase

ten-**eck**-teh-place
(TNKase)

CLASSIFICATION

Tissue plasminogen activator: thrombolytic

AVAILABILITY (Rx)

Powder for Injection: 50 mg

ACTION/*THERAPEUTIC EFFECT*

A tissue plasminogen activator (tPA) produced by recombinant DNA that binds to fibrin and converts plasminogen to plasmin, an enzyme that *degrades fibrin clots, fibrinogen, other plasma proteins.*

USES

Reduction of mortality associated w/acute myocardial infarction. (AMI).

INDICATIONS/DOSAGE/ROUTES

Note: Give as a single IV bolus over 5 sec. Precipitate may occur when given in an IV line containing dextrose. Flush with saline prior to and after administration.

Acute myocardial infarction:
IV: Adults: Dosage based on pt weight. Treatment to be initiated as soon as possible after onset of AMI symptoms.

WEIGHT (KG)	MG	ML
<60	30	6
≥60–<70	35	7
≥70–<80	40	8
≥80–<90	45	9
≥90	50	10

SIDE EFFECTS

FREQUENT: Bleeding (major: 4.7%; minor 21.8%).

thalidomide

thah-**lid**-owe-mide
(Thalomid)

CLASSIFICATION

Immunosuppressive

AVAILABILITY (Rx)

Tablets: 100 mg

ACTION/*THERAPEUTIC EFFECT*

Exact mechanism unknown. Has sedative, anti-inflammatory, and immunosuppressive activity. Action may be due to selective inhibition of the production of tumor necrosis factor alpha.

USES/*UNLABELED*

Treatment of leprosy. *Wasting syndrome of HIV or cancer, recurrent aphthous ulcers in HIV pts.*

INDICATONS/DOSAGE/ROUTES

AIDS-related muscle wasting:
Oral: Adults: 100–200 mg daily.

SIDE EFFECTS

FREQUENT: Drowsiness, dizziness, mood changes, constipation, xerostimia, peripheral neuropathy. **OCCASIONAL:** Increased appetite, weight gain, headache, loss of libido, edema of face and limbs, nausea, hair loss, dry skin, skin rash, hypothyroidism.

tinzaparin

tinn-zah-**pair**-inn
(Innohep)

CLASSIFICATION

Anticoagulant

AVAILABILITY (Rx)

Injection: 20,000 IU/ml.

ACTION/*THERAPEUTIC EFFECT*

Antithrombin; in presence of low molecular weight heparin, *produces anticoagulation* by inhibition of factor Xa. Tinzaparin causes less inactivation of thrombin, inhibition of platelets, and bleeding than standard heparin. Does not significantly influence bleeding time, prothrombin time (PT), activated partial thromboplastin time (APTT).

USES

Treatment of acute symptomatic deep vein thrombosis (DVT), w/ or w/o pulmonary embolism, when given in conjunction w/warfarin.

INDICATIONS/DOSAGE/ROUTES

Deep vein thrombosis (DVT):
SubQ: Adults, elderly: 175 IU/kg once daily. Continue at least 6 days and until pt is sufficiently anticoagulated w/warfarin (INR 2 or >2 consecutive days).

SIDE EFFECTS

OCCASIONAL (14%): Bleeding, pain, or irritation at injection site, nausea, asthenia (unusual tiredness or weakness), confusion, peripheral edema.

toremifene

tore-mih-feen
(Fareston)

CLASSIFICATION

Antineoplastic

AVAILABILITY (Rx)

Tablets: 60 mg

ACTION/*THERAPEUTIC EFFECT*

Interacts w/estrogen receptors to serve as an antiestrogen, depleting cytosolic estrogen receptors, resulting in *cytostatic effects on tumor growth.*

USES

Treatment of advanced breast cancer in postmenopausal women w/estrogen receptor-positive disease.

INDICATIONS/DOSAGE/ROUTES

Breast cancer:
Oral: Adults: 60 mg daily until disease progression is observed.

SIDE EFFECTS

FREQUENT: Nausea (14%), hot flashes (35%), sweating (20%), dizziness (9%), vaginal discharge (13%). **OCCASIONAL:** Anxiety, tremors, irritability, bone pain, insomnia, lethargy, headache, fatigue, skin rash, abdominal pain, weight gain, edema, vaginal bleeding.

trastuzumab

traz-**two**-zoo-mab
(Herceptin)

CLASSIFICATION

Monoclonal antibody, antineoplastic

AVAILABILITY (Rx)

Lyophilized Powder: 440 mg

ACTION/ *THERAPEUTIC EFFECT*

Inhibits proliferation of human tumor cells that overexpress HER-2 (HER-2 protein overexpression is seen in 25–30% of primary breast cancer pts). Mediates antibody-dependent cellular cytotoxicity.

USES

Treatment of metastatic breast cancer pts whose tumors overexpress HER-2 protein and who have received one or more chemotherapy regimens. May be used w/paclitaxel w/o previous treatment for metastatic disease.

INDICATIONS/DOSAGE/ROUTES

Note: Do not give as IV bolus or IV push. Dextrose solutions should *not* be used.

Breast cancer:
IV Infusion: Adults, elderly: Initially, 4 mg/kg as 90 min infusion, then weekly infusion of 2 mg/kg as 30 min infusion.

SIDE EFFECTS

FREQUENT (>20%): Pain, asthenia, fever, chills, headache, abdominal pain, back pain, infection, nausea, diarrhea, vomiting, cough, dyspnea. **OCCASIONAL (5–15%):** Tachycardia, CHF, flulike symptoms, anorexia, edema, bone pain, arthralgia, insomnia, dizziness, paresthesia, depression, rhinitis, pharyngitis, sinusitus. **RARE (<5%):** Allergic reaction, anemia, leukopenia, neuropathy, herpes simplex.

unoprostone

ewe-no-**pros**-tone
(Rescula)

CLASSIFICATION

Prostaglandin analogue, anti-glaucoma agent

AVAILABLITY (Rx)

Ophthalmic Solution: 0.15%

USE

Lower intraocular pressure (IOP) in pts w/open-angle glaucoma or ocular hypertension.

ACTION/ *THERAPEUTIC EFFECT*

Increases the outflow of aqueous humor, *lowering IOP.*

INDICATIONS/DOSAGE/ROUTES

Glaucoma, ocular hypertension:
Ophthalmic: Adults, elderly: 1 drop in affected eye(s) 2 times/day.

SIDE EFFECTS

Note: May cause permanent darkening of iris.
FREQUENT (10–25%): Burning, stinging, dry eyes, itching, increased eyelash length and redness. **OCCASIONAL (<10%):** Abnormal vision, eyelid disorder, foreign body sensation.

valrubicin

val-**rue**-bih-sin
(Valstar)

CLASSIFICATION

Antineoplastic

AVAILABILITY (Rx)

Solution for Intravesical Instillation: 40 mg/ml

ACTION/ *THERAPEUTIC EFFECT*

Following intracellular penetration, inhibits incorporation of nucleosides into nucleic acids, *causes chromosomal damage, arresting cell cycle in G2 phase, interfering w/DNA.*

USES

Intravesical therapy of BCG-refractory carcinoma in situ of urinary bladder in pts for whom cystectomy is unacceptable.

INDICATIONS/DOSAGE/ROUTES

Note: Not for IM/IV use.

Bladder cancer:
Intravesical: Adults, elderly: 800 mg once weekly for 6 wks.

SIDE EFFECTS

Local reaction: **FREQUENT (>10%):** Local bladder symptoms, urinary frequency, dysuria, urinary urgency, hematuria, bladder pain, cystitis, bladder spasms. **OCCASIONAL (<10%):** Nocturia, local burning, urethral pain, pelvic pain, gross hematuria. ***Systemic:*** **FREQUENT (5–15%):** Abdominal pain, nausea, urinary tract infection. **OCCASIONAL (2–5%):** Diarrhea, vomiting, urinary retention, microscopic hematuria, asthenia, headache, malaise, back pain, chest pain, dizziness, rash, anemia, fever, vasodilation. **RARE (1%):** Flatus, peripheral edema, increased glucose, pneumonia, myalgia.

zaleplon

zall-eh-plon
(Sonata)

CLASSIFICATION

Sedative hypnotic **(Schedule IV)**

AVAILABILITY (Rx)

Capsules: 5 mg, 10 mg

ACTION/ *THERAPEUTIC EFFECT*

Selectively binds to the benzodiazepine-1 receptor (omega-1), which is involved in sedation. Has little effect on normal stages of sleep and few, if any, anxiolytic, anticonvulsant, muscle-relaxant properties. *Produces hypnotic effect.*

USES

Short-term treatment of insomnia.

INDICATIONS/DOSAGE/ROUTES

Insomnia:
Oral: Adults: 10 mg/day. ***Elderly:*** 5 mg/day.

SIDE EFFECTS

FREQUENT (5–10%): Abdominal pain, asthenia, headache (28%), nausea, myalgia, dizziness. **OCCASIONAL (1–5%):** Fever, dyspepsia, amnesia, paresthesia, tremor, eye pain, dysmenorrhea. **RARE (<1%):** Malaise, photosensitivity, anorexia, edema, anxiety, vertigo, altered vision, ear pain.

zanamivir

zah-**nah**-mih-veer
(Relenza)

CLASSIFICATION

Antiviral

AVAILABILITY (Rx)

Powder for Oral Inhalation: 5 mg/inhalation

ACTION/*THERAPEUTIC EFFECT*

Selective inhibitor of influenza virus neuraminidase, an enzyme essential for viral replication. Activity against both influenza A and B viruses. *Suppresses spread of infection within respiratory system, reduces duration of clinical symptoms.*

USES

Symptomatic treatment of uncomplicated acute illness caused by influenza A or B virus in adults symptomatic no longer than 2 days.

INDICATIONS/DOSAGE/ROUTES

Influenza:
Oral Inhalation: Adults, children >12 yrs: 2 inhalations twice daily (approximately 12 hrs apart) for 5 days initiated within 2 days of onset of symptoms.

SIDE EFFECTS

OCCASIONAL (1.5–3%): Sinusitis, diarrhea, nausea, bronchitis, cough, ear, nose, throat infection, headache, vomiting, dizziness.

zonisamide

zoe-**niss**-ah-mide
(Zonegran)

CLASSIFICATION

Anticonvulsant

AVAILABILITY (Rx)

Capsules: 100 mg.

ACTION/*THERAPEUTIC EFFECT*

Mechanism of action unknown. May produce anticonvulsant effects through action at sodium and calcium channels, *stabilizing neuronal membranes and suppressing neuronal hypersynchronization.*

USES

Adjunctive therapy in treatment of patrial seizures in adults w/epilepsy.

INDICATIONS/DOSAGE/ROUTES

Partial seizures:
Oral: Adults, children >16 yrs: Initially, 100 mg/day for 2 wks. May increase by 100 mg/day at intervals of at least 2 wks. ***Maximum:*** 400 mg/day.

SIDE EFFECTS

FREQUENT (5–10%): Agitation, ataxia, confusion, depression, difficulty concentrating, fatigue, dizziness, headache, insomnia, somnolence, anorexia, abdominal pain, nausea, diplopia. **OCCASIONAL (2–5%):** Anxiety, nervousness, nystagmus, paresthesia, diarrhea, dyspepsia, altered taste, weight loss.

NAME/INDICATIONS	DOSAGE/ROUTES	SIDE EFFECTS
lidocaine (Xylocaine) Ventricular fibrillation, ventricular tachycardia, suppress PVCs, wide-complex tachycardias, wide complex PSVT	***Ventricular arrhythmias:*** ***IM: Adults, elderly:*** 300 mg (or 4.3 mg/kg). May repeat in 60–90 min. ***IV: Adults, elderly:*** Initially, 50–100 mg (1 mg/kg) IV bolus at rate of 25–50 mg/min. May repeat in 5 min. Give no more than 200–300 mg in 1 hr. ***Maintenance:*** 20–50 mcg/kg/min (1–4 mg/min) as IV infusion. ***Children, infants:*** Initially, 0.5–1 mg/kg IV bolus; may repeat, but total dose not to exceed 3–5 mg/kg. ***Maintenance:*** 10–50 mcg/kg/min as IV infusion.	Anxiety, seizures, nausea, vomiting, drowsiness, widening QRS complex
magnesium Refractory ventricular fibrillation, cardiac arrest associated with torsades de pointes, preeclampsia, eclampsia, life-threatening arrhythmias caused by digoxin toxicity, torsades de pointes	***IV:*** 1–2 g in 10 ml sodium chloride slow IVP over 1–2 min. ***Eclampsia:*** 1–4 g.	Drowsiness, bradycardia, dysrhythmia, decreased B/P, rash, hypothermia
methylprednisolone (Solu-Medrol) Treatment of asthma, status asthmaticus	***IV: Adults, elderly:*** Initially, 40–125 mg q4–6h. ***Children:*** I mg/kg.	Insomnia, heartburn, nervousness, abdominal distension, increased sweating, acne, mood swings, increased appetite, facial flushing, GI distress, delayed wound healing, increased susceptibility to infection, diarrhea/constipation
morphine Relief of severe, acute, chronic pain, preop sedation, anesthesia supplement, analgesia during labor. Drug of choice for pain due to myocardial infarction, dyspnea from pulmonary edema not resulting from chemical respiratory irritant	***Pain:*** ***IV: Adults, elderly:*** 4–10 mg, given very slowly. ***Myocardial infarction pain, keep SBP>90:*** ***IV: Adults, elderly:*** 2–4 mg for pain.	Sedation, decreased B/P, increased sweating, flushed face, constipation, dizziness, drowsiness, nausea, vomiting, respiratory depression
naloxone (Narcan) Diagnosis and treatment	***Opioid toxicity (IV route preferred):***	Too rapid reversal of narcotic depression may re-

(continued)

Name/Indications	Dosage/Routes	Side Effects
of opioid toxicity, treatment of opioid-induced respiratory depression, and other effects (e.g., sedation, coma, convulsions). Used in neonates to reverse respiratory depression caused by opioids given mother during labor and delivery. Adjunctive therapy to treat hypotension in management of septic shock	***IM/IV/SubQ: Adults:*** 0.4–2 mg as single dose. May repeat at 2–3 min intervals. ***Children:*** 0.01 mg/kg. May repeat w/0.1 mg/kg. **Note:** AAP recommends initial dose of 0.1 mg/kg for infants and children up to 5 yrs and weighing <20 kg. Children >5 yrs or >20 kg recommended initial dose is 2 mg. ***Opioid respiratory depression:*** ***IV: Adults:*** 0.1–0.2 mg q2–3 min until adequate ventilation and alertness w/o pain are obtained. May repeat dose at 1–2 hr intervals. ***Children:*** 5–10 mcg (0.005–0.01 mg) q2–3 min. ***Neonates:*** 10 mcg (0.01 mg)/kg. May repeat q2–3 min. ***Septic shock:*** ***IV: Adults:*** 0.03–0.2 mg/kg initially, then IV infusion of 0.03–0.3 mg/kg/hr for 1–20 hrs.	sult in nausea, vomiting, tremulousness, sweating, increased B/P, tachycardia. Hypotension or hypertension, ventricular tachycardia and fibrillation, pulmonary edema may occur in pts w/cardiovascular disease
nitroglycerin Acute ischemic coronary syndrome, angina, acute MI	***Sublingual: Adults:*** 0.4 mg. May repeat every 5 min as long as BP>90	Headache (may be severe) occurs mostly in early therapy, diminishes rapidly in intensity, usually disappears during continued treatment; transient flushing of face and neck, dizziness (esp. if pt is standing immobile or is in a warm environment), weakness, postural hypotension. Burning, tingling sensation at oral point of dissolution
procainamide (Pronestyl) Refractory ventricular fibrillation, ventricular tachycardia with a pulse, wide complex tachycardia, paroxysmal supraventricular tachycardia (PSVT)	30 mg/min, maximum total dose 17 mg/kg. ***Maintenance Infusion:*** 1–4 mg/min.	Confusion, dizziness, hypotension, conduction changes (50% widening of QRS complex, frequent ventricular premature contractions, ventricular tachycardia, complete AV block). Prolonged PR and QT intervals, flattened T waves occur less frequently

(continued)